W9-BSA-248

THE BASIC SCIENCE
OF
VASCULAR DISEASE

Edited by

Anton N. Sidawy, MD
Chief, Surgical Service
VA Medical Center
Professor of Surgery
George Washington University
Associate Professor of Surgery
Georgetown University
Washington, DC

Bauer E. Sumpio, MD, PhD
Chief, Vascular Surgery
Vice-Chairman of Surgery
Professor of Surgery
Yale University School of Medicine
New Haven, Connecticut

Ralph G. DePalma, MD
Chief, Surgical Service
VA Medical Center
Professor of Surgery
Associate Dean
University of Nevada
Reno, Nevada

**Futura Publishing
Company, Inc.**
Armonk, New York

Library of Congress Cataloging-in-Publication Data

The basic science of vascular disease / edited by Anton N. Sidawy,
    Bauer E. Sumpio, Ralph G. DePalma.
        p.   cm.
    Includes bibliographical references and index.
    ISBN 0-87993-627-4
    1. Blood-vessels—Pathophysiology.   I. Sidawy, Anton N.
II. Sumpio, Bauer E.   III. DePalma, Ralph G., 1931–   .
    [DNLM: 1. Vascular Diseases—physiopathology.   2. Vascular
Diseases—therapy.   WG 500 B311 1996]
RC691.4.B366   1996
616.1′3—dc20
DNLM/DLC
for Library of Congress   96-27629
                                                               CIP

Copyright © 1997
Futura Publishing Company, Inc.

Published by
Futura Publishing Company, Inc.
135 Bedford Road
Armonk, New York 10504

LC#: 96-27629
ISBN#: 0-87993-627-4

Printed in the United States of America.

Printed on acid-free paper.

Contributors

Elias J. Arbid, MD [14]
Assistant Professor of Surgery, West Virginia University, Charleston, West Virginia

Christopher E. Attinger, MD [37]
Associate Professor of Surgery, Section of Plastic and Reconstructive Surgery, Georgetown University Medical Center, Washington, DC

Mark Awolesi, MD [13]
Resident in Surgery, Yale University School of Medicine, New Haven, Connecticut

Jag Bhawan, MD [14]
Professor of Dermatopathology, Boston University Medical Center, Boston, Massachusetts

John J. Bergan, MD [15]
Scripps Memorial Hospital, La Jolla, California, Professor of Surgery, University of California, San Diego, California

Colleen M. Brophy, MD [13]
Associate Professor of Surgery, Medical College of Georgia, Augusta, Georgia

Nissage Cadet, MD [26]
Fellow, Vascular Surgery, Columbia Metrowest Medical Center, Framingham, Massachusetts

Elizabeth T. Clark, MD [30]
Assistant Professor of Surgery, University of Chicago, Chicago, Illinois

Alexander W. Clowes, MD [10]
Professor of Surgery, Division of Vascular Surgery, University of Washington, Seattle, Washington

Richard H. Dean, MD [29]
Professor of Surgery, Chairman of Department of General Surgery, Director of Division of Surgical Sciences, Bowman Gray School of Medicine/North Carolina Baptist Hospital, Winston-Salem, North Carolina

Ralph G. DePalma, MD [11,16,32]
Professor of Surgery, Associate Dean, University of Nevada, Chief of Surgical Service, Department of Veterans Affairs, Reno, Nevada

Philip B. Dobrin, MD, PhD [3,23]
Chief of Staff, Salt Lake City VA Medical Center, Associate Dean, Professor of Vascular Surgery, University of Utah School of Medicine, Salt Lake City, Utah

James M. Edwards, MD [22]
Assistant Professor of Surgery, Division of Vascular Surgery, Oregon Health Sciences University, Portland, Oregon

Michael M. Farooq, MD [33]
Resident, Department of General Surgery, Medical College of Wisconsin, Milwaukee, Wisconsin

Julie A. Freischlag, MD [33]
Associate Professor of Surgery, Department of Vascular Surgery, Medical College of Wisconsin, Milwaukee, Wisconsin

Gary L. Gallagher, MD [6]
Postdoctoral Fellow, Division of Vascular Surgery, Yale University School of Medicine, Yale University, New Haven, Connecticut

Numbers in brackets indicate chapters written or cowritten by the contributor.

Bruce L. Gewertz, MD [30]
Professor and Chairman, Department of Surgery, University of Chicago, Chicago, Illinois

Joseph M. Giordano, MD [1,19]
Professor and Chairman, Department of Surgery, George Washington University Medical Center, Washington, DC

Seymour Glagov, MD [4]
Professor of Pathology, University of Chicago, Chicago, Illinois

Peter Gloviczki, MD [34]
Consultant, Division of Vascular Surgery, Mayo Clinic and Foundation, Professor of Surgery, Mayo Medical School, Rochester, Minnesota

Anita K. Gregory, MD [27]
Assistant Professor of Surgery, Department of Surgery, Columbia University, St. Lukes'/Roosevelt Hospital Center, New York, New York

Howard P. Greisler, MD [8,25]
Professor of Surgery, Department of Surgery, Loyola University Medical Center, Maywood, Illinois

Sushil K. Gupta, MD [26]
Chairman, Department of Surgery, Columbia Metrowest Medical Center, Framingham, Massachusetts, Associate Clinical Professor of Surgery, Harvard Medical School, Boston, Massachusetts

Richard J. Gusberg, MD [31]
Professor of Surgery, Section of Vascular Surgery, Yale University School of Medicine, New Haven, Connecticut

Anil P. Hingorani, MD [27]
Research Fellow, Vascular Biology and Surgery, Department of Surgery, Columbia University, St. Lukes'/Roosevelt Hospital Center, New York, New York

Marsel Huribal, MD [36]
Division of Vascular Surgery, Department of Surgery, Millard Fillmore Hospital, Buffalo, New York

Bruce A. Jones, MD [17,35]
Research Fellow, Vascular Surgery Section, VA Medical Center, Washington, DC

Steven S. Kang, MD [25]
Assistant Professor of Surgery, Department of Surgery, Loyola University Medical Center, Maywood, Illinois

Mitchel Kanter, MD [16]
Clinical Instructor in Plastic Surgery, Johns Hopkins Hospital, Baltimore, Maryland

Larry W. Kraiss, MD [10]
Senior Fellow, Division of Vascular Surgery, Department of Surgery, University of Washington, Seattle, Washington

William C. Krupski, MD [9]
Professor of Surgery, Chief of Vascular Surgery, University of Colorado Health Sciences Center, Denver, Colorado

Joseph Kurantsin-Mills, PhD [21]
Associate Research Professor of Medicine and Physiology, Department of Medicine and Department of Physiology, George Washington University Medical Center, Washington, DC

Wayne W. LaMorte, MD, PhD, MPH [14]
Associate Professor of Surgery, Chief of Surgical Research, Boston University Medical Center, Boston, Massachusetts

John C. LaRosa, MD [18]
Chancellor, Tulane University Medical Center, New Orleans, Louisiana

Frank W. LoGerfo, MD [17]
Chief of Division of Vascular Surgery, New England Deaconess Hospital, Professor of Surgery, Harvard Medical School, Boston, Massachusetts

George H. Meier, MD [28]
Associate Professor of Surgery, Section of Vascular Surgery, Yale University School of Medicine, New Haven, Connecticut

James O. Menzoian, MD [14]
Professor of Surgery, Boston University School of Medicine, Chief of Vascular Surgery, Boston University Medical Center, Boston, Massachusetts

Ira Mills, PhD [7]
Research Scientist, Department of Vascular Surgery, Yale University School of Medicine, New Haven, Connecticut

Richard F. Neville, MD [24]
Assistant Professor of Surgery, Section of Vascular Surgery, Georgetown University Medical Center, Washington, DC

John A. Peyman, PhD [2]
Research Scientist, Department of Cardiothoracic Surgery, Yale University School of Medicine, New Haven, Connecticut

Tania J. Phillips, MD [14]
Associate Professor of Dermatology, Boston University Medical Center, Boston, Massachusetts

John M. Porter, MD [22]
Professor of Surgery, Head of Division of Vascular Surgery, Department of Surgery, Oregon Health Sciences University, Portland, Oregon

Max Rabinowitz, MD [12]
Senior Medical Officer, Division of Clinical Laboratory Devices, Food and Drug Administration, Clinical Professor of Pathology, Uniformed Services University of Health Sciences, Clinical Associate Professor of Pathology, Georgetown University, Washington, DC

John J. Ricotta, MD [36]
Professor of Surgery, Chief of Division of Vascular Surgery, Department of Surgery, Millard Fillmore Hospital, Buffalo, New York

David L. Robaczewski, MD [29]
Thoracic and Cardiovascular Fellow, University of Virginia Health Science Center, University Hospital, Charlottesville, Virginia

Anton N. Sidawy, MD [5,17,24,35,37]
Chief of Surgical Service, VA Medical Center, Professor of Surgery, George Washington University Medical Center, Associate Professor of Surgery, Georgetown University Medical Center, Washington, DC

Amy C. Sisley, MD [30]
Instructor of Surgery, Department of Surgery, Emory University, Atlanta, Georgia

Bauer E. Sumpio, MD, PhD [2,6,7,13]
Professor of Surgery, Chief of Vascular Surgery, Vice-Chairman of Surgery, Yale University School of Medicine, New Haven, Connecticut

Lloyd M. Taylor Jr., MD [22]
Professor of Surgery, Division of Vascular Surgery, Department of Surgery, Oregon Health Sciences University, Portland, Oregon

M. David Tilson, MD [27]
Professor of Surgery, Department of Surgery, Columbia University, St. Lukes'/Roosevelt Hospital Center, New York, New York

Rhonda Lee Travaglino-Parda, MD [37]
Chief of Plastic Surgery, VA Medical Center, Clinical Instructor of Surgery, Georgetown University Medical Center, Washington, DC

Bradford I. Tropea, MD [4]
Assistant Professor of Surgery, Department of Surgery, Division of Vascular Surgery, Stanford University Hospital, Stanford, California

Michael J. Tullis, MD [30]
Vascular Surgery Fellow, Department of Surgery, University of Washington, Seattle, Washington

Frank J. Veith, MD [26]
Chief of Vascular Surgery Services, Montefiore Medical Center, Professor of Surgery, Albert Einstein University, Bronx, New York

Thomas W. Wakefield, MD [20]
Associate Professor of Surgery, Section of Vascular Surgery, Department of Surgery, University of Michigan Medical School, Ann Arbor, Michigan

David Whitley, MD [34]
Fellow, Division of Vascular Surgery, Mayo Clinic and Foundation, Rochester, Minnesota

Christopher K. Zarins, MD [4]
Professor of Surgery, Department of Surgery, Division of Vascular Surgery, Stanford University Hospital, Stanford, California

Foreword

Vascular disease places an enormous burden on society, with its untold morbidity and disability which accompany pathologic changes that affect the circulation. Therefore, it is essential that advances in our scientific understanding of vascular disease be expeditiously applied to clinical care algorithms. The bridge from basic knowledge of events which affect the vessel wall to disease states which accompany alterations in blood flow in these vessels requires a clear dissemination of new knowledge to practitioners. This has been accomplished by Drs. Sidawy, Sumpio, and DePalma, who have done an admirable job in organizing, editing, and writing sections of *The Basic Science of Vascular Disease*. This has been an interdisciplinary accomplishment which bespeaks of the complexity surrounding the basic physiology and pathobiology of the vasculature.

Simple anatomy and physiology were the essence of medical knowledge during the early twentieth century. A more detailed understanding of normal and abnormal regulatory physiology evolved during the middle of this century, and allowed for tremendous strides in recognizing and treating disease states. Perhaps the most important intellectual advancement in the clinical discipline of surgery was the publication in 1959 of Francis D. Moore's *Metabolic Care of the Surgical Patient*. This single textbook altered clinicians' thinking and actions when treating patients, and provided a major impetus for many investigative and clinical advances during the decades that followed. *The Basic Science of Vascular Disease* offers a similar opportunity for those treating vascular disease.

As the close of the twentieth century approaches, our knowledge has evolved into more basic insights of cellular and molecular events, including genetic control mechanisms, that affect both normal organ physiology, as well as contribute to the pathophysiologic states of disease. In particular, it is the latter science that will have a profound impact on our understanding of vascular disease. This subject is a major focus of *The Basic Science of Vascular Disease*.

The contributors to this text have provided a core of contemporary information for students as well as practitioners who will use it as a guide in many investigative and clinical disciplines studying vascular diseases. Although the topics range from developmental anatomy to organ specific complications of vascular disease, the elements of scientific understanding represent a common interdisciplinary language that has supplanted the language of the more traditional disciplines of biochemistry, immunology, physiology, and pathology. *The Basic Science of Vascular Disease* is a well-conceived contribution to the intellectual ferment that will be the foundation for vascular medicine and surgery as we enter the next millennium. Like the practitioners and professors of a few decades ago who educated themselves in the elements of anatomy and physiology, today's wise students and teachers will serve themselves and their patients well if they assimilate the considerable wealth of information contained in *The Basic Science of Vascular Disease*.

James C. Stanley, MD
Professor and Head
Section of Vascular Surgery
University of Michigan
Ann Arbor, Michigan

Preface

A belief in causality . . . characterizes all valuable minds.

Ralph Waldo Emerson

A knowledge of basic science is critical for progress in patient care. The value of a text detailing the basic science of vascular disease becomes evident when one attempts a review of the voluminous literature on this subject. This book reflects the information available in this field, with special emphasis on recently introduced molecular biology methods. We have attempted to give the reader a complete and comprehensive review of the basic science of vascular disease, while satisfying the curiosity of the clinician interested in gaining knowledge in this area. In addition, the authors provide information detailed enough to allow students of vascular disease to use this text in planning and progressing in their vascular research career. To fulfill this purpose, we expanded the format of an earlier book entitled *The Basic Science of Vascular Surgery,* edited by Joseph M. Giordano, MD, Hugh H. Trout III, MD, and Ralph G. DePalma, MD. The current text describes, in more detail, disease processes and covers a wider variety of issues, especially at the level of cellular and molecular biology. Dr. Giordano provided the impetus for the current book, which the editors greatly appreciate.

This book is divided into three sections. *Section I. Fundamental Science: The Basic Disciplines* covers the embryology, physiology, and anatomy of the arterial, venous, and lymphatic systems. It includes an introduction to molecular biology and deals primarily with the basic science related to atherosclerosis and intimal hyperplasia. *Section II. The Science of Ancillary Disciplines: The Essential Tools for the Treatment of Vascular Disease* deals with the mechanisms of action of various risk factors as these influence the progression of the atherosclerotic and hyperplastic processes. In addition, the scientific basis of the methods used to treat the disease processes is presented, including vascular grafts, endovascular therapy, microcirculation and rheology, coagulopathies, and drugs used for the conservative treatment of vascular disease. A chapter is dedicated to statistics, as the knowledge of statistics is paramount in the critical evaluation of scientific literature. *Section III. The Science of Selected Entities: Physiology and Pathophysiology* elaborates on the basic science aspects of challenging clinical entities, such as renal hypertension, spinal cord ischemia with high aortic clamping, formation of aortic aneurysms, cerebral circulation, mesenteric ischemia, portal hypertension, male sexual function, skeletal muscle injury and its protection, dialysis arteriovenous fistulae, and vascular graft infections. A chapter covering the biomechanics and neuropathic etiology of foot ulcers is also included. All health care professionals dealing with foot problems require this information for the prevention and treatment of foot ulcers. These three sections contain 37 chapters written by authorities in the field of vascular disease.

It is our hope that this book will be useful to physicians dealing with vascular disease. Vascular surgeons, vascular medicine physicians, cardiologists interested in vascular disease and its management, and vascular interventional radiologists, in addition to their fellows and residents, will find it worthwhile to have this book as a basic science source to complement their clinical library. We are deeply indebted to the contributing authors who have given their time and effort to make this book a reality.

Anton N. Sidawy, MD
Bauer E. Sumpio, MD, PhD
Ralph G. DePalma, MD

Editors

Dedication

To our wives for the support they have provided us:

Mary Sidawy
Catherine Sumpio
Maleva DePalma

... and to our children for the inspiration they have given us:

Michelle and Nicholas Sidawy
Christina, Brett, and Brandon Sumpio
Ralph Lawrence, Edward, Lee, and Malinda DePalma

Table of Contents

I

Fundamental Science:
The Basic Disciplines

CHAPTER 1

Embryologic Development of the Vascular System

Joseph M. Giordano, MD

Initial Formation of the Vascular System

The vascular system is the first organ to assume a functional role in the developing embryo. During the first week after conception, the embryo receives its nourishment from inherent stores in the yolk sac. During the second week, the embryo depends on diffusion of oxygen and nutrients from maternal sources. By the third week, however, the size and complexity of the embryo make diffusion an ineffective process. Therefore, a functional vascular system must be established by the end of the third week.

Initial formation of the vascular system can be summarized as follows (Figure 1). Mesenchymal cells called angioblasts form in clumps throughout the developing embryo. Within these clumps, spaces develop and form cavities lined by cells. These cavities unite with each other so that by the third week, a network of endothelial-lined channels exist. This system establishes a connection to the developing heart, which at the end of the third week of gestation consists only of two tubes. At that time, circulation of blood begins.

Initially, capillaries are simply endothelial-lined tubes. Scattered cells resembling young fibroblasts attach themselves to the capillary wall. Although circulation of blood in the vascular system is well established at the beginning of the fourth week, there is no regulation of the circulation or contraction and dilatation of the peripheral arteries. Thus, definitive structure of the arterial wall is not established until the fourth month when the three divisions of the arterial wall begin to differentiate. The internal elastic membrane first appears just outside the endothelial cells. Small muscle cells proliferate, forming the tunica media. In the fifth fetal month, a poorly developed external elastic membrane separates the media from the developing tunica adventitia. The last layer develops slowly; it is not until the eighth month of gestation that characteristic collagenous bundles and elastic fibers appear. The vasa vasorum appears about the fourth month of gestation.

At the beginning of the fourth week, the functional cardiovascular system consists of two heart tubes connected to a dorsal aorta. This paired structure extends the entire length of the embryo and has: 1) segmental dorsal, ventral, and lateral branches to the body of the embryo; 2) umbilical arteries that establish connection to the vessels in the chorion (later the placenta); and 3) vitelline arteries that communicate with the yolk sac. The heart tubes then begin to fuse to form the heart. Just cephalad to the developing heart is the truncus arteriosus and the aortic sac.

Six pairs of arteries called aortic arches develop off the aortic sac, pass laterally around the developing gut, and connect to the paired dorsal aorta. During the sixth to eighth week of gestation, these six aortic arches and a seventh dorsal segmental artery develop into the aortic arch and its major branches (Figures 2A–2D).

Development of the Aortic Arch

The six pairs of aortic arches, together with the dorsal aorta and aortic sac, elongate, regress, disap-

From *The Basic Science of Vascular Disease*. Edited by Sidawy AN, Sumpio BE, and DePalma RG. Armonk, NY: Futura Publishing Company, Inc.; © 1997.

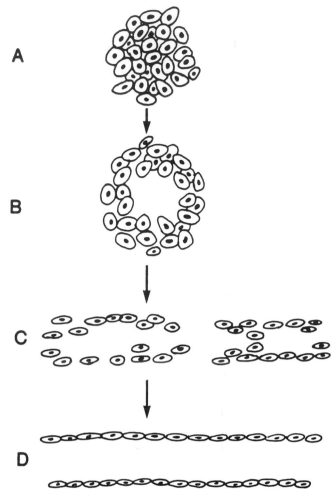

Figure 1. Initial development of vessels: **A.** clumps of cells form; **B.** cavities develop; **C.** channels form; **D.** channels unite to form primitive endothelial lined vessels.

axillary artery are formed from the right fourth arch, right dorsal aorta, and right seventh intersegmental artery. The left fourth arch and the left dorsal aorta distal to the fourth arch become part of the mature aortic arch. The left seventh intersegmental artery develops into the left subclavian artery. The proximal portion of

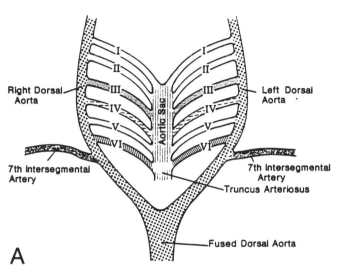

Figure 2A. The six primitive aortic arches. The first, second, and fifth arches disappear. The paired dorsal aortae fuse at the level of the seventh cervical vertebra to become the thoracic and abdominal aorta.

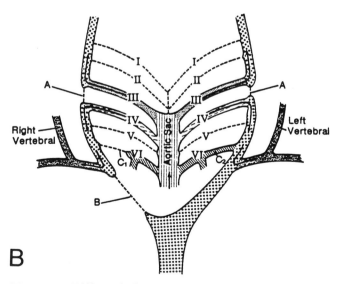

Figure 2B. Differentiation of aortic arches. The dorsal aorta between the third and fourth arches (**A**) involutes so that blood entering the third arch perfuses the head only. The third arch and its branches become the carotid system. The right dorsal aorta distal to the right seventh intersegmental artery (**B**) involutes so that blood entering the right fourth arch perfuses the right upper extremity. This system becomes the right subclavian artery. The distal part of the right sixth arch (**C-1**) involutes, but the distal part of the left sixth arch (**C-2**) persists, becoming the ductus arteriosus.

pear, and increase in size to become the fully developed aortic arch. In the following description, it may appear that all aortic arches are present at one time; this is not the case. Some of the arches are involuting, while others are developing. The first, second, fifth, and distal part of the right sixth arches disappear. The third aortic arch forms the common carotid artery. The connection of the third arch to the dorsal aorta and that part of the dorsal aorta that received the first two arches develop into the internal carotid artery. The dorsal aorta between the third and fourth arch involutes. Blood entering the third arch goes only to the head and neck. Blood entering the right fourth arch goes to the dorsal aorta and right seventh segmental artery, the vessel to the developing right arm. Because the aorta distal to the right seventh segmental artery completely involutes, blood entering the right fourth arch goes to the right arm. The right subclavian and

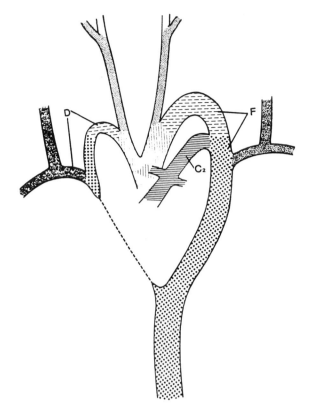

Figure 2C. Aortic arch development. The right fourth arch, the dorsal aorta distal to the right fourth arch, and the right seventh intersegmental artery become the right subclavian artery (**D**). The left fourth arch and the left dorsal aorta distal to it becomes part of the aortic arch (**F**). The left seventh intersegmental artery becomes the left subclavian artery. Pulmonary arteries are forming from the sixth arch with the ductus arteriosus (**C-2**) present.

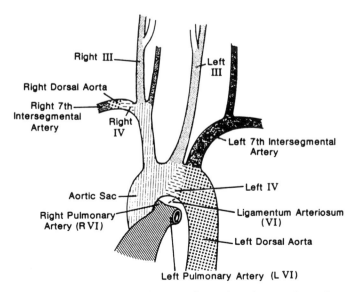

Figure 2D. Segments of the aortic arches that produce the adult aortic arch. Note that the patent ductus arteriosus has become the ligamentum arteriosum.

both sixth arches become the right and left pulmonary artery. However, unlike the involution that occurs in the distal part of the right sixth arch, the distal left sixth arch persists, connecting the left pulmonary artery to the aorta. In the fetus, this structure is the ductus arteriosus, which shunts blood away from the functionless lungs to the aorta. The innominate artery develops from the aortic sac.

In view of the complex events that change the six aortic arches to the mature thoracic aorta and its major branches, it is not surprising that anatomic variations and abnormalities occur.[1-5] Parts of the arch that normally disappear may persist, parts of the arch that normally persist might disappear, or a combination of these two processes can occur. Three types of "normal" variations of the aortic arch occur. Type A, present in 75% of white Americans and 50% of black Americans, is the most common arrangement in which the aortic arch gives off three major branches: the innominate artery, which divides into the right subclavian and right common carotid artery; the left common carotid artery; and the left subclavian artery. In type B, the innominate artery and left common carotid artery come off a common trunk. In type C, the left vertebral artery comes off the aortic arch instead of the left subclavian artery as in types A and B.

Aortic Arch Anomalies

Double Aortic Arch

The ascending aorta bifurcates with the right limb passing posterior to the esophagus to join the left limb that passes anterior to the trachea (Figure 3A). This forms a vascular ring around the esophagus and trachea, at times compressing them. The two aortas are not of equal diameter; the right is usually larger than the left. This anomaly is due to failure of the right dorsal aorta distal to the seventh intersegmental artery to involute (Figure 3B).

Right Aortic Arch

Two types of right aortic arch can occur. In the first type, right aortic arch with a retroesophageal component, the aortic arch passes posterior to the esophagus and with the ligamentum arteriosum, which in this anomaly connects the right pulmonary artery to the aorta, forms a vascular ring around the trachea and esophagus. The right aortic arch with a retroesophageal component may initially be a double aortic arch in which the left dorsal aorta later regresses. In the second type, the right aortic arch without a retroesophageal component, the arch originates in front of the trachea and no vascular ring is formed (Figure 4A).

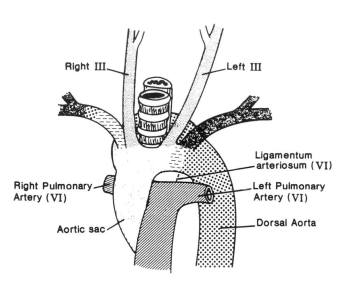

Figure 3A. Double aortic arch. The aorta passes anterior and posterior to the trachea and esophagus, forming a vascular ring.

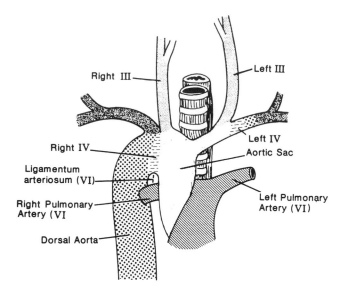

Figure 4A. The right aortic arch. One of the two types in which the right arch passes anterior to the trachea and esophagus so that no vascular ring is formed. If the right arch passes posterior to the trachea and esophagus, the ligamentum arteriosum and the right arch forms a vascular ring.

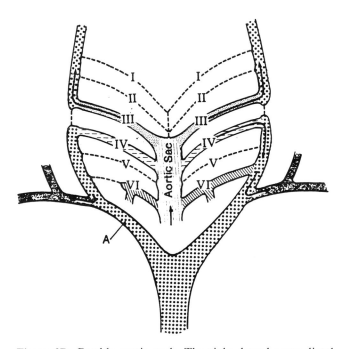

Figure 3B. Double aortic arch. The right dorsal aorta distal to the right seventh intersegmental artery (**A**) that normally involutes persists to become part of the double aortic arch.

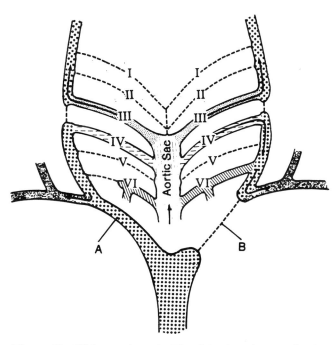

Figure 4B. Right aortic arch. The right dorsal aorta distal to the right seventh intersegmental artery persists (**A**), while the left dorsal aorta distal to the left seventh intersegmental artery involutes (**B**), the opposite of the normal occurrence.

The right aortic arch develops because the left dorsal aorta distal to the left seventh segmental artery involutes, while the right dorsal aorta distal to the right seventh segmental artery persists (Figure 4B). This is opposite to the sequence that normally occurs.

Retroesophageal Right Subclavian Artery

The retroesophageal right subclavian artery arises from the descending aorta distal to the left subclavian artery and passes posterior to the esophagus to supply the right upper extremity (Figure 5A). Most patients with this entity are asymptomatic, although difficulties with swallowing have been reported.[2] Normally, the right subclavian artery is formed by the right fourth aortic arch, the right dorsal aorta distal to the right fourth arch, and the right seventh intersegmental artery. In the formation of the retroesophageal right subclavian artery, the proximal right fourth arch and dorsal aorta involute so that the subclavian artery is formed from the seventh intersegmental artery (Figure 5B). The dorsal aorta distal to the right seventh intersegmental artery fails to involute and instead contributes to the formation of the right subclavian artery. As the arch of the aorta enlarges and migrates cranially, the right subclavian artery follows the left subclavian artery (Figure 5C), explaining the abnormal origin of the right subclavian artery distal to the left subclavian artery (Figure 5A).

Absence of the Internal Carotid Artery

The internal carotid artery is normally formed from the third arch and the dorsal aorta. If these vessels involute, the internal carotid artery fails to form. Most cases are unilateral and asymptomatic.

Patent Ductus Arteriosus

Patent ductus arteriosus is the most common congenital anomaly of the great vessels. The ductus arteriosus is formed from the distal portion of the left sixth aortic arch and connects the left pulmonary artery to the descending aorta during fetal development (Figures 2B and 2C). Immediately after birth, the high oxygen tension in the blood flowing through the ductus arteriosus causes it to contract. By 1 month, the ductus arteriosus has completely obliterated, becoming the ligamentum arteriosum (Figure 2D). If this does not occur, the ductus arteriosus remains patent, and blood from the high-pressure aortic system passes into the low-pressure system of the pulmonary circulation.

Coarctation of the Aorta

Coarctation of the aorta is a common malformation and is classified into postductal and preductal depending on the relation of the coarctation to the ligamentum arteriosum. In the common postductal type, the constriction is inferior to the ligamentum arte-

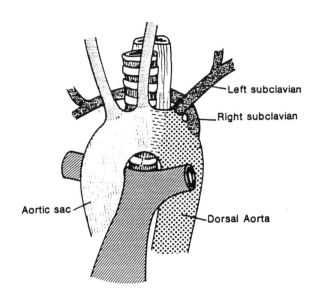

Figure 5A. Retroesophageal right subclavian artery. The right subclavian artery originates distal to the left subclavian artery, reaching the right upper extremity by passing posterior to the trachea and esophagus.

riosum, while the coarctation is superior to the ligamentum arteriosum in the less common preductal type. The cause of coarctation is unclear. The condition develops after birth and is thought to be caused by an unusual quantity of ductus arteriosus muscle tissue that is incorporated in the wall of the aorta. When the

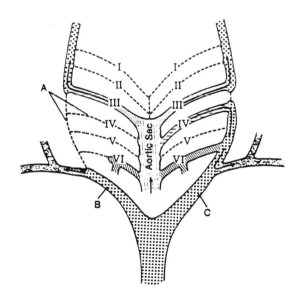

Figure 5B. Retroesophageal right subclavian artery. The right fourth arch and the dorsal aorta distal to the right fourth arch (**A**) abnormally involutes and, therefore, cannot contribute to the formation of the right subclavian artery. The right subclavian artery is then formed by the right dorsal aorta distal to the right seventh intersegmental artery (**B**) that normally involutes. (**C**) This becomes part of the thoracic aorta.

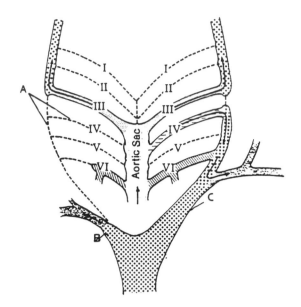

Figure 5C. Retroesophageal right subclavian artery. The left dorsal aorta (**C**) elongates, enlarges, and moves cranially to become the thoracic aorta. The right dorsal aorta (**B**) considerably shortens to become a branch of the thoracic aorta, leading to the subclavian artery. (**A**) This abnormally involutes (see Figure 5B).

ductus arteriosus contracts, the muscle in the aortic wall also contracts, causing the lumen to be narrowed. This area later becomes fibrotic and the narrowing becomes permanent. Clinically, the patient has easily palpable pulses in the upper extremities, but reduced pulses in the lower extremities. Extensive collateral circulation is developed to compensate for inadequate blood flow to the inferior part of the body.

Development of the Thoracic and Abdominal Aorta

Each of the paired dorsal aorta has lateral, ventral, and dorsal arteries supplying each segment of the embryo. At the fourth week, the paired dorsal aorta beginning at the level of the seventh cervical certebra fuse to become the single thoracic and abdominal aorta. The segmental branches, however, persist so that the fused aorta has bilateral dorsal, ventral, and lateral segmental branches. These segmental branches undergo changes by fusing or involuting. The paired dorsal segmental branches become the vertebral arteries in the neck, the intercostal arteries in the thorax, and the lumbar arteries in the abdomen. The fifth lumbar dorsal segmental arteries enlarge to become the common iliac arteries. The paired ventral segmental arteries become the vitelline arteries connected to the yolk sac. As the gut differentiates into the foregut, midgut, and hindgut, the vitelline arteries become its blood supply. Groups

of paired vitelline arteries fuse at three different levels of the aorta to become the celiac, superior mesenteric, and inferior mesenteric arteries. The umbilical arteries, which are also paired ventral arteries, join the fifth dorsal lumbar segmental arteries to become the internal iliac arteries.

The lateral segmental branches of the aorta provide arterial blood supply to the primitive urogenital system as it develops. At the seventh week of gestation, the metanephron (permanent) kidney ascends. The most caudal lateral segmental branches involute, and the cranial lateral segmental branches initially persist. Eventually, only one cranial lateral segmental branch remains to become the renal artery. This divides within the kidney into five segmental end arteries supplying the apical, upper, middle, lower, and posterior segments of the kidney. If involution of the cranial segmental branches is not complete, then multiple arteries arising independently off the aorta supply the kidney. This variation in blood supply to the kidney has been exhaustively studied by Merklin and Michaels whose findings are summarized in the Table.[6,7] If the kidney does not ascend and becomes ectopic, its blood supply frequently will form from multiple caudal segmental arteries or one artery distal to the usual location of the renal artery. Fusion of the caudal pole of the embryonic kidney prior to its cephalad movement causes a horseshoe kidney. As the joined kidney ascends, its cephalad movement is halted by the inferior mesenteric artery. Since the kidney does not assume a normal anatomic position, its blood supply may arise from multiple segmental branches off the aorta more distal to the usual location of the renal artery. It is important to note that both horseshoe and ectopic kid-

Table
Variations in the Arterial Supply
to the Kidney

Condition	Percent
1 Hilar artery	71.1
1 Hilar artery and 1 upper pole branch	12.6
2 Hilar arteries	10.8
1 Hilar artery and 1 upper pole aortic artery	6.2
1 Hilar artery and 1 lower pole aortic artery	6.9
1 Hilar artery and 1 lower pole branch	3.1
3 Hilar arteries	1.7
2 Hilar arteries, one with upper polar branch	2.7
Other variations	—

(Reproduced with permission from Reference 7.)

neys often exhibit an anomalous blood supply.[8] It is essential in patients with either of these entities who are undergoing aortic reconstruction to anatomically define the arterial blood supply to the kidney with a preoperative arteriogram.

Development of Arteries to the Extremities

Development of the extremities begins with the formation of a limb bud off the trunk of the embryo. Initially, the limb bud is nourished by a capillary plexus that coalesces to form a simple major artery as the limb enlarges. In the upper limb, the subclavian artery formed from the aortic arches attaches to the developing limb artery and its branches: axillary, brachial, and anterior interosseous artery. Later, the radial and ulnar arteries develop as branches of the brachial artery to become the major blood supply of the forearm. The anterior interosseous artery is reduced in size and significance.

The developing lower extremity receives its initial blood supply from the sciatic artery (ischiatic or axial artery), which develops off the umbilical artery.[9] As the name implies, the sciatic artery follows the course of the sciatic nerve along the posterior aspect of the lower extremity into the foot (Figure 6). At approximately the sixth week of gestation, the external iliac artery, which begins as a branch off the umbilical artery, develops into the femoral arterial system that supplies the thigh. The femoral arterial system terminates in the lower thigh into descending genicular and ramus communicans branches. This latter artery unites with the sciatic artery just above the knee, establishing continuity between the femoral arterial system and the sciatic artery. The femoral arterial system becomes the major blood supply to the thigh. The sciatic artery in the thigh regresses, atrophies, and eventually loses continuity with the umbilical artery. In the gluteal region, remnants of the sciatic artery form the internal iliac artery and the superior and inferior gluteal artery. In the leg, parts of the sciatic system remain and form sections of the popliteal and peroneal artery.

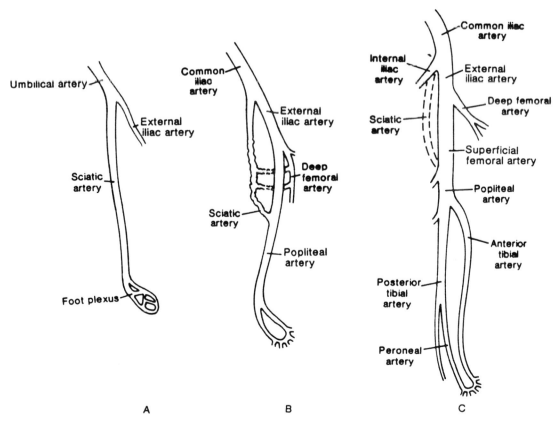

Figure 6. Arterial supply to the left lower extremity. **A.** Sciatic artery forming as a branch of the umbilical artery initially supplies the entire leg. **B.** The sciatic artery regresses, while the external artery develops into the common femoral artery to supply the thigh. Note that the sciatic artery communicates with the popliteal artery just above the knee. **C.** The sciatic artery disappears, although small portions remain to form the popliteal and peroneal artery.

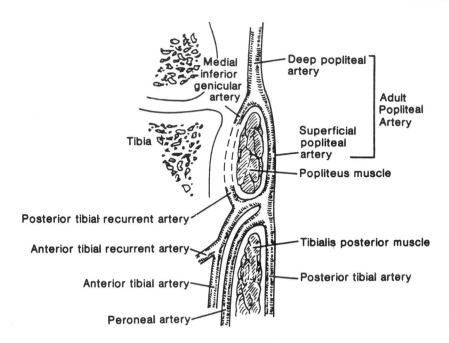

Figure 7. Embryologic development of the popliteal artery, modified from Senior.[9] The deep popliteal artery anterior to the popliteus muscle regresses, while the superficial popliteal artery posterior to the popliteus muscle becomes the mature popliteal artery. (Reproduced with permission from Reference 13.)

Formation of the popliteal artery is a complex process that occurs from the union of two embryonic vessels: the deep popliteal artery, which is part of the sciatic system, and the later developing superficial popliteal artery (Figure 7). The deep popliteal artery initially constitutes the blood supply to the lower leg. The part of the deep popliteal artery anterior to the popliteus muscle atrophies. The superficial popliteal artery develops posterior to the popliteus muscle and unites with the remaining deep popliteal artery at the knee to form the mature popliteal artery.

In summary, the mature arterial system of the lower extremity is derived from two embryonic systems: the primitive sciatic artery and the iliac femoral system. The sciatic system disappears, except for small branches in the gluteal area and parts of the popliteal and peroneal artery. The iliac femoral system, thus, becomes the dominant blood supply to the lower extremity. Three relatively unusual vascular anomalies of the lower extremity are important to vascular surgeons.

Lower Extremity Arterial Anomalies

Persistent Sciatic Artery

Persistent sciatic artery is a rare anomaly with an incidence of approximately 0.05%.[10] In this circumstance, the femoral system fails to develop completely, so that the vascular supply of the upper thigh occurs through the sciatic artery, which should atrophy. The sciatic artery usually is complete; that is, it is intact

from the internal iliac artery to the popliteal artery. A few cases have been reported in which the sciatic artery is incomplete, so that its connection to either the internal iliac or the popliteal artery is through small collateral vessels.

Anatomically, the persistent adult sciatic artery is a continuation of an enlarged internal iliac artery. It gives off superior gluteal and internal pudendal arteries in the pelvis, enters the thigh through the sciatic notch, and has a close relationship to the sciatic nerve in the thigh. It may be enclosed in the sheath of the nerve itself. At the insertion of the adducta magnus muscle, it enters the popliteal fossa to become continuous with the popliteal artery.

Patients with a persistent sciatic artery can present with aneurysm formation in the area of the buttocks, probably from repeated trauma and early atherosclerotic changes causing thrombosis or embolization.[11] At times, compression of the sciatic nerve by sciatic artery aneurysm causes neurologic symptoms as the presenting complaint. If the external iliac artery also fails to develop, as rarely occurs, the patient may exhibit absent femoral arterial pulses, but easily palpable popliteal and ankle pulses.

The Single Umbilical Artery

Normally the umbilical cord contains two arteries and one vein. The two arteries develop into the internal iliac arteries. Aplasia of one umbilical artery, which occurs in 0.75% to 1.1% of consecutive deliveries, is frequently associated with severe congenital malformations.[12] During gestation, the single umbilical artery carries the entire blood flow to the placenta. The internal iliac artery that develops from the single umbilical artery is frequently large and has a different microscopic structure when compared to normal iliac arteries. Calcification, subintimal hyperplasia, and early atherosclerotic changes have been reported in large iliac arteries of children who are born with a single umbilical artery.

Popliteal Entrapment Syndrome

This relatively uncommon developmental abnormality occurs either from an aberrant path of the popliteal artery or from an abnormal attachment of the medial head of the gastrocnemius muscle. Normally, the popliteal artery lies between the heads of the gastrocnemius muscle. In the popliteal entrapment syndrome, the popliteal artery lies medial to the medial head of the gastrocnemius muscle, becoming entrapped between this muscle head and the femur. Patients with this syndrome may present with claudication at a young age from compression of the artery during exercise. Repeated trauma to the artery from the gastrocnemius muscle can produce aneurysms of the popliteal artery with the complications of thrombosis and embolization.

Embryologically, the gastrocnemius muscle originates from the calcaneus and develops cephalad, dividing into a lateral and medial head.[9,13] The lateral head attaches first to the lateral epicondyle of the femur. The medial head attaches later. At the time of attachment of the medial head of the gastrocnemius, the development of the popliteal artery has occurred. The deep popliteal artery anterior to the popliteus muscle has atrophied, and the superficial popliteal artery has become the dominant artery below the knee. Either because of late development of the popliteal artery or early migration of the medial head of the gastrocnemius muscle, the movement of the medial head occurs at the time the popliteal artery is being formed. The popliteal artery is swept medially and impinged against the femur as the medial head of the gastrocnemius attaches. No case of entrapment of the popliteal artery has occurred from the lateral head, probably because this head attaches to the femur well before the popliteal artery changes from the anterior to the posterior surface of the popliteus muscle.

Development of the Venous System

The venous system, like the arterial system, initially develops from clumps of cells that form endothelial lined spaces. These spaces coalesce to form a capil-

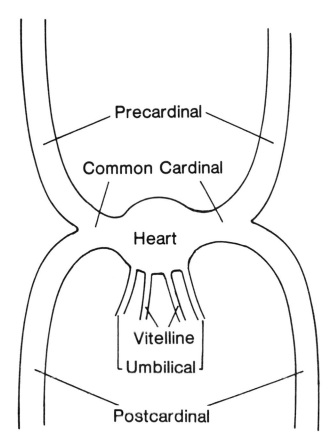

Figure 8. Venous system of 4-week-old embryo.

lary network. What distinguishes those clumps of cells that form arteries from those that form veins is not clear. As the embryo enlarges, certain channels of the capillary bed enlarge, eventually becoming the major veins of the embryo.

The 4-week-old embryo has three systems of paired veins that drain the embryo, the yolk sac, and the placenta—the vitelline, umbilical, and cardinal veins (Figure 8). The vitelline veins follow the yolk sac on either side of the intestinal canal, pass through the septum transversum that divides the thoracic from the abdominal cavity, and enter the sinus venosum of the heart. The developing liver breaks up the vitelline veins into a plexus of small capillary-like vessels called sinusoids. The vitelline veins cephalad to the developing liver that drain the sinusoid plexus become the hepatic veins, and the vitelline veins caudad to the developing liver become the portal vein and its major tributaries.

The umbilical veins bring oxygenated blood from the placenta into the heart. The veins fuse into one single trunk in the umbilical cord, but this single trunk divides into a right and left umbilical vein in the embryo. As in the case of the vitelline vein, the developing liver breaks up the umbilical venous system. The right umbilical vein disappears. The left umbilical vein between the liver and the heart also disappears. However, the left umbilical vein caudad to this enlarges rapidly and establishes a connection to the right hepatic vein. This connecting vein, the ductus venosus, brings oxygenated blood from the placenta directly into the heart without traversing the liver. The left umbilical vein and the ductus venosus atrophy after birth, forming the ligamentum teres and the ligamentum venosum of the liver.

The cardinal veins return blood from the body of the embryo. They both join to form the right and left common cardinal veins that empty into the heart (Figure 8). The precardinal veins eventually form the major veins of the head, neck, and thoracic cavity. The postcardinal veins, along with the subcardinal and supracardinal system, form the inferior vena cava.

Development of Superior Vena Cava

The precardinal and postcardinal veins unite to form the common cardinal veins that empty into the heart. The cephalad portion of the precardinal veins develop into the subclavian and internal jugular system. At the eighth week, the right and left precardinal veins become connected by an oblique anastomosis that develops into the left innominate vein (Figure 9A). The left precardinal vein caudal to the left innominate vein disappears. The right precardinal vein and the right common cardinal vein enlarge to become the superior vena cava that returns blood from the right and left innominate veins, draining the head and neck area (Figure 9B). The postcardinal veins, which previously united with the precardinal veins to form a common cardinal vein, assume a less important role and become the proximal part of the azygous system and hemiazygous system.

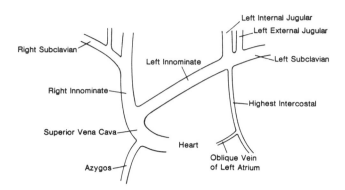

Figure 9B. Completed development of superior vena cava and major branches.

Superior Vena Cava Anomalies

Double Superior Vena Cava

The left precardinal system caudal to the left innominate vein together with the right precardinal system persist and drain independently into the right atrium, developing a double superior vena cava system.[14] The left innominate vein may or may not be present. It is apparent that if the left innominate vein does not form, the left precardinal vein must persist to become the left-sided part of the double superior vena cava.

Left-Sided Superior Vena Cava

The left precardinal vein does not regress, while the right precardinal vein regresses with an innominate vein carrying blood from the right to the left side that connects to the superior vena cava and into the heart.[15] While both double superior vena cava and left superior vena cava are clinically innocuous, they can produce unusual shadows on chest films that may be difficult to interpret.

Development of the Inferior Vena Cava

The inferior vena cava forms during the sixth to tenth week of gestation (Figures 10A to 10D). Three parallel pairs of veins appear during different periods of gestation, develop extensive anastomotic channels among themselves, and undergo partial regression. The remaining parts of these veins coalesce to form the adult inferior vena cava and the iliac bifurcation. The first set of veins to appear are the postcardinal veins. These veins are located on the posterior aspect of the fetus and empty into the common cardinal veins.

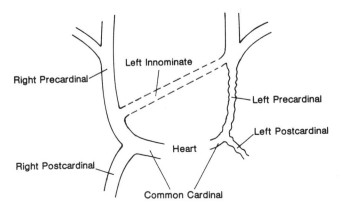

Figure 9A. Development of superior vena cava and major branches.

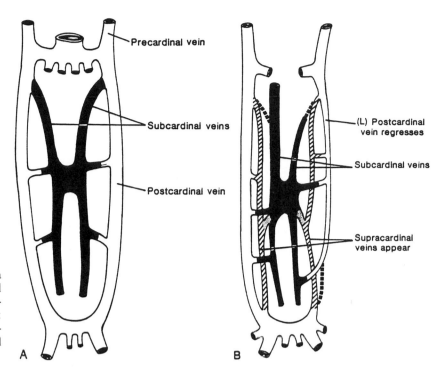

Figure 10. Development of inferior vena cava. **A.** Six-weeks gestation: postcardinal veins dominant with subcaudal system beginning to appear. **B.** Seven-weeks gestation: subcardinal veins dominant, and supracardinal system beginning to appear. Postcardinal veins are beginning to regress.

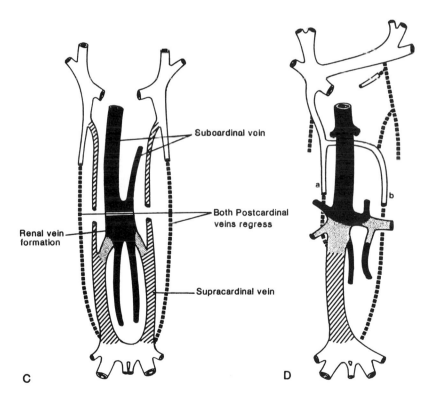

Figure 10 C. Eight-weeks gestation: subcardinal veins form prerenal inferior vena cava. Supracardinal veins form the postrenal inferior vena cava. Postcardinal veins regress. **D.** The adult inferior vena cava. Note that portions of the postcardinal veins persist to form the azygous system (**A**) and the hemiazygous system (**B**). ■ = subcardinal veins; □ = pre and postcardinal veins; ▨ = supracardinal veins; ⊠ = supra- and subcardinal veins. (Reproduced with permission from Reference 22.)

The postcardinal veins disappear except their most proximal sections, which form part of the azygous system, and the most distal section, which forms the iliac bifurcation. Next, the subcardinal veins located anterior and medial to the postcardinal veins appear. The left subcardinal vein completely regresses, while the right subcardinal vein forms the suprarenal inferior vena cava. The supracardinal veins located directly posterior to the aorta appear last. The left supracardinal system regresses and the right remains to form the infrarenal portion of the inferior vena cava. The suprarenal portion of the left and right supracardinal systems become connected to the proximal postcardinal veins to form the azygous system and hemiazygous system.

Both the subcardinal and the supracardinal systems form extensive anastomotic channels at the level of the renal vein. These channels coalesce to form a large vein anterior and posterior to the aorta that drains the left kidney and unites with the inferior vena cava. Eventually, the vein posterior to the aorta regresses, while the vein anterior to the aorta persists to become the left renal vein. In summary, the right subcardinal vein forms the suprarenal segment of the inferior vena cava, the right supracardinal vein forms the infrarenal segment, the postcardinal vein forms the iliac bifurcation, and the subcardinal and supracardinal systems contribute to the formation of the renal veins. The suprarenal right and left supracardinal veins and the proximal postcardinal veins form the azygous system and hemiazygous system. Variations in these developmental processes causes five uncommon, but important anomalies.[16–22]

Inferior Vena Cava Anomalies

Duplication or Double Inferior Vena Cava

Duplication or double inferior vena cava consists of large veins on both sides of the aorta that join anteriorly at the level of the renal arteries to become the infrarenal inferior vena cava. The cause of this anomaly is failure of the left supracardinal veins to regress.

Transposition or Left-Sided Inferior Vena Cava

Transposition or left-sided inferior vena cava consists of an inferior vena cava to the left of the aorta that crosses to its right side, usually anterior to the aorta at the level of the renal arteries. This anomaly is a true transposition so that the inferior vena cava on the left side is a mirror image of the normal right-sided inferior vena cava. Therefore, in a patient with left-sided inferior vena cava the left gonadal and adrenal veins, which normally empty into the left renal vein, instead empty into the inferior vena cava. The right gonadal and adrenal veins that usually drain into the inferior vena cava instead join the right renal vein in a patient with left-sided inferior vena cava. This anomaly occurs because the left supracardinal vein persists and the right supracardinal vein regresses, which is the opposite of normal.

Retroaortic Left Renal Vein

Retroaortic left renal vein consists of the left renal vein crossing posterior to the aorta to join the inferior vena cava. During gestation, the vein anterior to the aorta regresses while the vein posterior persists. This is the opposite of the normal occurrence.

Circumaortic Left Renal Vein

Circumaortic left renal vein consists of a left renal vein anterior and posterior to the aorta that join just before entering the inferior vena cava, thus forming a venous collar around the aorta. This anomaly occurs when the vein posterior to the aorta does not regress. It should be noted that both duplication and transposition of the inferior vena cava are associated with important anomalies of the renal veins. Although the inferior vena cava in both anomalies usually join or cross anterior to the aorta at the level of the renal arteries, either one can cross posterior with retroaortic left renal vein or might be associated with a circumaortic left renal vein.

Retrocaval Ureter

The right ureter lies anterior to the right supracardinal vein in the embryo. Since this vein forms the infrarenal inferior vena cava, the ureter anatomically is anterior to the inferior vena cava. The infrarenal inferior vena cava sometimes develops from the right subcardinal system. The ureter, which embryologically is behind the subcardinal system, then lies posterior to the inferior vena cava. The ureter must go to the left and in front of the inferior vena cava to attach to the bladder. When unsuspected, dissection of the inferior vena cava may cause injury to the ureter.

Absent Suprarenal Inferior Vena Cava

The suprarenal inferior vena cava is formed from the right subcardinal vein. If the right subcardinal system does not develop, then the suprarenal inferior vena cava is absent. Blood is returned to the heart through the azygous system and hemiazygous system that normally is formed by the suprarenal supracardinal veins and the proximal postcardinal veins. In this anomaly, blood from the lower body is returned to the heart through the supracardinal system that forms the infrarenal inferior vena cava and the azygous system. Because the azygous system becomes large, these veins may produce unusual shadows on chest x-rays.

Summary

Anomalies of the inferior vena cava are uncommon, but important entities to the vascular radiologist and the vascular surgeon. The radiologist must distinguish between an anomalous inferior vena cava and a pathologic process such as lymphadenopathy. He or she must also be aware of the anatomic variability of the renal veins in order to obtain blood samples for localization of adrenal tumors or the diagnosis of renovascular hypertension. The vascular surgeon needs to recognize anomalies of the inferior vena cava to perform safe dissections of the retroperitoneum in patients undergoing aortic reconstruction or sympathectomy, as well as to accurately interrupt or insert a filter in the inferior vena cava of patients with pulmonary embolism or deep venous thrombosis.

References

1. Arcinegas E, Hakima M, Hertzler JH, et al: Surgical management of congenital vascular rings. *J Thorac Cardiovasc Surg* 77:721, 1979.
2. Mahoney EB, Manning JA: Congenital abnormalities of the aortic arch. *Surgery* 55:1, 1964.
3. Richardson JV, Doty DG, Rossi NP, et al. Operation for aortic arch anomalies. *Ann Thorac Surg* 31:426, 1981.
4. Binet JP, Langlois J: Aortic arch anomalies in children and infants. *J Thorac Cardiovasc Surg* 73:248, 1977.
5. Lincoln JCR, Deverall PB, Stark J, et al: Vascular anomalies compressing the esophagus and trachea. *Thorax* 24:295, 1969.
6. Merklin RJ, Michaels NA: The variant renal and suprarenal blood supply with data on inferior phrenic, urethral, and gonadal arteries. *J Int Coll Surg* 29:41, 1958.
7. Gray SW, Skandalokis JE: *Embryology for Surgeons.* Philadelphia: WB Saunders, Co.; 486, 1972.
8. Anson BJ, Richardson GA, Minear WL: Variations in the number and arrangements of the renal vessels. *J Urol* 36:211, 1936.
9. Senior HD: The development of the arteries of the human lower extremity. *Am J Anat* 25:55, 1919.
10. Mayschak DT, Flye WM: Treatment of the persistent sciatic artery. *Ann Surg* 199:69, 1984.
11. McLellan GL, Morettin LB: Persistent sciatic artery: clinical, surgical, and angiographic aspects. *Arch Surg* 117:817, 1982.
12. Meyer WW, Lind J: Iliac arteries in children with a single umbilical artery. *Arch Dis Child* 49:671, 1974.
13. Gibson MHL, Mills JG, Johnson GE, et al: Popliteal entrapment syndrome. *Ann Surg* 185:341, 1977.
14. Nandy K, Blair CB Jr: Double superior venae cavae with completely paired azygous veins. *Anat Rec* 151:1, 1965.
15. Winter FS: Persistent left superior vena cava: survey of world literature and report of thirty additional cases. *Angiology* 5:90, 1954.
16. Babian RJ, Johnson DE: Major venous anomalies complicating retroperitoneal surgery. *South Med J* 72:1254, 1979.
17. Chaung VP, Mena CE, Hoskins PA: Congenital anomalies of the left renal vein: angiographic consideration. *Br J Radiol* 47:214, 1974.
18. Dardik H, Loop FD, Cox PA, et al: C-pattern inferior vena cava. *JAMA* 200:248, 1967.
19. Kolbenstvedt A, Kolmannskog F, Lien HH: The anomalous inferior vena cava—another structure between the aorta and the superior mesenteric artery. *Br J Radiol* 54:423, 1981.
20. Berner BJ, Darling C, Fredrick PL, et al: Major venous anomalies complicating abdominal aortic surgery. *Arch Surg* 108:160, 1974.
21. Mayo J, Gray R, St Louis E, et al: Anomalies of the inferior vena cava. *Am J Radiol* 140:339, 1983.
22. Giordano JM, Trout HH III: Anomalies of the inferior vena cava. *J Vasc Surg* 3:924, 1986.

CHAPTER 2

Molecular Biology and the Vascular Surgeon

John A. Peyman, PhD; Bauer E. Sumpio, MD, PhD

The Challenge of Molecular Surgery

Inherited single-gene defects, as well as multiple-gene products interacting with environmental factors, have been implicated in the initiation and progression of cardiovascular disease. The contributions of various genes and exogenous molecules are heterogeneous and complex, and the pathophysiologic changes can affect primary cells and also secondary associated cell types. Disturbances in cell-to-cell communication and intracellular signaling can lead to altered gene expression at the level of transcription of DNA into RNA in the cell nucleus, or in the translation of RNA into protein in the cell cytoplasm, or in post-translational processing steps along the protein biosynthetic pathway. Pinpointing the mechanisms responsible for the observed pathology, and understanding the molecules involved, should lead to more precise diagnostic tests and facilitate the development of incisive gene therapy, or "molecular surgery."

This chapter is a practical guide to molecular biology for the vascular surgeon. We introduce the basic concepts of the mechanism of gene expression and survey a spectrum of techniques in molecular biology that are useful in cloning and sequencing genes and studying their RNA and protein gene products. We have not furnished detailed protocols, which are amply described in the excellent laboratory manuals for gene cloning[1,2] and in specialized guides for specific experimental techniques,[3–6] or molecular diagnostic methods.[7] We review several of the available computer software packages which are useful for handling molecular sequence data. We point out appropriate reviews,[8–29] textbooks,[30–38] and videotapes[46–50] for the surgeon to gain a sense of the scope of molecular biology, and the reader is guided to the research literature[39–45] for specifics on several topics of molecular cell biology, molecular diagnostics, and gene therapy. For starters, we recommend the book by Berg and Singer which is a lucid and lively introduction to molecular biology, from its origins to its present-day expanding role in basic science and clinical practice.[31] We include glossaries of basic terms in molecular biology, in recombinant DNA technology, and in molecular genetics at the end of the chapter. We extend our discussion from methods in basic research that can provide analytical probes and preparative templates, to ideas on molecular diagnostic assays, and finally to a brief survey of gene therapy for disease caused by a single-gene defect and for disease with multifactorial inheritance. As molecular research leads to clinical trials with greater success, more and more patients will be treated with novel modes of gene therapy, cell therapy, and applications of recombinant DNA products. We attempt in this chapter to tie these ideas together and to encourage the reader to take on the challenge of molecular surgery.

The Central Dogma: DNA Makes RNA, and RNA Makes Protein

Human genes that encode proteins are composed of several basic elements (Figure 1). The messenger

From *The Basic Science of Vascular Disease*. Edited by Sidawy AN, Sumpio BE, and DePalma RG. Armonk, NY: Futura Publishing Company, Inc.; © 1997.

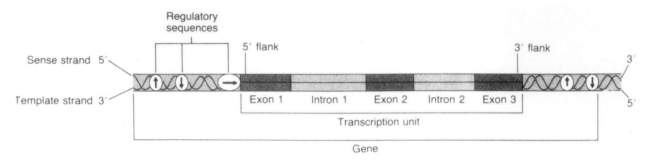

Figure 1. Structure of a representative human gene. (Reproduced with permission from Reference 31.)

RNA (mRNA)-encoding sequences (exons) are usually discontinuous and vary in number and size in different genes. Between the exons are the intervening noncoding sequences (introns). Sharp and Mullis recently received the Nobel Prize in medicine for their discovery of introns and the interrupted genes of eukaryotes. Some small human genes span 2 or 3 thousand base pairs (bp). Genes encoding large polypeptides can have over 100 exons, and some of these large genes have been found to extend over 1 million bp long! These genes include some large introns. The regions between separate genes (intergenic regions) do not code for protein, but these long stretches can be involved indirectly in gene expression, however, by taking part in the formation of higher order chromatin structures. These include open chromatin (euchromatin), the presence of which is a minimal requirement for expression of nearby genes, or condensed chromatin (heterochromatin) that is transcriptionally silent.

Each gene has a promoter that is the recognition site used by the RNA polymerase enzyme complex as it begins to interpret the genetic code that it encounters along the chromosome.[31,33] Regulatory proteins bind to promoter regions and guide the RNA polymerase complex to the start site; most stimulate initiation of transcription, but some suppress transcription. These proteins are encoded by genes at distant sites, and are thus *trans*-acting regulatory factors that function on the nearby, or *cis*-acting, regulatory DNA sequences of protein-encoding genes. Gene promoters are comprised of several short (5 to 10 bp) sequences. The promoter sequences that are found near genes expressed in a certain cell type or by a certain stimulus are often identical, and these common regulatory sequences give genes encoding unrelated proteins the capacity for coexpression. The promoter is located adjacent to the transcriptional start site at the 5′-end of a gene and is oriented in a particular direction.[33] Some regulatory sequences can act in either orientation and were originally called enhancers, but some promoters for one

gene act as enhancers for another. Some stimulatory sequences act as suppressors for other genes. A gene that is expressed in response to a combination of cytokines, steroids, neurotransmitters, and physical stimuli, for example, may utilize overlapping DNA regulatory sequences that interact with a battery of transacting factors to give the fine-tuning required. In general, sets of proteins are expressed due to localized activity of the RNA polymerase II complex that is facilitated by interactions with families of trans-acting transcription factors binding to groups of cis-acting DNA sequences.[13]

Estimates range between 10000 and 100000 for the number of genes coding for proteins along the 22 human autosomes and the X and Y sex chromosomes.[33,37] In each cell type, a small percentage of these genes is expressed as proteins which produce the unique structure and functions of the tissue. Each cell type in an individual human has the same chromosome content, except for the rearrangements and deletions that occur naturally in the course of B lymphocyte immunoglobulin gene and T lymphocyte antigen receptor gene expression. Operationally, this means that one can use any convenient cell type to analyze the genome of a patient or experimental animal by probing a Southern blot, for example. The mRNAs produced by transcription of the genes in a particular cell type form a unique array for that cell type under those physiologic or experimental conditions. The mRNAs encode the unique proteins in addition to the common proteins of the cell. Thus, the analysis of cellular mRNA shows patterns of cell and tissue specificity.[33,36,37] Some proteins are maintained at constant concentrations in the cell under all circumstances and are encoded by the so-called "housekeeping" genes. For instance, the genes encoding the cytoskeletal protein γ-actin and the glycolytic pathway enzyme glyceraldehyde-3-phosphate dehydrogenase (GAPDH) are considered housekeeping genes. The steady-state concentrations of actin or GAPDH mRNA are quite constant in most cells, and their levels are commonly used to calibrate the differences in expression of other genes studied. Exceptions in specific cell types do occur, and more sensitive or specific tests of gene function are necessary to reveal subtle regulatory differences. For example, the α-actin gene is not a housekeeping gene in smooth muscle cells (SMCs). All cell types undergo changes in gene expression during their normal cellular functions, and very few genes are not modulated in one way or another. The expression of most proteins is regulated over tissue development, over the course of the cell cycle in normal growth, and under particular conditions in response to acute stimuli for cellular activation. Discussions of gene structure and expression are well presented in the textbooks of Zubay,[38] Lewin,[33] and Watson et al.[37]

Gene expression involves the transfer of coding information from DNA to mRNA by the process of transcription (Figure 2), and the decoding of the gene sequence by the process of translation leading to the production of a polypeptide chain. Transcription occurs in the nucleus of human cells, and translation occurs in the cytoplasm after maturation of the mRNA

(Figure 3) and transport of the message out of the nucleus.[30,32] A putative transcriptional promoter can be tested by preparing a synthetic construct that combines the DNA fragment with a previously characterized and easily detected reporter gene. Reintroducing the molecular construct into cells allows one to follow the production of the reporter mRNA and/or reporter protein and to determine whether the control sequence is sufficient to induce expression.[1,2] Conversely, when the putative promoter sequence is chopped back progressively in the preparation of a series of constructs (5'-deletion mutants) some of these artificial DNA sequences lose the capability of promoting the expression of an adjacent protein-encoding sequence if critical stimulatory regions are removed before they are tested in living cells. These functional tests (promoter analyses) indicate that the promoter can be both necessary and sufficient to drive the expression of the gene. The sequence of a promoter is often initially discernible because of its similarity to promoters from other previously characterized genes. However, most genes have not been cloned to date, and many new regulatory regions and their mechanisms of action remain to be elu-

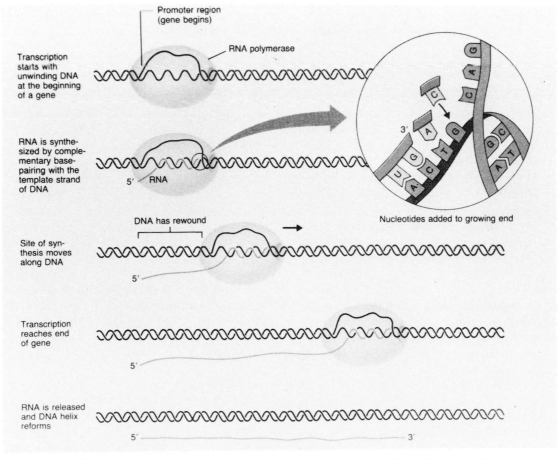

Figure 2. Transcription of a gene. (Reproduced with permission from Reference 31.)

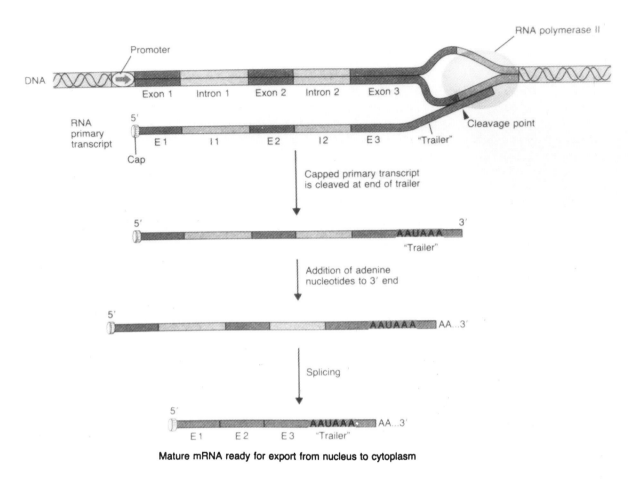

Figure 3. Sequence of steps in the maturation of a nascent RNA polymerase II transcript and the formation of a mature mRNA prior to its transport to the cytoplasm. (Reproduced with permission from Reference 31.)

cidated. The characteristics of a gene promoter can vary depending on the assay used: a promoter-reporter construct may be expressed at one level in vitro with cell extracts, at a different level when transferred into living cells, and differently still when engineered into the genome of a line of transgenic animals.[1,2,33,37] The gene's response to an applied stimulus in these assay systems may depend on its relationship to the neighboring DNA. The flux of intermediate forms of chromatin, which lie between the extremes of fully open and condensed,[33] as well as specialized organelles within the nucleus, likely represent additional mechanistic components operating to regulate gene expression.[39–41] These sites of interaction of multi-protein complexes with chromatin carry out DNA replication (Figure 4), repair, and transcription (Figure 2); sites of interaction of other multi-protein complexes with newly synthesized RNA carry out capping, polyadenylation, splicing, and transport (Figure 3). The basic dichotomy of cellular functions into growth and mitosis is reflected in the phases of the cell cycle: G0 cells are noncycling; G1-phase involves most protein biosyn-

thesis; S phase involves most DNA synthesis and some S-phase-specific protein synthesis; G2-phase involves some protein synthesis in preparation for mitosis; M-phase involves shutdown of protein and DNA synthesis, and chromosome condensation for mitosis.[30,32] The phases of the cell growth cycle besides mitosis are called interphase, and it is during interphase that gene expression is observed. There are functionally significant links between the transcription-translation systems that yield proteins and the replication systems that yield DNA.[32] There may be a specific spatial organization of these functional regions of the cell nucleus[14,39–41]; developmental regulation of these nuclear regions and implications for disease etiology have yet to be studied.

DNA Sequence Information

The sequence of a new gene provides digital information obtained from the sequencing ladders of a discrete set of A, C, G, and T data points. The orientation

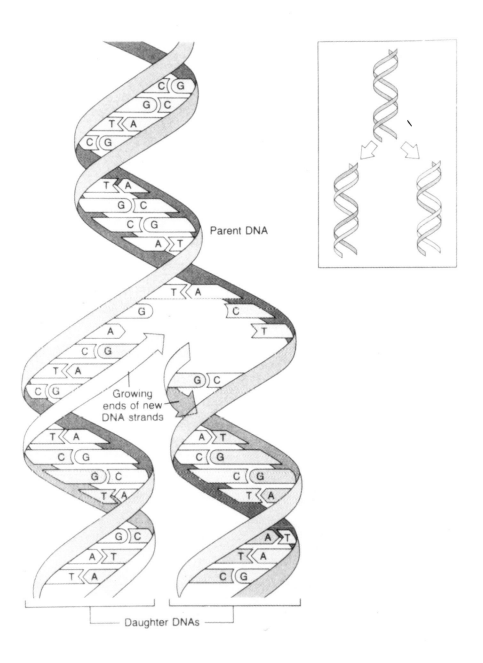

Figure 4. Replication of DNA. (Reproduced with permission from Reference 31.)

Parent DNA

Growing ends of new DNA strands

Daughter DNAs

of the sequence is usually known from the methodology used[1,2,4,6] and is written in the direction 5'-end . . . gene sequence . . . 3'-end. The orientation of the protein-coding regions is determined by testing each sequence of nucleotide triplets for the presence of codons that form a series long enough to encode the protein investigated and then end with one of three possible stop codons. Nascent polypeptides begin with an N-terminal methionine amino acid (AUG codon), and therefore the corresponding DNA triplet ATG marks the start of the open reading frame that yields the protein. The genetic code comprised of 64 codons for 20 amino acids and 3 termination signals is shown in Table 1.

The pattern of restriction endonuclease cleavage sites in a new gene is used to prepare samples for sequencing by cutting and religating conveniently sized pieces into carriers or vectors. These restriction enzyme sites are also important for identifying the overlapping fragments of a large gene that has been obtained by the cloning of a series of its component parts in separate experiments. The DNA bands in an agarose electrophoresis gel are visualized by staining with the fluorescent dye ethidium bromide and viewing on an ultraviolet light box. The sizes of the fragments provide rough structural information. The schematic representation of the data from restriction endonuclease diges-

Table 1
The Genetic Code

SECOND POSITION

FIRST POSITION		U			C			A			G			THIRD POSITION
	U	UUU UUC	Phe	(F)	UCU UCC	Ser	(S)	UAU UAC	Tyr	(Y)	UGU UGC	Cys	(C)	U C	
		UUA UUG	Leu	(L)	UCA UCG			UAA UAG	Stop Stop		UGA UGG	Stop Trp	(W)	A G	
	C	CUU CUC	Leu	(L)	CCU CCC	Pro	(P)	CAU CAC	His	(H)	CGU CGC	Arg	(R)	U C	
		CUA CUG			CCA CCG			CAA CAG	Gln	(Q)	CGA CGG			A G	
	A	AUU AUC	Ile	(I)	ACU ACC	Thr	(T)	AAU AAC	Asn	(N)	AGU AGC	Ser	(S)	U C	
		AUA AUG	Met	(M)	ACA ACG			AAA AAG	Lys	(K)	AGA AGG	Arg	(R)	A G	
	G	GUU GUC	Val	(V)	GCU GCC	Ala	(A)	GAU GAC	Asp	(D)	GGU GGC	Gly	(G)	U C	
		GUA GUG			GCA GCG			GAA GAG	Glu	(E)	GGA GGG			A G	

Abbreviations:

Ala:	alanine	His:	histidine	Stop:	termination codon
Arg:	arginine	Ile:	isoleucine	Thr:	threonine
Asn:	asparagine	Leu:	leucine	Trp:	tryptophan
Asp:	aspartic acid	Lys:	lysine	Tyr:	tyrosine
Cys:	cysteine	Met:	methionine	Val:	valine
Glu:	glutamic acid	Phe:	phenylalanine		
Gln:	glutamine	Pro:	proline		
Gly:	glycine	Ser:	serine		

The single-letter codes for the amino acids are given in parentheses.

tion and eletrophoresis is a ''restriction map.'' The sizes of the DNA fragments observed add up to the size of the intact linearized DNA molecule, and these data are accurate enough to be useful when added and subtracted during subsequent recombinant DNA manipulations like ligation, relinearization, and fragment isolation. This situation is in dramatic contrast to that of protein and peptide electrophoretic gels and chromatographic separations because of the physical heterogeneity of protein mixtures. This nonideal electrophoretic behavior of polypeptides is caused by large differences in the physical properties of the amino acids, and by additional post-translational modifications that add or remove charged residues or blocks of sugars to some amino acids. Most nucleic acids consist of sequences close to 50% A-T pairs and 50% C-G pairs, and, therefore, most nucleic acids, stripped of their associated proteins, have similar physical properties.

We can calculate the minimum size of DNA that is long enough to produce a certain protein. Determining the molecular mass of a protein usually involves data that are in analog form. The size of a protein can be experimentally determined as smaller than that of the encoded polypeptide because of post-translational clipping of a peptide or it can be larger due to the addition of polysaccharide, phosphate, sulfate, or lipid groups. Some proteins migrate faster or slower than average in electrophoretic gels, and their size is thus poorly estimated. The average molecular mass of an amino acid is 110 Daltons (Da). A small protein, for example, of molecular mass observed on a denaturing SDS-PAGE gel of 11,000 Da (11 kDa) would contain approximately 100 amino acids and, therefore, it would be the translation product of a mature mRNA of at least 300 nucleotides in length. A large protein of 110000 Da mass (110 kDa) would contain 1000 amino acids and require an mRNA of at least 3000 nucleotides in length.

The mRNAs in these examples would also contain a certain number of untranslated nucleotides at the 5'-end (5'-UT), and a requisite 3'-sequence including the termination codon and almost always a poly-adenylation signal sequence (usually 5'-AATAAA-3') followed by a variable number of nucleotides in the 3'-untranslated portion of the mRNA (3'-UT). The 5'-UT and the 3'-UT are specific sequences in each message that extend from the site of initiation of transcription to the site where transcription of the gene ends. The 3'-UT sequences can vary in size among different genes up to several thousand nucleotides in length. The primary transcript also includes introns that are removed by RNA splicing in the nucleus. Introns are not present in the mature mRNA found in the cytoplasm. A sequence of poly-A residues from about 50 to 200 nucleotides in length is added by a post-transcriptional mechanism in the nucleus to the extreme 3'-end of the mRNA. The 3'-UT can also contain repetitive sequences (such as Alu repeats in human genes) found in abundance throughout the genome (one every 6000 bp), that have no known function. In practical terms, the presence of an Alu sequence can create difficulties if the untranslated region of a cDNA clone is inadvertently used as a labeled probe to detect sequences related to the coding region of the cDNA. Such a probe would hybridize to many unrelated cDNAs or mRNAs or to hundreds of thousands of sequences of genomic DNA. Therefore, the use of protein-coding regions of genes and cDNAs as hybridization probes is recommended, unless sequence analysis confirms the absence of repetitive sequences.

Sequencing the fragments of the novel gene results in the accumulation of information that, when compiled, describes an mRNA long enough to code for the protein. Computer software has been designed to handle the overlapping sequence information and assemble a consensus. Several of the available programs will be discussed later in this chapter. The six possible reading frames, three on the sequenced strand, and three predicted on the complementary strand, are analyzed to find the longest open reading frame, i.e., from a methionine start codon to a termination codon. If more than one methionine codon occurs in the same long open reading frame at the 5'-end of the gene, additional experiments may be required to determine the precise starting point of translation in the cell. Utilization of alternate splice sites in some genes can also give rise to the production of distinct mRNAs in different tissues, although the mRNA in each tissue often has only one specific sequence.

There is more than one codon for each amino acid, except methionine and tryptophan (Table 1). This can be important in designing synthetic oligonucleotide hybridization probes[1,2] or polymerase chain reaction primers[3,4] that are based on amino acid sequencing in-

formation. In this type of situation, a gene sequence data bank and appropriate software are useful in determining which are the most prevalent codons utilized in previously sequenced genes from the species studied. Usage of the different codons for amino acids can vary among species, but is essentially constant in the different tissues of an individual. An oligonucleotide synthesis machine can be programmed to prepare a probe or pair of primers with the most likely DNA sequence corresponding to the polypeptide sequence of the new gene product.

Experimental Design: Specificity and Sensitivity of a Molecular Probe

Some important characteristics to consider when choosing experimental methods in molecular biology are their specificity, sensitivity, and technical complexity. Specificity of a molecular technique refers to the qualitative limits in the range of structurally related target molecules that are detected or isolated. For example, the detection of cellular RNA separated by size on a formaldehyde-agarose gel and transferred by blotting to the surface of a nylon membrane (a Northern blot) involves considerations of specificity in the binding of the labeled probe.[1,2] Another example is the case of bacterial colonies grown on an agar plate and these separate clones transferred to a nitrocellulose filter (a colony lift) for detection of the recombinant plasmid DNA produced by the bacteria. The bacterial clones yielding the DNA that anneals to the gene probe are identified and subsequently removed individually, and their content of identical plasmid molecules (cloned DNA) is amplified by further bulk cultures in suspension. The detection of the DNA on the colony lift similarly requires considerations of specificity.[1,2] A small fragment (400 to 1000 bp) of a previously cloned gene is often used as a DNA probe. It is radiolabeled or labeled with another small molecular tag to allow simple detection. The probe binds to the complementary RNA or DNA strand by base pairing in the process of hybridization. The binding to other dissimilar molecules would produce one or more background signals in the experiment. By adjusting the temperature and the NaCl concentration in hybridization procedures with DNA, RNA, or oligonucleotide probes, the binding to complementary DNA targets in Southern blots or mRNA targets in Northern blots can be enhanced and background binding can be reduced to an undetectable level. High salt concentration (150 mM to 1 M) at low temperature (25 to 50°C) forces a DNA probe used in molar excess over target sites to bind to DNA molecules in a sample that have short regions of complementarity in their structure. These conditions are called "low stringency" and are used to saturate the target sites with detectable probe. When the unbound probe solution is removed and the filter treated with a fresh solution of low salt concentration (15 mM to 1.5 mM) at an elevated temperature (50 to 80°C), the non-specifically bound molecules dissociate ("melt") and the DNA probe remains bound only to long stretches of target DNA that contain precisely complementary sequences. Treating the filters under these conditions is called "high-stringency" washing. Given a certain concentration of target mRNA or DNA in the samples used in the above examples, therefore, the conditions of probe binding and the stringency of the subsequent washing steps determine the specificity of the results obtained by the subsequent visualization of the bound probe. The concentration of target molecules of mRNA or DNA in the sample analyzed is the other principal contributor to the specificity of detected signals: abundant mRNAs of each tissue can be detected with a high level of signal specificity and low level of noise. In establishing a new method in the laboratory, the confirmation of the identity of detected target molecules is paramount in importance, and positive control samples from several cell types, tissues, species, or related molecular forms are extremely useful (see discussion of control experiments below). It is also important to rule out trivial reasons for the observation of detected signals by characterizing the detected molecules in several independent ways (discussed below).

The sensitivity of procedures in molecular biology ranges from the ability to detect single molecules by polymerase chain reaction[1-4,7] or fluorescence (high sensitivity with low to high accuracy,[39-41] to the accurate determination of concentrations of bulk solutions of DNA, RNA, or protein by spectrophotometry (low sensitivity with high accuracy).[1,2] The most sensitive techniques increase the product concentration exponentially by repeated DNA polymerase-catalyzed geometric doublings in reactions carried out with automated equipment, or increase the product concentration arithmetically by the use of two or three layers of detection reagents topped off with an enzyme-catalyzed increase in product.

The standard method used to detect DNA probes in the past has been labeling with a radioactive isotope and scintillation counting for liquid samples, or autoradiography for gels and blots (Southern blots for DNA and Northern blots for RNA).[1,2] Nearly all molecular methods can be adapted for use with radioactive nucleic acid probes. A [^{32}P]-deoxyribonucleoside triphosphate is incorporated into a DNA probe, or [^{32}P]-ribonucleoside triphosphate is incorporated into an RNA probe. For finer spatial resolution in in situ hybridization procedures, a [^{35}S]-ribonucleoside triphosphate is incorporated into an ^{35}S-labeled antisense RNA probe for detection after binding to cellular mRNA by the autoradiographic exposure of an overlaid photographic emulsion. Direct quantitation of radioactive signals on solid matrices like gels and blots can now be accomplished by use of electronic autoradiographic detectors and image processors that boost sensitivity and provide digital output (PhosphorImager SI, Molecular Dynamics, Sunnyvale, CA; InstantImager, Packard Instrument Co., Meriden, CT).

Recently a number of equally sensitive nonradioactive methods have been established that involve the use of multiple biotin tags, multiple digoxigenin tags, multiple fluorescent tags, or other small molecules on the synthetic DNA or RNA probe.[1,2] These side-groups do not necessarily interfere with sequence-specific annealing of probes in hybridization procedures, and are also tolerated by DNA polymerases used in DNA labeling, amplification, and sequencing reactions. Nonradioactive methods have not replaced radioactive probes in all applications, but the trend toward increased use of nonradioactive probes will continue because of their improved safety and convenience.

Detection of fluorescently labeled DNA probes or small aliquots of preparative samples can be accomplished by using a sensitive spectrofluorimeter for samples in solution, and by videocamera recording of fluorescent images of samples in gels or in the laser-scanning confocal microscope of images of cells or tissues. The digital images can be computer-enhanced to maximize signal and minimize noise. With these methods, the overall sensitivity of fluorescent detection is close to that of isotope detection. Moreover, the spatial resolution afforded by detection of the molecules in situ provides another advantage of fluorescence over a radioactive method.[39-41] Three-dimensional resolution of signals is lost when a two-dimensional image is produced on x-ray film or in an overlaid photographic emulsion.

Detection of chemically modified DNA probes usually takes advantage of the high-affinity binding of a small ligand to a polypeptide, such as biotin to avidin (or streptavidin).[1,2] One assumes that there is little biotin in the sample, and the labeled probe is detected subsequently by use of biotin-labeled horseradish peroxidase or biotin-labeled alkaline phosphatase in the multiple avidin-biotin complexes formed. In another sensitive method, a high-affinity antibody raised against the digoxigenin molecule is used to detect the modified DNA probe. Digoxigenin is a steroid not found in animal cells. An antibody specific for any type of derivatized DNA itself can be pre-labeled with the enzyme horseradish peroxidase or the enzyme alkaline phosphatase, each of which, in turn, has an armamentarium of detection methods that includes enzyme substrates that form soluble dyes, colored precipitates, fluorescent products, and light-emitting chemicals. Alternatively, the antibody bound onto the modified

DNA can be detected with even greater sensitivity by binding a second antibody that then becomes the object to be measured, by the same methods described.

The complexity of a method involves the precision with which the component operations must be carried out to ensure success. In contradistinction, the robustness of a method refers to the lack of critical manipulations in its successful operation. It is difficult to judge the complexity of a technique without applying it to a specific preparative or analytical system and testing the robustness of its components. This is true of the minor component methods, as well as the overall scheme. Some new methods have revolutionized molecular biology, and techniques are continually described as improvements. However, an old, time-consuming method sometimes outperforms a new, quick method due to the lack of productivity during the start-up and testing for sensitivity, specificity, and reproducibility of results with the new method. However, when the long-term benefits in cost, time, safety, or other aspects of productivity outweigh the start-up factors, then the effort invested in developing a new procedure may pay off. Consideration of the complexity is of prime importance when planning a project on a new experimental approach to the study of a disease mechanism, or on an analytical plan for more specific molecular diagnosis, or on a novel strategy for treatment by modulation of gene expression. Many of the binding techniques described in this chapter are commonly used as building blocks to form combination methods, and in addition are easily adapted with similar specificity and sensitivity, and with little or no added complexity to a wide range of samples and conditions. Thus, a labeled DNA, RNA, or oligonucleotide probe can be used to detect and even to isolate its specific binding partner in a bacterial cell extract or in a frozen section of human tissue, for example. The universality of the genetic code and the conservation of structures in cells of many organisms over the course of evolution provide investigators with the opportunity to study human genes and their RNA and protein products by using probes from other species.

Antibodies are proteins produced by cells of the immune system that recognize differences between self and nonself. The immunogenic regions of proteins drive the formation of these antibodies and are rarely those sequences common to all proteins in a family in one species or across species. In addition, recombinant proteins produced in bacterial cells are often aggregated and the epitopes of naturally biosynthesized proteins that bind antibodies can, therefore, be inaccessible. For these reasons, antibody probes are seldom used as general molecular screening reagents, although immunochemical analysis is very important in many areas of research and in clinical diagnosis. Antibodies have been used to isolate the cDNAs encoding their antigens from bacterial expression libraries with the λgt11 vector (see the discussion of prokaryotic expression vectors below).[1,2] Heteroantisera are generally more powerful than monoclonal antibodies as tools for expression cloning because the spectrum of epitopes recognized by polyclonal antisera gives a higher probability of detecting the desired polypeptide antigen produced by bacteria.

The chemistry of proteins is extremely diverse, and an interaction between a protein and other molecules often reflects specific properties of a region of the surface of the protein involved.[30,32] A greater understanding of the nature of protein structures and their functions is one of the principal goals of modern biology. DNA technology has the capability to precisely detect similarities and differences between biomolecules from changes of a single base to rearrangements of an entire gene region.[1-7] The resulting differences in the proteins encoded can be predicted by comparison to known structural motifs, and can also be observed in the test tube or experimental animal by actual production of natural and mutant recombinant molecules. Some of the most elegant protein studies are currently performed directly with molecular methods or indirectly with the use of recombinant molecules. These include structure-function correlations to show the effects of changing molecular structures, cell and tissue and animal expression studies to determine the physiologic significance of recombinant molecules, gene knockout experiments to show the results of the complete absence of specific proteins, and crystallographic studies mapping each atom in proteins overproduced and purified with the aid of recombinant techniques.

Many of the preparative methods described in this chapter can also be combined in various ways and adapted for use with a wide range of samples. In some cases, the tissues, cells, organelles, and molecules have unique preparations and general methods cannot be applied. These facets of a preparation or an analysis can be advantageous in providing an added dimension of selectivity. The tendency of a component of any mixture, of cells or molecules, for example, to separate or break down, or aggregate, or solubilize, by a certain treatment can help significantly in the isolation of that component or of the remaining components of the mixture.

Experimental Design: Controls, Replicates, and Independent Analyses

Positive controls are samples that have been shown to give a detectable signal in an assay. Negative controls are samples that give no signal because of absent target molecule or because of the intentional omis-

Table 2
Design of Preparative or Analytical
Experiments

Independent dimensions in sample preparation
- Normal and pathologic states.
- Human and other model systems.
- Fresh tissue and cultured cell lines.
- Whole cells and isolated organelles.
- Mixed samples and purified molecules.
- Electrophoretic and chromatographic separations.
- Homogenization and solubilization.
- Equilibrium methods, steady state methods, and rapid sampling methods.
- Isolation of components from active system and reconstitution of activity.

Independent dimensions in **DNA analysis**
- DNA clones and fresh genomic samples.
- Polymerase chain reaction amplified fragments and mini-prep DNA.
- Genomic sequence and cDNA sequence.
- Promoter-binding proteins in footprinting and gel shift assays.
- Footprinting with cell extracts and in intact cells.
- Spacing and sequence of components of gene promoter.

Independent dimensions in **RNA analysis**
- RNA on Northern blots and in situ hybridization.
- cDNA clones and fresh mRNA.
- Total cellular RNA and polyA$^+$-RNA.
- Nascent RNA transcript and mature mRNA.
- Transcription in original cell type and heterologous system.

Independent dimensions in **protein studies**
- Recombinant protein and natural protein.
- Native protein and denatured protein.
- Intact protein and deletion mutants.

Independent dimensions in **gene therapy**
- Interference with expression of mRNA and of protein.
- Addition and deletion of gene function.
- Delivery by retroviral vector, DNA viral vector, and liposomes.
- Use of constitutive gene promoter and inducible promoter.
- Targeting of single gene and two or more genes.

sion of one of the detection reagents. Standards are samples of known concentration or activity that are used to calibrate an assay in a quantitative manner as a measure of accuracy. Replicate determinations from the same preparation are used to determine the usual scatter in the assay results as a measure of precision. Independent preparations are used on different days with as many separately prepared reagents as possible to show the reproducibility of the results. Independent analyses are completely different methods used to confirm the data and also the conclusions obtained from one line of experiments. The inclusion of each of these controls is of ultimate importance to demonstrate that the results are valid, and not the outcome of a trivial difference between samples.

Sometimes, one cannot detect the most critical variable in an experiment while one varies a condition along a supposedly important dimension, and only when one investigates another aspect of the system does one uncover large differences produced by variations along this independent dimension. This may be important when attempting to confirm the results of a certain preparation or analytical procedure. A number of pairs of independent dimensions of preparation or analysis are listed in Table 2.

Experimental Design: Study of Normal and Mutant Genes by Classic and by Molecular Techniques

Human genes have a complex composition with several structural levels of compaction (Figure 5). Model systems using nonhuman species have provided most of the advances in molecular biology to date.[35] Indeed, much of our knowledge about human genes has been derived from studies of bacteria, viruses, yeast, fruit flies, frogs, and mice. The use of mutants in classic genetic analysis was the key to many early advances.[36] However, the study of gene structure and function in humans is no longer limited to mutant alleles for well-characterized proteins, such as those occurring in the α- and β-globin gene loci that cause thalassemia.[36] Several factors have contributed to this change. First, most diseases are not caused by mutations in the genes encoding abundant proteins in each cell (like hemoglobin in erythrocyte precursors). Proteins that regulate cellular activities are often present at low concentrations. Second, many diseases are multifactorial, with genetic predisposition superimposed on other precipitating factors; no single mutation in a structural protein of cells in the affected tissues has been implicated.[36] Third, and perhaps most significantly, the functions of newly discovered genes can be determined without the use of mutant sequences (Table 3).

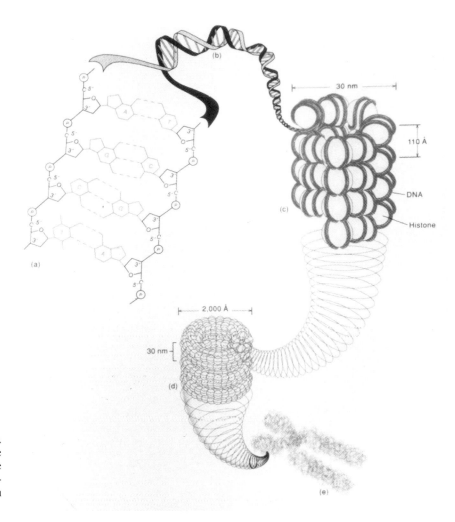

Figure 5. Levels of compaction of DNA in the double helix, in nucleosomes, in the 30 nm fiber, in the 2000Å fiber, and in the condensed chromosome undergoing mitosis. (Reproduced with permission from Reference 37.)

The ability to isolate genes, disassemble and reassemble them in all conceivable ways, and to produce replenishable supplies of the DNA, encoded RNA, and recombinant protein from each of these constructions (Figure 6), is due largely to the commercial availability of hundreds of purified and well-characterized enzymes.[1,2] Of singular importance is the growing family of restriction endonucleases that cleave double-stranded DNA at specific recognition sites of known sequence. Twenty-four restriction endonucleases, divided into three categories of cleavage product and five categories of recognition sequence, of the several hundred available, are listed in Table 4.

Also critical to the success of biotechnology is the availability of many other DNA modifying enzymes that join (ligate) DNA molecules (T4 DNA ligase), phosphorylate the 5'-ends of DNA (T4 polynucleotide kinase), dephosphorylate DNA (calf intestinal alkaline phosphatase), add methyl groups to cytosine or adenosine residues within specific recognition sites (various DNA methylases), add nucleotides exclusively to the 3'-ends of double-stranded DNA (terminal deoxynucleotidyl transferase), cleave single-stranded tails at

the ends of double-stranded DNA or at small regions of single-stranded structure (S1 nuclease), polymerize DNA from monomeric nucleotides along a single-stranded region of a DNA template forming double-stranded DNA (Klenow enzyme, Taq polymerase, and T4 DNA polymerase), produce single-stranded cDNA from an mRNA template (reverse transcriptase), or synthesize single-stranded RNAs from a double-stranded DNA template (SP6, T3, and T7 RNA polymerases).[1,2]

With these powerful methods of handling DNA (Figure 6), the molecular biologist does not require naturally occurring mutants to correlate structure and function. Additional methodologies for studying gene structure-function relationships will undoubtedly be developed in the future.

Experimental Design: Human Tissue, Cell Lines, and Animal Models

The design of molecular experiments using animals as models for human cardiovascular disease can take advantage of the intact cardiovascular system.

Table 3
Strategies for Determining Gene Functions

• Comparison of sequence information among related genes for correlation of structure and putative function.

• Transfer and expression of the gene with its natural promoter or a heterologous promoter to other cells or other species to observe an increase in function.

• Inhibition of the function of the natural mRNA by transfer and expression of synthetic constructs of the gene encoding partial or full-length RNA that is complementary to the natural mRNA (antisense RNA) or transfer of single-stranded antisense DNA or phosphorothioate analogs of antisense DNA.

• Production of gene products using cell extracts (in vitro transcription and translation) and characterization of the structure and function of the protein produced.

• Transfer and expression of mutant genes modified in the promoter or structural regions by point mutations, deletions, and insertions of sequence of supposed function, and observation of the decreases in molecular or cellular function.

Animal studies are suitable for following the induction of pathologic conditions at the molecular level, and are needed to test procedures involving gene therapy that can then be extended to human clinical trials. Whole animal experiments also include the production of transgenic rodents or other animals, with an added gene construct, or the preparation of knockout mice, with a gene deleted by homologous recombination with a deletion construct. The two latter methods demand a large investment in time and resources.

Studies with cells isolated from normal or pathologic experimental animals or from human organs have their advantages and disadvantages. The tissue studied can be assessed routinely by use of short-term cultures or cell preparations that are reasonably reproducible from animal to animal or from human donor to donor. Experimental studies of cells freshly isolated versus those that have been treated for a period of time in tissue culture similarly have their respective advantages and disadvantages. Cells isolated from tissues often contain minor cell types that must be taken into account in interpreting the results assumed to be due to the major cell population.

The use of continuously growing cell lines as models for the biology of normal cells is quite convenient. This source of human or animal cells is a generally reliable one, and one that can lead to results that are more easily reproduced in the laboratory and transferred from lab to lab than are studies using preparations of cells from whole organs. A basic disadvantage of using cell lines is the difference in control of growth and differentiation state seen in transformed cells. A cell line consists of a clone of cells recovered after the transforming events of tumorigenesis, and subsequently selected biologically for survival in the host until pathology develops. The cell line that is then produced experimentally from a tumor isolate, in addition, is further selected for growth in tissue culture. The gene expression regulating the cell cycle can, therefore, be subtly changed, as can be the gene expression controlling cellular adhesion, intercellular communication, cell membrane production, and organelle biosynthesis, and in general all aspects of cell physiology. A cell line arises from the oncogenic transformation of a cell at a specific stage of maturation of a precursor cell or end-stage cell of a certain lineage in a tissue, and this cell type can comprise a small or large percentage of the cells in the normal tissue. The differences between the cells of the normal tissue, as isolated in bulk preparations, and any one cell line isolated experimentally from a tumor originating in that tissue, therefore, might represent the sum of all these differences. These properties of cell lines, on the other hand, have been used to advantage as models for the study of differentiation itself.

When cell lines are grown in tissue culture media, the addition of blood serum is especially important because of its content of polypeptide growth factors. Bovine serum is the traditional additive, although sera from other animal species is sometimes substituted for specific reasons. Autologous serum alone or mixed with a less expensive heterologous serum is rarely used, but since the discovery of species-specificity in the binding of many growth factors and cytokines to receptors, the inclusion of autologous components in an experiment is understood to be a significant variable. For this reason, and because of the batch-to-batch variability of any serum preparation, several serum substitutes have been developed commercially. These consist of defined mixtures of purified or recombinant peptide growth factors.

It is important to balance the day-to-day convenience, the reliability of the source of material, and the reproducibility of the results produced with fresh tissue versus cell lines. The costs involved in preparing cells from tissues or the expenses of continuous culture for the experimental use of cell lines can be significantly different. These practical factors in a project's design should be considered together with an understanding of the basic differences between heterogeneous normal

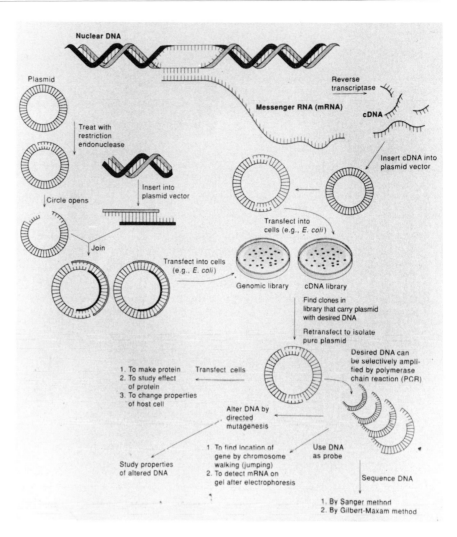

Figure 6. Recombinant DNA technology. (Reproduced with permission from Reference 37.)

tissues and homogeneous transformed cell lines. In most cases, the choice of a source of molecular material is straightforward because of one or more overwhelming factors. In the best possible situation, a suitable cell line or two are available, and normal cell preparations from human and animal sources are also reasonably homogeneous and well characterized. Molecular studies using all these related cell sources can be quite fruitful.

Analysis of biomolecules in situ is valuable because of the positional information that the subcellular, cellular, or tissue compartments afford.[30,32] Histologic sections can be analyzed for gene localization with chromosomal in situ hybridization, for mRNA localization to cell types in a tissue with in situ hybridization, as well as for antigen localization with immunocytochemistry. However, accurate doses of drugs, hormones, or other added substrates or macromolecules are sometimes difficult to deliver to particular cells in intact tissues, and experimental variables such as treatment time, cell temperature, pH, and ionic environment are, in some cases, more difficult to regulate

in whole tissue preparations. These problems can be overcome by using single cells dissociated by enzyme treatment of tissue homogenates,[30,32] but then cellular orientation is usually lost. The polarity of some cell types provides evidence of vectorial transport or other exclusively directional functions, often with an apical surface and a basolateral cell surface. The orientation of polarized cells and their different cell membrane domains in intact tissues can provide experimental methods for manipulating molecular processes at one cell surface, for gene targeting to a cell facing the lumen, and for the preparation of specific cellular membranes, organelles, and molecules that would be randomly sampled in a total tissue preparation. Examples of polarized cells are intestinal enterocytes, acinar and ductal cells of exocrine glands and tubules of other organs, chorionic villous epithelial cells, bronchiolar and alveolar epithelial cells, and vascular endothelial cells.[30,31]

While much has been learned from bacterial genetics and from the biology of bacterial viruses (the bacteriophages), important differences to keep in mind between prokaryotic and eukaryotic gene functions are

Table 4
Example of Restriction Endonucleases

Enzyme	Recognition Sequence	Cleavage Products

Both strands depicted:

*Bam*H I
```
5'......G↓GATC   C......3'          Fragments with 5'-overhangs:
       |  | | | |  |          ............G-3'           +        5'-GATCC...........
3'......C   CTAG↑G......5'                    |                              |
                                     ............CCTAG-5'                    3'-G...........
```

One strand depicted for each enzyme:

*Eco*R I   5'-G↓GATT C-3'
*Hin*d III 5'-A↓AGCC T-3'

*Eco*R V
```
5'......GAT↓ATC......3'           Fragments with blunt ends:
       | | |   | | |          ............GAT-3'          +        5'-ATC...........
3'......CTA↑TAG......5'                    | | |                     | | |
                                  ............CTA-5'                 3'-TAG...........
```

Hinc II 5'-GT(C orT)↓(A or G)AC-3'
Sma I   5'-CCC↓GGG-3'

Bgl I
```
5'...GCCN   NNN↓NGGC...3'         Fragments with 3'-overhangs:
    | | | |     | | |  | | | |    ............GCCNNNN-3'      +        5'-NGGC...........
3'...CGGN↑NNN   NCCG...5'                    | | | |                   | | | |
                                  ............CGGN-5'                 3'-NNNNCCG...........
```

Pst I   5'-CTGCA↓G-3'
Pvu I   5'-CGAT↓CG-3'

Palindromic 4-base pair sequences:

Alu I
```
5'......AG↓CT......3'          ............AG-3'          +        5'-CT...........
       | |  | |                         | |                       | |
3'......TC↑GA......5'          ............TC-5'                 3'-GA...........
```

Hae III 5'-GG↓CC-3'
*Hin*f I   5'-G↓ANTC-3'

Palindomic 6-base pair sequences:

Aat I
```
5'......G   ACGT↓C......3'          ............GACGT-3'       +        5'-C...........
       |    | | | |  |                       |                              |
3'......G↑TGCA   G......5'          ............C-5'                 3'-TGCAG...........
```

Kpn I   5'-GGTAC↓C-3'
Xho I   5'-C↓TCGAG-3'

Palindomic 8-base pair sequences:

Asc I
```
5'......GG↓CGCG   CC......3'          ............GG-3'          +        5'-CGCGCC...........
       | |   | | | |   | |                     | |                       | |
3'......CC   GCGC↑GG......5'          ............CCGCGC-3'              3'-GG...........
```

Not I   5'-GC↓GGCC   GC-3'
Pac I   5'-TTAAT↓TAA-3'

Non-palindomic sequences:

Alw I
```
5'...GGATCNNNN↓N   NN...3'          .........GGATCNNNN-3'      +        5'-NNN......
    | | | | | | | | |   |  |  |                | | | | | | | | |                | | |
3'...CCTAGNNNN   N↑NN...5'          .........CCTAGNNNNN-5'              3'-NN......
```

Ple I   5'-GAGTCNNNN↓-3'
*Sfa*N I   5'-GCATCNNNNN↓-3'

Multiple sequences:

Acc I
```
5'..GT↓(A or C)(G or T)   AC..3'          ......GT-3'          +     5'-(A or C)(G or T)AC......
    | |                    | |                  | |
3'..CA   (T or G)(C or A)↑TG..5'          ......CA(T or G)(C or A)-5'        3'-TG......
```

Ban I   5'-G↓G(C or T)(A or G)CC-3'
Dde I   5'-C↓TNAG-3'

those associated with the cell nucleus and the organelles of glycoprotein biosynthesis and turnover (the endoplasmic reticulum, the Golgi apparatus, and the trans-Golgi network, endosomes, and lysosomes) that are not found in prokaryotes.[30,31] These membrane-bound compartments in human cells play critical roles in isolating various communication signals from each other and from their response systems. Signal transduction pathways extend into the cell from the extracellular environment through one or more domains of the cell membrane and the cytoplasm to the nucleus where responses are carried out in terms of gene expression. Specific membrane receptors are linked to signaling systems at the inside face of the cell membrane, and consist of GTP-binding proteins, second messenger generating enzymes, protein kinases, nucleotide, lipid, and cation substances, and their associated regulatory proteins.[8] Responses involve immediate cell activation as well as long-term growth and differentiation programs. The particular subcellular localizations of molecular events in the pathophysiology of the cardiovascular system will be key factors to take into account in designing improved diagnostic and therapeutic procedures involving the SMCs, endothelial cells, macrophages, T lymphocytes, and platelets.[8] The modulation of gene expression in these cells is intimately involved with the normal and pathologic responses to external events, and the control points regulating gene expression provide numerous specific targets for novel diagnostic and therapeutic approaches to cardiovascular disease.

The goal of this chapter is to provide information and assistance in selecting materials and methods in molecular techniques that might be applied to the study of cardiovascular medicine.

DNA Analysis and Gene Structure

Analytical techniques in molecular biology can double as preparative methods, because molecular biology is the study of the mechanisms of transmission of genetic information. Modeling of this information transfer in living cells and in enzyme-catalyzed reactions generates both experimental data and molecular products useful in other procedures. The desired products of biochemical reactions and cellular processes are called signals, and the unwanted materials are called noise. The experimental use of DNA-dependent DNA polymerases (DNA replication), RNA-dependent DNA polymerases (reverse transcription), and DNA-dependent RNA polymerases (gene transcription) allows the investigator to take advantage of the information generation and the molecular production by various cellular and viral gene machines. We will point out in this section several methods that are in

the mainstream of DNA technology and indicate their advantages, as well as their limitations. These include cDNA cloning, genomic cloning, eukaryotic expression vectors, amplification of DNA by polymerase chain reaction, labeling and detection of probes, restriction endonuclease digestion and gel electrophoresis, subcloning methods, in vitro mutagenesis, and DNA sequencing.

Use of pH Buffers in Molecular Biology

The pH of solutions in which cells grow and reactions take place varies with the addition or removal of solutes, with temperature, and with atmospheric CO_2 absorption unless pH buffers are used. It is not only enzyme-catalyzed reactions that have pH optima, but so do each of the many parts of molecular isolation procedures and probe-binding procedures.[1-7] Care must always be taken to check if the pH of solutions is as expected. The pH of solutions used in preparation of DNA, RNA, and proteins is maintained constant with buffers such as a mixture of aqueous solutions of sodium phosphate monobasic and sodium phosphate dibasic, or a solution of sodium citrate neutralized by citric acid or HCl, or a solution of sodium acetate acidified by acetic acid. A series of nonbiological organic salts with different pH buffering ranges are commonly used because of their enzymatic unreactivity and convenience of preparation. These include Tris-HCl (for pH 7-9.5), HEPES-NaOH (for pH 6.5-8), and a variety of others with different pH buffering ranges.[1-7] Concentrated stock solutions of buffers, salts, and other enzyme reaction components can be stored for months if sterilized by autoclaving, and these make the preparation of working solutions quite convenient.

Quantitation of DNA and RNA

DNA is quantitated in solution by determining the UV absorption at a wavelength of 260 nm (A_{260}) of pure DNA in water or TE buffer (Tris-HCl-EDTA, pH 8).[1,2] The conversion factor is: 1 A_{260} unit is produced by a solution of 50 mg/mL DNA. With UV (quartz window) cuvettes that can be used with small volumes ($>50 \mu L$) (Beckman Instruments) the lower limit of detection at an arbitrary lower limit for the usual UV spectrophotometer of 0.005 is, therefore, (0.005 A_{260} unit) $\times$ (50 mg DNA/mL-A_{260} unit) $\times$ (0.05 mL) = 12.5 ng DNA in the 50-μL sample. Small amounts of DNA are thus readily quantitated. Another simple method of quantitation, specifically for restriction endonuclease fragments of DNA, involves applying the unknown sample in one lane of an agarose gel and several samples of linear DNA covering a range of known concentrations in adjacent lanes. After electrophoresis and staining of the DNA with ethidium bromide, the relative intensities of the fluorescent bands are compared by visual inspection to the intensity of the standards. A fluorescent assay for DNA in the presence of Hoechst dye is more sensitive than UV spectrophotometric detection. It is performed using quartz cuvettes in a spectrofluorimeter.[1,2]

Spectrophotometric quantitation of RNA is carried out like that of DNA except for two differences: the conversion factor is 40 mg/mL per 1 A_{260} unit, and the small RNA aliquots used for quantitation are usually discarded since RNA is labile when contaminated by trace amounts of the ubiquitous degrading enzymes RNAases.[1,2] Since Mg^{++} ion is a cofactor for essentially all DNA modifying enzymes, including DNAases, the Mg^{++} chelating agent EDTA is always used at 1 mM in solutions of DNA for storage. Prior to subsequent enzymatic manipulations, this inhibiting concentration of EDTA is usually counteracted by addition of sufficient Mg^{++} ion to saturate the EDTA and provide the required free concentration of Mg^{++} for the enzyme. RNAases have no such universal cofactor, and complete avoidance of possible contamination from biologic sources is the best strategy for maintaining a solution of pure RNA intact.

Methods of DNA Preparation

The types of DNA molecules used in molecular biology can be conveniently categorized by size (Table 5). Each of these molecular forms of DNA can be used as substrates or analytical probes in several specialized techniques.[1-7]

Oligodeoxynucleotides (oligos) are short DNAs of 10 to 100 bases in length that are chemically synthesized by automated instruments (Applied Biosystems, Inc.). Oligos can be purchased from a number of commercial sources ready-made for one of the routine applications, or they can be specially prepared for a particular purpose. Some of the important uses of oligos

---

Table 5
DNA Reagents Used in Molecular Biology

- Synthetic oligodeoxynucleotides (oligos)
- Plasmids
- Bacteriophage DNA
- Single-stranded phage and phagemid DNA
- Linear fragments of DNA constructs (gel bands)
- Genomic DNA
- Linear fragments of genomic DNA (gel bands)
- Chromatin
- Chromosomes

---

are listed in Table 6. Oligos can be separated from single nucleotides under nondenaturing conditions of buffer and temperature by gel filtration chromatography on spin columns containing BioGel P-6 or Sephadex G-25, or resolved from impurities differing by only one or two bases in length on denaturing urea-polyacrylamide electrophoresis gels (sequencing gels).[1,2] Double-stranded oligos can be prepared by mixing two individual samples that have partial or complete complementarity; they can be ligated to the ends of DNAs to add a recognition sequence for a particular restriction enzyme (blunt-ended linkers) or modify the end of a DNA molecule forming a pre-cut restriction endonuclease site (adapters).[1,2]

Plasmids are circular DNA molecules that have many uses as vectors for cDNA or genomic DNA. Most popular plasmids are approximately 3000 bp in size. Plasmids replicate independently of chromosomal DNA inside bacteria due to the plasmid sequence encoding a bacterial origin of replication. Many strains of E. coli have been characterized in terms of genotype with special reference to the properties that are important for the growth and faithful replication of plasmid DNA, and certain strains are recommended for use with certain plasmids.[1,2]

The "mini-prep" is a one-day experiment in which a dozen or two bacterial colonies taken from antibiotic-containing agarose plates can be used to determine which of these colonies contain recombinant plasmids of interest.[1,2] Basically, a colony is picked from a plate, and grown overnight in 5 mL of liquid medium. This "overnight" culture is divided into a small aliquot to save for possible subsequent use in a large preparation of plasmid DNA, and a large aliquot that is destructively analyzed to confirm that the plasmid that gave antibiotic resistance is the construct expected. Bacteria are lysed in boiling detergent solution with lysozyme added to break down the bacterial cell walls, and bacterial chromosomes are precipitated and aggregated by the addition of salt to the lysate. The soluble plasmid DNA is cleaned up by one or more phenol extractions. Residual contaminating phenol in the aqueous layer of the separated phases is removed by a chloroform extraction, and the DNA is precipitated with ethanol and salt. At the end of the mini-prep procedure, aliquots of the DNA solution can be cut with either: 1) a restriction endonuclease predicted to linearize the plasmid-insert construction for detection of the full length of the construct; or 2) with one or two restriction enzymes predicted to excise the insert or a portion of the insert for confirmation of the vector and insert sizes; or 3) with no enzyme to observe the supercoiled and circular forms of plasmid DNA. These three samples from each mini-prep can then be loaded onto an agarose gel with known DNA standards, run for 1 to 2 hours or until sufficient resolution of the components is observed, and stained briefly with ethidium bromide either simul-

Table 6
Uses of Synthetic Oligodeoxynucleotides

- **Hybridization** probes are used to detect complementary DNA or RNA in many experimental situations. They are labeled with a radioisotope or with a small molecular tag. A disadvantage of oligo probes is the low T_m of the resulting hybrids. An advantage is the convenience of automated synthetic DNA preparations without cloning. Labeled double-stranded oligos can serve as protein-binding probes to detect DNA-binding proteins isolated from the cell nucleus and to study their sequence specificity of binding.

- Two oligos are used as a pair of **primers for amplification** of DNA (routinely in the range of 100–1000 bp) by the polymerase chain reaction (PCR). Templates for amplification can be one cDNA, a cDNA library, a gene fragment, or any other DNA construct bordered by sequences complementary to the primers selected. The principal advantage and limitation of the PCR technique is the exponential increase in DNA product synthesized from the starting material, resulting in both exquisite sensitivity and possibly catastrophic spurious signals. The use of PCR to amplify a new cDNA related to a known gene can be accomplished overnight while the isolation of cDNA clones by screening a library can take several weeks.

- **Mutagenic primers** are used for the preparation of a series of DNA constructs that have variant sequences related to the natural sequence. Any combination of point mutation, deletions, and insertions can be produced from a known sequence. A mutagenic oligo is designed that anneals to two 20-base sites flanking the target region. DNA polymerase fills in the remaining natural sequence.

- **Sequencing primers** that anneal to known sequences adjacent to the target DNA for sequencing. The primers provide a double-stranded initiation site for any one of the DNA or RNA polymerases used in sequencing by the Sanger dideoxynucleotide chain-termination method.

- Two complementary oligos or a self-complementary oligo annealed to form blunt-ended double-stranded **linkers** can be used for ligation to blunt-ended DNA constructs. Excess linkers are concatamerized at both ends and then the designed restriction site is cleaved in each copy yielding a novel restriction endonuclease recognition sequence for further annealing and ligation to other DNA fragments. Dissimilar complementary oligos that directly anneal to form the product of a restriction enzyme cleavage reaction are called **adapters.**

taneously with electrophoresis or after halting DNA migration. The gel is then viewed and photographed on a UV light box, and the picture is analyzed to determine if the restriction digest of each sample matches the pattern predicted.[1,2]

Those colonies harboring the expected plasmids can be used to seed a larger plasmid preparation that will be used as the long-term laboratory stock of the DNA. The standard "plasmid prep" method[1,2] which yields several mg of plasmid DNA makes use of the difference in equilibrium density of supercoiled plasmid DNA and chromosomal DNA from the bacterial host in the presence of a high concentration of ethidium bromide. Ethidium bromide intercalates between the strands of DNA and allows fluorescent detection of the band of plasmid DNA below the chromosomal DNA in the centrifuge tube. Cellular RNAs form a pellet or ribbon at the bottom or edge of the tube. The plasmid DNA prepared in this way is of suitable purity for any type of further manipulation, but the procedure is laborious, time-consuming, expensive,

and generates solutions of mutagenic ethidium bromide as waste products.

A number of methods have been developed that are convenient alternatives to the isolation of small batches of plasmid DNA by the mini-prep method or the preparation of large batches of plasmid DNA on gradients of CsCl. While the maxi-prep can take 3 days, some of the alternatives take as little as 1 minute for isolation of each sample of plasmid DNA from overnight bacterial culture samples; the savings in time is so significant that it is well worth testing one or more rapid methods for suitability for an application. Three fast plasmid preparative procedures, from among a large and growing number, are carried out with Insta-Prep gel (5Prime-3Prime Corp.), PlasmidQuik columns (Stratagene Corp., La Jolla, CA), and Qiagentip columns (Qiagen Corp., Chatsworth, CA). Manufacturers have improved these plasmid prep kits to the point that purity is equal to that obtained by standard methods, and rapid plasmid preps have essentially replaced the older techniques for most purposes.

The principal means of preparing specific restriction endonuclease digestion fragments[1,2] is by the direct excision of the fluorescent gel bands with a razor blade while viewing on a UV light box. A long wavelength filter is used on the source to avoid molecular damage to the DNA. The DNA is then extracted from the gel band by one of several methods. A simple procedure calls for melting the agarose (use of special low melting agarose gel facilitates this procedure) and recovering the DNA in Tris-EDTA-NaCl layer over the added hot phenol solution.[1,2] Special electrophoretic devices are commercially available for recovery of DNA in gel bands; one makes use of a salt bridge that traps the DNA (Unidirectional Electroeluter, IBI/Kodak Corp., New Haven, CT), and another utilizes a permeable membrane next to an impermeable membrane for electroelution (Elutrap, Schleicher and Schuell, Inc., Keene, NH). Another method of recovering a DNA gel band involves incubating the gel slice with a hot NaI solution and binding and elution of the DNA from finely divided glass powder (GeneClean, Bio101 Corp., Vista, CA). The latter method also concentrates the DNA.

Concentration of samples of DNA is routinely accomplished by precipitation with ethanol or with other solvents.[1,2] These methods require a certain concentration of NaCl or other salts for precipitating amounts of DNA in the low μg up to mg range and give good recoveries for all but short oligodeoxynucleotides. Smaller amounts of DNA require lengthy incubations at $-20°C$ for efficient precipitation, or the addition of carrier tRNA or glycogen to aid quantitative recovery if these materials do not interfere with subsequent manipulations.

Single-stranded f1 bacteriophage DNA can be generated[1,2] by bacteria harboring a plasmid vector that contains an f1 filamentous phage origin of replication adjacent to the cloned DNA insert. Co-infection of these bacteria with a specific helper phage provides the molecular machinery to allow the production and export from the bacterial cells of encapsulated single-stranded phage DNA. Single-stranded DNA of this type can be, therefore, much longer than the synthetic oligodeoxynucleotides mentioned above and can span the entire sequence of a cDNA. It is useful for DNA sequencing and also for in vitro mutagenesis procedures that create any desired modification to a DNA sequence. These specifically designed mutations are extremely useful, in turn, for studies correlating DNA structure and gene expression or polypeptide sequence and protein function.

Linear (noncircular) fragments of double-stranded DNA that are produced by restriction endonuclease cleavage of cloned genes in plasmids or other vectors are routinely separated by electrophoresis on agarose gels and recovered by the methods described above.

Linear fragments are often handled from several hundred bp up to several million bp. The use of linear DNA in forming novel constructs is the central operation of molecular engineering. DNA is cleaved from known constructs, separated into component fragments, and after ligation to new desired components of a novel construct, the molecular assembly is introduced into a convenient strain of bacteria. Isolation of a single bacterial clone on agarose plates can be followed by a mini-prep for small-scale applications, or followed by further amplification by growth in bulk bacterial culture and isolation of a large batch of recombinant DNA.[1,2] Linear DNA up to several hundred bp can also be routinely prepared by amplification in the polymerase chain reaction by the use of two oligonucleotide primers, a small sample containing the DNA sequence to be prepared, and Taq polymerase. The polymerase chain reaction can be used for the amplification of fragments of several kb in length when steps are taken to optimize the Mg^{++} concentration and the pH of the reaction buffer.[3,4]

Genomic DNA is prepared as the starting material for the cloning and sequencing of genes themselves, as opposed to the cDNAs derived from the mRNAs expressed in a cell or tissue. The genes cloned do not need to be expressed. Genes include flanking regions, exons, and introns, and the sizes of genes is quite diverse. Human genes range in size from a few thousand bp to millions of bp. In the nucleus the chromatin is compact, but upon release from its native configuration by removal of histones and other DNA-associated structural and regulatory proteins by the action of proteinases or extraction by the denaturing solvent phenol, the DNA uncoils to very great lengths. This treatment yields mechanically fragile molecules that are sheared by vortex mixing or aspiration into pipette tips. Dilute solutions of high molecular weight DNA are viscous before restriction endonuclease digestion, and their viscosity decreases dramatically after linearized restriction fragments are formed.[1,2] Special techniques to prevent mechanical shearing are used to form intact genomic DNA for "mega-base mapping" with restriction endonucleases that recognize rare eight-base sequences. For these analyses intact cells or tissue are embedded while alive in low-melting agarose, and the subsequent detergent extraction and deproteinization steps, as well as the restriction endonuclease digestion are carried out directly in the agarose plugs. The resulting DNA is suitable for analysis by pulse-field gel electrophoresis of fragments of several million base pairs in length.[1,2]

Linear fragments of genomic DNA can be prepared by either of the methods described above. After separation by electrophoresis or other techniques, genomic fragments can be used for analytical or preparative methods that include the formation of genomic

DNA libraries and cloning of specific genomic sequences, or the analysis of specific genes by probing Southern blots with labeled DNA probes.[1,2]

Chromatin is the native material found in the cell nucleus and also can be reconstituted in vitro by supplying histones and other sequence-specific DNA-binding proteins to purified DNA. This approach can help to characterize the functions of a cloned gene in its native configuration.[1,2] Chromatin can be visualized in special preparations for the electron microscope[37,33]; studies using hybridization with fluorescently labeled specific gene probes have also visualized transcriptionally active loci on interphase chromatin in situ along with the encoded mRNA in individual cell nuclei.[39–41]

Chromosomes are readily visualized by chemical staining of those cells of a mixture that are in metaphase, and specific labeled gene probes can be used to localize genes to identifiable chromosomes.[1,2] At other points in the cell cycle of growing and dividing cells, most regions of the chromosomes are decondensed and undergoing all of the nonmitotic activities associated with normal metabolism.[33,37] The morphology of interphase chromosomes and the structure-function relationships of the genes and intergenic regions with the nuclear matrix and the soluble nuclear factors are complex. Much remains to be learned about genes in cell nuclei and the interrelated functions of replication and transcription.

cDNA Cloning

Screening a cDNA library with a labeled probe is a preparative method that provides a pure population of DNA molecules with a sequence similar or identical to at least part of the probe sequence.[1,2] The single cDNA species isolated is called a clone, since one recovers the vector DNA with its insert cDNA from a single clone of bacteria. The cDNA clone (gene clone) may also include sequences that are not necessarily contained in the probe's sequence.

The form the cDNA library takes determines the method of screening. Libraries consisting of inserts in phage or plasmid vectors are displayed as bacterial plaques or colonies, respectively, on agarose plates, and filter replicas are tested for specific content of DNA sequences using a labeled probe. Expression libraries in bacterial vectors are screened by determination of the presence of the engineered protein product by binding to an antibody or by some other characteristic of the protein molecule produced. Expression libraries in eukaryotic cells, such as insect cells, yeast cells, or mammalian cells, can be grown under their particular conditions and then screened for protein production by antibodies, or for any other functional property resulting from the production of the desired gene product. These types of expression cloning experiments are discussed below.

The probe can be a labeled, synthetic oligonucleotide, a labeled fragment of a related, cloned cDNA, or a labeled fragment of a related, cloned genomic DNA that includes part of at least one exon. Cloned genes are double-stranded DNA molecules that need to be dissociated (melted) in order to hybridize to a complementary target molecule, and the preparations of gene fragments used as probes are usually heated in a boiling water bath for several minutes before addition to the sample to be tested by hybridization. The labeled probe can anneal to both the single-stranded sites in the target sequences, as well to its original partner, the complementary strand of the probe preparation. Use of an excess amount of labeled probe over the amount of target molecules in the sample is important for maximization of signal generation. A synthetic oligonucleotide probe is a short single-stranded DNA molecule (20 to 50 nucleotides) that does not self-anneal; the design of proposed oligo probes can be checked by eye or by a computer program for secondary structure (self-annealing) before actual synthesis is carried out. Labeled RNA (riboprobes) made in the test tube from specialized in vitro transcription vectors are also single-stranded molecules. RNA probes bind with greater affinity to DNA target molecules than DNA probes. The use of an RNA probe can produce a greater signal than the corresponding DNA probe, but also gives greater background binding to sequences composed of short complementary stretches in other nontarget molecules. DNA, RNA, and oligo probes can each be used for detecting nucleic acids in samples, and the decision of which kind of labeled probe to prepare often rests on the sensitivity required and on the availability of a certain probe construct. DNA and RNA probes generally function the same in probing Southern blots and Northern blots and in colony and plaque screening. Use of RNA probes has certain advantages in the techniques of in situ hybridization and the RNAase protection assay that are discussed below in the section on RNA analysis. Oligos are advantageous since they can be synthesized up to approximately 100 nucleotides long and in large amounts (hundreds of microgram batches) by an automated DNA synthesizer with only the knowledge of the specific sequence desired. The production of oligos, therefore, does not require any cloned genes or cDNAs, and the use of oligos has become commonplace in a range of preparative and analytical procedures. The specificity of binding of an oligonucleotide probe or primer to a target sequence may be significantly lower than that of a longer cloned probe. The temperature at which the probe melts or dissociates from the target sequence, Tm, is lower for oligos than for cloned gene fragments since oligos are shorter sequences binding usually to 20 to 50 bases of DNA. The design of an oligo probe for hybridization, or a pair of oligo primers for the polymerase chain reaction, is critical, therefore, for the specificity of the signals generated.

cDNA Libraries

A cDNA (complementary DNA) library consists of a collection of DNA molecules composed of the chosen vector sequence and any one of the thousands or millions of cDNAs representing the genes expressed in the cells used for the original RNA source.[1,2] cDNAs are prepared from mixtures of mRNAs by the action of the enzyme reverse transcriptase, deoxynucleoside triphosphates (dATP, dCTP, dGTP, and dTTP), and a short stretch of double-stranded DNA-RNA hybrid formed by the addition of a primer oligonucleotide, usually oligo-dT[15-20]. Other primers can be used to initiate cDNA synthesis at sites other than the 3'-poly-A tail of mRNAs. Random hexanucleotide primers can be used in other related preparations to form many randomly distributed initiation sites for cDNA synthesis in order to assure equal representation of sequences distant from the 3'-end of the mRNA in the final batch of cDNA produced.[1,2] All cDNA vectors include a sequence that functions as a bacterial origin of DNA replication, and this allows the production in bacteria of a large number of copies of the entire plasmid construct, independent of bacterial cell growth. The vector also always carries a gene coding for antibiotic resistance (ampicillin resistance or tetracycline resistance) to provide for selective growth of only those bacteria in a mixed culture that have successfully incorporated the desired set of vector-insert molecules. If vector-insert molecules are not recircularized in their preparation, linear molecules result that are not replicated when introduced into bacteria. The cDNAs are linked to the vector structures at a cloning site that is often designed with multiple restriction endonuclease recognition sequences to facilitate the ligation of cDNAs that are produced with various restriction sites at their ends.

DNA with protruding ends produced by a certain restriction enzyme can in general be ligated to any other fragment with an end created by the same enzyme (Table 4). These sites are generally symmetrical, and 5'-ends and 3'-ends of any construct can be ligated to any other that has the same end. The suppliers of restriction endonucleases provide extensive information in their catalogs concerning the compatibility of DNA sequences produced by the various restriction enzymes for self-religation and for ligation with other related sequences, as well as the precision of the above sequence-specific maneuvers as shown by the repeated cutting of religated sites with each enzyme. Some enzymes cut downstream of the recognition sequence and, thus, cannot, in general, be ligated to any sequence except that next to the original unique cut site.

If nonidentical sites are present at the 5'- and 3'-ends of each DNA molecule in the cDNA batch, after cutting the DNA simultaneously or sequentially with two restriction enzymes, then these cDNAs can be inserted in a unique orientation into those same nonidentical sites in the vector. Such directional cloning in the preparation of the cDNA library can increase twofold the efficiency of the subsequent process of library screening if the expression of the cDNA is required, since all of the cDNAs are downstream of the gene promoter designed into the plasmid. The expression of the reversed cDNA gives an artificial RNA with a reversed sequence that does not code for the protein. In special cases, reversed RNA products (antisense RNAs) can be used as labeled probes for hybridization and as pharmacologic tools for interference with the normal function of mRNA in cells.[1,2]

Plasmid cDNA vectors are convenient for quick transfer of DNA fragments from one vector to another, for preparing labeled DNA probes, labeled RNA probes, nested sets of deletion mutants, and for use in both bacteria and human cells (shuttle vectors).

The preparation of a cDNA library is a straightforward, but tedious task that can take an experienced worker several weeks or months. The benefit of preparing one's own libraries is that a series of cDNA collections can be produced that take advantage of the differences between cell or tissue culture conditions such as drug, hormone, or cytokine treatments. One can prepare specialized libraries that contain cDNAs of any chosen range of sizes (size-selected libraries). One can enrich the population of cDNAs for those expressed predominantly in a cell under one condition, but not under another condition (subtraction libraries). One can also try various vectors (such as bacterial or mammalian expression vectors), several gene promoters (SV40, RSV, or CMV mammalian viral promoters or endogenous human promoters), or a number of mRNA sources. The specific cell types used in other related work can form the basis of cloning experiments with custom-made libraries. These variables in the design of a library can be important when one considers the time and effort it takes to isolate a particular gene from a library. If the gene is expressed at a high or moderate level in the cell sample that was used to build the cDNA library, then one can quite readily fish out cDNAs corresponding to the gene with a labeled probe. However, many genes encode proteins that have important physiologic functions, but are expressed at low levels as mRNA and protein. Enrichment for a low-level cDNA by specialized production of the library may be crucial, therefore, to success in isolating rare clones.

The most common method of screening a library is by the observation of signals from the labeled probe after binding of the probe (and washing off the excess unbound probe) to membrane filters blotted briefly on the bacterial cultures carrying the vector with inserts.[1,2] The vector can be a plasmid or a bacteriophage. The properties of various vectors are discussed below. The filters form a reversed image of the live bacteria or phage plaques on the plates. During the screening process, the original plates are saved for eventual physical removal of those plaques or colonies that give rise to reproducible signals on two replica filters made in succession from the plate. The bacterial or bacteriophage samples removed are the primary positive screening results, and these live cells or infectious phage samples alone are kept for further display on similar culture plates for secondary screening. The selected plasmid-containing bacteria or selected phage-infected bacteria are plated out again and replica filters are screened with the same probe. Several spots with equal positive signals on the second round of screening are observed if the samples picked after the first round were true positive signals. After the third or fourth round, all of the bacteria in each sub-sample are consistently positive for the observed hybridization signal, and at this point, the plate contains bacteria or phage with only one recombinant gene clone. Recovery of any of these bacteria or phage gives the same vector-insert construction and, thus, each of these recombinant clones of DNA has the same sequence. Other original colonies of bacteria or plaques of phage that gave positive signals in the first round of screening are carried through parallel procedures, and after these bacteria or phage have also been cloned, the restriction maps of DNA isolated from these parallel samples are compared to decide which have the proper structure. The structure of the plasmid or phage used to make the library is known, and an additional insert DNA fragment is expected.

Vectors for Cloning in Prokaryotic and Eukaryotic Cells

Vectors carry foreign DNA within cells and provide for self-replication with or without the expression of the foreign DNA as RNA and protein.[1,2,5] The non-recombinant vector structures originated in naturally occurring bacterial plasmids, in bacteriophage, or in eukaryotic viruses with an RNA genome (retroviruses) or a DNA genome (DNA viruses). Since the discovery and use of the original plasmids and phage, many specialized vectors have been designed, making use of the ever-increasing knowledge of gene promoters and structural sequences. Numerous advances have made the techniques of gene cloning, sequencing, and

expression more convenient. These vector sequences encode a few important functions that give the cell containing the foreign DNA certain reproductive advantages: an origin of replication in E. coli; bacterial resistance to the antibiotics ampicillin, tetracycline, or kanamycin; eukaryotic resistance to the antibiotics hygromycin, neomycin, or puromycin; or particular phage, viral, or chromosomal functions involving replication or expression or integration into host DNA. Table 7 describes a selection of commercially available vectors. This listing is by no means exhaustive; many other recombinant vectors have been described to carry out these functions, and new vectors are continually designed that can perform intricate molecular manipulations with DNA, RNA, or protein. Some eukaryotic vectors based on eukaryotic viruses replicate episomally within the host cells, but other eukaryotic vectors do not replicate unless integrated into the cell's genome by a type of DNA repair process. An integrated sequence may be lost unless the function it encodes, such as drug selection, gives a selective advantage that forces maintenance of the foreign DNA within the genome.

One selects a particular vector for a certain purpose because the properties of the vector provide the means of experimental selection or preparation of clones containing those insert sequences of interest.[1,2] This may require, for example, unbiased representation of all clones of a library in a screening process to isolate clones binding to a labeled probe. Another common use of particular vectors is the high-level expression in bacteria or eukaryotic cells of the recombinant DNA, or the production of a protein attached to a polypeptide tag for subsequent purification. Expression may be required under the control of a certain tissue-related promoter that allows discrimination between the desired clones and all others in a gene library. A vector may be selected to provide molecular interactions in a particular host cell, convenient RNA preparation in vitro, or unique ligation to a set of DNA molecules for study. Some of these properties and others are described in Table 7.

The foreign DNA can consist of small or large fragments. Each vector has a limitation on the size of insert DNA it can accommodate and still function in host cells.[1,2] Bacteriophage have absolute size limitations on the DNA that can be inserted at their cloning sites and still assemble within the capsid structure to form infectious particles. Plasmids often have a limit between 7 and 10 kb for inserts, and coincidentally, most cDNAs are less than 10 kb in length, often in the 1 to 3 kb range. Plasmids transform bacteria to express novel antibiotic resistance, and grow as bacterial colonies on antibiotic-containing culture plates. Phage can hold moderate sized genomic inserts, usually up to 15 kb or

(text continues on p. 42)

Table 7
Examples of Vectors Used in Recombinant DNA Techniques

Vector	Supplier	Size (kb)	Antibiotic Resistance	Characteristics
Bacterial cDNA Vectors				
pGEM series	Pr	2.8	Amp	Multifunctional vectors for cloning, sequencing, RNA preparation from either strand from SP6 or T7 promoters, single-stranded DNA preparation, expression of *lac z* fusion protein, series of multiple cloning sites.
pBLUESCRIPT II series	St	3.0	Amp	Multipurpose vectors, same as above, but T7 and T3 promoter sites, 19 site polylinker.
pMal-c2	Ne	6.7	Amp	Expression of fusion protein with maltose binding protein tag allowing amylose affinity chromatography purification, factor Xa proteolytic release of tag from recombinant protein at IEGR tetrapeptide site.
pGEX series	Ph	4.9	Amp	Expression of fusion protein with glutathione transferase, factor Xa or thrombin-specific release of recombinant protein, series of vectors with various multiple cloning sites.
pRIT2T	Ph	4.3	Amp	Protein A fusion protein binds IgG for purification.
pEZZ	Ph	4.6	Amp	Bacterial secretion of recombinant protein.
pRSETA, pRSETB, pRSETC series	In	2.9	Amp	M13 phage infection provides T7 RNA polymerase for high-level expression, T7 promoter drives recombinant protein production, T7 leader fused to His6 sequence for purification by Ni^{++}-chelate affinity chromatography, specific cleavage of recombinant protein from leader-His6 by enterokinase, series with all three reading frames.
pET series (3 to 25)	No	—	Amp or Kan	Multipurpose cloning and expression vectors with His6 tag for Ni^{++}-chelator purification, T7 gene 10 tag for antibody purification, OMP T leader for bacterial export to periplasmic space where signal peptidase releases recombinant protein, or factor Xa or enterokinase proteinases cleave recombinant protein from peptide after purification.

Table 7 (*continued*)

Vector	Supplier	Size (kb)	Antibiotic Resistance	Characteristics
Bacterial λ Phage cDNA Vectors				
λgt11	Pr, In, Ph.	40	—	Fusion protein with β-galactosidase allows blue/white detection of recombinants.
λgt10	Pr, In, Ph.	40	—	Selection for recombinants.
λZAP	St	40	—	Automatic subcloning into pBLUESCRIPT plasmid by phage-specific recombination event, directional cDNA ligation, multiple cloning site.
λExCell	Ph	40	—	Automatic subcloning, SP6 and T7 RNA polymerase sites flank β-galactosidase.
λEX*lox*	No	40	—	Directional ligation of cDNA, automatic subcloning.
Bacterial λ Phage Genomic DNA Vectors				
EMBL3, EMBL4	Pr	40	—	9–23 kb inserts can be cloned, specific selection for recombinants.
LambdaGEM-12	Pr	40	—	9–23 kb inserts, flanking T7 and SP6 promoters, allow preparation of RNA probes for selection of additional genomic clones adjacent to end sequences (chromosome walking).
Baculovirus Transfer Vectors				
pAcUW31	Cl	8.5	Amp	Polyhedrin promoter with a *Bam*H I cloning site, and p10 promoter with *Eco*R I and *Bgl* II cloning sites, for co-expression of 2 proteins in the same cell, flanking AcMNPV sequences allow recombination with viral DNA to transfer the dual expression cassette to the polyhedrin locus of baculovirus.
pAcAB3	Pn	10.1	Amp	Polyhedrin promoter and two copies of the p10 promoter drive simultaneous expression of three foreign genes in the same cell.
pAcGP67A, pAcGP67B, pAcGP67C	Pn	9.8	Amp	Polyhedrin promoter and gp67 leader sequence, multiple cloning site, fusion protein that is produced at high levels and secreted by cultured insect cells infected with baculovirus.
pAC360	In	9.8	Amp	High level expression of inserts having no transcription or translation start sites by fusion with the polyhedrin protein N-terminus.
pBacPAK8	Cl	5.5	Amp	Polyhedrin promoter, multiple coning site, m13 origin for single-stranded DNA sequencing of inserts.

(continued)

Table 7 (*continued*)

Vector	Supplier	Size (kb)	Antibiotic Resistance	Characteristics
Yeast Artificial Chromosome (YAC) Vector				
pYACneo	CI	15.7	Amp Neo	1000 kb inserts, *Eco*R I cloning site.
cRNA Probe and mRNA Vectors				
pGEM series	Pr	2.8	Amp	SP6 and T7 RNA polymerase promoters.
pBLUESCRIPT II series	St	3.0	Amp	T7 and T3 RNA polymerase promoters.
pT7T3 18U	Ph	2.9	Amp	T7 and T3 RNA polymerase promoters.
pcDNA II	In	3.0	Amp	T7 and SP6 RNA polymerase promoters.
pT3/T7-LUC	CI	4.7	Amp	T7 and T3 RNA polymerase promoters, luciferase reporter gene.
Eukaryotic Expression Vectors				
pCDNAIneo	In	7.0	Amp Neo	Cytomegalovirus promoter drives expression of insert, flanking T7 and SP6 sites allow preparation of RNA probes from either strand of insert, downstream splice donor/splice acceptor increases expression, Rous sarcoma virus long terminal repeat drives expression of neomycin resistance gene,
pSVK3	Ph	3.9	Amp	SV40 promoter drives expression of insert, multiple cloning site, downstream splice site, poly A signal.
pMSG	Ph	7.6	Amp Neo	Mouse mammary tumor virus long terminal repeat drives expression of insert multiple cloning site, splice site downstream, SV40 promoter drives expression of neomycin resistance gene.
pREP4	In	10.1	Amp Hyg	Rous sarcoma virus long terminal repeat drives expression of insert, multiple cloning site, poly A signal, oriP and Epstein-Barr nuclear antigen-1 sites, thymidine kinase promoter drives expression of hygromycin resistance gene.
Eukaryotic Promoter-Reporter Gene Expression Vectors				
pNASSβ	CI	6.5	Amp	β-Galactosidase reporter gene without promoter.
pCMVβ	CI	7.2	Amp	Cytomegalovirus promoter drives β-galactosidase gene, control construct or vector for replacement of CMV with unknown promoter sequences.

Table 7 (continued)

Vector	Supplier	Size (kb)	Antibiotic Resistance	Characteristics
pADβ	CI	7.1	Amp	Adenovirus promoter drives expression of β-galactosidase reporter gene, for control transfections or replacement of promoter sequence.
pGEM-Luc	Pr	4.9	Amp	Luciferase reporter gene without promoter.
pCAT-Basic	Pr	4.4	Amp	Chloramphenicol acetyltransferase reporter gene without promoter.
pKK232-8	Ph	5.1	Amp	Chloramphenicol acetyltransferase reporter gene without promoter.
pNEO	Ph	5.5	Amp Neo	Neomycin resistance reporter gene functions as a dominant selectable marker, without a gene promoter.
Single-Stranded DNA Vectors				
pXPRS	Un	3.75	Amp	Eukaryotic expression of insert driven by SV40 promoter/enhancer, splice site, and poly A addition signal, multiple cloning site, f1 intergenic region for preparation of single-stranded DNA.
pAX series	Un	6.2	Amp	Bacterial expression, β-galactosidase fusion protein in all three reading frames, purification by APTG-affinity chromatography, cleavage or recombinant protein by factor Xa, multiple cloning site, f1 origin of replication for single-stranded DNA preparation.
pBLUESCRIPT II	St	3.0	Amp	(See above.)
pTZ18R, pTZ19R	Ph	2.9	Amp	Multifunctional phagemid.
In Vitro Mutagenesis Vectors				
pALTER	Pr	5.7	Tet, Amp	f1 origin or replication for the preparation of single-stranded DNA for in vitro mutagenesis.
pMEX series	Un	3.6	Amp	(See above.)
pBLUESCRIPT	St	3.0	Amp	(See above.)
Exon Trapping Vector				
pET01	Un	—	Amp	Expression of any ligated exon is selected for by splicing of premRNA, transcription driven by Rous sarcoma virus long terminal repeat, poly A signal, bacterial origin allow use as shuttle vector.

(continued)

Table 7 (continued)

Vector	Supplier	Size (kb)	Antibiotic Resistance	Characteristics
PCR Product Cloning Vectors				
pGEM-T	Pr	3.0	Amp	*Eco*R V ends and 3'-T overhangs allow efficient ligation of the PCR product containing the non-template-directed 3'-A nucleotides at both ends, caused by the activity of the thermostable DNA polymerase.
pTOPE	No	4.0	Amp	(Same scheme.)
pCR II	In	3.9	Amp	(Same scheme.) *lac z* fusion protein, f1 origin of replication for production of single-stranded DNA, multiple cloning site.

Suppliers of vector DNA: Pr: Promega Corp., Madison, WI; Cl: Clontech Laboratories, Inc., Palo Alto, CA; Ph: Pharmacia Biotec, Inc., Piscataway, NJ; St: Stratagene, Inc., La Jolla, CA; Ne: New England Biolabs, Inc., Beverly, MA; No: Novagen, Inc., Madison, WI; In: Invitrogen, Inc., San Diego, CA; Un: United States Biochemical Corp., Cleveland, OH; Pn: Pharmingen, Inc., San Diego, CA.

so, and after infecting bacteria, grow as lysed bacterial plaques on a lawn of live bacteria. Cosmids are modified l phage that can contain approximately 40 kb inserts, but cosmids do not lyse bacteria and are grown as colonies of E. coli. Yeast artificial chromosomes (YACs) can hold up to a 1000 kb of DNA and are grown in yeast cells.

Characterization of a DNA region regulating expression of a human gene is a commonly sought goal of a project, and, for this purpose, a well-characterized reporter gene (chloramphenicol acetyltransferase, β-galactosidase, or luciferase) can be ligated at the 3'-end, or "downstream" of the DNA studied for its putative regulatory function. Various constructs can be compared for their ability to induce the expression of the reporter gene. Chloramphenicol acetyltransferase can be detected by a simple thin layer chromatographic assay of cell extracts. β-Galactosidase can be assayed by detection of a colored or fluorescent enzyme reaction product in live cells, in cell extracts, or in tissue sections. Luciferase can be assayed by detection of the formation of a luminescent reaction product in cell extracts.[1,2,5] Study of the relative levels of expression of a nested set of deletion mutants spanning the region hypothesized to control expression would allow one to correlate expression of the reporter gene with the presence of various promoter sequences of unknown function, compared to positive and negative control sequences. Discrimination of the cells that express added DNA from those that do not is required at the outset. A mammalian antibiotic resistance gene driven by a constitutive viral promoter would be useful in this example, and the dominant positive-selection construct could be transferred simultaneously as an independent molecule or recombined into the same plasmid as the promoter-reporter constructs. The batch of constructs with active and inactive regulatory sequences would be first prepared in bacterial cells and the purified DNA then introduced into mammalian cells in culture. The standard means of delivering DNA to the cytoplasm of mammalian cells are calcium phosphate-DNA coprecipitate-mediated transfection,[1,2] electroporation,[1,2,5] and lipofection.[1] The transfer of DNA into mammalian cells is inefficient. Cells that receive functional DNA constructs are selected by survival in medium containing antibiotic. The expression of the reporter gene is then monitored in the surviving fraction of cells. If a set of defined constructs were initially introduced, then the identity of the active regions could be ascertained by correlation of structure and function. If a large collection of randomly prepared fragments were introduced, then DNA rescue and characterization of the functional sequences would be required.[5]

Figure 7 depicts the structures of vectors that are designed for cDNA cloning, bacterial expression, expression in insect cells, expression in mammalian cells, in vitro mutagenesis, specific cloning of exons from genomic DNA, and cloning of polymerase chain reaction products. These types of vectors are also the starting materials for specialized constructions used for many purposes.

Expression Cloning

cDNA clones can also be isolated by using a screening method that depends on the expression in bacteria or mammalian cells of the encoded RNA or protein.[1,2,5] A vector is chosen to include a bacterial promoter, a transcription start site, a translation start site, and a stop codon (Figure 7). The λgt11 phage produces recombinant gene products that are fusion proteins with β-galactosidase of E. coli encoded by the phage lac z gene, and the cDNA can be screened with antibodies against the expressed protein, or with other ligands that bind proteins expressed by clones in the cDNA library. The maximum sizes of inserts with the λgt11 vector is approximately 7.2 kb. This phage vector and other plasmid vectors based on it take advantage of the interruption of the lac z gene at the fourth amino acid of β-galactosidase with concomitant loss of enzyme activity upon insertion of any cDNA at the cloning site. The recombinant phage grow as colorless plaques and nonrecombinant phage as blue plaques on agarose plates containing the chemical isopropylthiogalactoside (IPTG) that induces expression of the lac z gene and the enzyme substrate X-gal that is cleaved forming a blue color with active β-galactosidase. Picking white plaques ensures that recombinant phage are analyzed. The bacterial expression of proteins can provide not only a useful method of originally isolating a gene encoding a protein product for which there is an established detection system, but also can yield large amounts of pure recombinant protein when the desired bacterial clone is grown in a large batch. The limitations of production of recombinant proteins in bacteria include the facts that glycosylation of glycoproteins does not occur in prokaryotes, and that many proteins are produced in a denatured and aggregated form in bacteria that requires special means of renaturation or solubilization for function to be restored.

Bacterial cloning using either phage or plasmid vectors is always preferred when a previously characterized gene probe can be used. Procedures for bacterial growth and storage are relatively simple.[1,2] Bacterial cultures can be handled conveniently on the lab bench without problems of contamination. The short cell cycle (<1 hour) and small size allow the preparation of large quantities of bacteria in a short time.

The use of human or other mammalian cell lines as hosts for expression cloning of cDNAs has significant advantages when certain characteristics of gene expression are considered. For example, expressed glycoproteins can be glycosylated normally in appropriate human cell lines. Multi-subunit human proteins can be produced as hybrids between recombinant protein and natural human protein subunits.[30,32] Regulation of expression that is cell- or tissue-specific, or related to development or disease states, can be studied in tissue culture, by reintroduction of genes or cells with recombinant DNA into experimental animals, and eventually into humans for gene therapy.[1,2]

Insect cell lines are useful host cells for cDNA expression, and baculovirus transfer vectors give high-level expression of inserted DNA. Secretion of glycosylated recombinant products from the cultured cells is possible, and this is attractive because of both simplicity of purification and retention of native structure of the glycoprotein produced. Vectors specific for insect cell lines are commercially available (Figure 7).

Yeast cells are important host cells for cloning large genomic fragments by using recombinant chromosomal constructs as cloning vectors. This method is outlined below in the discussion of genomic cloning. Yeasts are also eukaryotes that process glycoproteins through their endoplasmic reticulum and Golgi apparatus, and can secrete proteins like human cells. Vectors are also available commercially (Figure 7) for yeast cell protein production.

The elimination of the time-consuming process of library screening for the initial identification of a fragment of a cDNA, or a small region of a genomic gene, is feasible by application of one of the methods of the polymerase chain reaction if DNA sequence information is available from at least one or two 20 to 30 bp regions of the gene sought. These methods are described below.

In mammalian cell expression cloning experiments, a plasmid with an appropriate mammalian gene promoter is ligated to a preparation of cDNA and used as an expression library in the host cells. There are a number of commercially available plasmids that can be introduced into mammalian cells in culture and function as expression vectors. Constructs can be prepared that incorporate a mammalian gene promoter upstream from the cDNA cloning site, which is itself upstream from a polyadenylation signal. An RNA splice donor-splice acceptor pair with a small intron either upstream or downstream of the insert site is often included, since the splicing process can increase expression of stable mRNAs in eukaryotic cells, depending on the promoter (Figure 7). Ampicillin is inappropriate for mammalian cell selection, since it specifically inhibits bacterial cell wall synthesis. A gene encoding a mammalian antibiotic resistance function driven by a viral promoter (neomycin resistance or hygromycin resistance, for example, with the powerful SV40 promoter or cytomegalovirus promoter) can be included in the same vector to provide a selective advantage for those cells incorporating the construct. If there is no resistance gene in the expression vector, then a small quantity (1/10 to 1/100 of the amount of cDNA) of a second independently prepared plasmid is transferred simultaneously. This construct consists of a viral promoter driving the antibiotic resistance gene. In this case, cells that take

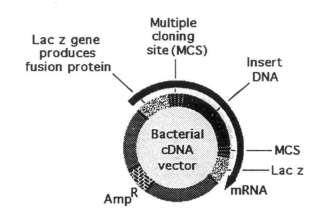

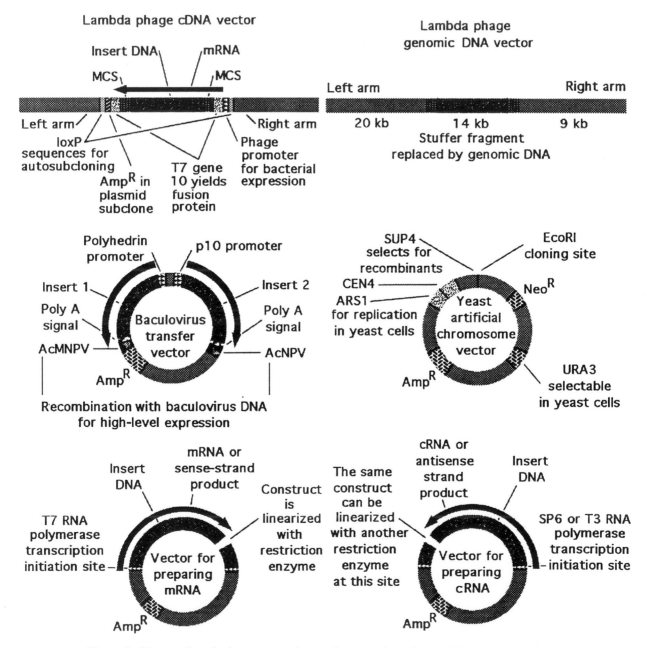

Figure 7. Vectors for cloning, sequencing, and expression of recombinant molecules.

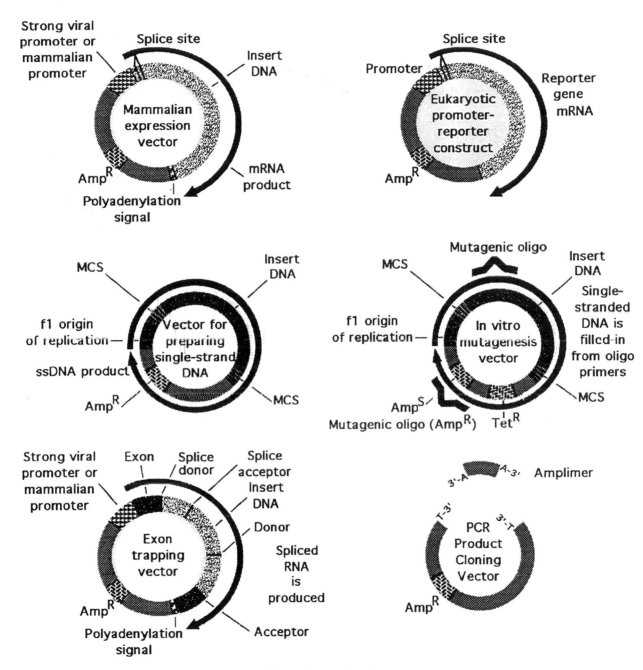

Figure 7. (*continued*)

up the antibiotic resistance gene are highly likely to take up the other DNA also and express antibiotic resistance. This provides for positive selection by growth of the cells in medium containing the appropriate drug. Two stages in the process of expression cloning are called for: preliminary selection of those cells that have taken up new DNA and become antibiotic resistant, and secondary selection of those cells exhibiting the special characteristics resulting from the production of the gene product under study. In general, a bacterial origin of replication and an ampicillin resistance gene are also necessary in all these constructs in order to be able to prepare batches of the expression library in bacteria prior to their use by transfer to mammalian cells. Plasmids such as these that are propagated in two species are known as shuttle vectors. DNA is transferred to the eukaryotic cells by transfection, a process that involves endocytosis of calcium phosphate-DNA co-precipitates, by electroporation using a transient electric shock to cause DNA in solution to enter cells through transient pores, or by lipofection with a polycationic lipid reagent that complexes with DNA and also dissolves in the cell membrane for internalization upon membrane turnover.[1,2,5]

Mammalian Gene Promoters and Enhancers

Well-characterized promoters and enhancers of gene expression can be utilized in the design of an effective mammalian expression vector.[1,2,5] There are a number of retroviral promoters, for example, Rous sarcoma virus 5′-long terminal repeat (RSV LTR) and Moloney murine leukemia virus LTR (MoMuLV LTR). DNA viral promoters, such as simian virus 40 (SV40) enhancer, adenovirus E1A (Ad E1A) promoter, polyoma virus (Py) enhancer, and cytomegalovirus enhancer (CMV) that can also be used for high-level constitutive expression of genes ligated downstream. In some instances, a promoter isolated from a genomic clone of a mammalian gene is useful for cloning genes functionally related to the promoter chosen.

Several serious drawbacks, on the other hand, of mammalian expression cloning include the large size and the slow growth of cell lines in tissue culture and the resulting inefficiency of screening large numbers of gene constructs in these cells relative to bacterial cultures, and the need to avoid microbial infections that quickly overgrow and ruin the mammalian cultures. The reader is referred to the laboratory manual of Kriegler[5] for a description of mammalian expression vectors, including eukaryotic promoters, for methods suitable for preparation of libraries and constructs, for gene transfer, and for analysis of the resulting expression. Some representative mammalian expression vectors that are available commercially are listed in Table 7.

There are a number of methods that are useful for the study of gene promoters and enhancers. The functional characteristics of a particular region of a gene are commonly determined by their stimulation of gene expression in cells or in cell extracts, and the resulting RNA or protein gene products are detected by a specific assay. Several important methods of RNA analysis are described below. The structural characteristics of a gene promoter or enhancer can often be observed in experimental systems by the binding of particular proteins. Two methods that can give complementary information about the DNA sequences involved in protein binding are the electrophoretic mobility shift assay (also called gel shift assay) and the footprinting assay.

In the gel shift procedure, a labeled double-stranded oligonucleotide probe corresponding to the DNA region believed to participate in DNA-protein interactions is mixed with proteins from cells, cell nuclei, or recombinant sources, and the bound protein-probe complexes are separated from the free labeled probe on a vertical acrylamide gel or a vertical agarose gel under nondenaturing conditions.[1,2] For example, a 30 bp oligo probe has a molecular weight of approximately 19kDa, and with two associated proteins of 50 kDa each the molecular weight becomes 119,000 Daltons. The probe migrates faster through the gel matrix than the protein-probe complex, and the difference in migration of free probe and protein-bound probe is the "gel-shift." The binding is reversible, saturable, and sequence- and protein-specific. Thus, the conditions for separation of probe from probe-protein complex(es) cannot include denaturing agents like SDS detergent or urea. The sizes of these complexes cannot be determined from the electrophoretic mobility, but sequence-specificity can be observed by the use of a series of probes varying in sequence. Saturable binding of protein to the probe indicates the relative affinity of interaction, as in protein to protein binding. The source of DNA-binding proteins for these experiments is usually a high-salt extract of cell nuclei from cells that are known to utilize the promoter or enhancer. Protein purification steps are often carried out to further characterize the nuclear components involved. Some DNA-binding proteins are ubiquitously expressed, while others are cell type-specific. Some DNA-binding proteins are constitutively expressed in the cell, while others are expressed following certain stimuli. A particular protein factor that is involved in regulation of gene expression by protein to protein binding may also be identified in a gel shift assay by a supershift of the probe upon formation of a protein antibody probe complex that migrates slower than the protein probe complex. The binding of isolated proteins to synthetic double-stranded oligo probes can provide information on the structure of a promoter or enhancer sequence, but there are many arbitrarily controlled conditions in the analysis, such as the sequence size and configuration of the pure DNA, and the reduction or the complete absence of other natural components of the cell nucleus or cytoplasm. The sequence used in the assay is predetermined to be important and single-base resolution of protein binding requires a whole set of mutant oligos.

Footprinting techniques are so-called because of the appearance of blank regions in a DNA sequencing ladder when the DNA is complexed with proteins that leave their "footprints."[1,2] Sequencing reactions are performed in the absence or presence of DNA-binding proteins that cover specific sites along the DNA and, therefore, enzymatic or chemical cleavage is inhibited differentially. The DNA sequencing gel is then run in the usual way with DNA purified free of proteins. In one variation of footprinting, the DNA samples with or without protein are treated with dimethyl sulfate to modify the accessible guanosine bases and then the Maxam-Gilbert sequencing reaction for guanosine is carried out with hydrazine to cleave at every modified guanosine, with the resulting blank sequences (methylation interference) for guanosine indicating that protein complexes had covered those sites. A disadvantage to methylation interference analysis is that results are determined only for the guanosine bases in a sequence; an important advantage, however, is the applicability of the technique to chromosomal DNA in the intact cell, as well as isolated DNA in the test tube. In another variation of the technique, the DNA region is hydrolyzed at every base by hydroxyl radical treatment, and the footprint is a blank region surrounded by a dense ladder of bands for each base in the DNA fragment. The sequence that forms the footprint must be identified by size markers in another lane of the gel. These chemical cleavage techniques are complementary to methods involving nuclease-sensitivity of chromosomal DNA, which has been used to characterize some of the features of genes and promoters.[1,2] A recent advance has been achieved by the combination of methylation interference in intact cellular DNA with detection of the resulting footprints at the level of one gene per cell by the use of the polymerase chain reaction. This method is called in vivo footprinting.[42] The in vivo footprints are compared to in vitro footprints produced by protein extracts of cell nuclei added to cloned gene fragments, and both of these kinds of results can be used to support arguments for or against a functional role for certain DNA-binding proteins in the physiologic regulation of gene expression. In vivo footprinting has also been used to correlate specific promoter occupancy in living cells with experimental treatments known to stimulate or suppress gene expression in those cells.

Polymerase Chain Reaction

The polymerase chain reaction is a method for producing a specific cDNA or genomic DNA in solution using a pair of oligonucleotide primers complementary to the 3'-ends of both strands of the template sequence of interest together with nucleoside triphosphates and a heat-stable DNA polymerase (Figure 8).[3,4] At the completion of each cycle of this repetitive production of the DNA located between the primer-binding sites, the original DNA template and the DNA product are melted apart, becoming substrates for each subsequent reaction. The overall yield approximates an exponential increase in product until nucleotide and primer substrates are depleted. The polymerase chain reaction can be applied to the routine preparation of DNA fragments of previously sequenced genes to use as reagents in other experiments. The polymerase chain reaction is also suitable for the detection and quantitation of mutant alleles or variant alleles of a known gene by the use of pairs of primers that hybridize to invariant DNA sequences flanking the region of interest.

The technique called reverse transcriptase-polymerase chain reaction can be used as a fast and simple alternative to some parts of screening cDNA libraries.[3,4] This method combines reverse transcription of RNA into cDNA using a reverse transcriptase enzyme, such as murine Moloney virus reverse transcriptase or acute myeloblastosis virus reverse transcriptase, with the standard polymerase chain reaction to amplify the amount of the cDNA product. One convenient universal primer for all poly-A$^+$-RNA is oligo-dT. A number of possibilities exist for the priming of unknown sequences, such as a mixture of cDNAs derived from cellular mRNA, including the ligation of an oligo linker to one or both ends of the template.

The mechanism of the polymerase chain reaction relies on the continued functioning of a DNA polymerase through a number of cycles of denaturation and re-annealing of the DNA. The discovery of the metabolic enzymes of thermophilic bacteria that thrive in thermal vent ecosystems on the sea floor[3,4] gave the impetus for developing this method and the automated thermal cyclers to carry it out conveniently. The addition of one of the thermostable DNA polymerases (e.g., Taq polymerase) that functions optimally at 72°C causes the extension of the product along the DNA template towards the opposite end. Repeated melting at 92 to 95°C of the double-stranded products, re-annealing of the primers at 42 to 55°C, and extension by the thermostable DNA polymerase at 72°C causes the concentration of the segment between the two chosen primer sites to approximately double each cycle (Figure 8). Reactions with 20, 30, or 40 cycles are usually performed. Exquisite sensitivity and good specificity of priming yield results with the polymerase chain reac-

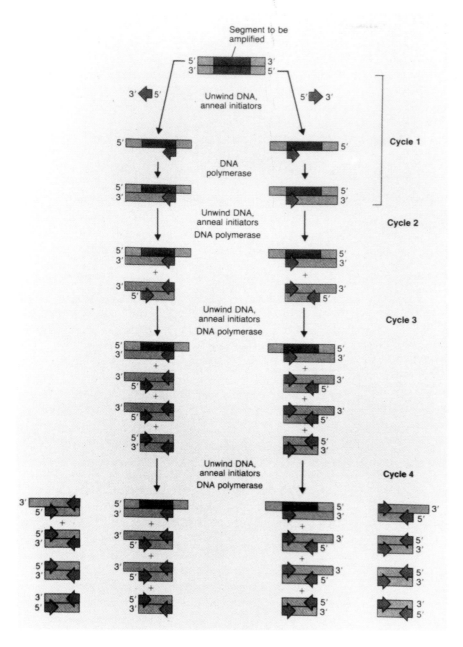

Figure 8. Amplification of DNA in the polymerase chain reaction. (Reproduced with permission from Reference 31.)

tion and the reverse transcriptase-polymerase chain reaction technique in situations unattainable by other methods of DNA and mRNA detection, respectively.[3,4]

The design of the primers used is important for the specificity of amplification, and for the avoidance of high background signals due to annealing to alternative genomic or cDNA priming sites, or the trivial annealing to the other primer to give primer-dimer product only.[3,4] Contamination of analytical polymerase chain reactions with template molecules derived from cloned genes used in the laboratory must be avoided or else false-positive signals will be generated.[3,4,7] Amplification of fragments longer than several hundred or one thousand base pairs is not always possible without

additional specific optimization. The concentration of free Mg^{++} in the reaction is one of the critical variables to optimize, since the thermostable DNA polymerase exhibits a sharp optimum for concentration of Mg^{++}, and the free Mg^{++} varies with total concentration of DNA template supplied.[3,4] The pH of the buffer used affects the specificity of the amplification as well, and pH between 8.5 and 10.0 have been used for optimal amplifications.[4] By adjusting the reaction conditions, amplified product bands of 2, 4, or 6 kb or longer can be produced.[3,4]

The polymerase chain reaction takes several hours to perform, and results can be analyzed by electrophoresis and staining with ethidium bromide the same day. Therefore, amplification of an initial gene fragment using a polymerase chain reaction method can speed up a cDNA cloning project by several weeks for each successful amplification. The sequence isolated can be used immediately as a labeled probe to screen a cDNA library for clones containing larger fragments, with extensions of this sequence at one or both ends. For this purpose, specialized cloning vectors (TA-vectors) have been designed that allow cloning of polymerase chain reaction products without any further treatment (Figure 7 and Table 7).

Other uses of the polymerase chain reaction include clinical assays for the detection of viral sequences, oncogene mutations, and other disease-associated or normal alleles of any gene that has been previously cloned and sequenced.[3,4,7] Also, many preparative and analytical procedures for research have been designed based on the polymerase chain reaction, and a few important types are: anchored polymerase chain reaction with one specific and one general primer, inverse polymerase chain reaction with primers facing outward in a circularized DNA construct to extend to an unknown sequence region, and multiplex PCR for the simultaneous detection of a number of related alleles in patient samples.[3,4]

Genomic DNA Cloning

Figure 7 depicts generalized structures of several types of bacterial vectors that are designed for genomic cloning, such as λ phage vectors and yeast artificial chromosome vectors. Table 7 lists several vectors that can be utilized for this purpose and are commercially available. YACs are especially useful as vectors for genomic cloning since the sizes of foreign DNA inserted can be several hundred thousand bp. Bacteriophage λ vectors are convenient and efficient carriers of eukaryotic genomic DNA, and genomic libraries prepared with phage vectors can be screened in large numbers with labeled nucleic acid probes in order to clone rare genes.[1,2]

A commercial firm offers genomic clone isolation from a number of species with a rapid turn-around time at a reasonable cost (Genome Systems, Inc., St. Louis, MO).This type of service may be attractive for those investigators who need to isolate genomic clones related to a known probe sequence, but who have not already made a significant investment in genomic library purchase, preparation, or screening.

Genomic DNA fragments are generally many kb in size, and many genomic genes span 20, 50, or 100 kb. The use of plasmid vectors is, therefore, inappropriate for these types of DNA in intact form. There are a number of related methods that make use of synthetic oligonucleotide probes or primers for the polymerase chain reaction, specially for the analysis of samples of genomic DNA to determine the presence of certain sequence regions, short sequence motifs, or even single-base differences from a previously cloned gene.[3,4] While these methods only highlight very small regions of genomic DNA, and are not designed for the cloning of novel genes, they are significant in the analysis of identified mutations in clinical samples.

Mapping of Restriction Endonuclease Cleavage Sites

Restriction mapping is the experimental determination of the enzyme recognition sites present in a purified DNA sample or in a natural mixture of DNAs. Separate aliquots of the DNA are incubated for 1 hour or overnight with a particular restriction endonuclease under its optimal conditions of salt concentration, pH, and temperature. The restriction digest is separated into bands of DNA on a horizontal agarose gel that is stained by ethidium bromide, and a pattern of fragments observed and compared to the expected pattern.[1,2] The DNA substrate is an intact plasmid or an intact large fragment and is cut into a number of smaller pieces by the action of the enzymes when one or more recognition sequences for the enzyme are present (Table 4).

Restriction mapping of recombinant constructs is performed routinely to confirm that the components are present in the correct positions, orientations, and sizes. Restriction enzyme cleavage sites are used that discriminate the proper configuration from other possible molecular outcomes. Any commercially available restriction enzymes can be chosen in designing the mapping process, with the purpose of definitively identifying the fragments of the DNA in the sample by sizes that can be clearly discerned from each other and also sized relative to known standards.[1,2] The most suitable enzymes, of the hundreds available, are those that cut at critical sequence sites, are on hand in the laboratory freezer, and are known to have functioned properly in other experiments. Next, are enzymes that cut at critical sites and have previously functioned properly, but need to be purchased specially for the job needed. Last, are those restriction enzymes that cut at specific sites needed to identify a fragment or construct, but have not been utilized before. Any new enzyme should be tested on another construct or vector DNA of a similar purity, that is, from a similar type of DNA preparation.

There are four or five buffers supplied by the manufacturers for use in restriction digests. The suppliers' catalogs are generally used as reference guides for the details of pH and salt concentration in each buffer, as well as the temperature and number of enzyme units required to completely cleave a standard type of DNA (usually bacteriophage λ DNA). The simultaneous use of two restriction endonucleases can give the same result as sequential digestion with the same two enzymes if their respective buffer and temperature requirements are similar. These conditions vary widely, and only some enzymes can work in double digests. Tables of restriction enzyme buffer compatibility are provided in cloning manuals and in the catalogs of several suppliers.[1,2] From a DNA sequence that is experimentally determined, or one that is accessed in a database, the theoretical restriction endonuclease cleavage map is quickly and easily calculated by using an available computer program. Some appropriate software for molecular biology is discussed below. Since in actual enzyme reactions care is taken to use purified plasmids or DNA fragments, and since the commercial vendors test their restriction enzymes for sequence-specificity and for contaminating exonuclease activities, the predictions based on computer-calculated restriction endonuclease maps are generally reliable.[1,2]

DNA Subcloning

Subcloning is a rapid manipulation for transferring a DNA fragment from one vector to a plasmid vector with specialized properties. Subcloning is performed to prepare samples for further manipulations, such as preparation of probes, sequencing, or joining to promoters or enhancers, reporter sequences, or deleted regions, hybrid regions, or experimental tags for subsequent expression of the construct.[1,2] The handling of DNA fragments is made simpler by use of comprehensive restriction endonuclease maps, although partial mapping and sequence information can be used successfully to produce subclones for the preparation of probes. When subclones are used for detailed analysis of the regulation of expression of a gene or of the function of a domain of a recombinant protein, then the sequence of the constructs is required to confirm that the observed effects are due to the assumed sequences. A computer-generated restriction map of a 3000 bp cDNA, for example, provides hundreds of restriction sites that can be used for planning a strategy for isolation and religation of fragments that is the most straightforward.

The length of these recognition sequences determines the frequency with which they occur in biological DNA samples. Short recognition sequences are more common and long sequences occur rarely in any average stretch of DNA. Enzymes that cut at a 4-base sequence (Table 4) may cleave a DNA molecule into fragments of tens to hundreds of bp with very few thousand bp pieces. 6-Base cutters are very useful in molecular biology (Table 4) because their sites are infrequent enough to provide one, two, or three fragments of a

cDNA, or a series of sites within a genomic clone that are convenient locations for recombining with other vectors for subsequent studies. Often protein domain-encoding regions, for example, or entire coding regions of a cDNA can be manipulated by isolating a fragment with one or two 6-base cutters, as can a 5'-upstream region of a genomic clone studied for its promoter activity. At the other extreme, a growing number of 8-base cutters is available commercially, and these enzymes yield fragments averaging several hundred thousand bp. These enzymes are very important in the restriction mapping of large chromosomal segments, such as the fragments of the human chromosomes that are studied in the human genome project.

To recombine DNA fragments with compatible ends, the enzyme T4 DNA ligase is used. This enzyme uses ATP as a cofactor and can only ligate fragments containing 5'-phosphate groups. All restriction endonuclease products have such ends, but chemically synthesized oligos need to phosphorylated with ATP and T4 polynucleotide kinase before ligation to any other DNA.

DNA Sequencing

Sequence information is obtained by reading the positions of electrophoretic gel bands generated from a DNA sample by either the Sanger dideoxynucleotide method[1,2,6] (Figure 9) or the Maxam-Gilbert chemical sequencing method[1,2] that correspond to the four bases A, C, G, and T. In the Sanger method of DNA sequencing, the addition of nucleotides along the template DNA actually stutters and stops in each of the four reactions for the template sequenced. In the A reaction, the four nucleotides (dATP, dCTP, dGTP, and dTTP) are supplemented with a chain-terminating nucleotide analog, dideoxyadenosine triphosphate (ddATP). Because of the absence of its 3'-OH group, the ddATP cannot be ligated to the 5'-phosphate of the next nucleotide in the chain, and the chain terminates for those molecules, incorporating a dideoxynucleotide analog at that position. The whole population of DNA product molecules consists of some that stopped at the first occurrence of an A nearest the priming site, some that stopped at the second A, and so on. A balance of natural ATP and the chain-terminating ddATP is struck so that the DNA polymerase enzyme can proceed from the primer all the way to the other end of the template, with a small, constant fraction of the product dropping off at each A, but continuing smoothly with each of the other nucleotides, dCTP, dGTP, and dTTP. One can separate the DNA product molecules precisely by size by electrophoresis on a denaturing polyacrylamide gel at 50 to 60°C in the presence of 4M urea. The image of the separation of these hundreds of DNA molecules

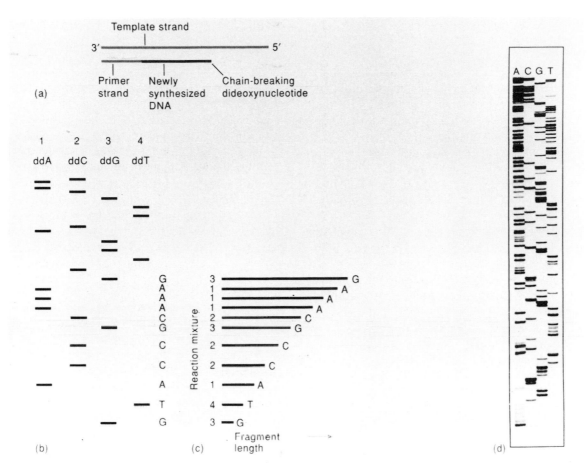

Figure 9. DNA sequencing by the Sanger dideoxynucleotide method. **(a)** Extension of some chains is halted in each reaction by incorporation of a dideoxy base. **(b)** Separate reactions for A, C, G, and T yield product mixtures ending with their respective dideoxynucleotides. **(c)** Together the four reactions contain fragments with every base in the sequence represented. **(d)** The four sets of product mixtures are separated into sequencing ladders on a urea-polyacrylamide electrophoresis gel.

in the A gel lane resembles the rungs of a ladder, and the results, usually on autoradiographic film detecting the ^{35}S-labeled DNA product, are known as sequencing ladders. In the three other parallel sequencing reactions, the other nucleotides (dCTP, dGTP, and dTTP) are likewise replaced by their dideoxynucleotide analogs (ddCTP, ddGTP, and ddTTP, respectively). Those reactions use the same DNA template and yield patterns of termination corresponding to the presence of a C, or a G, or a T in various positions along the template DNA. Samples from the four reactions are separated on the hot urea-polyacrylamide gel in adjacent lanes. The template DNA to be sequenced gives four related patterns starting with the set of product molecules at the bottom of the gel that are the smallest and were terminated nearest the primer, continuing up the gel to the DNA molecules that continued their extension to form products with lengths of 3-500 bases from the primer. The results from the gel are read by detecting bands from the bottom of the gel in succession from

the alternate lanes marked A, C, G, or T and recording the sequence of these signals in a linear array, the DNA sequence (Figure 9). Sequence determination using four-color fluorescent-labeled primers in thermal cycler reactions with automated sequence data acquisition (Applied Biosystems) has greatly increased overall efficiency.

Any region of a new gene that is related to a known gene can be readily sequenced by preparing a sequencing primer to initiate the sequencing reactions at the known sequence and to extend the dideoxynucleotide reaction into the unknown sequence. Primer design is greatly aided by the use of one of the computer programs described below.

In Vitro Mutagenesis of Cloned DNA

The routine modifications of a single nucleotide, a short region of sequence, or kilobases of DNA are feasible by the approach of in vitro mutagenesis using a cloned gene as a template in a plasmid vector and a specifically designed synthetic oligodeoxynucleotide as the mutagenic primer.[1,2] The oligonucleotide is designed to include perfect matches to sequences flanking the modified site. If one base is deleted or mutated, then the mutagenic oligo contains 20 nucleotides that anneal perfectly on either side of this base, leaving a 1 bp mismatch. When the mutagenic oligo is hybridized to the melted template and subsequently filled in with a DNA polymerase, the products are the original sequence plus a mutated sequence. Several sophisticated variations provide for direct selection of mutated plasmid sequences (Figure 7 and Table 7).

If a region of the cloned gene is to be replaced with a new sequence of any chosen design, then flanking sequences are similarly designed containing perfect-matches at the 5'- and 3'-ends of the mutagenic oligo and the mutated sequence is contained in the center.

With these procedures, essentially any variation of the original cloned gene can be readily prepared in large quantities. These types of preparations are critical for the precise mapping of DNA functions and are often required in the construction of multi-component DNA constructs for special uses. Otherwise, the design of DNA constructions would be limited to cutting and pasting sites at naturally occurring restriction endonuclease sites. Restriction fragments are usually satisfactory for the routine preparation of hybridization probes, but cannot begin to replace the finesse possible by the method of oligonucleotide-directed in vitro mutagenesis.

DNA Sources

American Type Culture Collection can provide purified DNA and live bacteria containing recombinant DNA to researchers for a small fee. The selection includes several thousand genes and cDNAs that have been provided by the original investigators for redistribution. (For information, contact ATCC, 12301 Parklawn Drive, Rockville, MD 20852, Tel. 800-638-6597.) A large number of commercial suppliers sell DNA, RNA, and protein reagents for research. The availability of reliable supplies of size standard DNA, plasmids, phage, oligonucleotide, cDNA, and genomic DNA in a wide array of forms makes many intricate manipulations in molecular biology quite convenient. These suppliers are listed in the laboratory manuals,[1-7] and they each provide technical information in their catalogs and fliers about their products. Detailed technical support from these companies is often available.

The DNA encoding a recently cloned gene or constituting a novel vector will often be provided by the original investigator following publication, if a reasonable request is made directly by telephone. Materials are usually shared free of cost, except for shipping when required; plasmid DNA can arrive in perfect condition in a small plastic tube in a normal first class letter. A humorous footnote to the acquisition of DNA reagents is the story of a certain competitor requesting a sample of recombinant bacteriophage from a colleague. The request was denied, but the return letter itself was extracted with phage buffer and live phage were recovered that encoded the desired construct anyway! Fragments of cloned genes for use as hybridization probes can be obtained by amplifying a desired sequence using synthetic PCR primers based solely on the published sequence information. This may, in some cases, eliminate the need to obtain cloned genes.

Computer Software for Molecular Biology

DNA, RNA, and protein sequence analysis includes a number of operations with large amounts of data that can only be handled reasonably by a computer. There are several types of programs available: large general-use molecular biology programs, small specialized sequence analysis programs, and shareware and freeware. Large-scale mapping and sequencing projects, like the human genome project, have additional requirements that we will not address. The principal software available that can perform all or nearly all of the functions necessary to analyze molecular sequence information includes The Genetics Computer Group's (GCG) programs for VAX computers and other mainframes, and four packages that include Kodak/IBI's MacVector and AssemblyLIGN, DNASTAR's LaserGene, Intelligenetics' GeneWorks, and Hitachi's MacDNASYS. OLIGO is a smaller computer program that is commercially available and designed for primer design. The programs with the complete range of functions cost several thousand dollars, the smaller programs cost several hundred dollars, and the shareware and freeware are distributed over computer networks as their names imply. The freeware program Authorin for transfer of novel sequence information to databases is also described below. The Macintosh versions of these programs will be considered here.

We have used the GCG programs for a number of years on the VAX computer including remote access by modem from home and lab Macintosh computers with consistently acceptable results. The GCG programs have grown over the last decade in response to the increased need for number-crunching ability, but require patience while learning and care during routine entry of commands by precise keystrokes. There are also now a number of hardware items, such as electronic autoradiograph digitizers, that are dedicated to automated sequence entry for laboratories with sequence-intensive requirements.

Each of the computer programs discussed here was found to be quite satisfactory for its designed purpose, and yet each has functional limitations and inconveniences. Ease of operation and differences in output formats set them apart, to some extent, from each other. For the purposes of this review, we tested full working versions of three major programs for Macintosh: 1) MacVector version 4.1 with AssemblyLIGN version 1.05; 2) LaserGene; and 3) GeneWorks version 2.2.1. These programs are each supplied with a compact disk that contains several entire DNA and protein sequence databases and requires the use of a CD-ROM drive. We also tested demonstration versions of MacD-NASYS version 2.0 and OLIGO version 4.1. While the demonstration versions give an overview of the functions and highlight the positive aspects of any program, it is not possible to determine the nature and frequency of problems that could occur when the full version is used for larger jobs. The demonstration versions of GeneWorks, MacDNASYS, and MacVector have small databases and cannot save results or download sequence files of particular interest to the prospective customer. The demonstration version of LaserGene, on the other hand, is fully functional for a period of a month after which it becomes nonfunctional. Other manufacturers might follow DNASTAR's good example in this regard.

It is feasible to utilize molecular probes and primers for the study of previously cloned genes without analyzing DNA, RNA, or protein sequences, and, in that case, computer software would not necessarily be needed. This could be accomplished by comparing data to published restriction maps and by following the advice of the commercial or academic providers of the DNA. However, most procedures with cloned DNA, synthetic RNA, and recombinant protein require the generation of detailed sequence information and restriction mapping data that is only attainable by the routine handling of sequences with many thousands of nucleotides and by determining the sites of DNA modification that would be predicted for hundreds of possible enzymes.

The determination of an unknown DNA sequence of several kb in length, in particular, involves the assembly of a number of overlapping, partial sequences derived from various sequencing gels into a contiguous sequence. These sequences are matched and aligned with their inconsistencies identified and resolved, and then a consensus sequence that is derived from clear sequencing data of both strands of the fragment is produced. This results eventually in the compilation of the sequence for the whole gene, cDNA, or construct. These tasks are beyond the capability of visual inspection. Each of the large computer programs is designed to handle the theoretical assembly of DNA sequences of all kinds and their analysis.

The advantages of personal computers for running sequence analysis programs are the convenience of using a familiar machine with new software, and the ability to move information easily from the analytical program to other graphics or word-processing programs. However, considerable RAM is needed to process large jobs on a personal computer with reasonable speed. Personal computers generally provide access to only one user at a time, although networking of high-end personal computers may solve this problem for some research groups. The use of larger computing platforms to handle sequence information allows simultaneous access for many users. The GCG programs are designed for use on a mainframe computer with the possibility of multiple user access. Extensive documentation accompanies the software, and on-screen help is also available. This group of programs is installed in our institution on a Digital Equipment Corporation (DEC) Vax computer using the VMS operating system. The GCG programs can also be installed on other computing platforms with the following configurations of hardware and operating systems: AXP/OpenVMS, Silicon Graphics (RISC)/IRIX, Sun (Sparc)/Solaris, and Convex/UNIX. The GCG programs are the standard against which all of the newer, more user-friendly programs that run on Mac or DOS systems are compared. The GCG programs have been upgraded repeatedly over the last decade and can perform essentially all of the operations required to handle DNA, RNA, and protein sequence data, perhaps with the exception of rapid design of PCR primers. There are several dozen separate programs that cover nucleic acid and protein sequence editing, sequence mapping, sequence conversion, sequence comparison, sequence alignment, compositional analysis, codon frequency analysis, secondary structure, and pattern recognition. The GCG programs also include periodically updated Genbank, EMBL, PIR-Protein, PIR-Nucleic, SWISS-PROT, VecBase, and PROSITE data banks. Files are included that contain the genetic code, specific DNA sites recognized by restriction endonucleases, and polypeptide sites cleaved by proteinases or chemical proteolysis. Several means of outputting the data are available from many of the programs, including lists, linear and circular maps, analytical graphs, and structural plots. A text editor is part of the VMS system. At our institution, there is a software support individual employed full-time who assists researchers with the GCG programs, and the system is also backed up by support in Madison, WI. Access is permitted by password at centralized and remote computer terminals and from personal computers with terminal-emulation software both on the university network or from elsewhere by modem. Data are stored in, manipulated by, and outputted from the central computer, and any public files and one's own files can also be downloaded to personal computers on the university network or by modem. Individual investigators may use the system for a nominal monthly fee, plus access time, modem time if applicable, processing time, disk storage of files, and printing costs. The GCG programs function admirably well, although entering commands and handling files is somewhat more tedious than with the point-and-click software for Macintosh. The programs were recently upgraded in GCG Version 8 with additional user-friendly characteristics. The GCG programs are especially attractive for organizations that can justify the higher initial costs of licensing and service, already have one or more VMS or UNIX system computers in place, and intend to provide service for a large group of users. In this way, the individual user fees would be minimized. For more information contact Genetics Computer Group, 575 Science Drive, Madison, WI 53711, Tel. 608-231-5200, Fax. 608-231-5202.

The MacVector/AssemblyLIGN combination of programs is designed to handle all of the sequence analysis needs of the molecular biologist. MacVector is a pleasure to use, and its convenient sequence editing functions, the adaptability of its menu-driven design, and its sensible graphics recommend it. The Macintosh interface makes the common operations extremely simple and convenient. A limitation to the database "browsing" feature is that only code numbers are shown until the individual sequences are opened. This makes scanning long lists tedious when searching for possibly interesting sequences with known characteristics. The PCR primer facility of MacVector allows one to control each critical variable of sequence range, melting temperature, self-annealing, and G-C content. In a test of the ability of the program to design a useful PCR primer pair for a known gene, results were generated in less than 5 minutes from start to finish. The additional criterion of possible cross-hybridization of the primer pair to other sequences in biologic samples was tested theoretically by searching for similarities in the database. Searching the approximate 176 Mb of data in the primates, rodents, other mammals, other vertebrates, organelles, and viral database portions of the CD with the test 21-mer oligo in the selected region of the known gene to find 20 of the best matches resulted 1 hour, 35 minutes later with at least 20 perfect matches to a wide variety of genes. This outcome indicated that this primer was, in fact, part of an Alu repetitive sequence and one of the worst choices to ever pick for a PCR primer or probe. This was already known from the sequence annotations. The program designers acknowledge that searching the database is faster if the desired parts are downloaded to the hard drive. The entire CD in this release contains 331 Mb of information, and consideration of the use of large capacity storage devices is important with these programs. MacVector includes a transcription factor database. The

MacVector/AssemblyLIGN system functioned on the Macintosh Quadra in this trial run very well with a convenient, automated installation procedure, and the program was easy to learn. Results were obtained within half an hour of installation. Restriction mapping of fragments with MacVector and displaying the results was quick and easy. Enzyme subsets could be used and previous settings for mapping were retained. There are conveniently linked windows showing related mapping results. Searching the database for specific cloned genes by author, locus, or keywords, was straightforward. The tutorial in the manual gives a nice introduction to the program. For further information on MacVector/AssemblyLIGN, contact Kodak/IBI, Inc., 25 Science Park, New Haven, CT 06511, Tel. 203-786-5600, 1-800-243-2555, Fax. 203-624-3143.

The LaserGene program installation is completely automatic and the program has a convenient main screen to jump from one function to another: sequence editing and analysis, restriction analysis and mapping, multiple sequence alignment, sequencing project management, biologic database resource, and protein analysis. The databases included on the CD-ROM disk with the LaserGene system are EMBL/GenBank, NBRF-PIR, Berlin RNA Data Bank, AIDS HIV Sequences, Brookhaven Protein Data Bank, SwissProt, Genetic MedLine, Translated GenBank, and Prosite. LaserGene, like MacVector and GeneWorks, is designed for keyboard entry of sequences, as well as entry from film scanners (not included), and automated sequencers (not included), as well as digitizing palettes (not included). Database searching with LaserGene was quite straightforward and rapid, with a helpful "dictionary" facility to aid in selecting keywords related to the word chosen. Pattern searching is possible, as are the operations of sequence comparison, sequence assembly, and restriction mapping. Protein sequence analysis by the standard methods of calculation, and several additional methods, can be performed with ease. Outputs in protein mode can be modified to include specific features and calculation results. Calculated protease digestion results were not included in the version tested, although pull-down menus listed them. The restriction mapping facility in LaserGene is adaptable and can provide a working map with gene features selected that can print at the single-base level on standard paper. Tables, lists, and a number of graphic output styles of restriction maps are also possible. Open reading frame analysis is not as adaptable and can run off the page if printed full size. The quick and flawless operation of LaserGene on the Macintosh Quadra right from the start attests to this program's usefulness. The absence of a PCR primer design facility is a limitation, as is the lack of linked windows between sequence view and map views. The graphic display and the output functions for the DNA analysis features are well-designed, and the protein analysis features are well thought out. For more information about LaserGene, contact DNASTAR, Inc., 1228 South Park Street, Madison, WI 53715, Telephone. 608-258-7420, Fax. 608-258-7439.

GeneWorks is a program that performs each of these functions: sequence editing, sequence comparison, sequence analysis, multiple sequence alignment, contig management, restriction site analysis, site tables, maps, simulated gels of digests, DNA secondary structure, open reading frame analysis, protein secondary structure, protein compositional analysis, protease maps as table or map or simulated gel, PCR primer design, dot matrix similarity, database searching, and locating patterns from the Prosite protein database. The PCR primer table parameters dialog box takes into account all the important factors. GeneWorks comes with a large user manual and a large reference manual, but these are not as helpful as the on-screen help in learning how to operate the myriad menus and buttons. The procedure found in the help screen for "Retrieving a sequence from a databank," for example, is not printed in the manual. Familiarization with "query" operations, referring to "a set of database search conditions," takes time. The molecular term "extract" here has the meaning "download in a form suitable for access, but only after re-saving," and the molecular term "restrict" signifies here "limit a search." Title words of sequence files are not included as keywords in searches, and as with any Boolean operations, there are sometimes surprises. GeneWorks draws restriction maps with a wide range of variables taken into account, and the linked windows handle all sorts of information simultaneously, such as the map, sequence features, motifs, literature citations, sequence name with keywords, and open reading frames. Merging these files for quick comparison of several related sequences is difficult, and although these limitations are minor compared to GeneWorks' overall functioning, additional upgrades will be appreciated of this big program for Macintosh computers. For additional information, contact IntelliGenetics, Inc., 700 East El Camino Real, Mountain View, CA 94040, Tel. 415-962-7300, 1-800-876-9994; Fax. 415-962-7302.

The MacDNASYS program is designed as a complete DNA, RNA, and protein analysis system and can perform the functions of sequence editing, sequence comparison, multiple sequence alignment, contig management, restriction site analysis, DNA secondary structure, protein structure, protein analysis, PCR primer design, and RNA folding prediction. For more information, contact Hitachi Software Engineering America, Ltd., 1111 Bayhill Drive, Suite 395, San Bruno, CA 94066, Tel. 415-615-9600, Fax. 415-615-7699.

The Oligo program searches for and analyzes oligonucleotides for the polymerase chain reaction, DNA sequencing and hybridization applications such as site-directed mutagenesis and Northern or Southern blots. The sources of oligonucleotides are keyboard entries, sequence files, or, importantly, sequences determined by searching the target sequence for primers and probes. The analysis of each oligonucleotide chosen or resulting from a search includes listing of the sequence, the length, and the sequence position at the 5'-end of the oligo, a calculation of the melting temperature (T_m), a measure of the stability of the duplex DNA (ΔG [25°C]), and a determination of the mass of DNA in a stock solution of known optical density (1/E [+strand]). In the Oligo program, the results of a search for primers and probes results in the design of oligonucleotides which are within the selected stability limits (T_m or ΔG), are not homo-oligomers, are highly specific, are free of duplex-forming structure (dimer and hairpin), and have 3'-ends which are unique within the search ranges and amplification region (will not false-prime). For additional information, contact National Biosciences, Inc., 3650 Annapolis Lane, Plymouth, MN 55447, Tel. 612-550-2012, 1-800-747-4362, Fax. 612-550-9625, 1-800-369-5118.

Authorin is a program used to enter new nucleic acid or protein sequence data into any of the major data banks, including GenBank, the European Molecular Biology Laboratory (EMBL) Data Library, the DNA Data Bank of Japan (DDBJ), the Protein Information Resource (PIR) data bank of the National Biomedical Research Foundation, the Martinsried Institute for Protein Sequence Data (MIPS), or the International Protein Information in Japan (JIPID). The software is available for Macintosh and for IBM-PC and permits direct entry by electronic means from the authors who have determined the new sequence information, avoiding manual entry by these organizations. Authorin is distributed free of charge by the National Center for Biotechnology Information, National Library of Medicine, National Institutes of Health, Bldg. 38A, Room 8N-803, 8600 Rockville Pike, Bethesda, MD 20894, Fax. 301-480-9241.

These programs and others that are not described here can be used to check the data that are produced in one's own molecular biology experiments, and to compare results to published work at the DNA, RNA, and protein levels. The future looks bright for further advances in automated sequence determination and analysis, in molecular modeling, and in sharing of molecular information over the Internet and the World Wide Web.

RNA Analysis and Gene Expression

Determination of mRNA quantity, size, and cellular localization demonstrates the varying status of expression of the gene encoding the RNA. There are a number of standard methods of determining the level of expression of a previously cloned and sequenced gene.[1,2] Most gene regulation apparently occurs at the point of initiation of transcription, but all of the subsequent steps in mRNA capping, polyadenylation, splicing, transport to the cytoplasm, and mRNA degradation may be regulated for a particular gene. Initiation of transcription is the most difficult aspect of mRNA biosynthesis to monitor directly, because of its dependence on several multi-subunit protein complexes within the nucleus. It is clear that initiation of transcription also differs for many genes under conditions of constitutive or basal expression and expression in response to extracellular stimuli.[13] The resulting steady state levels of mRNA and polypeptide encoded by a gene are more readily detectable, and most analyses of gene expression deal with differences in steady state levels of gene products under varying physiologic or pharmacologic conditions.

In Vitro Transcription Assay

Determination of the relative rates of initiation of transcription by an in vitro transcription assay involves the use of a set of recombinant transcription substrates consisting of various regions and lengths of the gene promoter in question and a detectable reporter gene. The transcription product can be either part or all of the natural gene or any mRNA for which a sensitive and specific assay is available. Often a portion of the 5'-end of the mRNA is suitable for detection by a sensitive RNAase protection assay developed to discriminate authentic initiation at the natural start site from other products derived by initiation at other sites on the mRNA. An active preparation of the enzyme complex RNA polymerase II and its associated transcription factors are required components in an in vitro transcription assay.[13] Preparation of enriched or isolated transcription factors that are specific or selective for the gene studied are major variables in this type of assay.[13] These nuclear proteins are often relatively unstable and found at low levels in the cell. Additional transcription factors and modifying enzymes that take part in inducible expression may be critical in the cell, and development of an assay for transcription initiation under inducible conditions would be a major undertaking.

Transcriptional Run-On Assay

Cells are maintained or treated under different experimental conditions, and freshly isolated nuclei are then used to follow ongoing transcriptional activity, usually by addition of a radioactive RNA polymerase substrate such as [^{32}P]-CTP. Natural transcription, therefore, "runs on" for a short time after disruption of the cells and isolation of the nuclei. This type of assay requires less sophistication than the in vitro transcription assay above, and can yield information on relative levels of transcription of natural mRNAs under various experimental conditions.

Determination of the Steady State Level of Expression of a Promoter-Reporter Construct

The definition of those sequences, usually at the 5'-end of a gene, that promote expression can be aided by the preparation of a nested set of deletion mutant constructs in which the predicted promoter regions are ligated to a reporter gene. The set of genes is reintroduced into living, mammalian cells by transfection, electroporation, or other techniques.[1,2,5] Differences in level of production of the reporter gene product are correlated with the presence or absence of the sequences in each construct. Essentially all of the mechanisms naturally occurring in the regulation of endogenous genes in the nucleus of these transfected cells are mirrored in the expression of transfected genes. Transfection of promoter-reporter constructs is useful for providing basic information on gene regulation in different cell types and in response to different cell treatments. Differences do exist, however, between the expression of exogenous gene sequences introduced into differentiated cells in culture, and the expression of genes that undergo differential regulation over the course of development in transgenic mice.

Determination of the Steady State Level of mRNA by In Situ Hybridization

Those cells in a tissue or in an animal that express a particular gene can be directly observed by hybridization of a labeled gene probe to the mRNA in the cytoplasm of the cells under study Care must be taken to avoid mRNA degradation due to endogenous nucleases or exogenous contamination. A procedure that is generally successful entails snap-freezing the tissue and preparation of frozen sections that are acetone-dehydrated and subsequently paraformaldehyde-fixed before application of the probe.[1,2] Hybridization of the mRNA retained in the lysed cells is performed using a labeled antisense cRNA probe. The probe is detected by autoradiographic or enzyme histochemical methods and the cells exhibiting the hybridization signal are identified morphologically. The use of positive-control probes allows one to discern signal from noise in this procedure. Thus, a minor cell population of a tissue can provide a strong signal in situ by hybridization for expression of a gene, whereas in a total tissue extract this same signal could be undetectable due to dilution by molecules representing the nonexpressing majority of cells. An advantage of in situ hybridization histochemistry over immunohistochemistry is that very specific sequence differences in related cloned genes can be used as the basis for selective detection of gene expression. Labeled oligonucleotide probes of 20 to 40 nucleotides can also be conveniently used in this method, as can long cloned probes up to several kb in size.

Determination of the Steady State Level of mRNA by Northern Blot Analysis

The preparation of intact RNA from cells[1,2] is not a trivial feat, due to its extreme lability and the ubiquitous degradative activity of RNAses. Once purified away from cell proteins and kept away from human fingers and common laboratory containers in a RNAase-free environment, RNA is completely stable and can be stored as frozen stock solutions or as ethanol precipitates for many years. RNA samples free of protein have an A_{260}/A_{280} ratio of ~2.0, like pure DNA. This ratio, however, gives no indication of the intactness of the RNA. Total cellular RNA consists mainly of the abundant ribosomal subunits 28S rRNA and 18S rRNA. These major RNA molecules of all human cells appear as broad bands in a stoichiometric ratio of 2 to 1. Degraded RNA samples show a reduced ratio of rRNAs of less than 2 to 1, and have little high molecular weight RNA.

In well-prepared samples of cellular RNA, the thousands of mRNAs expressed in most cells appear as an even smear along the whole lane of a formaldehyde-agarose gel stained with acridine orange, extending from sizes of less than 1 kb to greater than 5 kb. Major mRNAs may show up as distinct bands. The process of preparing and probing a Northern blot involves the separation of the RNA on an electrophoretic gel, blotting the RNA to a membrane filter, UV-fixation, and hybridization of target mRNA sequences with a labeled gene probe.[1,2] Equal loading of perhaps 10 μg of total cellular RNA in adjacent lanes from cells grown under different conditions can provide direct comparison of the relative steady state levels of the mRNA. Detection of the labeled probe is accomplished by autoradiography or by one of the nonradioactive methods available.[1,2] Quantitation depends on both titrating the sample loadings and demonstrating a series of signals that is linear with time. Since linearity is rarely achieved, semi-quantitative results are acceptable.

The isolation of mRNA in the form of poly-A$^+$-RNA is helpful for rare mRNAs to be detected. Poly-A$^+$-RNA can be prepared from total cellular RNA by a method using streptavidin-paramagnetic particles for recovery of mRNA-biotinylated oligo-dT hybrids, or by the traditional oligo-dT cellulose column chromatography. Up to 100 μg of the purified mRNA can be loaded per lane on a formaldehyde-agarose gel in order to boost the signal generated on the Northern blot.

Determination of the Steady State Level of mRNA by RNAase Protection Assay

Solution hybridization of a radiolabeled synthetic antisense RNA to target mRNA forms the basis of this sensitive detection method. Excess probe is completely removed by cleavage of single-stranded RNA with RNAase A and RNAase T$_1$. Radiolabeled probe when annealed to target mRNA is resistant to degradation, and this is quantitated with gel electrophoretic confirmation of the predicted size of the protected fragment. Alternatively, the protected probe is quantitated directly by liquid scintillation counting.[2]

Determination of the Steady State Level of mRNA by Reverse Transcriptase-Polymerase Chain Reaction

mRNA specific for one gene is detected by conversion of the batch of RNA to cDNA and amplification of the target sequence using a pair of specific oligodeoxynucleotide primers. Due to the exquisite sensitivity of the method, the possibility of contamination by genomic sequences must be corrected for by designing the primers to amplify a sequence that spans an intron in the genomic gene producing a larger amplimer band on the analytical gel. A modification that includes competing input targets as internal standards can give better quantitation, and several types of controls and precautions are recommended to insure reasonable results.[4]

Molecular Diagnosis of Cardiovascular Diseases

The recent book on molecular diagnosis[7] provides a thorough discussion of the practical aspects of establishing and operating a molecular biology laboratory in a clinical pathology setting. The suggestions for planning for equipment, supplies, space, and personnel are especially useful, as is the consideration of laboratory safety. The important subject of quality control of clinical molecular assays is emphasized throughout this guidebook.[7] Specific current applications of molecular biologic techniques to clinical assays are also described.

Specific tests for the molecular diagnosis of multifactorial cardiovascular diseases are not yet available. Molecular diagnostic methods are established in other areas, such as in the detection of monoclonality of lymphomas with B or T cell gene rearrangements by Southern blot analysis.[7] PCR is now used for the identification of human immunodeficiency virus, hepatitis B virus, genital papillomaviruses, and cytomegalovirus in patient samples. Molecular methods are used to diagnose the specific defects in Duchenne and Becker muscular dystrophy.[7] The single-gene defects in the LDL receptor gene in patients with familial hypercholesterolemia (FH) lead to premature heart disease in both homozygotes and heterozygotes, due to the formation of atheromas, xanthomas, and arcus cornea.[12] Experimental overexpression of apolipoprotein A-II in transgenic mice[43] or overexpression of the cholesteryl ester transfer protein in other transgenic mice[44] also cause atherosclerosis. However, it is likely that patients inherit several predisposing factors in addition to the factors of diet and hypertension that contribute to the pathogenesis of most cases of myocardial infarction, pulmonary embolism, and stroke.

In general, many kinds of mutations are found in the various alleles that constitute the range from normal to disease genes. Point mutations in a gene include amino acid substitutions or missense mutations, premature termination codons or nonsense mutations, and new RNA splice sites and missing RNA splice sites. DNA insertions and deletions include frameshift mutations that yield a new reading frame of codons for protein expression, codon insertions and deletions, and large scale deletions and duplications.[11] For example, since the cloning of the cystic fibrosis transmembrane conductance regulator gene (CFTR gene), more than 200 individual mutations in this gene have been reported.[9] The molecular mechanisms leading to expression of the defective membrane channel in cystic fibrosis patients have been grouped into four classes: 1) reduced protein production because of nonsense, frameshift, or splice mutations; 2) reduced intracellular processing and transport from the endoplasmic reticulum through the Golgi apparatus and transport vesicles to the plasma membrane; 3) defective regulation of activity by the protein at the cell surface; and 4) defective ion conduction by the CFTR protein.[9] Mutations of all four types—production, transport, regulation, and function—are also observed in the LDL receptor gene in FH.[12]

These ideas can serve as a paradigm for the defects in each of the affected cells in cardiovascular disease, with two modifications: 1) cells exhibiting one of these primary defects can also influence other cells through modulated production of cytokine, growth factor, and vasoregulatory molecules,[8] and 2) localized and systemic prothrombotic defects can be superimposed on these intracellular and intercellular phenomena.[10] The picture that emerges of the spectrum of cardiovascular disease is one of the cellular interactions normally taking part in wound healing, inflammation, or response

Table 8

Coagulation and Fibrinolytic Pathway Components Whose Genes Are Candidates for Prothrombotic Mutations

Loss of Function	Increased Function
Antithrombin III	Plasminogen activator inhibitor 1
Protein C	
Protein S	Factor VIII
Fibrinogen	Fibrinogen
Tissue plasminogen activator	Factor VII
	Tissue factor
Factor XII	von Willebrand factor
Thrombomodulin	Lipoprotein
Tissue factor pathway inhibitor	Histidine-rich glycoprotein
Heparin cofactor II	α_2-Plasmin inhibitor
β_2-Glycoprotein 1	Protein C inhibitor
(Pro)urokinase	Factor IX
α_2-Macroglobulin	Factor X
α_1-Antitrypsin	Factor V
Prekallikrein	

to other injury now going astray. These changes are due to inherited predispositions toward pathogenesis and due to other environmental factors. Growth factors, cytokines, and vasoregulatory molecules are produced by activated endothelial cells, and the effects on these cells of products of adherent macrophages, aggregating platelets in concert with plasma coagulation factors, as well as stimulated SMCs may contribute to atherogenesis.[8] These extracellular signaling molecules and their intracellular transduction machinery are suitable for investigation as possible disease-causing mutant alleles.

Table 8 indicates the known genes in the coagulation cascade and fibrinolytic pathway the mutations of which may contribute to prothrombotic lesions and increased incidence of cardiovascular disease.[10]

The presence of normal and mutant alleles of a particular gene can be determined by a number of related methods. These techniques either give new sequence information or else confirm a previously observed sequence variant. For example, multiplex sequencing involves use of PCR to generate many DNA sequencing samples within the regions of the gene of interest to compare normal and mutant alleles at many positions at once.[4]

Gene Therapy, Cell Therapy (Ex Vivo Gene Therapy), and Therapy with Recombinant Protein

The addition of function provided by an introduced gene, cell, or recombinant product forms the basis of nearly all current approaches to molecular biologic therapy of vascular disease.[15] Somatic gene replacement and somatic gene correction have yet to be implemented in human clinical trials, although these methods are powerful research techniques used in experimental cells and animals. Germ-line gene therapy is not desirable due to ethical considerations and social implications. Systemic gene therapy or local gene therapy can be envisioned for a number of vasculopathies, as summarized in Table 9.[15]

The clinical trials using gene therapy that are underway at the present time make use of the sophisticated medical and scientific resources found at large medical centers, but for these proposed molecular approaches to have a major impact on medical care in the future, gene therapy will have to be included among the routine procedures carried out by primary care

Table 9
Applications of Gene Therapy in Cardiovascular Disease

Indication	Target Gene
Systemic Gene Therapy	
Familial hypercholesterolemia	LDL receptor
Atherosclerosis	High-density lipoprotein
Hypercoagulable states	Tissue plasminogen activator
Refractory diabetes mellitus	Insulin
Local Gene Therapy	
Restenosis after angioplasty	Cell-cycle regulatory genes
Transplant rejection	Leukocyte adhesion molecule
Transplant vasculopathy	Cytokine
Myocardial infarction:	
Cardiac remodeling	Fibroblast growth factor
Angiogenesis	Transforming growth factor β
Myocarditis	Cytokine
Congenital heart disease	Myocyte differentiation factors
Thrombosis	Tissue plasminogen activator
Glomerular disease	Cytokine, cell-cycle regulatory gene
Aortic aneurisms	Protease

physicians with no special equipment or training.[21] Delivery of genes to sites of vascular pathology will then be considered as part of an overall strategy for treatment and not a separate therapeutic modality.[24] The initial pricing of these commercially produced therapeutic materials and associated diagnostic and follow-up tests by the biotech industry will have to be arrived at in light of the growing worldwide concern about the management of health care delivery. As an alternative to physician-operated therapeutic schemes, several companies are proceeding with plans to establish specialized clinics at which ex vivo gene transfer with patients' cells would be performed by highly-trained technical staff for reintroduction into the patients.[25]

Review of clinical gene therapy protocols is mandated by the U.S. National Institutes of Health for those investigators supported by NIH funds.[26] The major factors are concern for the clinical benefit to the research subject, informed consent, fair subject selection, and special safety precautions when partially characterized potentially biohazardous materials are involved. In addition, the U.S. Food and Drug Administration has established its own guidelines that recommend particular quality control procedures in the preparation and utilization of the recombinant materials in gene therapy protocols, including specifications for cell culture materials, characterization of cell identity and heterogeneity, and testing for the possible presence of adventitious agents.[26]

Somatic cell gene therapy in the treatment of serious disease is considered to be an ethical therapeutic option.[21] Modification of the germ-line of an individual is not ethical, for several reasons: the possibility exists of long-term side effects that are not predictable at present; and other philosophical, ethical, and religious questions arise, such as the rights of an unborn human to inherit his or her natural genome, the idea of informed consent for unborn patients to undergo experimentation, and the difficult question of "playing God."[21] The additional problem of the possible use of gene therapy for "enhancement" and not for treatment of serious illness is cause for concern.

The practical demonstration that exogenous genes can cause improvement in the clinical picture of human patients was seen in pilot studies in which a mutated adenosine deaminase gene was replaced with a normal gene in lymphocytes of children with severe combined immunodeficiency.[21] Genes introduced like this function essentially normally upon random integration into the genome, and insertional mutagenesis or inactivation of endogenous genes appear to be an extremely rare event.[21]

The use of potentially lethal retroviruses or adenoviruses causes one to reserve judgment as to the absolute safety of these procedures. The relative risks of iatrogenic oncogenesis and insertional inactivation of normal genes need to be determined by continued careful study in model systems and patients with the application of each new delivery system for gene therapy. Remarkably, the accumulated experience of 106 monkey-years and 23 patient-years shows the complete absence of retroviral-derived pathology, side effects, or malignancy.[21] The contamination of a retroviral vector preparation with helper virus in one bone marrow transplantation-gene transfer protocol in monkeys led to the development in three animals of malignant T cell lymphomas. The helper virus was deemed directly responsible for the lymphomas, and this emphasizes the need for strict quality control.[21]

Gene Delivery Systems

Methods are available for gene delivery to vascular cells, and their characteristics are compared in Table 10.[15] Expression of transfected foreign genes in endothelial cells that were subsequently returned to the vascular wall of animals has been observed to continue for 3, 4, or 5 weeks in several studies.[15] Lipofection of intact blood vessels has been achieved, although gene expression was found to be quite low.[15] HIV-mediated and adenovirus-mediated transfer of genes to vascular cells in situ succeeded in causing expression of the recombinant DNA. Antisense oligonucleotides that can anneal to and cause the turnover of specific mRNA molecules involved in vascular cell mitogenesis

after angioplasty were shown to inhibit neointimal formation for several weeks after a single treatment.[15]

The use of retroviral vectors is attractive because of their nearly quantitative conversion of target cells to expressing cells, but they can only infect dividing cells.[16] Replication-defective retroviral vectors are, therefore, extremely efficient DNA delivery vehicles.

Replication-defective adenovirus is a useful vector for infection of nondividing host cells with recombinant expression constructs, as are the herpes viruses. The disadvantage to working with adenovirus or herpes virus is that their genomes do not integrate into the chromosomes, but remain as episomes in the cell nucleus. Thus, these replication-defective DNA viruses are eventually lost by dilution from dividing cells.[16] The adeno-associated virus integrates stably into one region of chromosome 19, and its use as an expression vector is believed to reduce the risk of insertional mutagenesis of cellular genes that could lead to oncogenic transformation. However, this region is also involved in chromosomal abnormalities associated with chronic B cell leukemias,[24] and it is unclear that this site-specific integration would provide an extra margin of safety.

There is significant potential for the advancement of medical treatment using gene therapy, cell therapy, and targeting of recombinant DNA products to specific disease foci. The cardiovascular surgeon is in a uniquely favorable position to play a major role in these

Table 10
Gene Transfer Methods for the Cardiovascular System

Gene-Transfer Technique	Advantages	Disadvantages
Retrovirus-mediated transfer	High efficiency of gene integration.	Inefficient in vascular cells. Activates oncogenes? Limited insert size. Requires dividing cells.
Adenovirus	High efficiency. No requirement for mitosis.	Undefined risk of infection. Inflammation?
Myoblast implantation	Long-term expression ex vivo with relatively low risk. Need immunosupression?	Undefined risk of implantation. Tumorigenesis? Limited application (only somatic diseases).
Liposome-mediated transfer	Easy Safe	Low efficiency. Long incubation time.
Hemagglutinating virus of Japan	High efficiency. Easy	Nonspecific binding to red blood cells.

improvements in the prevention, diagnosis, and treatment of cardiovascular and other disease. The most significant improvements in management of cardiovascular disease in the near future will come from the molecular characterization of additional multifactorial disease traits and from the implementation of novel assays to correlate gene expression with clinical diagnosis and prognosis. The molecular modulation of the disease state will be feasible with this new information.

Conclusion

The technology of molecular biology has changed what vascular biologists do and perhaps even more importantly, the way they think. Armed with these powerful tools, the modern-day vascular surgeon, who is contemplating investigative study of a research problem, still has so much to do, and so much to learn.

Glossary

Basic Terms in Molecular Biology

Alpha helix A characteristic helical secondary structure seen in many proteins. The alpha helix allows maximum intramolecular hydrogen bond formation between C=O and H—N groups. One turn of the helix occurs for each 3.6 amino acid residues.

Amino acid sequence The linear order of the amino acids in a peptide or protein.

Backbone In biochemistry, the supporting structure of atoms in a polymer from which the side chains project. In a polynucleotide strand, alternating sugar-phosphate molecules form such a backbone.

Base-pairing rules The rule that adenine forms a base pair with thymine (or uracil) and guanine with cytosine in a double-stranded nucleic acid molecule.

Base pairs A partnership of nucleotide bases, such as adenine with thymine or cytosine with guanine, in a DNA double helix held together by hydrogen bonding.

Central dogma The concept describing the functional interrelations between DNA, RNA, and protein; that is, DNA serves as a template for its own replication and for the transcription of RNA which, in turn, is translated into protein. Thus, the direction of the transmission of genetic information is DNA→RNA→protein. Retroviruses violate this central dogma during their reproduction.

Chromosome 1) In prokaryotes, the circular DNA molecule containing the entire set of genetic instructions essential for life of the cell. 2) In the eukaryotic nucleus, one of the thread-like structures consisting of chromatin and carrying genetic information arranged in a linear sequence.

Coding region of DNA Gives rise to an RNA molecule of similar sequence (i.e., part of an exon).

Coding region of RNA Gives rise to a peptide whose amino acid sequence is determined by the nucleotide sequence of the mRNA.

Codon (also coding triplet) A group of three nucleotides that codes for either an amino acid, termination or initiation signal.

Complementary base sequence A sequence of polynucleotides related to the base-pairing rules. For example, in DNA a sequence AGT in one strand is complementary to TCA in the other strand.

Deoxyribonucleic acid A long polymer of linked nucleotides having deoxyribose as their sugar. They can form double-stranded or helical structures and are the fundamental substance forming genes.

Exons Exons generally occupy three distinct regions of genes that encode proteins. The first region signals the beginning of RNA transcription and contains sequences that the mRNA to the ribosomes for protein synthesis. The second region contains the information that is translated into the amino acid sequences of the proteins. The third region's exons are transcribed into the part of the mRNA that contains the signals for the termination of translation and for the addition of a polyadenylate tail.

Exon shuffling The creation of new genes by bringing together, as exons of a single gene, several coding sequences that had previously specified different proteins or different domains of the same protein, through intron mediated recombination.

Gene A segment of DNA involved in production of an RNA chain and sometimes a polypeptide. It includes regions preceding and following the coding region, as well as intervening sequences (introns) between coding segments (exons).

Gene expression The manifestation of the genetic material of an organism as a collection of specific traits.

Gene product For most genes, the polypeptide chain translated from an mRNA molecule, which in turn is transcribed from a gene; if the RNA transcript is not translated (e.g., rRNA, tRNA), the RNA molecule represents the gene product.

Genetic code The set of correspondences between nucleotide triplets in DNA and amino acids in proteins.

Genome All of the genes of an organism or individual.

Hydrogen bonding The formation of weak bonds involving sharing of an electron with a hydrogen atom. They are important in the specific base pairing in nucleic acids.

Intron In split genes, a segment that is transcribed into nuclear RNA, but is subsequently removed from within the transcript and rapidly degraded. Most genes in the nuclei of eukaryotes contain introns and so do mitochondrial genes and some chloroplast genes. The number of introns per gene varies greatly, from one in the case of rRNA genes to more than 30 in the case of yolk protein genes of Xenopus. Introns range in size from less than 100 to more than 10,000 nucleotides. There is little sequence homology among introns, but there are a few nucleotides at each end that are nearly the same in all introns. These boundary sequences participate in excision and splicing reactions.

Messenger RNA (mRNA) An RNA molecule transcribed from the DNA of a gene and from which a protein is translated by the action of ribosomes.

Molecular biology A modern branch of biology concerned with explaining biologic phenomena in molecular terms. Molecular biologists often use biochemical and physical techniques to investigate genetic problems.

Nucleotide The portion of nucleic acid composed of a deoxyribose or ribose sugar combined with a phosphate group and nitrogen base (purine or pyrimidine).

Nucleotide pair A hydrogen-bonded pair of purine-pyrimidine nucleotide bases on opposite strands of a double-helical DNA molecule. Normally, adenine pairs with thymine and guanine pairs with cytosine; also called complementary base pairs. See Deoxyribonucleic acid.

One gene—one polypeptide hypothesis The hypothesis that a large class of genes exists in which each gene controls the synthesis of a single polypeptide. The polypeptide may function independently or as a subunit of a more complex protein. This hypothesis replaced the earlier one gene—one enzyme hypothesis once heteropolymeric enzymes were discovered. For example, hexosaminidase is encoded by two genes.

Peptide A compound formed of two or more amino acids.

Polypeptide A polymer made up of amino acids linked together by peptide bonds.

Post-translational modification Change in chemical structure of a newly formed polypeptide, usually by addition of glycosyl, acyl, phosphate, sulfate, or amide residues, prior to its use.

Protein structure The primary structure of a protein refers to the number of polypeptide chains in it, the amino acid sequence of each, and the position of interchain and intrachain disulfide bridges. The secondary structure refers to the type of helical configuration possessed by each polypeptide chain resulting from the formation of intramolecular hydrogen bonds along its length. The tertiary structure refers to the manner in which each chain folds upon itself. The quaternary structure refers to the way two or more of the component chains may interact.

Proto-oncogene A cellular gene that functions in controlling the normal proliferation of cells and either 1) shares nucleotide sequences with any of the known viral oncogenes, or 2) is thought to represent a potential cancer gene that may become carcinogenic by mutation, or by overactivity when coupled to a highly efficient promoter. Some proto-oncogenes (e.g., c-src) encode protein kinases that phosphorylate tyrosines in specific cellular proteins. Others (e.g., c-ras) encode proteins that bind guanine nucleotides and possess GTPase activity. Still other oncogenes encode growth factors or growth factor receptors.

Purine Type of nitrogen base; adenine or guanine.

Pyrimidine Type of nitrogen base; cytosine or thymine.

Ribosome One of the ribonucleoprotein particles, 10 to 20 nm in diameter, that are the sites of translation. Ribosomes consist of two unequal subunits bound together by magnesium ions. Each subunit is made up of roughly equal parts of RNA and protein. Each ribosomal subunit is assembled from one molecule of ribosomal RNA that is noncovalently bonded to 20 to 30 smaller protein molecules to form a compact, tightly coiled particle. In eukaryotes, the rRNAs of cytoplasmic ribosomes are formed by cistrons localized in the nucleolus organizer region of chromosomes. At lease four classes of ribosomes exist that can be characterized by the sedimentation constants of their component rRNAs. Animal ribosomes also contain 5.8S rRNA, which is hydrogen-bonded to the 28S rRNA and is derived from the same intermediate precursor as the 28S rRNA.

Transcription The formation of an RNA molecule upon a DNA template by complementary base pairing; mediated by RNA polymerase.

Transfer RNA (tRNA) An RNA molecule that transfers an amino acid to a growing polypeptide chain during translation. Transfer RNA molecules are among the smallest biologically active nucleic acids known.

Translation The formation of protein directed by a specific messenger RNA (mRNA) molecule. Translation occurs in a ribosome. A ribosome begins protein synthesis once the 5'-end of an mRNA tape is inserted into it. As the mRNA molecule moves through the ribosome, much like a tape through the head of a tape recorder, a lengthening polypeptide chain is produced. Once the leading (5') end of the messenger tape emerges from the first ribosome, it can be attached to a second ribosome, and so a second identical polypeptide can start to form. When the 3'-end of the mRNA molecule has moved through the first ribosome, the newly formed protein is released, and the vacant ribosome is available for a new set of taped instructions.

Basic Terms in Recombinant DNA Technology

Agarose A linear polymer of alternating D-galactose and 3,6-anhydrogalactose molecules. The polymer, fractionated from agar, is often used in gel electrophoresis because few molecules bind to it and, therefore, it does not interfere with electrophoretic movement of molecules through it.

Antisense The DNA strand having the same sequence as messenger RNA (mRNA); there is a nucleotide substitution of thymidine (T) for uracil (U) found in RNA.

Antisense RNA or complementary RNA (cRNA) An RNA molecule with a nucleotide sequence complementary to a specific mRNA. Some bacteria generate antisense RNA as a mechanism for gene regulation. In the laboratory, cRNA is synthesized by splicing the gene under study in a reverse orientation to viral promoter. The coding strand is now transcribed. Once isolated and purified, the cRNA can be injected into an egg or embryo, where it will combine with natural messages to form duplexes. These block either the further transcription of the message or its translation.

Autoradiography Detection of images created by the effects of radioactively labeled molecules on X-ray film.

Bacteriophage (phage) Viruses that infect bacteria; these include lambda phage, among others. Usually used as cloning vectors.

Blotting The general name given to methods by which electrophoretically or chromatographically resolved RNAs, DNAs, or proteins can be transferred from the support medium (e.g., gels) to an immobilizing paper of membrane matrix. Blotting can be performed by two major methods: 1) capillary blotting, which involves transfer of molecules by capillary action (e.g., Southern blotting, Northern blotting); and 2) electroblotting, which involves transfer of molecules by electrophoresis.

cDNA clone A duplex DNA sequence complementary to an RNA molecule of interest carried in a cloning vector.

cDNA library A collection of cDNA molecules, representative of all the various mRNA molecules produced by a specific type of cell of a given species, spliced into a corresponding collection of cloning vectors such as plasmids of lambda phages. Since not all genes are active in every cell, a cDNA library is usually much smaller than a gene library. If it is known which type of cell makes the desired protein (e.g., only pancreatic cells make insulin), screening the cDNA library from such cells for the gene of interest is a much easier task than screening a gene library.

Chromosomal library Collection of cloned fragments together representing the DNA of an entire chromosome.

Chromosome walking The sequential isolation of clones carrying overlapping restriction fragments to span a segment of chromosome that is larger than can be carried in a phage or a cosmid vector. The technique is generally needed to isolate a locus of interest for which no probe is available, but that is known to be linked to a gene that has been identified and cloned. This probe is used to screen a genomic library. As a result, all fragments containing the marker gene can be selected and sequenced. The fragments are then aligned, and those segments farthest from the marker gene in both directions are subcloned for the next step. These probes are used to rescreen the genome library to select new collections of overlapping sequences. As the process is repeated, the nucleotide sequences of areas farther and farther away from the marker gene are identified, and eventually the locus of interest will be encountered. If a chromosomal aberration is available that shifts a particular gene that can serve as a molecular marker to another position on the chromosome or to another chromosome, then the chromosome walk can be shifted to another position in the genome. The use of chromosome aberrations in experiments of this type is referred to as chromosome jumping.

Clone 1) A group of genetically identical cells or organisms all descended from a single common ancestral cell or organism by mitosis in eukaryotes or by binary fission in prokaryotes. 2) Genetically engineered replicas of DNA sequences.

Cloned DNA Any DNA fragment that is passively replicated in the host organism after it has been joined to a cloning vector. Also called passenger DNA.

Cloned library A collection of cloned DNA sequences representative of the genome of the organism under study.

Cloning DNA cloning is the insertion of a chosen DNA fragment into a plasmid of a bacterium or a chromosome of a phage with subsequent replication to form many copies of that DNA.

Complementary DNA (cDNA) Single-stranded DNA copy of a messenger RNA made with the use of the enzyme reverse transcriptase; cDNA contains only the coding sequences of a gene.

Cosmid Plasmid vectors designed for cloning large fragments of eukaryotic DNA. The term signifies that the vector is a plasmid into which phage lambda cos sites have been inserted.

Cosmid vectors Plasmids into which lambda phage cos sites have been inserted. As a result, the plasmid DNA can be packaged in vitro into the phage head and can be used to infect a bacterium, after which it behaves like a plasmid.

DNA hybridization A technique for selectively binding specific segments of single-stranded DNA or RNA by base-pairing to complementary sequences on single-stranded DNA molecules that are trapped on a nitrocellulose filter. 1) DNA-DNA hybridization is commonly used to determine the degree of sequence identity between DNAs of different species. 2) DNA-RNA hybridization is the method used to select those molecules that are complementary to a specific DNA from a heterogeneous population of RNAs.

DNA restriction enzyme Any of the specific endonucleases present in many strains of Escherichia coli that recognize and degrade DNA from foreign sources. These nucleases are formed under the direction of genes called restriction alleles. Other genes called modification alleles determine the methylation pattern of the DNA within a cell. It is this pattern that determines whether or not the DNA is attacked by a restriction enzyme. See Restriction endonuclease.

DNA-RNA hybrid A double helix consisting of one chain of DNA hydrogen-bonded to a complementary chain of RNA.

DNA vector A replicon, such as a small plasmid or a bacteriophage, that can be used in molecular cloning experiments to transfer foreign nucleic acids into a host organism in which they are capable of continued propagation.

Electrophoresis The movement of the charged molecules in solution in an electric field. The solution is generally held in a porous support medium such as filter paper, cellulose acetate (rayon), or a gel made of starch, agar, or polyacrylamide. Electrophoresis is generally used to separate molecules from a mixture, based upon differences in net electrical charge and also by size or geometry of the molecules, dependent upon the characteristics of the gel matrix. The SDS-PAGE technique is a method of separating proteins by exposing them to the anionic detergent sodium dodecyl sulfate (SDS) and polyacrylamide gel electrophoresis (PAGE). When SDS binds to proteins, it breaks all noncovalent interactions so that the molecules assume a random coil configuration, provided no disulfide bonds exist (the latter can be broken by treatment with mercaptoethanol). The distance moved per unit time by a random coil follows a mathematical formula involving the molecular weight of molecule, from which the molecular weight can be calculated.

Ethidium bromide A compound used to separate covalent DNA circles from linear duplexes by density gradient centrifugation. Because more ethidium bromide is bound to a linear molecule than to a covalent circle, the linear molecules have a higher density at saturating concentrations of the chemical and can be separated by differential centrifugation. It is also used to locate DNA fragments in electrophoretic gels because of its fluorescence under ultraviolet light.

Genomic DNA DNA contained in chromosomes in the nucleus of a cell.

Genomic library A random collection of DNA fragments obtained from the total genetic material of a cell and carried in a suitable cloning vector.

Genomic probes Defined nucleic acid segments that can be used to hybridize (and therefore identify) specific DNA clones or fragments bearing the complementary sequence.

Hybridization The reannealing of single-stranded nucleic acid molecules; the formation of double-stranded regions indicating complementary sequences.

In situ hybridization A technique utilized to localize, within intact chromosomes, eukaryotic cells, or bacterial cells, nucleic acid segments complementary to specific labeled probes. To localize specific DNA sequences, specimens are treated so as to denature DNAs and to remove adhering RNAs and proteins. The DNA segments of interest are then detected via hybridization with labeled nucleic acid probes. The distribution of specific RNAs within intact cells or chromosomes can be localized by hybridization of squashed or sectioned specimens with an appropriate RNA or DNA probe.

Library A set of cloned fragments of DNA together representing a sample or all of the genome.

Molecular hybridization Base-pairing between DNA strands derived from different sources or of a DNA strand with an RNA strand.

Northern blotting A technique for transfer of RNA from agarose gel to a nitrocellulose or nylon filter on which it can be hybridized to a complementary nucleic acid. It is generally used to examine size and abundance of mRNA.

Oligonucleotide Single-stranded linear sequence of nucleotides (up to twenty or thirty nucleotides typically).

Plasmid An extrachromosomal, autonomously replicating, circular DNA segment.

Polyacrylamide gel A gel prepared by mixing a monomer (acrylamide) with a cross-linking agent (N,N′-methylenebisacrylamide) in the presence of a polymerizing agent. An insoluble three-dimensional network of monomer chains is formed. In water, the network becomes hydrated. Depending upon the relative proportions of the ingredients, it is possible to prepare gels with different pore size. The gels can then be used to separate biological molecules like proteins of a given range of sizes.

Polymerase chain reaction An in vitro method for the enzymatic synthesis of specific DNA sequences by repetitive cycles of template denaturation, primer annealing, and extension of annealed primers. This method uses two synthetic oligonucleotide primers flanking the region of interest in the target DNA and DNA polymerase (Taq polymerase) to amplify these sequences.

Probe In molecular biology, any biochemical labeled with radioactive isotopes or tagged in other ways for ease of identification. A probe is used to identify or isolate a gene, a gene product, or a protein. Examples of probes are a radioactive mRNA hybridizing with a single strand of its DNA gene, a cDNA hybridizing with its complementary region in a chromosome, or a monoclonal antibody combining with a specific protein. See Complementary DNA.

Recombinant DNA A composite DNA molecule created in vitro by joining a foreign DNA with a vector molecule.

Recombinant DNA technology Techniques for joining DNA molecules in vitro and introducing them into living cells where they replicate. The techniques make possible: 1) the isolation of specific DNA segments from almost any organism and their amplification in order to obtain large quantities for molecular analysis; 2) the synthesis in a host organism of large amounts of specific gene products that may be useful for medicine or industry; and 3) the study of gene structure-function relationships by in vitro mutagenesis of cloned DNAs.

Restriction endonuclease An enzyme that recognizes specific short sequences of (usually) unmethylated DNA and cleaves the duplex. Cleavage is sequence-specific and both DNA strands are cleaved, leaving either blunt or overhanging ends.

Retroviruses RNA viruses that utilize reverse transcriptase during their life cycle. This enzyme allows the viral genome to be transcribed into DNA. The name retrovirus alludes to this ''backwards'' transcription. The transcribed viral DNA is integrated into the genome of the host cell, where it replicates in unison with the genes of the host chromosome. The cell suffers no damage from this relationship unless the virus carries an oncogene. If it does, the cell will be transformed into a cancer cell. Among the oncogenic retroviruses are those that attack birds (such as the Rous sarcoma virus),

rodents (the Maloney and Rauscher leukemia viruses and the mammary tumor agent), carnivores (the feline leukemia and sarcoma viruses), and primates (the simian sarcoma virus). The virus responsible for the current AIDS epidemic is the retrovirus HIV. Retroviruses violate the central dogma during their replication.

Reverse transcriptase RNA-dependent DNA polymerase.

Southern blotting Procedure for transfer of denatured DNA from agarose gel to a nitrocellulose or nylon filter where it can be annealed with a radiolabeled complementary nucleic acid.

Transfection A term originally coined to describe the incorporation by a cell or protoplast of DNA or RNA isolated from a virus and the subsequent production of virus particles by the transfected cell. ''Transfection'' was used subsequently to refer to the incorporation of foreign DNA into cultured eukaryotic cells by exposing them to naked DNA. Such transfection experiments are directly analogous to those performed with bacteria during transformation experiments. However, the term ''transfection'' has been adopted rather than ''transformation'' because transformation is used in another sense in studies involving cultured animal cells (i.e., the conversion of normal cells to a state of unregulated growth by oncogenic viruses).

Transgenic animals Animals into which cloned genetic material has been experimentally transferred. In the case of laboratory mice, one-celled embryos have been injected with plasmid solutions, and some of the transferred sequences were retained throughout embryonic development. Some sequences became integrated into the host genome and were transmitted through the germ line to succeeding generations. A subset of these foreign genes expressed themselves in the offspring.

Vector 1) A self-replicating DNA molecule that transfers a DNA segment between host cells; also called a vehicle. 2) An organism (such as the malaria mosquito) that transfers a parasite from one host to another.

Basic Terms in Molecular Genetics

Allele One of several alternative forms of a gene that occupies a given locus on the chromosome.

Autosome A chromosome other than a sex chromosome. The genes residing on autosomes follow the mode of distribution of these chromosomes to the gametes during mitosis. This pattern (autosomal inheritance) differs from that of genes on the X or Y chromosomes, which show the sex-linked mode of inheritance.

Centimorgans (cM) The genetic unit used to measure

the distance between markers on a chromosome as derived from linkage analysis. Placement of chromosomal loci by such a technique is referred to as a genetic map, in contrast to a physical map where the actual distance is measured in base pairs. One centimorgan approximates 1 kb. The unit is derived from the recombination fraction (percentage of crossover where each 1% crossover or 0.01 recombination fraction = 1 cM).

Chromosome set A group of chromosomes representing a genome, consisting of one representative from each of the pairs characteristic of the somatic cells in a diploid species.

Complete linkage A condition in which two genes on the same chromosome fail to be recombined and, therefore, are always transmitted together in the same gamete.

Complete penetrance The situation in which a dominant gene always produces a phenotypic effect or a recessive gene in the homozygous state always produces a detectable effect.

Gene locus The position on a chromosome at which the gene for a particular trait is located; the locus may be occupied by any of the alleles for the gene.

Gene mapping Assignment of a locus to specific chromosome and/or determining the sequence of genes and their relative distances from one another on a specific chromosome.

Genetic distance 1) A measure of the numbers of allelic substitutions per locus that have occurred during the separate evolution of two populations of species. 2) The distance between linked genes in terms of recombination units or map units.

Genotype The genetic constitution of an individual at one or more given loci.

Hereditary disease A pathologic condition caused by a mutant gene.

Homologous chromosomes Chromosomes that pair during meiosis. Each homologue is a duplicate of one of the chromosomes contributed at syngamy by the mother or father. Homologous chromosomes contain the same linear sequence of genes and as a consequence each gene is present in duplicate.

Linkage map A chromosome map showing the relative positions of the known genes on the chromosomes of a given species.

Locus The position that a gene occupies in a chromosome or within a segment of a genomic DNA.

LOD score This abbreviation for log odds ratio is a measure of the confidence in establishing a putative genetic linkage. Numerically this signifies the ration of the logarithm of the odds for linkage versus the logarithm of the odds against linkage at different recombination fractions. Lod scores of three or more may be interpreted as establishment of linkage.

Molecular genetics The subdivision of genetics including studies on the structure and functioning of genes at the molecular level.

Pedigree A diagram setting forth the ancestral history or genealogical register. Females are symbolized by circles and males by squares. Individuals showing the trait are drawn as solid figures. Offspring are presented beneath the parental symbols in order of birth from left to right. Arrows point to the propositus.

Penetrance The proportion of individuals of a specified genotype that show the expected phenotype under a defined set of environmental conditions. For example, if all individuals carrying a dominant mutant gene show the mutant phenotype, the gene is said to show complete penetrance.

Phenocopy The alteration of the phenotype, by nutritional factors or the exposure to environmental stress during development, to a form imitating that characteristically produced by a specific gene. Thus, rickets due to a lack of vitamin D would be a phenocopy of vitamin-D-resistant rickets.

Phenotype Observable characteristics of an organism, resulting from interaction of its genes and the environment in which development occurs.

Polymorphism The existence of two or more genetically different classes in the same interbreeding population (Rh-positive and Rh-negative humans, for example).

Restriction fragment length polymorphism (RFLP) Inherited variations in the recognition sequences of restriction enzymes that produce different sizes of genomic fragments on Southern blotting.

References

Laboratory Guides:
1. Ausubel FM, Brent R, Kingston RE, et al: *Current Protocols in Molecular Biology.* New York: John Wiley & Sons; 1987.
2. Sambrook J, Fritsch EF, Maniatis T: *Molecular Cloning: A Laboratory Manual.* 2nd ed. Cold Spring Harbor, NY: Cold Spring Harbor Laboratory; 1989.
3. Erlich HA (ed): *PCR Technology: Principles and Applications for DNA Amplification.* New York: Stockton Press; 1989.
4. Innis MA, Gelfand DH, Sninsky JJ, White TJ (eds): *PCR Protocols: a Guide to Methods and Applications.* San Diego: Academic Press, Inc.; 1990.
5. Kriegler M: *Gene Transfer and Expression: A Laboratory Manual.* New York: Stockton Press; 1990.
6. United States Biochemical Corporation: Sequenase version 2.0. *Step-by-step protocols for DNA sequencing with sequenase version 2.0.* 7th ed. Cleveland, OH: 1992.
7. Farkas DH (ed): *Molecular Biology and Pathology: a Guidebook for Quality Control.* New York: Academic Press, Inc; 1993.

Reviews:
8. Ross R: The pathogenesis of atherosclerosis: a perspective for the 1990s. *Nature* 362:801–809, 1993.

9. Welsh MJ, Smith AE: Molecular mechanisms of CFTR chloride channel dysfunction in cystic fibrosis. *Cell* 73: 1251–1254, 1993.

10. Miletich JP, Prescott SM, White R, Majerus PW, Bovill EG: Inherited predisposition to thrombosis. *Cell* 72: 477–480, 1993.

11. Antonarakis SE: Diagnosis of genetic disorders at the DNA level. *N Engl J Med* 320:153–163, 1989.

12. Goldstein JL, Brown MS: Familial hypercholesterolemia. In: Scriver CR, Beaudet AL, Sly WS, Valle D (eds). *The Metabolic Basis of Inherited Disease*. 6th ed. New York: McGraw-Hill; 1215–1250.

13. Roeder RG: The complexities of eukaryotic transcription initiation: regulation of preinitiation complex assembly. *Trends Biochem Sci* 16:402–408, 1991.

14. Strauss PR: Dynamic hierarchies of chromatin organization and small soluble DNA: an overview. In: Strauss PR, Wilson SH (eds). 1990. *The Eukaryotic Nucleus: Molecular Biochemistry and Macromolecular Assemblies*. vol. 2. Caldwell, NJ: The Telford Press; 659–686, 1990.

15. Dzau VJ, Morishita R, Gibbons GH: Gene therapy for cardiovascular disease. *Trends Biotech* 11:205–210, 1993.

16. Mitani K, Caskey CT: Delivering therapeutic genes: matching approach and application. *Trends in Biotech* 11:162–166, 1993.

17. Williamson R: From genome mapping to gene therapy. *Trends Biotech* 11:159–161, 1993.

18. Friedmann T: Gene therapy: a new kind of medicine. *Trends Biotech* 11:156–159, 1993.

19. Dillon N: Regulating gene expression in gene therapy. *Trends Biotech* 11:167–173, 1993.

20. Porteous DJ, Dorin JR: How relevant are mouse models for human diseases to somatic gene therapy? *Trends Biotech* 11:173–181, 1993.

21. Anderson WF: Human gene therapy. *Science* 256: 808–813, 1992.

22. Chien KR: Molecular advances in cardiovascular biology. *Science* 260:916–917, 1993.

23. Langer R, Vacanti JP: Tissue engineering. *Science* 260: 920–926, 1993.

24. Mulligan RC: The basic science of gene therapy. *Science* 260:926–932, 1993.

25. Dodet B: Commercial prospects for gene therapy: a company survey. *Trends Biotech* 11:182–189, 1993.

26. Wivel NA: Regulatory considerations for gene-therapy strategies and products. *Trends Biotech* 11:189–191, 1993.

27. Kessler DA, Siegel JP, Noguchi PD, Zoon KC, Feiden KL, Woodcock J: Regulation of somatic-cell therapy and gene therapy by the Food and Drug Administration. *N Engl J Med* 329:1169–1173, 1993.

28. Sherman-Gold R: Companies pursue therapies based on complex cell adhesion molecules. *Genet Eng News* 13(13):6, July, 1993.

29. Heil M: Gene therapy conference highlights rapid development of delivery systems/vehicles. *Genet Eng News* 13(14):1, August, 1993.

Textbooks:

30. Alberts B, Bray D, Lewis J, Raff M, Roberts K, Watson JD: *Molecular Biology of the Cell*. 2nd ed. New York: Garland; 1989.

31. Berg P, Singer M: *Dealing With Genes: The Language of Heredity*. Mill Valley, CA: University Science Books; 1992.

32. Darnell J, Lodish H, Baltimore D: *Molecular Cell Biology*. New York: Scientific American Books; 1990.

33. Lewin B: *Genes IV*. New York: Oxford University Press; 1990.

34. Roberts R (ed). *Molecular Basis of Cardiology*. Oxford, England: Blackwell Scientific Publications, Inc.; 1992.

35. Russo VEA, Brody S, Cove D, Ottolenghi S (eds). 1992. *Development: The Molecular Genetic Approach*. Berlin: Springer-Verlag; 1992.

36. Thompson MW, McInnes RR, Willard HF: *Genetics in Medicine*. 5th ed. Philadelphia: WB Saunders, Co.; 1991.

37. Watson JD, Hopkins NH, Roberts JW, Steitz JA, Weiner AM: *Molecular Biology of the Gene*. 4th ed. Menlo Park, CA: Benjamin/Cummings; 1987.

38. Zubay G: *Biochemistry*. 3rd ed. Dubuque, IA: Wm. C. Brown; 1993.

Research Articles:

39. Xing Y, Johnson CV, Dobner PR, Lawrence JB: Higher level organization of individual gene transcription and RNA splicing. *Science* 259:1326–1330, 1993.

40. Carter KC, Bowman D, Carrington W, et al: A three-dimensional view of precursor messenger RNA metabolism within the mammalian nucleus. *Science* 259: 1330–1335, 1993.

41. Wansink DG, Schul W, van der Kraan I, van Steensel B, van Driel R, de Jong L: Fluorescent labeling of nascent RNA reveals transcription by RNA polymerase II in domains scattered throughout the nucleus. *J Cell Biol* 122:283–293, 1993.

42. Mueller PR, Wold B: In vivo footprinting of a muscle specific enhancer by ligation mediated PCR. *Science* 246:780–786, 1989.

43. Warden CH, Hedrick CC, Qiao J-H, Castellani LW, Lusis AJ: Atherosclerosis in transgenic mice overexpressing apolipoprotein A-II. *Science* 261:469–472, 1993.

44. Marotti KR, Castle CK, Boyle TP, Lin AH, Murray RW, Melchior GW: Severe atherosclerosis in transgenic mice expressing simian cholesteryl ester transfer protein. *Nature* 364:73–75, 1993.

45. Rosenfeld MA, Yoshimura K, Trapnell BC, et al: In vivo transfer of the human cystic fibrosis transmembrane conductance regulator gene to the airway epithelium. *Cell* 68:143–155, 1992.

Other Educational Media:

46. *DNA Sequencing Program* is a 65-minute videotaped live-action technical presentation from United States Biochemical Corporation, 1990. The narrator of the video program explains many practical aspects of DNA sequencing by the Sanger dideoxynucleotide chain termination method.

47. *Molecular Cloning: A Tutorial* is a computer floppy disk from Pharmacia LKB Biotechnology, Inc., 1988. This is an introductory on-screen demonstration program in Hypercard Stack format. The discussion includes some computer animation and sound effects, and it illustrates more than a dozen basic operations of molecular biology.

48. *Winding Your Way Through DNA* is a set of videotapes of lectures on molecular biology presented by renowned scientists. The total viewing time is approximately 8 hours. Published by Cold Spring Harbor Laboratory (Cold Spring Harbor, NY).

49. Videotaped training films are available from Videos for Science, Inc. (Logan, UT), on several dozen individual techniques of molecular and cell biology. These short presentations show actual laboratory personnel performing the manipulations with their own materials and equipment. The verbal descriptions are brief and to the point,

and a printed protocol summary is provided with each procedure. There are plans to continue updating these tapes and to add to the range of experimental techniques described. For more information call 1–800–995–1110; Fax 801–752–5615.

50. *Molecular Cardiology: Unlocking the Secrets of the Heart* (1993) is an hour-long videotape presentation by three molecular cardiologists, Dr. Robert Roberts, Dr. Victor Dzau, and Dr. Judith Swain. Following a brief introduction by Dr. Timothy Johnson to the functions of DNA in cells and the basic manipulations using DNA in molecular biology, four areas of current interest are discussed. Dr. Roberts outlines several aspects of the molecular genetics of cardiomyopathies, including the recent mapping of the genes for seven cardiomyopathies to specific loci of certain human chromosomes. These disease associations may lead to the cloning and sequencing and, thus, the identification of the gene involved in each disorder. Dr. Dzau then discusses the implications of mutations in the angiotensinogen and angiotensin-converting enzyme genes on hypertension and associations with increased risk of myocardial infarction. Dr. Roberts touches on possible treatments promoting new cardiac myocyte growth by the use of molecular mechanisms similar to those that function in skeletal muscle models. Finally, Dr. Swain describes transgenic animal technology (addition of a gene), and the knockout mouse technique (deletion of a gene), as well as advances in gene transfer into human vascular cells. The videotape is accompanied by a glossary of terms. It was produced by The American College of Cardiology with an educational grant from Genentech, Inc.

CHAPTER 3

Physiology and Pathophysiology of Blood Vessels

Philip B. Dobrin, MD, PhD

Introduction

The physiologic survival of complex multicellular organisms depends on the integrity of their vascular systems for delivery of nutrients and removal of waste products. The conduit and large distributing arteries offer little resistance to blood flow. Moreover, because of their compliance, they accommodate the stroke volume ejected with each contraction of the heart, storing a portion of this volume during systole and draining it during diastole. This provides continuing flow to the peripheral circulation. The accommodation offered by the conduit arteries is termed a *Windkessel* effect or "air cushion," after the German word describing a device which performed a similar function on fire pumps at the turn of the century. The large arteries also propagate the pulse and offer vascular impedance, i.e., dynamic resistance to the oscillatory components of pulsatile flow. The conduit and distributing arteries are the site of atherosclerotic disease, especially at junctions and ostia. The arterioles are the chief source of vascular resistance, controlling the distribution of flow. When the arterioles constrict abnormally, they cause systemic hypertension. When they dilate abnormally, they cause hypotension and, if extreme, cardiovascular collapse. The capillaries are the segment of the circulation responsible for the transfer of nutrient material and waste products between the blood and tissues. The veins are mainly storage organs, holding as much as 70% of the blood volume as it is returned to the heart.

This chapter reviews the physiology and pathophysiology of arteries and veins. The mechanical properties and control of these vessels are first described qualitatively, and then are considered quantitatively. The mathematical analyses presented are entirely algebraic and are presented in simple steps. The reader is encouraged to review them as they will provide quantitative insight into the mechanical behavior of blood vessels. Extensive reviews of the literature and detailed quantitative analyses are available elsewhere.[1–6]

When blood vessels are subjected to pressure, they are distended in the *circumferential* and *longitudinal* directions. At the same time, they undergo *radial* thinning of the wall. These three directions are at 90° to one another (Figure 1). Deformation occurs with little twist or torsion of the vessel.[7] Therefore, deformations may be described as orthogonal. This chapter examines the properties and behavior of blood vessels in each of these three orthogonal directions. It then reviews the properties of blood vessels in certain pathophysiologic conditions relevant to vascular surgery. These include aneurysms, poststenotic dilatation, autogenous vein grafts, hypertension, and atherosclerosis.

Finally, some recent bioengineering developments regarding blood vessels are presented. Throughout this chapter, there is an emphasis on the mechanical aspects of blood vessels, as well as the relevant physiology and pharmacology that alter those properties.

From *The Basic Science of Vascular Disease*. Edited by Sidawy AN, Sumpio BE, and DePalma RG. Armonk, NY: Futura Publishing Company, Inc.; © 1997.

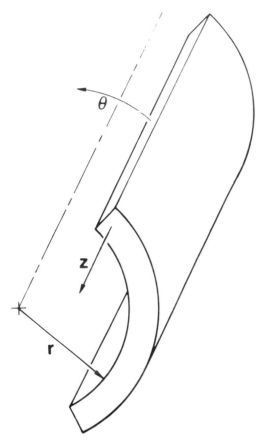

Figure 1. Diagram of segment of blood vessel illustrating circumferential (θ), longitudinal (Z), and radial (r) directions. Deformations and stresses are tensile in the θ and Z directions because the tissue is stretched in these directions when the vessel is pressurized. Deformation and stress in the r direction are compressive because the wall is forced to become thinner with pressurization.[1]

Circumferential Direction

Behavior of Arteries In Vivo

When arteries are subjected to arterial pressure, they deform in the circumferential direction. This manifests as an increase in circumference or diameter. All vessels are subject to continuous deformation by diastolic pressure and this is increased cyclically by the systolic-diastolic pressure oscillation. In fact, the diameter changes manifested by arteries closely resemble the configuration of the arterial pressure pulse, with little delay or phase lag between changes in pressure and changes in diameter (Figure 2).[8] The fact that the phase lag is small indicates that the vessel wall behaves largely as an elastic body with little viscosity. This also has been verified by detailed in vitro studies which demonstrate that, in relaxed vessels, only 5% to 10% of resistance to distention is attributable to viscosity.[9] The lower panel of Figure 2 also shows that the pres-

sure-diameter relationship is curvilinear. Numerous studies in normal animals and humans show that the carotid and femoral arteries oscillate 8% to 10% in external diameter with each pressure pulse.[1] However, simple surgical exposure of arteries may increase their measured stiffness.[10,11]

An 8% to 10% oscillation in external diameter corresponds to a 10% to 14% oscillation in internal diameter. The difference between external and internal diameter oscillations is due simply to geometry and the conservation of matter. In any incompressible cylinder, even a rubber tube, a given percent change in external diameter must be accompanied by a larger percent change in internal diameter. This is exemplified by the fact that as the cylinder increases in diameter, the wall becomes thinner, i.e., the internal diameter enlarges at a more rapid rate than does the external diameter. This seemingly academic point becomes important when one compares various methods of measurement of blood vessel deformation in patients. Angiographic and some ultrasonic techniques obtain measurements of internal dimensions. Other Doppler ultrasonic techniques, laser and optical methods, and linear displacement transducers may obtain external dimensions. Clearly, it is important to measure equivalent anatomic locations if one is to meaningfully evaluate and compare various interventions.

Unlike the systemic arteries, intrathoracic vessels exhibit larger changes in diameter during each cardiac cycle.[1] The intrathoracic aorta and pulmonary arteries undergo changes of 8% to 18% in external diameter during each cardiac cycle. During inspiration, the intrathoracic pressure which surrounds the vessels is decreased to negative values. This increases the transmural pressure, i.e., the difference between the intraluminal pressure and the pressure surrounding the artery. However, this increase in transmural pressure does not fully account for the increase in dimensional changes exhibited by intrathoracic vessels.

Relaxed Arteries

Relaxed arteries and veins exhibit characteristic pressure-diameter and volume-pressure relationships. At low pressures and small diameters, both arteries and veins are extremely distensible; at higher pressures, both vessels become very stiff (Figure 3).[12] This is due to the composition and architecture of the blood vessel wall. At very small dimensions and pressures up to 25 to 50 mm Hg, the elastic lamellae in the vessel walls are retracted and exhibit a corrugated appearance histologically. At pressures between 25 and 50 mm Hg, the elastic lamellae become fully straightened and confer their elastic characteristics to the vessel wall.[13,14] Elastin is a fibrous protein which acts mechanically

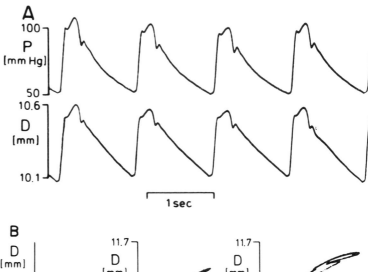

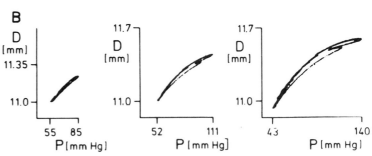

Figure 2. (**A**) Upper tracing shows simultaneous pressure (**P**) and diameter (**D**) recordings of the right common carotid artery in a 68-year-old man during surgery. Catheter manometer recorded pressure. A photoelectric measuring device using photocells measured diameter. (**B**) Pressure-diameter curves from a 64-year-old man during surgery. **Upper limbs of loops** correspond to rising aspect of pressure waves; **lower limbs of loops** correspond to falling aspect of pressure curves. Note that width of hysteresis loops increase with increasing pulse pressure. Note, also, that the pressure-diameter curves are curvilinear.[8]

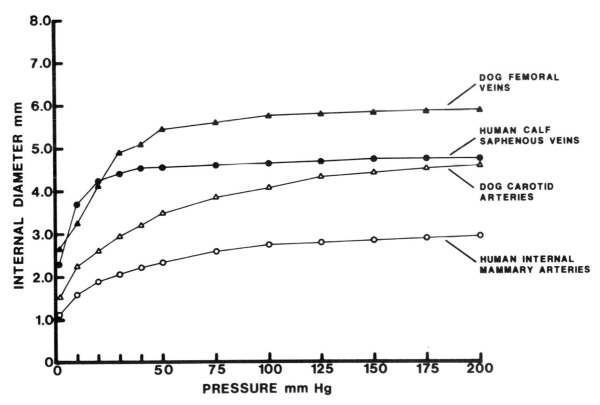

Figure 3. Pressure-diameter curves for dog and human arteries and veins. Curves are curvilinear, becoming stiffer with distention. Arteries stiffen at 80 to 100 mm Hg. Veins stiffen at 35 to 50 mm Hg.[12]

and thermodynamically like a folded chain. It is highly extensible and, when heated to a more entropic state, actually decreases in length. Rubber, another elastomer, also retracts when heated. When subjected to load at body temperature, single elastic fibers can be extended 50% to 70%. It has been computed that each individual elastic lamella in the aorta bears approximately 250 dyne or 0.0025 N, and this value applies for a large number of mammalian species from the mouse to the elephant.[15]

At pressures greater than 100 mm Hg, arteries exhibit great stiffness. This is associated histologically with fully stretched elastic lamellae and recruitment of, and orientation of, collagen fibers. Collagen is structurally different than elastin, as it is composed of tightly wound helical chains. These chains are tightly cross-linked, thereby restricting their extensibility. Studies of individual collagen fibers show that collagen can be stretched only 2% to 4%, as compared with the 50% to 70% exhibited by elastin. When elastin is stretched, it exhibits an elastic modulus, a measure of stiffness, of 4.5×10^5 N/m².[16–20] When collagen fibers are stretched, their elastic modulus fibers are approximately 1.0×10^9 N/m².[19–21] Thus, stretched collagen is several hundred to one thousand times as stiff as stretched elastin.

At least four types of collagen may be found in the vessel wall.[22] Smooth muscle cells (SMCs) are known to synthesize types I, III, and V. Types I and III are sometimes referred to as interstitial collagens and are the major collagen subtypes in the wall. They appear as striated fibers, and provide the great stiffness and tensile strength exhibited by arteries and veins at large deformations. Types I and III collagen are found in the media. Small amounts of type V collagen also may be found there. Type I collagen is the predominant type found in the adventitia. Type IV collagen is found mainly in basement membranes,[22] such as in the intima beneath the endothelial cells. Capillaries contain type III collagen organized as a reticular network. Venules and veins contain a similar network consisting of types I and III collagen.

Mechanical analysis suggests that only about 8% of collagen in the vessel wall is load-bearing in the dog carotid artery, and only 25% of the collagen is load-bearing in the renal, iliac, mesenteric, and coronary arteries.[23] These computations assume that elastin and collagen lie parallel with virtually no connections between them. Comparable values have not been estimated for human arteries. The shape of the pressure-diameter curve of arteries (Figure 3) shows that marked stiffening occurs at 80 to 100 mm Hg. In veins, marked stiffening occurs at 35 to 50 mm Hg. This has implications for the effect of arterial pressure on veins when they are used as arterial bypass grafts. When distended by arterial pressures, vein grafts exhibit nearly constant diameters, in spite of systolic-diastolic pressure oscillations.

Histometric,[18,20] enzymatic degradation,[24] and putrefaction studies[19] demonstrate that the physical properties of elastin and collagen largely determine the mechanical characteristics of both normal and diseased arteries. Elastin content correlates with the stiffness of large arteries at both small and large dimensions.[23,25] A similar correlation between collagen content and vessel stiffness has not been found. This is consistent with computations suggesting that much of the collagen in the wall is not load-bearing.[23] In fact, it is not surprising that there is a poor correlation when one considers the great stiffness of collagen relative to that of the vessel wall; very few collagen fibers contribute a great deal of stiffness. The elastic modulus of the vessel wall at physiologic pressures is about 4.5×10^5 N/m², whereas the elastic modulus of collagen is about 1.0×10^9 N/m². If most of the collagen in the wall were load-bearing, the wall would be about 200 times stiffer than it is. Nevertheless, collagen does influence wall properties. The abdominal aorta and most systemic arteries are stiffer than intrathoracic ones.[26] The arteries obtained from aged subjects are stiffer than those obtained from younger subjects.[27–29] The arteries obtained from hypertensive subjects are stiffer than those obtained from normotensive subjects.[30–33] All of these differences correlate with higher collagen-to-elastin ratios in the stiffer vessels.[32–38] As shown in Figure 4[39]

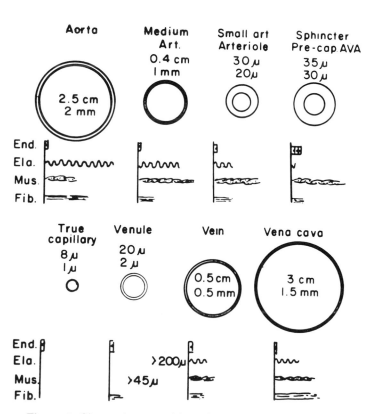

Figure 4. Size and composition of blood vessels. **End** is endothelium. **Ela** is elastin. **Mus** is vascular smooth muscle. **Fib** is fibrous connective tissue.[39]

Table 1
Constituents of Arterial Wall and Ratio of Collagen to Elastin in Dogs

Artery	No. of Specimens	Wet Tissue, %		Dry, Defatted Tissue, %			
		H_2O	Extracted fat +4.0	Collagen	Elastin	Collagen + Elastin	Collagen/ Elastin
Carotid	6	71.1 ± 0.1	71.2 ± 0.1	50.7 ± 2.1	20.1 ± 1.0	70.8 ± 2.5	2.55 ± 0.13
Coronary	9	63.2 ± 1.0*	71.5 ± 1.4	47.9 ± 2.6	15.6 ± 0.7	63.5 ± 2.7	3.12 ± 0.21
Aorta							
Ascending	9	73.8 ± 0.6	74.0 ± 0.5	19.6 ± 1.2	41.1 ± 2.1	60.7 ± 2.2	0.49 ± 0.04
Abdominal	10	70.4 ± 0.4	70.8 ± 0.3	45.5 ± 1.7	30.1 ± 1.7	75.6 ± 1.8	1.58 ± 0.15
Cranial mesenteric							
Proximal	10	70.8 ± 0.5	71.6 ± 0.4	38.1 ± 1.7	26.5 ± 1.7	64.6 ± 1.8	1.51 ± 0.15
Distal	9	71.4 ± 0.4	72.0 ± 0.4	37.4 ± 1.4	22.4 ± 1.5	59.8 ± 1.6	1.72 ± 0.11
Branches	10	69.5 ± 0.6	73.1 ± 0.7	36.1 ± 1.5	21.8 ± 0.9	57.9 ± 1.7	1.69 ± 0.10
Renal	9	70.4 ± 0.7	70.8 ± 0.7	42.6 ± 1.6	18.7 ± 1.8	61.3 ± 2.1	2.46 ± 0.27
Femoral	10	68.0 ± 0.3	68.1 ± 0.3	44.5 ± 1.4	24.5 ± 1.6	69.0 ± 2.1	1.89 ± 0.14

Percent values are mean ± standard deviation, weight/weight. Specimens were slightly dehydrated because of unavoidably long dissection.[10]

and Table 1,[40] the connective tissue composition of arteries, capillaries, and veins, and even different arteries, varies considerably. As noted above, the stiffness of the abdominal aorta is greater than that of the thoracic aorta, and this also corresponds with greater collagen content in the distal vessel. Interestingly, in the dog, the biochemical composition of the vessel changes within a few centimeters of the diaphragm.[34]

Histologic observations demonstrate that medial collagen fibers are stretched at physiologic pressures, but that adventitial collagen fibers are not.[13] Enzymatic degradation studies demonstrate that elastin bears loads in all three orthogonal directions, i.e., the circumferential, longitudinal and radial directions; collagen bears loads almost solely in the circumferential direction.[42,43]

Although the absolute content of connective tissue and collagen-to-elastin ratio are important, architectural arrangements involving the connective tissues also influence wall properties. For example, with aging, arteries dilate to larger diameters and develop thicker walls. Dilatation causes collagen fibers to become load-bearing at progressively lower pressures.[41] As a result of such dilatation, the arteries of aged humans become functionally stiffer at progressively lower pressures than those of young patients (Figure 5).[29] In addition, with age, elastic fibers become calcified,[44] further restricting the extensibility of these normally compliant elements. Collagen also plays a critical role in maintaining arterial integrity, as degradation of this connective tissue causes pressurized vessels to dilate aneurysmally and to rupture. This is true for normal dog and human arteries,[45] and also for aneu-

rysmal human arteries.[46] Rupture does not occur with degradation of elastin.[45,46]

Blood vessel walls also contain glycosaminoglycan ground substance. The electrolyte and water-binding properties of this material may be of chronic importance to the vessel wall; however, enzymatic degradation of ground substance demonstrates that this nonfibrous connective tissue has little acute effect on the mechanical characteristics of the vessel wall.

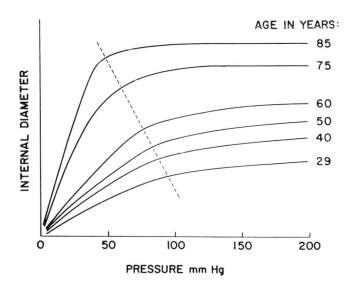

Figure 5. Pressure-diameter curves of thoracic aortas of humans ages 29 to 85 years. Reconstructed from data of Bader.[27] With age the aorta dilates, stiffening elastin and recruiting collagen fibers. This results in increasing vessel stiffness at progressively lower pressures. **Broken line** shows that transition from compliant to stiff vessel shifts to lower pressure with aging.[12]

Recently, a new possible function has been attributed to the glycosaminoglycans. Because of their viscoelastic properties and their sodium and water-binding properties, it has been hypothesized that the glycosaminoglycans may be the wall sensor of shear stress.[47]

Contracted Arteries

Another factor that can play a role in vascular mechanics is the activity of the vascular muscle. In large arteries and large veins, SMCs lie in the media arranged in a helical pattern, such that the majority of the force generated is exerted in the circumferential direction.[48–50] With excitation of the muscle, two mechanical effects occur: first, there is an increase in circumferential retractive force which tends to cause constriction. If smooth contraction occurs with a steady or only modestly rising blood pressure, contraction may lead to a decrease in vessel diameter. However, if vascular muscle excitation is part of a generalized pressor response, then the marked rise in blood pressure that results from constriction of the downstream resistance vessels may cause the large arteries to actually *increase* in caliber, in spite of activation of the muscle in their walls.[51] Thus, contraction can occur against falling pressure as in hypotension, against constant pressure ("isobaric contraction"), against rising pressure but with maintenance of constant diameter ("isometric contraction"), or against markedly rising pressure with increasing diameter in spite of activation of the muscle.

Figure 6A shows pressure-radius curves for an artery in the relaxed pretreatment state (Pre), after excitation of the muscle with norepinephrine (NE), and after relaxation of the muscle with potassium cyanide (KCN). During active shortening, the vascular muscle causes constriction of the vessel. During distention, marked hysteresis is observed indicating that the contracted muscle can bear more force applied to it than it can generate. The data shown in Figure 6A are for static steps. Much less hysteresis is seen in vessels subjected to pulsations over a relatively narrow pressure range. This indicates that most of the hysteresis seen in Figure 6A is the result of stress relaxation and not viscosity. The fact that there is little hysteresis in the relaxed (Pre) or chemically relaxed artery (KCN) indicates that most of the stress relaxation resides in the vascular muscle.

The horizontal distance between the curves for the relaxed (Pre) or inactivated (KCN) vessel and the contracted (NE) vessel is not constant. Instead, there appears to be a maximum at a given radius. If one assumes that the muscle and connective tissues are functionally parallel, then one may compute the stress at each radius for the vessel in contracted and relaxed

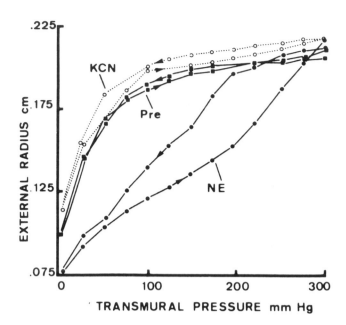

Figure 6A. Pressure-radius curves for a dog carotid artery in vitro in the relaxed state (**Pre**), after activation of the vascular muscle with norepinephrine (**NE**), and after inactivation of the muscle with potassium cyanide (**KCN**).

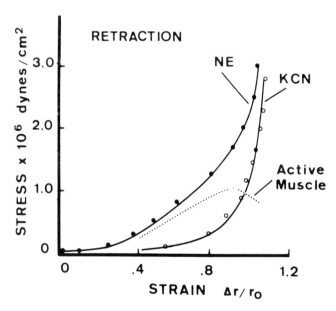

Figure 6B. Strain-stress relations for the vessel with the muscle active (**NE**) and relaxed with potassium cyanide (**KCN**). The difference between the two curves gives the unimodal active stress curve exerted by the vascular muscle.

state, and subtract the stress of the relaxed vessel from that of the contracted vessel to obtain the active stress exerted by the muscle. This is shown in Figure 6B. This clearly demonstrates that vascular muscle has a unimodal length-active stress curve. This is comparable to the "Starling curve" exhibited by heart muscle, and the length-active tension curve demonstrated by skeletal muscle. This is due, at least in part, to the overlap characteristics of actin and myosin. It is also evident that active isometric contraction exhibits a maximum over a broad range of physiologic pressures. This has been found for a large number of canine and rabbit arteries[52-54] and for human internal mammary artery.[55] In virtually all cases, the maximum isometric contraction occurs at pressures comparable to those to which the vessel is normally subjected.[52-54] Some vessels in the frog microcirculation are subject to pressures that are greater than those associated with maximum active contraction.[56]

Interestingly, when autogenous vein is subjected to arterial pressures, the vascular muscle is stretched to far above the maximum of its circumferential length-active tension relationship.[55] When smooth muscle is stretched to extreme lengths, it reversibly loses much of its contractility. This is seen in vascular smooth muscle,[57] in stomach following chronic gastric distention, and in urinary bladder following prolonged bladder distention.

The unimodal length-active stress curve of vascular muscle has important implications for investigators studying the responsiveness of vascular muscle following external interventions, such as radiation, exposure to hypertensive pressures, or various chronic drug treatments. In studying the contractility of the muscle, it is imperative to determine the peak in the active stress curve. External interventions may have effects on the connective tissues causing stiffening of the relaxed wall, so that unless precautions are taken one might inadvertently study the muscle at two different positions along the length-active stress curve. It is also important to differentiate strength of contraction from pharmacologic sensitivity of the muscle.

When a muscle contracts, it stretches all of the materials that are coupled in series with it. This functional "element" has been termed the "series elastic component" or SEC. The SEC temporarily stores energy and is stiffened with extension.[58,59] During maximum isometric contraction of vascular muscle, the SEC is stretched 7% in strips of artery[60] and 11% in cylindrical segments of artery.[61] This is 2 to 5 times greater than that observed for skeletal or cardiac muscle.[58,62] Enzymatic degradation studies show that the SEC in vascular muscle is largely elastin.[63] Thus, isometric contraction of the vascular muscle stiffens some portion of the wall elastin; but as discussed below, active constriction of the vessel also unloads the connective tissue in the wall.

A second mechanical function of vascular muscle is to alter arterial wall stiffness. Because the force generated by the muscle adds to that exerted by the connective tissue, activation of the muscle increases the stiffness of the wall, but this is more complicated than it first appears. Figure 7 plots the elastic modulus, a

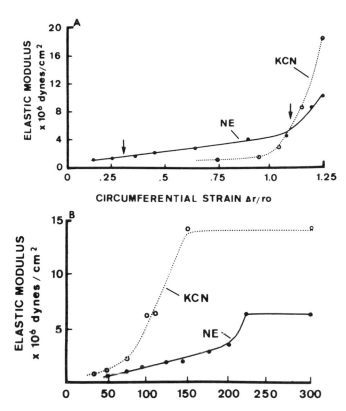

Figure 7. Elastic modulus, a measure of stiffness, for a dog carotid artery in which the vascular muscle was excited with norepinephrine (NE), then relaxed with potassium cyanide (KCN). Activation of the muscle increases wall stiffness if the data are plotted as a function of diameter or strain (top), but decreases wall stiffness if the data are plotted as a function of pressure (bottom).[64]

measure of wall stiffness, of a dog carotid artery after activation of the vascular muscle with NE, and after relaxation of the muscle with potassium cyanide (KCN). These data are plotted as a function of vessel deformation, in this case strain, i.e., the fractional increase in radius. These data show that at all, but the largest dimensions, activation of the muscle increases vessel stiffness as compared with that observed with the muscle relaxed. However, activation of the muscle also causes overall constriction; this unloads the connective tissue, decreasing the stiffness of the passive connective tissue elements. This is illustrated by the location of the arrows in the top panel of Figure 7. These points identify the strain or relative diameter of the vessel at 100 mm Hg in the contracted (left) and the relaxed (right) states. These arrows illustrate that constriction can decrease wall stiffness at 100 mm Hg if isobaric constriction is permitted to occur. This is further demonstrated by replotting the data points shown in the top panel of Figure 7 against pressure. This is shown in the lower panel of Figure 7. These data clearly show that, when plotted as a function of pressure, activation of the muscle *decreases* wall stiffness. As reviewed previously, examination of the published literature[64] reveals that virtually all of those investigators who reported that activation of vascular muscle *increases* wall stiffness plotted their data as a function of diameter or volume or strain, while all of those who reported that activation of vascular muscle *decreases* wall stiffness plotted their data as a function of pressure. Which effect then is applicable to the intact organism? In reality, activation of the muscle in vivo is usually neither isobaric nor isometric, but rather a mixture of the two, thus making it difficult to predict the effects of muscle contraction on wall stiffness. In any case, one must select the parameter against which stiffness will be examined—diameter or pressure.[4]

Control of Vascular Smooth Muscle

Vascular smooth muscle contractile activity is controlled by extrinsic and intrinsic mechanisms. Extrinsic control of blood vessel diameter is mediated through neural and humoral mechanisms. Sympathetic vasoconstrictor fibers innervate most blood vessels, releasing norepinephrine at their postganglionic terminals. This elicits vasoconstriction, and also maintains a basal level of tone. There are also sympathetic cholinergic fibers which vasodilate the blood vessels perfusing skeletal muscle. These fibers are influenced by cerebral activity and are thought to cause vasodilation with the very onset of muscle activity, even before nutritional requirements are increased or metabolic products are produced. Sympathetic activity is especially important in the case of the arterioles, less important in the case of the distributing arteries and capacitance (venous) vessels, and of little significance in the case of large elastic conduit arteries. There are also a few parasympathetic dilating nerves, such as those to the blood vessels supplying the salivary glands and the coronary vessels. The effects of these few fibers on the resistance of the overall circulation is minor, but they can have important effects on blood flow to the innervated vascular beds.

Humoral factors include epinephrine and NE released from the adrenal medulla under autonomic control. In low concentrations, epinephrine dilates the blood vessels of skeletal muscle (β-adrenergic stimulation); in high concentrations, the same hormone constricts the blood vessels of almost all vascular beds (α-adrenergic stimulation). The release of adrenergic agents from sympathetic nerves and from adrenal tissue is controlled by brain stem reflexes under the influence of such specialized afferent inputs as baroreceptors, chemoreceptors, and cardiopulmonary receptors.

Other important circulating vasoactive agents include angiotensin II (AII), vasoactive intestinal peptide (VIP), substance P, and the kinins, especially bradykinin. VIP, substance P, and bradykinin are believed to have their vasodilatory effects via the endothelium. Histamine is also a powerful vasodilator, but acts by means of H_2 receptors and appears to be independent of the endothelium. Calcitonin gene-related peptide (CGRP) is the most powerful dilator yet identified. It is found in perivascular nerves,[65] often in association with substance P, serotonin, and somatostatin. CGRP also may be in afferent neurons and play a role in local "axon reflexes." There is some evidence that CGRP may be co-released with acetylcholine from parasympathetic nerves to the coronary vessels.

A second major control system of vascular smooth muscle is by means of intrinsic mechanisms. The endothelium plays a critical role in this regard, releasing paracrine mediators. Prostacyclin, a vasodilator and inhibitor of platelet aggregation, is synthesized by endothelial cells from arachidonic acid precursors by cyclooxygenase. Thromboxane, a vasoconstrictor and promoter of platelet aggregation, is also synthesized from arachidonic acid precursors by cyclooxygenase, but in this case by platelets. These vasodilator and vasoconstrictor agents appear to maintain an equilibrium between their two opposing effects. Inhibition of cyclooxygenase with aspirin is short-lived in the endothelium, for these cells synthesize new cyclooxygenase within a few hours. By contrast, platelets are permanently acetylated by aspirin so that production of thromboxane is delayed until new platelets enter the circulation. Intrinsic mechanisms also include flow-sensitive regulation of muscle tone. The endothelium or subendothelial area is responsive to the shear stress exerted by the flowing blood. Shearing stresses cause the release of prostaglandin[66] and endothelial-derived relaxing factor (EDRF) from the endothelium.[67] Mechanical removal of the endothelium with a cotton swab or an embolectomy balloon abolishes these responses. As the endothelium repopulates the intima, EDRF synthesis returns.[68] Acetylcholine, adenosine triphosphate, bradykinin, and substance P all cause release of EDRF. Recent evidence demonstrates that EDRF is nitric oxide (NO). EDRF activates intracellular guanylate cyclase to increase cytosolic cyclic guanosine monophosphate. This substance causes vascular smooth muscle to relax. EDRF release is stimulated by shear stress, and by the endogenous agents enumerated above. Administration of exogenous nitroprusside, a powerful vasodilator, also increases intracellular cyclic guanosine monophosphate. Rhythmic digital compression of coronary arteries also causes the release of EDRF, suggesting that rhythmic contraction of the coronary arteries by the myocardium may facilitate flow through the coronary vessels.[67] Such a mechanism also may occur in skeletal muscle, contributing to increased blood flow to muscle during exercise. Endothelial-derived contracting factor (EDCF) and endothelin are constrictor agents produced by the endothelium, but little is known of their physiologic importance.[69,70] Thus, the release of relaxing and constricting factors from the endothelium in response to alterations in blood flow and shear stress provides tissues with a means of local control. Current evidence demonstrates that EDRF is an important determinant of vascular resistance[71] and regional blood flow.[72]

The control provided by local mechanisms is remarkably sensitive. Increased perfusion pressure to a specific vascular bed causes a brief increase in flow; this is followed by vasoconstriction and a subsequent reduction in flow approaching original levels. This is termed "autoregulation" and is operative over a wide range of physiologic pressures. In most tissues, this range is from 60 to 160 mm Hg. In addition to EDRF, EDCF, prostaglandins, and endothelin described above, several other mechanisms are thought to play a role in autoregulation. Stretching vascular smooth muscle, even in vitro, elicits a contractile response. This is termed a "myogenic" response. A second mechanism is termed "tissue pressure." An increase in perfusion pressure causes an increase in transmural pressure across the exchange vessels of the tissue being perfused. This provides a gradient for movement of fluid from the vascular space into the extravascular space. This results in elevation of extravascular tissue pressure which, in turn, compresses the vessels. This is especially important in muscle, wherein a compartment syndrome can develop. Fasciotomy releases the tissue pressure within the compartment that is compressing the vessels. It also occurs in the brain under extreme circumstances, as this structure is encased within the rigid skull. In the case of both muscle and brain, tissue pressure is not an important control mechanism under normal physiologic conditions. However, it may become important under pathophysiologic conditions such as reperfusion injury (muscle) and trauma (brain), when cerebrospinal pressure can rise to very high values. A third mechanism is termed "metabolic mechanism." There is a remarkable correlation between blood flow and metabolic requirements. This is seen in the heart where flow correlates closely with oxygen requirements, and in the case of the brain where flow correlates closely with carbon dioxide levels in the blood. Increased perfusion elevates the provision of nutritional elements such as oxygen and glucose, and provides removal of metabolic waste products such hydrogen ions, carbon dioxide, and potassium ions. This delivery/removal effect permits constriction after an initial distention and increased flow. Metabolic mechanisms are believed to be an important component of "active hyperemia," which occurs in muscle with activity. Metabolic mechanisms also are thought to play a role in "reactive hyperemia," wherein blood flow is increased through tissue following a period of ischemia. This is seen in skeletal muscle following release of an inflated constrictor cuff around a limb. Under physiologic conditions, extrinsic and intrinsic constrictor/dilator activity provides a fine balance of control that protects individual vascular beds and the organism as a whole. Not all vascular beds behave the same. The coronary circulation, the cerebral circulation, and blood flow through skeletal muscle, skin, and the viscera all vary in their response to specific stimuli and vary in the magnitude of their constriction or dilation. For example, the kidney and brain autoregulate very effectively. Skin exhibits very little autoregulation, with blood flow responding to the need for temperature regulation. Intestine autoregulates effectively, but blood flow varies profoundly depending upon whether or not the organism is postprandial.

Quantitative Aspects

The following computations describe quantitatively the mechanical properties of blood vessels in the circumferential direction. These computations are based on the assumption of equilibrium, i.e., that the force distending a vessel is at equilibrium with the force exerted by the wall in opposition to the distending force. Thus, at equilibrium, the vessel exhibits a steady diameter. From Newton's first law, force is given by:

$$^*F = M \times a \qquad (1)$$

where F is force, M is mass, and a is acceleration. When a vessel exhibits a steady, unchanging diameter, there is no acceleration and the *net* force on the wall is zero, i.e., distending and retractive forces are equal. Pressure (in liquids or gases) and stress (in solids) may generically be termed *stress*. Stress is force per unit area:

---

* Force in the CGS system is given in dynes (dyn) where 1 dyn = 1 gm mass accelerated 1 cm/sec^2. Force in the SI system is given in newtons, where 1 newton = 1 Kg mass accelerated 1 m/sec^2. Force can be converted from CGS to SI because force is exactly 5 orders of magnitude larger in the CGS system than it is in the SI system. For example, the force borne by each lamella is estimated to be 250 dyn or 0.00250 N.

Pressure and stress are given in units of force per unit area. In the CGS system stress is expressed in dyn/cm^2. For pressure, the density of mercury is 1.36 g/cm^2 for each millimeter of mercury. The acceleration due to gravity is 981 cm/sec^2. Therefore 1 mm Hg exerts 1×1.36 g/cm$^2 \times 981$ cm/sec^2 = 1,334 dyn/cm^2. Similarly, 100 mm Hg exerts 133,400 dynes/cm^2. In the SI system a pressure of 1 N/m^2 is also termed 1 Pascal.

Stress can be converted from the CGS system to the SI system because stress is exactly one order of magnitude larger in the CGS system than it is in the SI system. For example, the stress exerted by an artery wall at physiological pressures may be 1.33×10^6 dynes/cm^2 or 1.33×10^5 N/m^2.

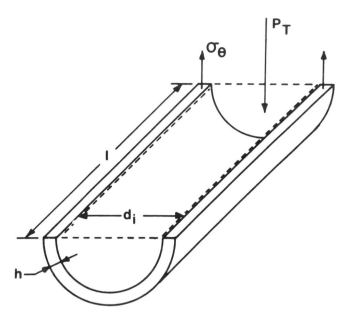

Figure 8. Free body diagram where a portion of the blood vessel has been removed and replaced with forces at equilibrium. Diagram illustrates computation of forces and stresses in the circumferential direction.[4]

$$\sigma \text{ or } P = \frac{F}{A} \tag{2}$$

where σ is stress, P is pressure, F is force, and A is the area over which that force is exerted.

Rearranging,

$$F = \sigma \text{ or } P \times (A) \tag{3}$$

where force may be computed as the product of stress or pressure and the area over which that force is exerted. One may use these principles to compute the circumferential distending and retractive forces present in a vessel wall at equilibrium (Figure 8).

The force distending a cylindrical blood vessel in the circumferential (θ) direction may be given by:

$$F_{D\theta} = P_T \times (D_i \times L) \tag{4}$$

where $F_{D\theta}$ is the distending force, P_T is the transmural pressure, i.e., the pressure within the lumen minus that surrounding the vessel, D_i is the internal diameter of the vessel, and L is the length of vessel under consideration. Note that pressure is the stress exerted against the vessel, and the product ($D_i \times L$) is the area over which that stress is exerted.

At equilibrium, the vessel wall exerts a retractive force in the circumferential direction:

$$F_{R\theta} = \sigma_\theta \times (h \times L \times 2) \tag{5}$$

where $F_{R\theta}$ is the retractive force, σ_θ is the stress exerted by the wall in the circumferential direction, h is the wall thickness, and L is the same vessel length considered in equation 4. The factor of 2 accounts for the two walls of the vessel.

Since the forces are at equilibrium, one may set equations 4 and 5 equal and solve algebraically for the stress exerted by the wall.

$$\sigma_\theta = P_T \times \frac{r_i}{h} \tag{6}$$

Note that for a vessel of infinitely thin wall thickness, equation 6 becomes the well-known law of Laplace.

One may now see that activation of the vascular muscle has complex effects, all leading to a new equilibrium condition. Activation of the muscle is the circumferential stress (equation 6). This causes constriction, which tends to decrease active stress as the muscle proceeds downward along its length-active stress curve. Constriction also increases the retractive force by increasing the wall thickness (equation 5) and decreases the distending force by decreasing the diameter. All of these factors change simultaneously until a new equilibrium is achieved. At that point, the actively contracted vessel will exhibit a new, stable diameter.

$$T = P_T \times r \tag{7}$$

The law of Laplace (equation 7) gives the tension (T) or retractive force ($F_{R\theta}$); equation 6 gives the stress or force percent area, for the wall at equilibrium.

When a vessel is subjected to pressure, it may distend. Deformation may be quantitated in several ways. Two of the simplest are strain and extension ratio:

$$\epsilon_\theta = \frac{\Delta D}{D_0} = \frac{D - D_0}{D} \tag{8}$$

where ϵ is strain in the circumferential direction, ΔD is the change in diameter, D is the diameter observed after deformation, and D_0 is the diameter before deformation. Thus, strain is the fractional change in dimensions. An even simpler measure of deformation is extension ratio:

$$\lambda_\theta = \frac{D}{D_0} \tag{9}$$

where λ_θ is extension ratio in the circumferential direction, D is observed diameter after deformation, and D_0 is the diameter before deformation. The units of strain and extension ratio are dimensionless quantities, e.g., cm/cm. The relationship between strain and extension ratio is simply:

$$\lambda_\theta = \epsilon_\theta + 1 \tag{10}$$

The use of strain or extension ratio permits one to compare the properties of vessels of different absolute dimensions.

As a vessel is deformed by distending force, the wall exerts increasing retractive force until equilibrium is achieved. The relationship between deformation and stress is given by stiffness:

$$E = \frac{\sigma}{\epsilon} \quad \text{or} \quad E = \frac{\sigma}{\lambda} \tag{11}$$

where E is the elastic modulus, a measure of stiffness, σ is stress, ϵ is strain, and λ is extension ratio. As shown by equation 11, the stiffer a vessel is, the greater the stress will be at any given level of deformation. This is also shown in Figure 9. However, equation 11 is applicable only for materials which have a linear strain-stress curve and for which a load is applied in only one direction. As demonstrated by the pressure-diameter curves for blood vessels (Figure 3), the strain-stress curve is very nonlinear. At low pressures and small diameters, a given pressure increment, say 25 mm Hg, produces a large amount of deformation. At high pressures and large diameters, a 25-mm pressure increment produces a much smaller amount of deformation. For this reason, a *tangent* elastic modulus or *incremental* elastic modulus more accurately depicts vessel stiffness. This is shown in Figure 9:

$$E_{inc} = \frac{\Delta\sigma}{\Delta\epsilon} \quad \text{or} \quad E_{inc} = \frac{\Delta\sigma}{\Delta\lambda} \tag{12}$$

where E_{inc} is the incremental elastic modulus, and $\Delta\sigma$, $\Delta\epsilon$, and $\Delta\lambda$ are the incremental changes in stress, strain, and extension ratio which accompany a given increase in deformation such as that produced by a pressure increase. Throughout the remainder of this chapter, the term elastic modulus will be used to refer to *incremental* elastic modulus.

The units of elastic modulus are the same as stress. The stiffness of the relaxed arterial wall is extremely low at 0 to 25 mm Hg; it increases to 2.0 to 6.0 $\times$ 10^5 N/m² at physiologic pressures, and approaches 1.0 $\times$ 10^6 N/m² at 200 mm Hg. For comparison, the stiffness of elastin is about 4.6 $\times$ 10^5 N/m² and the stiffness of collagen is about 1.0 $\times$ 10^9 N/m². Thus, it is clear that elastin, not collagen, must largely determine the stiffness of the artery wall at physiologic pressures. It is also apparent that only a small portion of collagen can be load-bearing even in the distended vessel, for if collagen were the chief determinant, then the vessel wall would be several hundred times as stiff as it really is.

The above discussion of elastic modulus treats the vessel as though it were deformed solely in the circumferential direction. In fact, with pressurization, the vessel is deformed in three directions simultaneously. Analysis of vessel stiffness under conditions of multidimensional stresses and deformations has been examined.[73–79] This is discussed in a later section of this chapter entitled *Multidirectional Aspects of Vessel Stiffness.*

Another, simpler estimate of stiffness is given by the "pressure elastic modulus,"[80] developed before

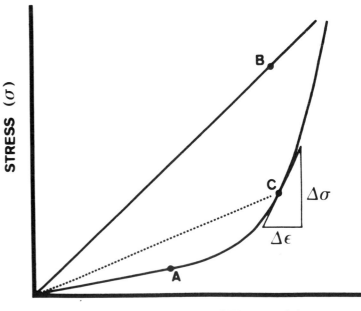

Figure 9. Strain-stress curves for a material that has a linear strain-stress relationship (**origin to B**) and for a material that has a nonlinear strain-stress relationship (**origin to C**). At any level of strain, a stiff material exerts more stress than does a less stiff one (B>C). For materials with a linear strain-stress curve, the elastic modulus (stiffness) may be determined by the stress/strain ratio (σ/ϵ) as from the origin to point B. However, for materials with a nonlinear strain-stress curve, this will give erroneous values, such as at point C. For nonlinear materials, one may compute an incremental elastic modulus, i.e., *change* in stress/*change* in strain ($\Delta\sigma/\Delta\epsilon$). This is shown at point C.[1]

technology permitted accurate and precise assessment of wall thickness.

$$E_P = \frac{\Delta P \times r}{\Delta r} \qquad (13)$$

where E_P is the pressure elastic modulus, ΔP is a change in pressure such as pulse pressure, r is the mean or diastolic radius, and Δr is the change in radius. Although the elements that contribute to the computation of E_P are similar to those that contribute to E_{inc}, E_P lacks the radius-to-wall thickness ratio (r_i/h). As a result, the value given by E_P is only 10% to 12% that given by E_{inc}.

Finally, one may compute the vessel compliance, again without requiring measurement of wall thickness.

$$C = \frac{\Delta r}{r \times \Delta P} \qquad (14)$$

where C is the compliance in the circumferential direction, Δr is the oscillation radius, r is the mean or diastolic radius, and ΔP is a change in pressure such as pulse pressure. Compliance is the inverse of pressure elastic modulus. Compliance is a measure of vessel distensibility, whereas the variously computed elastic moduli are measures of vessel stiffness.

Longitudinal Direction

Normal Arteries

The second major direction in which blood vessels are deformed is longitudinally. Unless they are transected, arteries exhibit little or no change in length. For example, during each cardiac cycle the intact descending thoracic aorta lengthens about 1%. Simultaneously, the abdominal aorta shortens by about the same amount.[81-83] The ascending thoracic aorta and pulmonary arteries extend 5% to 10%.[82] The latter deformations are due largely to motion of the heart. Most large arteries behave like the descending thoracic and abdominal aorta in that they exhibit negligible changes in length during each pressure cycle. Because arteries are held under traction, they do exhibit changes in length with alterations in body position. This is seen in the carotid artery with hyperextension of the cervical spine[4] and the femoral artery with extension of the knee joint.[84] Further evidence that arteries are held under traction is the fact that they retract when they are transected. Traction develops during neonatal development. Longitudinal traction is very low in the newborn. In the dog, it is about 23% at 1 week of age; it increases during the neonatal period to 34% at 16

weeks[85] as the body grows more rapidly than the vessels. During this time, traction increases linearly as a function of body weight.[85] Traction reaches a maximum at about 35% in the young adult,[86-88] and then decreases with age[28,86,88] as the vessels are invested with surrounding connective tissue and also as body height decreases slightly. The investment of connective tissue causes the vessels to be held at their in situ length irrespective of traction or pressure. Atherosclerosis also tends to fix the vessels.[89]

Tortuosity

When arteries are subjected to increased lengthening forces, they may buckle between constraining side branches. This presents clinically as tortuosity. Figure 10 illustrates the longitudinal forces acting on a blood vessel. Both the force due to pressure and the force

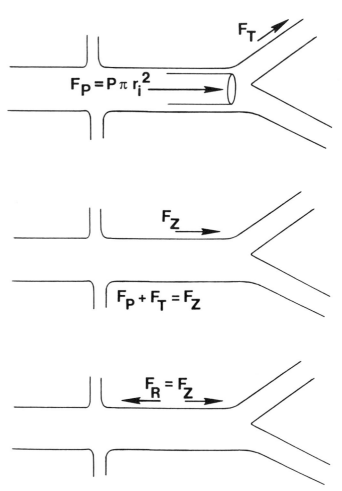

Figure 10. Forces acting on a blood vessel in the longitudinal direction. $\mathbf{F_P}$ is force due to pressure, $\mathbf{F_T}$ is force due to traction, $\mathbf{F_Z}$ is the net longitudinal force extending a vessel, i.e., the sum of $F_P + F_T$. $\mathbf{F_R}$ is the retractive force exerted by the wall. When $F_Z = F_R$, there is equilibrium and the vessel exhibits a stable length.[90]

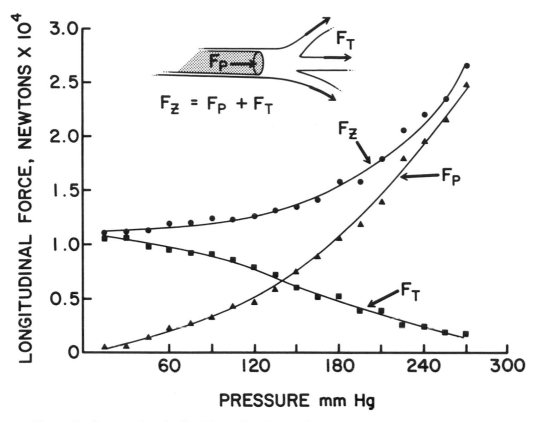

Figure 11. Pressure-longitudinal force data for arteries. At 0 mm Hg, all of the longitudinal force (F_Z) is due to traction (F_T). As pressure is increased, the force due to pressure (F_P) rises, but the traction force (F_T) declines. As a result, the net longitudinal force (F_Z) rises only slightly until very high pressures (160 to 180 mm Hg) are reached.[73]

due to traction are tensile in that they both cause the vessel to lengthen. As discussed above, the traction force (F_T) is due to stretch. Side branches also tend to hold the vessel at stretched lengths. The traction force cannot be determined analytically, but can be measured experimentally by grasping a vessel in situ with a force gauge and then transecting the vessel; the force gauge will then record the traction previously provided by the stretched vessel.[4,73] The second lengthening force is that due to pressure (F_P). This tends to push the vessel to greater lengths. The force due to pressure (F_P) can be determined analytically. It is equal to the product of pressure, π, and the square of the internal radius of the vessel. The middle panel of Figure 10 shows that the net force (F_Z) is the sum of the force due to traction (F_T) and the force due to pressure (F_P).

Figure 11 shows the normal interaction of the pressure force and the traction force on the arterial wall. In the artery without pressure, the net longitudinal force (F_Z) is due entirely to traction (F_T) with no longitudinal force due to pressure (F_P). With increasing pressure, the force due to pressure (F_P) rises and this causes the vessel to lengthen very slightly. With this slight increase in length, the force due to traction (F_T)

declines. Since the net longitudinal force (F_Z) is equal to the sum of the increasing force due to pressure (F_P) and the declining force due to traction (F_T), the net longitudinal force (F_Z) rises only slightly until very high pressures are encountered. This is evident by the nearly flat curve described by F_Z in Figure 11. As a consequence of the interaction between pressure and traction, the artery is subjected to almost constant longitudinal force, at least until very high pressures are encountered. This causes vessels to exhibit nearly constant length in vivo.

Returning to Figure 10, one may see in the lower panel that the net longitudinal force extending the vessel (F_Z) is opposed by an equal and opposite force, i.e., the longitudinal retractive force exerted by the stretched artery wall. In the diagram this is depicted as F_R. Under conditions of equilibrium where the vessel neither lengthens nor shortens, the net longitudinal force which tends to lengthen the vessel (F_Z) and the retractive force which tends to shorten the vessel (F_R) must be equal.

We may now consider conditions wherein a vessel is caused to lengthen. This occurs when the balance of forces described in the lower panel of Figure 10 is altered. This occurs in several common clinical conditions. It is seen in aged, hypertensive individuals, and may be evident on casual inspection of the superficial temporal artery. Hypertension causes increased longitudinal force due to pressure (F_P), while age is associated with decreased force due to traction (F_T), as the aging vessel is invested with surrounding connective tissue. In addition, the vessel exhibits decreased retractive force (F_R) with age. Enzymatic degradation studies of both healthy young animal arteries[90] and aged human arteries[91] demonstrate that the retractive force in the longitudinal direction exerted by the artery wall (F_R) is due largely to elastin. In the aged human vessels, there is a small contribution from collagen as the elastin in the wall is gradually replaced or augmented by collagen, but this is very slight.[91] Disruption of the elastic lamellae may, therefore, be expected to be associated with vessel lengthening. This connective tissue defect is in fact found in the vessel walls of patients with congenital kinking of arteries.[92] Tortuosity also is seen in ectatic and aneurysmal arteries and in arteries where the elastic lamellae are disrupted.[93,94] This is discussed below in the section entitled *Aneurysms*.

Longitudinal Shear Stress

The flow of blood over the endothelial surface also produces a longitudinal force. This is termed the blood-intima shear stress. Shear stress may be computed by the Hagen-Poiseuille formula.[95]

$$T_W = \frac{4\mu Q}{\pi r^3} \qquad (15)$$

where T_W is shear stress, μ is the viscosity of blood (0.035 Poise), Q is the rate of blood flow (mL/sec), and r is the internal radius of the vessel (cm). This force is several orders of magnitude smaller than the forces due to traction and pressure; however, shear stress plays a critical role in maintaining normal endothelial morphology and function. Endothelial cells exposed to normal shear stresses, i.e., about 15 dynes/cm², exhibit an elongated configuration with the long axis lying parallel to the flowing stream. If a segment of artery is excised, rotated 90°, and is reimplanted into the vessel wall, the orientation of the endothelial cells will change after several weeks to again conform to the direction of flow.[96,97] Thus, the artery wall is sensitive to shear stress. The endothelium releases prostaglandins and EDRF in response to shear,[66,98] this mechanism playing a critical local role in maintaining vessel dimensions.[98] Low or abnormal shear stresses that are associated with turbulence or stagnation predispose to the development of intimal hyperplasia in vein grafts,[99,100]

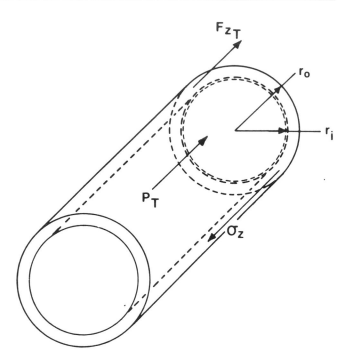

Figure 12. Free body diagram where a portion of the blood vessel has been removed and replaced with forces at equilibrium. Diagram illustrates computation of forces and stresses in the longitudinal direction.[4]

especially at the outflow of vein-artery anastomoses.[101] Low shear stress and disturbed flow also are associated with acceleration of atherogenesis.[102–104]

Quantitative Aspects

As with the presentation of quantitative aspects in the circumferential direction, the following computations for the longitudinal direction are for conditions of equilibrium, in this case where the length of a vessel is unchanging. As illustrated in Figure 12, the force extending a cylindrical vessel in the longitudinal direction is given by:

$$F_{DZ} = P_T \times (\pi r_i^2) \qquad (16)$$

where F_{DZ} is the extending force, P_T is transmural pressure, and r_i is the internal vessel radius. The area πr_i^2 is the area over which the pressure is exerted. At equilibrium, the retractive force exerted by the vessel wall is:

$$F_{RZ} = \sigma_Z \times (\pi r_o^2 - \pi r_i^2) \qquad (17)$$

where F_{RZ} is the retractive force in the longitudinal direction, σ_Z is the longitudinal stress exerted by the wall, and r_o and r_i are the outside and inside radii of the vessel. The term $(\pi r_o - \pi r_i)$ is the area of the "doughnut" on cross-section.

Since the forces are at equilibrium, equations 18 and 19 may be set equal. Solving for the longitudinal stress due to pressure one obtains:

$$\sigma_{ZP} = \frac{P_T \times \pi r_i^2}{\pi r_o^2 - \pi r_i^2} = \frac{P_T \times \pi r^2}{\pi(r_o^2 - r_i^2)} \qquad (18)$$
$$= \frac{P_T \times r_i^2}{(r_o + r_i)(r_o - r_i)}$$

The term $(r_o - r_i)$ is the wall thickness (h). Since the wall is very thin, about 10% to 15% of the radius, one may treat r_o as an approximation of r_i. Then,

$$\sigma_{ZP} = \frac{P_T \times r_i^2}{2r_i \times h} \cong \frac{P_T \times r_i}{2h} \qquad (19)$$

Comparing this relationship with equation 6, it may be seen that the longitudinal stress due to pressure (σ_{ZP}) is one half the circumferential stress (σ_θ). The longitudinal stress due to traction cannot be determined analytically, but must be obtained experimentally by measuring the traction force (F_T) and dividing this by the cross-sectional area of the vessel $(\pi r_o^2 - \pi r_i^2)$. Thus, the longitudinal stress due to traction is:

$$\sigma_{ZT} = \frac{F_T}{\pi r_o^2 - \pi r_i^2} \qquad (20)$$

Figure 11 shows the interaction of the longitudinal forces due to pressure (σ_{ZP}) and to traction (σ_{Z1}), and has been discussed in the preceding section on tortuosity.

Deformation in the longitudinal direction may be computed as:

$$\epsilon_Z = \frac{\Delta L}{L_0} \qquad (21)$$

where ϵ_Z is longitudinal strain, ΔL is change in vessel length, and L_0 is the original vessel length of the unloaded vessel.

Alternatively, one may compute extension ratio:

$$\lambda_Z = \frac{L}{L_0} \qquad (22)$$

where λ_Z is longitudinal extension ratio, L is the observed vessel length, and L_0 is the original length of unloaded vessel. The relationship between longitudinal strain and longitudinal extension ratio is:

$$\lambda_Z = \epsilon_Z + 1 \qquad (23)$$

The stiffness or elastic modulus (E_Z) in the longitudinal direction may be determined in the *unpressurized* artery where:

$$E_Z = \frac{\Delta \sigma_{ZT}}{\Delta \epsilon_Z} \quad \text{or} \quad \frac{\Delta \sigma_{ZT}}{\Delta \lambda_Z} \qquad (24)$$

Note that the stress used is that due to traction. One may not use stresses recorded in pressurized arteries because then one must account for the deformations and stresses that occur simultaneously in the circumferential and radial (wall thickness) directions. See the section entitled *Multidirectional Aspects of Vessel Stiffness* or more detailed sources[2-6] for further discussion.

Radial Direction

Normal Arteries

The third major direction in which blood vessels are deformed is radially. When a blood vessel is pressurized, it distends circumferentially and may extend slightly in the longitudinal direction. This is accompanied by narrowing of the wall thickness. Some of this narrowing is due directly to the compressive effects of pressure, but another portion is due indirectly to the deformations in the circumferential and longitudinal directions. Indeed, because arteries are held under constant longitudinal extension, even at 0 mm Hg, there is a constant level of narrowing in the radial direction, with further narrowing occurring as the vessel is distended circumferentially. Enzymatic degradation studies[43] demonstrate that the wall element that resists deformation in the radial direction is elastin. This was found for stretched vessel segments in which the elastic lamellae were lying flat, and also for unstretched vessel segments in which the elastic lamellae were retracted and corrugated in appearance.

Quantitative Aspects

The mean stress in the radial direction is given by:

$$\sigma_R = \frac{P}{2} \qquad (25)$$

where σ_R is the radial stress, and P is the transmural pressure. Note that because the radius-to-wall thickness ratio is a factor in the computation of circumferential and longitudinal stresses, but is not a factor in the computation of radial stress, the latter is only 5% and 10% of the stress in the circumferential and longitudinal directions, respectively. Deformation may be quantitated as strain or extension ratio:

$$\epsilon_R = \frac{h - h_0}{h_0} = \frac{\Delta h}{h_0} \quad \text{or} \quad \lambda_R = \frac{h}{h_0} \qquad (26)$$

where ϵ_R is radial strain, h is the wall thickness observed after deformation, h_0 is the original wall thickness, Δh is the change in wall thickness, and λ_R is extension ratio in the radial direction.

Note that unlike stresses in the circumferential and longitudinal directions, which are tensile, those in the radial direction are compressive. For this reason, radial stress is often shown with a negative sign. A possible role of the radial stress with regard to the patency of vasa vasorum is discussed at the end of this chapter in the section *Stress Distribution and Patency of Vasa Vasorum*.

Aneurysms

Aneurysmal dilatation of arteries is associated with disruption of the connective tissue in their walls.

Histologically, aneurysmal arteries exhibit a thinned media with overstretched and fragmented elastic lamellae.[94,105] It has been shown that, in the pig subjected to graded arterial crush injury, aneurysms formed only when fewer than 40 elastic lamellae remained intact; this may be compared with 75 intact lamellae in the normal artery.[106] The average tension borne by the lamellae in the aneurysmal arteries was 4087 to 4543 dyne/cm/lamella, as compared with 1316 dyne/cm/lamella in the uninjured control arteries.[106] Experimental enzymatic degradation of elastin in the vessel wall leads to about 30% increase in vessel diameter.[45] This is shown in Figure 13 (left). Following degradation of elastin, the vessel dilates and becomes stiffer as the distending load is shifted from elastin to stiffer collagen. Vessels treated in this way remain stable and do not rupture. By contrast, vessels treated with collagenase dilate more than they do after treatment with elastase (Figure 13, middle). They also become more compliant after treatment with collagenase, unlike the decreased compliance that they exhibit after treatment with elastase. In addition, they proceed rapidly to rupture. Vessels treated sequentially with elastase and then collagenase dilate profoundly and rupture very

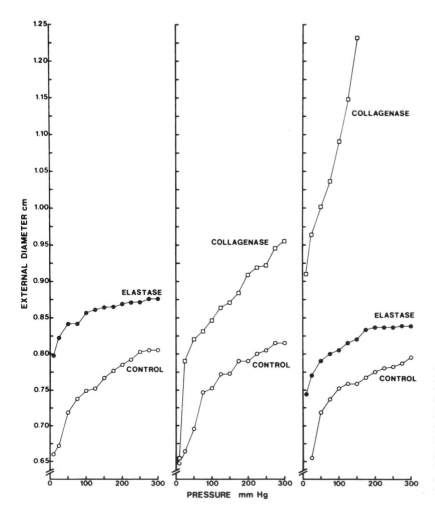

Figure 13. Pressure-diameter curves for three human internal iliac arteries treated with elastase (**left**), collagenase (**middle**), or the two enzymes in sequence (**right**). Treatment with elastase caused dilatation, stiffening of the vessel, but not rupture. Treatment with collagenase caused greater dilatation, decreased stiffness, and rupture. Sequential treatment with the two enzymes caused similar responses, but with gross dilatation before rupture.[45]

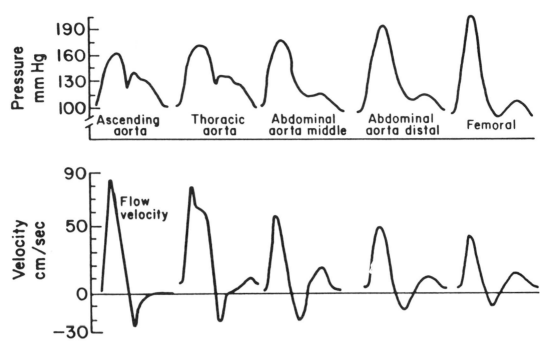

Figure 14. Pressure and flow waves in the dog aorta. Amplitude of pressure waves including systolic pressure increases distally, whereas amplitude of flow waves decreases distally.[114]

quickly (Figure 13, right). Enzymatic degradation studies show that aneurysmal human arteries behave in a similar fashion.[46] These data demonstrate that although disruption of elastin may be an early event in the formation of aneurysms,[94] collagen is the critical element in the wall preventing aneurysmal enlargement and rupture.

Studies of aortic tissue following excision demonstrate that aneurysms possess disorganized and tortuous elastic fibers,[94] and a higher collagen-to-elastin ratio than nonaneurysmal arteries.[107–109] In a recent study of aneurysmal tissue, elastin content was increased 2.3-fold, and collagen content was increased 5.7-fold.[110] The ratio of type I-to-type III collagen ratios was not altered.[109] Recently, it has been found that the collagen content also is increased in nonaneurysmal portions of the aorta in patients who have infrarenal aneurysms.[111] As noted earlier, aneurysmal vessels are stiffer than normal vessels in the circumferential direction.[45,107] Some of this increase in stiffness is due to vessel dilation with accompanying recruitment of remaining collagenous elements, and some apparently is due to increased synthesis of collagen. Propranolol has been reported to increase the cross-linking of connective tissues, and remarkably, administration of this agent has been reported to decrease the rate of enlargement of experimental aneurysms.[112]

Aneurysms occur most frequently in the infrarenal aorta, a unique vessel in many respects. It is subject to unusually large oscillating distending forces because it is one of the largest diameter arteries and is exposed to large pulsatile pressures with especially high systolic pressures (Figure 14). Increased pressure occurs because of at least three factors. First, the aorta decreases in the cross-sectional area because it gives off branches as it passes from the aortic valve to the bifurcation.[113] Second, it becomes stiffer distally, especially after it passes through the diaphragm.[26] This correlates with the fact that the abdominal aorta possesses a higher collagen-to-elastin ratio than does the thoracic aorta[34,40] (Table 1). Third, pressure waves passing down the aorta reflect off distal vessels. These reflections add to incoming pressure waves to amplify the systolic and pulse pressures in the abdominal aorta (Figure 14).[114] Mean pressure in the infrarenal aorta remains several mm Hg lower than that at the root of the aorta, thereby providing a pressure gradient to drive flow through the large, low resistance vessel. Wave reflection is least when the cross-sectional area of the iliac arteries is 1.1 to 1.2 that of the aorta.[115,116] In humans, this ratio is 1.1 early in infancy, but decreases to 0.75 by age 50.[117] This outflow-to-inflow ratio is decreased further by atherosclerotic narrowing of the iliac arteries and their ostia at the bifurcation.[118] The pressure wave in the infrarenal aorta also exhibits an increased rate of pressure rise, i.e., dP/dt. This is known to accelerate the rupture of aortic dissections, and recently has been reported to increase the rate of enlargement of vascular allografts placed in spontaneously hypertensive rats.[119] With increased pressure and increased dP/dt, the wall of the abdominal aorta is required to generate increased circumferential stress to maintain equilibrium. Recently, it has been shown that aneurysms in hypertensive rats undergo more rapid enlargement and exhibit a greater propensity to rupture than do aneurysms in normotensive rats.[120,121] In addition, in human aneurysms the portion of the circumference of the vessel which is flattest is the region most likely to rupture.[122] This region has the largest effective radius and, therefore, is subject to the largest distending force (equation 4). As a consequence, the largest amount of circumferential stress is required in this region of the wall in order to maintain equilibrium. Paradoxically, the abdominal aorta of humans has fewer elastic lamellae per unit thickness than other mammals[15] and fewer vasa vasorum per unit thickness than other mammalian arteries.[123] The number of vasa is probably not critical, because ablation of the vasa vasorum in experimental animals causes medial necrosis, but does not cause the formation of aneurysms.[106,124,125] Certain arteries are particularly susceptible to develop aneurysms. As noted above, the infrarenal aorta is the vessel that most frequently becomes aneurysmal. The popliteal artery and femoral arteries also are susceptible, perhaps because of flexure of the vessels with bending of the knee and hip joints. Aortic aneurysms often involve the iliac arteries. Isolated aneurysms may develop in iliac arteries, but do so in the internal iliac artery 10 times more frequently than they do in the external iliac artery.[126,127] There is no known explanation for this distribution. The visceral artery that most frequently becomes aneurysmal is the splenic artery. This occurs most often in women and is most likely to rupture during pregnancy, possibly because of the effects of the hormone relaxin.

Most aneurysms enlarge gradually, at an average rate of about 4 mm per year,[128] but aneurysms in individual patients may enlarge more slowly or more rapidly than this average value. Actuarial analysis of the rate of aneurysmal enlargement has demonstrated three independent determinants:[129] 1) anteroposterior dimensions at the time of diagnosis; 2) diastolic pressure; 3) the degree of chronic obstructive pulmonary disease. The size factor is readily apparent, as large aneurysms have already become large and, therefore, identify themselves to be at risk for further rapid enlargement. Diastolic pressure clearly is a factor in the distending force (equation 4). However, the degree of chronic obstructive pulmonary disease is more obscure. These patients cough frequently; this may influence venous return and, therefore, variations in blood pressure and dP/dt. In addition, patients with chronic obstructive pulmonary disease are known to possess elevated levels of neutrophil-derived elastase and elevated concentrations of the peptide products of elastin breakdown in plasma and urine.[130–132] This suggests that the aorta in these patients may be exposed chronically to elevated circulating proteinases. Similarly, patients with known stable aneurysms rupture at a much higher rate than expected after these patients have undergone laparotomy and procedures for diseases unrelated to the aneurysms. Rupture often occurs within the first 30 days after laparotomy.[133] This is the period when wound healing and collagen remodeling activity is high. Human aneurysms often contain inflammatory cells in the adventitia and the adventitia-medial junction.[134] The walls of aneurysms also exhibit measurable levels of elastase and collagenase,[135–141] with increased levels of elastase found in smokers.[137] The level of collagenase correlates linearly with the size of the aneurysm.[135] Proteinases are found in the aneurysmal wall, especially in proximity to the vasa vasorum.[140] Mechanically-induced aneurysmal-like poststenotic dilatation of arteries also is accompanied by increased collagenase levels, indicating that increased collagenase activity may be the *result* of aneurysmal enlargement.[142] Recently, an experimental model using infusion of crude elastase into the hydraulically-isolated aorta in rats has been shown to reliably produce aneurysms.[143] This is associated with an influx of inflammatory cells, principally macrophages and T-cells,[144] and the appearance of endogenous proteinases.[145] The appearance of inflammatory cells and endogenous proteinases correlates temporally with the sudden enlargement of the vessel as it becomes a true aneurysm.[144,145] Nonspecific activation of the immune system by infusion of thioglycolate and plasmin into the aorta also produces a gradually enlarging aortic aneurysm with the appearance of macrophages.[144] Macrophages and T-cells are known to secrete proteolytic enzymes. Using this same model, it was found that pretreating the animals with methylprednisolone or cyclosporine before aortic infusion with elastase limits the size of enlarging aneurysms to about one third that of saline-treated control animals, but does not completely prevent the aneurysms from occurring.[146] These data suggest that the inflammatory process may perpetuate the continued enlargement of aneurysms once it has begun. It thus appears that, once initiated, arterial aneurysms behave like healing wounds, with synthesis and remodeling of collagen and a high turnover of this protein; but because the "wound" is under tension, it continues to distract with progressive enlargement. The critical question then is what initiates the process of aneurysm formation?

It is unclear why most patients develop atherosclerotic *occlusive* disease whereas others, a smaller percentage, develop *aneurysms*. The classic view is that aneurysms result from atherosclerotic degeneration of the wall. Based on work in experimental animals and human specimens, it has been proposed that the local response of the media to injury in the presence of atherosclerosis may determine the outcome of the injury.[147] If the media heals completely, then an occluding atherosclerotic lesion will appear at the site of injury; if complete healing fails to occur, then the media will become atrophic and an aneurysm may develop.[147] A study was performed on cynomolgus and rhesus monkeys placed on an atherosclerotic diet, and then placed on a regression diet. Four of 31 cynomolgus monkeys (13%) and one of 107 rhesus monkeys (1%) developed aneurysms. Each had atrophy of the media.[148] These observations are consistent with the view that a small proportion of patients with atherosclerosis may develop aneurysms. In a clinical study of 250 patients who had undergone carotid endarterectomy for atherosclerotic disease, 12% also had dilatation of the aorta.[149] On the other hand, a clinical study of 100 consecutive patients who underwent aortic surgery showed that those with atherosclerotic occlusive aortic disease are different than those with aneurysmal aortic disease. The patients differed with respect to male-to-female ratio, age of onset of symptoms, and prognosis with respect to cardiovascular disease.[150] Patients with aneurysms may exhibit diffuse arteriomegaly which may progress to multiple aneurysms.[151,152] Moreover, epidemiologic studies demonstrate that in many cases aneurysms are familial, following a genetic pattern of predisposition.[152–155] This suggests a mechanism which may be independent of atherosclerosis. Several clinical studies have reported a high incidence of hernias in patients with aortic aneurysms.[156–158] Both lesions may be caused by connective tissue defects. Recently, a genetic defect was identified involving glycine/arginine amino acid substitutions in the synthesis of alpha-1-type III procollagen in a family in which several members developed nonmarfanoid aneurysms.[159] Although this family did not suffer from typical abdominal aortic aneurysms, this finding does illustrate the possibility of a link between a genetic abnormality resulting in a connective tissue defect and the propensity to develop arterial aneurysm-like lesions. Nevertheless, it is not uncommon for most patients who develop aneurysms to also have atherosclerosis, and it is possible that atherosclerosis and genetic factors interact to cause aneurysms in susceptible patients.

One of the fascinating observations regarding aneurysms is that once they develop, they do not rupture immediately. Clinical studies have demonstrated that the mean rate of aneurysmal enlargement is 4 mm/year.[128] As described previously, in order for a vessel to maintain stable dimensions, the wall must generate a circumferential force (equation 5) which opposes the distending force that results from pressure (equation 4). The retractive force required increases with enlarging diameter. Therefore, one may inquire as to how a vessel which could not provide sufficient tension to maintain equilibrium at normal dimensions can do so when the vessel enlarges aneurysmally. In other

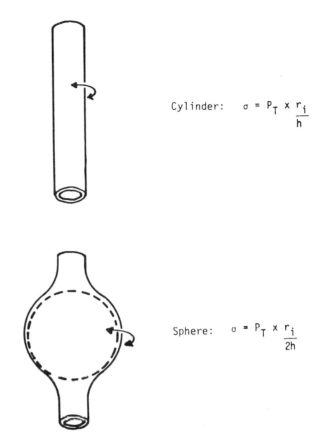

Cylinder: $\sigma = P_T \times \dfrac{r_i}{h}$

Sphere: $\sigma = P_T \times \dfrac{r_i}{2h}$

Figure 15. Circumferential stress for a cylindrical and spherical artery. By changing its shape from a cylinder to a sphere, an aneurysm reduces by about one half the stress required to maintain equilibrium.[45]

words, once enlargement begins, why does the vessel not proceed instantly to maximum dimensions and to rupture? There are several answers to this question. First, as aneurysms enlarge they recruit collagen fibers that had previously not been loaded. Evidence for this may be seen in Figure 13 which shows that the dilating vessel becomes stiffer. Computation of load distribution in these vessels suggests that only 1% to 8% of the collagen in the normal vessel is load-bearing.[45] Therefore, as aneurysmal dilatation occurs, previously unloaded collagen fibers may be recruited. Moreover, recent evidence suggests that increased collagen synthesis occurs as well.[110–111]

A second explanation as to why aneurysms gradually increase in size is related to their geometry. As a vessel dilates aneurysmally, it becomes fusiform, changing in shape from a cylinder to a sphere. As shown in Figure 15, this change in geometry reduces the wall stress required to maintain equilibrium by about 50%. Therefore, as the vessel changes in shape, it tends to stabilize itself. Finally, one may consider the role of the thrombus that is found in the lumen of the aneurysmal vessel. This thick layer of laminated thrombus usually leaves a luminal stream of normal dimensions. It readily transmits the pressure out to the wall acting as semisolidified blood. Therefore, the presence of the thrombus does not decrease the value for the radius or diameter, or the computation of distending force (equation 4). Intraluminal thrombus has little structural strength. This is readily apparent to the surgeon who easily scoops thrombus from within the lumen after an aneurysm has been opened. Therefore, the presence of the thrombus does not decrease the value for the radius in the computations of retractive force (equation 5) or retractive wall stress (equation 6). However, the thrombus may be important for accelerating vessel rupture. Fibrin liberated from the thrombus amplifies the production of plasminogen activator. In turn, plasminogen activator may activate collagenase, thereby facilitating degradation of the connective tissue elements remaining in the aneurysm wall. Such a mechanism has been described for the tissue destruction seen in rheumatoid arthritis and the invasive activity of tumor cells.[160] If the above hypothesis is correct, then the thrombus lining aneurysms may indirectly facilitate their enlargement. Administration of indium-labeled monoclonal antibody against human tissue plasminogen activator in patients demonstrates that plasminogen activator is, in fact, found in measurable quantities in the walls of aneurysms.[161] One of the serine proteinases found in aneurysmal tissue is plasmin,[162] raising the possibility that this agent may activate matrix metalloproteinases. It has been suggested that plasmin may leach into the aneurysm wall from the mural thrombus.[162] This notion is consistent with the observation that the presence and volume of mural thrombus is one of the best predictors of rapid aneurysmal enlargement.[163]

In summary, aneurysms do not enlarge instantaneously because of recruitment of collagen fibers that previously had not been load-bearing, the synthesis of new collagen fibers, and a change in geometry from a cylinder to a sphere. The relative contribution of each of these factors is unknown. The presence of laminated thrombus in the lumen does not appear to be important mechanically with regard to the maintenance of aneurysmal dimensions, but may have important biochemical effects which may accelerate enlargement.

Another mechanical feature of aneurysms is their tendency to become bowed and tortuous. Tortuosity is seen when the force applied to an artery causes it to lengthen, but the vessel is prevented from doing so by the presence of constraining side branches. The segment of vessel between branches then is forced to buckle. If buckling becomes excessive this appears clinically and radiographically as tortuosity. Tortuosity is seen in ectatic and aneurysmal arteries. Up to 44% of patients with aneurysms have tortuous carotid arteries as well.[93] Aneurysmal vessels dilate in part because of disrupted elastic lamellae,[45,94,105,106] and the loss of

elastin also results in decreased retractive force (F_R) exerted by the vessel wall in the longitudinal direction.[90,91,94] Because the force due to pressure in the longitudinal direction (F_P) is a function of the square of the vessel radius (equation 16), this force may be profoundly increased in aneurysmal and ectatic arteries. For example, the force extending a vessel in the longitudinal direction due to pressure (F_P) is 16 times as great in an 8-cm aneurysmal aorta, as it is in a normal 2-cm aorta. Thus, aneurysmal arteries become tortuous because of both greatly increased force due to pressure (F_P) which extends them, and decreased retractive force (F_R) that results from failure of elastin.

Poststenotic Dilatation

One of the most unexpected mechanical changes exhibited by arteries is the development of dilatation distal to an area of stenosis. This usually appears as a moderate increase in arterial dimensions 1 to 3 cm distal to a partial stenosis. Commonly, the dilated region of the vessel is 25% to 50% larger than normal dimensions. Poststenotic dilatation has been reported in the subclavian artery in association with thoracic outlet syndrome [164,165] in the aorta, with coarctation of the aorta,[166,167] and aortic valvular stenosis,[168,169] pulmonary valvular stenosis, [166,169] and stenosis of the vertebral, carotid,[170] and popliteal arteries.[171] In fact, 72% of normal common femoral arteries in humans exhibit some degree of dilatation where they emerge from under the inguinal ligament.[172] This suggests that the inguinal ligament may act as a partially stenosing structure, facilitated perhaps by motion of the hip joint. Thus, poststenotic dilatation is a common observation in arteries when they are subjected to partial, but persistent, narrowing. There is no correlation between the severity of stenosis and the magnitude of the dilatation. However, it has been found that patients with stenoses of the renal artery have *longer* areas of dilatation when the stenosis is tight than when it is mild.[173] Studies in dogs demonstrate that when experimental stenoses are too tight or too mild to produce turbulence, poststenotic dilatation does not occur. However, moderate stenoses that are associated with a bruit and a thrill do produce poststenotic dilatation. Several clinical papers demonstrate that poststenotic dilatation of the subclavian artery occurring in conjunction with thoracic outlet syndrome may be reversible after excision of a cervical rib.[164] This also has been observed in dogs following removal of experimentally applied stenoses.[174] Light and electron microscopic studies of the dilated region of vessels demonstrate that the fenestrations in the external elastic lamella are larger than in normal vessels and also occupy a larger proportion of the surface area. In some vessels, there is destruction

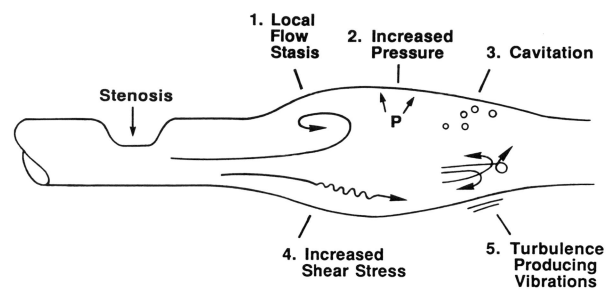

Figure 16. Five mechanical factors proposed to cause poststenotic dilatation.[180]

of the medial elastic tissue with fragmentation of the elastic lamellae and a decrease in the number of SMCs. If poststenotic dilatation has been present for 6 months or more, the wall may exhibit dissolution of elastin, with aggregation of collagen fibrils and a loss of SMCs.[175-178] Mechanical studies of vessels with poststenotic dilatation report that the wall is more distensible than normal, possibly reflecting damage to the connective tissue, especially elastin.[179] Dilatation is associated with damage to the vessel wall, and a loss of SMC volume density; this is correlated with increased wall stress in the dilated vessel.[178] Undoubtedly, these morphologic changes alter wall properties.

Five mechanical factors have been proposed as possible mechanisms for poststenotic dilatation (Figure 16).[180] These are: 1) stasis; 2) increased pressure; 3) cavitation; 4) high or abnormal shear stress; 5) turbulence producing vessel vibrations. Computational models of flow through cylindrical vessels with a stenosis demonstrate standing vortices distal to the stenosis.[181] However, these vortices rejoin the flowing stream without the formation of stasis at the wall. This suggests that stasis is not a critical mechanism.

It has been suggested that as flow exits a stenosis, the high kinetic energy is converted into high potential energy, i.e., increased transmural pressure.[182] It was suggested that the formation of jets striking the wall may cause poststenotic dilatation. However, as flow passes through a clinically significant stenosis, there often is a *decrease* in pressure, not an increase. Experimental studies using plaster casts of stenotic vessels demonstrate that cracks and fissures may occur in the casts.[183] However, these occurred where the casts were exposed to flow with high entrance pressures; cracks and fissures did not occur distal to the stenoses.

This suggests that the effect of jets is not a critical mechanism.

Studies of banded arteries in experimental animals have suggested that poststenotic dilatation may result from cavitation in the flowing stream.[184] Cavitation appears when fluids are greatly accelerated, producing local regions of low pressure (Bernoulli effect). When this occurs, dissolved nitrogen and oxygen may come out of solution to form gaseous bubbles. When flow velocity decelerates, these gas bubbles shrink as the gas returns to solution. However, they may contract unevenly to form microscopic jets which contain high kinetic energy. Such phenomena cause pitting and destruction of propellers of ships and impellers of pumps, and junctions of pipes of disparate size. However, several atmospheres of subatmospheric pressure are required to cause cavitation,[185] so it is unlikely that cavitation occurs in the cardiovascular system.

Evaluation of flow through the stenotic dog aorta,[186,187] plaster casts of stenotic arteries,[183] and mathematical models of flow through stenotic arteries[181] demonstrate the development of high shear stresses distal to stenoses. Measurement of shear stresses as fluids flow through transparent cylinders with stenoses demonstrates fluctuating shear stresses that increase more than eightfold distal to stenoses.[187] This observation suggests that vessels may dilate until an optimum level of shear stress is achieved, and then remain at that level. This has been demonstrated in atherosclerotic arteries.[95,188] The endothelium is sensitive to shear stress and may release agents that relax vascular smooth muscle.

It has been suggested that poststenotic dilatation may occur as the result of turbulence.[189] Turbulence can produce audible sounds and cause vessels to vibrate, producing a bruit and a thrill. Experimental studies of flow through stenoses show that flow is, in fact, turbulent and is associated with the development of poststenotic dilatation. Some investigators have reported that experimental vibration of human iliac arteries in vitro causes vessels to dilate when the vessel wall is exposed to 25 to 30 Hz. Frequencies of 80 to 1500 Hz had little effect.[190,191] However, other investigators[192] have been unable to produce poststenotic dilatation with vibrations in vivo with electromechanical vibrators glued to the aorta of chronic experimental animals. In vitro studies of flow through rigid transparent models containing a stenosis demonstrated that turbulence may occur, but does so remote from the region of dilatation.[193] It was hypothesized that it was not turbulence, but rather *variations* in shear stress which disturb the endothelium, stimulating it to release vasodilating agents. Just what vasodilating agent might be responsible is uncertain. Inhibition of NO synthesis in experimental animals with stenoses failed to alter the development of poststenotic dilatation,[193] but other agents might be involved. In addition, poststenotic dilatation increases wall collagenase even before marked dilatation has occurred.[142] As discussed in the preceding section on aneurysms, this may result from plasminogen or from plasmin derived from thrombus.[162] In conclusion, there is evidence to support abnormal shear stresses and possibly vibration as the stimuli for poststenotic dilatation. Although uncertain, it seems likely that abnormal shear stresses are an especially effective stimulus. Abnormal flow distal to the stenosis may induce biochemical changes that could affect the SMCs or the connective tissue, but these mechanisms remain to be clarified.

Although the dilated portion of the vessel may regress, it often exhibits aneurysmal changes histologically and remains dilated. Most surgeons resect the dilated region if it is large, saccular, or has produced thromboembolic complications. It is recommended that the dilated area be resected if it is dilated to twice the normal diameter, as the wall inevitably is thinned with aneurysmal changes in the media.[164]

Autogenous Vein Grafts

Autogenous vein is one of the most commonly used vascular grafts to bypass occluded arteries. As shown in Figure 3, veins are highly compliant at pressures up to 35 to 50 mm Hg; at higher pressures, they become exceedingly stiff with almost no change in caliber evident throughout the range of normal and hypertensive arterial pressures.[55,194] When a vein is used as a bypass graft, it is exposed continuously to arterial pressures. Under these conditions, vein grafts dilate approximately 30% over the course of 24 weeks, with

about 90% of this dilatation occurring within the first 4 weeks.[194] During this time, the vein develops increased intimal thickness that is hypercellular with increased quantities of connective tissue.[195] This occurs in the graft wall itself,[195-197] but is most exuberant in the host artery at and distal to the distal anastomosis.[101,198] At the same time as intimal hyperplasia develops, the vein wall undergoes medial thickening with increased numbers of SMCs and increased quantities of extracellular connective tissue matrix in the media.[197] When a vein is exposed to arterial pressures, it is subjected to at least nine altered mechanical parameters: deformations in the circumferential, longitudinal, and radial directions, stresses in each of these three directions, pulsatile pressures, possibly pulsatile deformations, and altered flow velocity and shear stresses.[100] A large number of studies[199] have been performed to alter these mechanical parameters in an attempt to identify which one or more of them is critically associated with the development of intimal hyperplasia and medial thickening. Investigators have deformed vein grafts by inserting plastic stents,[200] restricted vein grafts with sleeves,[100,201] with loose or tight fitting wraps,[201] and constructed vein grafts with arteriovenous fistulas[95,202] or with several outflow branches to alter volume flow and shear stress.[95,99,100,201-204] The angle of the anastomoses[205,206] and compliance mismatch[207-209] also have been investigated. It is important to recognize that when a vein is subjected to arterial pressure and flow, all of the nine deformations, stresses, and shear stress change simultaneously. Therefore, one may not conclude arbitrarily that one parameter and not another simultaneously altered parameter is the cause of histologic changes. Results of experiments designed specifically to separate these parameters from one another (Figure 17) show that intimal hyperplasia is best associated with low flow velocity, disturbed flow, and low shear stress,[99,100,203,210] with possibly some contribution from compliance mismatch.[207-210] Interposition of a short segment of vein at the anastomosis in a polytetrafluoroethylene (PTFE) graft-artery end-to-side anastomosis increases patency and diminishes intimal hyperplasia.[211] The vein cuff may: 1) decrease compliance mismatch between the PTFE and the artery; 2) reduce shedding of platelets, fibrin, etc., from the PTFE pseudointima onto the anastomosis; or 3) accommodate to the flow stream more readily than the less malleable PTFE. Wrapping the vein cuff with a jacket of PTFE to stiffen it does not increase intimal hyperplasia,[212] so that the beneficial effect of the vein cuff does not appear to be an alteration in compliance mismatch. In another study,[210] it was demonstrated that there are two distinct regions of anastomotic intimal thickening in end-to-side grafts: 1) intimal hyperplasia at the toe and heel of the graft and along the suture lines, and 2) intimal hyperplasia located on the

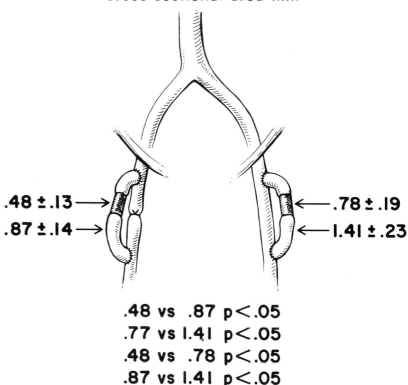

VEIN GRAFT INTIMA
Cross sectional area mm^2

.48 ± .13 →   ← .78 ± .19
.87 ± .14 →   ← 1.41 ± .23

.48 vs .87 p < .05
.77 vs 1.41 p < .05
.48 vs .78 p < .05
.87 vs 1.41 p < .05

Figure 17. Experiment in dogs to separate mechanical factors predisposing to the formation of intimal hyperplasia. Autogenous veins were reversed, partially cuffed, and used to bypass native femoral arteries. Femoral artery was ligated on one side. Intimal hyperplasia was maximum where flow velocity and shear stress were lowest, and was maximum where flow velocity was highest.[100]

bed of the recipient artery opposite the anastomosis (Figure 18). That along the heel and toe was greater with prosthetic grafts than with vein grafts, but the bed thickening was equal for prosthetic and vein graft anastomoses. The suture line thickening appears to be associated with vascular healing and may be associated with compliance mismatch. It also may be due to the deformity caused by the suture line protruding into the lumen. The arterial floor thickening, which was equal for prosthetic grafts and autogenous vein, correlated with regions of stagnant flow and low shear stress.[210]

Analysis of flow through anastomoses in vitro using a photochromic dye technique demonstrates a splitting of flow streams with those near the toe of the graft proceeding distally down the recipient artery, and those near the heel of the graft turning retrograde and recirculating in the proximal artery. An oscillating region of stagnation develops along the floor of the artery opposite the anastomosis (Figure 19). This is precisely

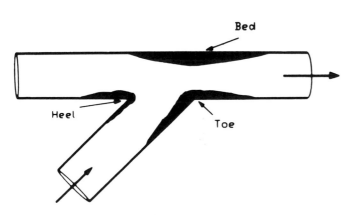

Figure 18. Distribution of intimal hyperplasia at the heel and toe of the graft, and along the bed of the recipient artery opposite the graft.[198]

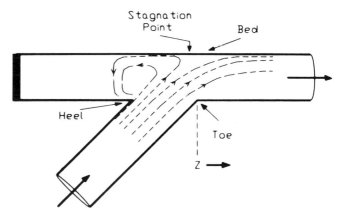

Figure 19. Flow streams from graft to artery in end-to-side anastomosis. An oscillating region of stagnation develops along the bed of the artery where intimal hyperplasia develops.[213]

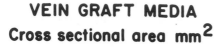

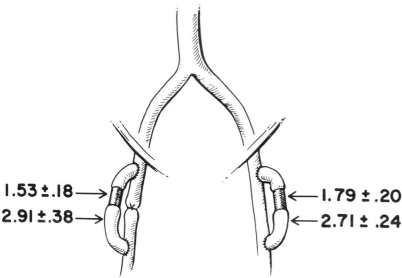

VEIN GRAFT MEDIA
Cross sectional area mm^2

1.53 ± .18 →

2.91 ± .38 →

← 1.79 ± .20

← 2.71 ± .24

1.53 vs 2.91 p < .05
1.79 vs 2.71 p < .05
1.53 vs 1.79 p = n.s.
2.91 vs 2.71 p = n.s.

Figure 20. Same experiment as shown in Figure 17, but here showing cross-sectional areas of the media. Medial thickening was greatest in dilated portions of the grafts, and was not dependent on flow velocity. This, and subsequent experiments, demonstrated that medial thickening best correlated with deformation, not stress, and specifically in the circumferential direction.

where intimal hyperplasia develops.[198,210] Intrusion of a mass on the bed of the artery to simulate intimal hyperplasia demonstrated that the mass acted as a flow divider, reducing the oscillations of the stagnant zone.[213–214] Abnormal oscillating flow can disturb the endothelium, initiating a cascade of cellular events that results in three histologic "waves": 1) proliferation of vascular SMCs in the media; 2) migration of these cells into the intima; and 3) proliferation of these "myointimal" cells in the intima. If this proliferation continues to excess it can narrow the lumen, and may cause graft occlusion.

By contrast with the effects of shear stress on the development of intimal hyperplasia, medial thickening is best associated with deformation. This is illustrated in Figure 20. Further experimental analysis demonstrated that medial thickening was best associated with deformation, not stress and, specifically, deformation in the circumferential direction.[100] Thus, intimal hyperplasia and medial thickening appear to be responses to separate stimuli. Treatment of animals with vein bypass grafts with aspirin and dipyridamole produces a reduction in the intimal thickness as compared with that in vein grafts in untreated control animals, but this treatment produces no reduction in medial thickening.[194] This substantiates the view that intimal hyperplasia and medial thickening are largely separate phenomena. An extensive review of the many studies

performed to evaluate mechanical factors associated with intimal hyperplasia and medial thickening is given elsewhere.[199] The cellular and molecular mechanisms underlying intimal hyperplasia and medial thickening of vein grafts are beyond the scope of this chapter, but are discussed in other chapters in this book.

Arteries of Hypertensive Subjects

Studies of patients and experimental animals with hypertension demonstrate that these subjects have elevated peripheral vascular resistance. However, the large arteries also are altered in these subjects. Four general mechanical changes have been described in the large arteries. The walls of these vessels are thickened.[215] This is thought to be adaptive because it is observed in arteries exposed to elevated arterial pressure, but is not observed in arteries in the same subjects when the vessels are protected from elevated pressure.[216] Increased wall thickness is associated with hypertrophy of medial SMCs, with increased connective tissue content[32,35,217,218] and increased water content.[219] The large arteries exhibit hypertrophy of SMCs[220] whereas the small arteries exhibit hyperplasia.[221] These morphologic changes result in an increased media-to-lumen ratio with narrowing of the lumen. Many studies of the mechanical properties of large arteries from hypertensive subjects demonstrate that these vessels offer increased resistance to distention, even in the relaxed state.[30–33,222,223] Moreover, both the dynamic elastic and viscous moduli are elevated in these vessels, further increasing their resistance to pulsatile pressures.[222] Analysis of mechanical factors indicates that the structural changes that occur in hypertensive arteries best correlate with increased pulse pressure.[223] This is consistent with the observation that cyclic stretching of SMCs in vitro stimulates them to synthesize extracellular matrix proteins.[224] In canine veins subjected to arterial pressure when used as bypass grafts, medial thickening is best correlated with deformation in the circumferential direction.[100] In rabbit veins exposed to arterial pressures as bypass grafts, the media is not histologically distinguishable from the intima. It is likely that much of the cross-sectional area is occupied by the media. In these grafts, the increase in cross-sectional area is best correlated with luminal area.[202] Luminal area is a manifestation of circumferential deformation, tension, and stress. Activation of vascular muscle in the large arteries of hypertensive subjects demonstrates unchanged or decreased strength of vascular smooth muscle contraction.[225,226] This surprising finding has been detected in a wide variety of animal models of hypertension, even when corrected for the relative position of the smooth muscle along its length-active tension relationship. However, pharmacologic studies demonstrate that although the muscle exhibits unchanged or decreased active stress, these vessels exhibit *increased* sensitivity to pharmacologic stimulation. This is manifested by a horizontal displacement of the dose-response curves.[227,228] In addition, there is evidence that hypertensive subjects have increased sympathetic autonomic discharge.[223,224,229,230] Increased pharmacologic sensitivity is apparently the result of systemic causes rather than exposure to elevated arterial pressure, because normotensive portal veins excised from animals with hypertensive arterial pressures also demonstrate increased pharmacologic sensitivity.[231] Moreover, whereas protection from elevated pressure prevents thickening of the artery wall, it does not prevent the development of increased sensitivity to pharmacologic agents.[216]

The above summary characterizes the large conduit arteries in hypertensive subjects. However, human essential hypertension is characterized by increased peripheral resistance, even when the subject is subjected to maximum vasodilatation.[232] Histologic evaluation of human intestinal arterioles demonstrates decreased luminal caliber[233] and increased media-to-lumen ratio.[233] In spontaneous hypertensive rats (SHR), the increased media-to-lumen ratio of the arterioles is associated with SMC hyperplasia,[234] whereas in one-kidney, one-clip Goldblatt hypertensive rats,

the increased media-to-lumen ratio of the arterioles is associated with SMC hypertrophy.[235] It will be recalled that the medial thickening of the large arteries is associated with SMC hypertrophy. In humans with essential hypertension, the increased media-to-lumen ratio of small subcutaneous arteries is associated with remodeling of the media with narrowing of the lumen and rearrangement of the medial SMCs, but not with statistically significant hyperplasia.[236] Remodeling of the media also is seen in the cerebral arterioles of hypertensive rats.[237] Studies of human digital arteries in vivo,[238] rat carotid arteries in vivo,[238] rat cerebral pial arteries in stroke-prone SHR,[239] and cerebral arteries of hypertensive rats[231] all show that the stiffness of these vessels is *decreased*, as compared with control vessels when they are suitably evaluated at comparable pressures. Because the pressure-diameter relationship of all arteries is markedly nonlinear, it is imperative that the vessels not be studied simply at their in vivo condition, but over a range of pressures and deformations. When studied in this way it is evident that, unlike the conduit arteries, the elastic modulus of the resistance vessels in hypertensive animals is decreased, not increased.[238–240]

The precapillary resistance vessels (500 μm or less) are responsible for the increased blood pressure in hypertensive subjects. There is evidence of abnormalities in the control of the resistance vessels in hypertensive subjects. Hypothalamic release of catecholamines is increased[230], and neuronal uptake of catecholamines is also increased in hypertensive animals and humans.[241–245] Sensitivity to vasoconstrictor agents is elevated[245] and relaxation in response to acetylcholine is reduced.[246–248] Recently, it has been demonstrated that the resistance vessels of SHR exhibit reduced endothelium-dependent relaxation of smooth muscle, but that endothelium-independent relaxation remains normal.[246–249] In normal blood vessels, an increase in intraluminal pressure stretches the vascular muscle and elicits myogenic constriction, whereas an increase in flow elicits release of EDRF which causes vessel dilation. These effects oppose one another, but appear to be poorly balanced in hypertension.[246–249] This suggests that, in hypertension, abnormalities of endothelium-dependent relaxing mechanisms may be a fundamental defect. In any case, it is important to recognize that the behavior of the resistance vessels is the predominant cause of hypertension, that the large vessels react histologically and mechanically to the chronic hypertensive load, and that both of these changes produce increased workload for the left ventricle.

Atherosclerotic Arteries

A number of studies have been undertaken to examine the effects of atherosclerosis on the mechanical properties of arteries. The presence of an atherosclerotic lesion leads to dilatation of the vessel, with maintenance of normal luminal dimensions until the atherosclerotic plaque occupies about 40% of the cross-sectional area of the lumen.[188] When the atherosclerotic lesion enlarges beyond this size, the vessel cannot dilate further and begins to exhibit histologic evidence of stenosis. This was found for the coronary arteries. Several investigators using cylinders, strips, and rings of artery have reported that atherosclerosis causes an increase in vessel stiffness.[250–252] Other investigators using similar methods have reported a decrease in vessel stiffness.[253–255] Still other investigators have reported no change in vessel stiffness.[255–258] Early atherosclerotic lesions are soft and occupy a small portion of the wall. As the lesion enlarges, it causes degeneration of the normal structural elements in the wall that are load-bearing. This may lead to a decrease in vessel stiffness. When the atherosclerotic plaque becomes calcified, this greatly increases the stiffness of the vessel wall, and this is readily recognized grossly at the time of surgery. Therefore, the contradictory reports of the effects of atherosclerosis on wall properties may simply reflect the stage of disease of the vessel that is being studied. Recently, high frequency intravascular ultrasound has been used to assess the stiffness of fibrous and nonfibrous atherosclerotic plaques. Results showed that fibrous plaques were twice as stiff as nonfibrous plaques, and calcified plaques were nine times as stiff as nonfibrous plaques.[259] Analytic models also have been used to predict the probability of plaque rupture. These studies show that the circumferential stress concentration is a critical determinant of plaque rupture. A plaque with thin fibrous cap overlying a lipid pool has a fourfold greater stress concentration than a plaque with a thick fibrous cap.[260] Therefore, the plaque with the thin fibrous plaque has the greater likelihood of rupturing, thrombosing the lumen of the vessel, and thereby producing an infarct of the dependent parenchyma.

Bioengineering Issues

Fundamental Assumptions

Certain key assumptions underlie the analysis of blood vessel mechanics. The first assumption is that the vessel wall is incompressible, i.e., that it remains isovolumetric upon pressurization. This assumption has largely been verified by radiographic volume analyses[64] and by studies of the bulk modulus of artery walls.[261] A second assumption is that the vessel is cylindrical. This appears generally to be correct. In spite of the fact that the arterial tree often is described as a set of tapered tubes, morphometric studies show that arteries usually are cylindrical, exhibiting a step decrease in diameter at sites just beyond where branches emerge.[262] Veins are clearly not cylindrical except at pressures greater than 35 to 50 mm Hg. A third assumption is that the arterial wall can be treated mechanically as a homogeneous material. Histologic studies,[13,15] as well as the results of biochemical (Table 1), putrefaction,[19] and enzymatic degradation experiments,[26] and studies of activation and inactivation of the vascular muscle,[64] demonstrate that the wall is composed of several different components and that these bear load differentially with distention and muscle activation. Nevertheless, detailed histometric studies demonstrate that, on a zonal basis, the inner, middle, and outer thirds of the wall exhibit elastic properties that are virtually equivalent.[14] In addition, when vessels are subjected to radial compression, the inner, middle, and outer thirds of the wall compress equivalently.[4] Therefore, it is reasonable to treat the wall of relaxed vessels as a mechanically homogeneous body. A fourth assumption is that the vessel is orthotropic, i.e., that deformations occur along three mutually perpendicular directions with little or no twist. Physiologic studies[7] demonstrate that this assumption is in fact true because arteries exhibit negligible twist when pressurized. Thus, these four fundamental assumptions are tenable.

Multidirectional Stresses

It is worthwhile to compare stresses computed above in the three directions. First, the *sense* of the three stresses is not the same. Whereas the stresses in the circumferential and longitudinal directions are tensile, that in the radial direction is compressive. Similarly, deformations in the circumferential and longitudinal directions are extension or stretch, whereas that in the radial direction is compression. The relative magnitude of stresses is also different. Because the radius-to-wall thickness ratio is 8:1 or 10:1, the relative stresses $\sigma\theta:\sigma_Z:\sigma_R$ are 20:10:1. Because the radial stress is only 5% of the circumferential stress and 10% of the longitudinal stress, many analyses of multidimensional properties of arteries have simply neglected stresses in the radial direction and all factors thereof. This greatly simplifies the mathematical solutions. However, the resistance to compression in the radial direction may prove to be significant in limiting deformations in the circumferential and longitudinal directions.

Multidirectional Aspects of Vessel Stiffness

It is important to recognize that the elastic modulus given in equations 11 and 12 is for a vessel deformed solely in the circumferential direction, as, for example,

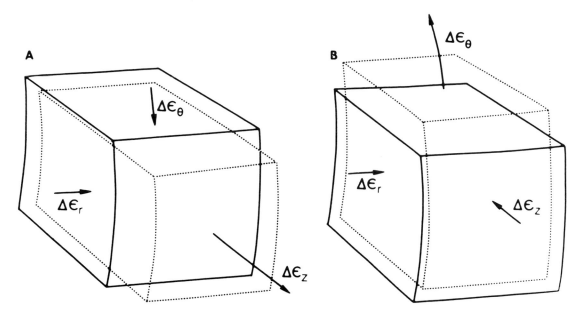

Figure 21. Illustration of computation of Poisson's ratio. **Left:** As tissue is made to extend in the longitudinal direction ($\Delta\epsilon_Z$), it must narrow in the circumferential ($\Delta\epsilon_\theta$) and radial ($\Delta\epsilon_r$) directions. **Right:** Similarly, when the tissue is made to extend in the circumferential ($\Delta\epsilon_\theta$) direction, it must narrow in the longitudinal ($\Delta\epsilon_Z$) and radial ($\Delta\epsilon_r$) directions. Poisson's ratio is ratio of deformations.[1]

for a ring of artery extended over two hooks. For a vessel which is pressurized, deformations occur in all three directions. Under these circumstances, extension in the longitudinal direction and thinning of the wall reduce the amount of deformation that occurs in the circumferential direction. The interaction of deformations that occurs in multiple directions (Figure 21) may be quantitated by using Poisson's ratio:

$$v_{\theta Z} = \frac{\Delta\epsilon_\theta}{\Delta\epsilon_Z} \quad \text{or} \quad \frac{\Delta\lambda_\theta}{\Delta\lambda_\theta} \qquad (27)$$

where $v_{\theta Z}$ is the Poisson's ratio describing the narrowing that occurs in the circumferential direction ($\Delta\epsilon_\theta$ or $\Delta\lambda_\theta$) when the vessel is extended in the longitudinal direction ($\Delta\epsilon_Z$ or $\Delta\lambda_Z$). Obviously, there are six Poisson's ratios, one that describes the narrowing that occurs in each direction as one imposes extension in each of the other directions (Figure 21). The directions are specified by the subscripts. The Poisson's ratio described by equation 27 is just one of the six.

If a material exhibits stiffnesses that are equal in all directions, then it is said to be *isotropic*. If the arterial wall were isotropic and were incompressible, then each of the Poisson's ratios would be 0.5. This would mean that when the vessel was extended in any one direction, *half* of the deformation would be accommodated by narrowing in each of the two remaining directions. For example, if a vessel were to be extended

10% in the longitudinal direction, then this would be accompanied by 5% narrowing in the circumferential direction, and 5% narrowing in the radial (wall thickness) direction. Concomitantly, if the vessel were isotropic, then the elastic moduli would be equal in all of the three directions. For a pressurized isotropic artery in which deformations may occur in all directions, the elastic modulus in the circumferential direction is given by:

$$E_{inc} = \frac{\Delta\sigma_\theta}{\Delta\epsilon_\theta}(1 - v_{\theta Z}^2) = \frac{\Delta\sigma_\theta}{\Delta\epsilon_\theta} \times 0.75 \qquad (28)$$

or

$$E_{inc} = \frac{\Delta\sigma_\theta}{\Delta\lambda_\theta}(1 - v_{\theta Z}^2) = \frac{\Delta\sigma_\theta}{\Delta\lambda_\theta} \times 0.75 \qquad (29)$$

where E_{inc} is the incremental elastic modulus for the condition where the wall is isotropic, $\Delta\sigma_\theta$ is the change in circumferential stress, $\Delta\epsilon_\theta$ is the change in circumferential strain, and $\Delta\lambda_\theta$ is the change in circumferential extension ratio. Thus, the elastic moduli in all three directions would be equal and would be given by 75% of the slope of the stress-strain curve (equation 28) or the stress-extension ratio curve (equation 29). The derivation of these relationships are given elsewhere in algebraic steps.[4]

A number of studies[64,73–78,261] have demonstrated that the vessel wall is incompressible, but is not isotropic. The Poisson's ratio $v_{\theta Z}$ of the dog carotid artery and the dog aorta is 0.3.[73-76] This means that if a vessel is extended 10% in the longitudinal direction ($\Delta\epsilon_Z$ = .10), then 3% of extension would be taken up by narrowing in the circumferential direction ($\Delta\epsilon_\theta$ = .03), the remaining 7% being taken up by narrowing in the radial (wall thickness) direction ($\Delta\epsilon_r$ = .07). Interestingly, the carotid artery approaches isotropy at typical arterial pressures,[77-79] but clearly is not isotropic over the full range of pressures and deformations possible under extreme physiologic conditions. The dog carotid artery is stiffer circumferentially than it is longitudinally,[73,74] whereas the dog aorta is stiffer longitudinally than it is circumferentially.[75,76] For an artery which is not isotropic, the elastic modulus in the circumferential direction may be computed as:

$$E_\theta = \frac{\Delta\sigma_\theta}{\Delta\epsilon_\theta + \dfrac{v_{\theta Z}\Delta\sigma_Z}{E_Z}} \tag{30}$$

where E_θ is the incremental elastic modulus, $\Delta\sigma_\theta$ is the increment in circumferential stress, $\Delta\sigma_Z$ is the increment in longitudinal stress, E_Z is the incremental longitudinal elastic modulus, and $v_{\theta Z}$ is the Poisson's ratio relating the degree of narrowing that occurs in the circumferential direction relevant to that which occurs in the longitudinal extension. Note that if one were to use equation 30 to compute the circumferential elastic modulus for an isotropic vessel, it would give the same values as that given by equation 28. The derivations of equations 28, 29, and 30 are given elsewhere.[4,73]

Finite Deformation Analysis

All of the above analyses employ the classic infinitesimal strain theory which assumes that the material studied undergoes very small deformations when subjected to load. This assumption is obviously incorrect since, when pressurized, arteries distend circumferentially up to 70% relative to the unstressed state. In addition, they are held in situ at 10% to 60% extension relative to their excised, retracted, unpressurized length. Moreover, vessels exhibit 4% to 18% changes in diameter and 1% to 2% changes in length with each pressure pulse. Thus, it is evident that vessel deformations are not infinitesimal. In order to circumvent this problem, analysis has been carried out using *incremental* elastic studies as exemplified by equations 12, 27–30, wherein small increments of stress and strain are taken. In the past few decades, the finite deformation theory also has been applied. This method deals more effectively with large deformations, the anisotropy, and the nonlinear features of arterial tissue. Use of this method utilizes the computation of the energy

stored in deforming the vessel. This deformation is expressed as strain energy density, i.e., the strain energy per unit volume. The derivative of the strain energy density with respect to deformation is then determined to obtain stress. From this, one readily obtains the stress-strain relationship. However, the empirical computation of the strain-energy and strain-energy derivative are complex exponential[3,263] or polynomial[3,264] expressions. Fung has argued persuasively that the exponential method is preferable, based on the following three observations. First, the mechanical properties of the constituent connective tissues, elastin and collagen, are best described by exponential relationships with less variability. Second, the data fits are better for exponential relationships. Third, the mathematical manipulation of the expressions is much easier if the strain energy density curves are fitted with exponentials rather than if they are fitted with polynomials. However, excellent fits may be obtained with both methods. Finite deformation methods and finite element models have been used to describe normal arteries,[3,263-265] aneurysmal arteries,[266,267] and arteries of hypertensive subjects.[268]

Stress Distributions and the Ideal Reference State

The stresses computed in all of the preceding analyses have been for the *mean* or *average* stress in each direction in the wall. In fact, these stresses are not uniform, but are distributed across the wall. If the wall is treated as a homogeneous body that is completely without stresses in the unpressurized state, then application of pressure will produce marked stress gradients across the thickness of the wall,[269,270] such as that illustrated in the left panel of Figure 22. The circumferential stress will be high at the lumen, declining to moderate values at the adventitia. The longitudinal stress is similarly distributed, but is about half that observed for the circumferential stress. The magnitude and distribution of the longitudinal stress also depend upon the component due to traction (σ_{ZT}, as is given in equation 20). The longitudinal stress is not shown in Figure 22 because it depends on the traction stress as well as pressure. The radial stress, being compressive, is distributed as follows. It is highest at the lumen, declining to vanish at the outer margin of the adventitia. Because it is compressive in sense, it is plotted with a negative sign; but, as noted previously, it is only about 5% of the circumferential stress. The left panel of Figure 22 shows a plot of circumferential and radial stress distributions across a vessel wall assuming a) that the wall behaves mechanically as a homogeneous body, and b) that it is free of stresses when it is not pressurized. In these computations, the unpressurized condition was used as the reference state. Recently, it has been shown

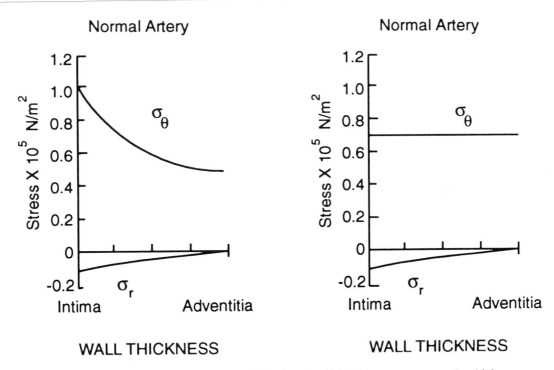

Figure 22. Distribution of circumferential (σ_θ) and radial (σ_r) stresses across the thickness of the wall. **Left panel** shows distribution of stresses estimated using 0 mm Hg as the unloaded reference state. **Right panel** shows distribution of the same stresses using 100 mm Hg as the unloaded reference state.

that when unpressurized cylindrical segments of arteries are incised longitudinally, they spring open in the circumferential direction.[5,6,271–273] This means that when the vessel is not pressurized, there actually is residual compressive stress at the intima, and residual tensile stress at the adventitia.[273] Accordingly, it has been proposed that the reference state should be at physiologic pressures, i.e., at 100 mm Hg.[5,6,274] However, this is quite complicated because there are residual longitudinal stresses,[275] as well as residual circumferential stresses.[275] Moreover, these vary along the length of the arterial tree,[275] and also vary with age and with arterial hypertrophy.[276,277] The large veins also exhibit residual stress.[278] Nevertheless, using the dimensions observed at 100 mm Hg pressure as a reference state dramatically alters the distribution of stresses across the thickness of the normal vessel wall.[274] Whereas using the vessel at 0 mm Hg as a reference produces extremely large tensile stress gradients across the wall (Figure 22, left), using the vessel at 100 mm Hg as a reference produces virtually uniform circumferential stresses across the wall (Figure 22, right). There are empirical data to support a uniform distribution of elastic properties in the circumferential direction.[14]

Stress Distribution and Patency of Vasa Vasorum

The distribution of stresses across the wall also have pathophysiologic implications. Figure 23 (left) shows the distribution of circumferential and radial stresses using 0 mm Hg as the reference state. The heavy broken curves repeat those shown in Figure 22 (left). Also, shown in Figure 23 (left) is an atheromatous plaque that occupies the inner 25% of the wall thickness. This is shown as a shaded area. This plaque is assumed to be twice as stiff as the remainder of the normal wall. The stress distributions obtained with the plaque are illustrated by the continuous curves. These curves show that, because of the load borne by the stiff plaque, the regions adjacent to the lesion are relieved of high stress. This distribution is of interest because it may explain the numerous vasa vasorum observed in atherosclerotic arteries.[279,280] In normal vessels, vasa vasorum are found only in the outer one third to one half of the wall; they are not found in inner regions of the wall.[279] This distribution may result from tissue distortion by the circumferential stress or compression by the radial stress. It would be unlikely for the vasa, which are perfused by pressures lower than mean arterial pressure, to remain patent if they were surrounded by circumferential stresses that were 8 to 10 times luminal pressure, and were subjected to the tissue distortion and compression that these stresses produce. In atherosclerotic arteries, vasa vasorum *are* found in the inner regions of the wall, especially in proximity to atherosclerotic plaques.[279,280] This suggests that 1) the vasa may develop in response to low tissue oxygen due to increased oxygen diffusion

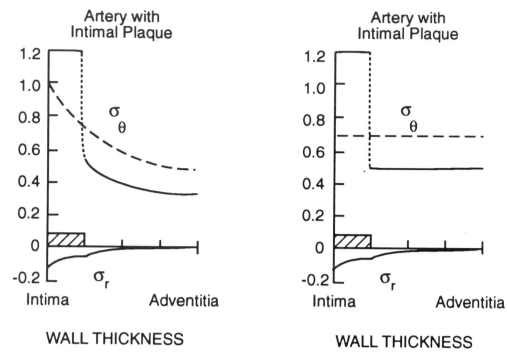

Figure 23. Distribution of stresses in the normal state (**heavy broken lines**) and when inner quarter of the wall contains a stiff atherosclerotic plaque (**continuous curves**). Plaque is shown as **shaded area**. Plaque bears a large portion of stresses unloading the adjacent tissue. This applies when stresses are estimated using 0 mm Hg as a reference state (**left panel**) and when estimated using 100 mm Hg as a reference state (**right panel**). Relieving the tissue beside the plaque of load may facilitate patency of the vasa vasorum.

distance from the lumen, the latter resulting from the thickness of the plaque; or 2) that the plaque, being stiffer than the remainder of the normal wall, acts as a stress-bearing member. If the latter hypothesis is true, then the plaque may permit the vasa vasorum to remain open by protecting the adjacent tissue from high stresses, local distortion, and compression. This is comparable to the role of steel rods embedded in concrete; the steel rods protect the adjacent more brittle concrete.

Figure 23 (right) again shows the distribution of stresses in the presence of a stiff plaque. In this graph, stresses were estimated using 100 mm Hg as a reference state. Note that without the plaque, circumferential stress is distributed uniformly across the wall. This is shown as a heavy broken curve and repeats that depicted in Figure 22 (right). Returning to Figure 23 (right), when one includes the plaque (solid curve), the stresses are redistributed with the plaque bearing a large portion of the load, relieving the adjacent tissue.

The mechanism of patency of vasa vasorum may have pathophysiologic significance. Disruption of an atherosclerotic plaque with hemorrhage into the lesion is often a sentinel pathologic event leading to vessel thrombosis. Whether the hypothesis presented above regarding the role of the plaque in facilitating patency

of vasa vasorum is important pathophysiologically remains to be demonstrated experimentally.

References

1. Dobrin PB: Mechanical properties of arteries. *Physiol Rev* 58:397–460, 1978.
2. Patel DJ: *Hemodynamics and Its Role in Disease Processes.* Baltimore: University Press; 1980.
3. Fung YCB, Fronek K, Patitucci P: Pseudoelasticity of arteries and the choice of its mathematical expression. *Am J Physiol* 237:H620-H631, 1979.
4. Dobrin PB: Vascular mechanics. In: Shepherd JT, Abboud FM (eds). *Handbook of Physiology: The Cardiovascular System.* Vol 3. Worthington, American Physiological Society; 65–102, 1983.
5. Fung YC: *Biomechanics.* Heidelberg: Springer-Verlag; 1984.
6. Fung YC: Stress, strain, and stability of organs. In: *Biomechanics.* Heidelberg: Springer-Verlag; 382–398, 1990.
7. Patel DJ, Fry DL: The elastic symmetry of arterial segments in dogs. *Circ Res* 24:1–8, 1969.
8. Busse R, Bauer RD, Schabert A, et al: The mechanical properties of exposed human carotid arteries in vivo. *Basic Res Cardiol* 74:545–554, 1979.
9. Bergel DM: The dynamic elastic properties of the arterial wall. *J Physiol Lond* 156:458–469, 1961.
10. Arndt JO, Kober G: Pressure diameter relationship of

the intact femoral artery in conscious man. *Pfleug Arch* 318:130–146, 1970.

11. Hasson JE, Megerman J, Abbott WM: Suture technique and para-anastomotic compliance. *J Vasc Surg* 3: 591–598, 1986.

12. Dobrin PB: Physiology of arteries and the pathophysiology of arterial disease: a mechanical perspective. In: Giordano JM, Trout HH, DePalma R (eds). *The Basic Science of Vascular Surgery.* Armonk, NY: Futura Publishing Company, Inc.; 183–210, 1988.

13. Wolinsky H, Glagov S: Structural basis for the static mechanical properties of the aortic media. *Circ Res* 14: 400–413, 1964.

14. Dobrin PB: Distribution of elastic properties across the thickness of the arterial wall. In: Vossoughi J (ed). *Biomedical Engineering Recent Developments.* Washington, DC: University of District of Columbia; 5–9, 1994.

15. Wolinsky H, Glagov S: Lamellar unit of aortic medial structure and function in mammals. *Circ Res* 20:99–111, 1967.

16. Ayer JP, Hass GM, Philpott DE: Aortic elastic tissue: isolation with use of formic acid and discussion of some of its properties. *AMA Arch Pathol* 65:519–544, 1958.

17. Azuma T, Hasegawa M: A rheological approach to the architecture of arterial walls. *Jap J Physiol* 21:27–47, 1971.

18. Reuterwall OP: Uber die elastizitat der Gefaswande und die Methode ihrer naheren Prufung. *Acta Med Scand* (suppl 2):1–175, 1921.

19. Remington JW, Hamilton WF, Dow P: Some difficulties involved in the prediction of the stroke volume from the pulse wave velocity. *Am J Physiol* 144:536–545, 1945.

20. Krafka JJ: Comparative study of the histo-physics of the aorta. *Am J Physiol* 125:1–14, 1939.

21. Stromberg DD, Wiederhielm CA: Viscoelastic description of a collagenous tissue in simple elongation. *Appl Physiol* 26:857–862, 1969.

22. Gay S, Miller EJ: Disposition of the collagens in connective tissues. In: Gay S, Miller EJ (eds). *Collagen in the Physiology and Pathology of Connective Tissue.* New York: Gustav Fisher Verlag; 57–62, 1978.

23. Cox RH: Passive mechanics and connective tissue composition of canine arteries. *Am J Physiol* 234:H533–H541, 1978.

24. Roach MR, Burton AC: The reason for the shape of the distensibility curves of arteries. *Can J Biochem Physiol* 35:681–690, 1957.

25. Ho HJ, Lin CY, Gaylash FT, et al: Aortic compliance: studies on its relationship to aortic constituents in man. *Arch Pathol* 94:537–546, 1972.

26. McDonald DA: Regional pulse-wave velocity in the arterial tree. *J Appl Physiol* 24:73–78, 1968.

27. Bader H: Dependence of wall stress in the human thoracic aorta on age and pressure. *Circ Res* 20:354–361, 1967.

28. Learoyd BM, Taylor MG: Alterations with age in the viscoelastic properties of human arterial walls. *Circ Res* 18:278–292, 1966.

29. Lanne T, Sonesson B, Bergvist D, et al: Diameter and compliance in the male human abdominal aorta: influence of age and aortic aneurysm. *Eur J Vasc Surg* 6: 178–184, 1992.

30. Aars H: Static load-length characteristics of aortic strips from hypertensive rabbits. *Acta Physiol Scand* 73:101–110, 1968.

31. Cox RH: Comparison of arterial wall mechanics in nor-

motensive and spontaneously hypertensive rats. *Am J Physiol* 237:H159–H167, 1979.

32. Feigl EO, Peterson LH, Jones AW: Mechanical and chemical properties of arteries in experimental hypertension. *J Clin Invest* 42:1640–1647, 1963.

33. Greene MA, Friedlander R, Boltox AJ, et al: Distensibility of arteries in human hypertension. *Proc Soc Exp Biol Med* 121:580–585, 1966.

34. Harkness MLR, Harkness RD, McDonald DA: The collagen and elastin content of the arterial wall in the dog. *Proc Roy Soc London Ser B* 146:541–551, 1957.

35. Ebel A, Fontaine R: Le collogene et hydroxyproline dans la parci aortique des berides et ses variations au cours du viellissement. *Pathol Biol Semaine Hop* 12: 842–843, 1964.

36. Karrer HE: An electron microscope study of the aorta in young and aging mice. *J Ultrastruct Res* 5:1–27, 1961.

37. Krafka J: Changes in the elasticity of the aorta with age. *AMA Arch Pathol* 29:303–309, 1940.

38. Fischer GM, Llaurado JG: Connective tissue composition of canine arteries: effects of renal hypertension. *Arch Pathol* 84:95–98, 1967.

39. Burton AC: Relation of structure to function of the tissues of the wall of blood vessels. *Physiol Rev* 34: 619–642, 1954.

40. Fischer GM, Llaurado JG: Collagen and elastin content in canine arteries selected from functionally different vascular beds. *Circ Res* 19:394–399, 1966.

41. Samila ZJ, Carter SA: The effect of age on the unfolding of elastin lamellae and collagen fibers with stretch in human carotid arteries. *Can J Physiol Pharmacol* 59: 1050–1057, 1981.

42. Dobrin PB, Canfield TR: Elastase, collagenase, and the biaxial elastic properties of dog carotid artery. *Am J Physiol* 247:H123–H131, 1984.

43. Dobrin PG, Gley WC: Elastase, collagenase, and the radial elastic properties of arteries. *Experientia* 41: 1040–1042, 1985.

44. Lansing AI, Alex M, Rosenthal TB: Calcium and elastin in human atherosclerosis. *J Gerontol* 5:112–119, 1950.

45. Dobrin PB, Baker WH, Gley WC: Elastolytic and collagenolytic studies of arteries: implications for the mechanical properties of aneurysms. *Arch Surg* 119: 405–409, 1984.

46. Dobrin PB, Mrkvicka R: Is failure of elastin or failure of collagen the critical connective tissue alteration underlying aneurysmal dilatation? *Cardiovasc Surg* 2: 484–488, 1994.

47. Bevan JA, Siegel G: Blood vessel wall matrix flow-sensor: support and speculation. *Blood Vessels* 28: 552–556, 1991.

48. Vonderlage M: Untersuchungen uber die mechanischen Eigenschaften von Streifenpraparaten verschiedener Schinittrichtung aus Aorta abdominalis des Kaninchens Pflugers. *Arch Gesamte Physiol Menchen Tierre* 301: 320–328, 1968.

49. Herlihy JT: Helically cut vascular strip preparation: geometrical considerations. *Am J Physiol* 238:H107–H109, 1980.

50. Vonderlage M: Untersuchungen über die mechanischen Eigenschaften von Streifenparaparaten verschiedener Schinittrichtung aus der Vena cava abdominalis des Kaninchens. *Pfluger's Arch* 303:71–80, 1968.

51. Gerova M, Gero J: Range of sympathetic control of the dog femoral artery. *Circ Res* 24:349–359, 1969.

52. Dobrin PB: Isometric and isobaric contraction of ca-

rotid arterial smooth muscle. *Am J Physiol* 225:
659–663, 1973.

53. Cox RH: Mechanics of canine iliac artery smooth muscle in vitro. *Am J Physiol* 230:462–470, 1976.

54. Pascale K, Weizsacker HW: In situ study of active and passive mechanical properties of rat tail artery. *Basic Res Cardiol* 82:66–73, 1987.

55. Dobrin PB, Canfield TR, Moran J, et al: Coronary artery bypass: the physiological basis for differences in flow with internal mammary artery and saphenous vein grafts. *J Thor Cardiovasc Surg* 74:445–454, 1977.

56. Gore RW: Wall stress: a determinant of regional differences in response of frog microvessels to norepirephrine. *Am J Physiol* 222:82–91, 1972.

57. Dobrin PB: Influence of initial length on length-tension relationship of vascular smooth muscle. *Am J Physiol* 225:664–670, 1973.

58. Sonnenblick EH: Series elastic and contractile elements in heart muscle: changes in muscle length. *Am J Physiol* 207:1330–1338, 1964.

59. Dobrin PB: Vascular smooth muscle series elastic element stiffness during isometric contraction. *Circ Res* 34:242–250, 1974.

60. Murphy RA: Mechanics of vascular smooth muscle. In: Bohr DF, Somlyo AP, Sparks HV Jr (eds). *Handbook of Physiology: The Cardiovascular System.* Sect 2, Vol II. Bethesda, MD: Bethesda Am Physiol Soc; 325–351, 1980.

61. Dobrin PB, Canfield TR: Series elastic and contractile elements in vascular smooth muscle. *Circ Res* 33: 454–464, 1973.

62. Close RI: Dynamic properties of mammalian skeletal muscles. *Physiol Rev* 52:129–197, 1972.

63. Dobrin PB, Canfield TR: Identification of smooth muscle series elastic component in intact carotid artery. *Am J Physiol* 232:H122-H130, 1977.

64. Dobrin PB, Rovick AA: Influence of vascular smooth muscle on contractile mechanics and elasticity of arteries. *Am J Physiol* 217:1644–1652, 1969.

65. Zaidi N, Breves PJ, Girgis SI, et al: Circulating calcitonin gene-related peptide comes from the perivascular nerves. *Eur J Pharm* 117:283–284, 1985.

66. Koller A, Sun D, Kaley G: Role of shear stress and endothelial prostaglandins in flow- and viscosity-induced dilation of arterioles in vitro. *Circ Res* 72: 1276–1284, 1993.

67. Lamontagne D, Pohl U, Busse R: Mechanical deformation of vessel wall and shear stress determine the basal release of endothelium-derived relaxing factor in the intact rabbit coronary vascular bed. *Circ Res* 70: 123–130, 1992.

68. Barone GW, Conerly IJM, Farley PC, et al: Endothelial injury and vascular dysfunction associated with the Fogarty balloon catheter. *J Vasc Surg* 9:422–425, 1989.

69. Furchgott RF, Vanhoutte PM: Endothelium-derived relaxing and contracting factors. *FASEB J* 3:2007–2017, 1989.

70. Feng Q, Hedner T: Endothelium-derived relaxing factor (EDRF) and nitric oxide. II. Physiology, pharmacology, and pathophysiological implications. *Clin Physiol* 10:503–526, 1990.

71. Vallance P, Collier J, Moncada S: Effects of endothelium-derived nitric oxide on peripheral arteriolar tone in man. *Lancet* 2:997–1000, 1989.

72. Gardiner SM, Compton AM, Bennett T, et al: Control of regional blood flow by endothelium-derived nitric oxide. *Hypertension* 15:486–492, 1990.

73. Dobrin PB, Doyle JM: Vascular smooth muscle and the anisotropy of dog carotid artery. *Circ Res* 27:105–119, 1970.

74. Cox RH: Anisotropic properties of the canine carotid artery in vitro. *J Biomech* 8:293–300, 1975.

75. Patel DJ, Janicki JJ, Carew TE: Static anisotropic elastic properties of the aorta in living dogs. *Circ Res* 25: 765–779, 1969.

76. Patel DJ, Janicki JS, Vaishnav RN, et al: Dynamic anisotropic viscoelastic properties of the aorta in living dogs. *Circ Res* 32:93–107, 1973.

77. Dobrin PB: Biaxial anisotropy of dog carotid artery: estimation of circumferential elastic modulus. *J Biomech* 19:351–358, 1986.

78. Weizsacker HW, Pinto JG: Isotropy and anisotropy of the arterial wall. *J Biomech* 21:477–487, 1988.

79. Dobrin PB, Mrkvicka R: Estimation of elastic modulus of nonatherosclerotic elastic arteries. *J Hypertension* (suppl 6)10:S7-S10, 1992.

80. Peterson LH, Jensen RE, Parnell R: Mechanical properties of arteries in vivo. *Circ Res* 8:622–639, 1960.

81. Lawton RW: Some aspects of research in biological elasticity: introductory remarks. In: Remington JW (ed). *Tissue Elasticity.* Washington, DC: *Am Physiol Soc* 1–11, 1957.

82. Patel DJ, Greenfield JC, Fry DL: In vivo pressure-length-radius relationship of certain blood vessels in man and dog. In: Attinger EO (ed). *Pulsatile Blood Flow.* Philadelphia: McGraw Hill; 293–306, 1963.

83. Patel DJ, Fry DL: In situ pressure-radius-length measurements in ascending aorta of anesthetized dogs. *J Appl Physiol* 19:413–416, 1964.

84. Browse NL, Young AE, Thomas ML: The effect of bending on canine and human arterial walls and on blood flow. *Circ Res* 45:41–48, 1979.

85. Dobrin PB, Canfield TR, Sinha S: Development of longitudinal retraction of carotid arteries in neonatal dogs. *Experientia* 31:1295–1296, 1975.

86. Hesse M: Uber die pathologischen veranderungen der arterien der oberen extremitat. *Virchows Arch Pathol Anat Physiol* 261:225–252, 1926.

87. Bergel DH: The static elastic properties of the arterial wall. *J Physiol Lond* 156:445–457, 1961.

88. Band W, Goedhard WJA, Knoop AA: Effects of aging on dynamic viscoelastic properties of the rat's thoracic aorta. *Pfluger's Arch* 331:357–364, 1972.

89. Band W, Goedhard WJA, Knoop AA: Comparison of effects of high cholesterol intake on viscoelastic properties of the thoracic aorta in rats and rabbits. *Atherosclerosis* 18:163–172, 1973.

90. Dobrin PB, Baker WH, Schwarcz TH: Mechanisms of arterial and aneurysmal tortuosity. *Surgery* 104: 568–571, 1988.

91. Dobrin PB, Schwarcz TH, Mrkvicka R: Longitudinal retractive force in pressurized dog and human arteries. *J Surg Res* 48:116–120, 1990.

92. Ochsner JL, Hughes JP, Leonard GL, et al: Elastic tissue dysplasia of the internal carotid artery. *Ann Surg* 185:684–691, 1977.

93. Mukherjee D, Mayberry JC, Inahan T, et al: The relationship of the abdominal aortic aneurysm to the tortuous internal carotid artery. *Arch Surg* 124:955–956, 1989.

94. White JV, Haas K, Phillips S, et al: Adventitial elastolysis is a primary event in aneurysm formation. *J Vasc Surg* 17:371–381, 1993.

95. Zarins CK, Zatina MA, Giddens DP, et al: Shear stress

regulation of artery lumen diameter in experimental atherogenesis. *J Vasc Surg* 5:413–420, 1987.

96. Flaherty JT, Pierce JE, Ferrans VJ, et al: Endothelial nuclear patterns in the canine arterial tree with particular reference to hemodynamic events. *Circ Res* 30: 23–33, 1972.

97. Sottiurai VS, Lim Sue S, Breaux JR, et al: Adaptability of endothelial orientation to blood flow dynamics: a morphologic analysis. *Eur J Vasc Surg* 3:145–151, 1989.

98. Pohl U, Herlan K, Huang A, et al: EDRF-mediated shear-induced dilation opposes myogenic constriction in small rabbit arteries. *Am J Physiol* 261:H2016-H2023, 1991.

99. Berguer R, Higgins RF, Reddy DJ: Intimal hyperplasia: an experimental study. *Arch Surg* 115:332–335, 1980.

100. Dobrin PB, Littooy FN, Endean ED: Mechanical factors predisposing to intimal hyperplasia and medial thickening in autogenous vein grafts. *Surgery* 105: 393–400, 1989.

101. Sottiurai VS: Distal anastomotic intimal hyperplasia: histocytomorphology and pathophysiology. In: Dobrin PB (ed). *Intimal Hyperplasia.* Austin, TX: Landes Publishing; 1994.

102. Hugh AE, Fox FA: The precise location of atheroma and its association with stasis at the origin of the internal carotid artery-a radiographic observation. *Br J Radiol* 43:377–383, 1970.

103. Friedman MH, Hutchins GM, Borgesson C, et al: Correlation of human arterial morphology with hemodynamic measurements in arterial casts. *Atherosclerosis* 39.425–536, 1981.

104. Zarins CK, Bomberger RA, Glagov S: Local effects of stenoses: increased flow velocity inhibits atherogenesis. *Circulation* 64 (part 2):221–227, 1981.

105. Glagov S: Pathology of large arteries. In: Abramson DI, Dobrin PB (eds). *Blood Vessels and Lymphatics in Organ Systems.* New York: Academic Press, Inc.; 39–53, 1984.

106. Zatina MA, Zarins CK, Gewertz BL, et al: Role of medial lamellar architecture in the pathogenesis of aortic aneurysms. *J Vasc Surg* 1:442–448, 1984.

107. Sumner DS, Hokanson DE, Strandness DE Sr: Stress-strain characteristics and collagen-elastin content of abdominal aortic aneurysms. *Surg Gynecol Obstet* 130: 459–466, 1970.

108. Menashi L, Campa J, Greenhalgh R, et al: Collagen in abdominal aortic aneurysm: typing, content and degradation. *J Vasc Surg* 6:578–582, 1987.

109. Rizzo RJ, McCarthy WJ, Dixit SN, et al: Collagen types and matrix protein content in human abdominal aortic aneurysms. *J Vasc Surg* 10:365–373, 1989.

110. Minion DJ, Davis VA, Nejezchleb BS, et al: Elastin is increased in abdominal aortic aneurysms. *J Surg Res* 1994. (In press.)

111. Baxter BT, Valerie A, Davis VA, Minion DJ, et al: Abdominal aortic aneurysms are associated with altered matrix proteins of the nonaneurysmal aortic segments. *J Vasc Surg* 19:797–803, 1994.

112. Slaiby JM, Ricci MA, Gadowski GR, et al: Expansion of aortic aneurysms is reduced by propranolol in a hypertensive rat model. *J Vasc Surg* 20:178–183, 1994.

113. Patel DJ, de Freitas FM, Greenfield JC, et al: Relationship of radius to pressure along the aorta in living dogs. *J Appl Physiol* 18:1111–1117, 1963.

114. McDonald DA: *Blood Flow in Arteries.* Baltimore: Williams & Wilkins, 90, 1974.

115. Newman DL, Gosling RG, Bowden NLR, et al: Pressure amplitude increase and matching the aortic iliac junction of the dog. *Cardiovasc Res* 7:6–13, 1973.

116. Womersley JR: Oscillating flow in arteries 2: the reflection of the pulse wave at junctions and rigid inserts in the arterial system. *Phys Med Biol* 2:313–323, 1958.

117. Gosling RG, Newman DL, Bowden LR, et al: The area ratio of normal aortic junctions. *Br J Radiol* 44:850–853, 1971.

118. Gosling RG, Bowden NLR: Changes in aortic distensibility and area ratio with the development of atherosclerosis. *Atherosclerosis* 14:231–240, 1971.

119. Petersen MJ, Abbott WM, H'Doubler PB Jr, et al: Hemodynamics and aneurysm development in vascular allografts. *J Vasc Surg* 18:955–964, 1993.

120. Anidjar S, Osborne-Pellegin M, Coutard M, et al: Arterial hypertension and aneurysmal dilatation. *Kid Int* 41(suppl 37)41:S61-S66, 1992.

121. Gadowski GR, Ricci MA, Hendley ED, et al: Hypertension accelerates the growth of experimental aortic aneurysms. *J Surg Res* 54:431–436, 1993.

122. Veldenz H, Schwarcz TG, Dobrin PB, et al: Morphology which predicts rapid growth of small abdominal aortic aneurysms. *Ann Vasc Surg* 8:10–130, 1994.

123. Wolinsky H, Glagov S: Nature of species differences in the medial distribution of aortic vasa vasorum in mammals. *Circ Res* 20:409–421, 1967.

124. Wilens SL, Malcolm JA, Vasquez JM: Experimental infarction (medial necrosis) of the dog aorta. *Am J Pathol* 47:695–711, 1965.

125. Heistad DD, Marcus ML, Larson GE, et al: Role of vasa vasorum in nourishment of the aortic wall. *Am J Physiol* 240:H781–H787, 1981.

126. Schuler JJ, Flanigan DP: Iliac artery aneurysms. In: Bergan J, Yao JST (eds). *Aneurysms: Diagnosis and Treatment.* New York: Grune & Stratton, Inc.; 469–485, 1982.

127. McCready RA, Pardero PC, Gilmore JC, et al: Isolated iliac artery aneurysms. *Surgery* 93:688–693, 1983.

128. Bernstein EF, Chan EL: Abdominal aortic aneurysms in high-risk patients. *Ann Surg* 200:255–263, 1984.

129. Cronenwett J, Murphy T, Zelenock G, et al: Actuarial analysis of variables associated with rupture of small abdominal aortic aneurysms. *Surgery* 98:472–483, 1985.

130. Ichikawa Y, Nonomiya H, Kogatt H, et al: Erythromycin reduces neutrophils and neutrophil-derived elastolytic-like activity in lower respiratory tract of bronchiolitis patients. *Amer Rev Respir Dis* 146:196–203, 1992.

131. Kucich U, Christner P, Lippmann M, et al: Utilization of peroxidase-antiperoxidase complex in an enzyme-linked immunosorbent assay of elastin-derived peptides in human plasma. *Amer Rev Respir Dis* 131:709–713, 1985.

132. Schriver EE, Davidson JM, Sutcliffe MC, et al: Comparison of elastin peptide concentrations in body fluids from healthy volunteers, smokers, and patients with chronic obstructive pulmonary disease. *Amer Rev Respir Dis* 145:762–766, 1992.

133. Swanson RJ, Littooy FN, Hunt TK, et al: Laparotomy as a precipitating factor in the rupture of intra-abdominal aneurysms. *Arch Surg* 115:299–304, 1980.

134. Koch AE, Haines GK, Rizzo RJ, et al: Human abdominal aortic aneurysms: immunophenotypic analysis suggesting an immune mediated response. *Am J Pathol* 137:1197–1213, 1990.

135. Busuttil RW, Abou-Zamzam AM, Machleder HI: Collagenase activity of the human aorta: comparison of pa-

tients with and without abdominal aortic aneurysms. *Arch Surg* 115:1373–1378, 1980.

136. Busuttil RW, Heinrich R, Flesher A: Elastase activity: the role of elastase in aortic aneurysm formation. *J Surg Res* 32:214–217, 1982.

137. Cannon DJ, Read R: Blood elastolytic activity in patients with aortic aneurysm. *Ann Thorac Surg* 34:10–15, 1982.

138. Brown SL, Blackstrom B, Busuttil RW: A new serum proteolytic enzyme in aneurysm pathogenesis. *J Vasc Surg* 2:393–399, 1985.

139. Cohen JR, Mandell C, Margolis I, et al: Altered aortic protease and antiprotease activity in patients with ruptured abdominal aortic aneurysms. *Surg Gynecol Obstet* 164:355–358, 1987.

140. Dubick MA, Hunter GC, Perez-Lizano E, et al: Assessment of the role of pancreatic proteases in human abdominal aortic aneurysms and occlusive disease. *Clin Chim Acta* 177:1–10, 1988.

141. Herron GS, Unemori E, Wong M, et al: Connective tissue proteinases and inhibitors in abdominal aortic aneurysms: involvement of the vasa vasorum in the pathogenesis of aortic aneurysms. *Arterioscler Thromb* 11:1667–1677, 1991.

142. Zarins CK, Runyon-Hass A, Lu CT, et al: Increased collagenase activity in early aneurysmal dilatation. *J Vasc Surg* 3:238–248, 1986.

143. Anidjar S, Salzmann JL, Gentric D, et al: Elastase-induced experimental aneurysms in rats. *Circulation* 82:973–981, 1990.

144. Anidjar S, Dobrin PB, Eichorst M, et al: Correlation of inflammatory infiltrate with the enlargement of experimental aortic aneurysms. *J Vasc Surg* 16:139–147, 1992.

145. Halpern VJ, Nackman GB, Gandhi RH, et al: The elastase infusion model of experimental aortic aneurysms: synchrony of indirection of endogenous proteinases with matrix destruction and inflammatory cell response. *J Vasc Surg* 20:51–60, 1996.

146. Dobrin PB, Baumgartner N, Anidjar S, et al: Inflammatory aspects of experimental aneurysms: effect of methylprednisolone and cyclosporine. *Ann NY Acad Sci,* 1996. (In press.)

147. Zarins CK, Glagov S: Aneurysms and obstructive plaques: differing local responses to atherosclerosis. In: Bergan JJ, Yao JST (eds). *Aneurysms: Diagnosis and Treatment.* New York: Grune & Stratton, Inc.; 61–82, 1982.

148. Zarins CK, Xu C, Glagov S: Aneurysmal enlargement of the aorta during regression of experimental atherosclerosis. *J Vasc Surg* 15:90–101, 1992.

149. Bengsston H, Ekberg O, Aspelin P, et al: Abdominal aortic dilatation in patients operated on for carotid stenosis. *Acta Chir Scand* 154:441–445, 1988.

150. Tilson MD, Stansel HC: Differences in results for aneurysms vs occlusive disease after bifurcation grafts: results of 100 elective grafts. *Arch Surg* 115:1173–1175, 1980.

151. Hollier HL, Stanson AW, Goviczki P, et al: Arteriomegaly: classification and morbid implications of diffuse aneurysmal disease. *Surgery* 93:700–708, 1983.

152. Clifton MA: Familial abdominal aortic aneurysms. *Br J Surg* 64:765–766, 1977.

153. Tilson MD, Seashore MR: Human genetics of the abdominal aortic aneurysm. *Surg Gynecol Obstet* 158:129–132, 1984.

154. Norrgard O, Rais O, Angquist K-A: Familial occur-

155. Johansen K, Koepsell T: Familial tendency for abdominal aortic aneurysms. *JAMA* 258:1934–1936, 1986.

156. Cannon DJ, Casteel I, Read RC: Abdominal aortic aneurysm, Leriche's syndrome, inguinal herniation, and smoking. *Arch Surg* 119:387–389, 1984.

157. Sterick CA, Long JR, Jamasbi B, et al: Ventral hernia following abdominal aortic reconstruction. *Amer Surg* 54:287–289, 1988.

158. Lehnert B, Wadoub F: High coincidence of inguinal hernias and abdominal aortic aneurysms. *Ann Vasc Surg* 6:134–137, 1992.

159. Kontusaari S, Kuivaniemi H, Tromp G, et al: A single base mutation in type III procollagen that converts the codon for glycine 619 to argianine in a family with familial aneurysms and mild bleeding tendencies. *Ann NY Acad Sci* 580:556–557, 1990.

160. Paranjpe M, Engel L, Young N, et al: Activation of human breast carcinoma collagenase through plasminogen activator. *Life Sci* 26:1223–1231, 1980.

161. Tromholt N, Jorgensen SJ, Hesse B, et al: In vivo demonstration of focal fibrinolytic activity in abdominal aortic aneurysms. *Eur J Vasc Surg* 7:675–679, 1993.

162. Jean-Claude J, Newman KM, Li H, et al: Possible key role for plasmin in the pathogenesis of abdominal aortic aneurysms. *Surgery* 116:472–478, 1994.

163. Wolf YG, Thomas WS, Brennan RJ, et al: CT findings associated with rapid expansion of abdominal aortic aneurysms. *J Vasc Surg.* (In press.)

164. Scher LA, Veith FJ, Haimovici H, et al: Staging of arterial complications of cervical rib: guidelines for surgical managment. *Surgery* 95:645–649, 1984.

165. Cormier JM, Amrane M, Ward A, et al: Arterial complications of the thoracic outlet syndrome: fifty-five operative cases. *J Vasc Surg* 9:778–787, 1989.

166. Wood P: *Diseases of the Heart and Circulation.* Eyre & Spottiswoode; 1005, 1956.

167. Zaroff LI, Kreel L, Sobel HJ, et al: Multiple and intraductal coarctations of the aorta. *Circulation* 20:910–917, 1959.

168. Rochoff SD, Austen WG: The hemodynamic significance of the radiologic changes in acquired aortic stenosis. *Am Heart J* 65:458–463, 1963.

169. Kincaid OW, Davis GD: Renal arteriography in hypertension. *Proc May Clinic* 36:689–701, 1961.

170. DeBakey ME, Crawford S, Morris GC Jr: Surgical considerations of occlusive disease of the innominate, carotid, subclavian, and vertebral arteries. *Ann Surg* 154:698–725, 1961.

171. Gedge SW, Spittel JA Jr, Ivins JC: Aneurysm of the distal popliteal artery and its relationship to the arcuate popliteal ligament. *Circulation* 24:270–273, 1961.

172. Lord JW Jr, Rossi G, Paula G: The inguinal ligament: its relation to poststenotic dilatation of the common femoral artery. *Bull NY Acad Sci* 55:451–462, 1979.

173. Roach MR, MacDonald AC: Poststenotic dilatation in renal arteries. *Invest Radiol* 5:311–315, 1970.

174. Roach MR: The reversibility of poststenotic dilatation in the femoral arteries of dogs. *Circ Res* 27:985–993, 1971.

175. Trillo A, Haust MD: Arterial elastic tissue and collagen in experimental poststenotic dilatation in dogs. *Exp Mol Pathol* 23:473–490, 1975.

176. Imataka K, Seki A, Tomona S, et al: Experimental production of poststenotic dilatation in the carotid arteries of rabbits. *Jpn Heart J* 22:127–133, 1981.

177. Legg MJ, Gow BS: Scanning electron microscopy of endothelium around an experimental stenosis in the rabbit aorta using a new casting material. *Atherosclerosis* 42:299–318, 1982.

178. Kukongviriyapan U, Gow BS: Morphometric analyses of rabbit thoracic aorta after poststenotic dilatation. *Circ Res* 65:1774–1786, 1989.

179. Roach MR: Changes in arterial distensibility as a cause of poststenotic dilatation. *Am J Cardiol* 12:801–815, 1963.

180. Dobrin PB: Poststenotic dilatation. *Surg Gynecol Obstet* 172:503–508, 1991.

181. Kawaguti M, Hamano A: Numerical study on poststenotic dilatation. *Biorheology* 20:507–516, 1983.

182. Holman E: The obscure physiology of poststenotic dilatation: its relation to the development of aneurysms. *J Thorac Surg* 29:109–133, 1954.

183. Rodbard S, Ikeda K, Montes M: An analysis of mechanisms of poststenotic dilatation. *Angiology* 18:349–367, 1967.

184. Robicsek F, Sanger PW, Taylor FH: Pathogenesis and significance of poststenotic dilatation in great vessels. *Ann Surg* 147:835–844, 1958.

185. Harvey EN: Bubble formation in liquids. In: Glasser O (ed). *Medical Physics*. Vol II. Chicago: Year Book Medical Publishers, Inc.; 137–150, 1950.

186. Talukder N, Fulenwider JT, Mabon RF, et al: Poststenotic flow disturbance in the dog aorta as measured with pulsed Doppler ultrasound. *J Biomech Eng* 108:259–265, 1986.

187. Ojha M, Johnston KW, Cobbold RSC: Evidence of a possible link between poststenotic dilatation and wall shear stress. *J Vasc Surg* 11:127–135, 1990.

188. Glagov S, Weisenberg BA, Zarins CK, et al: Compensatory enlargement of human atherosclerotic coronary arteries. *N Engl J Med* 316:1371–1375, 1987.

189. Halsted WS: Partial, progressive, and complete occlusion of the aorta and other large arteries in the dog by means of the metal band. *J Exp Med* 11:373–391, 1909.

190. Roach MR, Melech E: Effect of sonic vibration on isolated human iliac arteries. *Can J Physiol Pharmacol* 49:288–291, 1971.

191. Boughner DR, Roach MR: Effect of low frequency vibration on the arterial wall. *Circ Res* 29:136–144, 1971.

192. Gow BS, Legg MG, Yu W, et al: Does vibration cause poststenotic dilatation in vivo and influence atherogenesis in cholesterol-fed rabbits? *J Biomech Eng* 114:20–25, 1992.

193. Ojha M, Languille BL: Evidence that turbulence is not the cause of poststenotic dilatation in rabbit carotid arteries. *Arterioscler Thromb* 13:977–984, 1993.

194. Dobrin PB, Littooy FN, Golan J, et al: Mechanical and histologic changes in canine vein grafts. *J Surg Res* 44:259–265, 1988.

195. Imparato AM, Bracco A, Kim GE, et al: Intimal and neointimal fibrous proliferation causing failure of arterial reconstruction. *Surgery* 72:1007–1017, 1972.

196. Kern WH, Dermer GB, Lindesmith GG: Intimal proliferation in aortic-coronary saphenous vein grafts. *Amer Heart J* 84:771–777, 1972.

197. Fuchs JC, Mitchener JS, Hagen P-O: Postoperative changes in autogenous vein grafts. *Ann Surg* 188:1–15, 1978.

198. Sottiurai VS, Yao JST, Baston RC, et al: Distal anastomotic intimal hyperplasia: histological character and biogenesis. *Ann Vasc Surg* 3:26–33, 1989.

199. Dobrin PB: Mechanical factors associated with the development of intimal hyperplasia with respect to vascular grafts. In: Dobrin PB (ed). *Intimal Hyperplasia*. Austin, TX: Landes Publishing; 1994.

200. Pomposelli F, Schoen F, Cohen R, et al: Conformational stress and anastomotic hyperplasia. *J Vasc Surg* 1:525–535, 1984.

201. Kohler TR, Kirkman TR, Clowes AW: The effect of rigid external support on vein graft adaptation to the arterial circulation. *J Vasc Surg* 9:277–285, 1989.

202. Schwartz LB, O'Donohoe MK, Purut CM, et al: Myointimal thickening in experimental vein grafts is dependent on wall tension. *J Vasc Surg* 15:176–186, 1992.

203. Kohler T, Kirkman TR, Kraiss L, et al: Increased blood flow inhibits neointimal hyperplasia in endothelialized vascular grafts. *Circ Res* 69:1557–1565, 1991.

204. Rittgers SE, Karayannacos PE, Guy JE, et al: Velocity distribution and intimal proliferation in autologous vein grafts in dogs. *Circ Res* 42:792–801, 1978.

205. Bond MG, Hostetler JR, Karayannacos PE, et al: Intimal changes in arteriovenous bypass grafts: effects of varying the angle of implantation at the proximal anastomosis and of producing stenosis in the distal runoff artery. *J Thorac Cardiovasc Surg* 71:907–911, 1976.

206. Dennis JW, Baker WH, Dobrin PB, et al: The relationship between neointimal hyperplasia and distal anastomotic angles in vein bypass grafts. *Curr Surg* 43:202–205, 1986.

207. Abbott WM, Megerman J, Hasson JE, et al: Effect of compliance mismatch on vascular graft patency. *J Vasc Surg* 5:378–382, 1987.

208. Okuhn SP, Connelly DP, Calakos N, et al: Does compliance mismatch alone cause neointimal hyperplasia? *J Vasc Surg* 9:35–45, 1989.

209. Abbott WM, Megerman J: Does compliance mismatch alone cause neointimal hyperplasia? Letter to the editors. *J Vasc Surg* 9:507, 1989.

210. Bassiouny HS, White S, Glagov S, et al: Anastomotic intimal hyperplasia: mechanical injury or flow induced. *J Vasc Surg* 15:708–717, 1992.

211. Suggs WD, Henriques HF, DePalma RG: Vein cuff interposition prevents juxta-anastomotic neointimal hyperplasia. *Ann Surg* 207:717–723, 1988.

212. Sidawy AN, Trad KS, Sidawy MK, et al: Effect of vein cuff and ePTFE on the development of outflow intimal hyperplasia. *Surg Forum* 345–346, 1992.

213. Ojha M: Spatial and temporal variations of wall shear stress within an end-to-side arterial anastomosis model. *J Biomech* 26:1377–1388, 1993.

214. Ojha M: Wall shear stress temporal gradient and anastomotic intimal hyperplasia. *Circ Res*. (In press.)

215. Gariepy J, Massonneau M, Levenson J, et al: Evidence of in vivo carotid and femoral wall thickening in human hypertension. *Hypertension* 22:111–118, 1993.

216. Berecek KH, Bohr DF: Structural and functional changes in vascular resistance and reactivity in the deoxycorticosterone acetate (DOCA)-hypertensive pig. *Circ Res* (suppl 1)40:146–151, 1977.

217. Warshaw DM, Mulvany MJ, Halpern W: Mechanical and morphological properties of arterial resistance vessels in young and old spontaneously hypertensive rats. *Circ Res* 45:250–259, 1979.

218. Wolinsky H: Responses of the rat aortic media to hypertension: morphological and chemical studies. *Circ Res* 26:507–519, 1970.

219. Tobian L, Olson R, Chesley G: Water content of arteriolar wall in renovascular hypertension. *Am J Physiol* 216:22–24, 1969.

220. Owens GK, Schwartz SM: Alterations in vascular smooth muscle mass in the spontaneously hypertensive rat. *Circ Res* 51:280–289, 1982.

221. Lee RMKW, Forrest JB, Garfield RE, et al: Ultrastructural changes in mesenteric blood arteries from spontaneously hypertensive rats. *Blood Vessels* 20:72–91, 1983.

222. Bandick NR, Sparks HV: Viscoelastic properties of the aorta of hypertensive rats. *Proc Soc Exp Biol Med* 134:56–60, 1971.

223. Christensen KL: Reducing pulse pressure in hypertension may normalize small artery structure. *Hypertension* 18:722–727, 1991.

224. Leung DYM, Glagov S, Mathews MB: Cyclic stretching stimulates synthesis of matrix components by arterial smooth muscle cells in vitro. *Science* 191:475–477, 1976.

225. Bandick NR, Sparks HV: Contractile response of vascular smooth muscle of renal hypertensive rats. *Am J Physiol* 219:340–344, 1970.

226. Busse R, Bauer RD, Summa Y, et al: Comparison of the viscoelastic properties of the tail artery in spontaneously hypertensive and normotensive rats. *Pfleug Arch* 364:175–181, 1976.

227. Halloway ET, Bohr DF: Reactivity of vascular smooth muscle in hypertensive rats. *Circ Res* 33:678–685, 1973.

228. Hansen TR, Abrams GD, Bohr DF: Role of pressure in structural and functional changes in arteries of hypertensive rats. *Circ Res* (suppl 1)34:101–107, 1974.

229. Takeda K, Bunag RD: Augmented sympathetic nerve activity and pressor responses in DOCA hypertensive rats. *Hypertension* 2:97–102, 1980.

230. Pacak K, Vadid G, Jakab G, et al: In vivo hypothalamic release and synthesis of catecholamines in spontaneously hypertensive rats. *Hypertension* 22:467–478, 1993.

231. Greenberg S, Bohr DF: Venous smooth muscle in hypertension: enhanced contractility of portal veins from spontaneously hypertensive rats. *Circ Res* (suppl 1)36:208–215, 1975.

232. Sivertsson R: The hemodynamic importance of structural vascular changes in essential hypertension. *Acta Physiol Scand* (suppl 343):1–56, 1970.

233. Short D: Morphology of the intestinal arterioles in chronic human hypertension. *Br Heart J* 28:184–192, 1966.

234. Mulvany MJ, Baandrup U, Gundersen HJG: Evidence for hyperplasia in mesenteric resistance vessels of spontaneously hypertensive rats using a three-dimensional disector. *Circ Res* 57:794–800, 1985.

235. Korsgaard N, Mulvany MJ: Cellular hypertrophy in mesenteric resistance vessels from renal hypertensive rats. *Hypertension* 12:162–167, 1988.

236. Korsgaard N, Aalkjaer C, Heagerty AM, et al: Histology of subcutaneous small arteries from patients with essential hypertension. *Hypertension* 22:523–526, 1993.

237. Baumbach GL, Heistad DD: Remodeling of cerebral arterioles in chronic hypertension. *Hypertension* 13:968–972, 1989.

238. Hayoz D, Rutschmann B, Perret F, et al: Conduit artery compliance and distensibility are not necessarily reduced in hypertension. *Hypertension* 20:1–6, 1992.

239. Baumbach GL, Dobrin PB, Hurt MN, et al: Mechanics of cerebral arterioles in hypertensive rats. *Circ Res* 62:56–64, 1988.

240. Mulvany MJ: Biophysical aspects of resistence vessels studied in spontaneously hypertensive and renal hyper-

tensive rats. *Acta Physiol Scand* (suppl 571)133:129–138, 1988.

241. Webb RC, Vanhoutte PM: Sensitivity to noradrenaline in isolated tail arteries from spontaneously hypertensive rats. *Clin Sci* (suppl 5)57:31–33, 1979.

242. Mulvany MJ, Aalkjaer C, Christensen J: Changes in noradrenaline sensitivity and morphology of arterial resistance vessels during development of high blood pressure in spontaneously hypertensive rats. *Hypertension* 2:664–671, 1980.

243. Aalkjaer C, Heagerty AM, Petersen KK, et al: Evidence for increased media thickness, increased neuronal uptake, and depressed excitation-contraction coupling in isolated resistance vessels from essential hypertensives. *Circ Res* 61:181–186, 1987.

244. Kong JQ, Taylor DA, Fleming WW: Mesenteric vascular responses of young spontaneously hypertensive rats. *J Pharmacol Exp Therap* 258:13–17, 1991.

245. Folkow B: Physiological aspects of primary hypertension. *Physiol Rev* 62:347–504, 1982.

246. Konishi M, Su C: Role of endothelium in dilation responses of spontaneously hypertensive rat arteries. *Hypertension* 5:881–886, 1983.

247. Couvin C, Pegram B: Decreased relaxation of isolated mesenteric resistance vessels from 2 kidney 1 clip Goldblatt hypertensive rats. *Clin Exp Hypertension* 5:383–400, 1983.

248. Winquist RJ, Bunting PB, Baskin EP, et al: Decreased endothelium-dependent relaxation in New Zealand genetic hypertensive rats. *J Hypertension* 2:541–545, 1984.

249. Falloon BJ, Bund SJ, Tulip JR, et al: In vivo perfusion studies of resistance artery function in genetic hypotension. *Hypertension* 22:486–495, 1993.

250. Band W, Goedhard WJA, Knoop AA: Comparison of effects of high cholesterol intake on viscoelastic properties of the thoracic aorta in rats and rabbits. *Atherosclerosis* 18:163–172, 1973.

251. Pynadath TI, Mukherjee DP: Dynamic mechanical properties of atherosclerotic aorta: a correlation between the cholesterol ester content and the viscoelastic properties of atherosclerotic aorta. *Atherosclerosis* 26:311–318, 1977.

252. Hayashi K, Ide K, Matsumoto T: Aortic walls in atherosclerotic rabbits: a mechanical study. *J Biomech Eng.* (In press.)

253. Haut RC, Garg BD, Metke M, et al: Mechanical properties of the canine aorta following hypercholesteremia. *J Biomech Eng* 102:98–102, 1980.

254. Hudetz AG, Mark G, Kovach AGB, et al: Biomechanical properties of normal and fibrosclerotic human cerebral arteries. *Atherosclerosis* 39:353–365, 1981.

255. Farrar DJ, Bond MG, Sawyer JK, et al: Pulse wave velocity and morphologic changes associated with early atherosclerosis progression in the aortas of cynomolgus monkeys. *Cardiovasc Res* 18:107–118, 1984.

256. Farrar DJ, Green HD, Bond MG, et al: Aortic pulse wave velocity, elasticity and composition in a nonhuman primate model of atherosclerosis. *Circ Res* 43:52–62, 1978.

257. Cox RH, Detweiler DK: Arterial wall properties and dietary atherosclerosis in the racing greyhound. *Am J Physiol* 236:H790–H797, 1979.

258. Hayashi K, Takamizawa K, Nakamura T, et al: Effects of elastase on the stiffness and elastic properties of arterial walls in cholesterol-fed rabbits. *Atherosclerosis* 66:239–267, 1987.

259. Lee RT, Richardson G, Loree HM, et al: Prediction of mechanical properties of human atherosclerotic tissue by high-frequency intravascular ultrasound imaging: an in vitro study. *Arterioscler Thromb* 12:1–5, 1992.

260. Loree HM, Kamm RD, Stringfellow RG, et al: Effects of fibrous cap thickness on peak circumferential stress in model atherosclerotic vessels. *Circ Res* 71:850–858, 1992.

261. Carew TE, Vaishnav RN, Patel DJ: Compressibility of the arterial wall. *Circ Res* 23:61–68, 1968.

262. Sobin S, Tremer HM: Cylindricity of the arterial tree in the dog and cat (abstr). *Fed Proc* 39:269, 1980.

263. Doyle JM, Dobrin PB: Finite deformation analysis of the relaxed and contracted dog carotid artery. *Microvasc Res* 3:400–415, 1971.

264. Vaishnav RN, Young JT, Janicki JS, et al: Nonlinear anisotropic elastic properties of the canine aorta. *Biophys J* 12:1008–1027, 1972.

265. Simon BR, Kobayashi AS, Strandness DE, et al: Large deformation analysis of the arterial cross section. *J Basic Eng* 930:138–146, 1971.

266. Mower WR, Baroff LJ, Sneyd J: Stress distribution in vascular aneurysms: factors affecting risk of aneurysm rupture. *J Surg Res* 55:155–161, 1993.

267. Stringfellow MM, Lawrence PF, Stringfellow SM: The influence of aorto-aneurysm geometry upon stress in the aneurysm wall. *J Surg Res* 42:425–433, 1987.

268. Gaballa MA, Roya TE, Simon BR, et al: Arterial mechanics in spontaneously hypertensive rats: mechanical properties, hydraulic conductivity, and two-phase (solid/fluid) finite element models. *Circ Res* 71:145–158, 1992.

269. Vaishnav RN, Young JT, Patel DJ: Distribution of stresses and of strain-energy density through the wall thickness in a canine aortic segment. *Circ Res* 32:577–583, 1973.

270. Doyle JM, Dobrin PB: Stress gradients in the walls of arteries. *J Biomech* 6:631–639, 1973.

271. Vaishnav RN, Vossoughi J: Residual stress and strain in aortic segments. *J Biomech* 20:235–239, 1987.

272. Vaishnav RN, Vossoughi J: Estimation of residual strains in aortic segments. In: Hall CW (ed). *Biomedical Engineering II: Recent Developments*. New York: Pergamon Press; 330–333, 1983.

273. Vossoughi J, Hedjazi Z, Borris FS II: Intimal residual stress and strain in large arteries. *ASME BED Conference* 24:434–437, 1993.

274. Takamizawa K, Hayashi K: Strain energy density function and uniform strain hypotheses for arterial mechanics. *J Biomech* 20:7–17, 1987.

275. Vossoughi J: Longitudinal residual strain in arteries. *Proceedings of South Biomed Eng Conf.* 17–19, 1992.

276. Liu SQ, Fung YC: Relationship between hypertension, hypertrophy, and opening angle of zero-stress state of arteries following aortic constriction. *J Biomech Eng* 111:325–335, 1989.

277. Fung YC, Liu SQ: Change of residual strains in arteries due to hypertrophy caused by aortic constriction. *Circ Res* 65:1340–1349, 1989.

278. Xie JP, Liu SQ, Yang RF, et al: The zero-stress state of rat veins and vena cava. *Trans ASME* 113:36–41, 1991.

279. Geiringer E: Intimal vascularization and atheromatosis. *J Pathol Bact* 63:201–211, 1951.

280. Barger AC, Beewkes R III, Lainey LL, et al: Hypothesis: vasa vasorum and neovascularization of human coronary arteries: a possible role in the pathophysiology of atherogenesis. *N Engl J Med* 310:175–177, 1984.

CHAPTER 4

Hemodynamics and Atherosclerosis

Bradford I. Tropea, MD; Seymour Glagov, MD
Christopher K. Zarins, MD

Atherosclerosis is a generalized disease process that mainly affects large and medium-sized arteries. It is associated with well-recognized risk factors including hyperlipidemia, hypertension, and cigarette smoking. Although atherosclerosis is a lifelong disease process, morbidity and mortality usually result from localized plaque deposition rather than from diffuse disease. Certain vessels, such as the infrarenal abdominal aorta, carotid bifurcation, lower extremity arteries, and coronary arteries, are particularly susceptible to plaque formation; others, such as the upper extremity arteries and thoracic aorta, are rarely involved. Even in susceptible arteries, plaque deposition is focal. Observations that atherosclerosis tends to occur at arterial branchings, ostia, bifurcations, and bends suggest that modifications of flow dynamics may induce or potentiate plaque deposition.

Several hypotheses have been proposed to account for the unique and focal pattern of atherosclerotic plaque formation. The fact that blood flow exerts stress on the vessel wall and affects mass transport to arterial tissue has led to the hypothesis that fluid hemodynamic forces are localizing factors in atherogenesis. There are many alterations in the field flow that have been implicated in potentiating plaque formation, including increased velocity,[1] decreased velocity,[2] high-wall shear stress,[1] low-wall shear stress,[2–4] flow separation,[5,6] departures from unilaminar flow patterns,[7,8] and turbulence.[9] Altered mural tensile stress has been related to alterations in artery wall metabolism, thickness,[10] microarchitecture,[10,11] and compliance.[12]

Hemodynamic Forces

Flow in the human arterial tree is generally laminar; that is, fluid displacements follow predictable and stable linear paths. Blood flows in smooth layers, and a particle flowing in one layer tends to stay in that layer. If the rate of blood flow exceeds a critical level, the flow can be turbulent. In turbulent flow, particles disperse and follow an erratic and unpredictable pathway. There are random movements of elements in the flow field. Whether or not flow will be turbulent depends on viscosity, mean velocity, and the diameter of the vessel. The Reynolds number takes these into account and is given by:

$$\mathrm{Re} = \frac{pVd}{\mu}$$

where p is the density, V is the mean velocity (m/s), d is the diameter of the vessel lumen, and μ is the absolute viscosity (N·s/m^2). A Reynolds number exceeding a critical value for a given situation predicts the occurrence of turbulent flow. Abrupt changes in geometry distal to a stenosis, or other obstacles in the flow stream, may cause focal turbulence.

In straight vessels, blood flow is typically laminar and parabolic. Velocity is greatest in the center of the vessel and declines symmetrically toward the lumen surface because of the frictional resistance of the blood-endothelial interface (Figure 1). The distribution of velocities is displaced if there is an eccentric lesion in the vessel, or if the vessel curves. The velocity pro-

From *The Basic Science of Vascular Disease.* Edited by Sidawy AN, Sumpio BE, and DePalma RG. Armonk, NY: Futura Publishing Company, Inc.; © 1997.

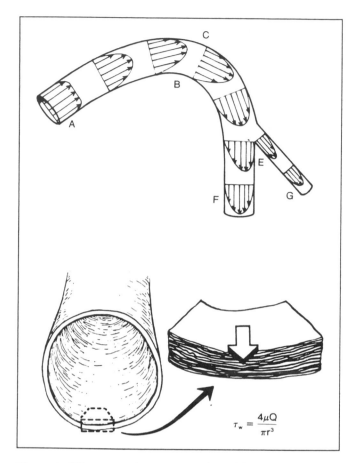

Figure 1. Diagrammatic representation of flow velocity profile and wall shear stress. **Top:** At entry region (**A**) profile reflects parabolic laminar flow particularly in straight portions of the vessel. At bends, high central velocities are skewed toward the outer or convex portion of the vessel (**C**) producing sharper gradients of near wall velocities than on the concave side (**B**). When flow reaches a branch point (**E**), the flow divider intercepts high velocities toward the center. Flow is restored to parabolic profile distal to the branch points (**F**) and (**G**). **Below:** Wall shear stress is the frictional force exerted by the flowing blood on the endothelial surface. Shear stress is related to the near-wall gradient of velocities and blood viscosity (μ). (Reproduced with permission from Reference 16.)

file returns to a symmetrical parabolic state when the vessel is again straight. The curvature of a vessel, branchings, and bifurcations, and the angle of branches all affect the velocity profile and can cause local flow disturbances. For example, the downstream edge of a branch vessel intercepts and divides the flow stream, and is exposed to higher flow velocities and shear stress than the upstream rim of the branch. Flow separation occurs when the flow velocity profile has been displaced away from the vessel wall. The flow velocity gradient is steeper on the inside of a flow divider, or on the convex or outer aspect of a curved vessel.

Shear stress has received much attention in the literature with respect to endothelial function and ath-

erosclerotic plaque formation. Wall shear stress is defined as the tangential drag force per unit area produced by blood moving along the endothelial surface (Figure 1). This force tends to displace the endothelium and inner layers of the artery wall in the direction of flow. The expression for wall shear stress for a parabolic blood flow in a cylindrical vessel is:

$$\tau_w = \frac{4\,\mu\,Q}{\pi\,r^3}$$

where τ_w is the wall shear stress (N/m^2), μ is the viscosity of blood, Q is the blood flow rate (L/s), and r is the vessel radius. Since shear stress is inversely related to the cube of the radius, small changes in the radius can have a significant impact on wall shear stress. Wall shear stress is also defined as the product of the viscosity and the velocity gradient of the fluid in the direction parallel to the blood-endothelial surface.

Intraluminal blood pressure exerts a distending and compressive force on the artery wall with a circumferential stretching force exerted in a direction tangent to the artery wall (Figure 2). This force is known as wall tension and is described by the law of Laplace ($T = Pr$), where T is tension (N/m), P is pressure (N/m^2), and r is the lumen radius. This equation is accurate if the thickness of the arterial wall is small compared to the diameter. Increasing wall tension is counterbalanced by increases in wall thickness to maintain a constant wall *tensile stress* as described by the equation $S = Pr/d$, where d is the wall thickness.

Mural tensile stress is modified in bends and curvatures, where the effective lumen radius is altered at bends, bifurcations, and stenoses. Thus, at the inner or concave side of a bend, the effective radius is increased with an increase in tangential tension and an equivalent increase in wall thickness; likewise, there is a decrease in tension at the convex portion of a bend and a decrease in wall tension.

The effective distending pressure of an artery is the difference between the intraluminal and peri-arterial pressure. Thus, the effects of distending pressure may be modified by surrounding organs or peri-adventitial tissue. Both the thickness and composition of the arterial wall are related to wall tension.[13] The close association between collagen and elastin in the wall of large arteries results in a modulus of elasticity lower than that of collagen alone and greater than that of elastin.[14] At blood pressures below diastolic, the modulus of elasticity is closer to elastin; as the pressure increases, the elasticity approaches that of collagen.[15]

Vessel Wall

It is well-known that the intima thickens in early atherosclerosis as a result of the proliferation and mi-

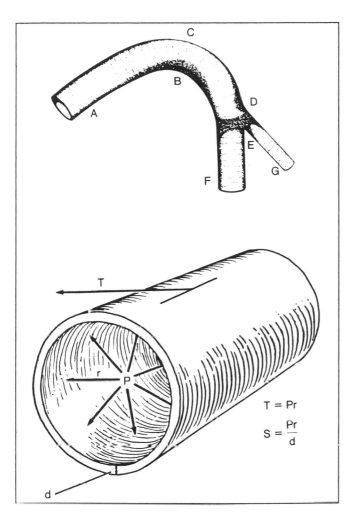

Figure 2. Representation of distribution of tensile stress (**top**). **Bottom**: Vector representing tangential tension (**T**) is shown diagrammatically. It is the product of the pressure (**P**) and radius for vessels with small thickness compared (**D**) to the radius. Tensile stress (**S**) in units of force per unit area takes wall thickness into account. **Top**: Distribution of tangential tension is represented by degree of prominence of shading in this model geometry. Wall tension is uniform in regions **A**, **F**, and **G**. Tension is larger in the concave side of the bend (**B**) because in this region, curvature of bend is opposite that of the vessel wall, producing a flattening (reduction of curvature) or large effective radius. At the convex aspect (**C**) of the bend, there is reduction of tensile stress. At the bifurcation (**E**), there is an increased region of tangential tension. Region (**D**) also exhibits increased tension similar to region (**B**) because of the concavity produced due to the angle of departure of the smaller branch. (Adapted with permission from Reference 16.)

gration of media smooth cells into the intima, and is modulated by the hemodynamic environment.[4,7,16] However, not all intimal thickening leads to lesion progression.[17] This thickening has been correlated with low and oscillatory shear stress.[2,7,18] The thicker intima may add a dense layer to the vessel wall, decreasing clearance of atherogenic substances.

Intraluminal pressure tends to promote diffusion of atherogenic substances into the vessel by convection.[19] Transit of particles from the intima to the adventitia is governed in part by the gradients of chemical activity and water flux across the wall in relation to local differences in wall composition.[20] The larger vessels tend to be thicker and have more fibrous walls, which may partially account for their predilection for atherosclerosis. With age, these larger vessels accumulate more connective tissue, become less compliant, and are more resistant to clearance of atherogenic particles across the wall from the intima. These conditions may be exacerbated by hypertension.[12,21] A few studies have suggested that increased wall stress correlates with higher risk for atherosclerosis. Differences in the depth of penetration of the vasa vasorum into the media and the condition of the perivascular lymphatics could also affect clearance of atherogenic substances through the artery wall. For example, the thoracic aorta, which usually has less atherosclerosis than the abdominal aorta, has an abundant supply of vasa vasorum; its abdominal counterpart is usually devoid of vasa vasorum.[22] Cyclic deformation of the media may be increased in the presence of hypertension, which may act to compress the vasa vasorum, and lead to decreased transmural clearance of atherogenic substances.[23]

The compliance or elasticity of the arterial wall may alter the hemodynamic characteristics of blood flow. Studies have demonstrated that elasticity modulates the propagating arterial pulse, and that impedance mismatching may contribute to atherosclerosis.[24] Cyclic stretching of the arterial wall may induce smooth muscle cells to synthesize extracellular matrix components.[25] Inhibition of atherosclerosis has been correlated with reduction of intramural tension and wall motion, which may be related to alteration in wall metabolism.[26,27]

Shear Stress and Endothelium

Wall shear stress has been considered an important determinant of atherosclerotic plaque formation. High shear stress was previously thought to potentiate plaque formation by producing endothelial injury and disruption, thereby exposing the underlying artery wall to circulating lipids and platelets.[28] In 1968, Fry constricted the canine aorta with a mechanical intraluminal device, increasing the wall shear stress proximal to the coarct. The shear stress was increased to 400 dynes/cm² from a normal of 15 to 20 dynes/cm².[28] Other studies have reported in vivo findings of damaged endothelial cells in high shear stress areas.[29] These findings were taken as evidence that high shear stress was an initiating factor in atherogenesis.

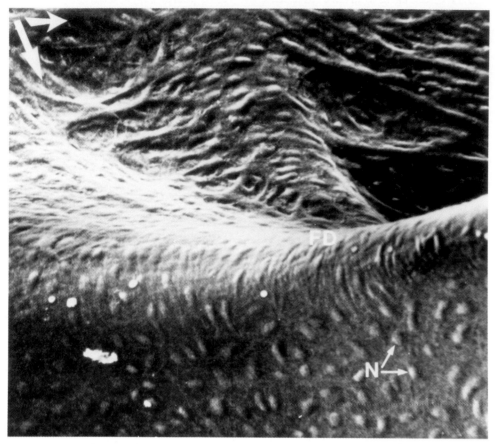

Figure 3. Scanning electron micrograph of a monkey artery ostium. Fixation was by controlled-pressure perfusion in situ and the aorta was dissected without distortion of the ostium. The region about the flow divider (**FD**) is the area with the highest flow velocity and shear stress, but there is no evidence of endothelial damage or desquamation. Endothelial nuclei (**N**) are visible. **Arrow** denotes the direction of flow (x 1000). (Adapted with permission from Reference 136.)

It is now generally recognized that high and low shear stress do not predispose to endothelial disruption in the arterial tree (Figure 3).[30] Shear stress elevated by aortic coarctation and studied at 10 days to several months, rather than acutely, showed no evidence of endothelial disruption in the high shear coarctation channel.[31] If endothelial damage occurred acutely, it healed rapidly without evidence of scarring or residual intimal thickening. Furthermore, atherosclerotic plaques tend to occur in areas of low, rather than high shear stress.[2]

The endothelium has received much attention with respect to initiation of atherosclerosis and lesion progression. The hemodynamic stress acts directly on the endothelium, because the endothelium is exposed to the distending pulsatile pressure, as well as shear stress. The endothelium thickens as smooth muscle cells replicate and invade the internal elastic lamina and, possibly, undergo a phenotypic change.[32] Low shear and oscillatory shear stress have been correlated with intimal thickening.[2,4,7] Shear stress has also been shown to alter endothelial cell structure and function.

Elevated shear elongates endothelial cells in the direction of flow.[33,34] Endothelial cells align themselves in the direction of flow, and the shape of a confluent layer of endothelial cells changes from polygonal to ellipsoid when exposed to unidirectional shear.[35,36] Elongated endothelial cells in pigeon coronary arteries were less likely to demonstrate early atherosclerosis after exposure to hyperlipidemia than endothelial cells that were less elongated.[37] Shear stress may also affect endocytosis and degradation of low density lipoproteins (LDL).[38] Rapid oscillations in flow and shear stress may cause cellular changes in the endothelium that increase lipid uptake. Areas of low and oscillatory shear tended to be stained with Sudan IV in hypercholesterolemic rabbits, suggesting that the local hemodynamic environment can enhance uptake of lipid particles.[39]

High shear may increase the number of stress fibers (F-actin), with an associated increase in stiffness.[40] Shear stress on endothelial function affects gene expression for proto-oncogenes.[41] It has also been shown that disturbed flow increases cell turnover,[42] particularly in areas with low shear, which could explain the loss of contact inhibition of cell growth. Evaluation of presumed low shear stress regions of the arterial tree in hypercholesterolemic rabbits suggests that these areas may possess an elevated number of mitochondria and rough endoplasmic reticulum with poorly developed stress fibers.[38] A thinner glycocalyx with elevated pinocytosis was also noted in the endothelium of these lower shear regions.

The endothelial layer must sense the arterial flow, and it is thought that these cells operate as a signal-transduction system for the hemodynamic forces associated with flow. Early atherogenesis occurs in areas with intact and functional endothelial cells, which indicates that the endothelium is an important modulator of atherogenesis.[43] Studies that have examined how the endothelium transduces the flow into a cellular signal indicate that shear stress affects the phosphoinositide system,[44] with elevated shear stress increasing intracellular calcium.[45] Second messengers have been implicated in flow-mediated alterations in endothelial function. Ion channels and cell surface glycoproteins may be altered by mechanical stresses, with convection-diffusion coupling of transport of atherogenic particles.[46,47] Shear stress acting on the endothelium is transmitted to the cytoskeleton, and transduction of signals may affect transmembrane integrins, adhesion proteins, and proteins linked to F-actin.[48]

Shear stress increases endothelial nitric oxide (NO) production. NO is responsible for increasing cyclic monophosphate (cGMP) levels (second messenger),[49] and cGMP levels can be modulated by calcium and ATP. NO production and cGMP levels increase in ex vivo confluent aortic bovine cells with increasing shear stress up to 40 dynes/cm^2.[50] The signal-transduction pathway may be mediated by a G-protein and a K + channel. Hyperpolarization of the endothelial membrane may alter the conformation of the NO synthase protein affecting NO production.[50] NO inhibits platelet aggregation, leukocyte and monocyte adhesion,[52] and it is able to scavenge free radicals. The hemodynamic milieu may alter NO production, which would modulate cellular adhesion, vessel relaxation, and the oxidative potential of certain blood-borne elements.

Monocyte adhesion and binding to the endothelium is important in atherosclerosis and is enhanced by chemotactic factors and upregulation of monocyte adhesion molecules on the endothelium.[53,54] Studies have demonstrated that monocyte adhesion can be affected by the hemodynamic environment. Low shear stress regions tend to increase monocyte adhesion, which correlates with areas of atherosclerosis.[37] Recent studies in our laboratory have shown that monocyte adhesion is enhanced proximal to a thoracic aortic coarctation (lesion-prone) as compared to the distal aorta (lesion-resistant) in a hypercholesterolemic rabbit model.[55] An ex vivo study of endothelial cells suggests that vascular cell adhesion molecule-1 (VCAM-1) is down-regulated with increasing shear stress.[56] Oxidized LDL enhances monocyte adhesion and enhances intercellular adhesion molecule (ICAM) upregulation in the presence of elevated shear stress, suggesting that hemodynamic factors may act along with other mediators in early atherogenesis.[57] Thinning of the glycocalyx at the endothelial membrane and increased monocyte adhesion with an intact endothelium has been noted, leading to conjecture that frictional forces at the glycocalyx can alter flow sensors.[58] This may lend credibility to the hypothesis that the hemodynamic environment can alter monocyte adhesion.

Plaque Localization

Atherosclerotic arterial degeneration involves many components and interactions including genetic and environmental factors. Artery wall responses are important in atherosclerosis, including endothelial and medial smooth muscle cell responses and interactions with blood-borne elements such as monocytes, leukocytes, and platelets. Atherosclerotic lesions are focal, and clinical disease is due to localized plaque complications such as thrombosis, plaque rupture, ulceration, or embolization. Hemodynamic factors are important determinants of plaque localization as well as artery adaptive responses and are likely to be important in influencing plaque complications and clinical consequences.

Human Carotid Bifurcation

Atherosclerotic plaques are particularly prone to form in the proximal internal carotid artery. Correlative studies of plaque localization in the human carotid bifurcation with quantitative flow model studies have demonstrated that intimal plaques form in the low shear stress region of the carotid sinus opposite the flow divider and not in the high shear stress region along the inner wall of the internal carotid artery.[2,7] Utilizing measurements on pressure-fixed vessels, the axial and circumferential location of intimal thickening was determined in a series of human carotid bifurcations obtained at autopsy.[2] Intimal thickening and plaque formation was greatest at the outer wall of the proximal segment and sinus of the internal carotid artery beginning at the origin of the vessel from the common carotid artery (Figure 4). Hemodynamic determinations were made in comparable glass scale models of the carotid bifurcation, which permitted qualitative

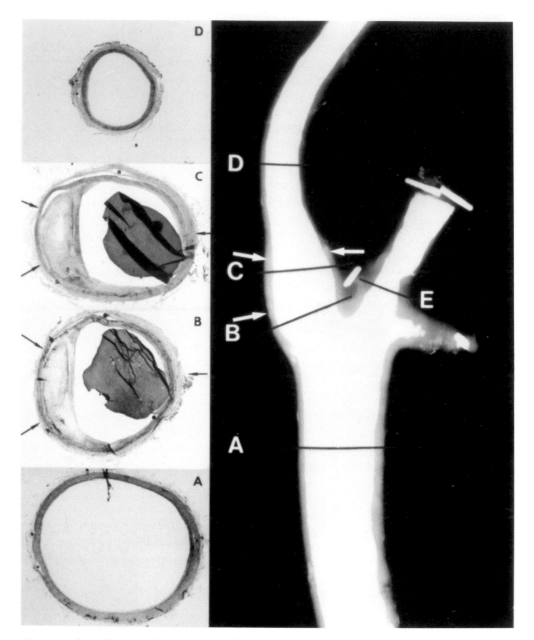

Figure 4. Localization of plaques at the human carotid bifurcation. Postmortem radiograph of a pressure-fixed human carotid bifurcation from an asymptomatic patient is shown at right. Lumen is regular and widened at the sinus. **Single white arrow** indicates the flow-divider side, while the **two white arrows** indicate the lateral wall opposite the flow divider. Sections shown to the left of the radiograph reveal well-developed atherosclerotic plaques at lateral wall (**two black arrows**), but little or no plaque at the flow-divider side (**single black arrow**). Proximal sinus (level **B**) and middle sinus (level **C**) demonstrate significant atherosclerosis, but the common carotid (level **A**) and the distal internal artery (level **D**) are spared. At all levels, lumen is circular and regular, and fibrous plaques are intact. (Adapted with permission from Reference 2.)

visualization and quantitative measurement and characterization of the flow field. Maximal intimal thickening, in autopsy specimens, occurred at the lateral wall which correlated with the region of flow separation, and formation of complex flow patterns and vortices. Along the inner wall of the carotid sinus, on the flow-

divider side, flow remained laminar and intimal thickening was minimal. Quantitative assessment of the flow field by laser-Doppler anemometry demonstrated that wall shear stress was lowest on the outer wall where intimal thickening was greatest.[2] Under conditions of pulsatile flow, oscillations in the direction of flow occurred along the outer wall of the carotid sinus in the region of flow separation and secondary vortex formation.[6] A reversal in shear stress direction occurred just after peak systole, and oscillatory shear stress was attenuated during diastole. Flow remained unidirectional with no oscillation of shear along the inner wall divider of the carotid artery. This was an area where plaque did not form.[59]

A number of field flow alterations have been implicated in plaque localization. These flow field changes are particularly prominent in the carotid bifurcation because of the widened area of the internal carotid sinus, and this may account for the vulnerability of this site to atherosclerosis. The carotid sinus has twice the cross-sectional area of the distal internal carotid artery, and this disparity, together with the effects of branching and angulation, results in a large area of flow separation and

stasis along the outer wall of the carotid sinus (Figure 5). Flow visualization studies demonstrate that flow streamlines are compressed toward the flow divider and inner wall of the internal carotid artery where flow is rapid, shear stress is high, and plaques tend not to form. There is flow reversal on the outer wall, which is not simply a zone of stasis and recirculation, but one of complex secondary patterns, including counter rotating helical trajectories (Figure 6).[2] The flow streamlines reattach distally in the carotid sinus and in the distal internal carotid, which are almost always free of plaque.

In phantoms, particles of dye are carried rapidly along the inner wall, but are cleared very slowly from the outer region of flow separation. Particles in the region of flow separation have increased particle residence time and, therefore, greater opportunity to interact with the vessel wall. Time-dependent lipid particle-vessel wall

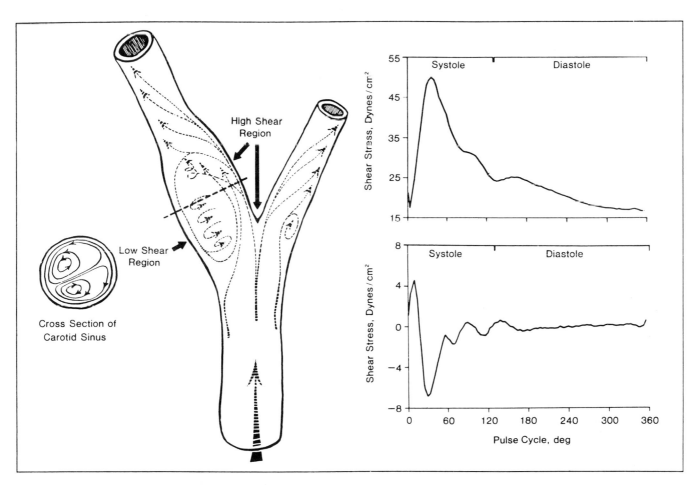

Figure 5. **Left**: Diagrammatic representation of flow features in a carotid bifurcation. Region of flow separation with formation of secondary vortices is present at low shear position at the lateral wall of internal carotid artery. Flow remains relatively laminar and mainly unidirectional at high shear flow-divider side. **Right**: Graphs show changes in wall shear stress in course of the cardiac cycle for the flow-divider region (**upper graph**) and for lateral wall (**lower graph**). The shear stress in the flow-divider side varies and remains unidirectional, but at the lateral wall where plaques form shear stress is low and there are oscillations in the direction of shear. Variations are marked during systole. (Adapted with permission from Reference 7.)

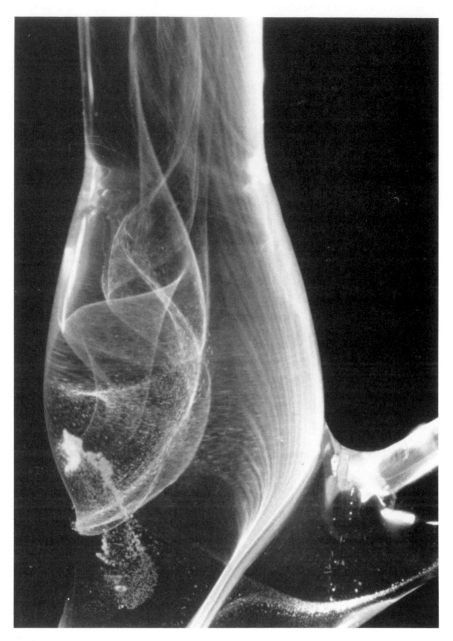

Figure 6A. Glass model of human carotid bifurcation. Hydrogen bubbles are generated in common carotid segment at wire oriented in plane of bifurcation angle. Under conditions of steady flow, there is flow stagnation and increased particle residence time at the lateral wall of sinus opposite flow divider.

interactions would, thus, be facilitated in the slow flow region, making it more likely for plaque to occur. Flow separation and low shear have been shown to favor deposition of platelets, monocytes, and granulocytes which may stimulate cell proliferation and induce intimal thickening and plaque formation.[60–62]

Coronary Arteries

Plaques are focal and tend to localize at branch points just distal to the bifurcation of the left main coronary artery into the LAD and circumflex. This is a region which is thought to experience relatively low blood flow velocity and low and oscillating shear stress,[63] hemodynamic conditions similar to the lesion-prone region of the carotid bifurcation. Angiographic studies of the right coronary artery have provided further evidence of the positive relationship between low shear and plaque formation.[64] A recent study suggested that focal low shear stress in the coronary artery tree correlates with progression of atherosclerosis.[65] Quantitative coronary angiography was obtained in

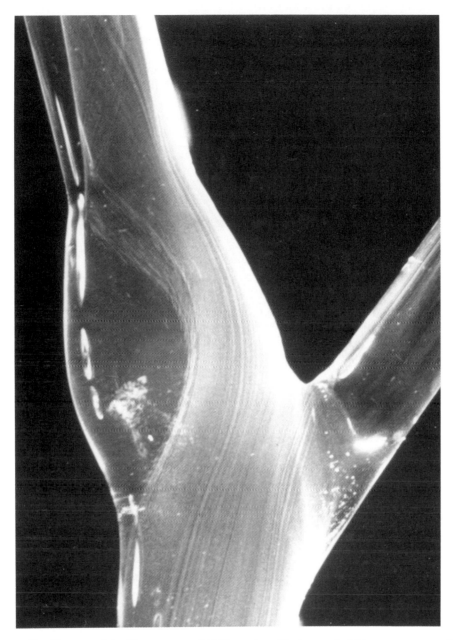

Figure 6B. Glass model of human carotid bifurcation. Hydrogen bubbles are generated in common carotid segment at wire oriented in plane of bifurcation angle. Under conditions of pulsatile flow, complex vortices are evident at lateral walls of sinus of internal carotid in the low shear separation region. At flow-divider side, flow remains laminar. (Adapted with permission from References 2 and 6.)

human subjects to calculate the change in arterial diameter over a 3-year period. When video imaging and finite-difference techniques were used to calculate shear stress in the original angiograms, there was a strong correlation between low shear stress and reduction of arterial diameter in the follow-up angiograms.

Frequently, the coronary arteries are extensively involved with atherosclerosis, whereas arteries with less complex flow, such as the renal and visceral arter-

ies, tend to be spared significant disease except at the ostia.[66,67] Hemodynamic factors, notably oscillatory shear stress and heart rate, have been implicated in the particular vulnerability of the coronary artery. The coronary arteries are subjected to two systolic phases and one diastolic flow episode during each cardiac cycle,[68] thus potentially placing them at greater risk than systemic arteries to atherosclerosis. Shear stress oscillation is directly influenced by heart rate since at higher heart rates, coronary arteries are exposed to more episodes of oscillatory shear stress.

An increase in mean heart rate, from 70 to 80 beats per minute, would result in an increase of approximately 5 million heart beats per year. The duration of the systolic phase is generally constant for varying heart rates, whereas the duration of the diastolic phase shortens with increasing heart rates.[69] At higher heart rates, the coronary arteries experience a larger percentage of time in systole, when they are exposed to oscillatory flow, than in diastole when steady flow conditions prevail. Experimental reduction in heart rate by sinoatrial ablation in cynomolgus monkeys[70] resulted in a 20% reduction in mean heart rate and a reduction in the magnitude of heart rate fluctuation. After 6 months on an atherogenic diet, animals with the lower heart rate had a 50% reduction in coronary plaque area, a 50% reduction in maximum lesion size, and a 50% reduction in percent stenosis compared to animals with a high heart rate. The evidence from this study indicated that reducing heart rate retards experimental plaque formation.

A number of prospective clinical trials have demonstrated that heart rate is a strong independent risk factor in human coronary artery disease.[71] High heart rates are predictive of future coronary atherosclerosis, and conversely, low heart rates are protective against the disease. Increased resting heart rate is associated with an atherogenic lipid profile in sedentary men, suggesting that the effect of heart rate on coronary artery disease may be mediated by alterations in metabolic pathways.[72] Thus, both theoretical and experimental data suggest that hemodynamic factors associated with cyclic myocardial contraction are associated with coronary artery disease. The effect of heart rate on atherosclerosis is not limited to the coronary arteries; studies have shown that high heart rates are also associated with carotid artery atherosclerosis.[73,74]

The Aorta

The infrarenal abdominal aorta is a preferential site for atherosclerosis, and this may be related to hemodynamic influences. The infrarenal abdominal aorta may be susceptible to early atherosclerotic disease because of the low flow velocities in this area compared to flow in the suprarenal portion. One quarter of the cardiac output is delivered to the renal arteries at rest.[75] The renal, celiac, and superior mesenteric arteries divert a significant percentage of flow from the proximal aorta, leaving the quantity of infrarenal blood flow greatly dependent on the muscular activity of the lower extremities. Recent flow visualization studies of the human abdominal aorta and its visceral branches have been utilized to assess the flow patterns above

and below the renal arteries.[76–78] In the lesion-prone infrarenal segment, there were vortices, increased particle residence time, flow reversal, stagnation and oscillating shear under rest, and postprandial simulations, particularly along the posterior wall. These hemodynamic profiles correlate with findings of early disease in the infrarenal abdominal aorta of pathologic specimens.[79] In contrast, these complex flow patterns were not seen in the suprarenal aorta. Under simulated exercise conditions, the flow in the infrarenal portion increased significantly. The complex flow patterns largely disappeared and were replaced by predominantly uniform laminar flow. The beneficial effects of exercise may be partly related to these hemodynamic modifications.

The curvature of the abdominal aorta may add to the flow separation seen in the infrarenal segment. The governing effects of the centrifugal forces to the viscous flow is described by the Dean number, $D = 4Re(d/R)^{1/2}$, where R is the radius of curvature. An increase in the Dean number generally indicates an increase in secondary flow for fully developed flow; however, at higher Reynolds numbers, the arc length of the infrarenal segment may be too short to permit development of curvature effects. Vessel curvature tends to displace the point of maximal axial velocity outwards and to decrease the shear stress along the inner curve.[80] Because there is anterior-posterior curvature of the abdominal aorta, it would be expected that there would be increased flow reversal and particle residence time along the posterior wall (inner curve) of the abdominal aorta.[77] This region of oscillatory shear and long particle residence time (posterior wall) approximately corresponds to the locations where lesions have been found in aortas from young individuals.[79,81]

The geometric conditions at the aortic bifurcation are somewhat analogous to that of the carotid bifurcation. Atherosclerosis at the aortic bifurcation is common and preferentially localized to the lateral walls opposite the central flow divider. Correlation of intimal thickening, flow characteristics, and plaque localization have been carried out using fixed postmortem human abdominal aortic bifurcations.[4,78] Flow separation was noted along the lateral walls of the aortic bifurcation in a cast of the abdominal aorta.[78] Retrograde flow was noted during the diastolic phase in the iliac arteries. Morphologic studies have also shown that plaques tend to form at the ostia of the major visceral branches, typically occurring at the inlet or proximal rim of the orifice and not at the distal edge of the flow divider.[3,82,83] However, the infrarenal aorta is significantly more susceptible to atherosclerosis than its major visceral branches.[67,83] Ultrasound examination of canine renal arteries suggests that there is separation of flow, low shear stress, and oscillatory shear stress at the cranial portion of the ostium of the renal artery.[84]

This study demonstrates that the flow is laminar and parabolic four diameters from the inlet to the renal artery, and it has been shown in autopsies that atherosclerotic lesions are prone to develop within 1 to 2 cm from the renal ostia.[66]

Turbulence

Turbulence is random or disordered flow produced by irregularities of the flow surface and by stenoses, and can occur at very high flow velocities. Direct evidence implicating turbulence in atherosclerosis is lacking. Experimental and theoretical models also fail to support the suggestion that turbulent flow is an independent risk factor for atherosclerotic plaque deposition. In monkeys, there was a twofold increase in turbulence velocity distal to a hemodynamically significant aortic coarctation in the area of post-stenotic dilatation.[85] When coarcted monkeys were fed an atherogenic diet, intimal plaque formed proximal to the coarct, but was inhibited distal to the stenosis in the region of higher turbulence, suggesting an inverse relationship between turbulence intensity and intimal plaque deposition.[86] In a separate study, lipid deposition was decreased distal to a stenotic rat caudal artery.[87] In the carotid bifurcation, glass models demonstrated zones of complex and secondary flow patterns but no evidence of turbulence.[6,88,89] No turbulence was present in the carotid bifurcation in normal human volunteers who underwent ultrasound examination.[59] These data suggest that turbulence is probably not a factor in atherosclerotic plaque formation, and that any turbulence in severe carotid stenosis may be a result of the stenosis rather than a cause of it.

Hypertension

Epidemiologic and postmortem studies have suggested that hypertension is associated with an increase in the severity of atherosclerosis.[90-93] Recent clinical trials have demonstrated an association between borderline hypertension and coronary artery disease.[94] Hypertension is a more important factor in cerebrovascular disease than in coronary artery and peripheral occlusive disease. The sites of atherosclerosis are typically in locations already predisposed to plaque formation; however, lesion-resistant arteries may form plaque in the presence of hypertension. For example, the pulmonary arteries are typically free of atherosclerotic disease, but in these arteries plaque may be seen in humans with pulmonary hypertension.[66]

There have been some explanations for the mechanism underlying the potentiation of atherogenesis by hypertension, but overall the mechanism is unknown. Several investigators have suggested that factors associated with hypertension may result in vascular injuries.[12,86,91-93] These include direct mechanical disruptive effects, actions on vasoactive hormones, effects of sodium influx, changes in blood rheology, and alterations in wall composition. Changes in wall metabolism and possible injury to the wall by angiotensin II are other described etiologic factors. Other changes noted in hypertensive animal models include endothelial cell changes, increased endothelial permeability, increased leukocyte adherence, smooth muscle cell proliferation, increased smooth muscle cell DNA, and intimal thickening.[95] Thickening of the arterial media is probably secondary to increased wall tension.[12] It is thought that although hypertension may potentiate or enhance atherogenesis, hypertension alone is probably not sufficient for atherogenesis.

When hypertension was induced in cynomolgus monkeys by the creation of mid-thoracic coarctations, there was increased atherosclerosis proximal to the coarctation, but decreased plaque distal to the coarctation (Figure 7). Both the proximal and distal aortic segments were exposed to hypertension since the aortic stenosis proximal to the renal arteries resulted in elevated renin production.[86,93] Other hemodynamic factors that may explain the difference between the proximal and distal aortic plaque deposition include pulse pressure, wall tension, and wall motion.[26] Inhibition of plaque, despite the presence of hypertension and marked hyperlipidemia, may be due to decreased pulse pressure and wall motion, and decreased arterial wall metabolism. Experimental findings suggest that hemodynamic factors other than hypertension may also be important in plaque pathogenesis. However, hypertension appears to enhance coronary artery plaque progression despite reduction of hypercholesterolemia in experimental animals.[96] The precise relationship and role of hypertension in plaque formation has yet to be elucidated.

Anatomy

Even though atherosclerosis is a generalized disease, the clinical manifestations are usually related to focal disease. The anatomic variants of blood vessels are known to alter the local hemodynamic environment and, consequently, may affect plaque pathogenesis. One study demonstrated that short left main coronary arteries favored proximal localization of coronary artery stenoses.[97] Diseased coronary arteries tended to favor a wider bifurcation angle of the LAD and circumflex arteries, but this tendency was not statistically significant. In a review of 100 consecutive abdominal aortograms, there was an average aortic bifurcation angle of 38° in those patients with occlusive disease and an average bifurcation angle of 52° in patients with normal or aneurysmal disease.[98]

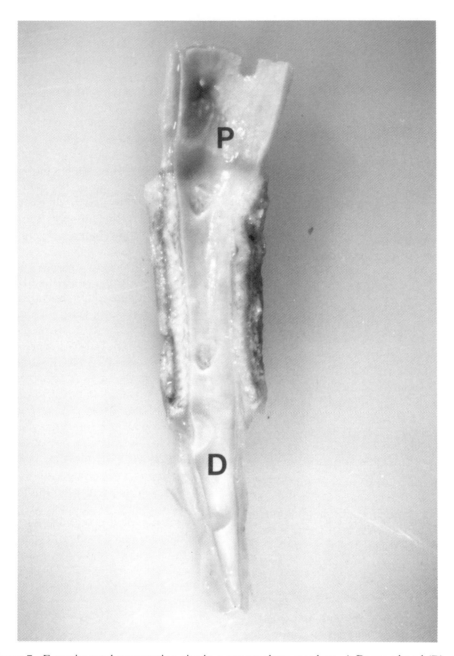

Figure 7. Experimental coarctation site in a cynomolgus monkey. A Dacron band (**D**) was wrapped around the aorta to cause a 50% luminal diameter reduction (75% cross-sectional area reduction). After 6 months on an atherogenic diet, the coarctation channel (high shear stress region) showed no evidence of endothelial damage or significant plaque deposition. However, in the hypertensive region proximal (**P**) to the coarctation, there was prominent plaque formation with reduction in atherosclerosis in the distal (D) segment. (Adapted with permission from Reference 136.)

Glass models of the aortic bifurcation were constructed with varying angles at the bifurcation, and the shear stress was calculated at the inner and outer walls.[98] The data from this experiment suggest that shear stress on the lateral wall correlates with increasing bifurcation angle and that there is a negative correlation between shear stress on the flow-divider side and bifurcation angle. It was also noted that the aortic

bifurcation takeoff was typically higher in patients with occlusive atherosclerotic disease. However, it is known that the aorta elongates with age and becomes more tortuous. The aortorenal angle did not have a significant impact on the blood flow velocities in ultrasound studies of the canine renal artery.[84] Increased recirculation and flow reversal were noted in a numerical simulation of the carotid artery bifurcation for geometries in which the carotid sinus was relatively wider.[99]

Hemodynamic Changes Associated with Stenoses

The hemodynamic and arterial changes attributed to a stenotic vessel can be significant. Plaques may initially develop fine luminal irregularities corresponding to the contours of subendothelial foam cells.[100] These irregular surfaces may cause focal flow disturbances and disrupt the endothelial cells, allowing penetration of foam cells. These flow disturbances, such as oscillatory shear stress, may favor accumulation of monocytes and platelets over surface interruptions.[101] Plaque enlargement occurs with accumulation of fibrin, and foam cells stimulate smooth muscle proliferation.[102] As plaques enlarge, the artery wall attempts to preserve the circular contour of the lumen by medial smooth muscle proliferation, matrix fiber synthesis, and formation of a fibrous cap.[16] The lumen surface tends to remain concave, whereas the arterial wall beneath the plaque bulges outward. As the plaque progresses, the geometric changes may predispose the vessel to flow instabilities, turbulence, and vibrations.

Most plaques in humans are eccentric, which results in field flow changes distal to a stenosis. These field flows may be altered with differing geometries of the stenotic regions.[103] There may be hemodynamic conditions distal to a stenosis favoring wall collapse with a decrease in lumen diameter. These factors may be partially responsible for the creation of stresses that lead to atherosclerotic plaque fracture, distal embolization, and post-stenotic dilatation.[104] Numerical simulations of pulsatile flow in an eccentrically constricted vessel predicted that the oscillatory shear is large, taking large positive and negative values, with peak shear stress highest for pulsatile flow distal to the stenosis.[105] The shear stress is complex, with eddies and reversed flow. This simulation showed that if there is a constriction or plaque on one side of the vessel, there will be flow separation immediately distal to the stenosis.

Our group performed thoracic aortic coarctations on cynomolgus monkeys that were fed an atherogenic diet.[31] Monkeys were separated into groups based on the type of constriction: circumferential banding, lateral plication, and combination of banding and plication. The lateral plication group showed plaque deposition immediately distal to the coarct on the side of the plication, as suggested by the numerical simulation. Plaque deposition was decreased immediately distal to the circumferential banding coarct. Some atherosclerosis was present further distal to the coarct, but was less than in the proximal segment. Using ultrasound, flow separation and systolic flow reversal were demonstrated immediately distal to coronary artery stenotic lesions.[106] Given that there are flow disturbances immediately distal to a coarct or stenosis, it is difficult to fully explain the decreased atherosclerosis in this location.

In our monkey model, atherosclerosis progressed with increasing distance from the coarctation, strongly suggesting that alterations in flow field are associated with plaque formation.[31] In another study of atherosclerosis in hypercholesterolemic monkeys who underwent aortic coarctation, an increase in plaque area was present distal to a mild or subcritical stenosis, in contrast to the presence of decreased plaque formation distal to a severe stenosis.[86] Subcritical stenosis represents about a 50% area reduction at the mid-thoracic aorta with no pressure gradient. Proximal to the coarctation, a tendency toward increased lesion severity was noted, but it was not statistically significant. The distal sites included the thoracic and abdominal aorta, indicating that hemodynamic effects are important far away from a stenosis. It is interesting to note that artery stenosis seemed to inhibit regression of diet-induced atherosclerosis when the diet was changed from hypercholesterolemic to normocholesterolemic.[107] Even without a pressure gradient, there may be modifications of the distal flow and boundary conditions.[105,108] Flow characteristics using laser-Doppler anemometry on plexiglass models of stenoses were studied by Giddens' group. They demonstrated that shear stress is low distal to the coarctation, but quite high in the throat of a stenosis. For moderate to severe stenoses, discrete frequency velocity oscillations were noted downstream from the constriction, but the degree of disorder gradually decreased distally.[108,109] Turbulence was noted only in the severe constriction model and was only present for a segment of the flow cycle.

Regulation of the Size of the Arterial Lumen

As plaques enlarge, arteries undergo enlargement and tend to conserve lumen diameter.[110] Studies on the coronary arteries of perfusion-fixed hearts have shown that the area delineated by the internal elastic lamina enlarges as plaque area increases.[111,112] The effective luminal area is maintained up to a certain point of plaque progression. The data from these studies suggest that the luminal area only decreases when plaque cross-sectional area exceeds 40% of the area encompassed by the internal elastic lamina (Figure 8). Some of the proposed mechanisms include direct effects of the enlarging plaque on the subjacent wall or effects of altered flow on the opposite wall. Outward extension of the artery wall beneath the plaque may be attributed

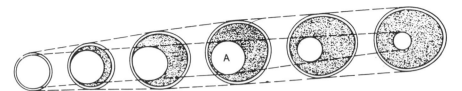

Figure 8. Diagrammatic representation of possible sequence of changes in atherosclerotic arteries leading eventually to lumen narrowing. The artery enlarges initially (**left to right**) as a response to enlarging plaque to maintain a normal lumen size. Early stages of lesion formation may be associated with overcompensation. At more than 40% stenosis, however, the plaque area continues to increase to involve the entire circumference of the vessel, and the artery no longer enlarges at a rate sufficient to prevent narrowing of the lumen. (Adapted with permission from Reference 111.)

to atrophy or degeneration of the arterial wall secondary to compression or inhibition of diffusion of certain nutrients.[16] Another possibility is that the connective tissue matrix may be degraded by enzymes.[112]

The arterial wall may circumferentially extend in response to the development of the enlarging plaque. This reaction may occur because of the increased flow velocity expected with narrowing of the lumen. Increased flow that occurs proximal to an arteriovenous (AV) fistula results in enlargement of the vessel diameter, whereas decreased flow may result in narrowing of the diameter by intimal thickening.[114–116] A quantitative study to determine the enlargement of the cynomolgus monkey iliac artery proximal to an AV fistula found that artery diameter increased with increased flow (Figure 9). This study suggests that this process occurs to normalize wall shear stress, because at the end of a 6-month period there was no difference in the shear stress between the control iliac arteries and those with fistulas. Although wall shear stress was calculated to be approximately 100 dynes/cm^2 for the newly created AV fistulas, 6 months after the operation shear stress proved to be about 15 dynes/cm^2 for both the control arteries and the AV fistula. This is the same level of shear stress as reported for normal arteries of several mammals.[114] Removal of the endothelium inhibited this adaptive enlargement to increased shear stress, demonstrating the importance of the endothelium in regulating vessel size.[117] In the monkey AV fistula study, no increase in intimal thickness or plaque deposition occurred in the vessels subjected to higher flow.[116] Other studies on development of atherosclerosis in AV fistula models have demonstrated both lower[118] and increased[119,120] atherosclerosis.

Hemodynamics Associated with Anastomoses

Intimal thickening is a normal healing response of arteries at graft anastomoses. However, progression of this response can lead to a hyperplastic occlusive lesion at the anastomotic graft site. Mechanisms postulated to cause this thickening include platelet activation,[121] injury,[122] cell migration, and extracellular matrix deposition,[123] and hemodynamic modifications.[124–126] Intimal thickening has been shown to be inversely correlated with shear stress and directly correlated with oscillatory shear[7] at arterial branch points and experimental stenoses. The anastomotic geometry engenders alterations in flow dynamics, wall shear, and wall tension which may play an important role in anastomotic intimal hyperplasia.

Vein and polytetrafluoroethylene (PTFE) end-to-side grafts implanted in dogs demonstrated suture-line thickening, particularly in the PTFE groups. There was also thickening on the floor of the artery in both the vein and PTFE groups.[124] Model flow visualization demonstrated flow stagnation, and low and oscillatory shear at the artery floor (Figure 10).[124–127] High shear and short particle residence time were noted at the hood of the graft where little intimal thickening occurred. The suture-line intimal thickening could be related to compliance mismatch, but there are conflicting data on this subject.[128] Another study suggested that blood flow in the proximal outflow segment leads to flow separation.[125] However, it is not known if the intimal thickening observed correlates with actual vessel stenosis or occlusion. More research in this area is probably warranted.

Aneurysms

Aneurysms have been associated with atherosclerosis, but the mechanism by which atherosclerosis induces or predisposes aneurysmal dilatation is not clear. A number of causes for aneurysm formation include increased proteolytic enzyme activity[129] (such as increased collagenase or matrix metalloproteinase activity),[130,131] normal trace metabolism,[132] and genetic deficiencies in connective tissue structure.[133] Studies have shown that diet-induced atherosclerosis in mon-

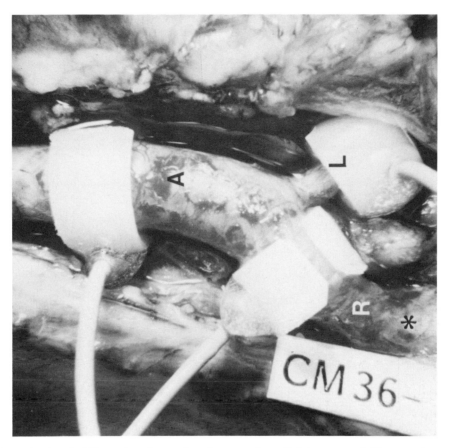

Figure 9. Aortic bifurcation 6 months after creation of right external iliac arteriovenous fistula. Electromagnetic flow probes are on the distal aorta (**A**), right (**R**), and left (**L**) common iliac arteries. Note enlarged right external iliac artery because of increased blood flow secondary to the fistula. **Asterisk** denotes the location of the arteriovenous fistula.

keys increases the incidence of aneurysm formation, with regression of plaque formation a particular risk factor for aneurysm formation.[134,135] Thinning of the media with atrophy and loss of architecture was noted in these experiments. The abdominal aorta suffered aneurysmal disease more than the thoracic aorta, possibly because fewer lamellar units are present in the abdominal aorta as compared to the thoracic aorta.[136] Proportionately, the thoracic aorta contains more elastin and less collagen than the abdominal aorta.[11] Pulse pressure is greater in the abdominal aorta than in the thoracic aorta which may lead to altered smooth muscle cell metabolism and increased plaque deposition. The outer two thirds of the thoracic aorta media is supplied by intramural vasa vasorum, whereas the abdominal aorta is devoid of vasa vasorum. The abdominal aorta would appear to be at a greater risk for intimal plaque deposition, which increases wall thickness and increases the diffusion distance from the lumen, promoting lipid trapping and media atrophy.

Hypertension is a well-known risk factor for aneurysm formation. Thinning of the media and dilation of

the arteries increase tensile stress. Weakening of the aortic wall by media destruction predisposes aortas to dilatation, ectasia, and aneurysm formation in relation to circumferential tensile stress. The fibrotic plaque in atherosclerosis may not be strong enough to support the weakened media. In cases of diet-induced regression, the fibrotic cap would recede. The resultant persistently weakened media would be susceptible to an increased incidence of aneurysms, as demonstrated in a monkey atherosclerosis model.[129] In human aneurysms, there is effacement of the normal lamellar structure,[136] with atrophic changes over the atherosclerotic plaque. These data suggest that hemodynamics, atherosclerosis, and aortic wall morphology are important in aneurysm formation.

Conclusion

Hemodynamic effects on the blood vessel wall are numerous and have been shown to correlate with atherosclerosis. As technology advances, we will be able

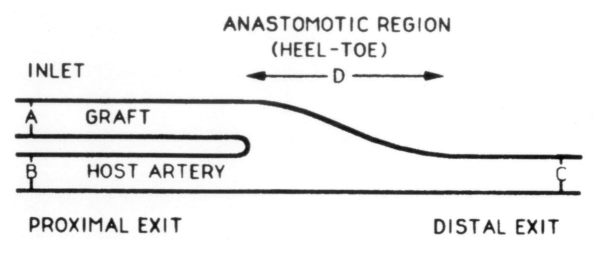

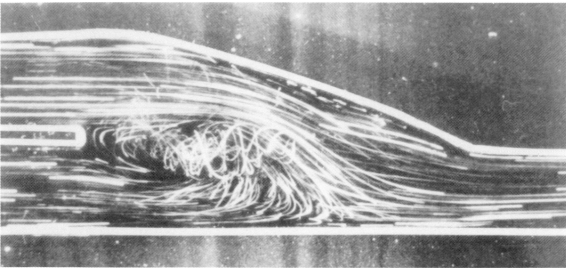

Figure 10. Model flow visualization study of an end-to-side anastomosis. **Top**: Diagrammatic representation of an end-to-side anastomosis. **Bottom**: Neutrally buoyant particles are illuminated in the pulsatile flow field by use of helium-neon laser sheet of light. A vortex is noted near the proximal outflow tract which started near the heel. (Adapted with permission from Reference 123.)

to better characterize the plaque composition, lumen and vessel wall changes, and the associated field flow modifications. The hemodynamic consequences of therapeutic interventions such as angioplasty, intra-arterial stent placement, surgical revascularization, and endarterectomy are important and may dictate the success of these procedures. Endothelial and medial responses to an altered hemodynamic environment are complicated, and the understanding of these mechanisms will require an interdisciplinary approach. Further research in the areas of cell biology, physiology, molecular biology, pathology, and fluid dynamics is essential to enhancing our knowledge in this area and integrating this knowledge into our understanding of the disease process.

References

1. Cornhill JF, Roach MR: A quantitative study of the localization of atherosclerotic lesions in the rabbit aorta. *Atherosclerosis* 23:489–501, 1976.
2. Zarins CK, Giddens DP, Bharadvaj, et al: Carotid bifurcation atherosclerosis: quantitative correlation of plaque localization with velocity profiles and wall shear stress. *Circ Res* 53:502–514, 1983.
3. Caro CG, Fitzgerald JM, Schroter RC: Arterial wall shear and distribution of early atheroma in man. *Nature* 223:1159–1161, 1969.
4. Friedman MH, Hutchins GM, Bargeron CB, et al: Correlation between intimal thickness and fluid shear in human arteries. *Atherosclerosis* 39:425–436, 1981.
5. Fox JA, Hugh AE: Static zones in the internal carotid artery: correlation with boundary layer separation and stasis model flows. *Br J Radiol* 43:370–376, 1976.

6. Ku DN, Giddens DP: Pulsatile flow in a model carotid bifurcation. *Arteriosclerosis* 3:31–39, 1983.

7. Ku DN, Giddens DP, Zarins CK, Glagov S: Pulsatile flow and atherosclerosis in the human carotid bifurcation: positive correlation between plaque location and low and oscillating shear stress. *Arteriosclerosis* 5: 293–302, 1985.

8. Davies PF, Remuzzi A, Gordon EJ, et al: Turbulent fluid shear stress induces vascular cell turnover in vitro. *Proc Natl Acad Sci USA* 83:2114–2117, 1986.

9. Gutstein WH, Farrell GA, Armellini C: Blood flow disturbance and endothelial cell injury in pre-atherosclerotic swine. *Lab Inves* 29:134–149, 1973.

10. Wolinsky H, Glagov S: Structural basis for the static mechanical properties of the aortic media. *Circ Res* 14: 400–413, 1964.

11. Clark JM, Glagov S: Transmural organization of the arterial wall: the lamellar unit revisited. *Arteriosclerosis* 5:19–34, 1985.

12. Wolinsky H: Long-term effects of hypertension on the rat aortic wall and their relation to concurrent aging changes. *Circ Res* 30:301–309, 1972.

13. Burton AC: Relation of structure to function of the tissues of the wall of blood vessels. *Physiol Rev* 34: 619–642, 1954.

14. Glagov S, Wolinsky H: Aortic wall as a "two-phase" material. *Nature* 199:606–608, 1963.

15. Roach MR, Burton AC: The reason for the shape of the distensibility curves of arteries. *Can J Biochem Physiol* 35:681–690, 1957.

16. Glagov S, Zarins CK, Giddens DP, Ku DN: Hemodynamics and atherosclerosis: insights and perspectives gained from studies of human arteries. *Arch Pathol Lab Med* 112:1018–1031, 1988.

17. Stary HC, Blackenhorn DH, Chandler AB, et al: A definition of the intima of human arteries and of its atherosclerosis-prone regions. *Arterioscler Thromb* 11: 120–134, 1992.

18. Friedman MH, Bargeron CB, Mark FF: Variability of geometry, hemodynamics, and intimal response of human arteries. *Monogr Arterioscler* 15:109–116, 1990.

19. Caro CG, Lever MJ, Laver-Rudich Z, et al: Net albumin transport across the wall of the rabbit common carotid artery perfused in-situ. *Atherosclerosis* 37: 497–511, 1980.

20. Weinbaum S, Caro CG: A macromolecule transport model for the arterial wall and endothelium, based on the ultrastructural specialization observed in electron microscopic studies. *J Fluid Mech* 74:611–640, 1976.

21. Newman DL, Lallemand RC: The effect of age on the distensibility of the abdominal aorta in man. *Surg Gynecol Obstet* 147:211–214, 1978.

22. Wolinsky H, Glagov S: Comparison of abdominal and thoracic aortic medial structure in mammals: deviation from the usual pattern in man. *Circ Res* 25:677–686, 1969.

23. Sacks AH: The vasa vasorum as a link between hypertension and arteriosclerosis. *Angiology* 26:385–390, 1975.

24. Holenstein R, Niederer P, Anliker M: A viscoelastic model for use in predicting arterial pulse waves. *J Biomech Eng* 102:318–325, 1980.

25. Leung D, Glagov S, Mathew MB: Cyclic stretching stimulates synthesis of matrix components by arterial smooth muscle cells in vitro. *Science* 191:475–477, 1976.

26. Cozzi PJ, Lyon RT, Davis HR, Sylora J, Glagov S, Zarins CK: Aortic wall metabolism in relation to susceptibility and resistance to experimental atherosclerosis. *J Vasc Surg* 7:706–714, 1988.

27. Thubrikar MJ, Baker JW, Nolan SP: Inhibition of atherosclerosis associated with reduction of arterial intramural stress in rabbits. *Arteriosclerosis* 8:410–420, 1988.

28. Fry DL: Acute vascular endothelial changes associated with increased blood velocity gradients. *Circ Res* 22: 165–197, 1968.

29. Reidy MA, Boyer DE: Scanning electron microscopy of arteries: the morphology of aortic endothelium in hemodynamically stressed areas associated with branches. *Atherosclerosis* 26:181–194, 1977.

30. Reidy MA: Biology of disease: a reassessment of endothelial injury and arterial lesion. *Lab Invest* 53:513–520, 1985.

31. Zarins CK, Bomberger RA, Glagov S: Local effects of stenosis: increased flow velocity inhibits atherogenesis. *Circulation* (suppl II)64:221–227, 1981.

32. Campbell GR, Campbell JH: Smooth muscle cell phenotypic changes in arterial wall homeostasis: implications for the pathogenesis of atherosclerosis. *Exp Mol Pathol* 42:139–162, 1985.

33. Levesque MJ, Liepsch D, Moravec S, Nerem RM: Correlation of endothelial cell shape and wall shear stress in a stenosed dog aorta. *Arteriosclerosis* 6:220–229, 1986.

34. Silkworth JB, Stehbens WE: The shape of endothelial cells in en face preparation of rabbit blood vessels. *Angiology* 26:474–487, 1975.

35. Dewey CF, Bussolari SR, Gimbrone MA, Davies PF: The dynamic response of vascular endothelial cells to fluid shear stress. *J Biomech Eng* 103:177–185, 1981.

36. Walpola PL, Gotlieb AI, Langille BL: Monocyte adhesion and changes in endothelial cell number, morphology, and F-actin distribution elicited by low shear stress in vivo. *Am J Pathol* 142:1392–1400, 1993.

37. Lewis JC, Taylor RG, Jones ND, et al: Endothelial surface characteristics in pigeon coronary artery atherosclerosis. I. Cellular alterations during the initial stages of dietary cholesterol challenge. *Lab Invest* 46:133–138, 1982.

38. Sprague EA, Steinbach BL, Nerem RM, Schwartz CJ: Influence of a laminar steady-state fluid-imposed wall shear stress on the binding, internalization, and degradation of low density lipoproteins by cultured arterial endothelium. *Circulation* 76:648–656, 1987.

39. Okano M, Yoshida Y: Endothelial cell morphometry of atherosclerotic lesions and flow profiles at aortic bifurcations in cholesterol fed rabbits. *J Biomech Eng* 114: 301–308, 1992.

40. Sato M, Levesque MJ, Nerem RM: Micropipette aspiration of cultured bovine aortic endothelial cells exposed to shear stress. *Arteriosclerosis* 7:276–286, 1987.

41. Hsieh HJ, Li NQ, Frangos JA: Pulsatile and steady flow induces c-fos expression in human endothelial cells. *J Cell Physiol* 154:143–151, 1993.

42. Caplan BA, Schwartz CJ: Increased endothelial cell turnover in areas of in-vivo Evans Blue uptake in the pig aorta. *Atherosclerosis* 17:401–417, 1973.

43. Goode TB, Davies PF, Reidy MA, Bowyer DE: Aortic endothelial cell morphology observed in situ scanning electron microscopy during atherogenesis in the rabbit. *Atherosclerosis* 27:235–251, 1977.

44. Nollert MU, Eskin SG, McIntire LV: Shear stress increases inositol triphosphate levels in human endothe-

lial cells. *Biochem Biophys Res Comm* 170:281–287, 1990.

45. Mo M, Eskin SG, Schilling WP: Flow-induced changes in Ca^{2+} signaling of vascular endothelial cells: effect of shear stress and ATP. *Am J Physiol* 260:H1698-H1701, 1991.

46. Lansman JB, Hallam TJ, Rink TJ: Single stretch activated ion channels in vascular endothelial cells as mechanotransducers? *Nature* 325:811–813, 1987.

47. Simon MI, Strathmann MP, Gautam N: Diversity of G proteins in signal transduction. *Science* 252:802–808, 1991.

48. Davies PF, Robotewskyj A, Griem ML, et al: Hemodynamic forces and vascular cell communication in arteries. *Arch Pathol Lab Med* 116:1301–1306, 1992.

49. Korenaga R, Ando J, Tsuboi H, Yang W, Sakuma I, Toyo-oka T, Kamiya A: Laminar flow stimulates ATP- and shear stress-dependent nitric oxide production in cultured bovine endothelial cells. *Biochem Biophys Res Comm* 198:213–219, 1994.

50. Ohno M, Gibbons GH, Dzau VJ, Cooke JP: Shear stress elevates endothelial cGMP: role of a potassium channel and G protein coupling. *Circulation* 88: 193–197, 1993.

51. Schultz SE, Klumpp S, Benz R, et al: Regulation of adenylylcyclase from paramecium by an intrinsic potassium conductance. *Science* 255:600–603, 1992,

52. Kubes P, Suzuki M, Granger DN: Nitric oxide: an endogenous modulator of leukocyte adhesion. *Proc Natl Acad Sci USA* 88:4651–4655, 1991.

53. Gerrity RG, Goss JA, Soby L: Control of monocyte recruitment by chemotactic factor(s) in lesion-prone areas of swine aorta. *Arteriosclerosis* 5:55–66, 1985.

54. Cybulski MI, Gimbrone MA Jr: Endothelial expression of a mononuclear leukocyte adhesion molecule in atherogenesis. *Science* 251:788–791, 1991.

55. Tropea BI, Huie P, Cooke JP, et al: Hypertension enhanced monocyte adhesion in experimental atherosclerosis. *J Vasc Surg* (In press.)

56. Ohtsuka A, Ando J, Korenaga R, et al: The effect of flow on the expression of vascular adhesion molecule-1 by cultured mouse endothelial cells. *Biochem Biophys Res Comm* 193:303–310, 1993.

57. Jeng JR, Chang CH, Shieh SM, Chiu HC: Oxidized low-density lipoprotein enhances monocyte-endothelial cell binding against shear-stress-induced detachment. *Biochimicas et Biophysica Acta* 1178:221–227, 1993.

58. Gerrity RG, Naito HK, Richardson M, Schwartz CJ: Dietary induced atherogenesis in swine: morphology of the intima in prelesion stages. *Am J Pathol* 95:775–792, 1979.

59. Ku DN, Giddens DP, Phillips DJ, et al: Hemodynamics of the normal human carotid bifurcation: in vivo and in vitro studies. *Ultrasound Med Biol* 1:13–26, 1985.

60. Schaffner T, Taylor K, Bartucci EJ, et al: Arterial foam cells exhibit distinctive immunomorphologic and histochemical features of macrophages. *Am J Pathol* 100: 57–80, 1980.

61. Parmentier EM, Morton WA, Petschek HE: Platelet aggregate formation in a region of separated blood flow. *Phys Fluids* 20:2012–2021, 1981.

62. Ross R, Harker L: Hyperlipidemia and atherosclerosis. *Science* 193:1094–1100, 1976.

63. Svindland A: The localization of sudanophilic and fibrous plaques in the main left coronary arteries. *Atherosclerosis* 48:139–145, 1983.

64. Sabbah HN, Khaja F, Brymer JF, et al: Blood velocity

in the right coronary artery: relation to the distribution of atherosclerotic lesions. *Am J Cardiol* 53:1008–1012, 1984.

65. Gibson CM, Diaz L, Kandarpa K, et al: Relation of vessel wall shear stress to atherosclerosis progression in human coronary arteries. *Arterioscler Thromb* 13: 310–315, 1993.

66. Glagov S, Ozoa AK: Significance of the relatively low incidence of atherosclerosis in the pulmonary, renal, and mesenteric arteries. *Ann NY Acad Sci* 149:940–955, 1968.

67. Glagov S, Rowley DA, Kohut RI: Atherosclerosis of human aorta and its coronary and renal arteries. *Arch Pathol Lab Med* 72:558–571, 1961.

68. Klocke FJ, Mates RE, Canty JM, et al: Coronary pressure-flow relationships: controversial issues and probable implications. *Circ Res* 56:310–323, 1985.

69. Boudoulas H, Rittgers SE, Lewis RP, et al: Changes in diastolic time with various pharmacologic agents. *Circulation* 60:164–169, 1979.

70. Beere PA, Glagov S, Zarins CK: Retarding effect of lowered heart rate on coronary atherosclerosis. *Science* 226:180–182, 1984.

71. Schroll M, Hagerup LM: Rosk factors of myocardial infarction and death in men aged 50 at entry. *Dan Med Bull* 24:252–255, 1977.

72. Williams PT, Haskell WL, Vranizan KM, et al: Associations of resting heart rate with concentrations of lipoprotein subfractions in sedentary men. *Circulation* 71: 441–449, 1985.

73. Beere PA, Stankunivicius R, Ku DN, et al: Low heart rates retards carotid atherosclerosis (abstr). *Arteriosclerosis* 6:524a, 1986.

74. Kaplan JR, Clarkson TB, Manuck SB: Pathogenesis of carotid bifurcation atherosclerosis in cynomolgus monkeys. *Stroke* 15:994–1000, 1984.

75. Guyton AC: *Textbook of Medical Physiology.* 2nd ed. Philadelphia: WB Saunders, Co; 356, 1961.

76. Ku DN, Glagov S, Moore JE, et al: Flow patterns in the abdominal aorta under simulated postprandial and exercise conditions. *J Vasc Surg* 9:309–316, 1989.

77. Moore JE Jr, Ku DN, Zarins CK, Glagov S: Pulsatile flow visualization in the abdominal aorta under differing physiologic conditions: implications for increased susceptibility to atherosclerosis. *J Biomech Eng* 114: 391–397, 1992.

78. Pedersen EM, Yoganathan AP, Lefebvre XP: Pulsatile flow visualization in a model of the human abdominal aorta and aortic bifurcation. *J Biomech* 25:935–944, 1992.

79. Cornhill JF, Herderick EE: Topographic distribution of human aortic atherosclerosis. *Proceedings of the 40th Annual Conference on Engineering in Medicine and Biology.* Niagara Falls, NY; 229, 1987.

80. Hamakiotes CC, Berger SA: Flow in curved vessels, with application to flow in the aorta and other arteries. *Monogr Atherosclerosis* 15:227–239, 1990.

81. Cornhill JR: Effects of risk factors on the localization of human aortic atherosclerosis. *First World Congress on Biomechanics.* vol 2, 184, 1990.

82. Roberts JC, Moses C, Wilkins RH: Autopsy studies in atherosclerosis: distribution and severity of atherosclerosis in patients dying without morphologic evidence of atherosclerotic catastrophe. *Circulation* 20:511–519, 1959.

83. Roberts JC, Wilkins RH, Moses C: Autopsy studies in atherosclerosis: distribution and severity of atheroscle-

rosis in patients dying with morphologic evidence of atherosclerotic catastrophe. *Circulation* 20:520–526, 1959.

84. Yamamoto T, Tanaka H, Jones CJ, et al: Blood velocity profiles in the origin of the canine renal artery and their relevance in the localization and development of atherosclerosis. *Arterioscler Thromb* 12:626–632, 1992.

85. Giddens DP, Khalifa AMA: Turbulence measurements with pulsed Doppler ultrasound employing a frequency tracking method. *Ultrasound Med Biol* 8:427–437, 1982.

86. Bomberger RA, Zarins CK, Taylor KE, Glagov S: Effect of hypotension on atherogenesis and aortic wall composition. *J Surg Res* 28:402–409, 1980.

87. Coutard M, Osborne-Pellegrin MJ: Decreased dietary lipid deposition in spontaneous lesions distal to a stenosis in the rat caudal artery. *Artery* 12:83–98, 1983.

88. Bharadvaj BK, Mabon RF, Giddens DP: Steady flow in a model of the human carotid bifurcation: II. Doppler anemometer measurements. *J Biomech* 15:363–378, 1982.

89. Bharadvaj BK, Mabon RF, Giddens DP: Steady flow in a model of the human carotid bifurcation: I. Flow visualization. *J Biomech* 15:349–362, 1982.

90. Kannel WB, Schwartz MJ, McNamara PM: Blood pressure and risk of coronary heart disease: the Framingham study. *Dis Chest* 56:43–52, 1969.

91. Bretherton KN, Day AJ, Skinner SL: Hypertension-accelerated atherogenesis in cholesterol-fed rabbits. *Atherosclerosis* 27:79–87, 1977.

92. Chobanian AV: The influence of hypertension and other hemodynamic factors in atherogenesis. *Cardiovasc Dis* 26:177–196, 1983.

93. Hollander W, Prusty S, Kirkpatrick B, Nagraj S: Role of hypertension in ischemic heart disease and cerebral vascular disease in the cynomolgus monkey with coarctation of the aorta. *Circ Res* (suppl I)40:70–83, 1977.

94. Julius S, Jamerson K, Mejia A, et al: The association of borderline hypertension with target organ changes and higher coronary artery risk: Tecumseh blood pressure study. *JAMA* 264:354–358, 1990.

95. Ram CVS: Hypertension and atherosclerosis. *Prim Care* 18:559–575, 1991.

96. Xu C, Glagov S, Zatina MA, Zarins CK: Hypertension sustains plaque progression despite reduction of hypercholesterolemia. *Hypertension* 18:123–129, 1991.

97. Saltissi S, Webb-Peploe MM, Cortart DJ: Effect of variation in coronary artery anatomy on distribution of stenotic lesions. *Br Heart J* 42:186–191, 1979.

98. Sharp WV, Donovan DL, Teague PC, et al: Arterial occlusive disease: a function of vessel bifurcation angle. *Surgery* 91:680–684, 1982.

99. Perktold K, Resch M: Numerical flow studies in human carotid artery bifurcations: basic discussion of the geometric factor in atherogenesis. *J Biomed Eng* 12:111–123, 1990.

100. Taylor K, Glagov S, Lamberti J, et al: Surface configuration of early atheromatous lesions in controlled-pressure, perfusion-fixed monkey aortas. In: Joharo O (ed). *Scanning Electron Microscopy*, part II. Chicago: Scanning Electron Microscopy, Inc.; 459–464, 1978.

101. Faggioto A, Ross R, Harker L: Studies of hypercholesterolemia in the nonhuman primate. I. Changes that lead to fatty streak formation. *Arteriosclerosis* 4:323–340, 1984.

102. Ross R: The pathogenesis of atherosclerosis: a perspective for the 1990s. *Nature* 362:801–809, 1993.

103. Prakash B, Gowda BHL, Singh M: Theoretical analysis of influence of shape and size of the stenosis on steady flow through tubes. *Monogr Atherosclerosis* 15:240–249, 1990.

104. Binns RL, Ku DN: Effect of stenosis on wall motion: a possible mechanism of stroke and transient ischemic attack. *Arteriosclerosis* 9:842–847, 1989.

105. Tutty OR: Pulsatile flow in a constricted channel. *J Biomech Eng* 114:50–54, 1992.

106. Kajiya F, Hiramatsu D, Kimura A, et al: Blood velocity patterns in poststenotic regions and velocity wave forms for myocardial inflow associated with coronary artery stenosis in dogs. *J Biomech Eng* 114:385–390, 1992.

107. Zarins CK, Bomberger RA, Taylor KE, et al: Artery stenosis inhibits regression of diet-induced atherosclerosis. *Surgery* 88:538–555, 1980.

108. Giddens DP, Mabon RF, Cassanova RA: Measurement of disordered flows distal to subtotal vascular stenoses in the thoracic aorta of dogs. *Circ Res* 39:112–119, 1976.

109. Ahmed SA, Giddens DP: Pulsatile post-stenotic flow studies with laser Doppler anemometry. *J Biomech* 17:695–705, 1984.

110. Armstrong ML, Heistad DD, Marcus ML, et al: Structural and hemodynamic responses of peripheral arteries of macaque monkeys to atherogenic diet. *Arteriosclerosis* 5:336–346, 1985.

111. Zarins CK, Weisenberg E, Kolettis G, et al: Differential enlargement of artery segments in response to enlarging atherosclerotic plaques. *J Vasc Surg* 7:386–394, 1988.

112. Glagov S, Weisenberg E, Zarins CK, et al: Compensatory enlargement of human atherosclerotic coronary arteries. *N Engl J Med* 316:1371–1375, 1987.

113. Davis HR, Glagov S, Zarins CK: Role of acid lipase in cholesterol ester accumulation during atherogenesis: correlation of enzyme activity with acid lipase containing macrophage in rabbit and human lesions. *Arteriosclerosis* 55:205–215, 1985.

114. Kamiya A, Togawa T: Adaptive regulation of wall shear stress to flow change in the canine carotid artery. *Am J Physiol* 239:H14-H21, 1980.

115. Guyton JR, Hortley CJ: Flow restriction of one carotid artery in juvenile rats inhibits growth arterial diameter. *Am J Physiol* 248:H540-H546, 1985.

116. Zarins CK, Zatina MA, Giddens DP, et al: Shear stress regulation of artery lumen diameter in experimental atherogenesis. *J Vasc Surg* 5:413–420, 1987.

117. Smiesko V, Kozik J, Dolezel S: Role of endothelium in the control of arterial diameter by blood flow. *Blood Vessels* 22:247–251, 1985.

118. Butterfield AB, Miller CW, Lumb WV, et al: Inverse effect of chronically elevated blood flow on atherogenesis in miniature swine. *Atherosclerosis* 26:215–224, 1977.

119. Towne JB, Quinn K, Salles-Cunha S, et al: Effect of increased arterial blood flow on localization and progression of atherosclerosis. *Arch Surg* 117:1469–1474, 1982.

120. Sako Y: Effect of turbulent flow and hypertension on experimental atherosclerosis. *JAMA* 179:39–44, 1962.

121. Hagen PO, Wang ZG, Mikat EM, et al: Antiplatelet therapy reduces aortic intimal hyperplasia distal to small diameter vascular protheses (PTFE) in nonhuman primates. *Ann Surg* 195:328–339, 1982.

122. Clowes AW, Reidy MA, Clowes MM: Kinetics of cellular proliferation after arterial injury. I. Smooth muscle

growth in the absence of endothelium. *Lab Invest* 49: 327–332, 1983.

123. Angelini GD, Bryan AJ, Williams HM, et al: Time-course of medial and intimal thickening in pig venous arterial grafts: relationship to endothelial injury and cholesterol accumulation. *J Thorac Cardiovasc Surg* 103:1093–1103, 1992.

124. Bassiouny HS, White S, Glagov S, et al: Anastomotic intimal hyperplasia: mechanical injury or flow induced? *J Vasc Surg* 15:708–717, 1992.

125. Crawshaw HM, Quist WC, Serrallach E, et al: Flow disturbances at the distal end-to-side anastomosis. *Arch Surg* 115:1280–1284, 1980.

126. Ojha M, Ethier CR, Johnston KW, et al: Steady and pulsatile flow fields in and end-to-side arterial anastomosis model. *J Vasc Surg* 12:747–753, 1990.

127. White SS, Zarins CK, Giddens DP, et al: Hemodynamic patterns in two models of end-to-side vascular graft anastomoses: effects of pulsatility, flow division, Reynolds number, and hood length. *J Biomech Eng* 115:104–111, 1993.

128. Wu MH, Shi Q, Sauvage LR, et al: The direct effect of graft compliance mismatch per se on development of host arterial intimal hyperplasia at the anastomotic interface. *Ann Vasc Surg* 7:156–168, 1993.

129. Menashi S, Campa JS, Greenhalgh RM, et al: Collagen in abdominal aortic aneurysm: typing, content, and degradation. *J Vasc Surg* 6:578–582, 1987.

130. Zarins CK, Runyon-Hass A, Zatina MA, et al: Increased collagenase activity in early aneurysmal dilatation. *J Vasc Surg* 3:238–248, 1986.

131. Newman KM, Ogata Y, Malon, et al: Identification of matrix metalloproteinases 3 (stromelysin-1) and 9 (gelatinase B) in abdominal aortic aneurysm. *Arterioscler Thromb* 14:1315–1320, 1994.

132. Dubick MA, Hunter GC, Casey SM, Keen CL: Aortic ascorbic acid, trace elements, and superoxide dismutase activity in human aneurysmal and occlusive disease. *Proc Soc Exp Biol Med* 184:138–143, 1987.

133. Johansen K, Koepsell T: Familial tendency for abdominal aortic aneurysms. *JAMA* 256:1934–1936, 1986.

134. Zarins CK, Glagov S, Vesselinovitch D, Wissler RW: Aneurysm formation in experimental atherosclerosis: relationship to plaque evolution. *J Vasc Surg* 12:246–256, 1990.

135. Zarins CK, Xu C, Glagov S: Aneurysmal enlargement of the aorta during regression of experimental atherosclerosis. *J Vasc Surg* 15:90–101, 1992.

136. Zatina MA, Zarins CK, Gewertz BL, Glagov S: Role of medial lamellar architecture in the pathogenesis of aortic aneurysms. *J Vasc Surg* 1:442–448, 1984.

137. Zarins CK, Glagov S: Aneurysms and obstructive plaques: differing local responses to atherosclerosis. In: Bergan JJ, Yao J (eds). *Aneurysms: Diagnosis and Treatment*. 1st ed. New York: Grune & Stratton, Inc.; 61–82, 1982.

CHAPTER 5

Peptide Growth Factors and Their Role in the Proliferative Diseases of the Vascular System

Anton N. Sidawy, MD

Growth factors are peptide molecules that influence the growth of human cells. They are produced by various cells and exert their effects on a variety of tissues. Platelet-derived growth factor (PDGF), for example, is not only released by platelets as its name indicates but, in response to endothelial injury, it is also released by endothelial cells, macrophages, and arterial smooth muscle cells (SMCs). It exerts its mitogenic effects on vascular SMCs; furthermore, PDGF has been found to be a growth factor for fibroblasts and glial cells. Growth factors play an important role in cellular proliferation and differentiation in normal development and in disease states. They exert their effects via specific receptors located on the cellular membrane. The interaction of various growth factors with their specific receptors unleashes a series of intracellular biochemical reactions that result in the specific effects of the growth factors; therefore, via their receptors, growth factors can positively or negatively affect the growth, multiplication, or differentiation of various cells. In proliferative vascular diseases, namely atherosclerosis and intimal hyperplasia, growth factors play an important role in the proliferation and migration of SMCs to form the atherosclerotic or hyperplastic lesion. Various growth factors act in concert to exert their specific functions. The addition of insulin-like growth factor I (IGF-I) to PDGF or fibroblast growth factor (FGF), for example, potentiates the effect of PDGF and FGF on the proliferation of SMCs in culture.[1] In addition, in vivo studies have demonstrated the importance of various growth factors on the progression of injury-induced intimal hyperplasia. Antibodies to PDGF were found to partially inhibit this process.[2] In this chapter, we discuss various growth factors, their receptors, and the importance of the growth factor-receptor interaction on cell metabolism and growth, in general, and vascular tissue, in particular.

Functions of Growth Factors

In order to multiply, the cell enters a specific cycle (Figure 1). The cell cycle consists of a distinct sequence of phases called G_1 phase (the first gap phase), S phase (DNA synthesis and chromosome replication), G_2 phase (the second gap phase) and, finally, M phase (mitosis phase). Cells are usually found in a resting quiescent phase called the G_0 phase. Peptide growth factors are divided into two groups based on their effects on the progression of the cell cycle: competence factors that advance the quiescent cell from the G_0 to the G_1 phase include PDGF, FGF, and epidermal growth factor (EGF); and progression factors, such as

From *The Basic Science of Vascular Disease*. Edited by Sidawy AN, Sumpio BE, and DePalma RG. Armonk, NY: Futura Publishing Company, Inc.; © 1997.

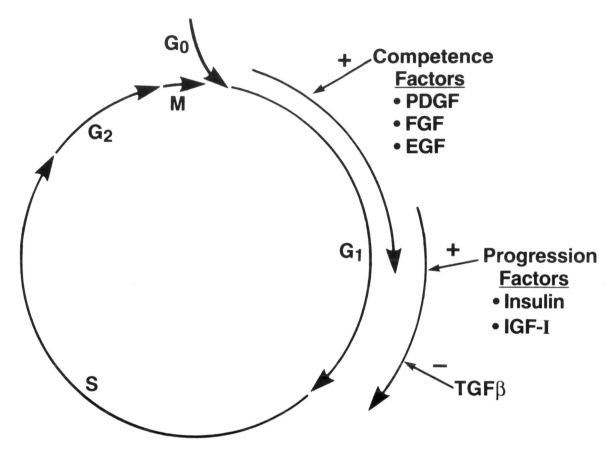

Figure 1. Schematic depicting the stages of the cell cycle and the effects that competence and progression growth factors have on the cell while progressing in the G_1 phase of the cycle. Note that the cell has to be under the influence of both groups in order to progress to the S phase. In addition, transforming growth factor β (TGF-β) exerts a negative effect on the cell in the later part of the cycle.

IGF-I and insulin, that commit the cell to the synthesis of DNA. During this process, simultaneous stimulation by both groups of factors is needed to keep the cell progressing in the G_1 phase of the cycle. The cell has to remain under the sustained influence of growth factors for an uninterrupted period of time; if the effect of growth factors is interrupted, the cell will revert back to the quiescent G_0 phase.[3] Not all growth factors have positive effects on the progression of the cell cycle; transforming growth factor β (TGF-β), for example, can inhibit the positive effects of growth factors even late in the G_1 phase.[3]

While some growth factors can only stimulate proliferation, others can also induce differentiation of the cell. FGF, for example, has been implicated in the proliferation and differentiation of endothelial cells during angiogenesis.[4] In addition, some growth factors, such as PDGF, play a chemotactic role to induce cells to migrate; after endothelial injury, PDGF release stimulates the proliferation and migration of medial SMCs

the subendothelial area to form the hyperplastic lesion. It has been found that endothelial cells in culture secrete a PDGF-like chemotactic factor which binds to specific mesenchymal cell receptors to result in their migration to the vicinity of forming capillaries.[5] These mesenchymal cells then organize in layers to form the cellular components of the vascular wall.[6]

Growth Factor Receptors and Mechanisms of Action

The mechanisms of action of growth factors vary (Figure 2).[7] Endocrine function is when a growth factor is released by an organ, and then is carried in the circulation by exerting its effect on cells of a distant organ. This situation is best illustrated by insulin production in the pancreas and its release in the circulation to affect distant target cells and exert its mitogenic function as a growth factor. A paracrine function is when the

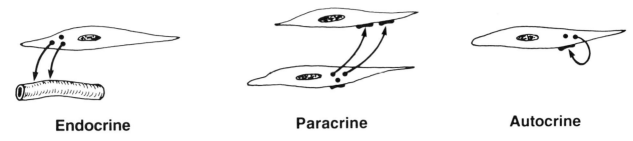

Endocrine   **Paracrine**   **Autocrine**

Figure 2. The modes of action of growth factors: endocrine, when the factor is released by the cell to travel in the circulation and exerts its effect on remote cells; paracrine, when the factor is released by the cell to exert its effect on a neighboring cell; and autocrine, when the growth factor exerts its effect on the cell which released it.

growth factor is secreted by cells located adjacent to its receptor containing target cells, a situation illustrated by the effect on arterial wall SMCs by PDGF, secreted by macrophages chemoattracted to an area of endothelial injury, or even by PDGF secreted by adjacent SMCs. An autocrine function occurs when the growth factor is produced by cells that, themselves, contain its specific receptor. Therefore, they are directly affected by their own production of the growth factor, such as when an injured SMC produces PDGF which binds to its specific receptor found on the same cell. This autocrine function is important when growth factor receptors support autonomous cell growth and differentiation.[7]

Whether the growth factor is secreted in a remote tissue, adjacent cells, or locally in the same cell, the presence of specific growth factor receptors in the cell wall determines the effect of the growth factor on that cell. The majority of growth factor receptors belong to a family of peptide receptors called receptor tyrosine kinases (RTKs). Once the ligand binds to the extracellular portion of the receptor, the kinase function becomes activated and phosphorylates specific cytoplasmic substrates to activate pathways required for the function of the growth factor. Various growth factor receptors use different substrates for their action. Finally, through poorly defined mechanism, these specific receptor substrates induce the activation of specific sets of genes to exert the specific effect of the growth factor.[3]

There are three subclasses or families of RTKs (Figure 3). Each may have a different molecular pathway to exert its effects. The first subclass is represented by the EGF receptor which contains two cysteine-rich residues in the extracellular domain. The second subclass, represented by the insulin and the IGF-I receptor, is characterized by 2 α and 2 β subunits; each α subunit contains only one cysteine-rich residue. The α subunits are connected to each other and to the β subunits with disulfide bonds. The third subclass of RTKs is represented by the PDGF recep-

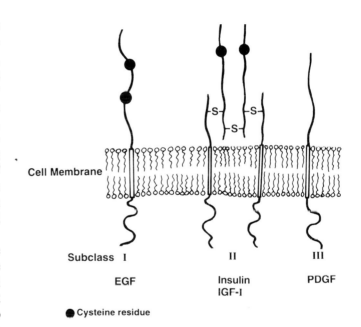

Figure 3. The three subclasses of the tyrosine kinase receptor. Subclass I, represented by the EGF receptor containing two cysteine-rich residues in its extracellular domain; subclass II, represented by the insulin and the insulin-like growth factor I (IGF-I) receptors which are formed of 2α and 2β subunits, each α subunit containing one cysteine-rich residue in its extracellular domain; and subclass III, represented by the platelet-derived growth factor (PDGF) receptor with no cysteine-rich residue in its extracellular domain.

tor; its extracellular domain contains no cysteine-rich residues (Figure 3).[8]

The RTKs are polypeptide structures found in the cell wall (Figure 4). Each RTK is formed of multiple domains[8]:

1. *Extracellular domain*: This domain is found outside the cell wall. It represents a large portion of the molecular mass of the receptor. It is a 500 to 850 amino acid glycoprotein. The polypeptide structures of various extracellular domains of growth factor receptors are different in their relative molecular mass, the location of glycolization sites, and the location of the cyste-

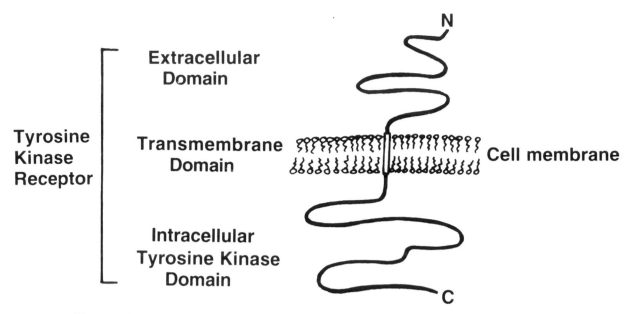

Figure 4. Schematic of the tyrosine kinase receptor with its extracellular, transmembrane, and intracellular tyrosine kinase domain. The N-terminal of the receptor protein molecule is in the extracellular domain and the C-terminal is located in the intracellular domain.

ine residues, if any. As described above, the presence, absence, and the number of cysteine-rich residues in the extracellular domain classify the RTKs into three distinct families. However, some growth factor receptors do not conform to any of the three families. The extracellular domain of the mannose-6-phosphate (Man-6-P) IGF-II receptor, for example, is formed of one single large mass glycoprotein without the α and β subunit structure present in the IGF-I receptor, despite the ability of cross-binding of IGF-I and IGF-II to each other's receptor. The extracellular domain has two important functions: high-affinity binding of the ligand, and the ability to convey the message to the cell that binding of the growth factor has occurred. The specific molecular changes related to these functions are poorly understood. High-affinity free serum receptors have been found and they represent the extracellular domain of truncated receptors. The function of these free plasma receptors is poorly understood; they may represent carrier molecules to the growth factor. Cross-binding of growth factors with each other's receptors is a known phenomenon. The affinity of a receptor to different ligands varies; in the case of IGF-I receptor, it reacts with almost the same high affinity for IGF-II as for its primary ligand IGF-I, whereas IGF-I receptor has very low affinity to insulin. This cross-binding is functional; insulin, for example, is believed to exert its metabolic effects via the insulin receptor and its growth-promoting effects via the IGF-I receptor.[9]

2. *Transmembrane domain*[8]: This 22 to 26 hydro-phobic amino acid segment of RTKs anchors the receptor to the cellular membrane. Similar to the extracellular domain, the transmembrane domain does not display primary structure conservation, in sharp contrast to the cytoplasmic tyrosine kinase domain which displays a high level of conservation when compared within the RTK group of receptors.[3] In addition to anchoring the receptor to the cellular wall, the transmembrane domain plays a role in signal transmission between the extracellular and cytoplasmic domains. This role is probably a passive one; the transmembrane domain is merely a link between the extracellular and the cytoplasmic domains.

3. *Cytoplasmic tyrosine kinase domain*[8]: This domain plays an important role in translating ligand binding into cellular response. The tyrosine kinase domain displays high amino acid sequence homology in receptors belonging to the same subclass. In addition, the cytoplasmic domain enjoys the highest degree of conservation, even when compared to other types of RTKs.[3] This domain contains specific amino acid sequences which define specific substrates unique to each growth factor receptor.

Endocrine hormones use tyrosine kinase receptors; however, these receptors have multiple extracellular, transmembrane, and cytoplasmic domains in contrast to the single domain structure of growth factor receptors. It is not yet known whether the simple structure of growth factor receptor influences the mechanism of action of the growth factor.[8]

The exact method by which ligand binding elicits

growth factor function is not completely understood; however, it is believed that once the ligand binds to the extracellular domain, adjacent cytoplasmic domains interact on the molecular level and the kinase function becomes activated. Specific substrates are then phosphorylated by various receptor kinases to activate pathways required for the mitogenic function of the growth factor. Some of the identified substrates are phospholipase-C (PLC), Ras guanosine triphosphatase activating protein (GAP), phosphatidylinositol 3' kinase (PI-3K), Src tyrosine kinases, and Raf protooncogene. Various growth factor receptors use different specific substrates for their actions, and the same growth factor may use a different substrate depending on the ultimate action required, whether it is cell division or differentiation. Finally, through poorly defined mechanism, these specific receptor substrates induce the activation of specific sets of genes to exert the specific effect of the growth factor.[3] Recently, various reports indicated the importance of the role of cyclic adenosine 3', 5'-monophosphate (cAMP) in growth factors' signalling pathways. cAMP effect is mainly one of inhibition of signal transmission through blocking the activation of Raf-1 by Ras and, therefore, preventing the activation of MAPK (mitogen activated protein kinase); the activation of MAPK induces gene activation.[10,11]

Signal transmission mechanism used by interferon α was recently elucidated by Schindler and his colleagues, who also predicted that the same pathway is used by other growth factors.[12] Once interferon binds to its receptor on the cell wall, the receptor becomes activated and the tyrosine kinase phosphorylates three large (113, 91, and 84 kD) cytoplasmic proteins which then link together and move toward the nucleus, in addition to a smaller protein (48 kD) also found in the cytoplasm. The three large proteins are all tyrosine kinase substrates for the interferon α receptor. In the nucleus, the linked-up larger proteins join the smaller protein to form a transcription factor. The smaller protein in the transcription factor comes in contact with a specific area in the gene called interferon-stimulated response element (ISRE); this contact activates the gene (Figure 5). In order for a gene to be activated by interferon, it has to carry the specific ISRE sequence. The formation and the movement of the transcription factor are instantaneous after interferon α binds to its receptor. In cells not exposed to interferon, all the pro-

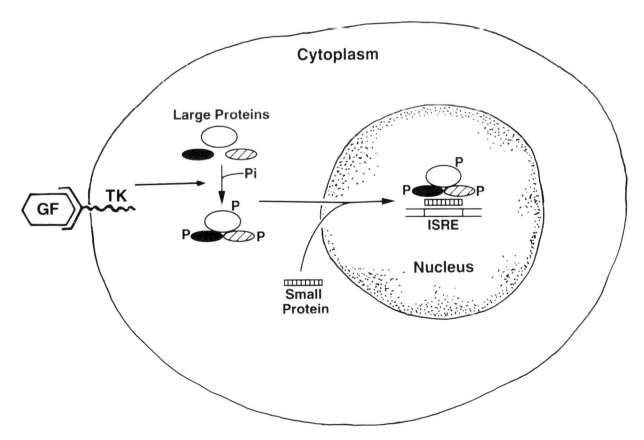

Figure 5. The role of the STAT family of proteins in signal transduction. The binding of the growth factor to its receptor activates the receptor to phosphorylate large cytoplasmic proteins which link together and move toward the nucleus where they join a smaller protein to form the transcription factor. STAT = signal transducers and activators of transcription.

teins forming the transcription factor were found free in the cytoplasm, in contrast to cells stimulated by interferon, in which the proteins were found linked together in the nucleus. Furthermore, these proteins were found to have SH2 domain which is commonly found in proteins phosphorylated by tyrosine kinase, and blocking phosphorylation caused the genes to no longer respond to stimulation by interferon-α.[12] The same researchers suggested that these proteins belong to a new protein family since they did not find any match in protein data banks. They later called them "signal transducers and activators of transcription" (STATs). The 91kD and the 84kD proteins were termed Stat1 α&β respectively and the 113kD protein was called Stat2. Recently, a Stat3 protein was described and was found to be activated via phosphorylation in response to EGF and interleukin-6.[13]

The changes in cell shape and motility triggered by some growth factors, such as EGF and PDGF, are also not completely elucidated. Recent data shed some light on the cellular mechanisms triggered by growth factors to cause the cell to change shape and to move toward a growth factor. How does binding of EGF to its receptor, for example, trigger the changes in cell skeleton leading to cell movement? It is known that the cell has a microcytoskeleton formed of actin microfilaments. Changes in cell shape and motility are thought to be caused by remodeling of the cell architectural skeleton. EGF is a growth factor that is known to trigger structural changes in the cell. However, the link between EGF binding to its receptor and the actual changes is not fully elucidated. Recently, the role of profilin, a protein which tightly binds to a cellular membrane phospholipid called phosphatidylinositol-4,5-biphosphate (PIP$_2$), was explored.[14] Profilin is a soluble actin-binding protein which causes the polymerization of actin to form the microfilaments. Once PIP$_2$ binds to profilin, it can only be broken down by the phosphorylated form of the enzyme phospholipase C-γ1 to liberate profilin. The binding of EGF to its receptor was found to cause the phosphorylation of the enzyme phospholipase C-γ1, thereby allowing the break down of PIP$_2$ bound to profilin. The free profilin can then interact with actin to form the skeletal microfilaments.[14]

Growth Factor Receptor Characterization

Growth factor receptors are characterized by their affinity and specificity to their ligands. The affinity of a receptor is determined by the equilibrium dissociation constant (K$_d$), derived from binding saturation experiments where the radiolabeled ligand and the unlabeled ligand bind to the receptors in a solution, cell culture, or tissue to form specific labeled ligand binding. The

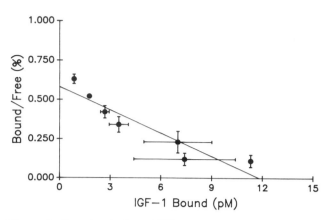

Figure 6. Scatchard plot of ^{125}I-IGF-I binding as a function of radiolabeled peptide concentration. Each value was determined in triplicate and the results are the mean ± SEM of three separate experiments. Calculated K$_d$ = 2 nM and B$_{max}$ = 11.5 pM (4.17 pmol/mg protein). (Reproduced with permission from Reference 16.)

graphical representation of binding saturation study is obtained by plotting the concentration of the bound ligand versus the free ligand as in Figure 6. The maximum binding capacity (B$_{max}$) is the maximum concentration of labeled ligand bound at saturation. The dissociation constant (K$_d$) is the concentration of labeled ligand which is bound to 50% of total binding sites. Both B$_{max}$ and K$_d$ are represented in Figure 6. A linear representation of the data can be obtained by using the Scatchard analysis method which was described by Scatchard to study the interaction of proteins with small molecules.[15] Regression analysis of the data produces a Scatchard analysis plot between bound/free and bound radiolabeled ligand. The point where the line intersects with bound represents B$_{max}$ and the point of intersection with bound/free represents B$_{max}$/K$_d$. Therefore, the dissociation constant K$_d$ in the Scatchard plot, and which is represented by the slope of the line, equals B$_{max}$ divided by the point of intersection with bound/free. The above is illustrated in Figure 6 which is a representation of a Scatchard plot of saturation data of IGF-I receptor binding in the normal arteries of the rabbit, where the B$_{max}$ is 11.5 pmol/L and K$_d$ is 2 nmol/L which represent high affinity binding sites for IGF-I in the tissue.[16] Analysis of the data can be performed using the Curve Fitting and Data Analysis Ligand Binding program (version 3.10 National Institutes of Health, Bethesda, MD.)[17] If the plot is nonlinear and it accepts a second degree regression analysis, it suggests that binding is taking place to more than one class of binding sites.[17] The lower the K$_d$, the higher the affinity of the binding sites.[17]

To study the specificity of the binding sites to a particular ligand such as IGF-I, for example, increased concentration of unlabeled IGF-I and similar growth factors, such as IGF-II and insulin, are added, in in-

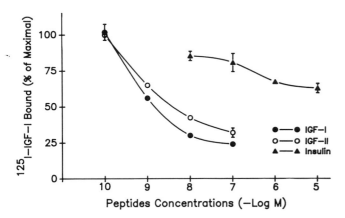

Figure 7. Binding inhibition curves of bound ^{125}I-IGF-I by IGF-I, IGF-II, and insulin. Each value was determined in triplicate and the results are the mean ± SEM of three separate experiments. Calculated IC$_{50}$ for IGF-I, IGF-II, and insulin were 1.75 nM, 5 nM and >100 uM respectively. (Reproduced with permission from Reference 16.)

creasing concentrations, to the buffer solution containing ^{125}I-IGF-I to compete for the binding sites.[16] As illustrated in Figure 7, the curves are then plotted between the concentrations of the peptides used and and the bound ^{125}I-IGF-I as a percentage of maximal binding. The concentration of peptide that inhibits 50% of maximum binding (IC$_{50}$) is calculated. In this example of binding inhibition studies in the normal arteries of the rabbit, the IC$_{50}$ of IGF-I, IGF-II, and insulin are 1.75 nM, 5 nM, and >100 nM respectively, which indicates that the binding sites are more specific to IGF-I than IGF-II and insulin. The difference in IC$_{50}$ between IGF-I and IGF-II is small, which indicates that IGF-II binds easily to IGF-I binding sites; it is known that IGF-I and IGF-II cross-react with each other's receptors. On the other hand, insulin is able to compete only partially with IGF-I receptors.[16]

Binding can be localized using autoradiography. A frozen section of the tissue is mounted on a slide and then incubated in a buffer solution containing the labeled peptide. Then the slide is exposed to film in a darkroom. The film is then developed and the autoradiograph is compared to an H&E-stained adjacent section of the tissue. An increased amount of the unlabeled peptide can be used to compete with the labeled peptide for its binding sites and confirm the specificity of these binding sites for that ligand. Figure 8 illustrates the localization of IGF-I binding to human greater saphenous vein.[18] The binding sites are specific to IGF-I, but not to insulin because an excess of IGF-I successfully competed for these binding sites as illustrated in Figure 8, whereas an excess of unlabeled insulin did not. The main advantage of this method is its ability to determine the in situ localization of binding in a tissue, a difficult task to accomplish using binding in cell

culture environment, and a very useful method when evaluating pathologic lesions.

Role of Peptide Growth Factors in the Proliferative Diseases of the Vascular Wall

The development of atherosclerotic arterial disease is a complex process as summarized in Chapter 11. In its early stages, the atherosclerotic lesion is made primarily of replicating SMCs of the media. These SMCs have the capability of secreting connective tissue components and accumulating variable amounts of lipids.[19,20] The intimal SMCs also multiply, but to a lesser degree. The SMCs of the media replicate and migrate to the subendothelial area.[21,22] The endothelial cells replicate, remaining in a monolayer.[23] Monocytes play a role in this process. In experimentally-induced atherosclerosis, monocytes were found attached to the surface of the arterial endothelium at numerous sites of the arterial tree.[20] These monocytes were found to migrate to the subendothelial area through the junctions between the endothelial cells. They accumulate lipids and, along with lipid-laden SMCs, form foam cells. This constitutes the early stage of the formation of so-called fatty streaks.[24] The endothelial cells overlying the fatty streaks separate and expose it; this promotes platelet adherence, aggregation, and possible thrombosis.[20,25] Growth factors, such as PDGF and FGF, have been found to play a role in stimulating the multiplication of arterial SMCs[21] and other cellular components of the atherosclerotic and hyperplastic lesions. The secretion of these growth factors is a response to injury, especially endothelial injury. This injury could be chemical, such as in hyperlipoproteinemia, where the increase in oxidized low density lipoprotein (LDL) promotes endothelial injury and, possibly, the development of the atherosclerotic plaque.[26,27]

Platelet-Derived Growth Factor

PDGF is a peptide growth factor originally discovered in 1974 by Ross et al who found that a platelet-rich serum stimulated the multiplication of arterial SMCs.[28] Despite its early discovery as a platelet product, and for which this factor was named "platelet-derived," PDGF was later found to be a ubiquitous mitogenic factor secreted by many cell types including arterial endothelial cells and arterial SMCs.[29,30] PDGF exerts its effects on cells of mesenchymal origin, such as arterial SMCs,[28] in normal growth and in disease conditions such as atherosclerosis, neoplasia, and the fibrotic response associated with many inflammatory diseases.

PDGF is a glycosylated protein with a molecular weight that varies from 28 kd to 31 kd. The carbohy-

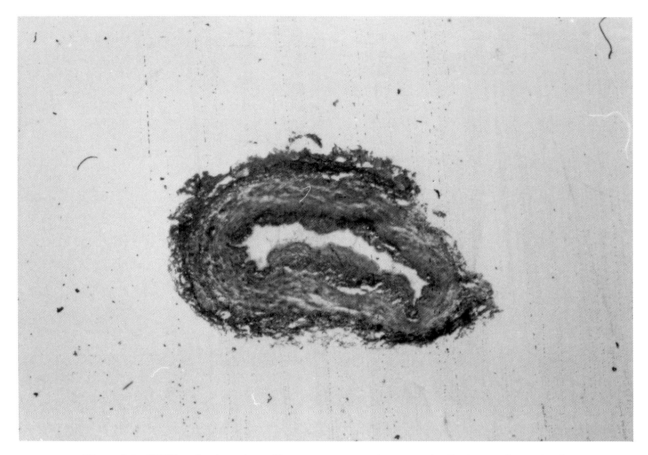

Figure 8 A. H&E-stained section of human greater saphenous vein. **B.** Autoradiograph of an adjacent section demonstrating ^{125}I-IGF-I grain density present over the venous wall. **C.** Nonspecific binding for insulin. **D.** Nonspecific binding for IGF-I. Note the difference in nonspecific binding between C and D. (Reproduced with permission from Reference 18.)

drate content of the PDGF molecule varies from 4% to 7% of the total mass. PDGF has been shown to be composed of two separate chains called A and B. PDGF has three isoforms, depending on the composition of the chains: PDGF-AA, PDGF-BB, and PDGF-AB. Each of these isoforms binds to a variety of PDGF receptors. These isoforms are expressed differently according to the species, in human 70% AB, 25% BB, and 5% AA,[31,32] compared to the pig, where 100% is of the BB dimer. The half-life of PDGF is only 2 minutes which suggests that it acts locally near the release site in an autocrine or paracrine fashion. Both SMCs and fibroblasts have been found to bind PDGF in culture. The gene for the A chain of PDGF is found on chromosome 7 and for the B chain on chromosome 22; each contains seven exons spanning 24 kilobases (kb) of the DNA.[33]

PDGF is expressed and secreted by many normal as well as abnormal animal cells. Normal cells found to express PDGF in a variety of combinations of A and B chains include endothelial cells of many origins (aortic, renal, umbilical vein, venous) and species, epi-

thelial cells, connective tissue cells such as fibroblasts, chondrocytes, and vascular SMCs, nerve tissue cells, and hematopoeitic cells such as lymphocytes, macrophages, and monocytes.[33] The amount of PDGF expressed or secreted depends on the environment of the cells and their state at the time of secretion. SMCs obtained from the vascular media of 2-week-old pup rats secreted increased levels of PDGF when compared to cells obtained from adult rats; this increased secretion was stable over multiple passages of the pup rat SMCs in culture.[30] This increase in PDGF secretion in cultured pup rat SMCs was mainly due to increase in PDGF B chain.[34] Furthermore, injury increased the secretion of PDGF; Walker and coworkers have shown that intimal SMCs isolated from balloon catheter-induced injury of the rat carotid arteries secreted higher amounts of PDGF.[35] Many mediators, including PDGF, induce the production of A and B chain transcripts; PDGF A or B chains are not expressed in fibroblasts in culture; however, the addition of PDGF to the fibroblast culture stimulated the production of PDGF A chain mRNA.[36]

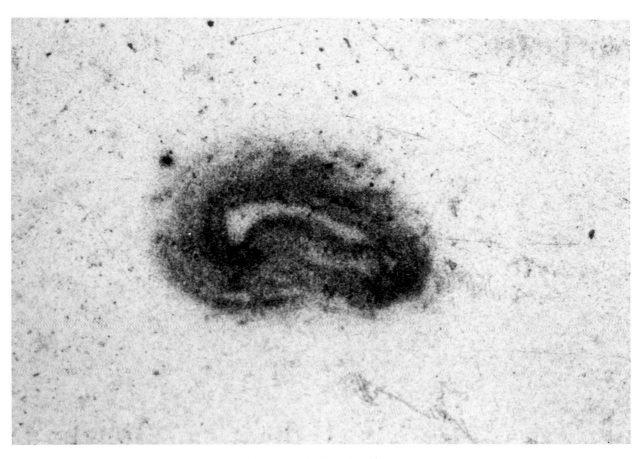

Figure 8 B. *(continued)*

PDGF Receptor

The PDGF tyrosine kinase receptor is a dimer of two subunits, α and β. The α subunit binds PDGF A and B, and the β subunit binds PDGF B only. Various combinations of α and β result in three types of PDGF receptors: $\alpha\alpha$-receptor which binds PDGF AA, AB, and BB, $\alpha\beta$-receptor which binds PDGF AB and BB, and $\beta\beta$-receptor which binds PDGF BB only. The α and β subunits are found in a monomeric form; binding of the ligand PDGF to these receptor subunits stimulates the formation of receptor dimers.[37] The PDGF receptor has high affinity to PDGF as shown by saturation binding experiments. This high affinity has been conserved during evolution, for the human ^{125}I-PDGF binds with similar affinity to human, fish, or rodent PDGF receptor.[33] A dissociation constant (K_d) of 10^{-11} M has been reported.[38] Binding of PDGF to its receptor is temperature- and time-dependent, reaching maximum binding at 37°C in 45 minutes.[39]

PDGF Effects

Most of the effects of PDGF are consistent with its positive effects on growth and tissue remodeling.

In addition, PDGF has been found to play a role in pathologic conditions affecting humans, such as neoplasia, inflammatory diseases, scleroderma, and proliferative diseases of the vascular wall.

PDGF is a competence factor. Progression factors such as IGF-I and insulin are needed to induce the progression of the cell in the G_1 phase and to commit the cell to DNA synthesis.[3] PDGF has been found to play a role in the production, destruction, and modification of connective tissue that constitutes cellular matrix; for example, PDGF increases collagen synthesis.[40] In addition, PDGF also stimulates the secretion of collagenase by dermal fibroblasts.[41] The contribution of PDGF to the secretion of collagen and collagenase, the enzyme responsible for the breaking down of collagen, may prove important in modeling the cellular matrix, an important step in wound healing. PDGF also induces a chemotactic effect in fibroblasts and SMCs as well as for monocytes and neutrophils[42] that may prove important in wound healing.

Lynch and coworkers have shown that adding PDGF to a wound site does not promote healing by itself. The addition of IGF-I to PDGF led to significant increase in the rate of DNA and protein synthesis and, histologically, the width of the new connective tissue

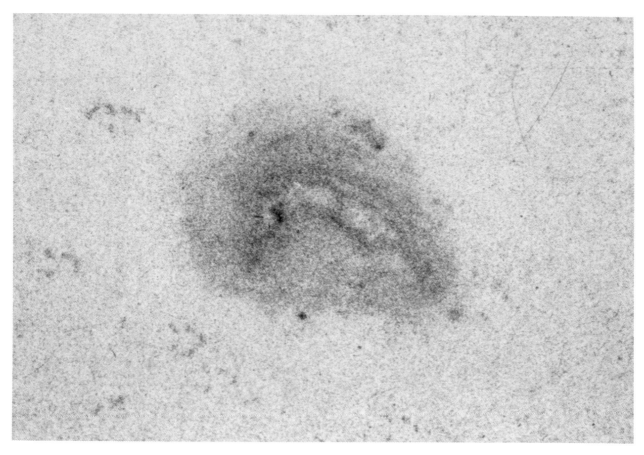

Figure 8 C. *(continued)*

increased by 2.4 times and the thickness of the epidermis increased by 95% in comparison to controls.[43] Furthermore, the addition of thrombin, usually available at vascular injury sites, increased the production of PDGF by endothelial cells, an additional evidence that PDGF aids in wound healing by recruiting and stimulating division of mesenchymal cells.[44]

PDGF has been found to be a potent vasoconstrictor causing contraction of strips of rat aorta. This vasoconstrictive effect was concentration-dependent and reversible; it occurred after a lag period and was more prolonged when compared to the effect of angiotensin II.[45] This effect has been shown to accompany intimal proliferation in balloon catheter-injured rabbit iliac artery, which may further decrease the lumen of the artery during the process of atherosclerosis.[46]

The Role of PDGF in the Proliferative Diseases of the Vascular System

Various growth factors play a role in stimulating the multiplication of vascular wall cells during the processes of atherosclerosis and intimal hyperplasia. PDGF has been found to promote multiplication of

SMCs.[28] It is secreted by platelets,[28] endothelial cells,[29] and SMCs,[30] that stimulate their own proliferation by producing this factor. Receptors for PDGF have been described in these cells.[47] Injury to the vascular wall, whether it is chemical caused by hypercholesterolemia, mechanical caused by hypertension, or physical caused by vascular angioplasty, stimulates the attachment of monocytes and platelets to the intimal surface; these monocytes convert to macrophages which, in addition to platelets, secrete multiple growth factors, the most prominent being PDGF.[25,48] PDGF gene expression in injured human arteries has been found to be markedly higher than its expression in control normal arteries.[49,50] Libby and colleagues[51] found B chain transcript in SMCs cultured from atherosclerotic lesions; furthermore, the cells released a PDGF-like material into culture medium. Similarly, Wilcox et al[52] used in situ hybridization to study advanced atherosclerotic lesions and found predominantly B chain expression in SMCs, but no detectable transcript in macrophages. However, Ross and colleagues were able to detect PDGF-B protein in macrophages in all stages of atherosclerotic lesions in humans.[53] Majesky et al have shown that balloon catheter injury of the rat

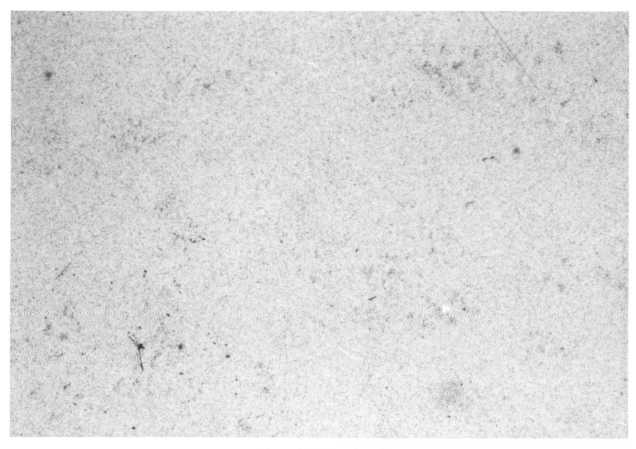

Figure 8 D. *(continued)*

carotid artery induced mRNA expression of PDGF A chain in addition to PDGF receptor subunits.[54]

To confirm the involvement of PDGF in the proliferation of SMCs of the vascular wall in response to injury, Ferns and colleagues[2] created a balloon catheter-induced intimal hyperplasia of rat carotid artery causing de-endothelialization and innermost layer cellular injury. They administered a goat polyclonal antibody to PDGF before and after balloon injury in one group of rats, and compared the results to controls which had the arterial injury without the administration of the antibody. Using neointimal measurement and labeling with [³H]thymidine, they found that the amount of neointimal hyperplasia was decreased, but [³H]thymidine labeling was not significantly different in the treated group when compared to controls. This led them to conclude that the administred doses of PDGF antibody inhibited SMC chemotaxis, but its effect on SMC replication was not significant. Whether higher doses of PDGF antibody inhibit SMC proliferation in vitro is not yet known.[2]

Fibroblast Growth Factor

The FGFs belong to a family of at least seven growth factors primarily involved in embryonic tissue induction. These growth factors have been found to promote the proliferation of mesoderm-derived cells.[55] They were called fibroblast growth factors because the first FGFs discovered, the acidic fibroblast growth factor (aFGF) and the basic fibroblast growth factor (bFGF), were described for their stimulation of fibroblast proliferation. The FGFs play an important role in cell maintenance, proliferation, differentiation, and motility. Their role is not limited to their physiologic actions, but extends to their involvement in disease states such as cancer and atherosclerosis. A consensus committee chaired by Baird and Klagsburn has proposed to change the nomenclature of the FGFs to account for the numerous FGFs described.[56] The committee proposed to give the FGFs numbers 1 to 7. Acidic FGF, also called endothelial cell growth factor (ECGF) or heparin-binding growth factor-1 (HBGF-1), was given the proposed name FGF-1. Basic FGF, also called heparin-binding growth factor-2 (HBGF-2), was given the proposed name FGF-2. The following names were proposed for the rest of the FGF family members: FGF-3 for the int-2 gene, FGF-4 for the kaposi sarcoma FGF (K-FGF, also called human stomach cancer transforming gene, hst-1), and FGF-7 for keratinocyte growth factor (KGF). The names FGF-5 and FGF-6 were proposed for the fibroblast growth factors 5 and 6, respectively.[56] All seven factors are homologous protein mitogens. The FGFs enjoy high sequence homology in different species including human, bovine, and rat. The high sequence homology is found in basic as well as acidic FGF.

Extract from brain and pituitary had been found to induce the proliferation of fibroblasts in culture as early as 1940.[57,58] The name fibroblast growth factor was coined by Gospodarowicz in 1974.[59] The first FGF discovered was about 12,000 Da in size and had a basic isoelectric charge, thus it was called basic FGF (bFGF). The bFGF is a 146 amino acid protein. Another substance was detected by Thomas in 1980 and had an acidic isoelectric charge, therefore called acidic FGF (aFGF).[60] The acidic molecule is a 140 amino acid protein with a size of 15,500 Da. The genes that encode for human aFGF and bFGF are located on chromosomes 5 and 4, respectively.[61] The FGF gene span about 38 kilobases of DNA. It has three exons.

As with other growth factors, many of the cells that are affected by FGFs also produce the growth factor (autocrine function, also seen in abnormal proliferation of cells such as in cancer and atherosclerosis). These cells include fibroblasts, endothelial cells, epithelial cells, SMCs, and adrenal cells. Some of these FGF-like growth factors are given different names when they are released by different tissues. For example, in the brain, the name heparin-binding growth factor (HDGF) is used.[62]

FGFs have been found to have high affinity for heparin. This feature distinguishes the FGFs from other growth factor families. This high affinity for heparin protects the FGFs from inactivation by enzymes, high temperature, or low pH.[63,64] In addition, when aFGF binds to heparin, its activity is potentiated and becomes as active as bFGF. This potentiating effect of heparin is mediated by its carbohydrate contaminants.[65] The maintenance of the structural integrity of aFGF is very important for its heparin dependence. All members of the FGF family share structure homology in 35% to 80% of their molecule, including two conserved cysteine residues. The loss of these cysteine residues affects the activity and heparin dependency of aFGF.[66]

FGF Receptor

Cells that respond to the stimulation of FGFs contain specific FGF surface receptors. These are high-affinity receptors specific for FGF. They have been identified on various cells including endothelial cells, SMCs, fibroblasts, and epithelial cells. This receptor is a tyrosine kinase receptor with high affinity to FGF with a Kd of 10 to 80 pM.[4] The receptor itself is a single chain peptide with a molecular weight of 110 to 150 kDa. Although this receptor binds both acidic and basic FGF, it has a higher affinity for the bFGF when compared to the aFGF. Once the growth factor binds to its receptor, phosphorylation of tyrosine occurs, triggering a cascade of biochemical reactions leading to cell division and proliferation. The FGF receptor has four different forms that differ mainly in their extracellular domain. The diversity of the FGF receptor resides at the gene level with different genes for the different forms of receptors.[67]

FGF Effects

In addition to its effect on the maintenance and proliferation of human cells, FGF has also been found to play a role in the abnormal proliferation of cells in pathologic conditions. FGFs induce the proliferation of cells derived from all three germ layers of the embryo: ectoderm, mesoderm, and endoderm.[68,69] Although bFGF is much more potent and active when compared with aFGF, the difference in potency depends on the target cell.[69] In addition, FGF can induce transformation in cell morphology. The effects of FGF on vascular endothelial cells in culture have been described. Endothelial cells in culture lost their morphologic characteristics after multiple passages, and they resembled fibroblast phenotype and grew in multiple layers. When FGF was initially added to the culture, this loss of differentiation was reversed, the cells continued to grow in confluence, and they maintained their nonthrombogenic apical surface.[70] In addition, this effect of FGF on the differentiation of cells was also described in myoblast, condrocytes, osteoblast, nerve, and glial cells.[69]

FGFs are important angiogenic factors. They were initially called tumor angiogenic factor (TAF) for their effect on angiogenesis.[71] They stimulate the formation of new capillaries in physiologic as well as pathologic models. The slow release of FGFs in the wall of the carotid artery of the rat induced the vascularization of the vasa vasora. This angiogenic effect of FGFs is important in the neorevascularization in disease states, such as the formation of collateral circulation in response to ischemia. This effect of angiogenesis is also important in tumor formation and various stages of reproduction (egg implantation and embryonic development).[67]

FGF has important interactions with extracellular matrix (ECM). Cells sensitive to bFGF have optimal growth, proliferation, and differentiation in the presence of ECM.[72] Further investigation has revealed that bFGF forms complexes with ECM heparan sulfate proteoglycan. These complexes protected bFGF from degradation. bFGF is, therefore, found in this insoluble state bound to ECM, acting as a local growth regulator and inducing the regeneration of tissue during the repair process.[73] The heparan sulfate-FGF complexes are biologically active. These complexes can be liberated from ECM by hydrolysis.[73]

FGF promotes wound healing and repair by inducing cellular responses important for these processes. FGF attracts cells important for wound healing.[74] In addition, as discussed above, FGF promotes the process of angiogenesis that is important to wound repair. FGF stimulates cells to release enzymes that degrade ECM. It also induces fibroblasts to produce ECM building materials, such as collagen and protein.[75,76]

The effect of bFGF on wound granulation tissue formation in the rat has been studied. DNA, protein, total collagen content, and relative collagen content (%) were measured. The amounts of DNA and protein were found to increase after treatment with bFGF; however, the total amount of collagen and the percentage of collagen in the wound decreased. This indicates a collagenolytic activity of cells that is increased by treatment with bFGF.[77] In addition, FGF has been found in increased amounts at the site of healing wounds and in wound fluids.[78,79]

The Role of FGF in the Proliferative Diseases of the Vascular System

bFGF has been found to be an important mitogen playing a significant role in the proliferation of the cellular components of the arterial wall following injury. After balloon catheter endothelial denudation, proliferation of endothelial cells takes place to cover the denuded area. This coverage is usually incomplete. In addition, in response to injury, medial vascular SMCs also proliferate and migrate to the subendothelial area. bFGF has been found to influence the proliferation of these two cellular components.[80]

The following highlights the importance of bFGF in the proliferation of these cells:

1. After endothelial injury, using an antibody raised against human bFGF, the proliferating endothelial cells near the denuded area showed strong staining for bFGF. This was in contrast to the endothelial cells adjacent to the nondenuded areas.[81]

2. In response to endothelial denudation and after the endothelial regeneration has stopped, the administration of bFGF has been found to once again stimulate the proliferation and regrowth of endothelial cells. This was in contrast to cells away from the injured area where the administration of bFGF has been found to show only minimal increase in replication.[82]

3. Vascular SMCs, themselves, have been found to produce aFGF and bFGF.[83,84] The administration of bFGF markedly increased the proliferation of SMCs in vivo after balloon catheter endothelial denudation in the rat.[85]

4. The administration of antibody to bFGF significantly reduced the proliferation of SMCs in response to balloon catheter denudation. However, the administration of antibody to bFGF did not significantly decrease the size of the intimal lesion.[86]

5. In the presence of high density lipoproteins (HDLs), vascular endothelial cells in culture have good response to FGF.[87]

The above citations suggest that bFGF plays an important role in the proliferation of endothelial and SMCs in response to injury, an important step in the processes of atherosclerosis and intimal hyperplasia.

Epidermal Growth Factor and Transforming Growth Factor α

Two important members of the epidermal growth factor family will be discussed: epidermal growth factor (EGF) and transforming growth factor α (TGF-α). EGF was first isolated by Cohen from the submaxillary glands of the mouse, and was first called the "tooth-lid factor" because when it was injected into newborn mice it caused the premature opening of eyelids and eruption of incisors.[88] Two years later, Cohen coined the term "epidermal growth factor" after studies showed that the tooth-lid factor promoted epidermal growth.[89,90] TGF-α was originally isolated from sarcoma preparations and was called "sarcoma growth factor." However, it was found to have EGF-like activity and EGF-like molecular sequence.[91] Purification of TGF-α showed that it was an analog of EGF with high affinity for the EGF receptor.[92] Because EGF and TGF-α share somewhat similar molecular structure and biologic activity they will be discussed together.

Human EGF and TGF-α share sequence homology in 42% of their molecular structure. The EGF molecule is rather small consisting of 53 amino acid residues. It is characterized by a folded configuration with three disulfide bonds connecting the cysteine residues.[93] In addition, the molecular structure of EGF contains aromatic side chains that are grouped together to form hydrophobic areas; these areas are thought to play a role in the growth factor-receptor interaction.[94] Members of the EGF family including TGF-α are similar in 11 amino acid residues, 6 of which are interconnected cysteine residues that define the structure of the EGF family of growth factors.[95]

The human EGF gene is located on chromosome 4; it spans approximately 120 kb and includes 24 exons and 23 introns. The gene for TGF-α is located on human chromosome 2 and it spans 70 to 100 kb, and contains 6 exons.[95]

The EGF Receptor

The EGF receptor is a tyrosine kinase receptor that mediates the activities of the members of EGF family of growth factors. Similar to other tyrosine kinase receptors, the EGF receptor also consists of three main domains, the N-terminal extracellular domain, a transmembrane receptor anchoring domain, and a C-terminal intracellular tyrosine kinase domain. The gene for the EGF receptor is located on chromosome 7 and spans about 110 kb and includes 26 exons. This receptor is expressed on all human cells except those of the hematopoietic system. Binding of the ligand to the receptor induces the formation of receptor dimers which have higher affinity for EGF than do the monomeric receptors.[8,95]

The Role of EGF and TGF-α in the Vascular System

EGF is a widely distributed growth factor. In addition, many cells have been found to produce it. EGF and TGF-α stimulate mitogenic, as well as nonmitogenic, responses in animal cells. The responses induced by both growth factors are somewhat similar. Like EGF, the administration of TGF-α to animals produces precocious eyelid opening.[96] The primary targets of these growth factors are epithelial cells. Normally EGF is an important factor in the continuation of the renewal and division process of epithelial cells.

EGF stimulates the migration and proliferation of cultured human omental microvascular endothelial cells. In addition, it induces the synthesis of tissue-like plasminogen activator (tPA) in these cells. Sato and colleagues examined the effects of various growth factors such as TGF-α and IGF-I and compared these effects to those of EGF. They found that IGF-I, comparable to EGF, induced the proliferation and migration of these cells, whereas TGF-α, similar to EGF, induced the expression of tPA in the omental microvascular endothelial cells. These investigators also found that EGF and TGF-α induced tube formation by these cells in type I collagen gel while IGF-I did not. This tube formation effect of EGF was blocked by the addition of anti-tPA antibody and aprotinin to the medium. The addition of exogenous tPA alone did not cause the induction of tube formation. However, with the addition of exogenous tPA and IGF-I, induction of tube formation in the gel was encountered. These experiments suggested that EGF and TGF-α have active angiogenic activity and could induce tPA, whereas IGF-I could induce angiogenesis only in the presence of tPA.[97] The effect of EGF on human omental microvascular endothelial cells is markedly decreased in late passaged senescent cells. These cells were found to have down-regulated EGF receptor that in turn decreased the responsiveness to EGF as an angiogenic factor.[98]

Gan and his colleagues have studied the effect of EGF and TGF-α administration on the blood flow in the femoral artery of the dog. They found that both EGF and TGF-α caused an increase in the femoral arterial blood flow; however, their administration did not affect the systemic blood pressure.[99] Therefore, these factors may have a localized vasodilator effect.

Pickering and colleagues evaluated the effect of a genetically engineered fusion protein called "DAB389 EGF," in which the receptor-binding domain of diphtheria toxin was replaced by human EGF. Incubation of proliferating vascular SMCs in culture with this protein caused a dose-dependent inhibition of protein synthesis. In addition, the incubation of human atherosclerotic plaque in DAB389 EGF inhibited the outgrowth of SMCs from the plaque. The authors concluded that DAB389 EGF may be of therapeutic value in vascular diseases characterized by SMC proliferation.[100] The use of human recombinant epidermal growth factor (h-EGF) in the healing of venous ulcers was investigated by Falanga and colleagues. A double-blind randomized study was conducted; 44 patients with venous ulceration of the lower extremities were treated. The size of ulcer and granulation tissue formation were followed. The results showed that topical application of h-EGF was safe with no untoward side effects related to its application. In addition, a greater reduction in ulcer size and increase of ulcer healing were encountered in the arm of the study in which h-EGF was used when compared to placebo.[101]

Heparin-binding EGF-like growth factor (HB-EGF) is a newly identified mitogen for SMCs. Dluz and colleagues explored the possibility of whether human vascular SMCs can also synthesize HB-EGF. They used human fetal vascular SMCs in cultures. They analyzed for the production of HB-EGF mRNA and the active growth factor. They found that growth factors that induced the proliferation of vascular SMCs, including HB-EGF, PDGF, or bFGF, stimulated the production of HB-EGF mRNA levels by the cultured cells; in addition, these cells were found to excrete a material that cross-reacted with anti-HB-EGF antibody.[102] Fluid obtained from porcine partial-thickness wounds contained HB-EGF-like growth factor, which indicates that HB-EGF may play an important role in the wound healing process.[103]

Transforming Growth Factor β

DeLarco and Todaro first described, in the late 1970s, the isolation of the sarcoma growth factor (SGF).[104] SGF had the ability to cause changes in cellular morphology and the transformation of non-neoplastic cells such as normal rat kidney (NRK) fibroblast. Therefore, the name of SGF was later changed to transforming growth factor.[105] Further characterization of the transforming growth factor revealed that there were two separate factors later termed α and β.[106] TGF-α was later found to be an analog of the EGF and it was discussed in the prior section. TGF-β is the subject of this section.

The TGF-β family consists of at least five growth factors. These growth factors are given the numbers 1 to 5 depending on their time of purification. These growth factors are 64% to 82% homologous. Structurally, they share some common features such as synthesis from a precursor and conservation of nine cysteine residues in each peptide. TGF-βs are highly conserved between species. The degree of conservation reaches almost 100% in some instances.[107] The first TGF-β purified from human platelets was called TGF-β 1. This peptide is a 25,000 molecular weight homodimer that is 71% homologous with TGF-β 2. TGF-β 2 was purified from porcine platelets, bovine bone, and cultured cells. TGF-β 1 and TGF-β 2 are interchangeable in most assays.[107] TGF-βs 3, 4, and 5 were later identified from cDNA libraries.[108] TGF-β 3 and TGF-β 5 have been found to bind to TGF-β receptors and share TGF-βs 1 and 2 activities.[109] The TGF-βs are produced first as precursors which are cleaved to produce the mature peptides. The shortest precursor is TGF-β 4; it consists of 308 amino acids compared to 382 to 412 for the rest of the TGF-βs.[108] The TGF-β 1 precursor is a 390 amino acid molecule, which when cleaved, gives rise to 112 amino acid monomeric of the TGF-β peptide.[110] Although the number of amino acids in the precursor complex of the TGF-βs varies, the number of amino acids in the TGF-βs themselves is almost the same. TGF-βs 1, 2, 3, and 5 are formed of 112 amino acids and TGF-β 4 is formed of 114. However, TGF-β 4's precursor is formed only of 304 amino acids. This suggests that TGF-β 4 may have a different biologic activity.[107]

The human gene for TGF-β1 is located on chromosome 19, the gene for TGF-β2 is located on chromosome 1, and that for TGF-β3 is located on chromosome 14.[111] The gene for the human TGF-β1 precursor is encoded by 7 exons. This gene is estimated to be greater than 100 kb.[112]

TGF-β Receptors

TGF-βs, as in other growth factors, exert their effect via specific receptors located in the cellular wall. TGF-β receptors have been found on almost all cell types. There are four types of TGF-β receptors. These types are named I through IV. TGF-β I, II receptors have a much higher affinity for TGF-β1 than TGF-β2. Type III has equal affinity to TGF-β1 and TGF-β2. These three types of receptors are ubiquitously found

on many cell lines. The molecular weight of these receptors are: 53 kd, 83 kd, 110 to 130 kd, and 60 kd, respectively. Type IV receptor is found mainly in pituitary gland cells. Most cell lines display all type I through III receptors in varying proportions. TGF-β receptor types I & II are glycoproteins and type III receptor is a beta-glycan complex.[113]

Functions of TGF-βs

TGF-βs exert their functions on almost every cell. TGF-β1 has the ability to inhibit the proliferation of normal and oncogenically transformed cells of epithelial, hemopoietic, and endothelial origin. The actions of the TGF-βs are complex; although TGF-β1 is known to promote the development of bone and cartilage, it does inhibit the differentiation of muscle as opposed to hemopoietic progenitor cells. In these actions and in most assay systems, TGF-β1 and TGF-β2 are indistinguishable. However, TGF-β1 has been found to be more potent at inhibiting the growth and multiplication of hemopoietic and aortic endothelial cells. These diverse functions are carried on by one receptor.[113] The nature of TGF-β actions on a particular target cell is dependent on many factors such as the cell type, its state of differentiation, growth conditions, and other growth factors present.[114] TGF-βs have been found to play a role in growth, multiplication, and differentiation of normal as well as abnormal cells.

TGF-β interferes with the signaling of receptors for other growth factors such as PDGF, EGF, FGF, and IGF-I. TGF-β itself does not use the tyrosine kinase mechanism in exerting its effects. The inhibitory effects of TGF-β are exerted on the late G_1 phase of the cell cycle; therefore, it interferes with the progression of the cell in the G_1 phase and delays its entry into the S phase.[3,107] However, the cells that are already in the S or G_2 phases are no longer inhibited by the effect of TGF-β.[115]

As alluded to earlier, TGF-βs are found in and exert their action on almost every tissue in the body. Although TGF-βs are found in high concentration in platelets, the bony skeleton represents the richest pool of TGF-β in the body. In bone, the function of TGF-β is thought to be one of repair and continuous remodeling. TGF-β has been found to act on chondrocytes, osteoblasts, and osteoclasts.[116] Furthermore, TGF-β has been found to be mitogenic for osteoblasts in culture despite its inhibitory effects on most other cells.[117] In addition, TGF-β has an effect on mesenchymal cells; therefore, it plays an important role in the control of ECM in most tissues including bone. In addition to its effect on chondrocytes, osteoblasts, and osteoclasts, TGF-β has an effect on the mesenchymal precursor cells in bone. It does stimulate ECM protein synthesis by increasing transcription of the genes for collagen and fibronectin. Furthermore, it inhibits ECM protein degradation by decreasing the secretion of proteases and increasing the secretion of protease inhibitors. In addition, TGF-β increases the transcription and processing of cellular receptors for collagen, fibronectin, and other matrix proteins.[107] Although the effect of TGF-β on most epithelial cells in culture is one of inhibition, it does promote the growth of some epithelial cells such as human mesothelial cells.[118] TGF-β inhibits the differentiation of skeletal muscle cells. The physiologic significance of this effect is poorly understood.[107]

TGF-βs affect the cells of the immune system. They inhibit the proliferation of lymphocytes and thymocytes, and counteract the actions of interleukins, tumor necrosis factor and interferons. In contrast, TGF-βs enhance the function of monocytes and macrophages and serve as a chemoattractant for monocytes. In turn, monocytes express TGF-β1 mRNA and secrete TGF-β1 in response to activation.[119]

TGF-β Effects on the Vascular Wall

TGF-βs have been found to play a role in the proliferation of all cellular components of the vascular wall, mainly the endothelium and SMCs. In culture, TGF-β1 and 2 have been found to inhibit the proliferation of endothelial cells. In that regard, the effect of TGF-β1 is much stronger than that of TGF-β2. In addition, TGF-β1 opposes the stimulatory effect of FGF on the growth and proliferation of endothelial cells in culture.[120] Furthermore, TGF-β1 antagonizes the effect of FGF on the migration of endothelial cells.[115] TGF-β1 stimulates the endothelial cells to increase the synthesis of mRNA of the A and B chains of PDGF.[121] In an in vivo study, Madri and colleagues injured the carotid artery of the rat using balloon catheter de-endothelialization. They found that there was increased TGF-β staining in the media of the de-endothelialized area of the vessel.[122]

TGF-β has been found to be produced by adult human aortic SMCs in culture. This production contributed to the inhibition of the growth and multiplication of these cells in culture. Addition of an antibody to TGF-β decreased population doubling time from 74 to 46 hours. This suggests that TGF-β acts in an autocrine fashion to inhibit the multiplication of SMCs.[123] Bovine aortic endothelial and SMCs have been found to have the same response to TGF-β1, 2, and 3 in terms of inhibition of proliferation, cell migration, and neovascularization.[124] The effect of TGF-β was examined on the proliferation and migration of the human saphenous vein SMCs. In a concentration-dependent manner, TGF-β inhibited the proliferation induced by

PDGF, b-FGF, EGF and serum. Furthermore, TGF-β inhibited the migration induced by PDGF and b-FGF.[125]

Therefore, the action of TGF-β on the arterial wall cellular component, including endothelial and SMCs, is mainly one of inhibition of proliferation and migration.

Insulin–Like Growth Factors

Insulin-like growth factors I and II are peptide growth factors that have metabolic effects similar to insulin, hence the name "insulin-like." In addition, IGF-I and IGF-II have potent mitogenic effects that lead to cell proliferation and differentiation. IGF-I is a 70 amino acid protein. IGF-II is a 67 amino acid peptide.[126] Originally, these two growth factors were named depending on their noted effects. IGF-I was initially called somatomedin A, or somatomedin C. IGF-II was initially called multiplication stimulating activity (MSA). The IGFs are secreted in different tissues, especially the liver, and circulate in the serum bound to IGF binding proteins. These binding proteins serve as a storage pool for IGFs. In order for the IGFs to exert their effects, they are released from their binding protein. IGF-I and IGF-II are highly conserved among species. Human, cow, and pig IGF-I is identical. IGF-I from rat and mouse are very closely similar to human IGF-I. IGF-II molecule is also highly conserved among species.[126] Each of the molecules of IGF-I and IGF-II is formed of four domains called A, B, C, and D. Both IGF-I and IGF-II are synthesized as a precursor peptide. These precursors have an E peptide domain in addition to the A, B, C, and D domains of the peptide. The mature IGF-I and IGF-II peptides are located on the amino terminal of the precursor. In humans, the gene for IGF-I is located on chromosome 12 and that for IGF-II on chromosome 11.[111] By comparison, the molecule of insulin contains only A and B domains, referred to as A and B chains.

The liver is a major source of IGF synthesis. Hepatic IGF secretion is growth hormone-dependent. The synthesis and secretion of IGF by the liver is continuous and steady. Schwander and colleagues used rat liver perfusion to study IGF synthesis. When they added ^{35}S-cysteine to the perfusion medium, this amino acid was incorporated in the IGF molecule. In 20 to 30 minutes, the secreted IGF contained ^{35}S-cysteine that reached a plateau in 1 hour. This steady slow synthesis and secretion of IGF from the perfused rat liver paralleled albumin secretion. The liver does not store IGF or its precursor; rather, IGF is synthesized rapidly and regularly secreted. In addition, the liver synthesizes IGF-binding protein.[127] Although the secretion of IGF by the liver is growth hormone-dependent, the secretion of IGF-binding protein by the liver is not. In hypophysectomized rats, the liver does not secrete any measurable amounts of IGF; it does secrete, however, normal amounts of IGF-binding protein.[127] It is estimated that 90% of the total IGF is secreted by the liver.[128] In addition to the hepatic synthesis of IGFs, they are also synthesized by various animal cells. Although the molecule and the metabolic effects of the IGFs closely resemble those of insulin, there are many differences in the metabolism of these peptides. Insulin is synthesized by the islet cells of the pancreas and not the liver; the rates of synthesis and secretion are not steady but change depending on its need; it is found free in the circulation, not attached to binding proteins; and the secretion of insulin is not growth hormone-dependent. In addition, insulin is stored in the β-granules of the pancreas; this prestored insulin is secreted in the circulation when the glucose level rises.[129] Complete absence of growth hormone in pituitary dwarfs leads to extremely low levels of IGF-I and moderately decreased IGF-II levels. The levels of IGF-II are usually one third to one half the normal concentration. Despite these levels of IGF-II, growth in these dwarfs is deficient; therefore, IGF-I is probably more active in stimulating growth than IGF-II. Growth hormone was found to markedly increase IGF-I mRNA in hepatocytes in normal as well as hypophysectomized rats, which suggests that growth hormone acts directly on the hepatocytes.[130] In addition, growth hormone treatment of hypophysectomized rats also increased IGF-I mRNA in many other tissues including muscle, heart, pancreas, and uterus.[131-133] Furthermore, other hormones such as estrogens and prolactin, and nonhormonal factors such as nutrition, diabetes, and injury, do affect the secretion of IGF.[126]

IGF Receptors

Although both IGF-I and IGF-II have similar mitogenic effects, they exert those effects via different receptors. There are two types of IGF receptors: type I and type II. There are major differences between the type I and type II receptors. Type I receptor, also called IGF-I receptor, binds IGF-I with high affinity and IGF-II with lower affinity. In addition, the type I receptor interacts weakly with insulin. The type II, also called IGF-II receptor, has a high affinity for IGF-II and interacts with IGF-I with lower affinity. The type II receptor does not recognize insulin. The receptor for IGF-I is a tyrosine kinase receptor, whereas that for IGF-II does not have an intracellular tyrosine kinase domain and is a Man-6-P receptor.[126] The type I IGF receptor molecular structure resembles that of the insulin receptor. It is a tyrosine kinase receptor organized as a heterotetramer, with two α binding subunits

with a molecular weight of 130,000 and two β subunits with a molecular weight of 95,000. This structure highly resembles the insulin receptor; however, the receptors can be distinguished from each other by ligand binding affinity and reactivity to anti-receptor antibodies. The type I IGF receptor has more affinity for IGF-I than for insulin, whereas the insulin receptor has much more affinity for insulin. The α subunit of the type I IGF receptor is smaller than that of the insulin receptor.[134] The α subunits of the insulin and IGF-I receptors represent the extracellular domain of these receptors and they contain cysteine-rich regions. The intracellular portion of the β subunits represent the cytoplasmic tyrosine kinase domains. The α and β subunits are connected with disulfide bonds (Figure 3).[126] The type I IGF receptor is a high affinity receptor to IGF-I with a dissociation constant (K_d) of 1.5×10^{-9}.[16,18,135] IGF-II binds to the type I receptor with about threefold less affinity than IGF-I, and insulin binds to the type I IGF receptor with about 100 times less affinity than IGF-I.[16]

The type II IGF receptor is a Man-6-P receptor. This receptor contains a very large extracellular domain when compared to its intracellular segment. The type II IGF receptor has high affinity for IGF-II and binds IGF-I with lower affinity. It does not recognize insulin. Interestingly, IGF-II mitogenic effects on cells in culture are carried via the type I IGF receptor.[136] However, in some instances, IGF-II does exert its effect via the IGF-II receptor. The type II IGF receptor does not possess an intrinsic tyrosine kinase activity.[134]

IGF–Binding Protein

IGFs have been found to travel in the circulation bound to specific carrier protein later termed "IGF-binding protein" (IGFBP). In 1989, for easier identification, the IGFBPs were given numbers. Originally, four binding proteins were discovered. Those were termed IGFBP 1, 2, 3, and 4.[137,138] Later on, two more binding proteins were identified by Shimasaki and colleagues and they were given the numbers 5 and 6.[139] These binding proteins share sequence homology. Their genes, however, are located on different chromosomes. The genes for IGFBP 1, 2, 3, 4, and 5 are located on the chromosomes 2, 7, 17, and 5, respectively. The IGFBPs have been isolated in a variety of biologic fluids such as human blood, amniotic fluid, cerebral spinal fluid, saliva, and lymph. Furthermore, these IGFBPs have also been found in a variety of tissues, including the liver where they are primarily synthesized.[127]

It is believed that the functions of the IGFBPs are many. While the IGFs are bound to their binding proteins in the plasma, they are protected from enzymatic degradation because the large molecular weight of the IGFBPs prevent them from crossing the capillary wall into the tissue where they are degraded. Furthermore, due to the high affinity of the IGFBPs to the IGFs, it is believed that these binding proteins decrease the availability of the IGFs to bind with their receptors to exert their functions; therefore, in a way, the IGFBPs act to control the effect of the IGFs. Clemmons and coworkers have shown that cells can secrete IGFBP to control the access of IGF-I or IGF-II to their own receptors.[140] In addition, the IGFBPs act as a storage pool for IGFs. The IGFBPs are synthesized and secreted by the liver and by a variety of cells including human fibroblasts that secrete predominantly IGFBP 3 and 4.[141]

IGF Functions

The functions of IGFs are twofold: metabolic effects that resemble those of insulin and mitogenic effects.

1. *Insulin-like effects of IGFs*: Intravenous injection of IGFs results in a drop of glucose level in the blood within 15 to 30 minutes. The simultaneous injection of anti-insulin serum did not block this effect of IGFs. This indicates that the hypoglycemic effect of IGFs is not mediated via insulin.[128,142] The fact that serum IGF is bound to carrier protein is important in preventing the hypoglycemic effects of the IGFs. When the IGF is released from the binding protein, it crosses the capillary barrier and reaches its target tissue to exert its effect. Like insulin, the IGF also has metabolic effects on adipose and skeletal tissue. However, insulin has a much more powerful effect on adipose tissue when compared to IGFs.[128]

2. *Mitogenic effects of IGFs*: Transcripts for IGF-II are expressed as early as the two-cell embryo, whereas those for IGF-I are not expressed at the pre-implantation stage. Furthermore, the transcripts for IGF-II receptor have been found in the two-cell embryo, whereas those for IGF-I have been found at the eight-cell embryo stage.[143] Through their effect on cellular proliferation there is great evidence to indicate that IGF-I and IGF-II have important roles in cellular differentiation and fetal growth.[144] In pituitary dwarfs, IGF-I levels were found to be very low, and they increased when these patients are treated with growth hormones.[145] This suggests that growth hormone effects are mediated via IGF-I.

IGFs play a role in wound healing. We have found that IGF-I receptor binding at day 7 after surgical wound has significantly increased when compared to day 0.[146] In addition, IGFs play an important role in tumor proliferation. In a small cell lung carcinoma cell line that produces IGF-I, IGF-I receptor antibody inhibited cell growth.[147] Furthermore, IGFs promote the differentiation of a variety of cells including myoblast, osteoblast, and chondroblast.[128] The IGFs have also been found to promote chemotaxis such as in endothelial cells.[148]

The Effects of IGFs on the Proliferation of Vascular Wall Cellular Components

Using autoradiography, we have demonstrated the presence of ^{125}I-IGF-I binding in the arterial wall of the rabbit[16] and in the wall of normal human saphenous vein.[18] In addition, we demonstrated increased ^{125}I-IGF-I binding in atherosclerotic plaques in rabbits fed a high cholesterol diet.[149] In the arterial wall, the dissociation constant (K_d) of IGF-I binding was 2 nmol/L. The binding sites in rabbit arteries and atherosclerotic plaques and in human saphenous veins have been found to be highly specific for IGF-I when compared to IGF-II and insulin, closely related peptides.[16,18,149] IGF-I has been found to induce SMC proliferation that was demonstrated by increased incorporation of [6-^{3}H]thymidine into the DNA of cultured cells.[150,151] In promoting the growth of rat aortic SMCs, IGF-I has been found to act in concert with other growth factors such as PDGF and FGF. When IGF-I was combined with PDGF or FGF, it markedly increased the incorporation of [6-^{3}H]thymidine in the DNA of cultured SMCs when compared to individual growth factors effect. This potentiation of PDGF and FGF effects by IGF-I is exerted via specific IGF-I receptors.[1] Not only does IGF-I act via the IGF-I receptor, insulin too may act via the IGF-I receptor to exert its mitogenic effect. Cultured capillary endothelial cells derived from diabetic rats exhibited markedly decreased insulin binding sites; the IGF-I binding sites were unchanged. The insulin growth-promoting effects were unchanged; however, its metabolic effects were markedly decreased.[152]

IGF-I has been implicated in the reaction of the arterial wall to injury and in arterial wall regeneration. Balloon catheter-denuded arterial endothelium showed regenerating endothelial cells expressing increased IGF-I immunoreactivity.[153] In addition, balloon de-endothelialization of rat aortas induced IGF-I mRNA within 24 hours after injury; IGF-I mRNA peaked at 7 days.[154] Increasing vascular load to one femoral artery by ligating the contralateral artery caused an increase in IGF-I immunoreactivity in the media of the nonligated artery; this suggests a role for IGF-I in the response of arterial wall to tension and to increase in vascular load.[155]

The role of IGF-I as an angiogenic factor has been studied by Grant and colleagues. They have examined the role of IGF-I and bFGF in rabbit cornea model. IGF-I induced angiogenesis in all rabbits studied. This

IGF-I effect was comparable to that of bFGF. In addition, the effects of IGF-I and bFGF were complementary.[156]

The interaction of IGF-I with other growth factors on the proliferation of vascular SMCs was further investigated. IGF-I, TGF-β, and angiotensin enhanced the mitogenicity of PDGF-BB, bFGF, and EGF.[157] In addition, angiotensin II has been found to regulate the transcription of IGF-I gene in vascular SMCs; the presence of IGF-I was necessary for angiotensin II-induced DNA synthesis. These findings implicated IGF-I in the effect of the renin-angiotensin system and vascular growth.[158]

In cultured capillary and large vessel endothelial cells, receptors for IGF-I have been described.[159,160] These endothelial cell receptors are thought to regulate the transport of IGF from the intravascular space to the subendothelial region to act on its target tissue.[160,161] Kwok and colleagues have implicated IGF-I in the development of diabetic vascular complications by the finding that the α-subunit of the IGF-I receptor increased by 50% in aortic endothelial cells cultured from diabetic rats when compared to cells cultured from nondiabetic controls.[162]

Other Growth Factors

In addition to the growth factors detailed above, that have been found to play an important role in the proliferation of vascular wall cellular components, there are other growth factors that directly or indirectly play a role in the vascular system. These growth factors are detailed in other areas of this book relating to a specific function of these factors. In addition to its metabolic effect, insulin, for example, has been found to be a mitogen and its role in that regard is detailed in Chapter 17 dealing with the effect of diabetes on the peripheral vascular system.

References

1. Pfeifle B, Broeder H, Ditscheuneit H: Interaction of receptors for insulin-like growth factor I, platelet-derived growth factor, and fibroblast growth factor in rat aortic cells. *Endocrinology* 120:2251–2258, 1985.
2. Ferns GAA, Raines EW, Strugel KH, Motani AS, Reidy MA, Ross R: Inhibition of neointimal smooth muscle accumulation after angioplasty by an antibody to PDGF. *Science* 253:1129–1132, 1991.
3. Aaronson SA: Growth factors and cancer. *Science* 254: 1146–1153, 1991.
4. Baird A, Bóhlen P: Fibroblast growth factors. In: Sporn MB, Roberts AB (eds). *Peptide Growth Factors and Their Receptors*. Vol I. New York: Springer-Verlag; 369–418, 1990.
5. Zerwes HG, Risau W: Polarized secretion of a platelet-derived growth factor-like chemotactic factor by endothelial cells in vitro. *J Cell Biol* 105:2037–2041, 1987.
6. Risau W, Drexler H, Zerwes HG, et al: Regulation of blood vessel growth and differentiation. In: Bellvé AR,

Vogel HJ (eds). *Molecular Mechanisms in Cellular Growth and Differentiation*. San Diego: Academic Press, Inc.; 207–222, 1991.
7. Sporn MB, Todaro GJ: Autocrine secretion and malignant transformation of cells. *N Engl J Med* 303: 878–880, 1980.
8. Yarden Y, Ullrich A: Growth factor receptor tyrosine kinases. *Ann Rev Biochem* 57:443–478, 1988.
9. King GL, Goodman AD, Buzney SM, Moses A, Kahn CR: Receptors and growth promoting effects of insulin and insulin-like growth factors on cells from bovine retinal capillary and aorta. *J Clin Invest* 75:1087, 1985.
10. Wu J, Dent P, Jelinek T, Wolfman A, Weber MJ, Sturgill TW: Inhibition of the EGF-activated MAP kinase signaling pathway by adenosine 3', 5'-monophosphate. *Science* 262:1055–1059, 1993.
11. Cook SJ, McCormick F: Inhibition by cAMP of Ras-dependent activation of Raf. *Science* 262:1069–1072, 1993.
12. Schindler C, Shuai K, Prezioso VR, Darnell JE: Interferon-dependent tyrosine phosphorylation of a latent cytoplasmic transcription factor. *Science* 257:809–813, 1992.
13. Zhong Z, Wen Z, Darnell JE: Stat3: a stat family member activated by tyrosine phosphorylation in response to epidermal growth factor and interleukin. *Science* 264: 95–98, 1994.
14. Goldschmidt-Clermont PJ, Kim JW, Machesky LM, Rhee SG, Pollard TD: Regulation of phospholipase C-γl by profilin and tyrosine phosphorylation. *Science* 251: 1231–1233, 1991.
15. Scatchard G: The attraction of proteins for small molecules and ions. *Ann NY Acad Sci* 51:660–672, 1949.
16. Sidawy AN, Termanini B, Nardi RV, Harmon JW, Korman LY: Insulin-like growth factor I receptors in the arteries of the rabbit: autoradiographic mapping and receptor characterization. *Surgery* 108:165–171, 1990.
17. Munson PJ: Ligand: a computerized analysis of lingand binding data. *Methods in Enzymol* 92:543,
18. Sidawy AN, Hakim FS, Neville RF, Korman LY: Autoradiographic mapping and characterization of insulin-like growth factor-I receptor binding in human greater saphenous vein. *J Vasc Surg* 18:947–953, 1993.
19. Burke JM, Ross R: Synthesis of connective tissue macromolecules by smooth muscle. *Int Rev Connect Tissue Res* 8:119, 1979.
20. Faggiotto A, Ross R, Harker L: Studies of hypercholesterolemia in the nonhuman primate. I. Changes that lead to fatty streak formation. *Arteriosclerosis* 4:323, 1984.
21. Ross R: The pathogenesis of atherosclerosis: an update. *N Eng J Med* 314:488, 1986.
22. Clowes AW, Schwartz SM: Significance of quiescent smooth muscle migration in the injured rat carotid artery. *Circ Res* 56:139, 1985.
23. Gimbrone MA: Culture of vascular endothelium. *Prog Hemost Thromb* 3:1, 1976.
24. Mcgill HC (ed): *The Geographic Pathology of Atherosclerosis*. Baltimore: Williams & Wilkins; 1968.
25. Faggiotto A, Ross R: Studies of hypercholesterolemia in the nonhuman primate. II. Fatty streaks conversion to fibrous plaque. *Arteriosclerosis* 4:341, 1984.
26. Cathcart MK, Morel DW, Chisolm GM: Monocytes and neutrophils oxidize low-density lipoprotein making it cytotoxic. *J Leuk Biol* 38:341, 1985.
27. Jackson RL, Gotto AM: Hypothesis concerning membrane structure, cholesterol, and atherosclerosis. In: Paoletti R, Gotto AM (eds). *Atherosclerosis Review*. vol I. New York: Raven Press; 1976.

28. Ross R, Glomset JA, Kariya B, Harker L: A platelet-dependent serum factor that stimulates the proliferation of arterial smooth muscle cells in vitro. *Proc Natl Acad Sci USA* 71:1207–1210, 1974.

29. Dicorleto PE, Bowen-Pope DF: Cultured endothelial cells produce a platelet-derived growth factor-like protein. *Proc Natl Acad Sci USA* 80:1919–1923, 1983.

30. Seifert RA, Schwartz SM, Bowen-Pope DF: Developmentally regulated production of platelet-derived growth factor-like molecules. *Nature* 311:669–671, 1984.

31. Hammacher A, Hellman U, Johnsson A, et al: A major part of platelet-derived growth factor purified from human platelets is a heterodimer of one A and one B chain. *J Biol Chem* 263:16493–16498, 1988.

32. Hart CE, Bailey M, Curtis DA, et al: Purification of PDGF-AB and PDGF-BB from human platelet extracts and the identification of all three PDGFs dimers in human platelets. *Biochemistry* 29:166–172, 1990.

33. Raines EW, Bowen-Pope DF, Ross R: Platelet-derived growth factor. In: Sporn MB, Roberts AB (eds). *Peptide Growth Factors and Their Receptors-I*. Heidelberg: Springer-Verlag; 173–262, 1990.

34. Majesky MW, Benditt EP, Schwartz SM: Expression and developmental control of platelet-derived growth factor A-chain and B-chain/sis genes in rat aortic smooth muscle cells. *Proc Natl Acad Sci USA* 85:1524–1528, 1988.

35. Walker LN, Bowen-Pope DF, Ross R, Reidy MA: Production of platelet-derived growth factor-like molecules by cultured arterial smooth muscle cells accompanies proliferation after arterial injury. *Proc Natl Acad Sci USA* 83:7311–7315, 1986.

36. Paulsson Y, Hammacher A, Heldin CH, Westermark B: Possible positive autocrine feedback in the prereplicative phase of human fibroblasts. *Nature* 328:715–717, 1987.

37. Seifert RA, Hart CE, Phillips PE, et al: Two different subunits associate to create isoform-specific platelet-derived growth factor receptors. *J Biol Chem* 264:8771 8778, 1989.

38. Bowen-Pope DF, Ross R: Platelet-derived growth factor. II. Specific binding to cultured cells. *J Biol Chem* 257:5161–5171, 1982.

39. Williams LT, Tremble PM, Lavin MF, Sunday ME: Platelet-derived growth factor receptors form a high affinity state in membrane preparations: kinetics and affinity cross-linking studies. *J Biol Chem* 259:5287–5294, 1984.

40. Owen AJ, Geyer RP, Antoniades HN: Human platelet-derived growth factor stimulates amino acid transport and protein synthesis by human diploid fibroblasts in plasma-free media. *Proc Natl Acad Sci USA* 79:3203–3207, 1982.

41. Bauer EA, Cooper TW, Huang JS, Altman J, Deuel TF: Stimulation of in vitro human skin collagenase expression by platelet-derived growth factor. *Proc Natl Acad Sci USA* 82:4132–4136, 1985.

42. Deuel TF, Sehior RM, Huang SS, Stroobant P, Waterfield MD: Chemotaxis of monocytes and neutrophils to platelet-derived growth factor. *J Clin Invest* 69:1046–1049, 1982.

43. Lynch SE, Nixon JC, Colvin RB, Antoniades HN: Role of platelet-derived growth factor in wound healing: synergistic effects with other growth factors. *Proc Natl Acad Sci USA* 84:7696–7700, 1987.

44. Harlan JM, Thompson PJ, Ross RR, Bowen-Pope DF: α-thrombin induces release of platelet-derived growth factor-like molecule(s) by cultured human endothelial cells. *J Cell Biol* 103:1129–1133, 1986.

45. Berk BC, Alexander RW, Brock TA, Gimbrone MA, Webb CR: Vasoconstriction: a new activity of platelet-derived growth factor. *Science* 232:87–90, 1986.

46. Baumgartner HR, Hosang M: Platelets, platelet-derived growth factor and arteriosclerosis. *Experientia* 44:109–112, 1988.

47. Bowen-Pope DF, Seifert RA, Ross R: The platelet-derived growth factor receptor. In: Boynton AL, Leffert HL (eds). *Control of Animal Cell Proliferation: Recent Advances*. Vol I. New York: Academic Press, Inc.; 1985.

48. Shimokado K, Raines EW, Madtes DK, Barrett TB, Benditt EP, Ross R: A significant part of macrophage-derived growth factor consists of at least two forms of PDGF. *Cell* 43:277–286, 1985.

49. Barrett TB, Benditt EP: Sis (platelet-derived growth factor B chain) gene transcript levels are elevated in human atherosclerotic lesions compared to normal artery. *Proc Natl Acad Sci USA* 84:1099–1103, 1987.

50. Barrett TB, Benditt EP: Platelet-derived growth factor gene expression in human atherosclerotic plaques and normal artery wall. *Proc Natl Acad Sci USA* 85:2810–2814, 1988.

51. Libby P, Warner SJ, Salamon RN, et al: Production of platelet-derived growth factor-like mitogen by smooth muscle cells from human atheroma. *N Engl J Med* 318:1493–1498, 1988.

52. Wilcox JN, Smith KM, Williams LT, Schwartz SM, Gordon D: Platelet-derived growth factor mRNA detection in human atherosclerotic plaques by in situ hybridization. *J Clin Invest* 82:1134–1143, 1988.

53. Ross R, Masuda J, Raines EW, et al: Localization of PDGF-B protein in macrophages in all phases of atherogenesis. *Science* 248:1009–1012, 1990.

54. Majesky MW, Reidy MA, Bowen-Pope DF, Hart CE, Wilcox JN, Schwartz SM: PDGF ligand and receptor gene expression during repair of arterial injury. *J Cell Biol* 111:2149, 1990.

55. Gospodarowicz D, Rudland P, Lindstom J, Benirschke K: Fibroblast growth factor: localization, purification, mode of action and physiological significance: Nobel symposium on growth factors. *Adv Meta Dis* 8:302–335, 1975.

56. Baird A, Klagsburn M: Nomenclature meeting, report, and recommendations, January 17, 1991. In: Baird A, Klagsburn M (eds). *The Fibroblast Growth Factor Family*. Ann NY Acad Sci 638:xiii-xvi, 1991.

57. Growell OA, Chirb E, Willemer EN: Growth of tissues in vitro. VI. The effects of some tissue extracts on the growth of periosteal fibroblast. *J Exp Biol* 16;60–70, 1939.

58. Hoffman RS: The growth-activating effect of extracts of adult and embryonic tissues of the rat on fibroblast colonies in cultures. *Growth* 4:361–376, 1940.

59. Gospodarowicz D: Localization of a fibroblast growth factor and its effect alone and with hydrocortisone on cell growth. *Nature* 249:123–127, 1974.

60. Thomas KA, Riley MC, Lemmon SK, Baglan NC, Bradshaw RA: Brain fibroblast growth factor: nonidentity with mild and basic protein fragment. *J Biol Chem* 255:5517–5520, 1980.

61. Jaye M, Hawk R, Burgess W, et al: The human endothelial cell growth factor: cloning nuclear type sequence, and chromosome localization. *Science* 233:541–545, 1986.

62. Lobb RR, Fett JW: Purification of two distinct growth

factors from bovine neural tissue by heparin affinity chromatography. *Biochemistry* 23:6295–6299, 1984.

63. Baird A, Schubert D, Ling N, Guillemin R: Receptor and heparin-binding domains of basic fibroblast growth factor. *Proc Natl Acad Sci USA* 85:2324–2328, 1988.

64. Gospodarowicz D, Cheng J: Heparin protects basic and acidic FGF from inactivation. *J Cell Physiol* 128:475–484, 1986.

65. Uhlirch S, Lagente O, Lenfant M, Courtois Y: Effect of heparin on the stimulation of nonvascular cells by human acidic and basic FGF. *Biochem Biophys Res Commun* 137:1205–1213, 1986.

66. Thomas KA, Ortega S, Soderman D, et al: Structural modifications of acidic fibroblast growth factor alter activity, stability and heparin dependence. *Ann NY Acad Sci* 6389–6417, 1991.

67. Dionne CA, Jaye M, Schlessinger J: Structural diversity in binding of FGF receptors. *Ann NY Acad Sci* 638:161–166, 1991.

68. Gospodarowicz D: Fibroblast growth factor and its involvement in developmental processes. *Curr Top Dev Biol* 24:57–93, 1990.

69. Gospodarowicz D: Biological activities of fibroblast growth factors. *Ann NY Acad Sci* 638:1–8, 1991.

70. Vlogasky I, Gospodarowicz, D: Structural and functional alterations in the surface of vascular endothelial cells associated with the formation of a confluent cell monolayer and with the withdrawal of fibroblast growth factor. *J Supramol Struct* 12:73–114, 1979.

71. Folkman J: Angiogenesis: new concepts in therapy. *Ann Surg* 175:409–416, 1972.

72. Gospodarowicz D, Lui GM: Effect of substrata and fibroblast growth factor on the proliferation in vitro of bovine aortic endothelial cells. *J Cell Physiol* 109:69–81, 1981.

73. Saksela O, Moscatelli D, Sommer A, Rifkin DB: Endothelial cell-derived heparan sulfate binds basic fibroblast growth factor and protects it from proteolytic degradation. *J Cell Biol* 107:743–755, 1988.

74. Sprugel KH, McPherson JM, Clowes WA, Ross R: Effects of growth factors in vivo. I. Cell ingrowth into porous subcutaneous chambers. *Am J Pathol* 129:601–613, 1987.

75. Chua CC, Barritault D, Geiman DE, Ladda RL: Induction and suppression of type I collagenase in cultured human cells. *Coll Relat Res* 7:277–284, 1987.

76. Davidson JM, Klagsbrun M, Hill KE, et al: Accelerated wound repair, cell proliferation, collagen and accumulation are produced by cartilage-derived growth factor. *J Cell Biol* 100:1219–1227, 1985.

77. Davidson JM, Broadley KN: Manipulation of the wound healing process with bFGF. *Ann NY Acad Sci* 638:306–315, 1991.

78. Finkelstein SB, Apostolides PG, Caday CG, Prosser J, Phillips MF, Klagsbrun M: Increased bFGF immunoreactivity at the site of local brain wounds. *Brain Res* 460:253–259, 1988.

79. Hamerman D, Taylor S, Kirschenbaum I, et al: Growth factors with heparin binding affinity in human synovial fluid. *Proc Soc Exp Biol Med* 186:384–389, 1987.

80. Reidy MA, Lindner V: Basic FGF and growth of arterial cells. *Ann NY Acad Sci* 638:290–299, 1991.

81. Lindner V, Reidy MA, Fingerle J: Regrowth of arterial endothelium: denudation with minimal trauma leads to complete endothelial cell regrowth. *Lab Invest* 61:556–563, 1989.

82. Lindner V, Majack RA, Reidy MA: Basic fibroblast growth factor stimulates endothelial regrowth and pro-liferation in denuded arteries. *J Clin Invest* 85:2004–2008, 1990.

83. Gospodarowicz D, Ferrara N, Haaparanta T, Neufeld G: Basic fibroblast growth factor: expression in cultured bovine vascular smooth muscle cells. *Eur J Cell Biol* 46:144–151, 1988.

84. Winkels JA, Friesel R, Burgess WH, et al: Human vascular smooth muscle cells both express and respond to heparin-binding growth factor I (endothelial cell growth factor). *Proc Nat Acad Sci USA* 84:7124–7128, 1987.

85. Lindner V, Lappi DA, Baird A, Majack RA, Reidy MA: Role of basic fibroblast growth factor in vascular lesion formation. *Circ Res* 68:106–113, 1991.

86. Lindner V, Reidy MA: Proliferation of smooth muscle cells after vascular injury is inhibited by and antibody against basic fibroblast growth factor. *Proc Natl Acad Sci USA* 88:3739–3743, 1991.

87. Tauber JP, Cheng J, Gospodarowicz D: Effect of high and low density lipoproteins on proliferation of cultured bovine vascular endothelial cells. *J Clin Invest* 66:696–708, 1980.

88. Cohen S: Isolation of a mouse submaxillary gland protein accelerating incisor eruption and eyelid opening in the newborn animal. *J Biol Chem* 237:155–162, 1962.

89. Cohen S: Isolation and biological effects of an epidermal growth-stimulating protein. In: Rutter WJ (ed). *Metabolic Controlled Mechanisms in Animals Cells.* National Cancer Institute Monograph 13; 13–27, 1964.

90. Cohen S: The stimulation of epidermal proliferation by a specific protein (EGF). *Dev Biol* 12:394–407, 1965.

91. Todaro GJ, De Larco JE: Transformation by murine and feline sarcoma viruses specifically blocks binding of epidermal growth factor to cells. *Nature* 264:26–31, 1976.

92. Marquardt H, Hunkapiller MW, Hoot LE, et al: Transforming growth factors produced by retrovirus transformed rodent fibroblast and human melanoma cells: amino acid sequence homology with epidermal growth factor. *Proc Natl Acad Sci USA* 80:4684–4688, 1983.

93. Mayo KH, Burke C: Structural and dynamical comparison of alpha, beta, and gamma forms of murine epidermal growth factor. *Eur J Biochem* 169:201–207, 1987.

94. Mayo KH, Schandies B, Savage CR, De Marco A, Kaptein R: Structural characterization and exposure of aromatic residues in epidermal growth factor from rat. *Biochem J* 239:13–18, 1986.

95. Carpenter G, Wahl MI: The epidermal growth factor family. In: Sporn MD, Roberts AB (eds). *Peptide Growth Factors and Their Receptors I.* Heidelberg: Springer-Verlag; 69–171, 1990.

96. Smith JM, Sporn MB, Roberts AB, Derynck R, Winkler M, Gregory H: Human transforming growth factor-α causes precoctious eyelid opening in newborn mice. *Nature* 315:515–516, 1985.

97. Sato Y, Okamura K, Morimoto Λ, et al: Indispensable role of tissue-type plasminogen activator in growth factor-dependent tube formation of human microvascular endothelial cells in vitro. *Exp Cell Res* 204:223–229, 1993.

98. Matsuda T, Okamura K, Sato Y, et al: Decreased response to epidermal growth factor during cellular senescence in cultured human microvascular endothelial cells. *J Cell Physiol* 150:510–516, 1992.

99. Gan BS, Hollenberg MD, MacCannell KL, Lederis K, Winkler ME, Derynck R: Distinct vascular actions of epidermal growth factor-urogastrone and transforming growth factor-α. *J Pharmacol Exp Ther* 242:331–337, 1987.

100. Pickering JG, Bacha PA, Weir L, Jekanowski J, Nichols JC, Isner JM: Prevention of smooth muscle cell outgrowth from human atherosclerotic plaque by recombinant cytotoxin specific for the epidermal growth factor receptor. *J Clin Invest* 91:724–729, 1993.

101. Falanga V, Eaglstein WH, Bucalo B, Katz MH, Harris B, Carson P: Topical use of human recombinant epidermal growth factor (h-EGF) and venous ulcers. *J Dermatol Surg Oncol* 18:604–606, 1992.

102. Dluz SM, Higashiyama S, Damm D, Abraham JA, Klagsbrun M: Heparin-binding epidermal growth factor-like growth factor expression in cultured fetal human vascular smooth muscle cells. *J Biol Chem* 268:18330–18334, 1993.

103. Marikovsky M, Breuing K, Liu PY, et al: Appearance of heparin-binding EGF-like growth factor in wound fluid as a response to injury. *Proc Natl Acad Sci USA* 90:3889–3893, 1993.

104. DeLarco JE, Todaro GJ: Growth factors from murine sarcoma virus-transformed cells. *Proc Natl Acad Sci USA* 75:4001–4005, 1978.

105. Roberts AB, Lamb LC, Newton DL, Sporn MB, Delarco JE, Todaro GJ: Transforming growth factors: isolation of polypeptides from viral and chemically transformed cells by acid efimnol extraction. *Proc Natl Acad Sci USA* 77:3494–3498, 1980.

106. Anzano MA, Roberts AB, Smith JM, Sporn MB, DeLarco JE: Sarcoma growth factor from conditioned medium is composed of both type α and type β transforming growth factors. *Proc Natl Acad Sci USA* 80:6264–6268, 1983.

107. Roberts AB, Sporn MB: The transforming growth factor-betas. In: Sporn MB, Roberts AB (eds). *Peptide Growth Factors and Their Receptors*. Vol 95. Heidelberg: Springer-Verlag; 419–472, 1990.

108. Roberts AB, Kim SJ, Kondaiah P, et al: Transcriptional control of expression of the TGF-βs. *Ann NY Acad Sci* 593:43–50, 1990.

109. Danielpour D, Dart LL, Flanders KC, Roberts AB, Sporn MB: Immuno-detection and quantitation of the two forms of transforming growth factor-beta (TGF-beta 1 and TGF-beta 2) secreted by cells in culture. *J Cell Physiol* 138:79–86, 1989.

110. Madisen L, Lioubin MN, Farrand AL, Brunner AM, Purchio AF: Analysis of proteolytic cleavage of recombinant TGF-β 1: production of hybrid molecules with increased processing efficiency. *Ann NY Acad Sci* 593:7–25, 1990.

111. Chromosomal locations of growth factors/growth factor receptors. In: Sporn MB, Roberts AB (eds). *Peptide Growth Factors and Their Receptors I*. Appendix B. Heidelberg: Springer-Verlag; 775–776, 1991.

112. Deroinck R, Rhee L, Chen EY, Van Tylburg A: Intron-exon structure of human transforming growth factor-beta precursor gene. *Nucleic Acids Res* 15;3188–3189, 1987.

113. Massague J, Cheifetz S, Boyd FT, Andres JL: TGF-β receptors and TGF-β binding proteoglycans: recent progress in identifying their functional properties. In: Transforming growth factor-βs: chemistry, biology, and therapeutics. KA Peiz and MB Sporn (Eds). *Ann NY Acad Sci* 593:59–72, 1990.

114. Sporn MB, Roberts AB, Wakefield LM, de Crombrugghe D: Some recent advances in the chemistry and biology of transforming growth factor-beta. *J Cell Biol* 105:1039–1045, 1987.

115. Heimark RL, Twardzik DR, Schwartz SM: Inhibition of endothelial cell regeneration by type-beta transforming growth factor from platelets. *Science* 233:1078–1080, 1986.

116. Centrella M, McCarthy TL, Canalis E: Skeletal tissue and transforming growth factor-beta. *FASEB J* 2:3066–3073, 1988.

117. Centrella M, McCarthy TL, Canalis E: Transforming growth factor beta is a bifunctional regulator of replication and collagen synthesis in osteoblast-enriched cell cultures from fetal rat bone. *J Biol Chem* 262:2869–2874, 1987.

118. Gabrielson EW, Gerwin BI, Harris CC, Roberts AV, Sporn MB, Lechner GF: Stimulation of DNA synthesis in cultured primary human mesothelial cells by specific growth factors. *FASEB J* 2:2717–2721, 1988.

119. Assoian RK, Fleurdelys BE, Stevenson SC, et al: Expression and secretion of type beta transforming growth factor by activated human macrophages. *Proc Natl Acad Sci USA* 84:6020–6024, 1987.

120. Baird A, Durkin T: Inhibition of endothelial cell proliferation by type beta transforming growth factor: interactions with acidic and basic fibroblast growth factors. *Biochem Biophys Res Commun* 138:476–482, 1986.

121. Starksen NF, Harsh GR, Gibbs VC, Williams LT: Regulated expression of the platelet-derived growth factor: a chain gene in microvascular endothelial cells. *J Biol Chem* 262:14381–14384, 1987.

122. Madri JA, Reidy MA, Kocher O, Bell O. Endothelial cell behavior following denudation injury is modulated by TGF-β1 and fibronectin. *Lab Invest* 60:755–765, 1989.

123. Kirschenlohr HL, Metcalfe JC, Weissberg PL, Grainger DJ: Adult human aortic smooth muscle cells in culture produce active TGF-beta. *Am J Physiol* 265:C571-C576, 1993.

124. Madri JA, Bell L, Merwin JR: Modulation of vascular cell behavior by transforming growth factor beta. *Mol Reprod Dev* 32:121–126, 1992.

125. Mii S, Ware JA, Kent KC: Transforming growth factor-β inhibits human vascular smooth muscle cell growth and migration. *Surgery* 114:464–470, 1993.

126. Rechler MM, Nissley SP: Insulin-like growth factors. In: Sporn MB, Roberts AB (eds). *Peptide Growth Factors and Their Receptors I*. Heidelberg: Springer-Verlag; 263–367, 1990.

127. Schwander J, Hauri C, Zapf J, Froesch ER: Synthesis and secretion of insulin-like growth factor and its binding protein by the perfused rat liver: dependence on growth hormones status. *Endocrinology* 113:297–305, 1983.

128. Froesch ER, Schmid C, Schwander J, Zapf J: Actions of insulin-like growth factors. *Ann Rev Physiol* 47:443–467, 1985.

129. Zapf J, Froesch ER, Humbel RE: The insulin-like growth factors (IGF) of human serum: chemical and biological characterization and aspects of their possible physiological role. *Curr Top Cell Regul* 19:257–309, 1981.

130. Norstedt G, Moller C: Growth hormone induction of insulin-like growth factor-I mRNA in primary cultures of rat liver cells. *J Endocrinol* 115:135–139, 1987.

131. Turner JD, Rotwein P, Novakofsky J, Bechtel PJ: Induction of mRNA for IGF-I and IGF-II during growth hormone stimulated muscle hypertrophy. *Am J Physiol* 255:E513-E517, 1988.

132. Roberts CT, Lasky SR, Lowe WL, Seaman WT, LeRoith D: Molecular cloning of rat insulin-like growth

factor I complementary deoxyribonucleic-acids: the differential mRNA ribonucleic acid processing and regulation by growth hormone and extrahepatic tissues. *Mol Endocrinol* 1:243–248, 1987.

133. Murphy LJ, Bell GI, Duckworth ML, Friesen HG: Identification, characterization, and regulation of a rat complementary deoxyribonucleic acid which encodes insulin-like growth factor-I. *Endocrinology* 121: 684–691, 1987.

134. Nissley ST, Haskell JF, Sasaki N, DeVroede MA, Rechler MM: Insulin-like growth factor receptors. *J Cell Sci* (suppl)3:39–51, 1985.

135. Steel-Perkins G, Turner J, Edman JC, et al: Expression and characterization of a functional human insulin-like growth factor I receptor. *J Biol Chem* 263:11486–11492, 1988.

136. Conover CA, Misra P, Hintz RL, Rozenfeld RG: Effect of an anti-insulin-like growth factor I receptor antibody on insulin-like growth factor II stimulation of DNA synthesis in human fibroblast. *Biochem Biophys Res Commun* 139:501–508, 1986.

137. Drop SLS, Hintz RL (eds). IGF-binding proteins. Amsterdam-New York: Excerpta Medica International Congress Series 881; 1989.

138. Drop SLS, Brinkman A, Kortleve DJ, Groffen CAH, Schuller A, Zwarthoff EC: The evolution of the insulin-like growth factor binding protein family. In: Martin Spencer E (ed). *Modern Concepts of Insulin-Like Growth Factors*. New York: Elsevier Science Publishing Co., Inc.; 1991.

139. Shimasaki S, Shimonaka M, Zhang HP, Ling N: Isolation and molecular characterization of three novel insulin-like growth factor binding proteins. In: Martin Spencer E (ed). *Modern Concepts of Insulin-Like Growth Factors*. New York: Elsevier Science Publishing Co., Inc.; 1991.

140. McCusker RH, Camacho-Hubner C, Bayne ML, Cascieri MA, Clemmons DR: Insulin-like growth factor (IGF) binding to human fibroblast and glyoblastoma cells: the modulating effect of cell released IGF binding proteins (IGFBPs). *J Cell Physiol* 144:244–254, 1990.

141. Clemmons DR, Camacho-Hubner C, Jones JI, McCusker RH, Busby WH: Insulin-like growth factor binding proteins: mechanisms of action at the cellular level. In: Martin Spencer E (ed). *Modern Concepts of Insulin-Like Growth Factors*. New York: Elsevier Science Publishing, Co., Inc.; 1991.

142. Froesch ER, Müller WA, Bürgi H, Waldvogel M, Labhart A: Non-suppressible insulin-like activity of human serum. II. Biological properties of plasma extracts with non-suppressible insulin-like activity. *Biochem Biophys Acta* 121:360–374, 1966.

143. Rappolee DA, Werb Z: Endogenous insulin-like growth factor II mediates growth in pre-implantation mouse embryos. In: Martin Spencer E (ed). *Modern Concepts of Insulin-like Growth Factors*. New York: Elsevier Science Publishing, Co., Inc.; 1991.

144. D'Ercole AJ: Somatomedins/insulin-like growth factors and fetal growth. *J Dev Physiol* 9:481–495, 1987.

145. Merrimee TJ, Zapf J, Froesch ER: Insulin-like growth factors (IGFs) in pygmies and subjects with the pygmy trait: characterization of the metabolic actions of IGF-I and IGF-II in man. *J Clin Endocr Metab* 55:1081–1088, 1982.

146. Hakim FS, Shetty S, Sidawy AN, Curcio LD, Korman LY, Harmon JW: Increased specific binding of insulin-like growth factor-I in healing cutaneous wounds. *Wound Repair and Regeneration* 3:492–499, 1995.

147. Nakanishi Y, Mulshine JL, Kasprzyk PG, et al: Insulin-like growth factor-I can mediate autocrine proliferation of human small cell lung cancer cell lines in vitro. *J Clin Invest* 82:354–359, 1988.

148. Grant M, Jerdan J, Merrimee GJ: Insulin-like growth factor-I modulates endothelial cell chemotaxis. *J Clin Endocrinol Metab* 65:370–371, 1987.

149. Sidawy AN, Termanini B, Harmon JW, Nardi RV, Korman LY: Autoradiographic mapping of insulin-like growth factor-I receptor binding in the atherosclerotic arteries of the rabbit. *Surgical Forum* 41:334–336, 1990.

150. Pfeifle D, Ditschuneit HH, Ditschuneit H: Binding and biological actions of insulin-like growth factors on human smooth muscle cells. *Horm Metab Res* 14: 409–414, 1982.

151. Clemmons DR: Interaction of circulating cell-derived and plasma growth factors in stimulating plasma smooth muscle cell replication. *J Cell Physiol* 121:425–430, 1984.

152. Kwok CF, Goldstein BJ, Muller Wieland D, Lee TS, Kahn CR, King GL: Identification of persistant defects in insulin receptor structure and function in capillary endothelial cells from diabetic rats. *J Clin Invest* 83: 127–136, 1989.

153. Hansson HA, Jennische E, Skottner A: Regenerating endothelial cells express insulin-like growth factor-I immunoreactivity after arterial injury. *Cell Tissue Res* 250: 499–505, 1987.

154. Cercek B, Fishbein MC, Forrester JS, Helfant RH, Fagin JA: Induction of insulin-like growth factor I messenger RNA in rat aorta after balloon denudation. *Circ Res* 66:1755–1760, 1990.

155. Hansson HA, Jennische E, Skottner A: IGF-I expression in blood vessels varies with vascular load. *Acta Physiol Scand* 129:165–169, 1987.

156. Grant MB, Mames RN, Fitzgerald C, Ellis EA, Aboufriekha M, Guy J: Insulin-like growth factor-I acts as an angiogenic agent in rabbit cornea and retina: comparative studies with basic fibroblast growth factor. *Diabetologia* 36:282–291, 1993.

157. Ko Y, Stiebler H, Nickenig G, Wieczorek AJ, Vetter H, Sachinidis A: Synergistic action of angiotensin II, insulin-like growth factor I, and transforming growth factor-beta on platelet-derived growth factor BB, basic fibroblast growth factor and epidermal growth factor-induced DNA synthesis in vascular smooth muscle cells. *Am J Hypertens* 6:496–499, 1993.

158. DeLafontaine P, Lou H: Angiotensin II regulates insulin-like growth factor I gene expression in vascular smooth muscle cells. *J Biol Chem* 268:16866–16870, 1993.

159. Bar RS, Boes M: Distinct receptors for IGF-I, IGF-II, and insulin are present on bovine capillary endothelial cells and large vessel endothelial cells. *Biochem Biophys Res Commun* 124:203–209, 1984.

160. Bar RS, Boes M, Dake BL, Booth BA, Henley SA: Insulin, insulin-like growth factor and vascular endothelium. *Am J Med* (suppl)85:59–70, 1988.

161. Banskota NK, Carpentier JL, King GL: Processing and release of insulin and insulin-like growth factor I by macro- and microvascular endothelial cells. *Endocrinology* 119:1904–1913, 1986.

162. Kwok CF, Ho LT, Jap TS: Insulin-like growth factor-I receptor increases in aortic endothelial cells from diabetic rats. *Metabolism* 42:1381–1385, 1993.

CHAPTER 6

Endothelial Cells

Gary L. Gallagher, MD; Bauer E. Sumpio, MD, PhD

Introduction

The vascular endothelium exists as a single, continuous layer of cells presenting a structural and functional interface between the blood and the vessel wall. Although it was once thought to be a passive, nonthrombotic barrier, the vascular endothelium is now known to be an active and influential participant in both normal and abnormal physiologic processes. The endothelium is uniquely situated in the vessel wall to come into contact with luminal signals, whether it be physical forces, chemical substances, or immunologic mediators. For these signals to be effective, they must be recognized by the endothelium, transduced into intracellular messages, and then transmitted as secreted moieties to the surrounding blood and vessel cells. The endothelium is now recognized as an important metabolic organ, capable of interacting with its cellular and acellular environment (Figures 1 and 2). For example, the endothelial cell is capable of producing vasoconstricting and vasorelaxing substances that, together with the influence of the sympathetic nerve stimuli, coordinate to provide a balanced system able to respond to local and systemic stimuli altering vascular tone. The endothelium participates in the process of new vessel development—as in embryogenesis and neovascularization—and chronic vascular remodeling by influencing the growth and migration of cellular elements, and by regulating the composition of the underlying extracellular matrix (ECM). Endothelial cells are also capable of synthesizing a number of stimulatory or inhibitory mitogens, which exert both autocrine and paracrine effects.

Normally, there exists a balance between the prothrombotic and antithrombotic/fibrinolytic character of the endothelial cell, favoring the anticoagulated milieu and keeping the blood fluid.

Perturbation or injury of the endothelium by various means alters this resistant state, setting into motion the cascades of plasma coagulation and platelet activation (Figure 2) during which the endothelial cell has a promoting and limiting role providing for an efficient coagulation response.

The endothelium also interacts with lymphocytes in specialized areas, providing for the targeting and recirculation of these cells in the normal process of immune surveillance. When stimulated by local inflammatory mediators, the endothelium responds to coordinate the overall immune response, leading to local vasomotor and vessel permeabilbity changes, and interacting with leukocytes, lymphocytes, and platelets to specifically direct the cellular response (Figure 2).

The goal of this chapter is to provide an introduction to the basic structure and function of the endothelial cell. Since much of what is known about endothelial cells comes from in vitro studies, the last section of this chapter introduces the techniques used to cultivate and grow endothelial cells from various sources. The endothelial cell's role in regulating vessel tone and growth, and its function in the process of plasma coagulation cascades, are covered extensively in other chapters.

Development

Vascular channels and capillary plexuses are among the first structures noted during embryonic morphogenesis of many organ systems. In general, there are two mechanisms by which vessels form during development: the budding and branching of existing vessels—angiogenesis—or the in situ differentiation of

From *The Basic Science of Vascular Disease*. Edited by Sidawy AN, Sumpio BE, and DePalma RG. Armonk, NY: Futura Publishing Company, Inc.; © 1997.

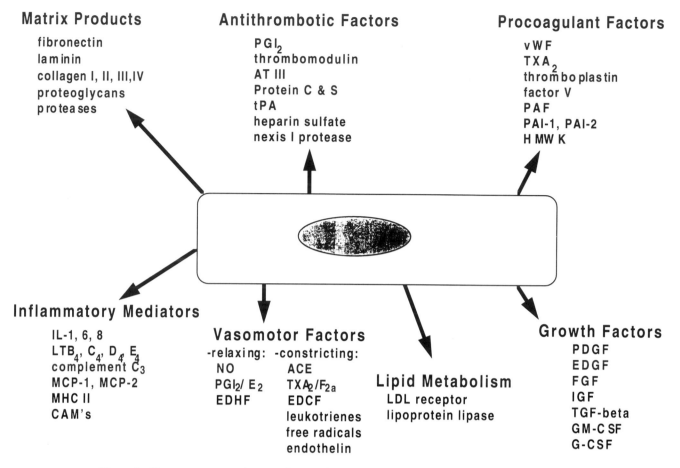

Figure 1. Known secretory/expression products of endothelial cells relating to vessel physiology.

endothelial cells from precursor cells—vasculogenesis.[1,2] Initially, it was thought that all vessels were derived from extraembryonic precursors, which formed vascular channels throughout the embryo through the mechanism of angiogenesis. This theory resulted from early observations that the first detectable signs of vessel developement occurred outside the embryo in the yolk sac, where aggregates of cells in the splanchnic mesoderm, called *blood islands*, formed channels through fusion of adjacent vesicles, and grew to invade the adjacent embryo. Subsequent studies separating the yolk sac and embryo prior to such invasion, however, failed to prevent embryonic vascular channels from forming,[3] indicating that intraembryonic endothelial cells could develop in situ as well. More recent studies, utilizing antibodies specific to endothelial cells,[4] have detected in some areas, the presence of intraembryonic precursor cells prior to vessel formation.[4,5] By transplanting quail embryo mesoderm into chick embryos, Noden et al[6] determined that all intraembryonic mesoderm, except the prechordal plate, contained angiogenic precursors. Furthermore, the transplanted angioblasts invaded the surrounding mes-

enchyme, taking part in vessel formation appropriate to the site through in situ formation of vesicles, and by angiogenesis (Figure 3). Since transplanted precursors become part of the site-appropriate vasculature, cues directing the organization of the vessels must reside within the surrounding cellular environment. It appears now that the adjacent endoderm promotes in situ vessel formation, or vasculogenesis, whereas ectoderm induces more angiogenesis.[2] Angiogenesis has also been reported as the predominant mechanism of vessel formation in kidney,[7] and brain.[1] Seifert et al[8] have shown that both mechanisms operate during limb bud vascularization in bird embryos. Thus, it appears that the process of vasculogenesis is limited to embryogenesis, while angiogenesis plays an important role throughout life in such processes as wound healing and placenta development after pregnancy. Angiogenesis also contributes to many pathologic conditions, such as in tumor vascularization and the neovascularization of diabetic retinopathy.

The signals directing early events of vessel morphogenesis are not well defined, but appear, in some part, to involve changes in the composition of ECM components. Initially, fibronectin is secreted, promoting endothelial cell migration and proliferation. Risau et al[1] were able to show that cells in the yolk sac blood islands, as well as early intraembryonic capillaries and dorsal aorta exist in a fibronectin matrix. In addition, sprouts of endothelial cells invade the embryonic neuroectoderm at day 4 of brain development, only when a fibronectin matrix is present on the abluminal side of the migrating cells. As the vascular channels proliferate, laminin begins to appear, concurrent with a down-regulation of endothelial cell proliferation and migration, and the onset cell differentiation and smooth muscle precursor aggregation.[9] Laminin appears in adult-like distribution in dorsal aorta between day 8 and 10, and codistributes with fibronectin in brain capillaries by day 6.[1] Arciniegas et al[10,11] have noted endothelial cell activation in the aorta of chick embryos between day 7 and 18, concomitant with qualitative and quantitative changes in ECM components, and a progression of intercellular junctions towards the focal tight junctions normally seen in mature arteries. Cell migration and vessel lumen formation occurring during the process of development appear to also require proteolytic digestion of the restraining matrix, possibly liberating matrix-bound growth factors. Microvascular endothelial cells are known to produce several proteolytic enzymes in response to angiogenic agents,[12] and a balance between proteolytic activity and protease inhibitors may be required for normal capillary morphogenesis.[13]

In addition to the potential role of matrix components in directing vessel morphogenesis, many growth-promoting substances are produced by the endothelium or adjacent cells. Many compounds have been identified which promote or inhibit angiogenesis both in vitro and in vivo (Table 1).[14,15] Acidic- and basic-fibroblast growth factor (aFGF, bFGF) are potent endothelial cell mitogens both in vitro and in vivo,[8] and are temporally expressed in conjunction with the onset of vascularization in the chick embryo.[1] bFGF is known to influence endothelial cell expression of matrix components, including collagen, proteoglycans, and fibronectin.[16] The spatial and temporal pattern of vascular endothelial cell growth factor (VEGA) expression correlates with the ingrowth of blood vessels into the developing neuroectoderm during brain angiogenesis.[17] Thompson et al [18] have been able to induce and sustain organoid vascular structures in vivo

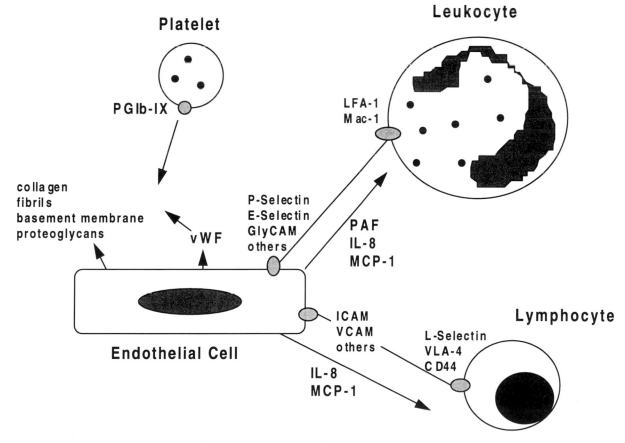

Figure 2. Molecules of importance in regulating the interactions of endothelial cells with platelets, leukocytes, and lymphocytes.

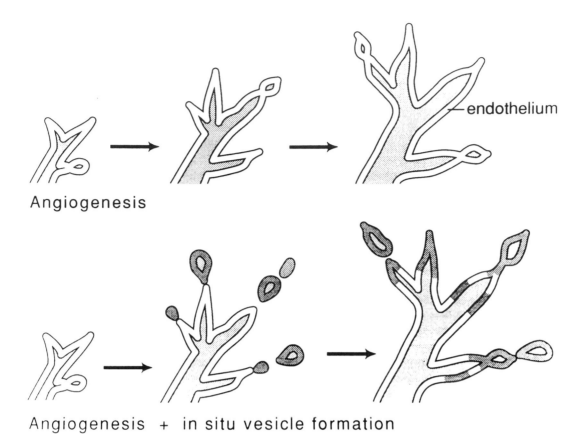

Figure 3. Schematic depiction of embryonic vasculogenesis based upon results of transplantation experiments. (Reproduced with permission from Reference 6.)

by implanting aFGF polypeptide, bound to collagen type I-coated polytetrafluoroethylene (PTFE), onto rat livers. Multiple vascular channels lined by endothelial cells, surrounded by layers of differentiated vascular smooth muscle cells (SMC) were induced. In addition, the organoid contained several neural-like structures, and was circumscribed by a monolayer of mesothelial cells. The ordered anatomic organoid suggests that the presence of a specific growth factor (such as aFGF) in the presence of a specific ECM component (such as collagen type I), can coordinate the differentiation of mesoderm- and perhaps neuroectoderm-derived cells. The early events in vessel formation and angiogenesis may be influenced by a variety of other growth substances, and later, by the hemodynamic forces of flowing blood.

Structure of the Endothelium

Extracellular Matrix

Endothelial cells lie atop a well-defined basement membrane in vivo. This layer is comprised of an electron-lucent zone, the lamina rara, and an electron-dense zone, the lamina densa, which lies next to the interstitial connective tissue. The basement membrane is a heterogeneous, highly specialized structure constructed from components of ECM proteins. They primarily serve to anchor adjacent cells, but can also regulate cell differentiation, migration, and phenotype. In addition, they act as barriers for filtration of macromolecules.

Endothelial cells attach to the basement membrane via specific cellular receptors. Interactions depend upon the existence of unique sequences and domains within the ECM molecules, and can involve matrix-bound growth factors. The ability to initiate the formation of new blood vessels and to repair existing damaged ones requires that the endothelium respond to appropriate stimuli by undergoing phenotypic changes that enable the endothelial cells to migrate, proliferate, and effect repair. It is not surprising then, that almost all cellular events occurring during development, angiogenesis, and wound healing are influenced by components of the ECM.

A continuous monolayer of endothelial cells attached to an underlying basement membrane represents a nonthrombogenic surface to the blood. Normally, the intact endothelium is a quiescent, contact-inhibited monolayer with a low mitotic index, reflecting the stability and integrity of the vessel wall. The endothelial cells form complex cell to cell junctions, synthesize and secrete ECM components, such as fibronectin, and secrete a basement membrane, comprised of laminin, proteoglycans, and several collagen species. The underlying reticular layer, when present, consists of collagen types I and III produced by the endothelial cells and SMCs. Evidence suggests that ECM components can influence cell phenotype in both endothelial cells and SMCs.

In culture, endothelial cells proliferate rapidly until a confluent monolayer is produced. As confluence is approached, the cells take on a characteristic cobblestone appearance, similar to in vivo, contact-inhibited layers. Endothelial cell phenotype is influenced by the growth media, growth surface, and the age of the cultures. Most culture procedures utilize serum or tissue extracts as a source of growth and attachment factors, and many culture vessels are coated with ECM elements (i.e., fibronectin, collagen, laminin) to promote attachment and growth. When endothelial cells are maintained at confluent densities for an extended duration, or when growth factors are withdrawn, capillary-like structures form spontaneously.[19] When microvascular endothelial cells are cultured on gelatin-coated culture vessels, they flatten, lose cellular contacts, and form tubular structures.[20] When endothelial cells are grown on interstitial collagens (types I and III), or fibronectin, they lose their tight junctions, express smooth muscle α-actin mRNA and protein, and form tubules.[21,22] When grown on natural (e.g., amnion), or reconstructed basement membranes (e.g., Matrigel), basal lamina collagens (types IV and V), or laminin, endothelial cells are more differentiated, having a low proliferative rate, exhibiting intercellular tight junctions, and luminal and abluminal membrane specializations. Laminin, the principle glycoprotein in Matrigel, a reconstituted basement membrane preparation from murine Engelebreth-Holm-Swarm (EHS) mouse tumor cells, has been shown to induce the tubular growth pattern.[23]

Unlike endothelial cells derived from large vessels which are flattened, polygonal, two-dimensional monolayers, microvascular endothelial cells exist in a three-dimensional matrix. Two-dimensional cultures are, therefore, not likely to reflect the in vivo condition of these cells. Transforming growth factor-β_1 (TGF-

Table 1
Factors Known to Promote (top), and Inhibit (bottom) Angiogenesis In Vitro and In Vivo

Angiogenesis Factors

Name	MW	Heparin-Binding	Angiogenesis	EC Migration	EC Proliferation	EC Specific	Secreted
FGF	18,000	+	+	+	+	0	0
VEGF/VPF	46,000 (dimer)	+	+	+	+	+	+
PD-ECGF	46,000	0	+	+	+	+	0
TGF-α	5,500	0	+	+	+	0	+
Angiogenin	14,100	0	+	0	0	nd	+
Angiotropin	4,500	nd	+	+	0	+	+
TGF-β	25,000 (dimer)	0	+	−	−	0	+
TNF-α	17,000	0	+	+	−	0	+

Angiogenesis Inhibitors

Factor	MW	Heparin-Binding	Angiogenesis	EC Migration	EC Proliferation
Angiostatic steroids	na	na	−	nd	−
Platelet Factor IV	28,000	+	−	nd	−
TNF-α	17,000	0	+	+	−
Thrombospondin	160,000	+	−	−	nd
TGF-β	25,000 (dimer)	0	+	−	−
γ-interferon	50,000	0	−	−	−
Protamine	43,000	+	−	nd	−

+: yes; 0: no; −: inhibitory; nd: not determined; na: not applicable; EC: endothelial cell.
(Reproduced with permission from Reference 63.)

β_1), when added to in vitro, two-dimensional cultures of endothelial cells, inhibits proliferation and induces profound increase in expression of smooth muscle α-actin mRNA, opposite to the cytokine's effect in vivo.[24] Two-dimensional culture (i.e., single mono-layer), also results in expression of platelet-derived growth factor (PDGF) receptors by microvascular endothelial cells, which can then respond to the growth factor by increasing cellular proliferation. Several three-dimensional culture systems and specific organ culture models have been developed in an attempt to approximate the in vivo milieu of microvascular endothelial cells.[25] In three-dimensional culture, microvascular endothelial cells show a lower proliferative rate, and the mitogenic effects of several growth factors, such as TGF and PDGF, are reduced. These effects may partially result from the loss of PDGF receptor in the three-dimensional system. Although TGF-β will not increase endothelial cell proliferation in this system, it will induce differentiation, as evidenced by the tubular aggregates, tight junctions, and the organization of a basal lamina.

The biochemical composition of basement membranes has been intensively studied using models which produce major components of the basement membrane, such as the EHS mouse tumor cell line[26,27] and embryonal carcinoma derived from endodermal cells.[28] The basement membrane components include heparan-sulfate proteoglycans, laminin, nidogen (entactin), and types IV and V collagen. Electron microscopy demonstrates that the components interact through spatially-specific binding domains, although different basement membranes are structurally unique. Nonetheless, the general molecular architecture appears to be based upon a three-dimensional network located in the lamina densa, consisting of collagen type IV surrounded by laminin, and further associated with double tracks of heparan sulfate proteoglycans (Figure 4).[29] The lamina rara displays a more amorphous appearance.

Proteoglycans are a complex and diverse set of ubiquitous macromolecules, which can influence a variety of arterial properties, such as viscoelasticity, permeability, lipid metabolism, hemostasis, and thrombosis.[15,30] Endothelial cells in culture primarily produce heparan sulfate-like proteoglycans, along with smaller amounts of dermatin and chondroitin sulfate. The heparan sulfate chains produced by endothelial cells contain heparin sequences which are chemotactic for endothelial cells. Heparin modulates endothelial cell growth factor (ECGF), increasing its mitogenic activity. Endothelial cells grown in the presence of heparin and ECGF have a decreased expression of collagen types I and IV, fibronectin, and the proteoglycan, decorin.[31] Three species of proteoglycans have been identified in cultured endothelial cells, beta-glycan, decorin, and versican.

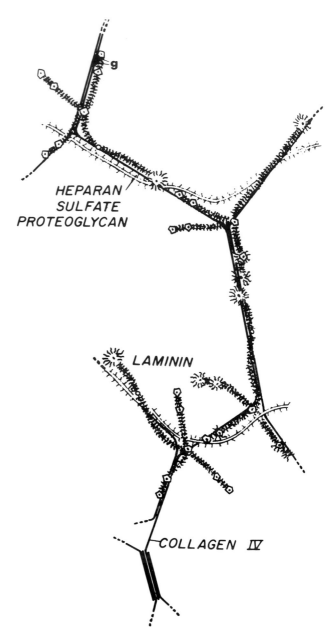

Figure 4. Proposed structure resulting from the interaction of collagen type IV, laminin, and heparan sulfate proteoglycans in the lamina-densa of the basement membrane. (Reproduced with permission from Reference 29.)

They are strongly bound within the basement membrane, and may be clustered by self-assembly. They interact with other ECM components, including laminin and collagen IV, and may influence serine protease activity, which is critical in basement membrane remodelling. Beta-glycan is a large polymorphic chondroitin sulfate/heparan sulfate proteoglycan, which can occur in either a soluble or membrane-bound form. Decorin is an abundant chondroitin sulfate/dermatin sulfate complex which is leucine-rich, and frequently associated with type I collagen fibrils in tissues.

Collagen plays an important role in endothelial cell attachment to the subendothelial matrix, contributing to monolayer integrity. Fourteen collagen types have been described to date, and have been divided into fibril (I, II, III, V, XI), or nonfibril-forming species (IV, X), depending upon whether they form networks or microfibrils.[32-34] In contrast to fibronectin or laminin, which possess few, well-defined binding sites, collagen has multiple cellular interaction sites along its structure. Type IV collagen is characteristic of the basement membranes and has been isolated from human aorta and the basal lamina of vascular SMCs. Cultured endothelial cells and SMCs will synthesize type IV collagen. Type IV monomers exhibit a triple helical structure with glycine in every third position, and a high content of proline and hydroxyproline.[35] The triple helix is 390 nm long and contains a triad of genetically distinct alpha chains (alpha$_1$-alpha$_5$), although the major ubiquitous isoform is composed of two alpha$_1$ chains associated with one alpha$_2$ chain. The identity of the molecules into which the minor chains, alpha$_{3-5}$, become incorporated has not yet been defined. The alpha-chains of type IV collagen differ from alpha-chains of fibril-forming collagens by virtue of the contained interruptions in their Gly-X-Y repeats by noncollagenous sequences. These are evenly distributed along the helix, imparting flexibility, and providing sites for proteolytic digestion. The C-terminus is bounded by a globular domain, NC1, which has a high degree of sequence homology with other alpha-chains. Furthermore, the alpha$_1$ and alpha$_2$ segments of collagen type IV possess internal repeats of cysteine residues, which create symmetric folding around the formed disulfide bonds. Dimers of type IV collagen are generated through association between the C-terminal domains. The N-terminal domain, 7S, can associate with other 7S segments, leading to tetramer formation (Figure 5).[26] These intramolecule interactions allow a complex, supramolecular structural network to be constructed (Figure 4).

Endothelial cell adhesion and migration, which are processes associated with cytoskeletal alterations, are preferentially enhanced by type IV collagen.[19,36] In organ culture models of angiogenesis, type IV collagen occurs predominantly at the most distal tip of the angiogenic sprout, whereas in the area of differentiation, type VI collagen, along with type V collagen, laminin, and fibronectin, is arranged into a diffuse envelope, surrounding the luminal structures.[37] Fibronectin and type V collagen are organized into cable-like structures, while laminin is located diffusely over the cell surface.[25] Type V collagen is a pericellular collagen produced by both endothelial cells and SMCs. It may function to bind interstitial collagen to cells or basal laminae.

As noted, the growth of endothelial cells on interstitial collagens elicits a proliferative phenotype. Of the interstitial collagens, types I and III are by far the most predominant in the vessel wall. Although type I is the major type present in human aorta intima-media, type III collagen is present in the subendothelium of younger individuals, and may be produced by the endothelium. Bovine endothelial cells have been shown to produce type III collagen in vitro. In variant "sprouter" cells, appearing spontaneously in endothelial cell cultures grown to confluence, type I collagen production can be induced concomitant with a shift in fibronectin RNA processing.[38] These cells are characterized by their elongation and formation of an interconnecting, reticular network underneath the monolayer from which they originated. The variant cells have altered polarity and increased fibronectin on their apical surface. Trypsinization or subculturing causes these cells to revert to their polygonal phenotype. Morphologically, normal endothelial cells from several sources exhibit a similar pattern of collagen gene expression. The cells are unable to produce collagen type I until activation or derepression of the type I gene occurs, an event associated with transformation to the elongated sprout. The proposed function of the sprout cell is to act as a lead cell, establishing a matrix that normal cells can follow, leading to the formation

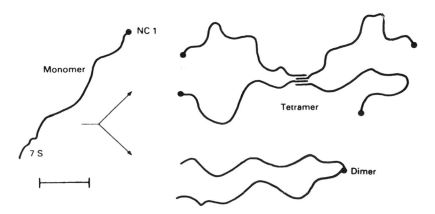

Figure 5. Model of type IV collagen and its modes of association. (Reproduced with permission from Reference 35.)

of new endothelium. The fibronectin isoforms may be required for normal collagen association, providing a scaffold for collagen types I and III.

Laminin is a noncollagenous basement membrane component with distinct cell binding properties, and has been one of the most extensively studied.[35,39,40] The most common isoform has a molecular weight of 900 kDa and consists of three peptide chains; an A chain (Mr = 400 k), a B1 chain (Mr = 210 k), and a B2 chain (Mr = 200 k). Their genes have been localized to the human chromosomes 18, 7, and 1, respectively.[41] The three chains form a triple-stranded, coiled-coil structure, corresponding to the long arm of the molecule (Figure 6). The long arm ends in a large, globular domain formed by folding of the A chain. Laminin can polymerize in vitro, in the presence of Ca + +, through the association of the globular domains. In vitro studies have demonstrated that laminin can accelerate the attachment of endothelial cells to type IV collagen. Multiple interaction with other extracellular components and with cells through their surface receptors, make laminin a key mediator of cell-base-ment membrane interactions. A portion of the A chain, fragment 1 (P1), contains the RGD sequence (arginine-glycine-aspartic acid) found in a number of protein-cell attachment sites, and mediates cellular binding to laminin (Figure 6).[35,37] Laminin has the ability to bind heparan sulfate and collagen type IV, which may be mediated by nidogen (entactin).[42] The nidogen-laminin complex, which can be extracted from basement membranes, is formed by the interaction of nidogens C-terminal, globular domains, with a short arm segment of laminin corresponding to fragment 1 (P1). Nidogen has a molecular weight of 148 kDa, and is 5% carbohydrate. It contains three globular domains, G1–3, which are easily cleaved by proteases; a sensitivity thought to be important in basement membrane remodelling. Nidogen promotes the formation of a ternary complex between laminin and collagen IV, both components interacting independently. The binding to collagen is promoted by the G2 domain of nidogen, whereas laminin binding occurs on the C-terminal G3 domain. In a similar fashion, it appears that nidogen also serves to mediate complex formation between laminin and proteoglycans, revealing the molecules important role in basement membrane organization and stabilization.

A second sequence on the short arm of the laminin B1 chain contains the sequence YIGSR (tyrosine-isoleucine-glycine-serine-arginine), which is thought to be involved in cell interaction, and is responsible for the adhesion of cultured endothelial cells to Matrigel.[37] Another sequence near the C-terminal end of laminin, on the B1 chain, contains the sequence SIKVAV (serine-isoleucine-lysine-valine-alanine-valine), which has been shown to promote adhesion, migration, and differentiation. Human umbilical vein endothelial cells (HUVEC) grown on Matrigel are induced to differentiate, forming a network of capillary-like structures, with polarized cells mimicking new vessel formation. Addition of cycloheximide, cytochalasin, or colchicine will inhibit tube formation, suggesting that protein synthesis and an intact cytoskeleton are necessary. In addition, antisera against laminin or nidogen, but not proteoglycans, collagen IV, or fibronectin, also inhibit tube formation. Addition of synthetic laminin-derived peptides containing the above mentioned sequences results in a variety of effects (Table 2). An RGD-containing peptide can block cell attachment to the matrix, whereas the YIGSRC-containing peptide will inhibit the morphologic changes associated with tube formation. The SIKVAV-containing peptide will induce cells to invade the substratum, increase their secretory proteolytic activity, and can cause new vessel formation in vivo. This suggests that laminin sequences can have substantial effects on endothelial cell behavior, and may be important in angiogenic activity in vivo.

Fibronectin is a large glycoprotein comprised of two disulfide-linked subunits, A and B chains, occur-

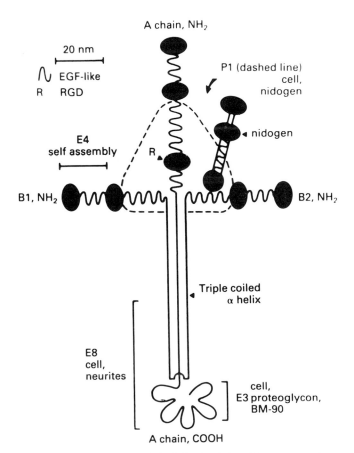

Figure 6. Structural model of the laminin-nidogen complex. The crucial structure of laminin is formed by the B1, B2, and A chains. The location of nidogen, as well as the proteolytically generated fragments P1, E3, E4, and E8, are shown. (Reproduced with permission from Reference 35.)

Table 2
The Relative Activities of Three Synthetic
Peptides Corresponding to Specific
Laminin Sequences (see text) for Several
Biological Assays

	Bioactivity of Laminin Peptides		
	YIGSR	RGD	SIKVAV
Adhesion	+ +	+ + +	+ +
Morphology	+ + +	+	+ + +
Migration	+	+	+ + + +
Growth	0	+	0
Differentiation	+ + +	0	+ +
Collagenase	+ +	0	+ + + +

(Reproduced with permission from Reference 88.)

ring in several spliced variants. It has a molecular weight of 200000, and can promote adhesion and spreading of mesenchymal and epithelial cells, the proliferation and migration of embryonic and tumor cells, and control cell differentiation, shape, and cytoskeletal organization. Microvascular and HUVECs preferentially attach to fibronectin as compared with laminin or collagen, and will migrate in greater numbers through fibronectin. Expression of the sprouter cell phenotype is associated with alterations in fibronectin RNA processing, preferentially producing a cellular form of the protein, over the plasma form, which is expressed by

morphologically normal endothelial cells. The plasma form lacks a 270 and 273 nucleotide exon in the A and B chain RNA. The presence of the A chain extra exon sequence in fibronectin correlates with developmental changes, wound healing, and acute tissue and endothelial cell injury. TGF-β, which stimulates angiogenesis in vivo, has been shown to increase fibronectin production in endothelial cells.[43] It binds microvascular endothelial cells through multiple cell surface integrin receptors in an RGD sequence-dependent fashion. Fibronectin has separate domains for binding to collagen, heparin, proteoglycans, and fibrin, demonstrating the importance of these molecules in matrix structure. It has also been suggested, that fibronectin regulates endothelial cell growth by modulating cell shape through an effect on cellular microfilaments (see below).

TGF-β has been shown to play a critical role in the synthesis and degradation of ECM,[44] as well in the response of cells to the ECM mediated through cell surface integrin receptors. It has been found to increase the mRNA levels and subsequent protein production of a number of matrix proteins in many different cell types (Figure 7).[43,44] In addition, the growth factor reduces the synthesis and secretion of several proteases that act upon the ECM, and can increase the secretion of protease inhibitors. Five different isoforms of TGF-β have been identified, all with significant identity and conserved cysteine residues. TGF-β_1 is the most abundant form. The factor is a potent, but reversible, inhibitor of endothelial cell growth, and antagonizes the mitogenic action of both FGF and

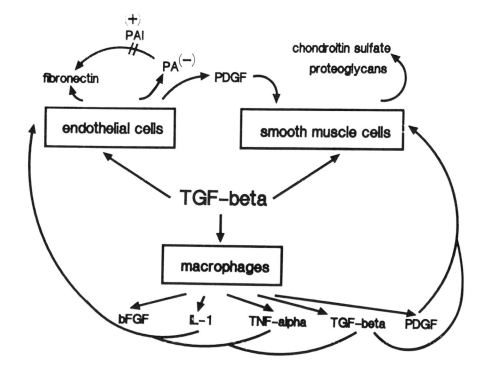

Figure 7. Complex effects of transforming growth factor-beta (TGF-β) on regulation of endothelial cells and vascular smooth muscle cells (SMCs). In addition to cell-specific modulation of matrix protein secretion, TGF-β induces endothelial cells to secrete platelet-derived growth factor (PDGF), a known SMC mitogen. The activation of growth factor expression in macrophages is thought to account for the effects of TGF-β on angiogenesis in vivo. (Reproduced with permission from Reference 44.)

PDGF on vascular cells. PDGF expression by endothelial cells, both A and B chains, is increased after stimulation with TGF-β. PDGF is chemotactic and mitogenic for SMCs. TGF-β also inhibits endothelial cell migration and capillary-tube formation in endothelial cells cultured on collagen gels. However, tube formation can be induced when microvascular endothelial cells are grown in three-dimensional collagen cultures, although their proliferation is not inhibited. It appears that the latter effect may be related to the inability of growth factors to modulate matrix protein synthesis in the three-dimensional system. In contrast, TGF-β_1 inhibits proliferation of endothelial cells grown on laminin, type IV collagen, or fibronectin-coated dishes. Such differences may result from either alterations of ECM proteins, or TGF receptor subtypes. TGF-β cell surface receptors comprise three distinct classes of proteins.[15] Class I and II receptors are glycoproteins, and evidence suggests that the inhibition of endothelial cell proliferation is mediated through the class I receptor. Class III receptor, now known to be the proteoglycan beta-glycan, is the most abundant, and is composed of heparan sulfate glycosaminoglycan chains with smaller amount of chondroitin and dermatin sulfate. It is found in membrane-bound and soluble forms, and may function to regulate the ability of TGF-β to bind to other receptors. HUVECs have only one binding site for TGF-β_1, whereas fetal bovine heart endothelial cell possess two. TGF-β_1 only slightly promotes HUVEC growth, whereas low concentrations stimulate the heart cells. High concentrations of TGF-β_1 inhibited heart endothelial cell proliferation.

Depending upon the endothelial cell culture surface, TGF-β has been shown to increase synthesis of fibronectin, and types IV and V collagen, with laminin synthesis being unaffected. The increase in fibronectin may mediate the inhibitory effect of TGF-β on the proliferation of endothelial cell monolayers, since soluble fibronectin has similar effects when added to cultures. In addition, TGF-β binds avidly to several matrix components, including type IV collagen and the proteoglycans, betaglycan and decorin; these interactions may subsequently deliver, inactivate, or clear the active factor.[44] Matrigel is able to deliver active TGF-β to cells, and its effects can be inhibited by the addition of anti-TGF antibodies. TGF-β induces the synthesis of decorin, which in turn antagonizes the activity of TGF-β by competing with the receptors for binding sites in TGF-β. The binding is reversible, and may serve as a local reservoir of the factor. TGF-β can also influence the expression of adhesive receptors on vascular cells. It has been shown to regulate the level of receptor mRNA and the rate of subunit processing, such as the alpha and beta subunits of the fibronectin receptor, thereby increasing cell adhesion to the matrix. As growth, migration, and the organization of the

endothelial cells are influenced by the composition of the ECM, it seems likely that TGF-β effects on the endothelial cells may play an important role in such processes as embryogenesis, angiogenesis, and endothelial cell response to injury and inflammation. TGF-β is highly angiogenic in a variety of in vivo assay systems,[43,44] and has been shown to increase the accumulation of matrix in wound beds. It has been implicated in the increases in fibronectin and collagen types I and III, occurring in the neointima of vessels following balloon angioplasty.[45] It has been co-localized with matrix components during branching morphogenesis in the mouse lung.

TGF-β is released from vascular cells in a biologically inactive form, consisting of a noncovalent complex which must be dissociated. The activation of the latent hormone in cultured vascular cells can only occur when cells are in contact with vascular pericytes. Pericytes (Rouget cells, mural cells) are intimately associated with endothelial cells, forming a discontinuous layer extending from the terminal arteriole to the postcapillary venule, sometimes lying within the endothelial cell-basement membrane. Like SMCs, they contain α-actin, and are thought to contribute to contraction, phagocytosis, and to serve as a source of undifferentiated mesenchymal cells. Co-culture experiments have shown that pericyte proximity correlates with endothelial cell growth inhibition, is cell specific, and requires only intermittent contact, suggesting a soluble mediator.[46] From media conditioned by co-cultures, investigators were able to attribute the inhibitory effect to active TGF-β. Evidence suggests that pericytes participate in the activation of locally derived TGF-β.

The Endothelial Cell Cytoskeleton

The endothelial cell cytoskeleton is a complex network of contractile proteins.[47] Actin is a major component and occurs in two forms: filamentous F-actin, or the monomeric G-actin. Reversible polymerization and cross-linking occurs in the course of many cellular functions. This shift of equilibrium between the monomeric and filamentous forms is regulated by a number of accessory proteins. The filamentous form can organize into either a diffuse network of short microfilaments or into prominent bundles. The former organization can be seen in the cell cortex and in cell extensions such as pseudopods. Actin bundles occur as central microfilament arrays, or in the periphery of the cell as prominent dense bands (Figure 8). A particular type of microfilament bundle, the stress fiber (Figure 8), contains other contractile proteins such as myosin, tropomyosin, and α-actinin. The actin filaments in the stress fiber are arranged in parallel alignment with non-

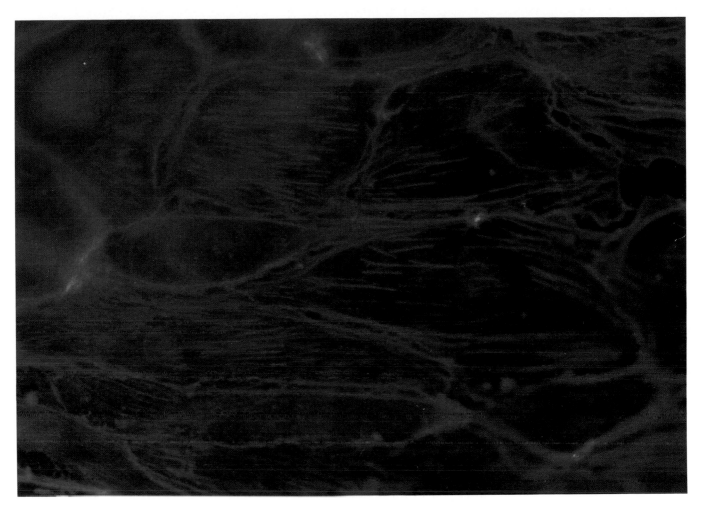

Figure 8. The F-actin filaments of cultured endothelial cells subjected to stationary or dynamic culture conditions are visualized with rhodamine phalloidin. Stationary cells show random central microfilaments and prominent dense peripheral band. After being subjected to stretch, stress fibers appear, aligned perpendicular to the stretch force vector. (Reproduced with permission from Reference 51.)

uniform polarity and are contractile and, therefore, can exert tension. Microfilaments emanate from the dense bands and course into the cytoplasmic side of the plasma membrane to attach to focal adhesion points, or plaques, on the basal surface (Figure 9). These plaques are comprised of intercellular adhesion molecules and junctional complexes in the periphery, and with integral membrane proteins at the apical surface and possibly at the nuclear membrane.[48] Actin structures within the endothelial cell have been visualized by a variety of techniques, including electron microscopy, immunofluorescence and fluorescence microscopy utilizing antibodies to actin, or derivatives of phallacidin, a phallotoxin isolated from mushrooms. Phallacidin is commonly employed in investigative studies because of its high affinity for F-actin. Perfusion-staining techniques have allowed in situ characterizations of endothelial cell cytoskeletal structure in

areas of normal flow, at branch points, and in regions of low and high shear forces.[47] In areas of normal flow, peripheral actin arrays are less visible than that observed in confluent endothelial cell cultures. Central bundles are oriented along the long axis of the cells, and are more prominent in the abdominal aorta than in the thoracic aorta. In low shear stress areas, endothelial cells have a cobblestone shape, with prominent peripheral actin bands, and thin, randomly oriented central fibers, similar to the morphology observed in cell cultures. In contrast, high shear stress areas contain elongated endothelial cells with thick actin stress fibers oriented in the direction of flow, with very little peripheral bundles.

Microtubules are concentrated and organized around centrosomes, which are randomly distributed in the perinuclear area, and become less prominent toward the cell periphery. The importance of the cen-

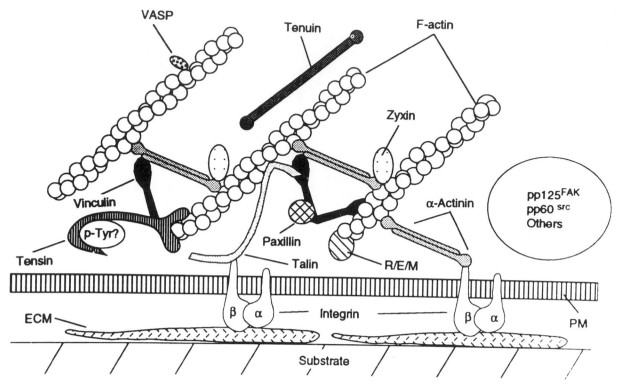

Figure 9. Working model of the protein-protein interaction in focal adhesions determined by in vitro binding experiments. ECM = extracellular matrix; PM = plasma membrane; p-Tyr-? = unknown phosphotyrosine-containing protein; R/E/M—ember of the radixin/ ezrin/moesin family of actin-binding proteins; VASP = vasodilator-stimulated phosphoprotein; pp125^{FAK} = a focal adhesion kinase. (Reproduced with permission from Reference 48.)

trosome in cell migration has been validated in an experimental wound model, in which endothelial cell centrosomes redistribute to an area between the nucleus and the leading lamellipodia prior to migration.[47]

Endothelial cells also contain intermediate filaments such as vimentin, which is found primarily in mesenchymal cells and desmin. Both are expressed in high endothelial venules of lymph nodes in rats. Their role in endothelial cell function is currently not known, although antibodies to the intermediate filaments result in filament coiling around the nucleus. Cell morphology and locomotion remain unaffected.

Endothelial cells are able to contract under certain circumstances, and are postulated to play an active role in regulation of vascular permeability, flow resistance, and blood cell migration. Cultured pulmonary endothelial cells have been shown to deform a flexible substratum in response to agents known to contract and relax SMCs. However, not all endothelial cells from different vascular beds have been able to show a similar substratum deformation. When peripheral actin filaments are disrupted with agents such as cytochalasin, intercellular gaps form and permeability increases. Increases in vascular permeability in response to throm-

bin occur with loss of the peripheral filament bundles. Endothelial gap formation is ATP-dependent, induced by increased intracellular calcium, and mediated by the interaction of actin and myosin. Recent reports have shown that cells can generate force within their intracellular skeleton, and this force is resisted by the surrounding structures through the extracellular contacts.[49] It is upon this force equilibrium that all external mechanical forces are imposed. The extracellular contacts regulate cellular tension based upon their ability to resist the mechanical load.

In order to maintain endothelial monolayer integrity, cells must form attachments to the subendothelium and to adjacent cells. The sensitivity of the endothelial cell to hemodynamic forces is manifested by growth and orientation changes in response to applied stresses.[47,49] F-actin redistribution varies according to the local pattern of stress, with high shear stress causing loss of peripheral dense bends and the appearance of central stress fibers (Figure 8). This adaptation is thought to protect the integrity of the endothelial cell monolayer. Cultured endothelial cells respond to uniform fluid shear stress, or to cyclic stretching, by changing from a polygonal to an ellipsoidal shape, and with reorientation in the direction of flow or stretch (Figure 8).[51,52] Cellular microfilaments undergo a corresponding reorganization, aligning with the major axis of the cell. Endothelial cells have been shown to decrease deformability in response to shear stress, and this effect can be blocked with microfilament disrupting agents. Active, directional remodeling of basal focal adhesion sites has been reported to occur in response to fluid shear stresses, as has an alteration in collagen and fibronectin synthesis. Cell wall tension varies with the density of extracellular membrane contact sites on the cell base. Furthermore, endothelial cell adhesion is impaired when F-actin network is disrupted with cytochalasin B.

Endothelial Cell Integrins

Of a number of membrane proteins that can anchor the cytoskeleton to the membrane and adjacent structures, the integrin family of cell surface proteins has been the most extensively studied.[49,53-57] Integrins are a group of heterodimeric, transmembrane proteins which link the cytoskeleton to the ECM and to adhesion molecules on other cells. They play a major role in platelet aggregation, immune functions, tissue repair, and tumor invasion. They are formed by two non-covalently linked subunits, designated alpha and beta, both of which span the plasma membrane (Figure 10). A subclassification of the integrin family has been suggested, based upon observations that the beta subunits seem to associate with multiple alpha-chains. Although there are many different heterodimeric integrins identified to date, the major integrins expressed by endothelial cells are five members of the B1 subtype, $a_v b_3$, and $a_v b_5$ varieties (Table 3). The extracellular domains bind to the matrix proteins laminin, fibronectin, and collagen, as well as vibronectin. The link to F-actin on the cytoplasmic side of the membrane occurs indirectly, via several actin-associated proteins (Figure 9). For instance, the b1 cytoplasmic domain has been shown to link to talin and α-actinin, both of which can be found at focal membrane contact points. Vinculin appears to bind via quaternary complexes with talin. Integrins and similar proteins may function by transmitting force changes to the underlying cytoskeleton, inducing coordinated changes in microfilament assembly in an effort to restore a force equilibrium.

Binding interactions between cytoskeletal filaments and cellular proteins may effect the observed functional responses. For example, the association of an actin-binding protein, profilin, with specific phosphoinositols has been shown to inhibit phospholipase C, revealing a direct interaction between the cytoskeletal assembly and inositol lipid metabolism. Further-

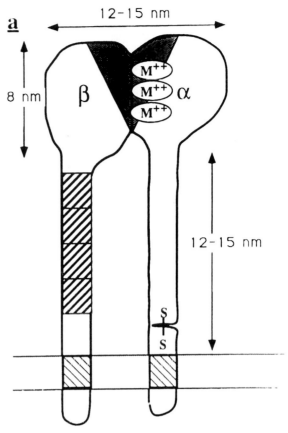

Figure 10. Structural features of the integrin receptors showing overall shape, as well as the locations of the cystine-rich repeats of the beta subunit (**crosshatched**) and metal-binding sites (M^{++}). The **shaded area** represents the proposed ligand-binding area. (Reproduced with permission from Reference 56.)

Table 3
Integrin Receptors in Human Endothelial Cells

Subunit	Ligand/Function
$\alpha^1 \beta_1$	lm, coll
$\alpha^2 \beta_1$	lm, coll, fn, cell-cell
$\alpha^3 \beta_1$	fn, lm, coll
$\alpha^5 \beta_1$	fn, cell-cell
$\alpha^6 \beta_1$	lm
$\alpha^v \beta_3$	vn, fg, vW, tsp, fn, lm, thr
$\alpha^v \beta_5$	vn

vn: vitronectin; vWF: von Willibrand factor; lm: laminin; fg: fibrinogen; tsp: thrombospondin; thr: thrombin; coll: collagen; cell-cell: endothelial cell contacts.

(Reproduced with permission from Reference 54.)

more, this interaction may be mediated through alterations in the cell to extracellular contacts. Another actin-associated protein, tubulin, can complex with membrane G-proteins, inhibiting adenylate cyclase. In addition to their role in cytoskeletal-transducer coupling, integrins may function as primary transducers. Recent studies have localized a cytoplasmic tyrosine kinase to integrin-associated focal contacts, suggesting the possibility of a force-induced phosphorylation mechanism. Indeed, tyrosine phosphorylation events as well as cytoplasmic alkalinization triggered via integrins have been described in a variety of cell types, suggesting that integrins can act as signalling receptors.

Endothelial Interactions

Endothelium and Platelets

In the intact endothelial monolayer, there exists a complex system of membrane related antithrombotic glycosaminoglycans, as well as transmembrane protein thrombomodulin, which resist fibrin formation. A major reason for the antithrombotic character of this layer has been attributed to the anionic surface charge from the high proportion of heparan sulfate and chondroitin sulfate. Endothelial cells prevent further platelet adherence and activation by possessing surface ADPase activity, synthesizing prostaglandins, such as PGI_2 and PGD_2, and promoting a vasodilatory state by basal release of nitric oxide (NO) (Figure 11).[58,59] In the undisturbed state, there is a normal balance between prothrombotic and antithrombotic/fibrinolytic mechanisms[60] of the endothelial cells, favoring the anticoagulated state. Perturbation of the endothelium by various stimuli may contribute to loss of this resistant state, contributing to the pathogenesis of a number of conditions.

Two separate systems, platelet aggregation and plasma coagulation, cooperate to provide for blood clotting. In the high flow arterial system, platelet acti-

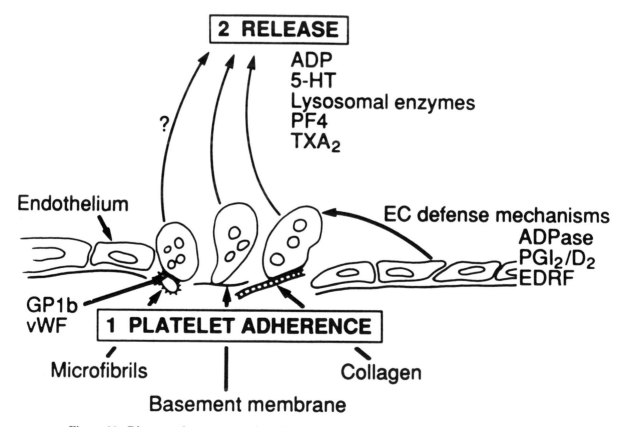

Figure 11. Diagramatic representation of the immediate adherence of platelets to exposed subendothelium after vascular damage. Platelets adhere to collagen, basement membrane, and microfibrils in the presence of von Willibrand Factor (vWF) and platelet membrane glycoprotein Ib. Collagen induces platelet degranulation, releasing ADP and serotonin (5-HT), and thromboxane A_2 (TXA_2) is formed from free arachidonic acid. Endothelial antithrombotic mechanisms function to limit the size of the thrombus. Later, formation of a platelet thrombus will initiate the release of tissue plasminogen activator from endothelial cells, beginning fibrinolysis. (Reproduced with permission from Reference 58.)

vation tends to predominate with formation of "white" thrombus, whereas in the venous circulation, platelets are less prominent and thrombi are comprised predominantly of fibrin. Regardless of which coagulation system predominates, endothelial cells play an integral role in coordinating and limiting clot formation.

In the unperturbed endothelium, platelets circulate without attaching. Endothelial cell production of prostacyclin (PGI_2), and possibly other prostanoids, is thought to account for the absence of platelet adhesion to the endothelium.[58-60] In some experimental models, such as virus infected cells, thrombin-activated endothelial cells and indomethacin-treated endothelial cells platelets do adhere. The latter case suggests an important role for the metabolites of arachidonic acid in the prevention of platelet adherence. The ability of PGI_2 to inhibit platelet activation is thought to be mediated by increasing cyclic adenosine monophosphate phosphodiesterase (cAMP) levels in the platelet cytoplasm. There is also evidence that NO is basally secreted in some vascular beds, leading to vasodilation. In addition, NO can inhibit platelet aggregation through the production of cyclic monophosphate (cGMP) in the platelet cytoplasm. cGMP interferes with the ability of platelet agonists to generate intracellular second messengers required to promote aggregation and release of prothrombotic substances. Thrombomodulin is present in high density on the endothelial cell surface, binding thrombin and preventing platelet activation and fibrin production. The complex also activates protein C. Both functions tend to maintain blood fluidity. The endothelial cell surfaces also possess an ADPase that breaks down ADP to AMP, adenosine, and inosine. ADP is an important cofactor in platelet aggregation induced by plasmin.

Platelets form plugs through a series of steps: adhesion, activation, and aggregation.[61] In the vasculature, platelets first recognize areas of altered endothelium, then arrest and attach to the endothelial cell. von Willebrand Factor (vWF) on the endothelial cell surface and subendothelial matrix, as well as plasma vWF that is rapidly adsorbed onto exposed structures of the damaged vessels, interacts with the platelet glycoprotein (GP) Ib-IX-V receptor complex, initiating adhesion, activation, and aggregation (Figure 11).

Platelets appear to adhere to arterial subendothelium through a process of contact, followed by activation and spreading along the subendothelial surface. Contact depends upon the composition of the blood and the rate of flow, as platelet contact will not occur unless there are high shear rates. This appears to be a unique feature of platelet thrombus formation, in that adhesion depends upon a mechanical force to affect specific surface molecules. Binding of GPIb to vWF does not occur in the absence of shear. In addition, high shear forces can directly activate platelets in

vitro.[61] It is not clear how shear affects the individual molecules involved. Nevertheless, understanding the mechanism underlying the shear-dependent adhesion mechanism may lead to the developement of methods for inhibiting arterial platelet adhesion and for treating thrombotic diseases.

Contact occurs through the receptor ligand interaction of the platelet molecule GPIb and vWF.[61,62] Deficiency of either molecule results in abnormal arterial platelet adhesion. GPIb:Bernard-Solier syndrome, and von Willibrand disease, both result in excessive bleeding. GPIb belongs to the integrin family of cell surface receptors, composed of alpha and beta subunits linked via disulfide bonds. The receptor is associated with a separate gycoprotein, GPIX. The GPIb-IX complex constitutes the surface receptor for arterial platelet adhesion. The binding site for vWF occurs on the largest member of the complex, the alpha chain (GPIb-alpha). All three surface peptides of the complex are absent in patients with Bernard-Solier syndrome. The disease is characterized by large, circulating platelets, and defective adhesion. Patients with this disease also lack a 92 kDa surface glycoprotein, GPV. The underlying defect which results in the deficiency of these platelet surface receptors is unknown. All four of the subunits contain leucine-rich segments, which are often present in molecules as tandem repeats, and are known to mediate a variety of cell interactions. However, the presence of these segments in the GPIb-V-IX complex suggests a functional significance. The vWF binding site within GPIb-alpha lies outside of the leucine-rich regions and represents a second domain rich in O-linked carbohydrates. The intervening residues, linking the leucine-rich regions and vWF binding site, are termed the "hinge" region.

Mature vWF is a multimeric glycoprotein, and exists as a series of oligomers containing a variable number of subunits.[62] The variable organization provides for a multitude of possible contact sites for platelets and subendothelial structures. Individual species range from 500 to 10000 kDa in size, the largest soluble human plasma protein. The larger oligomers are the most effective in promoting platelet adhesion and aggregation, and are stored in intracellular granules within the endothelial cells, the Weibel-Palade bodies. They are detected only transiently in the blood of normal adults. This sequestration ensures participation of highly active vWF multimers in hemostasis, while limiting their presence in the blood where they would cause unregulated thrombus formation. The nature of the limiting mechanism has not been fully elucidated. Mature vWF produced by endothelial cells contains 2050 amino acid residues, and a variable carbohydrate content representing 10% to 19% of the total molecular mass. A characteristic structural feature of vWF is a high cysteine content, which manifests as intramolecular disulfide bridges, imparting a highly ordered structure. After translocation of the vWF mRNA, the product undergoes extensive processing to produce the multimeric species. The primary translation product consists of a 22 residue signal peptide, an unusually large 741 residue pro-peptide, and the mature subunit of 2050 residues. The pro-peptide, identical to a previously described von Willibrand antigen II, is diminished in patients with von Willibrand disease. It contains active collagen binding domains, and inhibits collagen-induced platelet aggregation. This pro-peptide is thought to regulate the size of the platelet thrombus at areas of arterial injury, thereby balancing the prothrombotic effects of vWF.

The pro-vWF monomers associate through intramolecular disulfide bonding in the carboxy-terminal region. The pro-peptide drives the association of dimers to form highly ordered structures linked through cysteine residues in the amino terminal domain of each subunit. The mature subunit is further modified by addition of carbohydrate side-chains. The noncovalent association of factor VIII with vWF is the final step in the processing. It becomes apparent only after endothelial cell-derived vWF is released into the circulation. Lack of demonstrable co-localization suggests that the interaction occurs after they have been released from adjacent endothelial cells. The pro-peptide of vWF appears to play a significant role in the formation of a functional factor VIII binding site. Persistence of the uncleaved pro-peptide impairs the ability of vWF to bind to factor VIII.

Unlike other proteins, vWF can be secreted by a number of routes.[62] In endothelial cells, the majority of vWF is secreted through a constitutive pathway, which is directly linked to the synthesis of the molecule. The endothelial cells release vWF in both the luminal and abluminal directions. Secretion can also occur through a regulated pathway via the storage of mature vWF in Weibel-Palade bodies in endothelial cells, or in alpha-granules in megakaryocytes and platelets. Weibel-Palade bodies are derived from the Golgi apparatus and are composed of longitudinally oriented tubules enclosed within a surrounding membrane. The longitudinal arrays most likely represent organized, multimeric vWF. The mechanism by which vWF is stored is unknown, although it is thought that stored vWF represents the larger multimeric species. Regulated secretion occurs in response to several agonists, including histamine, estrogens, thrombin, and heparin. Local vWF secretion also occurs in areas of inflammation where gamma-interferon (γ-IFN) and tumor necrosis factor (TNF) may modulate the response. Vasoactive substances also cause the release of vWF, but are not active on cultured endothelial cells. Up to 20% of the total blood vWF may be carried in alpha-granules of platelets. Weibel-Palade bodies

also contain a P-selectin, GP-140, also called PADGEM; a cell adhesion molecule involved in the interaction of leukocytes with endothelial cells and platelets.

In mediating the platelet adhesion to endothelial cells, vWF acts as a bridge between components of the vessel wall, and specific receptors on the platelet surface. Although subendothelial vWF alone can cause platelet adhesion, plasma vWF is necessary for optimal initiation of hemostasis. vWF binding interactions to other elements such as those to type VI collagen, and the platelet receptor GP1b, have distinct binding domains for each interaction. The structures of the matrix involved in anchoring vWF at the site of injury have not yet been fully defined. It is clear, however, that vWF can bind to different types of collagen.[62] Type I collagen, found in deeper layers of the vessel, and exposed only after extensive injury, binds vWF avidly, as does type III collagen found in the subendothelial matrix. Type VI collagen, present in the microfibrillar extracts from vascular tissue, and resistant to bacterial proteolytic cleavage, is also a potential binding site for vWF. Proteoglycans may also contribute to the binding in subendothelium, as demonstrated by the interaction of vWF with heparin. VWF also contains a distinct heparin binding site located in the loop region. A second site of lower affinity exists within the subunit domain containing the factor VIII binding site. Heparin-like glycosaminoglycans are ubiquitous in the ECM and may represent structures onto which the vWF becomes insolute at the site of injury.

Platelets have two distinct receptors for vWF: GP1b in the GP1b-V-IX complex, and GPIIb-IIIa.[61] As noted, mechanical forces are necessary for the interaction of vWF with GP1b, as binding will not occur in the absence of shear. The mechanism of shear effect upon the molecular conformation of the proteins is unknown at present. Congenital defects of both vWF and GP1b have been described, resulting in loss of the shear-dependence of binding and a hypercoaguable state. Structural changes within the "hinge" domain of GP1b, or the vWF "loop" region, can result in hyperfunctional receptor:ligand interaction. Evidence indicates that several discontinuous residues on vWF participate in the binding to GP1b. The disulfide loop in the A1 domain is responsible for the conformation which binds GP1b with high affinity. It is thought that the limited sequences involved in GP1b recognition lay in proximity to the two cysteine residues forming the loop, whereas those modulating the affinity of the interaction reside more toward the center. Structural elements such as carbohydrate side-chains may also be involved in affinity modulation. Ten O-linked carbohydrates flank the A1 loop structure and are of sufficient proximity to effect binding. Normal glycosylation, however, does not appear to be necessary for binding to the GP1b receptor.

When contact and adhesion have occurred, the process of platelet activation and spreading takes place. Activation involves transmembrane signalling, oxygen consumption, and cytoskeletal reorganization, accompanied by granule secretion. The GP1b-V-IX receptor is exposed only on unactivated platelets, and is internalized once activation begins. Upon activation, the platelet GPIIb-IIIa surface receptor changes conformation and binds several glycoproteins including vWF. The vWF:GPIIb-IIIa interaction occurs only after activation. The GPIIb-IIIa binding site on the vWF molecule involves a ubiquitous tetrapeptide sequence (arg-glc-asp-ser), which exists in several moieties involved in cell adhesion. Antibodies to this region inhibit the interaction with GPIIb-IIIa, and block shear-induced platelet aggregation. The tetrapeptide sequence appears to be essential for binding. The functional integration of the GP1b and GPIIb-IIIa binding sites on vWF is demonstrated by the fact that shear-induced aggregation at high wall shear rate requires vWF interaction with both the receptors. The binding of vWF to GP1b complex may lead directly to interaction of GPIIb-IIIa with either surface bound vWF, or soluble vWF, in order to support adhesion and aggregation. Therefore, vWF can both initiate and mediate platelet thrombus formation. The GPIIb-IIIa receptor, and probably several vascular ligands (vibronectin, fibrinogen), contribute to the process of platelet spreading.

Fibrin deposition from the plasma coagulation system strengthens the developing platelet plug by providing additional fibrous links between individual platelets. Factor VIII of the coagulation cascade has a functionally significant half-life only when complexed to vWF. The binding site for factor VIII on vWF comprises an area formed by discontinuous residues held in approximation by intramolecular disulfide bridges. Amino acid substitutions at specific residues in the region result in reduced binding affinity. The vWF may serve as a cofactor, accelerating the thrombin catalyzed cleavage of light chain factor VIII, leading to dissociation of the complex. This separation may be necessary for activated factor VIII (VIIIa) to perform its cofactor function in the activation of factor X. Additionally, the association of vWF to factor VIII, protects the latter from the proteolytic effects of activated protein C, allowing activation to occur before degradation can occur. The larger vWF multimers bind preferentially to fibrin, whether cross-linked or not. They bind to the alpha-chain of fibrin via covalent linkage brought about by a transglutamination reaction catalyzed by factor XIII. The exact site involved on the VWF is unknown, but the interaction helps stabilize the forming clot, especially since vWF is constitutively present in the subendothelium.

Endothelium and Lymphocytes

Lymphocytes circulate throughout the body in a process of immune surveillance, travelling through the blood stream, moving into tissues, and returning to the circulatory system via the lymphatic channels. Discrete mechanisms exist which regulate lymphocyte movement into tissues, and are critical for the generation of an immune response. The interaction with endothelial cells represents the first step in lymphocyte trafficking. Unlike the mechanisms for neutrophils and platelets which cause binding to endothelial cells in inflammatory situations, lymphocytes also interact with normal endothelium. The interaction of lymphocytes with endothelium during recirculation, as well as during inflammation, has been the subject of intensive research in recent years. Many adhesion molecules of endothelial cells and lymphocytes have been identified through the use of monoclonal antibodies that block lymphocyte binding to endothelium.

Early histologic studies demonstrated that lymphocytes in circulation leave the blood stream to enter lymph nodes and Peyer's Patches by passing through the endothelium of specialized, postcapillary venules.[63,64] They are termed *high endothelial venules* because of their more columnar and cuboidal appearance in comparison to the more flat endothelium lining of other postcapillary venules in the circulation. They also display distinctive histochemical and ultrastructural features. Circulating lymphocytes recognize and extravasate via these specialized cell segments in lymph nodes and mucosal lymphoid tissues, such as Peyer's Patches and the appendix, and at sites of chronic inflammation. In vivo experiments demonstrate that recirculation of lymphocytes is not a random process, and that lymphocytes vary in their ability to enter different lymphoid organs through the high endothelial venules. Using in vitro homing assays, Stamper and Woodruff,[65] in 1976, were among the first to show that rat lymphocytes would preferentially adhere to endothelial cells of high endothelial venules when overlaid on frozen tissue sections of various lymphoid organs.

Lymphocyte subsets vary in their level of binding to the high endothelial venules, but corresponding to the cells ability to migrate into secondary lymphoid organs in vivo. Certain murine and human lymphomas or normal lymphocyte subsets like the gut-homing immunoblasts, gut intraepithelial leukocytes, or lamina propria lymphoblasts, bind to high endothelial venules in mucosal lymphoid tissues, but not to peripheral lymph node high endothelial venules. Alternatively, other lymphoid lines bind selectively to peripheral lymph node high endothelial venules. The binding of normal lymphocyte populations to peripheral—versus mucosal—lymph node high endothelial venules is precisely regulated by complex mechanisms, and at various stages of lymphocyte differentiation.[63–66,68]

The complexity of the lymphocyte interaction with the endothelium stems from the multiplicity of molecules that mediate the cell-to-cell interactions.[64,66,67] Cells of different lineage differ in their interaction with endothelial cells resulting in the distinct patterns of migration. In general, it seems that most virgin B and T lymphocytes express "homing" receptors for both peripheral and mucosal high endothelial venules, allowing a wide dispersement of immunologically naive cells. In addition to the lineage-specific and the intralineage (naive versus mature cell) variable migration patterns of lymphocytes, certain subpopulations preferentially migrate into particular anatomic sites. There is a substantial number of anatomic compartments served by specialized T cell subsets, including gut, synovium, and skin. Homing patterns are the result of specific pairs of molecules on the endothelial cells and lymphocyte that confer this regional specificity. The interaction of lymphocytes with endothelial cells is dramatically modified in the course of inflammation. Specific T cell adhesion molecules, that mediate homing under unstimulated circumstances (such as L-selectin and VLA-4 discussed below), also contribute to adhesion under inflammatory circumstances. This suggests that many of the ligands that participate in normal homing and recirculation can be induced at sites where they are not normally expressed. The mature effector and memory cell lines, however, appear to display a more highly selective tracking and tissue-specific recognition. Virtually all T cells found in tissues such as skin, gut lamina propria, and bronchial surfaces are of the memory phenotype, suggesting a preferential migration of these cells to normal and inflamed nonlymphoid tissues. Naive T cells account for most of the cells entering the lymph nodes. Memory T cells are biased to return to tissue in which they were originally stimulated, where they would most likely reencounter the same antigenic threat. The experimental basis comes from studies where the fate of lymphocytes derived from different anatomic sites were monitored following reinduction into the host, clearly establishing a tissue-specific migratory pattern. Molecules on lymphocytes and their counterparts on endothelial cells include structures belonging to distinct adhesion receptor families (Table 4), such as the selectins, integrins, the Ig superfamily, and CD44, a hyluronate receptor generated by alternative splicing.[66–68]

Memory T cells (CD4 +) express higher levels of several adhesion molecules (Leukocyte Function-associated Antigen-1, Very Late Antigen-4, 5, 6; see below) than do their naive counterparts, and display a correspondingly higher capacity to bind the relevant ligands (Intercellular Adhesion Molecule-1, Vascular Cell Adhesion Molecule-1, laminin, fibronectin). Preferential migration of naive T cells, assays of T cell binding to high endothelial venules in frozen lymph node sections, and monoclonal antibody blocking of in vivo migration, have implicated the peripheral lymph node homing receptor, termed L-selectin, as the responsible receptor on high endothelial cell venules responsible for the regulation of lymphocyte recirculation when the lymphocytes are in an unstimulated state.

The Ig superfamily of cell adhesion molecules consists of a number of molecules having at least one globular protein domain containing an intradomain disulfide bridge as in the immunoglobulin molecules. Three members of the Ig superfamily are involved in lymphocyte-endothelial cell interactions, namely Intramolecular Cell Adhesion Molecule I and II (ICAM-1, ICAM-2), and Vascular Cell Adhesion Molecule (VCAM). They serve as endothelial cell surface ligands for the integrins LFA-1 (Leukocyte Function-associated Antigen-1) and VLA-4 (Very Late Antigen-4), among others, expressed by activated lymphocytes. ICAM-1 (Figure 12), contains five extracellular immunoglobulin domains anchored by a transmembrane domain with a short cytoplasmic tail by which it may interact with the endothelial cytoskeleton. Its expression on endothelial cells can be increased after cytokine stimulation with interleukin-1 (IL-1), TNF, γ-IFN, or lipopolysaccharide (LPS). It is remarkable for its large number of known counter-structures, and can bind members of the beta$_2$ integrin family (LFA-1, Mac-1), found on activated lymphocytes. In contrast to ICAM-1, which is only weakly expressed on resting endothelium, ICAM-2 is constitutively expressed at high levels on resting endothelial cells, is not augmented by endothelial cell activation, nor does it bind Mac-1. ICAM-2 is truncated, possessing only two of the five Ig domains found on ICAM-1. It appears that differential regulation of ICAM-1, ICAM-2, and VCAM expression plays a critical role in the use of various adhesion pathways by lymphocytic cells. Expression of ICAM-1 by endothelial cells in vitro is protein dependent, peaking 12 hours after cytokine stimulation, and remains elevated for at least 36 hours.

VCAM-1 is a 100 to 150 kDa cell surface glycoprotein expressed on endothelium and follicular dendritic cells. Basal expression is considerably lower than ICAM-1, and is increased after stimulation of the endothelial cells by some of the same nonspecific inflammatory mediators (IL-1, TNF, LPS), but not by γIFN. VCAM-1 occurs as a variable spliced product of either six or seven Ig-like domains, and is the major endothelial cells ligand for the beta$_1$ integrin, VLA-4, found mainly on lymphocyte and monocytes. VCAM expression is protein synthesis-dependent and can be induced upon endothelial cell stimulation with IL-4, peaking after 6 to 10 hours of cytokine treatment, and is sustained in some cases for as long as 72 hours. VCAM-

Table 4
Families of Adhesion Molecules and Their Counter-Structures

Family	Adhesion Molecule (CD Nomenclature)	Chain Composition	Alternative Name(s)	Counter-Structure(s)
Ig superfamily	CD2		LFA-2	LFA-3
	LFA-3 (CD58)			CD2
	ICAM-1 (CD54)			LFA-1; Mac-1
	ICAM-2			LFA-1
	VCAM-1		INCAM-110	VLA-4
	CD4			MHC class II
	CD8			MHC class I
	NCAM (CD56)			NCAM; heparan sulfate
	PECAM-1 (CD31)			?
Integrin family	VLA-1 (CD49a/CD29)	α^1/β_1		laminin; collagen
	VLA-2 (CD49b/CD29)	α^2/β_1	gpla/lla; ECMRII	laminin; collagen
	VLA-3 (CD49c/CD29)	α^3/β_1	ECMRI	fibronectin; laminin, collagen
	VLA-4 (CD49d/CD29)	α^4/β_1	LPAM-1	fibronectin; VCAM-1
	VLA-5 (CD49e/CD29)	α^5/β_1	FNR; gplc/lla; ECMRVI	fibronectin
	VLA-6 (CD49f/CD29)	α^6/β_1	gplc/lla	laminin
	CD51/CD29	α^V/β_1		fibronectin
	LFA-1 (CD11a/CD18)	α^L/β_2		ICAM-1; ICAM-2; ICAM-3
	Mac-1 (CD11b/CD18)	α^M/β_2	CR3	ICAM-1; C3bi; factor X; fibrinogen
	p150,95 (CD11c/CD18)	α^X/β_2	CR4	ICAM-1; C3d
	CD41/CD61	α^{llb}/β_3	gpllb/llla	fibronectin, fibrinogen. von Willebrand factor
	CD51/CD61	α^V/β_3	VNR	vitronectin; fibrinogen; von Willebrand factor
	CD49f/CD-	α^6/β_4		?
	CD51/CD-	α^V/β_5		vitronectin; fibronectin
	CD49d/CD-	α^4/β_p	LPAM-2	?
Selectin family	L-selectin		LAM-1; PLN-HR	carbohydrate moiety
	P-selectin (CD62)		GMP-140; PADGEM	carbohydrate moiety
	E-selectin		ELAM-1	sialyl-Lewis^x antigen
Unclassified	CD44		Hermes; ECMRIII; Pgp-1	hyaluronic acid

(Reproduced with permission from Reference 121.)

1 expression is both locally and temporally correlated with the development of atherosclerotic lesions in animal models, possibly recruiting monocytes into the area.

Selectins, previously termed LECAM (Leukocyte-Endothelial Cell Adhesion Molecule), appear to play specialized roles in cell-to-cell adhesive interactions in the vasculature. The molecular structure of this family of transmembrane receptors is characterized by an N-terminal domain, similar in structure to Ca+ +-dependent animal lectins. An epidermal growth factor-like domain is then followed by a variable number of complement regulatory domains (so noted because their 62 amino acid sequences are homologous to a number of complement regulatory proteins that bind C3b or C4b of the complement cascade), a transmem-

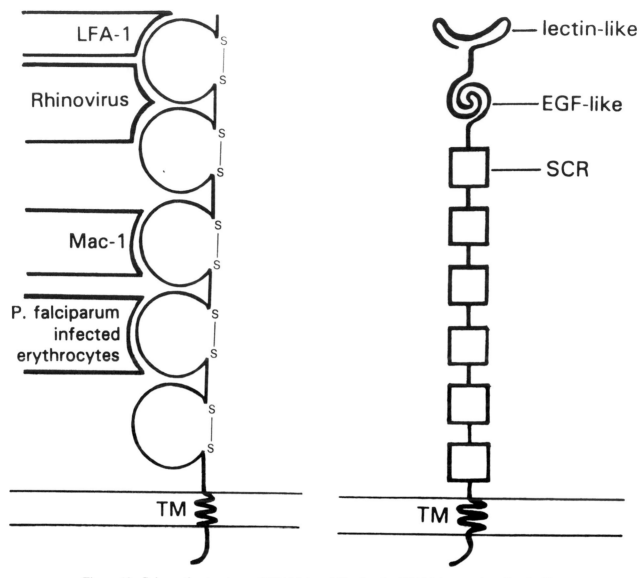

Figure 12. Schematic structure of ICAM-1 and E-selectin. ICAM-1 comprises five Ig-like domains, each containing a disulfide bond (S-S). The domains to which severl ligands bind are indicated. E-selectin consists of six short consensus repeats (SCR), an EGF-like domain, and a lectin-like domain, which interacts with carbohydrate moieties on other cells. TM = transmembrane. (Reproduced with permission from Reference 67.)

brane domain, and a short cytoplasmic tail. The lectin-like region appears to be essential for cell adhesion, while the EGF domain likely has a regulatory role. Members of this family of adhesion molecules (L-selectin, E-selectin, and P-selectin) are involved in leukocyte adhesion.

L-selectin was first recognized as a lymphocyte homing receptor when murine lymphocytes binding to peripheral lymph node high endothelial venules could be blocked with the addition of a monoclonal antibody, MEL-14. The antibody also partially blocked adhesion of lymphocytes to mesenteric lymph node high endothelial venules, but did not effect the interaction with

Peyer's Patches high endothelial venules. MEL-14 recognizes an 85 to 95 kDa, two-complement regulatory domain, glycoprotein on murine lymphocytes, whose gene has been cloned and sequenced. The N-terminal region of 118 amino acids is homologous to various animal lectins, suggesting that it might recognize a carbohydrate determinant on endothelial cells. Treatment of peripheral node-, but not Peyer's Patches-high endothelial venules, with sialyladenase enzyme, destroys their ability to bind lymphocytes. The EGF-like domain is homologous to sequences found in the beta$_2$ integrin subunit (CD18), found on leukocytes and lymphocytes (LFA-1). The remaining extracellular portion of the molecule includes two identical repeats, the complement regulatory domains. There is a hydrophobic transmembrane region and a hydrophilic cytoplasmic tail, similar in structure to the E-selectin molecules (see below). Both murine peripheral lymph node endothelial cell receptors and the human homologues have been included in the L-selectin class of receptors. In addition to mediating lymphocyte homing to peripheral lymph nodes, L-selectin appears to be involved in both neutrophil and lymphocyte adhesion to activated endothelial cells. The high endothelial venules ligands for the lymphocyte L-selectins and other homing receptors have been referred to as vascular "addressins," signifying their role in the tissue-specific trafficking of lymphocytes.

E-selectins, previously termed endothelial-leuko-cyte adhesion molecules 1 and 2 (ELAM-1, ELAM-2), are inducible cell surface molecules first described as the mediators of neutrophil adhesion to activated endothelial cells. E-selectins can also mediate the adhesion of a subpopulation of resting CD4 + memory T cells to activated endothelial cells. E-selectins (Figure 12), are a 95 to 115 kDa, six-complement regulatory domain, glycoprotein expressed exclusively on endothelium activated by IL-1, TNF-β, and LPS. The receptor is not constitutively expressed, and the appearance on the endothelial cell surface is protein synthesis-dependent, occurring 4 to 6 hours after cytokine stimulation, and returning to basal levels within 24 hrs.

Both E- and L-selectins bind to specific sialylated carbohydrates. The peripheral lymph node high endothelial venule addressin has been defined by a functional inhibitory antibody, MECA-79, in both mice and humans. MECA-79 directly inhibits lymphocyte adhesion to peripheral lymph node sites in vivo, but does not inhibit binding to the Peyer's Patches high endothelial venules. MECA-79 antigen can be detected in Western blots and immunoprecipitates as lymph node-specific, binding to heterogenous set of glycoproteins. These antigens are predominately O- and N-glycosylated glycoproteins, between 50 and 150 kDa. Ligands for E-selectin include sialyl-Lewis X and Lewis X which are alpha-(1–3)-fucosylated derivatives of polygalactosamine, and are expressed on neutrophils and macrophages. Similar carbohydrates exist on the surface of a subset of memory T cells. Anti-silayl-Lewis-X monoclonal antibody inhibits neutrophil binding to E-selectin, and cells can be converted to E-selectin-adhesive cells by expressing a single sugar transferase (alpha-1,3-fucosyltransferase).

P-selectin is a 140 kDa, nine CRP domain, glycoprotein located in secretory granules of platelets and endothelial cells. It is an activation-dependent, external membrane protein, and has been given the cluster designation, CD62. It is expressed within minutes of endothelial cell stimulation by thrombin or histamine, but is not expressed in response to the cytokines IL-1 and TNF. Anti-P-selectin monoclonal antibody inhibits the leukocyte adhesion induced by thrombin and histamine. Thrombin-induced expression of platelet activating factor (PAF) may affect neutrophil adhesion in response to thrombin. P-selectin, like the E-selectins, can recognize the sialyl-Lewis X antigen.

The mucosal lymph node high endothelial venule vascular addressin has been defined through the use of monoclonal antibody MECA-367 and MECA-87, and is selectively expressed by vessels involved in lymphocyte trafficking into mucosal tissues, including Peyer's Patches, mesenteric lymph nodes, the lamina propria, small and large intestine, and the mammary gland. MECA-367 blocks lymphocyte binding to mucosal high endothelial venules, and completely prevents lymphocyte extravasation into Peyer's Patches. Extravasation of gut-homing lymphoblasts into the lamina propria or Peyer's Patches is only partially blocked, suggesting additional mechanisms may function at these sites. A number of glycoprotein species of varying molecular weights bear epitopes for this antibody and are adhesion molecules for lymphocytes.

CD44, a widely expressed cell surface protein with homology to cartilage-link proteins, binds to the addressin defined by monoclonal antibody MECA-367. CD44, previously referred to as H-CAM, or Hermes antigen, is another class of lymphocyte homing receptor defined by antibody inhibition studies. CD44-specific monoclonal antibodies have been shown to inhibit lymphocyte binding to all high endothelial venule classes previously mentioned, including synovial high endothelial venules. It has been shown to be increasingly expressed by memory lymphocytes in murine and human models. Originally, it was described as a polymorphic antigen of mesenchymal cells and used as a marker of thymocyte maturation, since anti-CD44 antibodies inhibit homing of bone marrow cells to the thymus. The amino-terminal portion of this transmembrane molecule is homologous to several animal cartilage-link proteins and a rat cartilage proteoglycan core protein. CD44 does not share homologous regions with the MEL-14 antigen, nor the CD11/CD18 integrin subfamily (LFA-1, Mac-1). It binds to the glycosaminoglycan, hyaluronic acid, and its binding to cultured endothelial cells can be blocked by the addition of hyaluronidase. N-terminal sequences are highly conserved in mouse and humans, but a more proximal, extracellular domain, is only 40% identical. The function of this domain may be determined by carbohydrate modifications, and most monoclonal antibodies against CD44 appear to recognize epitopes within this region. The mucosal high endothelial venules addressin, identified by MECA-367, bind CD44 in solution in a saturable, reversible manner, suggesting that the molecule is one lymphocyte surface receptor for mucosal vascular endothelial cells. CD44 is a ubiquitous entity, expressed on diverse cell types, and it has also been implicated in T cell adhesive interaction involving the integrins LFA-3 and CD2. Like other cartilage link proteins, CD44 may also serve as a receptor for ECM components. It can be co-precipitated with ECM receptor type 4, which binds collagen I and IV, and is associated with the cytoskeletal protein, lamentin. Its increased expression on activated memory cells may serve as a receptor for ECM proteins similar to the expression of certain VLA integrins on activated human T cells, known to have ECM receptor function.

In addition to the vascular addressins, selectins, and CD44, many members of the integrin family of cell surface receptors have been implicated in the recirculation of lymphocytes, in a nonorgan specific manner. Both the Leukocyte Function Associated Antigen (LFA-1) and VLA-4 play major roles in lymphocyte adhesion to activated endothelium. LFA-1 is a member of the beta$_2$ integrin subfamily, which is composed of three distinct, but related alpha-chain peptides—CD11a, CD11b, and CD11c—expressed on the cell surface in noncovalent association with a common beta subunit, CD18. These three heterodimers are known respectively as LFA-1, Mac-1, and P150/95 (Table 4). LFA-1 is expressed on the majority of leukocytes and related leukemic cell lines, and binds to the endothelial cell adhesion molecule ICAM-1, as noted. Both Mac-1 and P150/95 have affinity for ICAM-1, as well as for certain proteolytic fragments of compliment component C3. LFA-1 is expressed by all T cells, but at one- to twofold higher levels on memory than the naive cells. Anti-LFA-1 monoclonal antibody decreases adhesion of lymphocytes to viable monolayers of endothelial cells in vitro, suggesting a general role in nonorgan specific strengthening of adhesion. VLA-4 is a member of the beta$_1$ integrin family consisting of one of six distinct alpha-polypeptide chains in association with a common beta$_1$ subunit, CD29. VLA-4 is found mainly on hematopoietic cells, such as lymphocytes, monocytes, and related leukemic cell lines, and serves to mediate cell-to-cell interactions, as well as functioning as a receptor for fibronectin. It demonstrates a heterogenous pattern of expression, being minimally expressed on naive cells.

Endothelium and Leukocytes

In contrast to lymphocyte homing and recirculation, the adhesion of polymorphonuclear leukocytes (PMN) is an early and requisite event in acute inflammation, and does not occur under unstimulated circumstances.[68–72] Adhesive interactions of PMNs are spatially-specific, occurring at sites adjacent to bacterial invasion or tissue trauma. While leukocytic infiltration is a necessary response, and is beneficial to the immune response and wound healing, it may be deleterious if persistent or unregulated, as occurs with organ reperfusion after hypoxia, or after transplantation, where tissue injury may be compounded by activated leukocytes. Acute inflammation begins with leukocyte margination, the displacement of leukocytes along the lining of postcapillary venules caused by the rheologic interactions with erythrocytes. The leukocytes appear to adhere transiently to the endothelium, producing a "rolling" phenomena that has been observed in most tissues. It represents a process of early inflammation. Reported rolling velocities are of the order of 50 um/s, and can only occur in flowing blood if the cell is impeded by adhesion. In addition, higher shear rates have been shown to cause considerable deformation of rolling leukocytes, suggesting the presence of active adhesion. It appears that arterial and arteriolar endothelium are unable to support rolling, even at reduced flow rates. Leukocytes, like lymphocytes, constitutively express adhesion molecules on their plasma membranes. They can rapidly alter their functional state or number in response to stimuli. The three beta$_2$ integrins previously discussed are constitutively present on PMN membranes. Heritable deficiencies in expression of beta$_2$ integrins, resulting from mutations of the beta$_2$ (CD18) chain, dramatically reduce PMN accumulation at extravascular sites of infection, and impair wound healing in patients with the disorder, known as leukocyte adhesion deficiency (LAD). Upon endothelial cell activation by various compounds, PMN's rapidly become adhesive for endothelium.

Adhesion molecules of the L-selectin and beta$_2$ integrin class are involved in tethering the PMN to endothelial cells.[69,70] They participate in the initial interactions, such as rolling and tight adhesion, prior to emigration (Figure 13). The initial adhesive interaction is transient, mediated by LFA-1 and Mac-1. The beta$_2$ integrins are constitutively expressed on circulating leukocytes, without conferring adhesiveness in the unstimulated state. Mac-1 is present in subcellular granules, and translocates to the PMN surface within minutes of endothelial cell activation. Increased expression, however, is not necessary nor sufficient for adhesiveness. The primary mechanism of increased adhesiveness appears to be an alteration in the heterodimers already present on the plasma membrane, suggesting cytoskeletal attachment. PMNs are stimulated by the peptide FMLP, or PAF, and adhere to endothelial cells through a Mac-1-dependent mechanism, before recruitment of new copies to the surface is maximal. In addition, inhibition of the up-regulation of Mac-1 does not block adhesion or aggregation. LFA-1 mediates adhesion, but does not appear to be quantitatively up-regulated when the cell is activated. In pa-

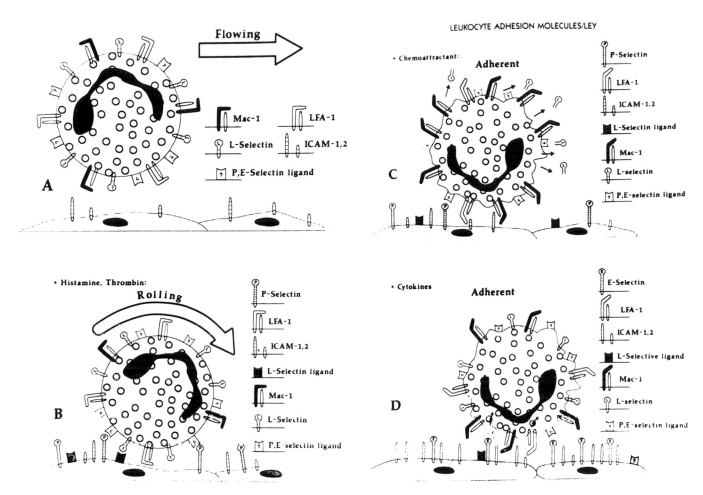

Figure 13. The sequence of events in granulocyte adhesion. **A.** In the absence of inflammation, the granulocyte does not interact with the endothelium. Leukocyte integrins LFA-1 and Mac-1 (**shaded**) are in a resting, nonadhesive conformation. Endothelial cells express ICAM-2 and some ICAM-1, but no selectins or selectin ligands. L-selectin and carbohydrate ligands for P- and E-selectin containing sialyl-Lewis X are present on the leukocyte, but the endothelium does not possess corresponding counterstructures. **B.** On stimulation by inflammatory mediators, such as thrombin or histamine, endothelial cells rapidly express P-selectin (along with PAF [see text]), and a ligand for L-selectin, causing the granulocyte to begin rolling along the endothelium. **C.** When a chemoattractant reaches the granulocyte, the integrins convert to an adhesive conformation, binding to ICAM-1 and ICAM-2. ICAM = intramolecular cell adhesion molecule; PAF = platelet activating factor. (Reproduced with permission from Reference 70.)

tients with hereditary LAD, a hereditary mutation prevents the surface expression of the beta$_2$ molecule. The patient suffers recurrent bacterial infections, being unable to recruit granulocytes.

ICAM-1, but not ICAM-2, is the counter-receptor for Mac-1, whereas LFA-1 recognizes both. Mac-1 binds to the third Ig repeat of ICAM-1, whereas LFA-1 binds the first repeat. The oscillation of ICAM-1 effects binding of Mac-1, but not of LFA-1. It seems that binding of the surface integrins of activated PMNs to the ICAM species on endothelial cells facilitates transendothelial migration. Although ICAM-1 is increasingly expressed on cytokine-activated endothelial cells, the increased number alone does not enhance adhesion of leukocytes. Up-regulation of the beta$_2$ integrins of the PMN is also required.

L-selectins are abundant on granulocytes, monocytes, and many circulating lymphocytes. The lectin domain of the molecule is critically involved in adhesion, and is rapidly shed by proteolytic cleavage near the transmembrane span when leukocytes are activated. Rapid enhancement of adhesiveness of L-selectin for its counter-receptor on endothelial cells occurs prior to the shedding process (Figure 13). Blocking leukocyte L-selectin with monoclonal antibodies impedes rolling along stimulated, cultured endothelial cells layers in the presence of flow. Recombinant L-selectin, as well as monoclonal antibodies, have been shown to

Table 5
Evolution of the Inflammatory Response

Phase	Event	Consequence	Mediators
A. Immediate (5–30 minutes)	1. Endothelial secretion of prostacyclin, EDRF	1. Vasodilation and increased leukocyte delivery	1. Histamine, thrombin, LTC$_4$, etc.
	2. Endothelial contraction	2. Vascular leak and local blood stasis	2. Histamine, thrombin, LTC$_4$, etc.
	3. Endothelial expression of GMP-140	3. Neutrophil (monocyte) adhesion	3. Histamine, thrombin, LTC$_4$, etc.
	4. Endothelial synthesis of PAF	4. Neutrophil activation and chemokinesis	4. Histamine, thrombin, LTC$_4$, etc.
	5. β_2 integrin-dependent transmigration of activated neutrophils	5. Neutrophil infiltration	5. PAF, C5a, LTB$_4$, etc.
B. Early (2–6 hours)	1. Augmented endothelial secretion of prostacyclin (?EDRF)	1. Sustained vasodilation and increased leukocyte delivery	1. IL-1, TNF
	2. Endothelial reorganization	2. Vascular leak and local blood stasis	2. IL-1, TNF
	3. Endothelial expression of ELAM-1	3. Neutrophil (monocyte) adhesion	3. IL-1, TNF
	4. Endothelial secretion of IL-8/ MCP-1	4. Neutrophil/monocyte activation and chemokinesis	4. IL-1, TNF
	5. β_2 integrin-dependent transmigration of activated neutrophils	5. Neutrophil infiltration	5. IL-8, PAF, C5a, LTB$_4$, etc.
C. Delayed (12–48 hours)	1. Augmented endothelial secretion of prostacyclin	1. Sustained vasodilation and leukocyte delivery	1. IL-1, TNF
	2. Continued endothelial reorganization	2. Increased vascular leak and local blood stasis	2. IL-1, TNF, IFN-γ
	3. Increased endothelial expression of ICAM-1, INCAM-110/VCAM-1; diminished ELAM-1	3. Lymphocyte/monocyte adhesion; diminished neutrophil adhesion	3. IL-1, TNF, IFN-γ
	4. Endothelial secretion of IL-8/ MCP-1	4. Lymphocyte/monocyte chemokinesis	4. IL-1, TNF, IFN-γ
	5. β_2 integrin dependent and independent (VLA-4 or CD44-dependent?) transmigration of lymphocytes/monocytes	5. Mononuclear cell infiltration	5. IL-8, MCP-1, others?

(Reproduced with permission from Reference 127.)

reduce rolling along endothelial venules in rat and rabbit mesentery by as much as 80%. L-selectin may interact with E-selectin (ELAM), which is expressed on cytokine-activated endothelial cells. Binding, however, to TNF-α-stimulated endothelial cells appears to be independent of E-selectin expression. In addition, shear forces may be necessary for L-selectin mediated PMN binding. The exposed N-terminal lectin domain results in a high forward rate of binding in the selectin family. The dissociation is also high, and may be increased as the bond becomes stressed. This could be important in accounting for the rolling behavior in the presence of shear forces.

The selectins display a broad, carbohydrate specificity, including the common recognition of sialyl-Lewis X. The N-terminal, C-type, lectin domain ex-

hibits considerable homology among the selectins, as well as with other C-type lectins. Immunoprecipitation of an L-selectin ligand from high endothelial venules from peripheral lymph nodes reveal a sulfated, fucosylated and sialylated glycoprotein with a molecular mass of 50 kDa, and O-linked carbohydrate side chains. Cytokine-activated endothelial cells may express a similar ligand.

Endothelial cells express leukocyte signalling molecules when activated (Figure 13, Table 5).[70,71,73] PAF is not constitutively present on resting endothelial cells, but is synthesized within minutes of endothelial cell stimulation by thrombin, histamine, leukotriene C4, and other agonists. PAF is not released into the fluid phase by endothelial cells but, rather, is expressed on the cell surface. The cellular enzymes required for its synthesis, Ca^{++}-dependent phospholipase A2, and a specific acetyltransferase, are regulated by phosphorylation. PAF associated with endothelial cells activates polymorphonuclear leukocytes by binding to a surface receptor linked to membrane G-proteins. Ligation of this receptor by PAF induces up-regulation of LFA-1 and Mac-1 on leukocytes. This mechanism appears to mediate adhesion and emigration of leukocytes in situ vascular segments, and in inflamed vessels in vivo, as well as in cultured endothelial cells.

P-selectin is translocated from the endothelial cell secretory bodies, Weibel Bodies, within seconds of stimulation by thrombin or histamine. It then becomes rapidly reinternalized, resulting in a transient surface expression that parallels polymorphonuclear leukocyte adhesion to endothelial cells. In vitro, PAF-unresponsive granulocytes detach from the endothelium after the shedding of P-selectin, whereas PAF-sensitive granulocytes remain attached. It has been shown that P-selectins mediate transient, reversible adhesions of leukocytes to thrombin- or histamine-activated endothelial cells in cooperation with PAF. This transient expression contrasts to the sustained surface expression of the P-selectin on activated platelets. The reinternalization mechanism provides a means of temporal regulation of adhesive interactions. Certain pathologic agonists, such as oxidants, may impair the reinternalization pathway, sustaining the activation of polymorphonuclear leukocytes. The receptor on leukocytes for P-selectin has not yet been fully identified, however, the isolation of cDNA products has predicted variants of the molecule, including a soluble protein lacking the transmembrane domain. The soluble form may inhibit the CD11/CD18 adhesiveness of PMNs. Other experiments have shown no such effect, and the role of the soluble P-selectin remains to be determined.

E-selectin is found exclusively on cytokine-activated endothelial cells,[69–71] and occurs via induction of mRNA for the protein, preceded by activation of NF-kB or related transcription factors. Expression, in response to agonists TNF-α, IL-1, and LPS, requires roughly 1 hour, reaching a peak at 4 to 8 hours, and declines by 24 to 48 hours. E-selectin (Figure 12) contains six complement regulatory domains, and originally was thought to bind only granulocytes, but more recently has been shown to bind monocytes and highly selected populations of T cells. PMN adhesion appears to parallel the endothelial cell, E-selectin time course, but also exhibits a residual enhanced adhesiveness after E-selectin decline. Antibodies against E-selectin partially inhibit PMN adhesion, and can inhibit myeloid cell binding to E-selectin transfected cells and to recombinant E-selectin constructs. Transfected cells deficient in the lectin or EGF-like domain do not support adhesion, suggesting that the EGF domain is important in maintaining conformation of the lectin region. Neither PMN activation nor beta$_2$ integrins, is required for E-selectin dependent adhesion. Antibodies to beta$_2$ integrins inhibit PMN adhesion to cytokine-activated endothelial cells expressing E-selectin, to a variable degree. Binding of PMN to cytokine-activated endothelial cells results in the activation of the Mac-1-dependent functions. In addition, a soluble E-selectin mutant, lacking the transmembrane and cytoplasmic domains, induces Mac-1 activation and is chemotactic for PMN. Ligation of the E-selectin receptor by the complete molecule expressed by endothelial cells may both tether PMNs, and mediate activation contributing to the migration into the extravascular tissues. The counter-receptors for E- and P-selectin appear to have sialic acid as part of their structure, and both molecules recognize sialyl-Lewis X, found in leukocyte glycolipids and glycoproteins. Fucosylation may be the step that distinguishes the receptors from other carbohydrate structures. L-selectin may be a candidate for a sialyl-Lewis-X-bearing structure that is recognized by the other two selectins. Undifferentiated HL60 cells, lacking L-selectin, bind to both P- and E-selectin. Monoclonal antibody to P-selectin, and treatment of PMN with soluble P-selectin, does not inhibit their binding to endothelial cells expressing E-selectin, suggesting that they recognize different receptors.

The first observable events of acute inflammation are the hemodynamic changes at the site of injury (Table 5).[73] Vessels become extensively dilated, increasing blood flow and the delivery of blood components to the tissue site. Occurring within minutes of the onset of inflammation is the release of mediators which then act upon the endothelium. These include thrombin, histamine, and leukotriene C_4 which stimulate the endothelial cells immediately, resulting in the increased levels of intracellular free Ca^{++} concentration. The increased Ca^{++} in turn activates phospholipase A2, leading to the release of arachidonic acid from the plasma membrane phospholipid, and converted via the cyclooxygenase pathway into PGI_2. The amount produced depends upon the presence of the cellular enzymes responsible for the conversion. The relevant enzymes can be increased by endothelial cells stimulation with IL-1 or TNF, releasing markedly more PGI_2 in response to the same degree of thrombin or histamine stimulation. NO is also released from arginine through a Ca^{++}-dependent enzyme. The result is a vasodilation causing an increase in local blood volume and a decrease in blood flow velocity at the inflammatory site. The increased cytoplasmic free Ca^{++} also leads to endothelial cell contraction and cell separation, via an intracellular pathway involving calmodulin and myosin light chain kinase. The contraction is rapid, leading to a fluid leak contributing to blood stasis. The effect is transient, and depends upon the agonist used. Cytokines also result in increased vascular permeability, but a more prolonged structural reorganization within the cell is required, usually developing over a 4- to 6-hour period. Unlike contraction, it involves a protein synthetic event. Leukocytes and lymphocytes may cause endothelial cell injury, leading to cell retraction or lysis, and vascular leakage. The net effect of the vasodilatation and permeability is a reduction in the shear force, favoring leukocyte adhesion to the cell surface. The first leukocyte adhering to the stimulated endothelial cells is the granulocyte, or PMN, using P-selectin as an anchor.[70,73] The intracellular free Ca^{++} levels cause fusion with the plasma membrane of P-selectin containing Weibel-Palade Bodies, which also releases highly polymerized vWF. PAF synthesis is also increased. Expression of both molecules is required for maximal PMN adhesion to endothelial cells activated by histamine and thrombin. The tethering step mediated by P-selectin is required for efficient interaction of PAF with its receptor on leukocytes. PMN activation results in recruitment of CD11/CD18 integrins, enhancing the tightness of the adhesion event. This is necessary since the binding by P-selectin is weak, and the molecule is only transiently expressed. CD11/CD18-deficient PMNs bind weakly. PAF-stimulated polarization of the PMN up-regulates the beta$_2$ integrins and primes the leukocytes for enhanced response to fluid phase chemotactic factors that may be critical in migration, and in other functional responses. The enhancement of PMNs caused by PAF may be caused by other activators, such as FMLP, C5a, and LTB$_4$. If enough activator is introduced, the interaction with P-selectin becomes unnecessary, and adhesion proceeds directly through the CD11/CD18 pathway. In response to the cytokines IL-1 and TNF, endothelial cells begin de novo synthesis and expression of E-selectin and the cytokine IL-8. IL-8 stimulates neutrophil chemotaxis and chemokinesis, and can activate PMN degranulation and the respiratory burst. IL-8 down-regulates adhesion through MEL-14 antigen, while activating the CD11/CD18 system. The granulocyte adhesion molecule L-selectin is rapidly shed when the cell is activated by this cytokine. Concomitant with this "loosening" effect, the IL-8-induced cell movement may serve as an early step in transmigration. Transmigration depends upon the granulocyte integrin/endothelial cell ICAM interaction.[74] As noted, ICAM-1 expression is markedly augmented by IL-1 or TNF-mediated endothelial cells activation in vitro or in vivo. In patients with LAD, granulocytes readily adhere to endothelial cells, but fail to extravasate through the vessel wall, and instead begin recirculating. The co-expression of E-selectin and IL-8 potentially regulates the avidity of the PMN binding, since IL-8 may alter E-selectin by virtue of its adhesion-inhibitory activity. IL-1- and TNF-mediated PMN adhesion at several hours after the onset of in-

flammation may be similar to the histamine and leukotriene C$_4$-mediated adhesion occurring immediately via PAF/P-selectin co-expression. The PMN activator in each case, IL-8 and PAF, respectively, may cause bound PMNs to switch to lower affinity leukocyte CD11/CD18-ICAM-1 dependent mechanism to stimulate transmigration. The importance of the CD11/CD18-ICAM interaction in granulocyte migration and accumulation can be seen by the effects of monoclonal antibodies to the molecules.[69,72] In vitro monoclonal antibodies to CD18, such as 60.3 and IB4, inhibit PMN accumulation. Administration of 60.3 dose dependently depresses the accumulation of neutrophils into subcutaneous, chemoattractant soaked sponges, and into skin sites injected with similar agents. Incubation of PMNs with 60.3 before injection blocks their accumulation in response to C5a, LTB4, FMLP, and IL-1 in rabbit models. Other studies demonstrate the ability of the antibodies to block accumulation in areas or reperfusion following ischemia. Although transmigration is affected in these studies, neutrophil rolling behavior remains intact. Antibodies to L-selectin block rolling in vivo and P-selectin have also been implicated in in vitro studies. IB4 has been shown to reduce tissue damage in rabbit models of meningitis. 60.3 also has been shown to protect against ischemia-induced injury of the gut. The antibodies are similarly effective in models of myocardial and whole body reperfusion injury. Lung injury, however, does not appear to be prevented by these monoclonal antibodies. These observations point to the importance of the CD11/CD18 adhesion of leukocytes as a key determinant of leukocyte accumulation in inflammatory sites. Anti-ICAM monoclonal antibodies have also been shown to be a blocking agent of PMN accumulation, reducing migration into air spaces of rabbits induced by PMA. Antibodies to ICAM also have reduced injury to ischemic hearts after reperfusion. It has also been successfully utilized as the sole immunosuppressant agent in renal allograft transplanted monkeys, improving graft survival. Anti-ICAM antibodies also attenuate antigen-induced bronchial hyperresponsiveness and eosinophil influx in primate models of asthma.

After 4 to 6 hours from the first inflammatory stimulus, the leukocytic infiltrate shifts from a granulocyte rich one to an accumulation of lymphocytes and monocytes. The change correlates with the alteration in expression of endothelial cells-adhesion molecules. P-selectin expression is transient, the molecule becoming rapidly internalized. By 6 to 8 hours, E-selectin expression has begun to recede, involving both a decrease in synthesis and a reinternalization. In contrast, ICAM-1 expression continues to increase, reaching plateau levels only after 24 hours. Correspondingly, VCAM is synthesized and expressed. VCAM-1 is absent on resting endothelial cells and is up-regulated by

IL-1, TNF, but not γ-IFN. L-selectin expressed by monocytes and T-cells, and endothelial cells E-selectin have, in vitro, been shown to be involved in the initial adhesion of monocytes and T-cells to endothelial cells. Lymphocytes, unlike neutrophils, do not exhibit rolling behavior, and in contrast appear to collide several times with the endothelial cells and then rapidly stop. Most lymphocytes of the circulation are in a resting state, and would bind weakly via integrins, which require cell activation for expression and strong binding. Evidence suggests that the T-lymphocytes that migrate into inflammatory sites are memory cells, which may have been previously stimulated by antigen. Memory T-cells have a higher surface expression of CD44 compared to naive cells. Integrins on T-cells mediate adhesion only when the cells receive an activating stimulus. A multitude of cell surface molecules can activate T cell integrin expression, including the CD3, CD2, CD7, CD28, CD31, and VLA-4 T cell surface receptors. The binding of VLA-4 to endothelial VCAM can amplify its own adhesion, since monoclonal antibody ligation induces expression. This autoregulation appears similar to that of the platelet GPIIb-IIIa. VLA-4 and CD31 are expressed only on some T cells. L-selectin is also a potential triggering molecule since it regulates Mac-1 function on neutrophils. Integrin regulation on T cells by E-selectin has not been reported, however. Integrins, once induced and expressed on T cells induce strong adhesion predominantly through the VLA-4/VCAM, LFA-1/ICAM pathway. Transendothelial migration requires the LFA-1/ICAM interaction. In individuals lacking LFA-1, lymphocytes can enter inflammatory sites, whereas neutrophils cannot. In vitro migration assays demonstrate an inhibition of T cell migration through endothelial monolayers by LFA-1 and CD44 monoclonal antibodies. Decreased migratory capacity of T cells has also been demonstrated in LFA-1 deficient clones. It has been suggested that T cell migration involves a reduction in adhesion such as shedding of L-selectin upon T cell activation, or a signal that induces integrin function, then decays rapidly, followed by orderly migration. Lymphocytes and monocytes enter inflamed tissues in increased numbers at later times. Monocytes do not respond to IL-8, but rather to a structurally related cytokine or monocyte chemotactic protein, induced by IL-1 and TNF. Monocytes, via LFA-1, Mac-1, and VLA-4, appear to recognize ligands on endothelial cell surfaces.

Culture of Endothelial Cells

Endothelial cells forming the inner lining of blood vessels are involved in a myriad of physiologic processes. The ability to grow pure cultures of endothelial cells has resulted in greater understanding of their structure and function. However, there is considerable species-dependent variation in morphology and function of endothelial cells harvested from different vascular beds. In addition, the methods used to obtain pure endothelial cell cultures can vary depending upon the anatomy of the vascular bed and the composition of the surrounding tissue. A number of techniques have been reported for harvest and isolation of large vessel endothelial cells, from human umbilical vein,[75,76] bovine aorta,[77] porcine aorta,[78] and pulmonary artery,[79] as well as for microvascular endothelial cells from various organs. Several of these techniques have been extensively reviewed elsewhere.[80,81] Described here are selected techniques for the isolation of endothelial cells from human umbilical vein and bovine aorta utilizing enzyme dispersion and mechanical harvesting, respectively, and a brief examination of primary culture of microvascular endothelial cells.

Large Vessel Endothelial Cells

Human Umbilical Vein (Enzyme Dispersion Techniques)

The first successful method of isolating large vessel endothelial cells involved the instillation of proteolytic enzyme solutions into the vessel lumen to disrupt intra- and subcellular protein attachments. Early studies using trypsin as the proteolytic agent resulted in poor endothelial cell growth and viability. Collagenase was then utilized and enabled successful long-term culture of endothelial cells from both human umbilical artery and vein,[75,76,82–85] as well as from other sources. However, several studies have suggested that exposure of endothelial cells to the proteolytic enzymes used for harvesting and passaging cells, can result in damage to the cell membrane proteins, alterations in surface receptors and responsiveness to agonists, reduced areas of junctional contacts, and possibly alteration of DNA structure. Despite these critiques, the enzyme dispersion technique remains widely utilized because of its effectiveness in procuring endothelial cells from large vessel, including human umbilical vein, which is resistant to the alternative mechanical methods of harvesting these cells for culture (see below).

Umbilical cords are collected after delivery, stored at 4°C for up to 48 hours in a prepared buffer solution (140 mM NaCl, 4 mM KCl, 11 mM D-glucose, 10 mM HEPES [N-2-hydroxyethylpiperozine-N′-ethane sulfonic acid], pH 7.3, 100 IU/mL penicillin, 0.10 mg/mL streptomycin). Other groups,[86] utilize phosphate-buffered saline (PBS), supplemented with penicillin, streptomycin, gentamicin, and mycostatin, and claim good endothelial cell yields up to 72 hours of umbilical cord storage. Clamped or otherwise damaged segments of the cord are not used, as this allows for fibroblast and SMC contamination. A metal cannula or plastic three-way tap is inserted into one end of the umbilical vein, secured, and then flushed slowly with buffer to remove red cells and debris. The free end is tied off and the vessel is distended with the proteolytic solution. A collagenase (Worthington Biochemical Corp., CLS type 1) solution is commonly used and is prepared in 0.1 to 0.5 g/mL concentration using sterile PBS, or PBS supplemented with 25 mM HEPES, filtered (0.45 μm), and stored at $-20°C$ until needed. Van Hinsbergh et al[85] recommends diluting the collagenase solution with medium (Medium 199 with 25 mM HEPES and penicillin/streptomycin), to a final concentration of 0.10% prior to use. Alternatively, a 0.05% collagenase/dipase (Boehringer Mannheim) solution can be utilized.

The umbilical vein filled with proteolytic enzyme is incubated for 15 minutes at 37°C in an oven or water bath. The contents are then drained into a 50 mL centri-

fuge tube by flushing the vein segment with 20 to 25 mL of PBS or Medium 199. The flask should contain 10 mL of culture medium with 10% fetal calf serum (FCS) to neutralize the protease. The cell suspension is centrifuged for 5 minutes at 200 to 500 g, the supernatant discarded, and the pellet resuspended in culture media. The cells are seeded into T-25 flasks and incubated at 37°C under 5% CO_2 atmosphere. Endothelial cells attach to the flask, producing an adherent, confluent monolayer within 3 to 7 days (Figure 14). The culture medium is replaced every 2 to 3 days to get rid of metabolic wastes and to renew nutrients. The endothelial cells are passaged when confluent.

HUEVC retain their epithelioid morphology, growing to confluent monolayers of densely packed (approx. 100000 cells/cm2) polygonal cells, resulting in a characteristic cobblestone appearance (Figure 14). In cultures maintained at confluence for prolonged periods, elongated, "sprouting" cells appear (the significance of which will be discussed later), as well as multi-

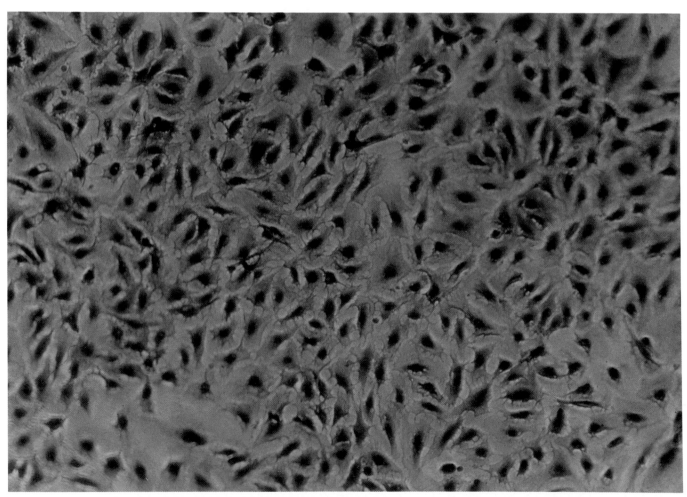

Figure 14. Phase contrast photomicrograph of confluent human umbilical vein endothelial cells.

nucleated giant cells (Figure 3), which have also been observed in vivo at the edge of intimal lesions and in aortas from older people. Ultrastructurally,[87] the cultured HUVECs retain the structural characteristics of the in vivo endothelium,[88] forming intercellular junctions, and displaying Weibel-Palade bodies.

Bovine Aorta (Mechanical Harvest Techniques)

Ryan and collegues[89] reported a technique of lightly scraping calf pulmonary artery luminal surface with a scalpel to collect endothelial cells for culture. Intact sheets of endothelium are obtained relatively free from contaminating fibroblasts and SMCs, and are not exposed to the possible adverse effects of proteolytic enzymes on cell structure. In addition, the cells retain their three-dimensional polarity and remain connected by junctional complexes, including tight junctions, which are generally absent from cells treated with proteolytic enzymes. Given the simplicity of this technique and the resulting efficiency of the primary cultures, mechanical methods of endothelial cell harvesting have been utilized to obtain cells from most large vessels.[86,90] For bovine aorta, thoracic aortas are removed aseptically at the time of slaughter, from the heart-lung block. The intrathoracic aorta extending from the aortic valve to the diaphragm, together with the surrounding fat, is placed in a sterile saline solution containing antibiotics (300 U/mL penicillin, 300 ug/mL streptomycin and transferred on ice to the tissue culture facility. Typically, endothelial cells are harvested within 1 to 3 hours of procurement. Within a laminar flow biosafety hood, the aorta is cleaned with 70% ethanol, and is transferred to a sterile 150 mm tissue culture plate. The surrounding periaortic fat is removed using sterile technique, and the vessel is opened lengthwise. The intimal surface is gently scraped with a sterile #10 scalpel, with care being taken not to scrape too deeply or too close to the cut edge, which could lead to contamination by other cell types. The scraped cells are dispersed in culture dishes containing Dulbecco's Modified Eagle's Medium with nutrient medium F12 (D-MEM/F12, Gibco Laboratories, Grand Island, NY) supplemented with 10% heat-inactivated calf serum, 5 ug/mL deoxycytidine, 5 ug/mL thymidine, and 1% penicillin-streptomycin and fungizone. The cells are incubated at 37°C, in 5% CO_2 atmosphere.

Microvascular Endothelial Cells

In contrast to early success in obtaining primary cultures of large vessel endothelium, the isolation and culture of microvessel endothelial cells has proven to be a formidable task. The difficulty arises from the diverse architecture of various microvascular sources, and the varied characteristics of differentiated endothelial cells obtained from these different sources. Primary cultures of capillary endothelial cells were obtained in 1975 by Wagner and Matthews,[91] by treating epididymal fat pads with collagenase. Endothelial cells were isolated by floatation followed by filtration through a 200 um mesh. The first successful, long-term serial culture of microvascular endothelial cells was reported by Folkman and Haudenschild,[92] utilizing a combination of mechanical and collagenase disruption of adrenal tissue. Only by tediously eliminating contaminating cells and by adding feeder cells to condition the medium, were the investigators able to obtain pure cultures of endothelial cells. Techniques for isolation and culture of endothelial cells from brain, heart, and lung, were soon reported.

Significant advances have been made in obtaining pure microvascular endothelial cell cultures from various sources.[80,81] The techniques vary, but generally involve one of three methods: tissue mincing and dispersion, followed by cell separation and selective growth (Figure 15); whole organ protease perfusion to obtain mixed cell suspensions; or organ perfusion of microcarrier polystyrene beads of known dimensions to obtain adherent cells from vessels in which the beads lodge (Figure 16). The latter method, has been utilized by Ryan[93] for the isolation of pulmonary microvascular cells, and involves the initial nonenzymatic loosening of endothelial cells by cold shock and EDTA perfusion of lung preparations, followed by the introduction, then recovery, of 40 to 80 um diameter, polystyrene microcarrier beads (Figure 16). Cells from either the arteriolar or postcapillary endothelium can be obtained, depending upon whether the microcarriers are introduced and collected from the arterial or venous side of the preparation. This technique has also been utilized to successfully isolate capillary endothelial cells from hearts.[94] The advantage of the method is the selective harvest of endothelial cells from specific-sized vessels, from either the arterial or venous side of the circulation, and the avoidance of tissue proteolysis.

Identification of Endothelial Cells

Phase contrast microscopy of early confluent monolayers of cultured endothelial cells from all sources reveal tightly-packed polygonal cells with central, ovoid nuclei, resulting in a recognizable, cobblestone pattern (Figure 14). The uniformity of this layer, however, is dependent on the serum content of the culture medium and the amount of time the cells remain at confluence. The uniformity can also vary with the content of contaminating cells. After reaching confluence, many authors report a progressive disorganization of the endothelial cell architecture, with the ap-

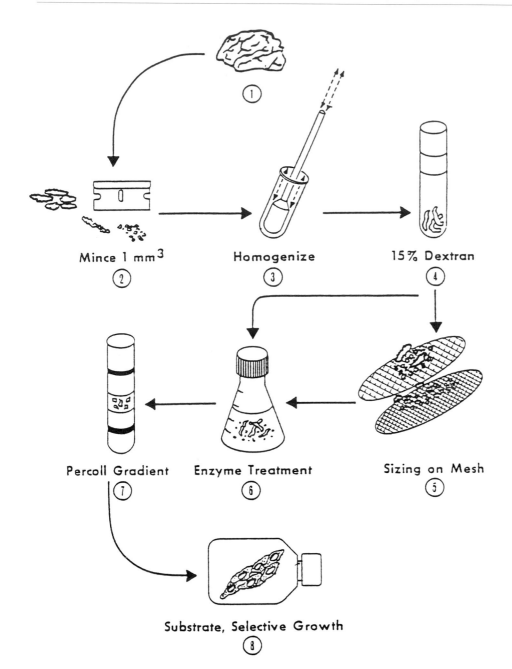

Mince 1 mm³
②

Homogenize
③

15% Dextran
④

Percoll Gradient
⑦

Enzyme Treatment
⑥

Sizing on Mesh
⑤

Substrate, Selective Growth
⑧

Figure 15. General scheme used for isolating and cultivating microvascular endothelial cells, in this case from brain, using tissue mincing/dispersion, gradient and mesh separation, then selective growth. (Reproduced with permission from Reference 80.)

pearance of ''sprouter'' cells and multinucleate giant cells. The sprouter cells have been shown to leave the monolayer, growing atop the cell culture, and can stain positive for SMC α-actin, complicating the process of assessing culture purity by visual criteria. Fibroblasts are generally easy to recognize in early confluent cultures as spindle-shaped cells.

A number of cell types, depending upon the vessel source, can grow in the usual 10% to 30% serum-containing culture medium typically used for growing endothelial cells, and can overgrow confluent cultures when endothelial cell growth rate slows. This problem can be overcome to some extent by the passage of endothelial cell cultures shortly after confluence. How-

ever, due to the ability of endothelial cultures to demonstrate a variable pattern of growth, and the ability of some cells of mesodermal origin to display a cobblestone appearance in culture, the development of other markers specific for endothelium has been necessary to confirm the endothelial origin of the cultured cells.

Jaffe et al[76] used immunofluorescence techniques and rabbit antihuman factor VIII:vWF serum to distinguish HUVECs from contaminating fibroblasts and SMCs, which do not express the complex. The complex stains endothelial cells in a granular pattern (Figure 17), corresponding to the location of the factor in intracellular storage organelles, termed Weibel-Palade bodies. However, the Weibel-Palade bodies and asso-

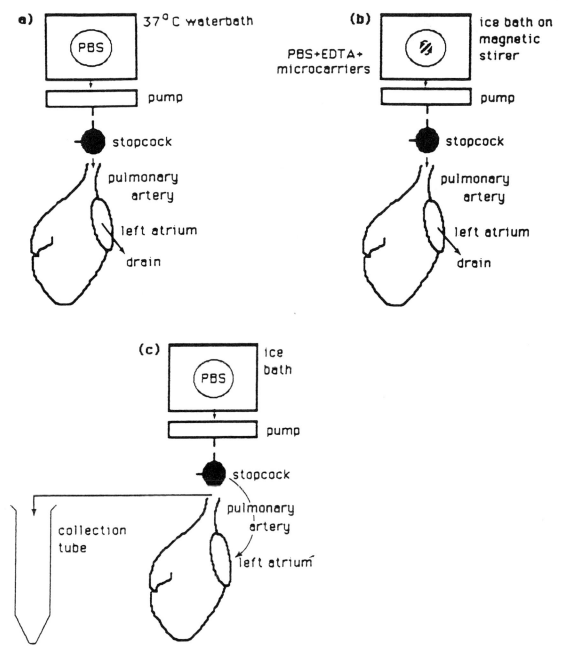

Figure 16. General method used for isolation of microvascular endothelial cells from rabbit lung using microcarrier beads. **a)** Lungs are perfused blood-free using warm PBS with added antibiotics. **b)** Then the preparation is perfused with a Ca^{++}- and Mg^{++}-free solution containing 40–80 um microcarrier beads. **c)** The flow direction is reversed and the perfusate from the arterial side is collected. The flow direction is reversed again to collect perfusate from the venous side. (Reproduced with permission from Reference 80.)

ciated immunoreactivity for factor VIII:vWF are not present in all endothelial cells. The markers are present in reduced numbers in endothelial cells from bovine sources, and are rare in pigs, rat, and rabbit vessels. They are variably present in microvascular endothelial cells, including human glomerular capillaries, splenic endothelium, lung and adrenal capillaries, and some lymphatic sources.

Other antibodies have been raised against putative endothelial cell antigens. Their use as markers has been recently reviewed.[95] ACE is localized to the luminal surface of endothelium, and has been used as an immunohistochemical and functional marker in cultures of endothelial cells from different vessels and species.[96,97] Its usefulness is limited, however, by the immunologic heterogeneity of the enzyme in several species, as well

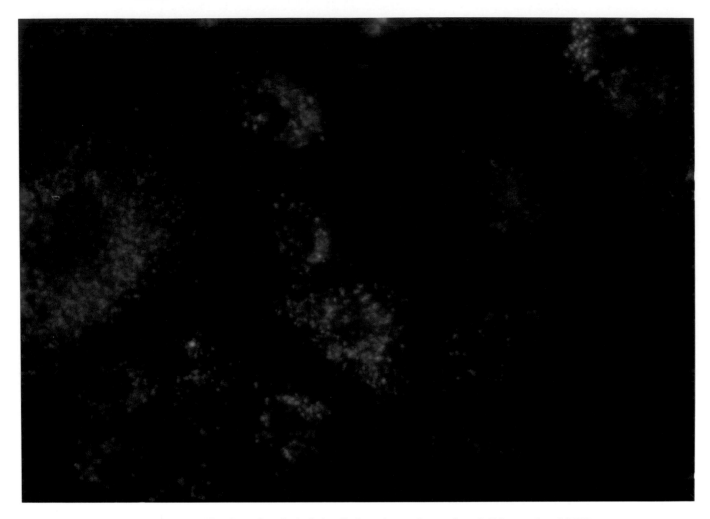

Figure 17. Identification of endothelial cells in culture via uptake of di-I-acetylated LDL. LDL = low density lipoproteins.

as its absence in some tissues. In addition, some mesodermal cells can express ACE activity, and the enzyme can be significantly reduced on endothelial cells exposed to proteolytic enzymes during harvesting and passage.

Many investigators have taken advantage of the endothelial cell's ability to bind and take up various chemically modified forms of low density lipoprotein (LDL).[80,98,99] Cells are grown on glass coverslips to confluence, then incubated with a solution of LDL, labelled with 1,1-diododecyl,1–3,3,3,3-tetramethyl-indocarbocyanine pechlorate (Di-I-LDL; Biomedical Technologies) for 4 hours. The cover slips are washed three times at room temperature with PBS, then fixed in 3% formaldehyde. The Di-I-LDL uptake can be visualized using fluorescence photomicroscope equipped for epi-illumination, using standard excitation and emission filters (350 to 560 nm for rhodamine; 340 to 380 nm for bisbenzamide). Di-I-LDL accumulates around the nucleus (Figure 17). Neither fibroblasts, SMCs, or pericytes take up LDL.

Alternatively, the number of SMCs and pericyte contamination of the cultures can be determined by using antibodies against SMC α-actin, an isoform not expressed in endothelial cells (see Chapter 7).

Endothelial Cell Culture Media

The two most commonly used solute solutions for culture endothelial cells are Dulbecco's Modified Eagle's Minimum Essential Medium (DMEM; Sigma Chemical), or Medium 199 (various suppliers). In our laboratory, we prefer DMEM, supplemented with Ham's F12 nutrient supplement (DMEM-F12, Gibco Laboratory) to grow bovine aortic endothelial cells. DMEM is a complete formula, containing the following (g/L): inorganic salts [Calcium Chloride (0.265), Ferric Nitrate (0.0001), Magnesium Sulfate (0.09767), Potassium Chloride (0.400), Sodium Bicarbonate (3.700), Sodium Chloride (6.400), and Sodium Phosphate Monobasic (0.109)]; amino acids [L-arginine (0.084), L-cysteine (0.0626), glycine (0.030), L-histidine (0.042), L-isoleucine (0.105), L-leucine (0.105), L-lysine (0.146), L methionine (0.030), L phenylalanine (0.066), L-serine (0.042), L-threonine (0.095), L-tryptophan (0.016), L-tyrosine (0.10379), and L-valine (0.094)]; vitamins oline chloride (0.004), folic acid (0.004), myoinositol (0.0072), niacinamide (0.004), D-pantothenic acid (0.004), riboflavin (0.0004), and thiamine (0.004)]; and other ingredients [D-glucose (4.5), phenol red (0.0159), and added glutamine (0.584)]. The final pH is adjusted to 7.3 + 0.3 with 15 mM HEPES buffer, and the final osmolality is 334 + 5%. Addition of L-glutamine appears to be required, having a half-life of 9 days at 35°C. In addition, the culture medium is supplemented with 10% heat-inactivated fetal calf serum (Hyclone Laboratories, Utah), 5 ug/L each of deoxycytidine and thymidine, and 1% antibiotic solution (penicillin, streptomycin, and fungizone).

Serum is a necessary component of the culture medium needed to support growth and viability of cells. HUVEC will not attach to culture substratum, nor will established cultures grow in serum-free medium.[75] As little as 1% to 2% added serum could restore these activities; 10% serum was shown to be sufficient to maintain endothelial cultures, although initial growth rates could be enhanced by increasing the serum concentration to 30%. Any incremental change gained above 30% was small. Similar effects have been demonstrated with other cell types, although the serum type and amount necessary depend somewhat upon the tissue of origin. For bovine aortic endothelial cells, we have found the use of 10% heat-inactivated fatal calf serum adequate to sustain cell cultures. The serum is electrophoretically scanned, and pre-filtered through 40 nm filters before use. Our culture medium ingredients are combined in a laminar hood, aseptically, filtered through 0.45 μm acetate filters, and stored at 4°C for serial use.

Growth of human endothelial cells in fetal calf serum or fetal bovine serum is dependent upon the presence of added ECGF, which originally referred to a crude extract derived from brain tissue.[100] It has been found to contain growth factors of the heparin-binding growth factor family (HBGF), namely, aFGF and bFGF. To date, a number of ECGF (Table 1) known to trigger endothelial cell proliferation in vitro and in vivo have been identified.[15,101,102] Much effort has gone into the development of semi-synthetic, and synthetic media for the culturing of endothelial cells. For human lines, in addition to ECGF, cells appear to require epidermal growth factor (EGF) as well. The further addition of human lipoprotein, and heparin, have been shown to improve growth with such media. Recently, Gorfin and colleagues[103] were able to utilize serum-free media (Endothelial-SFM, Gibco BRL, Gaithersburg, MD), with added vibronectin at the initial plating, to grow and maintain long-term cultures of endothelial cells from bovine, porcine, and canine large vessel sources. The cells retained their characteristic appearance, were positive for factor VIII:vWF and Di-I-LDL uptake, and were able to produce PGI_2 and PDGF. HUVECs could be grown for up to four passages with hydrocortisone, pituitary extract, and epidermal growth factor added to the medium.

Summary

Far from a passive barrier, the vascular endothelium is now known to actively influence many physiologic processes. Much of what we know about endothelial cell behavior has resulted from the developement of harvest and culture techniques to isolate endothelial cells from many tissue sources. The techniques continue to evolve, demonstrated by the advent of three-dimensional culture for microvascular endothelial cells, and the developement of serum-free culture medium, allowing for better characterization of cell behavior.

From embryogenesis onward, the endothelium is constantly responding to signals in the surrounding environment, be they physical, chemical, inflammatory, or immunologic. Components of the basement membrane and surrounding ECM can influence cell growth, differentiation, and migratory capacity. Interactions with these components and with blood cells occur via specific transmembrane receptors, such as the integrins, which lead to coordinated responses effecting coagulation, immune surveillance, and inflammation.

Dysfunction of the endothelium is thought to contribute to the developement of a number of pathologic entities, including atherosclerosis, hypertension, sepsis, and vessel stenosis following angioplasty or grafting. A better understanding of endothelial cell function and dysfunction may lead to therapeutic interventions to slow or prevent these conditions.

References

1. Risau W, Lemmon V: Change in the vascular extracellular matrix during embryonic vasculogenesis and angiogenesis. *Devel Bio* 125:441–450, 1988.
2. Pardanaud L, Yassine F, Dieterlen-Lievre F: Relationship between vasculogenesis, angiogenesis, and hemopoiesis during avian ontogeny. *Development* 105:473–485, 1989.
3. Reagen FP: Vascularization phenomena in fragments of embryonic bodies completely isolates from yolk-sac entoderm. *Anat Rec* 9:329–341, 1915.
4. Pardanaud L, Altman C, Kitos P, Dieterlen-Lievre F, Buck CA: Vasculogenesis in the early quail blastodisc as studied with a monoclonal antibody recognizing endothelial cells. *Development* 100:339–349, 1987.
5. Coffin JD, Poole TJ: Embryonic vascular development:

immunohistochemical identification of the origin and subsequent morphogenesis of the major vessel primordia in quail embryos. *Development* 102:735–748, 1988.

6. Noden DM: Embryonic origins and assembly of blood vessels. *Am Rev Respir Dis* 140:1097–1103, 1989.

7. Ekblom P, Sariola H, Karkinen-Jaakelainen M, Saxon L: The origin of the glomerular endothelium. *Cell Differ* 121:35–39, 1982.

8. Seifert R, Zhao B, Christ B: Cytokinetic studies on the aortic endothelium and limb bud vascularization in avian embryos. *Anat Embryol* 186:601–610, 1992.

9. Navaratnam V: Organization and reorganization of blood vessels in embryonic development. *Eye* 5: 147–150, 1991.

10. Arciniegas E, Servin M, Arguello C, Mota M: Development of the aorta in the chick embryo: structural and ultrastructural study. *Atherosclerosis* 76:219–235, 1989.

11. Arciniegas E, Sanchez F, Candelle D, Villegas GM: Concomitant changes in endothelial cell junctions and extracellular matrix components in the chick embryo aorta. *Anat Embryol* 183:461–473, 1991.

12. Mascatelli D, Rifkin DB: Membrane and matrix localization of proteases: a common theme in tumor invasion and angiogenesis. *Biochim Biophys Acta* 948:67–85, 1988.

13. Pepper MS, Mantesaro R: Proteolytic balance and capillary morphogenesis. *Cell Differ Develop* 32:319–328, 1990.

14. Klagsburn M: The fibroblast growth factor family: structural and biological properties. *Prog Growth Factor Res* 1:207–235.

15. Bobik A, Campbell JH: Vascular derived growth factors: cell biology, pathophysiology, and pharmacology. *Pharmacol Rev* 45(1):1–42, 1993.

16. GodPodarowicz D, Ferrara N, Schweigerer L, Neufield G: Structural characterization and biological functions of fibroblast growth factor. *Endocrinol Rev* 8:95–114, 1987.

17. Breier G, Albrecht U, Sterrer S, Risau W: Expression of vascular endothelial growth factor during embryonic angiogenesis and endothelial cell differentiation. *Development* 114:521–532, 1992.

18. Thompson JA, Haudenschild CC, Anderson KD, DiPietro J, Anderson WF, Maciag T: Induction of organoid neovascular structures in vivo. *Proc Natl Acad Sci USA* 86:7938, 1989.

19. Madri JA, Pratt BM: Endothelial cell matrix-interactions: in vitro models of angionenesis. *J Histochem Cytochem* 34:85–91, 1986.

20. Madri JA, Bell L, Marx M, Merwin JR, Basson CT, Prinz C: The effects of soluble factors and extracellular matrix composition on vascular cell behavior in vitro: models of deendothelialization and repair. *J Cell Biochem* 45:1–8, 1991.

21. Merwin JR, Anderson J, Kocher O, van Itallie C, Madri JA: Transforming growth factor β_1 modulates extracellular matrix organization and cell-cell junctional complex formation during in vitro angiogenesis. *J Cell Physiol* 142:117–128, 1990.

22. Kocher O, Madri JA: Modulation of actin mRNAs in cultured capillary endothelial and aortic endothelial and smooth muscle cells by matrix components and TGF-β_1. *In Vitro* 25:424–434, 1989.

23. Grant DS, Lelkes PI, Fukuda K, Kleinman HK: Intracellular mechanisms involved in basement membrane-induced blood vessel differentiation in vitro. *In Vitro Cell Devel Biol* 27A:327–336, 1991.

24. Madri JA, Pratt BM, Tucker AM: Phenotype modulation of endothelial cells by transforming growth factor beta depends upon the composition and organization of the extracellular matrix. *J Cell Biol* 106:1375–1384, 1988.

25. Madri JA, Marx M: Matrix composition, organization, and soluble factors: modulators of microvascular cell differentiation in vitro. *Kidney Int* 41:560–565, 1992.

26. Timpl R: Structure and biological activity of basement membrane proteins. *J Biochem* 180:487–502, 1989.

27. Kleinman HK, McGarvey ML, Liotta LA, Robey PG, Tryggvason K, Martin GR: Isolation and characterization of type IV procollagen, laminin, and heparan sulfate proteoglycan from the EHS sarcoma. *Biochem* 24: 6188–6193, 1982.

28. Chung AE, Freeman IL, Braginski JE: A novel extracellular membrane elaborated by a mouse embryonal carcinoma-derived cell line. *Biochem Biophys Res Comm* 79:859–868, 1977.

29. Leblond P, Inque S: Structure, composition, and assembly of basement membrane. *Am J Anat* 185: 367–390, 1989.

30. Wight TN: Cell biology of arterial proteoglycans. *Arteriosclerosis* 9:1–20, 1989.

31. Nader HB, Dietrich CP, Buonassisi V, Colburn P: Heparin sequences in the heparan sulfate chains of on endothelial cell proteoglycan. *Proc Natl Acad Sci USA* 84: 3565–3569, 1987.

32. Kuhn K: The collagne family: variations in the molecular and supermolecular structure. *Rheumatology* 10: 29–69, 1986.

33. Mayne R, Burgeson RE (eds). *Structure and Function of Collagen Types*. Orlando: Academic Press; 1987.

34. Furthmayr H, Wiedemann H, Timpl R, Odermatt E, Engel J: Electron-microscopical approach to a structural model of intima collagen. *Biochem J* 211:303–311, 1983.

35. Weber N: Basement membrane proteins. *Kidney Int* 41: 620–628, 1992.

36. Ingber DE, Folkman J: Mechanochemical switching between growth and differentiation during fibroblast growth factor-stimulated angiogenesis in vitro: role of extracellular matrix. *J Cell Biol* 109:317–330, 1989.

37. Schnaper HW, Kleinman HK, Grant DS: Role of laminin in endothelial cell recognition and differentiation. *Kidney Int* 43:20–25, 1993.

38. Myers JC: Differential expression of type I collagen and cellular fibronectin isoforms in endothelial cell variants. *Kidney Int* 43:45–52, 1993.

39. Beck K, Hunter I, Engel J: Structure and function of laminin: anatomy of a multidomain glycoprotein. *FASEB J* 4:148–160, 1990.

40. von der Mark K, von der Mark H, Goodman S: Cellular responses to extracellular matrix. *Kidney Int* 41: 632–640, 1992.

41. Olsen DR, Nagayoshi T, Fazio N, et al: Human laminin: cloning and sequence analysis of cDNAs encoding A, B1, and B2 chains, and expression of the corresponding genes in human skin and cultured cells. *Lab Invest* 60: 772–782, 1989.

42. Aumailley M, Wiedemann H, Mann K, Timpl R: Binding of the laminin-nidogen complex to basement membrane collagen type IV. *Eur J Biochem* 184:241–248, 1989.

43. Roberts AB, Sporn MB: Regulation of endothelial cell

growth, architecture, and matrix synthesis by TGF-β_1. *Am Rev Resp Dis* 140:1126–1128, 1989.

44. Roberts AB, McCune BK, Sporn MB: TGF-β: regulation of extracellular matrix. *Kidney Int* 41:557–559, 1992.
45. Majewsky MW, Lidner V, Twardzik DR, Schwartz SM, Reidy MA: Production of Transforming growth factor-1 during repair of arterial injury. *J Clin Invest* 49:904–910, 1991.
46. Antonelli-Orlidge A, Smith SR, D'Amore PA: Influence of pericytes on capillary endothelial cell growth. *Am Rev Resp Dis* 140:1129–1131, 1989.
47. Gottlieb AI, Langille BL, Wong MKK, Kim DW: Biology of disease: structure and function of ecdothelial cytoskeleton. *Lab Invest* 65(2):123–137, 1991
48. Luna EJ, Hitt AL: Cytoskeleton-plasma membrane interactions. *Science* 258:955–964, 1992.
49. Ingber D: Integrins as mechanotransducers. *Curr Opin Cell Biol* 3:841–848, 1991.
50. Nerem RM, Harrison DG, Taylor WR, Alexander RW: Hemodynamics and vascular endothelial biology. *J Cardiovasc Pharmacol* 21(suppl 1):S6-S10, 1993.
51. Iba T, Sumpio BE: Morphological response of human endothelial cells subjected to cyclic strain in vitro. *Microvasc Res* 42:245–254, 1991.
52. Dewey CF, Bussolari SR, Gimbrone MA, Davies PF: The dynamic response of vascular endothelial cells to fluid shear stress. *J Biomech Eng* 103:177–185, 1981.
53. Smyth SS, Janeckis CC, Parise LV: Regulation of vascular integrins. *Blood* 81(11):2827–2843, 1993.
54. Dejana E: Endothelial cell adhesive receptors. *J Cardiovasc Pharmacol* 21(suppl 1):S8-S21, 1993.
55. Dejana E, Raiteri M, Lampugnani MG: Endothelial integrins and their role in maintaining the integrity of the vessel wall. *Kidney Int* 43:61–65, 1993.
56. Hynes RO: Integrins: versatility, modulation, and signaling in cell adhesion. *Cell* 69:11–25, 1992.
57. Lampugnani MG, Resnati M, Dejana E, Marchisio PC: The role of integrins in the maintenance of endothelial monolayer integrity. *J Cell Biol* 112(3):479–490, 1991.
58. Marcus AJ, Safier LB: Thromboregulation: multicellular modulation of platlet reactivity in hemostasis and thrombosis. *FASEB J* 7:516–522, 1993.
59. Ware JA, Herstad DD: Platlet-endothelilum interactions. *N Engl J Med* 329(9):628–635, 1993.
60. Gertler JP, Abbott WM: Current research review: prothrombotic and fibrinolytic function of normal and perturbed endothelium. *J Surg Res* 52:89–95, 1992.
61. Rothe GJ: Platelets and blood vessels: the adhesion event. *Immunol Today* 13(3):100–105, 1992.
62. Ruggeri ZM, Ware J: Von Willibrand factor. *FASEB J* 7:308–316, 1993.
63. Stoolman LM: Adhesion molecules controlling lymphocyte migration. *Cell* 56:907–910, 1989.
64. Cavender DE: Interactions between endothelial cells and the cells of the immune system. *Int Rev Exper Pathol* 32:57–94, 1991.
65. Stamper HB, Woodruff JJ: Lymphocyte homing into lymph nodes: in vitro demonstration of the selective affinity of recirculation lymphocytes for high endothelial venules. *J Exp Med* 144:828–833, 1976.
66. Shimizer Y, Newman W, Tanaka Y, Shaw S: Lymphocyte interactions with endothelial cells. *Immunol Today* 13(3):106–112, 1992.
67. Westphal JR, de Waal RMW: The role of adhesion molecules in endothelial cell accessary function. *Mol Bio Reports* 17:47–59, 1992.
68. Williams TJ, Hellewell PH: Endothelial cell biology: adhesion molecules involved in the microvascular inflammatory response. *Am Rev Resp Dis* 146:S45-S50, 1992.
69. Zimmerman GA, Prescott SM, McIntyre TM: Endothelial cell interactions woth granulocytes: tethering and signaling molecules. *Immunol Today* 13(3):93–97, 1992.
70. Ley K: Leukocyte adhesion to vascular endothelium. *J Reconstr Microsurg* 8(6):495–503, 1992.
71. Butcher EC: Cellualr and molecular mechanisms that direct leukocyte traffic. *Am J Pathol* 156(1):3–11, 1990.
72. Redl H, Schlag G, Dinges HP, Kneidinger R, Davies J: Leukocyte-endothelial interactions in trauma and sepsis. In: Faist E, Meakus J, Schildberg FW (eds). *Host Defense Dysfunction in Trauma, Shock, and Sepsis*. Berlin: Springer-Verlag; 277–286, 1993.
73. Pober JS, Cotran RS: The role of endothelial cells in inflammation. *Transplantation* 50(4):537–554, 1990.
74. Rothelein R, Wegner C: Role of intercellular adhesion molecule-1 in the inflammatory response. *Kidney Int* 41:617–619, 1992.
75. Gimbrone MA, Cotran RS, Folkman J: Human vascular endothelial cells in culture: growth and DNA Synthesis. *J Cell Biol* 60:673, 1974.
76. Jaffe EA, Nochman RL, Becker CG, Minick CR: Culture of human endothelial cells dericed from umbilical vein. *J Clin Invest* 52:2745, 1973.
77. Booyse FM, Sedlak BH; Rafelson ME: Culture of arterial endothelial cells: charactcrization and growth of bovine aortic endothelial cells. *Thromb Diath Haemorrh* 34:325–839, 1975.
78. Slater DN, Sloan JM: The porcine endothelial cell in culture. *Atherosclerosis* 21:259–272, 1975.
79. Ryan US, Clements E, Habliston D, Ryan JW: Isolation and culture of pulmonary artery endothelial cells. *Tissue Cell* 10:535–554, 1978.
80. Piper HM (ed). *Cell Culture Techniques in Heart and Vessel Research*. Berlin: Springer-Verlag; 1990.
81. Warren JB (ed). *The Endothelium: An Introduction to Current Research*. New York: Wiley-Liss; 1990.
82. Gimbrone MA Jr, Shefton EJ, Cruise SA: Isolation and primary dulture of endothelial cells from human umbilical vessels. *Tissue Culture Assoc* 4:813–817, 1979.
83. Jaffe EA: Culture of human endothelial cells. *Transplat Proc* 1249–1253, 1980.
84. Maciag T, Kadish J, Wilkins L, Stemerman MB, Weinstein R: Organizational behavior of human umbilical vein endothelial cells. *J Cell Biol* 94:511–520, 1982.
85. Van Hinsbergh VWM, Scheffer MA, Langeler EG: Macro- and microvascular endothelial cells from human tissues. In: Piper HM (ed). *Cell Culture Techniques in Heart and Vessel Research*. Berlin: Springer-Verlag; 178–204, 1990.
86. Warren JB: Large vessel endothelial isolation. In: Warren JB (ed). *The Endothelium: An introduction to Current Research*. New York: Wiley-Liss; 263–272, 1990.
87. Haudenschild CC, Cotran RS, Gimbrone MA Jr, Folkman J: Fine structure of vascular endothelium in culture. *J Ultrastruc Res* 50:22–32, 1975.
88. Parry EW, Abramovich DR: The ultrastructure of human umbilical vessel endothelium from early pregnency to full-term. *J Anat* 111(1):29–42, 1972.
89. Ryan US, Mortara M, Whitaker C: Methods for microcarrier culture of bovine pulmonary artery endothelial cells avoiding the use of enzymes. *Tissue Cell* 12(4):619–635, 1980.
90. Rosenthal AM, Gotlieb AI: Macrovascular endothelial cells from porcine aorta. In: Piper HM (ed). *Cell Culture*

Techniques in Heart and Vessel Research. Berlin: Springer-Verlag; 117–129, 1990.

91. Wagner RC, Matthews MA: The isolation and culture of capillary endothelium from epididymal fat. *Microvasc Res* 10:286–297, 1975.

92. Folkman J, Haudenschild CC: Long-term culture of capillary endothelial cells. *Proc Natl Acad Sci USA* 76:5217–5221, 1979.

93. Ryan US: Microvascular endothelial cells from the lungs. In: Piper HM (ed). *Cell Culture Techniques in Heart and Vessel Research.* Berlin: Springer-Verlag; 130–139, 1990.

94. Schelling ME, Meininger CH, Hawker JR Jr, Granger HJ: Venular endothelial cells from bovine heart. *Am J Physiol* 254:H1211-H1217, 1988.

95. Ruiter DJ, Schlingemann RO, Rietveld FJR, de Waal RMW: Monoclonal antibody defined human endothelial antigens as vascular markers. *J Invest Dermatol* 93:25S-32S, 1989.

96. Caldwell PRB, Seegel BC, Hsu KC: Angiotensin-converting enzyme: vascular endothelial localization. *Science* 191:1050–1051, 1976.

97. Seitz RJ, Neunen E, Henrich M, Schrader J, Wechsler W: Angiotensin I-converting enzyme (ACE): a marker for vascular endothelium. In: Cervos-Navarro J, Ferszt R (ed). *Stroke and Microcirculation.* New York: Raven Press; 111–115, 1987.

98. Voyta JC, Via DP, Butterfield CE, Zetter BR: Indentification and isolation of endothelial cells based on their increased uptake of acetylated-low density lipoprotein. *J Cell Biol* 99:2034–2040, 1984.

99. Gaffney J, West D, Arnold F, Sattar A, Kumar S: Differences in the uptake of modified low density lipoproteins by tissue cultured endothelial cells. *J Cell Sci* 79:317–325, 1985.

100. Maciag T, Cerundolo J, Ilsley S, Kelley PR, Forand R: An endothelial cell growth factor from bovine hypothalamus: identification and partial characterization. *Proc Natl Acad Sci USA* 76:5674–5678, 1979.

101. Gospodarowicz D: Growth factors for vascular endothelial cells. In: Piper HM (ed). *Cell Culture Techniques in Heart and Vessel Research.* Berlin: Springer-Verlag, 230–244, 1990.

102. Klagsbrun M, D'Amore PA: Regulators of angiogenesis. *Ann Rev Physiol* 53:217–239, 1991.

103. Gorfien S, Spector A, DeLuca D, Weiss S: Growth and physiological functions of vascular endothelial cells in a new serum-free medium (SFM). *Exp Cell Res* 206:291–301, 1993.

CHAPTER 7

Vascular Smooth Muscle Cells

Ira Mills, PhD; Bauer E. Sumpio, MD, PhD

Introduction

This chapter serves as an overview of the smooth muscle cell (SMC) and the recent studies performed using cultured vascular SMCs. The reader is also referred to the many excellent reviews that are available in the current literature on SMC biology, particularly as it relates to the pathophysiology of atherosclerosis.[1-15] The focus of this chapter is, first, to introduce SMC histology and function in vivo and, second, to present the phenotypic modulation of cultured SMCs with reference to contractile protein expression, Na$^+$ pump activity, plasma membrane receptor expression, and the contribution of the extracellular matrix (ECM) (Figure 1). Studies describing contraction of cultured SMCs are briefly discussed; third, the major focus is signal transduction in cultured SMCs. This segment includes a description of signaling pathways, as well as the effects of individual SMC agonists and growth factors (Figure 2). Lastly, the utility of SMCs as a model system to examine vascular cell biology is presented, particularly in relation to SMC hypertrophy versus hyperplasia. Specifically, studies are presented that characterize SMCs obtained from vessels of both hypertensive (hypertrophic) and atherosclerotic (hyperplastic) animals. There is also a brief discussion of recent studies that employ novel molecular techniques to selectively interfere with the genetic expression of SMCs that may lead to the treatment of patients with atherosclerosis and other vascular diseases associated with SMC pathophysiology.

Finally, the SMC phenotype in culture is presented. Several methodologies available for the isolation and culturing of SMCs are described. These include classic techniques such as enzymatic digestion and explant methodologies, as well as a novel procedure of magnetic selection of SMCs from preglomerular arterioles.

Smooth Muscle Cells (In Vivo)

Histology

The vascular wall is composed of three layers including the tunica intima (innermost layer), tunica media (middle layer), and adventitia (outermost layer) (Figure 3).[16] The intima is composed of a single layer of endothelial cells and a subendothelial layer of collagenous bundles, elastic fibrils, occasional SMCs and fibroblasts, as well as a thin basal lamina. The media is a collection of SMCs, elastic sheets, bundles of collagenous fibrils, and a network of elastic fibrils. SMCs form the primary and, in some cases, the sole cell type found in the tunica media of blood vessel walls. SMCs found in muscular arteries are spindle-shaped cells and measure approximately 2 μM in width and 60 μM in length.[17] In contrast, SMCs present in elastic arteries exhibit irregular shapes and form numerous branch processes.[18,19] SMCs are not present in the adventitia except in large veins such as the vena cava.[16]

SMC nuclei are large and centrally located with peripheral chromatin clumping and moderately developed nucleolar material. The cytoplasm is notable for containing plentiful tracts of myofibrils with associated dense bodies. The composition of the contractile apparatus has been well studied in freshly isolated amphibian SMCs which resemble mammalian, vertebrate smooth muscle.[20] The actin filaments are packed in small bundles in a hexagonal arrangement. Myosin filaments with a 25 to 30 nm cross-sectional diameter fill the spaces surrounding the actin bundles. The ratio of

From *The Basic Science of Vascular Disease*. Edited by Sidawy AN, Sumpio BE, and DePalma RG. Armonk, NY: Futura Publishing Company, Inc.; © 1997.

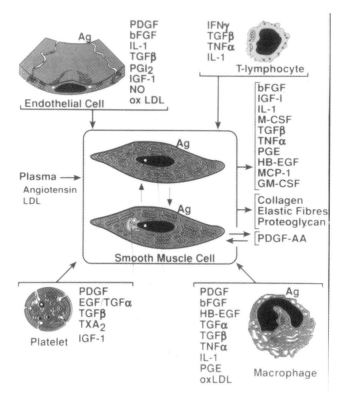

Figure 1. Two potentially different phenotypic states of smooth muscle cells (SMCs). In the synthetic phenotype, it is presumed that SMCs can form connective tissue molecules as well as growth factors such as PDGF-AA, and can stimulate themselves as well as their neighbors. In their interactions with the overlying endothelium and neighboring T lymphocytes, platelets, and macrophages, SMCs can respond to the different cytokines, grown-regulatory molecules, and vasodilator and vasoconstrictor substances that can be generated from these cells, as well as substances from the plasma, such as angiotensin. Thus, the genes that are expressed in the different phenotypic states by the smooth muscle (**listed to the right**), as well as those expressed by the neighboring cells (**listed next to each cell**) in the artery wall that result from these cellular interactions will determine the outcome as to whether a lesion will progress or regress. (Reproduced with permission from Reference 29.)

actin to myosin is 50 to 1. Another prominent feature of the contractile apparatus is the presence of dense bodies containing a high concentration of α-actinin.

Bond and Somlyo[21] examined the arrangement of dense bodies and their relationship to thin filaments in permeabilized SMCs from rabbit vas deferens and portal vein. Cytoplasmic dense bodies of circular or oval shape were surrounded by transverse profiles of 10-nm filaments. A chain of dense bodies connected by the 10-nm filaments was sometimes observed. Dense bodies serve as anchoring sites for thin filaments. This was confirmed by attachment of actin by myosin subfragment 1 which showed that the thin filaments insert into the dense bodies with opposite polarity. In skeletal muscle, the Z-band in isolated I-bands performs a similar function and it was concluded that thin filaments,

thick filaments and dense bodies form the smooth muscle contractile unit.[21]

The structural basis of muscle contraction is not clear. However, most investigators favor a sliding filament model analogous to that observed in skeletal muscle.[22] Both muscle types contain interdigitating thick and thin filaments. However, vascular smooth muscle differs from skeletal muscle in having a less precise arrangement of contractile filaments, attachment of actin filaments to dense bodies instead of Z lines, and calcium binding to calmodulin instead of troponin.[23]

In an attempt to determine how contractile proteins interact during contraction, Cooke and colleagues[20] examined single, isolated SMCs fixed during a partial contraction. They observed a change from a uniform axial orientation in relaxed areas of the cell to axial disoriented filaments in shortened regions. They concluded that a simple, uniform interdigitation of filaments is unlikely to occur in SMCs undergoing contraction.[20]

More precise examination of the structural basis of contraction was obtained in in vitro studies. For instance, Sellers and colleagues[24] quantitated the rate of phosphorylated and nonphosphorylated myosin on ordered actin cables of the giant alga, *Nitella*. They found that phosphorylated myosin moved at a velocity of 0.15 to 0.4 μm/s. This was confirmed by Cooke and colleagues[20] who demonstrated a similar rate of movement of 0.3 μm/sec of dense bodies in contracted SMCs dynamically followed by optical microscopy.

SMCs form gap junctions with other SMCs, endothelial cells, and form attachments with elastic fibers. Gap junctions are aqueous channels that connect adjoining cells for the transfer of ions and small molecules.[25] Blennerhassett and colleagues[26] studied gap junction occurrence and function in rat aortic SMCs. They observed extensive areas of gap junctions in SMCs. Impaling a ''source'' cell with a current pulse was followed by a deflection in membrane potential in neighboring cells. In addition, intercellular transfer of a fluorescent compound, 5(6)-carboxyfluorescein, was detected within 15 seconds of injection. Lash and colleagues[25] recently isolated a cDNA from vascular smooth muscle that encodes a 43 kD connexin homologous to cardiac connexin43. Microinjection of in vitro transcribed vascular SMC connexin43 mRNA in two-cell B6D2 mouse embryos induced intercellular coupling in previously uncoupled blastomeres. Coupling between SMCs and endothelial cells was supported by the observation of connexin43 in both cell types.

Function

SMCs exist in two phenotypic states that dictate their function: a contractile and a synthetic phenotype. In vivo, under normal conditions, proliferation of SMCs is very slow and the contractile state predomi-

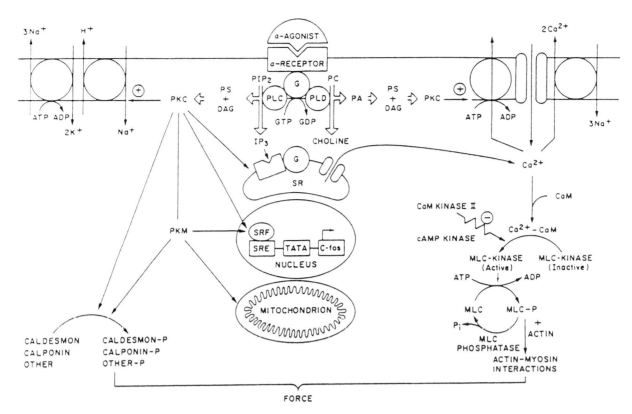

Figure 2. Schematic representation of the different excitation-contraction coupling pathways in vascular smooth muscle. Putative targets and substrates of protein kinase C (PKC) are also shown. DAG = diacylglycerol; IP₃ = inositol 1,4,5–trisphosphate; PIP₂ = phosphatidylinositol 4,5-bisphosphate; G = G protein; SR = sarcoplasmic reticulum; SRF = serum response factor; SRE = serum response element; PS = phosphatidylserine; PLC = phospholipase C; PLD = phospholipase D; PC = phosphatidylcholine; PA = phosphatidic acid; MLC—yosin light chain; CaM = calmodulin. (Reproduced with permission from Reference 31.)

nates. Thymidine index was assessed by autoradiographic localization of tritiated thymidine. Clowes labeled SMCs undergoing DNA synthesis within a 24-hour period by injecting rats with ^{3}H-thymidine at 17, 9, and 1 hour prior to fixation. The group calculated a thymidine labeling index of (0.06%).[27,28] In this contractile state, SMCs respond to numerous agonists that cause either vasoconstriction or vasorelaxation (Figure 1). Norepinephrine, angiotensin II (AII), vasopressin, and even platelet-derived growth factor (PDGF) can induce vasoconstriction. Atrial natriuretic polypeptide (ANP) and nitric oxide (NO) are examples of agonists that can promote vasorelaxation. SMCs in the contractile phenotype respond to agonists that cause either vasocontraction or vasorelaxation.[29] For instance, AII can promote vasoconstriction via binding to specific, high-affinity receptors on the SMC plasma membrane.

The key event in the initiation of vascular smooth muscle contraction is myosin light chain phosphorylation.[23] Upon phosphorylation of the serine-19 of the 20-kDalton myosin light chain, myosin ATPase activity increases which promotes cross-bridge cycling and contraction.[22] Phosphorylation of myosin light chain is caused by the enzyme myosin light chain kinase (MLCK). In the absence of calcium, MLCK is inactive. Activation of the enzyme occurs via increased levels of intracellular calcium from either the extracellular space or intracellular stores of calcium-calmodulin. The activity of this enzyme is modulated by protein kinases including cyclic adenosine monophosphate (cAMP)-dependent protein kinase, cyclic monophosphate (cGMP)-dependent protein kinase, Ca^{2+}/calmodulin-dependent kinase II, and protein kinase C (PKC).[22]

Characteristic of smooth muscle is the maintenance of tension despite the reduction in intracellular calcium levels and the phosphorylation of the myosin light chain. This has been termed the "latch state" by Murphy and colleagues and is characterized by the presence of attached, noncycling cross-bridges.[30]

Vascular SMC contraction is thought to involve pathways in addition to Ca^{2+}-dependent myosin light chain phosphorylation of myosin light chain.[31] One candidate pathway is that of PKC. For example, Morgan and colleagues showed contraction of vascular smooth muscle in response to phenylephrine, prosta-

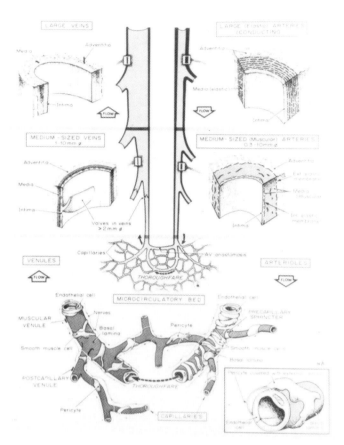

Figure 3. Schematic drawing summarizing major structural characteristics of principal segments of blood vessels in mammals. (Reproduced with permission from Reference 16.)

glandin $F_{2\alpha}$, and phorbol esters in the absence of changes in intracellular calcium.[32–34] In addition, Rasmussen and colleagues have demonstrated the phosphorylation of caldesmon, intermediate filaments (synemin, α- and β-desmin, synemin), and five cytosolic proteins[35] with sustained contraction caused by phorbol ester.

Caldesmon and calponin are both PKC substrates that have been postulated to play a role in the regulation of SMC contraction.[22,31] Both caldesmon (145000 kD) and calponin (34000 kD) are actin-binding proteins present in vascular smooth muscle that have been shown to inhibit actomyosin ATPase in vitro.

SMCs involved in the development, repair, and pathologic conditions such as atherosclerosis or intimal hyperplasia have a synthetic phenotype. It has been postulated that injury to the endothelium promotes the differentiation of SMCs from the contractile to the synthetic phenotype in vivo.[36] In the synthetic state, SMCs express a variety of growth factor and cytokine genes including bFGF, IGF-1, M-CSF, TGF-β, and IL-1.[29] The secretions of these factors act in an autocrine fashion to affect SMC proliferation (e.g., PDGF) and also stimulate the neighboring endothelium

or vascular channels within atherosclerotic lesions.[29] Thus, as recently reviewed by Ross,[29] the synthetic SMC is a major player in the fibroproliferative component of atherosclerosis.

Many of the characteristics of SMCs with the synthetic phenotype have been delineated by the study of SMCs that transform after 6 to 8 days in culture. Typical of these modulated SMCs are a greatly reduced number of filaments and abundance of secretory protein organelles such as the endoplasmic reticulum and Golgi apparatus.[29,36,37] Lysosomal content and enzymes such as acid phosphatase and N-aceyl-β-glucosaminidase are also increased in SMCs with a synthetic versus contractile phenotype. Other enzymes including cytochrome C and nicotinamide adenine dinucleotide phosphate (NADPH)-dependent cytochrome C reductase are increased 2.3- and 12.8-fold, respectively, in synthetic versus contractile SMCs. In addition, the accumulation of lipid is enhanced in synthetic SMCs; after a 24-hour incubation with β-very low density lipoprotein, many more droplets are found in synthetic SMCs versus contractile-like SMCs. ECM production is also increased in synthetic SMCs as shown by an increase in collagen and sulfated glycosaminoglycans.[38]

The conversion of SMCs from the contractile to the synthetic state is reversible. SMCs generally show phenotypic modulation after 6 to 8 days in culture. However, if the cells are seeded densely enough to result in less than five cumulative population doublings or are immediately confluent (or 5 to 7 days postmodulation), the SMCs can revert back to the contractile phenotype.

Chamley-Campbell and colleagues[39] have described a heparin-sensitive glycosaminoglycan extract from the artery wall that can inhibit smooth muscle phenotypic modulation. These findings have led Campbell and colleagues to postulate that a heparin-like glycosaminoglycan in the basal lamina of SMCs maintains the cells in the contractile phenotype.[38] Co-culture with endothelial cells in a noncontact-dependent manner can also prevent phenotypic modulation of SMCs.

Phenotypic Modulation of Smooth Muscle Cells in Culture

Under serum-fed preconfluent conditions, SMCs are known to undergo phenotypic modulation in culture from a contractile toward a synthetic state[36] (Figure 1). The morphologic characteristics of the synthetic SMC phenotype include a euchromatic nucleus, a prominent endoplasmic reticulum, and Golgi complex. Synthetic SMCs can proliferate actively in culture and are capable of synthesizing and secreting ECM components. In vivo counterparts to the synthetic SMC phenotype are SMCs obtained from developing vessels and atherosclerotic lesions. For example, Moose et al[40] found a twofold increase in the content of synthetic organelles in the cells of diffuse intimal thickenings as compared to the adjacent media. The similarity between SMCs of the synthetic type in culture and in atherosclerotic lesions extends to the nature of contractile proteins. Gabbiani et al[41] observed a switch in actin isoform expression from the α- to the β- and γ-actin forms.

In contrast, the contractile SMC phenotype is characterized by a heterochromatic nucleus and abundant actin and myosin filaments. The contractile SMC contracts in response to both chemical and mechanical stimulation. In vivo counterparts of the contractile phenotype are SMCs obtained from media of vessels of normal adults. These cells are highly differentiated with abundant filaments and are quiescent.

As suggested by Campbell and Campbell,[42] as well as Gordon and Schwartz,[28] the identification of SMCs as belonging to either of these two phenotypes is a gross simplification and may actually represent extreme culture conditions. The behavior of SMCs is not locked into a particular phenotype such that SMCs classified as belonging to the "synthetic" phenotype are not able to contract and vice versa. Chamley and Campbell[43] noted that single SMCs from newborn guinea pig vas deferens, observed by time-lapse photography, underwent mitosis despite the fact that the cells were in a morphologically-defined differentiated state. This finding emphasized the need to examine biochemical parameters, in addition to morphologic characteristics, to better define the phenotypic state of SMCs in culture.[28]

Outlined below are some of the important gross biochemical changes that occur in cultured SMCs, with emphasis on contractile protein expression, Na^+ pump activity, plasma membrane receptors, and ECM formation.

Contractile Protein Expression

Myosin Heavy Chain

Phosphorylation of myosin heavy chains is thought to affect myosin interaction with actin and the assembly of myosin into filaments.[44] Furthermore, SMCs from human atherosclerotic plaques can be stained with antisera directed against myosin despite the fact that these cells are "synthetic-like."[45] Thus, it is of interest to determine the expression of myosin heavy chains in cultured vascular SMCs under various conditions.

Expression of myosin heavy chain in cultured cells is different from that observed in freshly isolated cells.[46,47] In freshly isolated vascular SMCs from rat aorta, two myosin heavy chains (204 and 200 kDa) that

cross-react with antibodies against smooth muscle myosin were found. In actively growing cultured cells, a myosin heavy chain of 196 kDa was observed that cross-reacted with antibodies raised to platelet myosin and not smooth muscle myosin. The accumulation of nonmuscle myosin in rat vascular SMCs is thought to occur via decreased degradation of the protein at first entry into the M phase,[48] despite the fact that Id gene expression does not appear to be involved in the myosin heavy chain dedifferentiation of these cells[49]; Id protein is known to form heterotrimers with basic helix-loop-helix proteins which act as transcriptional activators for myosin heavy chain-like genes. In postconfluent cultured cells, both the smooth muscle myosin (204 and 200 kDa) and the nonmuscle myosin (196 kDa) were present.

Actin

As described for myosin, expression of smooth muscle α-actin is modulated by the state of differentiation of vascular SMCs in culture.[41,50] Owens et al[50] noted that in both freshly isolated vascular SMCs from rat aorta as well as native tissue, approximately 70% of the actin was in the α isoform. Although levels of the α isoform remained high as late as 36 hours postplating, the fractional synthesis of this protein was decreased markedly. As expected, the decreased fractional synthesis of α-actin was accompanied by a decrease in the levels of this protein in the cell as well as an increase in the amount of β-nonmuscle actin and γ-smooth and nonsmooth muscle actin isoforms. Upon confluence, the synthesis and amount of α-actin in SMCs was restored to levels observed in freshly isolated cells. This was associated with decreased levels of β-actin, but no change in the amount of the γ isoform of actin. The above changes in actin isoform expression were detected regardless of whether primary or subcultured SMCs were studied. Subconfluent SMCs switched from serum-supplemented to serum-starved conditions exhibited increased synthesis of the α-actin isoform. This response was reversible since replenishment of the serum to the growth medium led to a decrease in α-actin synthesis. In summary, α-actin isoform expression associated with a differentiated, contractile phenotype was observed under either postconfluent or serum-starved conditions. Similar results were obtained in cultured BC_3H1 cells by Strauch et al.[51] In their study, contractile protein expression was dictated by the growth conditions. Elevated α-actin isoform expression was observed in either serum-free or postconfluent conditions.

Alterations in α-actin fractional synthesis and content in SMCs are thought to be controlled by translational and/or post-translational controls, since α-actin mRNA was unchanged in postconfluent density arrested cultures as compared to proliferating subconfluent cultures.[52] Furthermore, in postconfluent arrested SMCs, serum-induced growth and PDGF both caused a decrease in fractional α-actin synthesis under conditions of enhanced proliferation. Under these conditions, PDGF caused a dramatic decrease in α-actin mRNA and did not alter nonmuscle β-actin, whereas serum replacement did not affect α-actin mRNA but increased nonmuscle β-actin.[52]

Gabbiani et al[41] demonstrated marked changes in actin isoform expression in SMCs obtained from human atheromatous plaque as compared to normal tissue. Although total actin levels remain unchanged, in plaque-derived SMCs there is a switch in actin isoform from the alpha to the beta and gamma forms. Specifically, the ratio of α-smooth muscle actin:β-cytoplasmic actin in normal media is 2 to 1. In atheromatous plaques, the ratio of cytoplasmic β to γ actin is 7 to 2, with less than 10% present as α-smooth muscle actin.

Na$^+$ Pump

Allen et al[53,54] hypothesized that regulation of intracellular Na$^+$ is an important signal in the mitogenic reponse of vascular SMCs. In their studies, they utilized serum-fed[53] primary cultures of adult canine coronary artery. Characteristic of this cell line is a prolonged duration of the G$_1$ phase, which is the phase critical to controlling the rate of the cell cycle. During the G$_1$ phase, they measured an increase in the intracellular sodium content (Na$_i^+$), and cell volume prior to the appearance of nonmuscle myosin and a shift in the cell cycle. They subsequently observed an increase in the number of Na$^+$ pumps and a concomitant decrease in both (Na$_i^+$) and cell volume. In the presence of ouabain, the Na$^+$ pump was inhibited and cells arrested in G$_1$ without upregulation of nonmuscle myosin. After removal of ouabain, the Na$^+$ pump number was increased, (Na$_i^+$) decreased, and progression into the S and G$_2$ + M phase and upregulation of nonmuscle myosin occurred. They concluded that compensatory increases in the number of Na$^+$ pumps in response to elevated (Na$_i^+$) may be an important regulatory step in the mitogenic response of SMCs.

Receptor Changes

ANP receptor expression provides an excellent model for the phenotypic changes that occur to receptors on vascular SMCs in culture.[55] In intact aorta, the two guanylate cyclase coupled receptors are expressed, with the ANP-A receptor at a much greater level than ANP-B receptor. In contrast, the C receptor, that is involved in the clearance of ANP, is barely de-

tectable. In cultured aortic SMCs, the expression of the guanylate cyclase receptors are reversed such that the ANP-B receptor is dominant compared to the ANP-A receptor. Furthermore, the C receptor mRNA levels and numbers are significantly increased as compared to the intact tissue. Although ANP peptides have been shown to exert antimitogenic effects via the clearance receptor,[56] the physiologic significance of these changes is not clear.

Since enhanced contractile sensitivity to serotonin is observed in proliferating SMCs in vivo, Corson et al[57] postulated that phenotypically-modulated SMCs had an increased gene expression of phospholipase C-coupled 5-HT serotonin receptor. Phenotypic modulation was confirmed by examination of actin isoform expression which demonstrated that the β- and γ-actin were increased compared to α-actin. Northern blot analysis demonstrates that, indeed, 5-HT receptor (i.e., 5-HT$_2$ subtype) mRNA was expressed at fiftyfold greater levels in cultured cells as in intact aortic SMCs.[57]

Extracellular Matrix

The ECM can have a profound influence on the phenotypic expression of SMCs. This was demonstrated in a recent study by Hedin et al[58] who examined the influence of various substrates (fibronectin fragments, type IV collagen, and laminin) on SMC morphology. Both fibronectin and a 105-kD cell-binding fragment caused modulation of SMCs from a contractile to a synthetic phenotype. The SMCs were deficient in myofilaments, flattened with numerous free ribosomes, had an extensive rough endoplasmic reticulum, and stacked Golgi cisternae. Associated with SMC modulation under these conditions was enhanced attachment and spreading of SMCs and stimulated uridine incorporation, protein accumulation, and DNA synthesis. SMCs, when cultured on fibronectin or the 105-kD binding fragment, secrete fibronectin fibrils, which is speculated to arise from de novo synthesis and not from the coated substrate itself.[58] Formation of fibronectin fibrils could be prevented by the addition of a GRGDS (Gly-Arg-Gly-Asp-Ser) peptide that contains the cell-attachment sequence (RGDS) of fibronectin, but not by a control peptide GRGES (Gly-Arg-Gly-Glu-Ser).[58]

A delayed phenotypic modulation of SMCs was observed when they were grown on laminin. SMCs remained in the contractile phenotype for approximately 6 days, after which a slow and incomplete "catch-up" modulation was noted. Since this later modulation of SMCs could be prevented by GRGDS, the response was thought to be due to the production of fibronectin in these cells. In fact, SMCs cultured on laminin substrate produced a much greater amount of fibronectin than SMCs grown on fibronectin substrate. Furthermore, SMC-secreted fibronectin was just as effective as plasma fibronectin in inducing SMC differentiation from a synthetic to a contractile state.

In this regard, Liau and Chan[59] examined the relationship between ECM and the induction of quiescence in SMCs by different means, including confluence, low serum, and heparin. They observed that mRNA levels were increased for $\alpha 1(III)$, $\alpha(IV)$, $\alpha 2(I)$, $\alpha 2(V)$ collagens, thrombospondin and fibronectin (from five- to one and a halffold, respectively) in postconfluent SMCs compared to proliferating SMCs. In contrast, only $\alpha 1(III)$ collagen mRNA was elevated in growth-arrested SMCs as compared to an actively proliferating fibroblast cell line. Examination of the time course of these changes revealed that $\alpha 1(III)$ and $\alpha 2(V)$ collagen mRNA did not significantly increase until postconfluency, whereas the other ECM mRNA levels rose progressively with increased cell/cell and/or cell/matrix contact.[59] Under low-serum quiescent conditions, only $\alpha 1(III)$ collagen mRNA was increased compared to proliferating, preconfluent SMCs. Similarly, in the presence of heparin at a dose which inhibits SMC proliferation, $\alpha 1(III)$ collagen mRNA was increased two and a halffold. Thus, the expression of certain ECM proteins, most notably $\alpha 1(III)$ collagen, can be affected by the SMC phenotype.

In a related study, LeBaron et al[60] coated culture wells with several different ECM proteins including types I to VI collagen, fibronectin, and laminin, and measured the binding of heparin/heparan sulfate to these substrates. Type V collagen bound to heparin/heparan sulfate with the greatest affinity suggesting that it might be an important substrate for glycosaminoglycan-mediated cell attachment. They also demonstrated that Chinese hamster ovary cell mutants had a deficiency in glycosaminoglycan synthesis and attached with less affinity to the collagen substrate than control, wild-type cells. In addition, they also showed that SMC attachment to type V collagen could be hampered by the addition of exogenous heparin.

Several studies have confirmed that the ECM plays a substantive role in determining the phenotypic expression of cultured SMCs. For example, epidermal growth factor (EGF)-stimulated DNA synthesis in quiescent SMCs could be markedly enhanced by plating the cells onto plasticware coated with ECM and could be prevented by the addition of antibodies to thrombospondin.[61] In this study, flasks were previously seeded with SMCs incubated with ascorbic acid to promote collagen deposition.

Proteoglycans are an important macromolecular component of the ECM and are composed of polysaccharides and protein. Proteoglycans, along with collagen and elastin, act to maintain the structural integrity of vessel walls.[62] In human aorta,[63] the polysaccha-

rides include glycosaminoglycans of at least four classes, including 67% chondroitin sulfate, 22% dermatan sulfate, 8% heparan sulfate, and 4% hyaluronidate. The accumulation of proteoglycans, particularly of the chondroitin and sulfate classes, is considered by many as a hallmark of atherosclerosis.[64] Inhibition of proteoglycan synthesis causes a reduction in α-actin and in the synthesis of ECM elements such as chondroitin sulfate, fibronectin, thrombospondin, and laminin, that mediate the inhibition of postconfluent SMC growth.[65] These phenomena were not observed when SMCs were grown on preformed SMC ECM.

Tenascin is a newly discovered ECM protein that is expressed in proliferating SMCs.[66] In serum-starved SMCs, Sharifi et al[67] demonstrated a ninefold increase in the synthesis of the antiadhesive protein tenascin that was preceded by an increase in tenascin mRNA levels. This effect was specific to tenascin, as other ECM proteins such as fibronectin and laminin showed only a minimal response to AII. In addition, several intracellular Ca^{2+}-binding proteins have been shown to be released from cultured SMCs which are capable of binding ECM proteins. Watanabe et al[68] described one such constitutively expressed protein, calvasculin, that is secreted by cultured bovine aortic SMCs. Calvasculin is an 11 kDa EF-hand protein (intracellular Ca^{2+}-binding protein) that binds to microfibril-associated glycoproteins (MAP) in a Ca^{2+}-dependent manner. The physiologic implication of this interaction is not clear. However, the interaction is specific for the 36 kDa MAP and calvasculin does not associate with types I to V collagen and fibronectin. Furthermore, calvasculin could only be demonstrated in SMCs obtained from vascular, but not nonvascular, sources.[68]

Approximately 50% of the volume fraction of freshly isolated vascular SMCs is composed of myofilaments. The volume fraction of myofilaments decreases to 15% in SMCs which were seeded on type I and type III collagen and increases twofold by growing the cells on types I and IV collagen or Matrigel (a solubilized extract of the EHS tumor containing predominantly type IV collagen and laminin). These findings support the thesis that the ECM components can modulate the phenotype of subconfluent SMCs in culture and may suggest a role of ECM in the maintenance of the contractile state of SMCs in vivo.[69]

Contraction of Smooth Muscle Cells

Several investigators have been able to demonstrate contraction of vascular SMCs in culture. For instance, Warshaw et al[70] studied by digital video microscopy the electrical stimulation of *Bufo marinus* SMCs, tagged with marker beads on the cell surface.

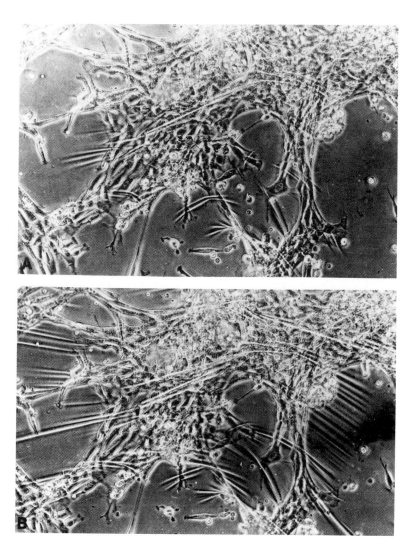

Figure 4. Contractile response of pulmonary artery smooth muscle cells to angiotensin II (AII). A primary culture seeded onto polymerized polydimethyl siloxane is shown before (**A**) and 2 minutes after (**B**) exposure to 320 nM AII. Basal tension in the cell, as indicated by the wrinkling of the substrate under the unstimulated cells, is markedly increased by this treatment. Changes were documented by phase-contrast microscopy at 37°C. Magnification = × 112. (Reproduced with permission from Reference 71.)

Corkscrew-like contractions were observed with a pitch of 1.4 cell lengths and at a rate of 27° per second. The authors concluded that the contractile apparatus and/or the cytoskeleton of smooth muscle was arranged in a helical orientation in the cell.[70]

Murray et al[71] grew both pulmonary artery and aortic cell cultures on microscope coverslips coated with polydimethyl siloxane. In response to a number of contractile agonists including AII, they could detect the tension forces generated by the SMCs by the wrinkling and distortion of the novel flexible growth surface (Figure 4). The tension force responsiveness of cultured vascular SMCs could be maintained over a prolonged time and with multiple passages in culture. The

wrinkling phenomenon could be reversed by treatment of SMCs with isoproterenol.

Gunther et al[72] demonstrated hormone-induced contraction of enzymatically dissociated rat mesenteric SMCs. The SMC contraction caused by AII or alpha$_1$-adrenergic agonists was present during the first 3 days in culture, then lost during the proliferative phase, and later restored in postconfluent cells (7 to 9 days). Smooth muscle culture contractility persisted in postconfluent cultures for as long as 2 months.[72]

As described in detail in Chapter 13, myosin light chain phosphorylation is the critical biochemical step associated with the initiation of SMC contraction. However, there are only a few studies that characterize this event in cultured vascular SMCs. Lobaugh and Blackshear[73] demonstrated phosphorylation of myosin light chain by neuropeptide Y. Neuropeptide Y is a 36-amino acid polypeptide present in postganglionic sympathetic neurons and is a known effector of vasoconstriction. Application of neuropeptide Y resulted in a transient stimulation of myosin light chain phosphorylation that was not accompanied by changes in cAMP and cGMP, phosphatidylinositol turnover, or PKC activation. However, neuropeptide Y could reverse the inhibitory effect of forskolin on myosin light chain phosphorylation, presumably by preventing inhibition of forskolin-stimulated cAMP accumulation.[73]

Vasoconstrictor prostanoids are also capable of stimulating myosin light chain phosphorylation in vascular SMCs. U46619 (a thromboxane A_2 receptor agonist), $PGF_{2\alpha}$, and PGE_2 all stimulated phosphorylation of the 20 kDa myosin light chain in rat aortic SMCs.[74] Blockade of the thromboxane receptor with the thromboxane A_2 receptor antagonist, SQ29548, prevented the phosphorylation response for all three prostanoids. The data suggest that $PGF_{2\alpha}$ and PGE_2 stimulate phosphorylation of myosin light chain by cross-agonism at the thromboxane A_2 receptor. In addition, the data suggest that thromboxane A_2 is a potent stimulator of vascular SMC contraction with an EC_{50} of 10 nm, whereas $PGF_{2\alpha}$ and PGE_2 are much less potent with EC_{50} values of 4800 nm and 8500 nm, respectively.[74]

Rabbit aortic SMCs in long-term culture also showed both mono- and diphosphorylation of myosin light chain by $PGF_{2\alpha}$. The stimulation of myosin light chain diphosphorylation by $PGF_{2\alpha}$ was mediated by PKC, since both staurosporine or protein kinase down regulation blocked the response.[75] The phosphorylation of SMCs was also found in the presence of concanavalin A and fetal calf serum which may be involved in their ability to promote cell rounding.[75]

Smooth Muscle Cell Signal Transduction

Signaling Pathways

Calcium

The signal transduction pathways which result in the elevation of intracellular Ca^{2+} are complex and are a critical event in the final response of the SMC whether it involves contraction, growth, or proliferation (Figure 5).[22,76] Transient events, such as short-term contraction, involve the release of Ca^{2+} from intracellular stores, whereas maintained contraction or tone requires a balance between the entry of Ca^{2+} from external stores and extrusion from the cell.[77]

The mobilization of Ca^{2+} from intracellular sources involves the release of Ca^{2+} from the sarco-plasmic reticulum from either inositol-1,4,5-trisphosphate (IP_3)-activated channels or from ryanodine receptor-like Ca^{2+} channels.[22] Somlyo et al[78] demonstrated IP_3-mediated Ca^{2+}-release and tension development in rabbit main pulmonary artery smooth muscle permeabilized with saponin or digitonin. Hashimoto et al[79] also showed that norepinephrine causes the elevation of inositol phosphates, and that exogenous IP_3 can cause Ca^{2+} release and contraction in rabbit mesenteric artery. In saponin skinned primary cultured rat aortic SMCs, Yamamoto and van Breemen[80] demonstrated IP_3 stimulation of both ^{45}Ca uptake and ^{45}Ca efflux, suggesting that IP_3 acts as the messenger molecule transducing receptor activation and intracellular calcium release in vascular smooth muscle. Although ATP is essential for IP_3-mediated calcium release from the sarcoplasmic reticulum, this process is not affected by low temperatures, suggesting the involvement of a ligand-binding mechanism and not a metabolic reaction.[81] Recent data show that the Ca^{2+} content of the sarcoplasmic reticulum of the cultured A7r5 aortic SMC line appears to modulate agonist-stimulated synthesis of inositol phosphates in these cells in an inverse manner.[82] Depletion of sarcoplasmic reticulum Ca^{2+} stores, with either thapsigargin (an irreversible specific inhibitor of the Ca^{2+}-ATPase that depletes the IP_3-sensitive Ca^{2+} store) or by briefly depleting the extracellular Ca^{2+} concentration, causes an increase in vasopressin synthesis of inositol phosphates. Conversely, elevation of sarcoplasmic reticulum Ca^{2+} stores with 40 mM K^+, BAY 8644, or low Na^+ solution results in a decrease in vasopressin-induced inositol phosphate production.

A ryanodine-like channel in sarcoplasmic reticulum was demonstrated by ryanodine-blockade of Ca^{2+}-release from the sarcoplasmic reticulum in response to either norepinephrine or caffeine.[83] The contribution of the Ca^{2+} from the sarcoplasmic reticulum appears to depend on the vascular bed of study since the ability of caffeine to cause Ca^{2+}-release from the sarcoplasmic reticulum as well as its blockade by ryanodine was more pronounced in rat thoracic aortic smooth muscle as compared to bovine tail artery smooth muscle. Ryanodine stimulates passive release of Ca^{2+} from the sarcoplasmic reticulum such that if Ca^{2+} extrusion is inhibited by blockade of Na^+-Ca^{2+} exchange, tension will be generated.[83]

Ca^{2+} entry to the cytoplasm from the extracellular space is mediated by either voltage-dependent Ca^{2+} channels, receptor-operated channels, or by Na^+-Ca^{2+} exchange. The predominant voltage-dependent Ca^{2+} channel is the dihydropyridine-sensitive "L-type" Ca^{2+} channel.[77] L-type Ca^{2+} channels are known to inactivate slowly and incompletely during prolonged depolarizations.[77] Depolarization of vascular SMCs from their resting membrane potential of -60

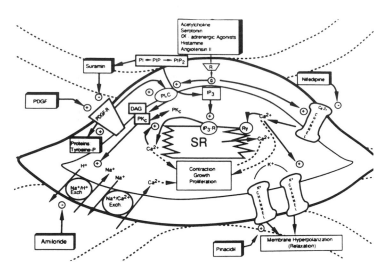

Figure 5. Schematic of signal transduction mechanisms in vascular smooth muscle. Ca^{2+} mobilization is affected by many pathways in the vascular myocyte. Various hormones acting through receptors (R) coupled to G-proteins (G) activate membrane-bound phospholipase C (PLC), which converts L-α-phosphatidyl inositol diphosphate (PIP_2) to diacylglycerol (DAG) and inositol-1,4,5 triphosphate (IP_3). The IP_3 stimulates release of Ca^{2+} from sarcoplasmic reticulum (SR) via an IP_3-receptor protein (IP_3-R), which is a type of Ca^{2+} channel. Synthesis of DAG in the membrane and an increase in intracellular Ca^{2+} result in translocation of protein kinase C from cytoplasm (PK_C) to sarcolemma. PK_C phosphorylates many sarcolemmal proteins and, via this mechanism, stimulates activity of the Na^+-K^+ exchanger (Na^+-K^+ exch.) and the open time of L-type Ca^{2+} channels. The PK_C pathway is also activated by growth factors such as platelet-derived growth factors (PDGF). PDGF binds to a specific receptor (PDGF-R), which is also a tyrosine kinase, that transfers phosphate from ATP to various proteins (tyrosine-P). Two other mechanisms for Ca^{2+} entry into the cytoplasm include Na^+-Ca^{2+} exchange (Na^+-Ca^{2+} exch.) and release of Ca^{2+} from SR via specialized Ca^{2+}-release channels, also known as ryanodine receptors (Ry) because of their capacity to bind this plant alkaloid. Na^+-Ca^{2+} exchange occurs in response to increases in intracellular Na^+, whereas Ca^{2+} release via Ry is stimulated by Ca^{2+}. Ca^{2+} is extruded from the myocyte by a sarcolemmal Ca^{2+} pump and is imported into SR via a different kind of Ca^{2+} pump. Many pharmacologic agents modulate various activities or functions of vascular muscle, including contraction, growth, and proliferation, by affecting Ca^{2+} transport or mobilization. For example, amiloride can indirectly modulate intracellular Ca^{2+} by inhibiting Na^+-H^+ exchange or directly inhibit Na^+-H^+ exhange. Suranim, an antihelmintic drug, blocks the PDGF receptor. Nifedipine, a dihydropyridine, inhibits activity of L-type or voltage-dependent Ca^{2+} channels. Pinacidil activates ATP-sensitive K^+ channels, resulting in membrane hyperpolarization; this leads to relaxation due to inactivation of voltage-dependent Ca^{2+} channels. (Reproduced with permission from Reference 22.)

to -75 mV (-40 to -55 mV in vivo) by either electrical stimulation, potassium chloride, or neurotransmitters such as norepinephrine or serotonin will activate inward calcium current by L-type Ca^{2+} channels.[22,77] For instance, in rat mesenteric artery, norepinephrine-induced contraction was observed in the presence of depolarization and an increase in the open probability of single voltage-dependent Ca^{2+} channels.[84]

Receptor-operated Ca^{2+} channels are postulated to occur in vascular SMCs based on the observation that agonists may stimulate ^{45}Ca influx with concomitant contraction in the absence of depolarization.[85] Benham and Tsien[86] first demonstrated ligand-gated Ca^{2+} current in freshly dispersed SMCs from rabbit ear ar-

tery with patch-clamp techniques. ATP activated Ca^{2+} channels at very negative potentials which was further characterized as being distinct from voltage-operated channels based on the failure of cadmium and nifedipine to block the Ca^{2+} channels.

Na^+-Ca^{2+} exchange is thought to play a role in calcium homeostasis in vascular SMCs. Nabel et al[87] showed that in response to a low external sodium concentration $[Na]_o$, transmembrane Ca^{2+} uptake was increased in rat aortic SMCs. In fact, Ca^{2+} content varied inversely with $[Na]_o$ under steady-state conditions. AII-stimulated Ca^{2+} efflux was also enhanced in the presence versus the absence of extracellular Na^+.[87]

A variety of agonists stimulate SMC contraction

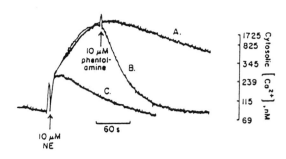

Figure 6. Norepinephrine-induced Ca^{2+} transients in DDT$_1$ cells. Cytosolic [Ca^{2+}] was measured in quin 2-loaded cells incubated in normal balanced salt solution (BSS) (**A,B**) or in BSS which was supplemented with 2 mM EGTA (**C**) for 30 seconds prior to the addition of 10 uM norepinephrine. In (**B**), 10 uM phentolamine was added 90 seconds after the norepinephrine addition. (Reproduced with permission from Reference 88.)

by increasing the concentration of intracellular calcium. Norepinephrine activation of alpha$_1$-adrenergic receptors can mobilize calcium from intracellular stores, as well as through an influx of extracellular calcium through receptor-operated channels in DDT$_1$ cells (a SMC line derived from rat vas deferens) (Figure 6).[88] The intracellular mobilization of cytosolic calcium is accompanied by alpha$_1$-adrenergic-induced inositol phosphate production in these cells.[88]

Protein Kinase C

PKC is a family of molecules that comprises more than 10 subspecies (Table 1).[89] Common to all protein kinases that have been cloned or purified is the activation by phosphatidylserine. However, the Ca^{2+} and phospholipid metabolites required for its activation vary greatly. Three distinct groups of PKC have been described. The conventional protein kinase subspecies include the α-, β_1-, β_2-, and γ-subspecies. The conventional subspecies of PKC are activated by Ca^{2+}, diacylglycerol, phosphatidylserine, as well as cis-unsaturated fatty acid and lysophosphatidylcholine. Four new protein kinase subspecies (δ-, ϵ-, η-, and θ-forms) have been described that are insensitive to Ca^{2+}, but are sensitive to diacylglycerol and phosphatidylserine. An atypical group of protein kinases has also been described including the ζ- and λ-forms of the enzyme. The ζ-subspecies is unique in that it does not respond to either Ca^{2+}, diacylglycerols, or phorbol esters, but is activated by phosphatidylserine and cis-unsaturated fatty acids.

The activation of PKC has been postulated to affect either transient or sustained responses depending on the source of diacylglycerol (Figure 7).[89] Acute responses are linked to the production of diacylglycerol and inositol phosphate associated with phospholipase C-mediated breakdown of phosphatidylinositol 4,5-bisphosphate. Recent studies indicate that phosphatidylcholine serves as the primary donor of sustained diacylglycerol production and is, therefore, linked to late cellular responses such as proliferation and differentiation. Activation of phospolipase A$_2$ can lead to the generation of cis-unsaturated fatty acids, as well as lysophosphatidylcholine which can modulate both transient and sustained cellular responses by activating different subspecies of PKC.

Table 1
PKC Subspecies in Mammalian Tissues

Group	Subspecies	Apparent Molecular Mass (kDa)	Activators[b]	Tissue Expression
cPKC	α	76 799	Ca^{2+}, DAG, PS, FFA, LysoPC	Universal
	βI	76 790	Ca^{2+}, DAG, PS, FFA, LysoPC	Some tissues
	βII	76 933	Ca^{2+}, DAG, PS, FFA, LysoPC	Many tissues
	γ	78 366	Ca^{2+}, DAG, PS, FFA, LysoPC	Brain only
nPKC	δ	77 517	DAG, PS	Universal
	ϵ	83 474	DAG, PS, FFA	Brain and others
	η(L)[a]	77 972	?	Lung, skin, heart
	θ[a]	81 571	?	Skeletal muscle (mainly)
aPKC	ζ	67 740	PS, FFA	Universal
	λ[a]	67 200	?	Ovary, testis and others

[a] The detailed enzymologic properties of the η(L)-, θ-, and λ-subspecies have not yet been clarified (Akimoto et al, unpublished).

[b] The activators for each subspecies are determined with calf thymus H1 histone and bovine myelin basic protein as model phosphate acceptors.

DAG: diacylglycerol; PS: phosphatidylserine; FFA: cis-unsaturated fatty acid; LysoPC: lysophosphatidylcholine. (Reproduced with permission from Reference 89.)

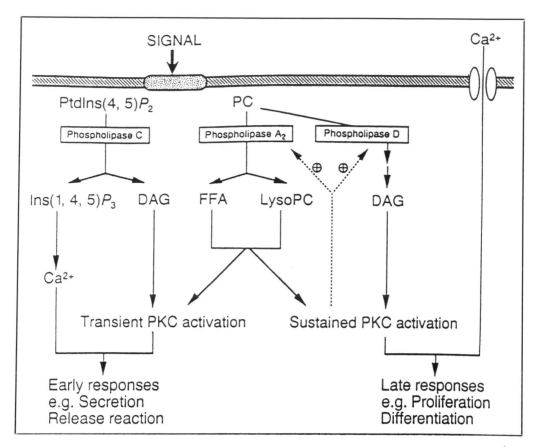

Figure 7. Signal-induced degradation of membrane phospholipids and cellular processes. **Dashed lines** and **crosses inside the circles** indicate the positive feedback effect of PKC on the activities of phospholipases. PtdIns $(4,5)P_2$ = phosphatidylinositol 4,5-bisphosphate; PC = phosphatidylcholine; Ins $(1,4,5)P_3$ = inositol 1,4,5–trisphosphate; DAG = diacylglycerol; FFA = *cis*-unsaturated fatty acid; LysoPC = lysophosphatidylcholine; PKC = protein kinase C. (Reproduced with permission from Reference 89.)

Morgan and colleagues have demonstrated that phenyephrine, prostaglandin $F_{2\alpha}$, and phorbol esters cause SMC contraction in the absence of changes in the levels of intracellular Ca^{2+}.[32–34] The involvement of PKC in these events was inferred by the observation that the PKC pseudosubstrate inhibitor could block the phenylephrine response. The pseudosubstrate inhibitor is a specific inhibitor of PKC based on its peptide sequence that is identical to the pseudosubstrate region of the enzyme with an amino acid substitution (alanine instead of serine).[31] Khalil and Morgan[90] used a fluorescent BODIPY derivative of active phorbol ester, 12-(1,3,5,7-tetramethylBODIPY-2-propionyl)phorbol-13–acetate to dynamically monitor the distribution and translocation of PKC in ferret portal vein SMCs by imaging techniques. The advantage of using this inert probe is that one can dynamically measure PKC localization in intact cells. They observed an intense signal in the perinuclear membrane, with a small fraction translocating from the cytosol to the surface membrane in the presence of phenylephrine (Figure 8).

This group[91] also examined the distribution of Ca^{2+}-independent PKC isoforms in ferret aorta SMCs. Under control conditions, the PKC isoforms ϵ and ζ were observed in the cytosol and the perinuclear space, respectively. Upon stimulation with phenylephrine, ϵ-PKC translocated to the plasma membrane and ζ-PKC to the intranuclear compartment. Their findings suggest that the translocation of ϵ-PKC to the plasmalemmal surface may be critical for Ca^{2+}-independent agonist stimulated contraction since it did not occur in ferret aortic cells, which only produce Ca^{2+}-dependent agonist contraction.

In rat aortic SMCs, activation of PKC by phorbol esters causes a shape change (i.e., contraction).[92] This effect is maximal after a 40-minute exposure to 10^{-9}-10^{-7}M PMA. In contrast, vasopressin, which unlike PMA causes an increase in $[Ca^{2+}]_i$, attains peak contraction at 20 minutes.[92] SMC contraction induced by PMA can be reproduced by dioctanoylglycerol, a diacylglycerol mimetic, but not with the non-PKC activating 4-a-phorbol, and inhibited by the protein kinase

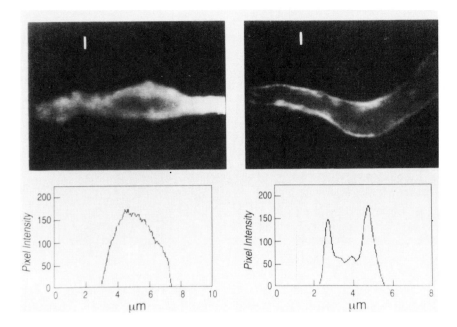

Figure 8. Distribution of ε-PKC in isolated ferret aorta cell. **Left:** ferret aorta cell treated with staurosporine (10⁻⁶M) and fixed at rest. **Right:** ferret aorta cell treated with staurosporine (10⁻⁶M) for 15 minutes and phenylephrine (10⁻⁵M) for 10 minutes before fixation. **Bottom: line scans** across cell at position indicated by **white bar.** Bar = 2μm. (Reproduced with permission from Reference 91.)

inhibitor, H7, or by downregulation of PKC, suggesting that the contractile effect of PMA occurs through a PKC-mediated pathway. Removal of extracellular Ca^{2+} or treatment with a Ca^{2+} channel blocker, such as verapamil, significantly attenuate the PMA-induced contraction of SMC implicating an important role for transmembrane Ca^{2+} flux in PKC activation. The Ca^{2+} ionophore, ionomycin, potentiates the effect of low concentrations of PMA to induce SMC contraction while the calmodulin antagonist, calmidazolium, is ineffective. In cells preincubated in serum-free medium, PMA results in intracellular alkalinization; treatment with amiloride, a Na^+ transport antagonist, partially inhibits the PMA-induced contraction of SMCs.[92] In patch clamp experiments in porcine coronary artery SMCs, Minami et al[93] demonstrated that PKC inhibits the Ca^{2+}-activated K^+ channel. Both PMA and 1-oleoyl-2-acetylglycerol decreased the open probability of A23187-, dibutyryl cAMP-, or caffeine-activated K_{ca} channels. Presumably, PKC activation causes membrane depolarization prior to SMC contraction. PKC has also been demonstrated to modulate the conductance of dihydropyridine-sensitive Ca^{2+} channels in vascular SMCs.[94] In A7r5 rat aortic SMCs, glucocorticoid stimulation of Ca^{2+} uptake via these channels can be blocked by staurosporine, a PKC inhibitor.[95]

PKC translocation from the cytosol to a membrane fraction has been detected in porcine coronary artery SMCs exposed to medium with high glucose (25 mM).[96] The elevated glucose was found to promote a concomitant increase in total cell protein, cell volume, DNA synthesis, and cell number. The relevance of the PKC response of SMCs exposed to high glucose with the global changes in cell growth and division is unknown, but has been speculated to be important in understanding some of the vascular complications found in patients with diabetes mellitus.

Mitogenic stimulation of vascular SMCs is also associated with an activation of Na^+-H^+ exchange. Both the acute[97] and long-term regulation[98] of Na^+-H^+ exchange is known to be regulated by PKC. The acute serum stimulation of Na^+-H^+ exchange is predominantly controlled by PKC, while the AII-,[97] thrombin-,[99] and PDGF-[99] induced stimulation of Na^+-H^+ exchange involves both PKC-dependent and PKC-independent pathways. Addition of serum or phorbol 12,13-dibutyrate to SMCs caused a significant decrease in long-term ethylisopropylamiloride (EIPA)-sensitive Na^+ influx which could be prevented by sphingosine, a naturally occurring lysophingolipid inhibitor of PKC.[100]

In certain vascular SMCs, PKC can exert an antiproliferative response.[101,102] For instance, in neonatal rat vascular SMCs, α-thrombin-induced DNA synthesis could be inhibited by a phorbol ester.[101] Curiously, the expression of the immediate-early growth related gene, c-myc, was inversely related to SMC growth; c-myc expression was maximal under conditions where PKC maximally inhibited thrombin-induced DNA synthesis and reduced upon downregulation of PKC.[100] In rabbit aortic SMCs, the inhibition of proliferation by a phorbol ester was demonstrated to result from a block in the cell cycle from the late G_1 to the S phase.[102] In fact, phorbol ester inhibited whole blood serum-induced DNA synthesis even if added 12 hours after the blood. However, prolonged treatment with phorbol ester caused downregulation of PKC and the loss of its anti-proliferative response. Weiss et al[100] found that PMA inhibits thrombin-induced DNA synthesis in neonatal vascular SMCs. The effect of PMA was mimicked by DiC8, a synthetic diacylglycerol, and reversed by sphingosine.[100]

In other SMCs, PKC exerts mitogenic properties. One interesting example involves the response of porcine pulmonary vascular SMCs to hypoxic conditions, in which these cells exhibit a proliferative response in vivo but not in vitro.[103] However, in cultured cells "primed" with phorbol ester, hypoxia stimulated proliferation of SMCs. Both downregulation of PKC and treatment with the dihdrosphingosine prevented the hypoxic response, suggesting an important role of PKC in the response of SMCs to hypoxia.

Phospholipase D catalyzes the hydrolysis of phosphatidylcholine to phosphatidic acid and choline. Phosphatidic acid is then converted to the PKC activator, diacylglycerol, by phosphatidic acid phosphomonoesterase.[104] The sustained levels of diacylglycerol generated by phospholipase D action are thought to play a role in the long-term responses (e.g., mitogenesis) in vascular SMCs. In rat vascular SMCs incubated with [³H] myristate, phospholipase D activity, as assessed by the formation of [³H] phosphatidylethanolamine in the presence of alcohol, was increased in response to tissue plasminogen activator (tPA) and PDGF.[105,106] EGF, A23187, AII, vasopressin, and endothelin modestly stimulated phospholipase D activity while bradykinin was ineffective.[105,107] The activation of phospholipase D by TPA could be blocked by downregulation of PKC or chelation of extracellular Ca^{2+}.[105] In a subsequent study by these investigators, treatment of vascular SMCs with exogenous phospholipase D from *S. chromofuscus* caused choline release, phosphatidic acid production, and DNA synthesis analogous to the phenomenon shown for PDGF.[105] These data suggested that activation of phospholipase D by PDGF is a significant pathway in its mitogenic action.

Tyrosine Kinase

Tyrosine kinase activity is thought to play a key role in SMC mitogenic activity. For example, the mitogenic activity of α-thrombin can be blocked by the tyrosine kinase inhibitor, herbimycin A.[108] A confluent, quiescent R22D clone of SMCs was preincubated for 24 hours with 0.1 to 5 μM herbimycin. Thrombin (1 U/mL) stimulation of ³H-thymidine incorporation was inhibited by 50% at 0.1 μM herbimycin and > 90% at 5 μM herbimycin. Furthermore, the mitogenic activity of a number of growth factors, such as PDGF, EGF, bFGF, is also thought to involve the intrinsic tyrosine kinase activity of their receptors in SMCs.[109] The cytoplasmic portion of the PDGF receptor contains a sequence homologous to other tyrosine kinases (e.g., macrophage colony stimulating factor receptor) that is interrupted by a kinase insert domain.[109] To assess the role of tyrosine kinase, Williams et al[109] prepared transfectants containing mutants deficient in tyrosine kinase activity. In the absence of tyrosine kinase activity, the ability of PDGF to stimulate autophosphorylation, phosphatidylinositol turnover, Ca^{2+} mobilization, pH change, phosphatidylinositol kinase, conformational change of the receptor, and DNA synthesis were all lost. Only PDGF-stimulated downregulation of the PDGF-receptor was not affected by loss of tyrosine kinase activity.

Recent reports have begun to elucidate the identity of the tyrosine phosphorylated substrates in vascular SMCs.[110,111] Tsuda et al[111] demonstrated by Western blot with antityrosine antisera that at least nine proteins with molecular weights ranging from 190 to 40 kDa were phosphorylated at tyrosine residues by a variety of "vasoconstrictors" in cultured rat aortic SMCs. These include AII, vasopressin, serotonin, and norepinephrine. Phorbol esters or ionomycin, an activator of Ca^{2+} influx, mimicked the effects of these agonists. Although the tyrosine phosphorylated substrates are undefined proteins, the data suggest that these vasoconstrictors cause tyrosine phosphorylation through activation of Ca^{2+} signaling pathways in SMCs.[111] In rat aortic SMCs, Molloy et al[110] described the phosphorylation of several cellular proteins (42, 44, 75, and 120 kD) by AII. A cascade of interaction between different classes of protein kinases was indicated by the identification of 42 and 44 kD tyrosine-phosphorylated proteins as p42[mapk] and p44[mapk] mitogen-activated protein kinases.

Wijetunge et al[112] showed that tyrosine phosphorylation may be involved in excitation-contraction coupling in SMCs. In their study, two tyrosine phosphorylation inhibitors, tyrphostin 23 and genistein, blocked voltage-operated calcium channel currents in rabbit ear artery SMCs. However, they could not exclude the possibility of a direct effect of these inhibitors on the voltage-operated calcium channels.[112]

Cyclic AMP

cAMP accumulation in SMCs is caused by the conversion of ATP to cAMP by the enzyme adenylate cyclase. Adenylate cyclase is a well-characterized G protein effector (Figure 9).[113] Upon agonist binding to stimulatory G protein coupled receptors, such as the β-adrenergic receptor, the heterotrimeric G protein (G_s)

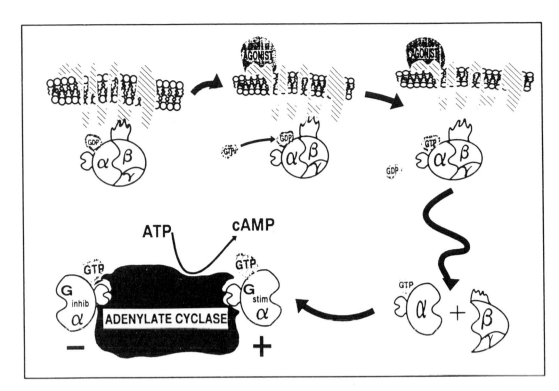

Figure 9. G proteins consist of a heterotrimer with α, β, and γ subunits. Depicted are members of the G_s/G_i families. In the resting state, the subunit normally binds GDP; upon receptor activation the GDP is replaced by GTP which leads to dissociation of the trimer into α and $\beta\gamma$ subunits. The α subunit can now activate or inhibit the effector (adenylate cyclase in this case). The α subunit contains intrinsic GTPase activity, and upon hydrolysis of GTP to GDP the response is terminated. (Reproduced with permission from Reference 263.)

undergoes a conformational change such that guanosine diphosphate (GDP) is released from the guanine nucleotide binding site. Guanosine triphosphate (GTP) binds to the empty site causing both the dissociation of the G protein coupled receptor from the G protein (thereby reducing the affinity of hormone for the receptor) and the dissociation of the α subunit from the $\beta\gamma$ subunit of G_s. The released α subunit of G_s then activates the adenylate cyclase effector.

The tetrameric enzyme protein kinase A is stimulated by elevation of cAMP levels. cAMP binds to the regulatory subunits of the enzyme resulting in release of the catalytic subunits. The released catalytic subunit causes the phosphorylation of many cytosolic and membrane substrates, as well as the nuclear protein CREB, the cAMP-regulated transcription factor (Figure 10). CREB protein controls gene expression by binding to the cAMP response element (CRE) located in the promoter region. CREB is phosphorylated on serine 133 by 30 minutes with declining phosphorylation present by 24 hours.[114] Upon phosphorylation, the transcriptional activity of CREB is enhanced ten- to twentyfold.

cAMP is known to cause SMCs to relax, presumably via phosphorylation of the MLCK[115] and/or reducing $[Ca^{2+}]_i$.[116] In addition, the stimulation of cAMP

accumulation in vascular SMCs is associated with a decrease in cell proliferation and a trend toward a more differentiated state. Jonzon et al[117] found an increase in cAMP accumulation and a decrease in DNA synthesis in rat aortic SMCs treated with either forskolin or adenosine analogs that act via the A_2 receptor subtype. Liau et al[118] found that ferritin gene expression is a marker for growth-arrested and differentiated SMCs, whose mRNA was enhanced fivefold in the presence of forskolin and dibutryl cAMP. Elevation of cAMP by forskolin also inhibited SMC migration.[119] In a recent study, cAMP was demonstrated to stimulate the synthesis and function of low density lipoproteins (LDL) in human umbilical SMCs.[120]

The effect of cyclic strain on adenylate cyclase activity has been examined extensively in coronary vascular SMCs. In contrast to that described above for endothelial cells, coronary vascular SMCs exhibit a reduction in adenylate cyclase activity in response to acute cyclic strain.[121] Both basal and maximal stimulation in the presence of forskolin and Mn^{++} were reduced by approximately 30% in membranes obtained in stretched versus unstretched cells. Interestingly, basal adenylate cyclase activity was inversely related to the degree of cyclic strain. A pressure of -20 kPa

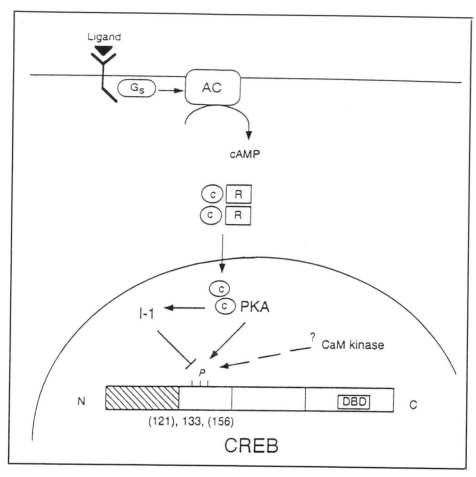

Figure 10. The regulation of CREB activity in response to extracellular signals that elevate cAMP levels. The pathway that leads to the activation of PKA activity can be viewed as a simple two-component system as shown. cAMP binds to the regulatory subunit of PKA (**R**), allowing the catalytic subunit (**C**) to dissociate and translocate to the nucleus where it phosphorylates CREB on Ser133. The phosphorylation of Ser133 is attenuated by protein phosphatase 1, which is itself a substrate of PKA. The function of other potential phosphorylation sites of CREB is unknown. Also, the calmodulin-dependent kinase has been shown to phosphorylate CREB in vitro, but the physiologic significance of this event has not been established. Ser133 is located within a regulatory domain that affects the conformation and activity of the *trans*-activation domain (**hatched box**) located nearer the amino-terminus. (Reproduced with permission from Reference 114.)

was required to demonstrate a statistically significant effect although a trend in the reduction of adenylate cyclase activity was observed at -15 kPa.

Similar findings were obtained in coronary vascular SMCs exposed to chronic stretch.[122] Basal, Gpp(NH)p, and forskolin-stimulated adenylate cyclase activity were all inhibited significantly in stretched (1 day) versus unstretched cells. The reduction in adenylate cyclase activity observed after 1 day of stretch was associated with a significant reduction in the levels of $G_{s\alpha45}$, the alpha subunit of the stimulatory G protein. In contrast, the alpha subunit of the inhibitory G protein, $G_{i\alpha1,2}$, remained unchanged after 1 day of cyclic strain. With continued cyclic strain of 7 days, a significant

reduction in $G_{s\alpha45}$ levels remained as compared to unstretched cells. However, strain-induced inhibition of adenylate cyclase activity was not observed at this later time. Thus, while strain-induced changes in $G_{s\alpha45}$ levels may play an important role in temporarily modulating adenylate cyclase activity, over time, other factors are effective in restoring adenylate cyclase activity to control levels.

Second Messenger Crosstalk

Activators of phosphoinositide turnover are known to potentiate agonist-stimulated cAMP accumulation in vascular SMCs. For example, AII caused a two- to threefold potentiation of isoproterenol, PGI₂, and adenosine-stimulated cAMP accumulation in rat aortic SMCs.[123] AII is thought to promote G_s-adenylate cyclase interaction since it doubled cholera toxin-stimulated cAMP accumulation, but increased forskolin-stimulated cAMP by only 40%. Since phorbol esters, Ca^{++} chelators, and calmodulin antagonists prevent the AII potentiation of agonist-stimulated cAMP, a Ca^{++}-calmodulin-dependent mechanism is thought to be involved.

Another example of second messenger cross talk was presented by Lincoln et al.[124] In primary rat aortic SMCs, forskolin was found to inhibit vasopressin-induced stimulation of Ca^{2+}. However, in passaged SMCs, forskolin caused an increase in Ca^{2+} levels by stimulating Ca^{2+} uptake accompanied by a diminution of its modulation of vasopressin-induced stimulation of Ca^{2+}. Likewise, the levels of cGMP-dependent protein kinase were normal in primary SMCs and diminished in passaged cells. Interestingly, the addition of purified cGMP-dependent protein kinase to passaged cells restored forskolin actin to that observed in primary cells. The data suggest that forskolin-stimulated cAMP accumulation causes the activation of both cAMP- and cGMP-dependent protein kinases in vascular SMCs. Furthermore, with regard to Ca^{2+} levels, the data suggest that cAMP-dependent protein kinase stimulates Ca^{2+} uptake from extracellular sources, whereas cGMP-dependent protein kinase activation by cAMP leads to a reduction in intracellular Ca^{2+}.

Smooth Muscle Cell Agonists

ATP

Neurotransmission is the principal route of delivery of adenine nucleotides to SMCs.[125] Extracellular ATP/ADP mediate either vasoconstriction or vasodilation in vascular SMCs by binding to the purinergic receptors P_{2Y} or P_{2x}, respectively. ATP appears to exert mitogen-like effects in SMCs since its binding to the P_{2Y} receptor subtype leads to the induction of both immediate-early genes (e.g., c-fos, KC, c-myc, and JE) as well as delayed-early genes (e.g., 2F1, M11) in rat aorta SMCs (Figure 11).[126] In addition to its native mitogenic effect, ATP can act synergistically with insulin, IGF-1, EGF, PDGF, and other mitogens, as well as AII, phospholipase C, serotonin, or carbachol, to stimulate DNA synthesis in porcine aortic SMCs.[127] The mitogenic effect of ATP is thought to involve both arachidonic acid metabolism and PKC.

Serotonin (5-HT)

Serotonin is released into the general circulation from central or peripheral nerves and chromaffin

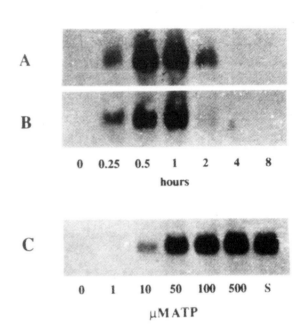

Figure 11. ATP-mediated induction of c-fos protooncogene. Quiescent aortic smooth muscle cells (SMCs) were stimulated for different times either by fetal calf serum (FCSA) or 100 uM ATP (**B**). **C**: Cells were submitted to different ATP concentrations for 30 minutes. After stimulation period, RNA was extracted from 10⁶ cells and tested for specific mRNA detection. (Reproduced with permission from Reference 126.)

cells.[128] Serotonin is deaminated by monoamine oxidase in endothelial cells and liver. Nondeaminated serotonin accumulates in dense granules found in platelets. Upon platelet aggregation, serotonin is released by platelets, after which it binds to 5-HT₂ receptors found on SMCs, causing contraction. Normal endothelium can counteract the vasoconstrictor action of serotonin via 5-HT₁ receptors that mediate the release of vasodilating agents such as NO and prostacyclin.[128] Serotonin acting via the 5-HT₂ receptor subtype caused both a fivefold increase in the mobilization of intracellular calcium as well as a tenfold induction in c-fos mRNA in SMCs (Figure 12).[57] Both weak[57] and strong[129,130] SMC mitogenic activity has been ascribed to serotonin. As shown by Lee et al, 5-HT can regulate SMC growth[131] as well as cell morphology[132] by two different regulatory mechanisms. These include stimulation of DNA synthesis by an intracellular mechanism of an undefined nature and an inhibition of DNA synthesis when serotonin or 5-HT₁ₐ agonists are exposed to cells in the presence of agents that increase cAMP accumulation.

Pertussis toxin-sensitive G proteins play an important role for some mitogens (bombesin, thrombin), but

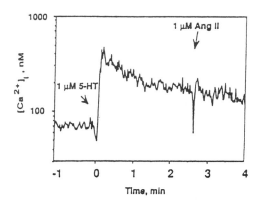

Figure 12. Mobilization of intracellular Ca^{2+} $[Ca^{2+}]_i$ by 5-HT in rat aortic smooth muscle cells (RAsmooth muscle cells). RAsmooth muscle cells were growth arrested in 1% platelet-poor plasma (PPP), loaded with 2 uM fura-2/acetoxymethyl ester (AM), and studied in suspension. $[Ca^{2+}]_i$ level is depicted on ordinate and determined by calibration of 340/380 fluorescence signals. A single aliquot of cells was stimulated with 1 uM 5-HT (**first arrow**) and then 1 uM angiotensin II (**second arrow**). (Reproduced with permission from Reference 57.)

not others (PDGF). In contrast, serotonin-induced mitogenesis occurs through a distinct mechanism.[130] In bovine aortic SMCs, Kavanaugh et al[130] observed pertussis toxin inhibition of 5-HT stimulation of DNA synthesis. However, pertussis toxin exerted its effect in the absence of any alteration in 5-HT stimulation of cAMP, phosphatidylinositol turnover, or increased intracellular calcium.[130]

Angiotensin II

Local production of AII is thought to play a critical role in the control of vascular tone. Both vascular SMCs[133] and endothelial cells[134] possess renin activity. Renin causes the hydrolysis of angiotensinogen to the decapeptide angiotensin I (AI), which is then cleaved by angiotensin-converting enzyme to form AII. High-affinity binding sites for AII are present on cultured vascular SMCs.[72,135–137] AII binding to its specific receptors in cultured vascular SMCs has been reported to cause an increase in intracellular calcium[138,139] inositol phosphate production,[139] and PKC activation.[140] AII (10^{-8}M) stimulated an increase in $[Ca^{2+}]_i$ by 15 seconds that declined gradually and was blocked by pretreatment with the AII antagonist [Sar^1, Ile^8]. In the absence of extracellular calcium, AII caused a twofold increase in $[Ca^{2+}]_i$, but reduced the peak AII response and blocked the plateau phase of the response, implicating a mechanism involving both mobilization of intracellular calcium and influx of extracellular calcium. In addition, a high concentration of AII (> 10 nM), could release Ca^{2+} from intracellu-

lar pools.[139] The increase in cytosolic-free calcium caused by AII is associated with an intracellular acidification in vascular SMCs.[97,141]

Lang and Vallotton[140] characterized the effect of AII on PKC activity in rat aortic SMCs. PMA caused a translocation of PKC activity from the cytosolic to the membrane fraction, but in the presence of 50 nM AII, they observed an increase in both the cytosolic and membrane-associated PKC activity. Another contrast between AII and PMA stimulation of SMCs is in the Ca^{2+} sensitivity of the stimulated membranous PKC activity. Membranous PKC activity stimulation was highly $[Ca^{2+}]_i$-dependent for AII and largely $[Ca^{2+}]_i$-independent for PMA. In the presence of both AII and PMA, the activation of membranous PKC was additive and the cytosolic PKC was depressed as seen with PMA alone.[140] The additive response of membranous PKC to AII and PMA correlated with the stimulation of prostacyclin release.[140] AII activation of PKC suppressed AII-induced phosphatidylinositol turnover; downregulation of PKC potentiated the AII-stimulated IP$_3$ formation in rat aortic SMCs.[142] Conversely, acute stimulation with TPA caused a reduction in AII-stimulated IP$_3$ formation.[142]

AII stimulation of PKC has been demonstrated to affect nuclear events. Tsuda and Alexander[143] observed phosphorylation of nuclear lamins A (70 kDa), B (67 kDa), and C (60 kDa) in rat aorta SMCs exposed to AII. This response was inhibited by downregulation of PKC and could be mimicked by phorbol esters. In addition, AII can induce parathyroid hormone-related protein (PTHrP) mRNA in vascular SMCs.[144] This action of AII can be viewed as autoregulatory since PTHrP has been shown to inhibit AII-stimulated DNA synthesis.

Takeuchi et al[145] transfected SMCs with a thymidine kinase promotor chloramphenicol acetyl transferase (CAT) construct containing an AP-1 binding element. AII stimulated CAT expression nearly threefold in rat aortic SMCs transfected with a minimal promoter from the herpes simplex virus thymidine kinase gene containing a 3X tandem repeat of the TPA responsive element (TGACTAA). The AII antagonist, Sar^{1}Ile^8 AII, significantly reduced CAT expression as did the PKC inhibitor, staurosporine.[145]

In a recent study, Anderson et al[135] demonstrated internalization and degradation of AII in cultured rat aortic SMCs. After diffuse binding of AII to the cell surface, they observed aggregation of AII receptors in coated pits. These membrane areas were transformed into small intracellular vesicles and AII was subsequently localized within large lysosomal-like vesicles in the cell interior.[135] Previous studies by Griendling et al[146] suggested that these early events in the internalization of AII may be critical in the sustained activation of diacylglycerol by AII. They found that either low temperature or phenylarsine oxide, an agent that prevents receptor internalization, could inhibit the AII-sustained diacylglycerol response. In contrast, both monesin and chloroquin, drugs that interfere with lysosomal degradation, were ineffective.

The synthesis of ECM molecules is also affected by AII. In rat aortic SMCs, Sharifi et al[67] demonstrated a ninefold increase specifically in tenascin synthesis, with mild stimulation or no change in fibronectin and laminin synthesis, respectively. This was accomplished at the level of transcription with AII stimulation of tenascin mRNA synthesis evident by 2 hours.

AII, as well as other vasoconstrictor agents such as vasopressin, stimulates glucose transport in quiescent vascular SMCs both acutely (30 minutes) and chronically (hours).[147] The acute activation of glucose transport is thought to involve the translocation of glucose transporters, whereas the chronic stimulation appears to involve induction of GLUT-1 mRNA, the insulin-insensitive glucose transporter.[147]

AII at a threshold concentration of 0.3 nM can also promote reversible contraction of rat mesenteric artery SMCs.[72] Contraction was observed after 30 to 45 seconds of exposure, maximal at 1 to 5 minutes, and can be blocked by the specific antagonist, (Sar$_1$, Ile$_8$)-AII.

AII is also a potent stimulator of vascular SMC hypertrophy, but not hyperplasia, in most[148,149] but not all studies.[136,150] Vascular SMCs which hypertrophy with AII stimulation also have enhanced Na/K/2Cl cotransport.[151] In rat aorta SMCs exposed to 100 nM AII for 24 hours, Berk et al[148] noted an 80% increase in protein synthesis in the absence of alterations in cell number. The stimulation of protein synthesis is thought to be mediated by mitogen-activated protein (MAP) kinases. Duff et al[152] demonstrated that AII led to the tyrosine phosphorylation of pp42^{mapk} and pp44^{mapk}, two kinases involved in protein synthesis through a phosphorylation cascade involving ribosomal S6 protein. AII stimulation of protein synthesis is unaffected by agents which prevent Na^+/H^+ exchange, alkalinization, or PKC activation. However, an elevation of intracellular Ca^{2+} appears to be critical since chelation of Ca^{2+} with quin 2-AM blocked AII activation of protein synthesis. Induction of PDGF A-chain and c-myc gene expression has also been implicated in the hypertrophic activation of SMCs.[153,154]

In addition to its role in stimulating vascular SMC hypertrophy, AII has been shown to prevent basic fibroblast growth factor (bFGF) and TGF-β_1-induced DNA synthesis.[155,156] The ability of AII to promote hypertrophy, but not hyperplasia, may be explained by recent studies in vascular SMCs which demonstrate AII stimulation of TGF-β_1 gene expression, as well as its conversion to a biologically active form.[149] Using antisense oligomers complementary to bFGF, PDGF-A, and TGF-β_1, Itoh et al[157] recently confirmed the

hypothesis that AII is nonmitogenic in vascular SMCs as a consequence of the activation of a proliferative pathway involving bFGF (and not PDGF-AA) and an antiproliferative pathway mediated by TGF-β_1.

Endothelin

Endothelin-1 (ET-1) is a potent vasconstrictor of vascular SMCs secreted by endothelial cells.[158] Three forms of endothelin (ET) have been described including endothelin-2 (ET-2), ET-1, and endothelin-3 (ET-3), in order of potency.[158] Specific receptors for ET with a maximal binding capacity (Vmax) of approximately 10000/cell and an apparent Kd of 126 pM have been described in human[159] and rat[160] vascular SMCs. The ET receptor on vascular SMCs is of the ET$_A$ class. ET binding to this receptor causes the activation of phospholipase C, generation of inositol phosphates (Ca^{2+}), and diacylglycerol (PKC) (Figure 13).[158] In some vessels, the ET$_A$ receptor is linked to voltage-operated Ca^{2+} channels through a G protein.[158]

cAMP stimulates the induction of ET$_A$ receptor mRNA and greatly enhances the ability of ET to increase intracellular Ca^{2+}.[161] ET produces a dose-dependent, biphasic increase in intracellular Ca^{2+} in primary cultures of human umbilical artery[162] and in rabbit aortic SMCs.[163] ET stimulates PKC activity in rat aortic SMCs.[164] Blockade of ET-induced PKC activation results in an inhibition of ANP-stimulated cGMP accumulation. The different isoforms of ET increase SMCs [Ca^{2+}] by distinct mechanisms. For instance, neomycin, a phospholipase C inhibitor, has been shown to inhibit ET-1-induced mobilization of Ca^{2+} but not that of ET-3. The findings suggest that ET-1 increases intracellular Ca^{2+} via an IP$_3$-mediated release of calcium from intracellular stores, whereas ET-3 induces elevation of intracellular Ca^{2+} by a IP$_3$-independent mechanism.[165] In A10 SMCs, ET has been shown to stimulate phosphatidylinositol turnover, diacylglycerol release, and mobilization of intracellular Ca^{2+}.[166] ET-induced Ca^{2+} efflux from rat aortic SMCs is not abrogated in the presence of Ca^{2+}-free medium and EGTA, thereby implicating ET mobilization of intracellular Ca^{2+}.[167] Komuro et al[168] demonstrated that ET can stimulate SMC mitogenic activity. Incubation of serum-deprived rat aortic SMCs with 10^{-7}M ET led to enhanced c-fos and c-myc expression by 30 and 120 minutes, respectively. In addition, in the presence of insulin, ET stimulated thymidine incorporation to 35% of that observed with fetal calf serum and 65% of that observed with PDGF.

Alpha$_1$-Adrenergic Agonists

Alpha$_1$-adrenergic agonists cause cultured vascular SMCs to contract reversibly.[72] Both α_{1A} and α_{1B}

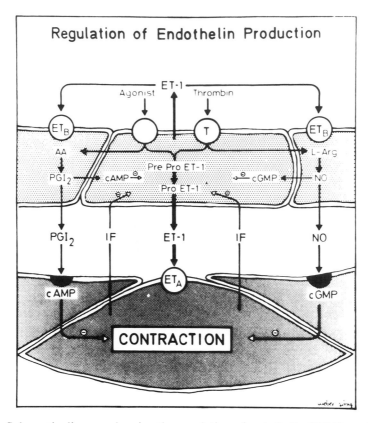

Figure 13. Schematic diagram showing the regulation of endothelin-(ET-1) production and action. Production of ET-1 is stimulated by thrombin and other receptor-operated agonists (**open circles**). Released ET-1 can activate receptors on vascular smooth muscle mediating contraction and on endothelial cells releasing nitric oxide (NO) and prostacyclin (PGI$_2$). Increase in cyclic GMP (cGMP) and cyclic AMP (cAMP) in endothelial cells evoked by the latter inhibits the production of ET-1. In addition, vascular smooth muscle cells produce inhibitory factor (IF) that reduces ET-1 production. At the level of vascular smooth muscle, both NO and PGI$_2$ blunt or prevent ET-1-induced contraction. (Reproduced with permission from Reference 264.)

receptor subtypes have been observed in rat vascular smooth muscle.[169] It appears that the α_{1A} receptor subtype when activated causes the influx of extracellular Ca^{2+}, whereas activation of the α_{1B} receptor prduces the mobilization of intracellular Ca^{2+} stores.[169,170] The α_1-adrenergic receptor subtype that mediates the contractile response to norepinephrine varies between vascular beds. For example, rat aorta contains primarily α_{1B} receptors, renal artery contains α_{1A}, and portal vein a combination of the two receptor subtypes. In the presence of 10^{-8}-10^{-6}M epinephrine, rat mesenteric SMC contraction could be blocked by the alpha-adrenergic antagonist, phentolamine. Colucci et al[171] demonstrated the presence of alpha$_1$-adrenergic agonists on cultured rabbit aorta SMCs. Norepinephrine binding to this receptor caused Ca^{++} efflux from cells preloaded with ^{45}Ca. Long-term exposure of vascular SMCs to norepinephrine led to a reduction in α_1 as well as $\beta2$ adrenergic receptor density.[172] Norepinephrine activation of the α_1-adrenergic receptor caused a transient

decrease in α_1-adrenergic receptor mRNA.[173] This effect is mediated by both a reduction in the level of transcription and an increased destablization of α_1-adrenergic receptor message.[173]

Prolactin

In addition to its well-characterized lactogenic action, prolactin has been reported to lower blood pressure in rats,[174] stimulate plasminogen activator in rat aorta,[175] and stimulate the proliferation of vascular SMCs.[176] A possible proximal source of prolactin to the vasculature are mononuclear cells, which have been shown to be capable of secreting a prolactin-like molecule in response to conacanavalin A.[177] To date, we are not aware of any study that has characterized prolactin receptors in vascular smooth muscle. Prolactin (10^{-11} to 10^{-7}M) increased both cell number and ^{3}H-thymidine incorporation in both low-serum and PDGF-stimulated A10 aortic SMCs.[176] Prolactin stimulated PKC activity which could be inhibited by either prolactin antiserum or the prolactin receptor antibody. Prolactin activation of PKC may be responsible for its mitogenic response, since PKC inhibitors (staurosporine, sphingosine, and H-7) prevent the prolactin-induced proliferation.[176]

Atrial Natriuretic Polypeptide

The major source of atrial natriuretic polypeptide (ANP) is the cardiac atria.[178] ANP receptors consist of a guanylate cyclase-free (65 kDa) and a guanylate cyclase-containing form (135 kDa). In vascular smooth muscle, 99% of the receptor is the guanylate cyclase-free form and is thought to play a role in the clearance of excess ANP from the circulation.[178] ANP acts as a potent antimitogenic and antihypertrophic factor in vascular SMCs.[179] Likewise, ANP inhibited proliferation and DNA synthesis in bovine aortic ET cells.[157] Thus, ANP may act as a general growth modulator in the vasculature.[157,179] In rat aortic SMCs, ANP caused a reduction in all of the following: 1) 1% and 5% serum-stimulated proliferation, and DNA synthesis; 2) basal and TGF-β_1-stimulated ^{3}H-uridine and ^{3}H-leucine incorporation; and 3) AII-stimulated RNA and protein synthesis.[179] The effects of ANP can be mimicked by cGMP and are not affected by down-regulation of PKC.[179] Furthermore, down-regulation of PKC enhances ANP-stimulated cGMP accumulation in rat aortic SMCs.[180] In contrast to heparin, however, ANP inhibits serum-stimulated proliferation of not only SMCs, but also ET cells.[181]

Heparin

Guyton et al[182] showed that heparin administration to rats subjected to balloon de-endothelialization of the carotid artery could inhibit the resultant proliferation of SMCs in vivo. Hoover et al[183] subsequently demonstrated that heparin inhibits SMC proliferation and DNA synthesis in vitro. This response to heparin was specific to SMCs and not endothelial cells, and was related to its anticoagulant property. Heparin has also been shown to be a potent inhibitor of rat aortic SMC migration.[184] In fact, heparin, nonanticoagulant heparin fragments, and heparin-like glycosaminoglycans are all potent inhibitors of SMC migration. In contrast, the nonheparin-like glycosaminoglycans are unable to inhibit SMC migration. Both endothelial cells[185] and postconfluent SMCs[186] produced antiproliferative heparan sulfate.

Reilly et al[187] demonstrated that heparin inhibited SMC proliferation by blocking the mid-G$_1$ phase of the cell cycle and not the G$_o$ to G$_1$ transition. In phorbol ester activated rat SMCs[188] and murine fibroblasts,[189] heparin blocked the induction of c-fos and c-myc mRNA via a PKC-dependent pathway. Clowes et al[190] have postulated that heparin inhibits SMC proliferation and migration by preventing the expression and activity of plasminogen activators such as tissue-type plasminogen activator (tPA) and urokinse-type plasminogen activator (uPA). Presumably, heparin prevents the protease action and resultant breakdown of ECM by these chemicals. In support of this hypothesis, Au et al[190] demonstrated that heparin prevents serum or phorbol ester-stimulated tPA, but not uPA mRNA expression and protein in baboon SMCs via a PKC pathway.

Thrombin

Coughlin et al[191,192] have recently cloned the human thrombin receptor and have shown that it belongs to the seven transmembrane domain receptor family. The thrombin receptor exhibits a novel mechanism of activation involving the proteolytic cleavage of a portion of the amino-terminal extracellular domain (Figure 14). The new unmasked portion of the amino terminus thereby functions as a ligand-like activator of the receptor. In fact, they have shown that a peptide analog corresponding to the unmasked amino terminus is capable of stimulating both thrombin receptor and platelet activation.

α-Thrombin is a procoagulant that exerts mito-

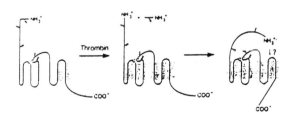

Figure 14. Mechanism of thrombin receptor activation: working model. The amino-terminal extracellular extension of the intact and unactivated thrombin receptor is cleaved by thrombin, revealing a new amino terminus and releasing a short receptor fragment. The newly exposed amino terminus then functions as a receptor agonist, binding to an as yet undefined region of the thrombin receptor and activating it. The thrombin receptor is thus activated by a mechanism analogous to zymogen-enzyme conversion. The mechanism depicted above as well as the relatedness of the thrombin receptor to the seven transmembrane domain receptors suggest that the thrombin receptor may be viewed as a peptide receptor that contains it own ligand, the sequence S$_{42}$F$_{43}$. Whether the intramolecular rearrangement that mediates thrombin receptor activation represents an evolutionary specialization of earlier peptide receptors or a more primitive mechanistic heritage from which peptide receptors have evolved is unknown. (Reproduced with permission from Reference 192.)

genic activity in rat neonatal vascular SMCs.[101] α-Thrombin also stimulates early responses in these cells, including inositol phosphate release and a spike in Ca^{2+} release. Interestingly, phorbol ester was found to specifically inhibit both the early and late responses caused by α-thrombin.[101] Furthermore, the ability of phorbol esters to inhibit α-thrombin-induced DNA synthesis was not related to its blockade of α-thrombin-induced early responses. In fact, the maximal inhibition of DNA synthesis is observed 4 hours after phorbol ester addition, suggesting involvement of the G_1 phase or at the G_1-S transition of the cell cycle.[101]

Berk et al[193] examined the effect of thrombin on cultured vascular SMCs and noted: 1) a biphasic change in intracellular pH; a rapid acidification followed by a sustained alkalinization (Figure 15); 2) increased $[Ca^{2+}]$; 3) activation of phospholipase C; 4) increase in inositol phosphate production; and 5) induction of c-fos message. In contrast to the observations in neonatal SMCs,[101] these changes were associated with an increase in protein synthesis in the absence of a proliferative response.

Thrombin also induces plasminogen activator inhibitor-1 (PAI-1) mRNA expression in serum-free vascular SMCs.[194] In addition, thrombin will act synergistically with TGF-β_1 to increase PAI-1 production.

Nitric Oxide

Interferon-γ inhibits proliferation of SMCs.[195] In rat aortic SMCs, interferon-γ inhibition of DNA synthesis is associated with cGMP accumulation. It appears that the ability of interferon-γ to stimulate cGMP is related to the production of NO, since the NO synthase inhibitor, N^G-nitro-L-arginine, blocked the response. NO inhibits SMC proliferation by activation of soluble cGMP.[196] Furthermore, cholesterol enrichment by cationized LDL upregulates both cytokine (e.g., IL-1a) and lipopolysaccharide (LPS) induction of NO synthase. Growth factors also play a role in cytokine induction of NO synthase. For example, PDGF-AB and PDGF-BB both inhibit and FGF and EGF synergistically increase IL-1β stimulation of NO production in SMCs.[197] In a recent study, an inducible NO synthase similar to that found in macrophages was cloned in rat vascular SMCs.[198]

Vasopressin

Vasopressin is an extremely potent vasoconstrictor of blood vessels at a physiologic concentration of 10^{-13} to 10^{-11} M.[199] In cultured rat vascular SMCs, Penit and colleagues[200] demonstrated vasopressin binding sites numbering 25000/cell with a Kd of 30 and 12 nM for Lys^8- and Arg^8-vasopressin, respectively. Vasopressin, like AII, has been shown to increase both phosphatidylinositol turnover and $[Ca^{2+}]_i$ in rat aortic vascular SMCs[139,201] and the established SMC line A-10.[202] Binding of these hormones to vascular SMCs through distinct receptors leads to an increase in $[Ca^{2+}]_i$ by mobilization of intracellular stores and by activation of receptor-operated Ca^{2+} channels.[139,201] In A-10 cells, vasopressin will bind specifically to the V_1 vasopressin receptor subtype (Kd = 6 nM; 100000 sites/cell)[203] leading to induction of c-fos protein.[204]

Other Smooth Muscle Cell Agonists

Lipoproteins have been shown to stimulate the increase of intracellular Ca^{2+}, elevate intracellular pH, and vasoconstrict and induce expression of immediate-early genes in rat aorta SMCs.[205] Lysolecithin, an oxidative product of LDL, will also markedly increase $[Ca^{2+}]$ and increase basal and PDGF-stimulated DNA synthesis, suggestive of a mechanism by which LDL promotes atherosclerosis.[206]

Growth Factors Produced by Smooth Muscle Cells

Platelet-Derived Growth Factor

PDGF causes many biochemical responses in SMCs including changes in ion flux, activation of several kinases, alterations in cell shape, increased gene

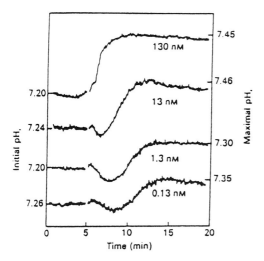

Figure 15. 2',7'-bis(carboxymethyl)-5(6)-fluorescein-loaded vascular smooth muscle cells on coverslips in Na^+ solution were treated with the concentrations of thrombin indicated. All tracings are drawn on the same pH scale. Calculated values for initial pH_i and maximal pH_i are indicated on the **left** and **right** respectively. Results are typical of three experiments. (Reproduced with permission from Reference 193.)

transcription, and activation of enzymes involved in phospholipid metabolism.[109] PDGF is also a potent mitogen for vascular SMCs released by SMCs, endothelial cells, macrophages, and platelets.[29] PDGF is a disulfide-linked dimer of two homologous peptides termed A and B.[109] PDGF forms include the AA, BB, and AB dimers of undefined specific biologic function.[109] The PDGF receptor is a 180 to 190 kD membrane glycoprotein present on SMCs, but not endothelial cells. The extracellular PDGF-binding domain of the receptor contains five immunoglobulin-like domains. The PDGF receptor also contains intrinsic tyrosine kinase activity as described above.

In cultured rat aortic SMCs, Berk et al[207] demonstrated that PDGF increases cytosolic free calcium concentration. This response occurred after a lag period and was more prolonged than the rapid increases observed with AII[207] or α-thrombin.[208] The increase in cytosolic calcium, as measured by quin2 fluorescence, was mediated by a release of calcium from intracellular pools as well as increased membrane permeability to extracellular calcium. Huang et al[209] demonstrated that the PDGF-mediated Ca^{2+} entry from the extracellular medium requires ongoing receptor occupancy by PDGF, is blocked by antibodies to PIP_2, and does not involve the heparin-sensitive IP_3 receptor.

Berk et al[207] made the seminal observation that growth factors, such as PDGF, could also constrict smooth muscle strips (Figure 16). Utilizing helical strips of rat aorta exposed to cumulative addition of PDGF, the investigators observed a concentration-de-

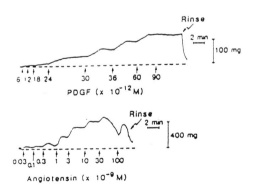

Figure 16. Contraction of isolated rat aorta induced by platelet-derived growth factor (PDGF) or angiotensin II (AII). Helical strips of rat aorta were prepared and allowed to equilibrate for 2 hours in a muscle bath. All strips had intact endothelium as assessed by vasodilation on exposure to acetylcholine. The strips were placed at an optimal length for the development of active force in response to norepinephrine. Contractile responses to PDGF or AII were recorded after sequential addition of increasing amounts of either agonist to the bath. Concentrations are expressed as the cumulative molar concentration. **Tracings** are representative of ten separate experiments. (Reproduced with permission from Reference 207.)

pendent increase in contractility. PDGF (0.09 nM) caused a contractile response equivalent to 30% of that observed with 100 nM AII. The response was reversible and unaffected by removal of the endothelium, but could not be observed in the absence of extracellular Ca^{2+}. They postulate that the ability of PDGF and other growth factors (EGF, FGF, TGF-β) to promote vasoconstriction may be responsible for the enhanced vasoreactivity of atherosclerotic vessels.[148,207]

The mechanism responsible for growth factor stimulation of vasoconstriction is probably not singular. Although EGF increased ^{45}Ca efflux from rat aortic SMCs, EGF does not elevate cytosolic-free calcium.[207] Nevertheless, PDGF and EGF cause contraction of rat aortic strips to approximately 40% of that induced by AII,[207,210] suggesting that multiple mechanisms are involved in growth factor-mediated vasoconstriction in SMCs.[207]

PDGF is a well-studied SMC mitogen. As described by Homma et al,[211] both PDGF-BB and -AB stimulated SMC proliferation, inositol phosphate production, and tyrosine phosphorylation of phospholipase C-γ2.[211] Sharma and Bhalla[212] suggest, however, that the PKC and c-fos pathway are not important since downregulation of PKC by 24-hour pretreatment with PMA does not affect PDGF-stimulated ^3H-thymidine incorporation in rat aortic SMCs. Consistent with these findings, Kihara et al[213] showed that inhibition of PKC acitivity with polymixin B did not affect PDGF-stimulated mitogenesis in rat aortic SMCs. Instead, the entry of calcium ions appears too critical in PDGF mitogenesis.[214] The homodimer PDGF-AA is a weak stimulator of these events, but can inhibit SMC migration stimulated by a number of growth factors including PDGF-AB, PDGF-BB, fibronectin, and SMC-derived migration factor. This inhibition can be blocked by the PKC inhibitor, staurosporine.[119]

Heparin-Binding Epidermal Growth Factor

Higashiyama et al[215] first described the secretion of a 22-kDa heparin-binding epidermal growth factor (HB-EGF) by SMCs and macrophages that acts as a SMC mitogen. Based on the predicted amino acid sequence from cDNA clones, the mitogen was classified as a new member of the EGF family. HB-EGF is an extremely potent mitogen for SMCs that does not exert mitogenic properties for capillary endothelial cells. HB-EGF was recently shown to be transcribed in SMCs.[216] Low levels of HB-EGF mRNA were detected in these cells. However, AII and TPA caused an eleven- and nearly fivefold increase in HB-EGF mRNA expression. Thus, HB-EGF may play an important autocrine role in the proliferative response of SMCs.

Fibroblast Growth Factor

Fibroblast Growth Factor (FGF) is synthesized in vascular SMCs and can act as an autocrine regulator of SMC growth.[217,218] In addition, bFGF is also produced by endothelial cells and macrophages in the vascular wall. Expression of FGF mRNA has been demonstrated in human aortic and umbilical vein SMCs, but not in human umbilical vein endothelial cells.[218] Both SMCs and endothelial cells possess receptors for FGF and both cells responded to FGF mitogenic activity.[218] Klagsbrun and Edelman[217] have postulated that FGF plays an important role in the pathogenesis of atherosclerosis based on its intricate involvement in macrophage, platelet, endothelial cell, and SMC autocrine and paracrine loops, and associated mitogenic and angiogenic properties. Folkman et al[219] demonstrated FGF localization in basement membranes of bovine cornea and suggested that abnormal release of FGF from this site may lead to neovascularization.

Insulin-Like Growth Factor

Insulin-like growth factor (IGF-1) is produced by platelets in the vascular circulation and exerts mitogenic actions on SMCs. Bovine aorta SMCs were found to contain high-affinity sites for both IGF-1 and multiplication stimulating activity (MSA).[220] Cultured human SMCs grown from explants exposed to insulin showed an enhanced proliferative response[220,221] between that observed with 0.1% and 1.0% fetal calf serum.[221] Bovine aorta SMCs were found to contain high-affinity sites for both IGF-1 and MSA.[220] IGF-1 and PDGF synergistically increased proliferation[222] and additively increased c-fos mRNA induction in aortic SMCs.[222]

Transforming Growth Factor β_1

Transforming growth factor β_1 (TGF-β_1) is secreted by SMCs as well as endothelial cells, T-lymphocytes, macrophages, and platelets.[29,223] Both SMC proliferation (with additional growth factors)[224] and migration[225] were shown to be enhanced by TGF-β_1. SMCs from injured carotid arteries were found to synthesize TGF-β_1.[226] The increase in TGF-β_1 levels was correlated with increased fibronectin, collagen α2(I), and collagen α1(III) gene expression.[226] Basson et al[227] and others[228] found an increase in both mRNA and surface pools of beta3 integrin classes in bovine aortic SMCs.

Smooth Muscle Cells as a Model to Study Vascular Cell Biology

Hypertrophy Versus Hyperplasia

Hypertrophy/Characterization of Smooth Muscle Cells Obtained From Hypertensive Animals

SMC growth is characteristic of hypertension and atherosclerosis, but the nature of the response is quite different in the two vascular disease states. In atherosclerosis, SMCs exhibit enhanced proliferation (hyperplasia) and migration from the medial to the neointimal zone, in the absence of a significant hypertrophic response. In contrast, SMC growth in hypertension involves a cellular hypertrophy within the media of the blood vessel with endoduplication of DNA and the formation of polyploid cells.[11] In arteries of spontaneously hypertensive as compared to normotensive Wistar-Kyoto and Sprague-Dawley rats, Owens et al[229] observed: 1) increased average DNA/cell ratios; 2) greater percentage of polyploid SMCs; and 3) no change in cell number. The DNA/cell ratio increased in aortic SMCs from spontaneously hypertensive rats compared to either Sprague-Dawley or Wistar-Kyoto control rats. Greater than 20% of the spontaneously hypertensive rats contained tetraploid (4C) DNA compared to 8% to 10% of the normotensive controls. Hyperplasia of hypertensive, polyploid SMCs has also been shown to occur under certain conditions.[11] For example, tetraploid SMCs from rat aorta were shown to proliferate in serum-supplemented medium in culture as viable tetraploid cells.[230] Thus, hypertrophied, polyploid SMCs are capable of dividing.

The mechanism responsible for SMC hypertrophy is not known, but could involve mechanical factors associated with the elevation of blood pressure.[11] In spontaneously hypertensive rats treated with a cocktail of anti-hypertensive drugs (reserpine, hydralazine, chlorathiazide), the accelerated SMC growth due to hypertrophy and polyploidy was prevented.[231] In a subsequent study, Owens[232] showed a correlation between blood pressure and the frequency of polyploidy and increased content of SMCs. Likewise, Lichtenstein[233] showed an increase in both SMC tetraploidy and size in rats treated with deoxycorticosterone-salt induced hypertension.

In SMCs subjected to cyclic strain in vitro, alignment of cells in an annular fashion perpendicular to the strain gradient was observed.[234] In addition, under low frequency, in cyclic strain conditions in which cell proliferation was inhibited,[234] ECM formation was enhanced, with increases observed for both collagen[235] and elastin synthesis.[236] In recent studies performed in our laboratory with bovine aortic SMCs, we have observed an increase in the proliferative response in response to high frequency cyclic strain (Sumpio et al, unpublished observations). Furthermore, cyclic strain caused an acute monophasic activation of phospholipid turnover that correlates with inositol phosphate production and activation of PKC in bovine aortic SMCs (Sumpio et al, unpublished observations). Further studies are necessary to determine whether cyclic strain can cause enhanced growth via hypertrophic- and/or hyperplasia-like programs in SMCs obtained from distinct vascular beds and species.

In rabbit aortic SMCs grown on purified elastin membranes, Leung et al[237] demonstrated synthesis of collagen, hyaluronate, and chondroitin 6-sulfate in response to cyclic strain. In another study, Kollros et al[238] demonstrated a stretch-induced increase in collagen and protein synthesis that could be prevented by elevation of cAMP in rabbit aortic SMCs grown on elastin membranes.

The involvement of AII in SMC hypertrophy was suggested by the greater efficacy of captopril as compared to hydralazine and propranolol in preventing polyploidy and increased cell content despite similar reductions in blood pressure.[232] Consistent with the in vivo data, AII has been demonstrated to promote hypertrophy in cultured SMCs.[239] In rat aortic SMCs, AII, unlike mitogen activators such as PDGF, causes an increase in protein synthesis, but not DNA synthesis and cell proliferation. Although AII shares with mitogen activators (PDGF) the ability to promote acute alkalinization of SMCs, Berk et al[239] tested the hypothesis that chronic changes in pH may differ in response to mitogenic versus nonmitogenic agents. In fact, mitogenic stimulators (PDGF, 10% serum, phorbol esters) exposure to SMCs for 24 hours caused significantly higher pH than that observed in either growth-arrested and AII-treated cells. The alkalinization caused by the mitogenic agents was related to a reduction in Na^+/H^+ exchange, whereas angiotensin and growth arrest of SMCs did not affect Na^+/H^+ exchange. Thus, intracellular pH regulatory mechanisms may play a role in determination of a hypertrophic versus a hyperplasia response in SMCs.[239]

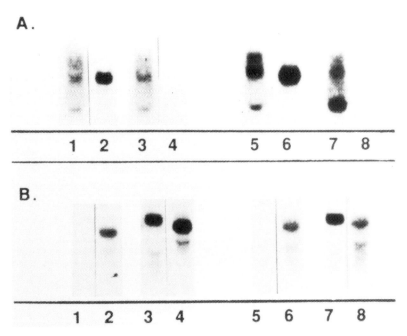

Figure 17. Platelet-derived growth factor (PDGF) ligand and receptor gene expression in adult carotid smooth muscle cells (SMCs). **Panel A:** Fifteen micrograms of total cellular RNA from paired cultures of neointimal (lanes 1 and 2) and medial (lanes 3 and 4) SMCs were electrophoresed, blotted, and hybridized for PDGF-A (lanes 1 and 3) and PDGF-B (lanes 2 and 4) transcripts. Neoinitimal and medial SMC cultures were used at the sixth passage. A similar analysis was performed for aortic SMC cultures from newborn (12-day-old, lanes 5 and 6) and adult (3-month-old, lanes 7 and 8) rats for PDGF-A (lanes 5 and 7) and PDGF-B (lanes 6 and 8) mRNAs. **Panel B:** The blots shown in panel A were reprobed for PDGF a-receptor (lanes 1,3,5, and 7) and PDGF b-receptor (lanes 2, 4, 6, and 8) transcripts. The PDGF mRNA phenotype of adult carotid neointimal SMCs in vitro resembles that of newborn rather than adult aortic SMCs. (Reproduced with permission from Reference 241.)

Hyperplasia/Characterization of Smooth Muscle Cells
Obtained From Atherosclerotic Lesions

In SMCs obtained from advanced lesions of the human superficial femoral artery, Ross et al[240] found a reduced in vitro proliferative response as compared to underlying medial cells. In fact, the inability of the lesion cells to respond normally to added serum in culture resembled the response these investigators observed in senescent cells. They hypothesize that the reduced proliferative response is a result of enhanced doublings of these cells in vivo, as compared to the sublesion medial SMC population.[240]

In SMCs cultured from the neointima of injured rat carotid arteries, Majesky et al[241] observed expression of PDGF-B gene and poor expression of PDGF-A receptor mRNA, similar to SMCs from 12–day-old rats. In contrast, in medial SMCs obtained from the contralateral carotid, the situation was reversed (i.e., expression of PDGF-A receptor mRNA and poor expression of PDGF-B), similar to SMCs from adult aorta (Figure 17). These findings and those of earlier studies by Walker et al[242] suggest that the process of neointimal formation may represent a re-expression of the sequelae associated with smooth muscle development. In support of this hypothesis, Majesky et al[241] identified two cDNA clones that encoded rat tropoelastin and α_1 procollagen whose cognate mRNA levels were both developmentally regulated in neonatal rat aorta and expressed abundantly in neointimal SMCs from injured carotid arteries. α-Thrombin was found to reproduce the effects of neointimal injury causing both a transient increase in PDGF-A and a decrease in PDGF β-receptor mRNA.[243]

Selective Interference of Atherosclerosis

As suggested by Ross,[12] the importance of inflammation, smooth muscle and monocyte replication, connective tissue formation, and lipid accumulation allows for selective interference in the atherosclerotic process. For example, Simons et al[244] used antisense c-myb oligonucleotide to selectively inhibit SMC proliferation in vivo. Antisense oligonucleotides were developed corresponding to c-myb, since it is was a previously described mitogen in SMCs. In a rat carotid artery injury model, antisense oligonucleotide was delivered as a pluronic gel immediately after balloon angioplasty from the region where the adventitia had been stripped (Figure 18). After 2 weeks, Northern blot analysis demonstrated that injury-induced expression of c-myb was blocked in antisense-treated animals. In addition, intimal SMC proliferation was also prevented in antisense-treated animals. This new strategy appears promising as a future direction for the treatment of ath-

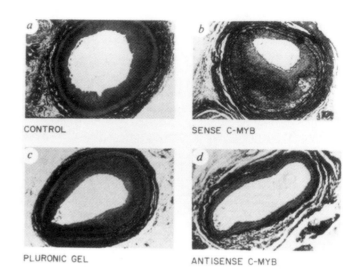

CONTROL   SENSE C-MYB

PLURONIC GEL   ANTISENSE C-MYB

Figure 18. Effect of antisense and sense c-myb oligonuceotides on neointimal formation in rat carotid arteries subjected to balloon angioplasty. Representative cross-sections from the carotid artery of an untreated rat (**a**), a rat treated with pluronic gel containing 200 μg antisense oligonucleotide (**b**), a rat treated with pluronic gel (**c**), and a rat treated with pluronic gel containing 200 μg antisense nucleotide (**d**). (Mason trichrome, magnification × 80.) Male Sprague-Dawley rats (average weight 500 g) were anesthetized with Nembutal (4 mg per 100 g), and the left carotid artery of each animal was isolated by a midline cervical incision, suspended on ties, and stripped of adventitia. A 2F Fogarty catheter was introduced through the external carotid artery of each rat, advanced to the aortic arch, the balloon was inflated to produce moderate resistance to catheter movement, and then gradually withdrawn to the entry point. The entire procedure was repeated three times for each animal. The oligonucleotides were added at a concentration of 1 mg mL^{-1} to 25% (w/v) solutions of F127 pluronic gels prepared as outlined by the manufacturer (BASF Wyandotte Corporation, Wyandotte, MI) and maintained at 4°C. Prechilled pipettes and tips were used to apply the solution to the left carotid artery of each animal with generation of a gel surrounding the exposed blood vessel, and the wounds were then closed. At the time of killing (2 weeks later), the animals were anesthetized with Nembutal and perfused with 150 cc normal saline under a pressurer of 120 mm Hg. The carotid arteries were removed, fixed in 3% formalin, and processed for light microscopy in a standard manner. (Reproduced with permission from Reference 244.)

erosclerosis, as do recent animal studies employing gene therapy.

Lynch et al[245] demonstrated gene transfer of recombinant retroviral vectors with an *E. coli* B-galactosidase gene or a human adenosine deaminase (ADA) reporter gene into vascular SMCs (Figure 19). Furthermore, rat carotid artery seeded with SMCs infected with human ADA were observed to express human ADA activity for up to 6 months. Attempts to directly transfer the gene into the rat carotid artery via virus infusion were unsuccessful. Nevertheless, the positive

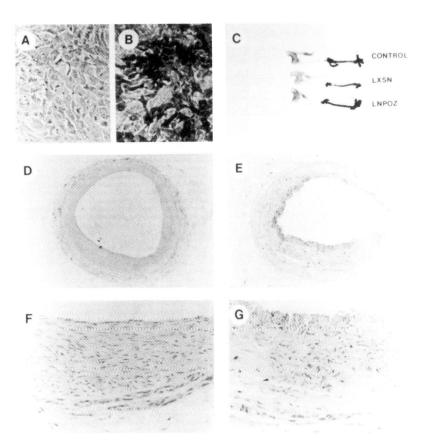

Figure 19. Analysis of b-gal activity. b-Gal activity was determined in cultured smooth muscle cells infected with LXSN (retroviral vector encoding neomycin phosphotransferase) (**A**), or LNPOZ (retroviral vector encoding neomycin phosphotransferase adn b-gal) (**B**), in rat carotid arteries 2 weeks after balloon catheter injury (control). (**C, top**) after injury and seeding with LXSN-infected cells (**C, middle**) or after injury and seeding with LNPOZ-infected cells (**C, bottom**). Also shown are microscopic cross-sections from the balloon-injured carotid (**D and F**) and the carotid seeded with LNPOZ-infected cells (**E and G**) at low-power magnification (**D and E**) and at high-power magnification after counterstaining with acridine saffronin O (**F and G**). (Reproduced with permission from Reference 245.)

results obtained via seeding of transduced cells shows great promise as a model for gene therapy. Plautz et al[246] also demonstrated catheter implantation of SMCs infected with a retrovirus transducing the B-gal gene into denuded arteries in vivo. In a recent study, DNA transfer directly in SMCs in vivo was demonstrated in canine coronary,[247,248] rabbit aorta,[249] and peripheral arteries.[247,248,250] In femoral arteries subjected to injury 3 days prior to transfection, activity of the luciferase marker gene was markedly enhanced.[250]

Isolation and Culturing of Smooth Muscle Cells

A variety of methodologies are described in the literature for the isolation and culturing of vascular SMCs,[72,136,251–255] and an exhaustive listing of the various techniques has been reviewed by Campbell and

Campbell.[37] We have chosen the four most pertinent which provide the basis for similar methodologies that have been adopted by numerous laboratories. As with any cell culture technique, the optimal goal is to balance yield with purity.

Enzyme Dispersion Method

Enzyme dispersion of vascular SMCs is particularly valuable since cells isolated in this manner have been shown to be capable of maintaining contractile function in culture. As described by Gunther et al[72] for harvesting SMCs from rat mesenteric artery, endothelium-denuded and adventitia-cleared media segments are digested for 90 minutes at 37°C in Hanks' balanced salt solution (Ca^{2+}, Mg^{2+}-free) with 0.2 mM added Ca^{2+}, 15 mM HEPES buffer (pH 7.2–7.3), 1.0 mg/mL collagenase (*C. histolyticum*, CLS Type I, Worthington Biochemical Corp., Freehold, NJ), 0.125 mg/mL elastase (pancreatopeptidase, E.C. 3.4.4.7; Sigma Chemical Co., chromatographically prepared, Type I-S), and 2.0 mg/mL crystallized bovine albumin. At the conclusion of the incubation period, the tissue has a fluffy appearance and the SMCs are rounded within the collagen matrix. The mixture is titurated through a sterile 12 g needle such that the shearing force acts to dissociate the cells from their matrix. The titurate is then filtered through a 100 μ filter. The filtrate is centrifuged at 200 × g for 5 minutes and resuspended in Dulbecco's Modified Eagle Medium supplemented with 10% heat-inactivated calf serum, 2 mM L-glutamine, 25 mM HEPES buffer, 100 U/mL penicillin, and 100 ug/mL streptomycin.

SMCs isolated by this technique display many of the morphologic aspects of native smooth muscle. Electron microscopy of freshly isolated SMCs confirms the presence of myofilament bundles in the cytoplasm as well as plasmalemmal vesicles along the plasma membrane (Figure 20). By the third day in culture, elongated spindle-shaped cells are already apparent and can be distinguished from nonproliferating islands of endothelial cells or fibroblast-like cells screened out via filtration (Figure 21). Despite the loss of thick myofilaments with prolonged (>24 hours) culture, these SMCs retain binding sites for AII binding sites. Notably, AII can cause contraction of these cells with little diminution for up to 3 days in culture, with contractility still present at 7 to 9 days (Figure 22).

Explant Method

Ross[254] first described an explant method to culture homogeneous, differentiated SMCs. With the aid of a dissecting scope, segments of inner media and intima are carefully dissected from immature guinea pig aorta. Segments of vessel measuring 1 mm square are placed on glass slides and inverted in Leighton tissue culture tubes bathed in 3 mL of Dulbecco-Vogt modification of Eagle's medium containing 7.5% sodium bicarbonate, 1 mL of nonessential amino acids, 1 mL of sodium pyruvate, 10% newborn calf serum, and 0.5 mL penicillin. Tubes are equilibrated with 95% air:5% CO_2 and left undisturbed in an incubator for 1 week when the explants are rebathed with fresh medium. After 4 weeks in culture, a confluent population of cells can be seen emanating from the explant.

Typical of SMCs grown in this manner is an overlapping "hill and valley" phenotype that distinguishes them from fibroblasts known to grow in a sworl-like fashion. Examination of these cells by electron microscopy shows a differentiated phenotype with the presence of numerous myofilaments (60 A in diameter), a well-developed endoplasmic reticulum and Golgi appa-

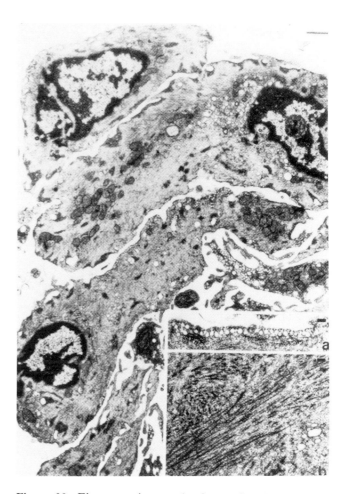

Figure 20. Electron micrograph of a section through a cell pellet obtained by enzymatic dissociation of rat mesenteric artery. Portions of several smooth muscle cells are seen. × 11,800. bar, 1 um. (**a**) Row of plasmalemmal vesicles (intracellular caveolae) at cell surface × 40,000. bar, 0.1 um; (**b**) myofilament bundles, visible in longitudinal and cross-section, contain prominent thick (12–18 nm) filaments surrounded by thin (5–8 nm) filaments × 37,500. bar, 0.1 um. (Reproduced with permission from Reference 72.)

ratus, dense bodies, mitochondria, and other organelles. Found around many cells is basement membrane-like material and the extracellular space contains numerous 110 A microfibrils.

Human Vascular Smooth Muscle Cells

The isolation of vascular SMCs from the umbilical artery as described by Gimbrone and Cotran[253] is a modification of the methodology used to isolate endothelial cells.[256] With this technique, mixed populations of endothelial cells and SMCs are obtained. SMCs are selectively subcloned and contain myofilament bundles and dense bodies characteristic of SMCs found in intact umbilical vessel.

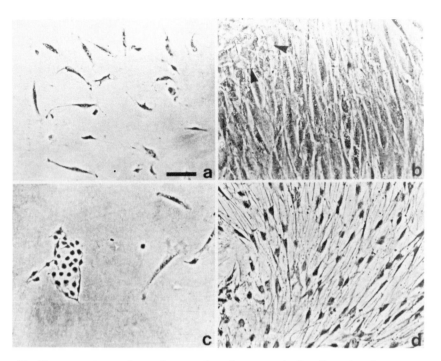

Figure 21. Phase-contrast photomicrographs of enzymatically dissociated rat mesenteric artery cells in primary culture × 350; bar, 30 um. (**a**) Primary culture of smooth-muscle-rich final cell pellet at 3 d. Most cells are elongated and contain an ovoid nucleus with 1–3 nucleoli and perinuclear collections of phase-dense granules. (**b**) Confluent primary culture at 7 d shows parallel alignment of cells with developing hillock (**arrows**) of intertwined, overlapping cells, a growth pattern characteristic of vascular smooth muscle cultures. Cell size and cytoplasmic/nuclear ratio appear increased compared with freshly isolated and 3-d cultured cells. (**c**) Island of small polygonal cells (presumably endothelium) in a sparse primary culture at 3 d. These focal contaminants failed to proliferate in culture. (**d**) Outgrowth of spindle-shaped fibroblast-like cells from explant of undigested tissue residue trapped on 100-um nylon mesh. Such cells were not observed in primary smooth muscle cultures. (Reproduced with permission from Reference 72.)

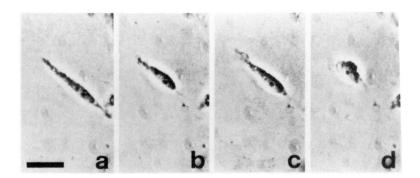

Figure 22. Sequential phase-contrast photomicrographs of contractile response of isolated rat mesenteric artery smooth muscle cells in primary culture. × 500. (**a**) 15-minute superfusion with control medium; (**b**) 1 min after infusion of 10 nM angiotensin II; cell has shortened to 65% of original length; (**c**) 10-minute washout with control medium: note partial relaxation to 86% of original length; (**d**) 3 min after rechallenge with 10 nM angiotensin II; cell has shortened to 42% of original length. (Reproduced with permission from Reference 72.)

The method consists of cannulating both ends of the vessel followed by digestion with type 1 collagenase (200 mg/mL) for a 60-minute period at 37°C. A 30 mL syringe is attached to each cannula at the end of the digestion to vigorously perfuse the luminal contents until the effluent appears turbid. After centrifugation, the pellet is resuspended and cultured in Medium 199 supplemented with 10% fetal calf serum, 15 mM HEPES buffer, 0.006% penicillin, and 0.012% streptomycin.

SMCs isolated by this technique exhibit numerous myofilaments (60 to 70 A) with associated dense bodies. With prolonged time in culture (2 weeks), extracellular fiber deposition is noted with the appearance of a distinct basal lamina. Palade bodies, characteristic of endothelial cells, are not observed in the SMC populations studied.

Renal Arteriolar Smooth Muscle Cells

In a recent study, Dubey et al[136] described an ingenious method for the isolation of rat renal preglomerular arterioles. A suspension of iron oxide particles are infused systemically through the left ventricle. Iron-laden microvessels of a kidney cortex dispersion are magnetically selected from nonvascular tissue. The microvessels are then digested with type I collagenase and further separated from glomeruli by filtration. Aliquots of the final suspension of microvessels are grown in culture medium containing Dulbecco's Modified Eagle Medium, 20% fetal calf serum, HEPES (25 mM), 13 mM sodium bicarbonate, 100 U/mL penicillin, and 1000 ug/mL streptomycin.

Oxide-filled renal preglomerular arterioles are seeded onto culture wells and within 3 to 4 days, SMCs are found to be proliferating from the explants. The SMCs displayed the following properties: 1) positive immuoreactivity to anti-smooth muscle α-actin, myosin and desmin, but not von Willebrand factor; 2) AII stimulation of DNA synthesis, proliferation, and c-fos expression; and 3) contraction to both AII and norepinephrine.

At confluence, a modification of the procedure of Aviv et al[257] is used to eradicate possible fibroblast contamination based on the greater avidity of fibroblasts to the culture dish than SMCs. Flasks are incubated with 0.01% trypsin in Hanks' balanced salt solution (without Ca^{2+} and Mg^{2+}) for 3 to 4 minutes, after which 75% to 80% of the trypsin solution is removed. After 10 additional minutes, fresh culture medium is added to the flasks and the cells are magnetically separated from the microvessels by agitation. The microvessel-free cell suspension is allowed to attach to a culture flask for 20 minutes at 37°C. SMCs (unattached cells) are aspirated and transferred to a separate flask and allowed to attach for 20 minutes again. The cells are subjected to this treatment four more times prior to the final plating of the cells.

Identification of Smooth Muscle Cells in Culture

In order to confirm the identity of SMCs in culture, there exist numerous requirements concerning their phase-contrast appearance, electron microscopic appearance, immunofluorescence reactivity to SMC-directed antisera, and functional properties that should be satisfied.[258] However, the hallmark used by most investigators is the growth of spindle-shaped cells in a hill-and-valley pattern coupled with the demonstration of positive immunofluorescence using a monoclonal antibody against smooth muscle α-actin.[259] Table 2 is a checklist of other SMC characteristics that, if confirmed, allow for more confidence in the identification of cultured cells as SMCs and not fibroblasts or some other cell type.

Many of the desired characteristics are based on differences between SMCs and fibroblasts. For in-

---

Table 2

I. Phase Contrast Appearance
  A. Spindle-shaped cells (hill and valley pattern)
  B. Oval nucleus with two or more nucleoli
  C. Phase dense cytoplasm
  D. Homogeneous cytoplasm; few visible inclusions

II. Immunofluorescence
  A. (+) Reactivity to anti-α-actin and γ-actin AB
  B. (+) Reactivity to smooth muscle anti-α-actin Ab
  C. (+) Reactivity to smooth muscle antimyosin Ab
  D. (+) Reactivity to smooth muscle antidesmin Ab

III. Electron Microscopic Appearance
  A. Defined basal lamina
  B. Plasmalemmal vesicles
  C. 100 Å filaments associated with dense bodies

IV. Functional Properties
  A. Heparin inhibition of proliferation
  B. Angiotensin II binding
  C. Contraction to angiotensin II/norepinephrine

stance, a defined basal lamina is characteristic of SMCs in vivo and in vitro, but is not present in fibroblasts.[258] It should be noted, however, that SMCs obtained via enzyme digestion lose their basal lamina for a few days.[258] A second distinguishing characteristic is the growth pattern of vascular SMCs compared to fibroblasts. SMCs typically grow in a hill-and-valley formation, whereas fibroblasts do not pile up in culture. Plasmalemmal vesicles are common to both SMCs and fibroblasts, but they appear as tracts in SMCs and singly in fibroblasts.[258] Finally, contractile filaments can be found in association with dense bodies in SMCs but not in fibroblasts.

α-Actin immunoreactivity is detected with monoclonal antisera directed against smooth muscle-derived α-actin. These antisera are available from many commercial sources. Two commonly used monoclonal antisera are from hybridomas HHF35 and CGA7 which recognize α and γ isoforms of actin from muscle (skeletal, cardiac, and smooth) and α and γ isoforms of smooth muscle, respectively. Antisera that solely recognize the α-actin isoform are also available commercially. We have successfully utilized clone no. 1A4 (Sigma Chemical Co., Cat. #A2547) to confirm the identity of SMCs in our laboratory. α-Actin immunoreactivity may be present, albeit weak, since α-actin content decreases in replicating SMCs.[259] However, even though staining intensity may be unimpressive, the population should display homogeneous positive reactivity. It is possible to complement α-actin staining with detection of either myosin or desmin in SMCs. A panel of antisera was studied by Dubey and colleagues,[136] in the study described above, to confirm the presence of SMCs in renal arterioles. In addition, it is advisable to perform a negative control with antisera against factor VIII to rule out endothelial cell contamination.

As described above, the demonstration of contractile properties associated with cultured vascular SMC is technically difficult and is not usually performed. A simpler assay for functional properties of SMCs is the demonstration of heparin inhibition of proliferation. However, we have experienced difficulty in reproducing the phenomenon in different primary cell lines from bovine aorta. The reason for this is not clear, but has been reported by other investigators. Based on the studies of Chan and colleagues, the sensitivity of human SMCs to heparin is a variable phenomenon that is inhibited in patients with restenosis as compared to normal patients.[260]

Smooth Muscle Medium

Dulbecco's Modified Eagle's minimal essential medium (DMEM) supplemented with 10% fetal calf serum and antibiotics constitutes the most commonly used medium for cultured vascular SMCs.[42] This is borne out in a random survey of 10 recent publications which examined different aspects of cultured SMC biology (Table 3). Another medium that is commonly utilized for growing SMCs in culture in Medium 199. However, before undertaking any study, it is critical to investigate the many ingredients of commercially available cell culture medium. For example, Medium 199 contains ATP which may be problematic if one wishes to study some aspect of adenine nucleotide metabolism in SMCs. In our laboratory, Dulbecco's Modified Eagle's Medium is the medium of choice for growing SMCs in culture. In contrast, we have observed that SMCs do not fare well in a 1 to 1 mixture of Dulbecco's Modified Eagle's Medium and Ham's F12, which is better suited for growing endothelial cells.

Dulbecco's Modified Eagle's Medium (Sigma

Table 3

Author	Reference	Medium	Serum	Supplements
Wang	250	DMEM	FCS (10%)	AB, G, B, H
Liau	145	M199	FCS (15%)	Ab, G
Berk	19	DMEM	FCS (10%)	Ab, G
Suga	237	DMEM	FBS (10%)	Ab
Kemp	124	M199	FCS (10%)	Ab, G
Goldberg	78	MEM	FCS (20%)	Ab, U, P
Kawamoto	123	M199	FCS (10%)	Ab
Tsuda	245	DMEM	FCS (10%)	Ab, G
Gibbons	75	DMEM/F12	FCS (10%)	Ab, G, U, H

DMEM: Dulbecco's Modified Eagle's Medium; F12: Ham's F12; M199: Medium 199; FCS; fetal calf serum; Ab: antibiotics (preferred concentrations = 100 U/mL penicillin and 100 μg/mL streptomycin); G: glutamine (preferred concentration = 2 mmol/L); U: glucose (0.9 mg/mL); P: pyruvate (6.6 μg/mL); H: Hepes (10 mmol/L).

Chemical Co., St. Louis: Cat. #D5530) is a complete formula that contains the following (g/L): 1) inorganic salts (calcium chloride (0.265), ferric nitrate (0.0001), magnesium sulfate (0.09767), potassium chloride (0.400), sodium bicarbonate (3.700), sodium chloride (6.400), and sodium phosphate monobasic (0.109); 2) amino acids (L-arginine (0.084), L-cysteine 0.0626), glycine (0.030), L-histidine (0.042), L-isoleucine (0.105), L-leucine (0.105), L-lysine (0.146), L-methionine (0.030), L-phenylalanine (0.066), L-serine (0.042), L-threonine (0.095), L-tryptophan (0.016), L-tyrosine (0.10379), and L-valine (0.094); 3) vitamins (choline chloride (0.004), folic acid (0.004), myoinositol (0.0072), niacinamide (0.004), D-pantothenic acid (0.004), riboflavin (0.0004), and thiamine (0.004); 4) other, D-glucose (4.5), phenol red (0.0159); 5) added glutamine (0.584). The final pH of the medium is 7.3 + 0.3 and the osmolality is 334 + 5%.

The selection of fetal bovine serum is a critical factor for the successful growth of SMCs in culture. Serum contains many molecules with both growth-promoting and growth-inhibiting activities that provide hormonal factors that stimulate cell growth and function, attachment and spreading factors and transport proteins that carry hormones, minerals, lipids, etc.[261] Major serum components include the following: 1) proteins (albumin, fibronectin, α_2-macroglobulin, fetuin, and transferrin); 2) polypeptides and growth factors (insulin, IGF-I and II, somatomedin A and C, multiplication stimulating activity, PDGF, EGF, FGF, EGF, eye-derived growth factor; 3) peptides (glutathione); 4) hormones (cortisol, estrogens, thyroid hormones); 5) lipids (linoleic acid, prostaglandins, cholesterol); 6) metabolites (amino acids, α-keto acids, polyamines; 7) minerals (Fe^{2+}, Zn^{2+}, Cu^{2+}, Mn^{2+}, SeO_3^{2+}, Co^{2+}).

The most obvious disadvantages of using serum for cell culture are the inherent differences between serum and the normal extracellular fluid that is in contact with the cell.[261] Second, serum contains cytotoxic elements such as bacterial toxins and lipids. Third, one must contend with lot-to-lot variation and must, therefore, carefully screen new lots as they become available. Fourth, serum may contain low levels of cell-specific growth factors that may need to be supplemented.[261]

In our laboratory, we use 10% heat-inactivated fetal calf serum (Hyclone Lab, Logan, Utah; Catalog #A-1111). This fetal calf serum is defined and has been tested negative for bacteria, fungus, virus, and mycoplasmas; endotoxin levels are < 10 EU/mL, hemoglobin concentration is < 10 mg/dL, and has been scanned electrophoretically. In addition, the fetal calf serum is prefiltered through 40 nm filters.

In the absence of serum, SMCs, or any diploid mammalian cell, will not grow in culture.[258] There is minimal growth at 0% to 0.5% serum, a significant in-

crease at 1% or 2.5% serum, and at 5%, 10%, and 20% serum, cells grow logarithmically for increasing periods of time.[258]

In the absence of injury or disease, SMCs do not proliferate to a great extent in the vascular wall. Therefore, attempts have been made to mimic the in vivo environment by providing a suitable quiescent medium for the growth of vascular SMCs in culture. In one study, Libby and O'Brien[262] found that supplementation of Dulbecco's Modified Eagle's Medium with insulin (10^{-6}M), selenium (10^{-9}M), transferrin (5 ug/mL), and ascorbic acid (10^{-4}M) was suitable to maintain SMCs in culture in a quiescent, noncatabolic state. Although transferrin and selenium had little or no effect on DNA or protein synthesis in this study, their use is recommended since they bind potentially toxic-heavy metal ions that may be present and enhance cell viability. DNA and protein synthesis decreased by greater than 50% in bovine aortic SMCs cultured for 3 days in the absence of supplements. However, in SMCs incubated for 3 days with insulin (10^{-6}M), transferrin (5 μg/mL) and ascorbate (0.2 mM) in the presence of the above-mentioned supplements, DNA and protein synthesis increased to levels comparable to those observed in the presence of 5% calf serum, but without an increase in cellular proliferation.[262]

Summary

The purpose of this chapter was to present an overview of cultured SMC biology. Major topics that have been outlined include the isolation and culturing of SMCs, phenotypic modulation of SMCs, SMC contraction, signal transduction pathways, SMC vasoactive agonists, growth factors, and hyperplasia versus hypertrophy. However, it should be emphasized, as described by Ross,[29] that SMC phenotype expression is controlled by a complex interaction between SMCs, circulating substances, and a number of other cell types including endothelial cells, macrophages, T-lymphocytes, and platelets.

References

1. Campbell GR, Campbell JH: The phenotypes of smooth muscle expressed in human atheroma. *Ann NY Acad Sci* 598:143–158, 1990.
2. Casscells W: Migration of smooth muscle and endothelial cells: critical events in restenosis. *Circulation* 86: 723–729, 1992.
3. Davies PF, Robotewsky A, Griem ML, Dull RO, Polacek DC: Hemodynamic forces and vascular cell communication in arteries. *Arch Pathol Lab Med* 116: 1301–1306, 1992.
4. Dzau VJ, Gibbons GH, Pratt RE: Molecular mechanisms of vascular renin-angiotensin system in myointi-

mal hyperplasia. *J Am Coll Cardiol* 18:II100-II105, 1991.

5. Hadrava V, Kruppa U, Russo RC, Lacourciere Y, Tremblay J, Hamet P: Vascular smooth muscle cell proliferation and its therapeutic modulation in hypertension. *Am Heart J* 122:1198–1203, 1991.

6. Ip JH, Fuster V, Badimon L, Badimon J, Taubman MB, Chesebro JH: Syndromes of accelerated atherosclerosis: role of vascular injury and smooth muscle proliferation. *J Am Coll Cardiol* 15:1667–1687, 1990.

7. Jackson CL, Schwartz SM: Pharmacology of smooth muscle replication. *Hypertension* 20:713–736, 1992.

8. Karnovsky MJ, Wright TC Jr, Castellot JJ Jr, Choay J, Lormeau JC: Heparin, heparan sulfate, smooth muscle cells, and atherosclerosis. *Ann NY Acad Sci* 556:268–281, 1989.

9. Libby P, Schwartz D, Brogi E, Tanaka H, Clinton SK: A cascade model for restenosis: a special case of atherosclerosis progression. *Circulation* 86:III47-III52, 1992.

10. Marks AR: Calcium channels expressed in vascular smooth muscle. *Circulation* 86:III61-III67, 1992.

11. Owens GK: Control of hypertrophic versus hyperplastic growth of vascular smooth muscle cells. *Am J Physiol* 257:H1755-H1765, 1989.

12. Raines EW, Ross R: Smooth muscle cells and the pathology of the lesions of atherosclerosis. *Br Heart J* 69:S30-S37, 1993.

13. Reidy MA: Factors controlling smooth-muscle proliferation. *Arch Pathol Lab Med* 116:1276–1280, 1992.

14. Reidy MA, Fingerle J, Lindner V: Factors controlling the development of arterial lesions after injury. *Circulation* 86:III43-III46, 1992.

15. Ross R, Masuda J, Raines EW: Cellular interactions, growth factors, and smooth muscle proliferation in atherogenesis. *Ann NY Acad Sci* 598:102–112, 1990.

16. Rhodin JAG: The cardiovascular system. Section 2: Circulation. In: Bohr DF, Somylo AP, Sparks HV Jr (eds). *Handbook of Physiology*. Vol II. Bethesda, MD: American Physiology Society; 1–31, 1980.

17. Cliff WJ: Blood vessels. In: Harrison RJ, McMinn RMH, Treherne JE (eds). *Biological Structure and Function*. Vol 6. Cambridge: Cambridge University Press; 214, 1976.

18. Cliff WJ: The aortic media in growing rats studied with the electron microscope. *Lab Inv* 17:599–615, 1967.

19. Cliff WJ: The aortic tunica media in aging rats. *Expt Mol Pharm* 13:172–189, 1970.

20. Cooke PH, Kargacin G, Craig R, Fogarty K, Fay FS: Molecular structure and organization of filaments in single, skinned smooth muscle cells. In: Siegman MJ, Somlyo AP, Stephens NL (eds). *Regulation and Contraction of Smooth Muscle*. New York: Alan R. Liss, Inc.; 1–25, 1987.

21. Bond M, Somlyo AV: Dense bodies and actin polarity in vertebrate smooth muscle. *J Cell Biol* 95:403–413, 1982.

22. Hathaway DR, March KL, Lash JA, Adam LP, Wilensky RL: Vascular smooth muscle: a review of the molecular basis of contractility. *Circulation* 83:382–390, 1991.

23. Adelstein RS, Sellers JR: Effects of calcium on vascular smooth muscle contraction. *Am J Cardiol* 59:4B-10B, 1987.

24. Sellers JR, Spudich JA, Sheetz MP: Light chain phosphorylation regulates the movement of smooth muscle myosin on actin filaments. *J Cell Biol* 101:1897–1902, 1985.

25. Lash JA, Critser ES, Pressler ML: Cloning of a gap junctional protein from vascular smooth muscle and expression in two-cell mouse embryos. *J Biol Chem* 265:13113–13117, 1990.

26. Blennerhassett MG, Kannan MS, Garfield RE: Functional characterization of cell-to-cell coupling in cultured rat aortic smooth muscle. *Am J Physiol* 252:C555-C569, 1987.

27. Clowes AW, Reidy MA, Clowes MM: Kinetics of cellular proliferation after arterial injury. *Lab Inv* 49:327–333, 1983.

28. Gordon D, Schwartz SM: Arterial smooth muscle differentiation. In: Campbell JH, Campbell GR (eds). *Vascular Smooth Muscle in Culture*. Boca Raton, FL: CRC Press; 1–14, 1987.

29. Ross R: The pathogenesis of atherosclerosis: a perspective for the 1990s. *Nature* 362:801–809, 1993.

30. Dillon PF, Aksoy MO, Driska SP, Murphy RA: Myosin phosphorylation and the cross-bridge cycle in arterial smooth muscle. *Science* 211:495–497, 1981.

31. Khalil RA, Morgan KG: Protein kinase C: a second E-C coupling pathway in vascular smooth muscle? *NIPS* 7:10–15, 1992.

32. Bradley AB, Morgan KG: Alterations in cytoplasmic calcium sensitivity during porcine coronary artery contractions as detected by aequorin. *J Physiol Lond* 385:437–448, 1987.

33. Collins EM, Walsh MP, Morgan KG: Contraction of single vascular smooth muscle cells by phenylephrine at constant [Ca^{2+}]$_i$. *Am J Physiol* 252:H754-H762, 1992.

34. Jiang MJ, Morgan KG: Agonist-specific myosin phosphorylation and intracellular calcium during isometric contractions of arterial smooth muscle. *Pfluegers Arch* 413:637–643, 1989.

35. Park S, Rasmussen H: Carbachol-induced protein phosphorylation changes in bovine tracheal smooth muscle. *J Biol Chem* 261:15734–15739, 1986.

36. Thyberg J, Hedin U, Sjolund M, Palmberg L, Bottger BA: Regulation of differentiated properties and proliferation of arterial smooth muscle cells. *Arteriosclerosis* 10:966–990, 1990.

37. Campbell JH, Campbell GR: *Vascular Smooth Muscle in Culture*. Boca Raton, FL: CRC Press, Inc.; 39–55, 1987.

38. Campbell GR, Campbell JH, Manderson JA, Horrigan S, Rennick RE: Arterial smooth muscle: a multifunctional mesenchymal cell. *Arch Pathol Lab Med* 112:977–986, 1988.

39. Chamley-Campbell JH, Campbell GR: What controls smooth muscle phenotype? *Atherosclerosis* 40:347–357, 1981.

40. Moose PRL, Campbell GR, Wang ZL, Campbell JH: Smooth muscle phenotypic expression in human carotid arteries. I. Comparison of cells from diffuse intimal thickenings adjacent to atheromatous plaques with those of the media. *Lab Inv* 53:556–562, 1985.

41. Gabbiani G, Kocher O, Bloom WS, Vandederckhove J, Weber K: Actin expression in smooth muscle cells of rat aortic intimal thickening, human atheromatous plaque, and cultured rat aortic media. *J Clin Inv* 73:148–152, 1984.

42. Campbell JH, Campbell GR: Methods of growing vascular smooth muscle cells in culture. In: Campbell JH, Campbell GR (eds). *Vascular Smooth Muscle in Culture*. Boca Raton, FL: CRC Press; 15–21, 1987.

43. Chamley JH, Campbell GR: Mitosis of contractile smooth muscle cells in tissue culture. *Exp Cell Res* 84:105–110, 1974.

44. Kamm KE, Hsu L, Kubota Y, Stull JT: Phosphorylation of smooth muscle myosin heavy and light chains: effects of phorbol dibutyrate and agonists. *J Biol Chem* 264:21223–21229, 1989.

45. Larson DM, Fujiwara K, Alexander RW, Gimbrone MA Jr: Heterogeneity of myosin antigenic expression in vascular smooth muscle in vivo. *Lab Inv* 50:401–407, 1984.

46. Kawamoto S, Adelstein RS: Characterization of myosin heavy chains in cultured aorta smooth muscle cells. *J Biol Chem* 262:7282–7288, 1987.

47. Rovner AS, Murphy RA, Owens GK: Expression of smooth muscle and nonmuscle myosin heavy chains in cultured vascular smooth muscle cells. *J Biol Chem* 261:14740–14745, 1986.

48. Grainger DJ, Hesketh TR, Metcalfe JC, Weissberg PL: A large accumulation of nonmuscle myosin occurs at first entry into M phase in rat vascular smooth muscle cells. *Biochem J* 277:145–151, 1991.

49. Kemp PR, Grainger DJ, Shanahan CM, Weissberg PL, Metcalfe JC: The Id gene is activated by serum but is not required for de-differentiation in rat vascular smooth muscle cells. *Biochem J* 277:285–288, 1991.

50. Owens GK, Loeb A, Gordon D, Thompson MM: Expression of smooth muscle-specific à-isoactin in cultured vascular smooth muscle cells: relationship between growth and cytodifferentiation. *J Cell Biology* 102:343–352, 1979.

51. Strauch AR, Rubenstein PA: Induction of vascular smooth muscle à-isoactin expression in BC$_3$H1 cells. *J Biol Chem* 259:3152–3159, 1984.

52. Corjay MH, Thompson MM, Lynch KR, Owens GK: Differential effect of platelet-derived growth factor-versus serum-induced growth on smooth muscle α-actin and nonmuscle β-actin mRNA expression in cultured rat aortic smooth muscle cells. *J Biol Chem* 264:10501–10506, 1989.

53. Allen JC, Navran SS, Seidel CL, Dennison DK, Amann JM, Jemelka SK: Intracellular Na$^+$ regulation of Na$^+$ pump sites in cultured vascular smooth muscle cells. *Am J Physiol* 256:C786-C792, 1989.

54. Feltes TF, Seidel CL, Dennison DK, Amick S, Allen JC: Relationship between functional Na$^+$ pumps and mitogenesis in cultured coronary artery smooth muscle cells. *Am J Physiol* 264:C169-C178, 1993.

55. Suga S-I, Nakao K, Kishimoto I, et al: Phenotype-related alteration in expression of natriuretic peptide receptors in aortic smooth muscle cells. *Circ Res* 71:34–39, 1992.

56. Cahill PA, Hassid A: Clearance receptor-binding atrial natriuretic peptides inhibit mitogenesis and proliferation of rat aortic smooth muscle cells. *Biochem Biophys Res Comm* 179:1606–1613, 1991.

57. Corson MA, Alexander RW, Berk BC: 5-HT$_2$ receptor mRNA is overexpressed in cultured rat aortic smooth muscle cells relative to normal aorta. *Am J Physiol* 262:C309-C315, 1992.

58. Hedin U, Bottger BA, Forsberg E, Johansson S, Thyberg J: Diverse effects of fibronectin and laminin on phenotypic properties of cultured arterial smooth muscle cells. *J Cell Biol* 107:307–319, 1988.

59. Liau G, Chan LM: Regulation of extracellular matrix RNA levels in cultured smooth muscle cells: relationship to cellular quiescence. *J Biol Chem* 264:10315–10320, 1989.

60. LeBaron RG, Hook A, Esko JD, Gay S, Hook M: Binding of heparin sulfate to Type V collagen: a mechanism of cell-substrate adhesion. *J Biol Chem* 264:7950–7956, 1989.

61. Scott-Burden T, Resink TJ, Burgin M, Buhler F: Extracellular matrix: differential influence on growth and biosynthesis patterns of vascular smooth muscle cells from SHR and WKY rats. *J Cell Physiol* 141:267–274, 1989.

62. Merrilees MJ: Synthesis of glycosaminoglycans and proteoglycans. In: Campbell JH, Campbell GR (eds). *Vascular Smooth Muscle in Culture*. Boca Raton, FL: CRC Press; 133–152, 1987.

63. Salisbury BGJ, Wagner WD: Isolation and preliminary characterization of proteoglycans dissociatively extracted from human aorta. *J Biol Chem* 256:8050–8057, 1981.

64. Wight TN: Cell biology of arterial proteoglycans. *Arteriosclerosis* 9:1–20, 1989.

65. Hamati HF, Britton EL, Carey DJ: Inhibition of proteoglycan synthesis alters extracellular matrix deposition, proliferation, and cytoskeletal organization of rat aortic smooth muscle cells in culture. *J Cell Biol* 108:2495–2505, 1989.

66. Hedin U, Holm J, Hansson GK: Induction of tenascin in rat arterial injury: relationship to altered smooth muscle cell phenotype. *Am J Pathol* 139:649–656, 1991.

67. Sharifi BG, LaFleur DW, Pirola CJ, Forrester JS, Fagin JA: Angiotensin II regulates tenascin gene expression in vascular smooth muscle cells. *J Biol Chem* 267:23910–23915, 1992.

68. Watanabe Y, Usuda N, Tsugane S, Kobayashi R, Hidaka H: Calvasculin, an encoded protein from mRNA termed pEL-98, 18A2, 42A, or p9Ka, is secreted by smooth muscle cells in culture and exhibits Ca^{2+}-dependent binding to 35-kDa microfibril-associated glycoprotein. *J Biol Chem* 267:17136–17140, 1992.

69. Stadler E, Campbell JH, Campbell GR: Do cultured vascular smooth muscle cells resemble those of the artery wall? If not, why not? *J Cardiovasc Pharm* (suppl 6)14:S1-S8, 1989.

70. Warshaw DM, McBride WJ, Work SS: Corkscrew-like shortening in single smooth muscle cells. *Science* 236:1457–1459, 1987.

71. Murray TR, Marshall BE, Macarak EJ: Contraction of vascular smooth muscle in cell culture. *J Cell Physiol* 143:26–38, 1990.

72. Gunther S, Alexander RW, Atkinson WJ, Gimbrone MA: Functional angiotensin II receptors in cultured vascular smooth muscle cells. *J Cell Biol* 92:289–298, 1982.

73. Lobaugh LA, Blackshear PJ: Neuropeptide Y stimulation of myosin light chain phosphorylation in cultured aortic smooth muscle cells. *J Biol Chem* 265:18393–18399, 1990.

74. Dorn GW 2d, Becker MW, Davis MG: Dissociation of the contractile and hypertrophic effects of vasoconstrictor prostanoids in vascular smooth muscle. *J Biol Chem* 267:24897–24905, 1992.

75. Sasaki Y, Seto M, Komatsu K-I: Diphosphorylation of myosin light chain in smooth muscle cells in culture: possible involvement of protein kinase C. *FEBS Lett* 276:161–164, 1990.

76. Rasmussen H: The complexities of intracellular Ca^{2+} signalling. *Biol Chem* 371:191–206, 1990.

77. Nelson MT, Patlak JB, Worley JF, Standen NB: Calcium channels, potassium channels, and voltage dependence of arterial smooth muscle tone. *Am J Physiol* 259:C3-C18, 1990.

78. Somlyo AV, Bond M, Somlyo AP, Scarpa A: Inositol

trisphosphate-induced calcium release and contraction in vascular smooth muscle. *Proc Natl Acad Sci* 82: 5231–5235, 1985.

79. Hashimoto T, Hirata M, Itoh T, Kanmura Y, Kuriyama H: Inositol 1,4,5-trisphosphate activates pharmaco-mechanical coupling in smooth muscle of the rabbit mesenteric artery. *J Physiol Lond* 370:605–618, 1986.

80. Yamamoto H, van Breemen C: Inositol-1,4,5-trisphosphate releases calcium from skinned cultured smooth muscle cells. *Biochem Biophys Res Comm* 130: 270–274, 1985.

81. Smith JB, Smith L, Higgins BL: Temperature and nucleotide dependence of calcium release by *myo*-inositol 1,4,5-trisphosphate in cultured vascular smooth muscle cells. *J Biol Chem* 260:14413–14416, 1985.

82. Berman DM, Goldman WF: Stored calcium modulates inositol phosphate synthesis in cultured smooth muscle cells. *Am J Physiol* 263:C535-C539, 1992.

83. Ashida T, Schaeffer J, Goldman WF, Wade JB, Blaustein MP: Role of sarcoplasmic reticulum in arterial contraction: comparison of ryanodine's effect in a conduit and a muscular artery. *Circ Res* 62:854–863, 1988.

84. Nelson MT, Standen NB, Brayden JE, Worley JF: Noradrenaline contracts arteries by activating voltage-dependent calcium channels. *Nature* 336:382–385, 1988.

85. van Breeman C, Saida K: Cellular mechanisms regulating [Ca^{2+}]$_i$ smooth muscle. *Ann Rev Physiol* 51: 315–329, 1989.

86. Benham CD, Tsien RW: A novel receptor-operated Ca^{2+}-permeable channel activated by ATP in smooth muscle. *Nature* 328:275–278, 1987.

87. Nabel EG, Berk BC, Brock TA, Smith TW: Na$^+$-Ca^{2+} exchange in cultured vascular smooth muscle cells. *Circ Res* 62:486–493, 1988.

88. Reynolds EE, Dubyak GR: Activation of calcium mobilization and calcium influx by alpha$_1$-adrenergic receptors in a smooth muscle cell line. *Biochem Biophys Res Comm* 130:627–632, 1985.

89. Asaoka Y, Nakamura S, Yoshida K, Nishizuka Y: Protein kinase C, calcium, and phospholipid degradation. *TIBS* 17:414–417, 1992.

90. Khalil RA, Morgan KG: Imaging of protein kinase C distribution and translocation in living vascular smooth muscle cells. *Circ Res* 69:1626–1631, 1991.

91. Khalil RA, Lajoie C, Resnick M, Morgan KG: Ca^{2+}-independent isoforms of protein kinase C differentially translocate in smooth muscle. *Am J Physiol* 263:C714-C719, 1992.

92. Caramelo C, Okada K, Tsai P, Schrier RW: Phorbol esters and arginine vasopressin in vascular smooth muscle cell activation. *Am J Physiol* 256:F875-F881, 1989.

93. Minami K, Fukuzawa K, Nakaya Y: Protein kinase C inhibits the Ca^{2+}-activated K$^+$ channel of cultured porcine coronary artery smooth muscle cells. *Biochem Biophys Res Comm* 190:263–269, 1993.

94. Fish RD, Sperti G, Colucci WS, Clapham DE: Phorbol ester increases the dihydropyridine-sensitive calcium conductance in a vascular smooth muscle cell line. *Circ Res* 62:1049–1054, 1988.

95. Kato H, Hayashi T, Koshino Y, Kutsumi Y, Nakai T, Miyabo S: Glucocorticoids increase Ca^{2+} influx through dihydropyridine-sensitive channels linked to activation of protein kinase C in vascular smooth muscle cells. *Biochem Biophys Res Comm* 188:934–941, 1992.

96. Natarajan R, Gonzales N, Xu L, Nadler JL: Vascular smooth muscle cells exhibit increased growth in response to elevated glucose. *Biochem Biophys Res Comm* 187:552–560, 1992.

97. Berk BC, Brock TA, Gimbrone MA, Alexander RW: Early agonist-mediated ionic events in cultured vascular smooth muscle cells. *J Biol Chem* 262:5065–5072, 1987.

98. Mitsuka M, Berk BC: Long-term regulation of Na$^+$-H$^+$ exchange in vascular smooth muscle cells: role of protein kinase C. *Am J Physiol* 260:C562-C569, 1991.

99. Lowe JHN, Huang C-L, Ives HE: Sphingosine differentially inhibits activation of the Na$^+$/H$^+$ exchanger by phorbol esters and growth factors. *J Biol Chem* 265: 7188–7194, 1990.

100. Weiss RH, Huang CL, Ives HE: Shingosine reverses growth inhibition caused by activation of protein kinase C in vascular smooth muscle cells. *J Cell Physiol* 149: 307–312, 1991.

101. Huang CL, Ives HE: Growth inhibition by protein kinase C late in mitogenesis. *Nature* 329:849–850, 1987.

102. Kariya K-I, Fukumoto Y, Tsuda T, et al: Antiproliferative action of protein kinase C in cultured rabbit aortic smooth muscle cells. *Expt Cell Res* 173:504–514, 1987.

103. Dempsey EC, McMurtry IF, O'Brien RF: Protein kinase C activation allows pulmonary artery smooth muscle cells to proliferate to hypoxia. *Am J Physiol* 260: L136-L145, 1991.

104. Nishizuka Y: Intracellular signaling by hydrolysis of phospholipids and activation of protein kinase C. *Science* 258:607–614, 1992.

105. Konishi F, Kondo T, Inagami T: Phospholipase D in cultured rat vascular smooth muscle cells and its activation by phorbol ester. *Biochem Biophys Res Comm* 179: 1070–1076, 1991.

106. Welsh CJ, Schmeichel K, McBride K: Platelet-derived growth factor activates phospholipase D and chemotactic responses in vascular smooth muscle cells. *Cell Dev Biol* 27A:425–431, 1991.

107. Welsh CJ, Schmeichel K, Cao H, Chabbott H: Vasopressin stimulates phospholipase D activity against phosphatidylcholine in vascular smooth muscle cells. *Lipids* 25:675–684, 1990.

108. Weiss RH, Nuccitelli R: Inhibition of tyrosine phosphorylation prevents thrombin-induced mitogenesis, but not intracellular free calcium release, in vascular smooth muscle cells. *J Biol Chem* 267:5608–5613, 1992.

109. Williams LT: Signal transduction by the platelet-derived growth factor receptor. *Science* 243:1564–1569, 1989.

110. Molloy CJ, Taylor DS, Weber H: Angiotensin II stimulation of rapid protein tyrosine phosphorylation and protein kinase activation in rat aortic smooth muscle cells. *J Biol Chem* 268:7338–7345, 1993.

111. Tsuda T, Kawahara Y, Shii K, Koide M, Ishida Y, Yokoyama M: Vasoconstrictor-induced protein-tyrosine phosphorylation in cultured vascular smooth muscle cells. *FEBS Lett* 285:44–48, 1991.

112. Wijetunge S, Aalkjaer C, Schachter M, Hughes AD: Tyrosine kinase inhibitors block calcium channel currents in vascular smooth muscle cells. *Biochem Biophys Res Comm* 189:1620–1623, 1992.

113. Hepler JR, Gilman AG: G proteins. *TIBS* 17:383–387, 1992.

114. Karin M, Smeal T: Control of transcription factors by signal transduction pathways: the beginning of the end. *TIBS* 17:418–422, 1992.

115. Sellers JR, Adelstein RS: *The Enzymes*. Orlando, Fl:

Academic Press, Inc.; 381–418, 1987. (Boyer PD, Krebs EG, ed. ; vol 18).

116. Scheid CR, Fay FS: β-Adrenergic effects on transmembrane ^{45}Ca fluxes in isolated smooth muscle cells. *Am J Physiol* 246:C431-C438, 1984.

117. Jonzon B, Nilsson J, Fredholm BB: Adenosine receptor-mediated changes in cyclic AMP production and DNA synthesis in cultured arterial smooth muscle cells. *J Cell Physiol* 124:451–456, 1985.

118. Liau G, Chan LM, Feng P: Increased ferritin gene expression is both promoted by cAMP and a marker of growth arrest in rabbit vascular smooth muscle cells. *J Biol Chem* 266:18819–18826, 1991.

119. Koyama N, Morisaki N, Saito Y, Yoshida S: Regulatory effects of platelet-derived growth factor-AA homodimer on migration of vascular smooth muscle cells. *J Biol Chem* 267:22806–22812, 1992.

120. Middleton B, Middleton A: Cyclic AMP stimulates the synthesis and function of the low-density lipoprotein receptor in human vascular smooth-muscle cells and fibroblasts. *Biochem J* 282:853–861, 1992.

121. Mills I, Letsou G, Rabban J, Sumpio BE, Gewirtz H: Mechanosensitive adenylate cyclase activity in coronary artery vascular smooth muscle. *Biochem Biophys Res Comm* 171:143–147, 1990.

122. Wiersbitzky M, Mills I, Gewirtz H: Stretch-induced reduction in G protein steady state levels in coronary vascular smooth muscle cells. *FASEB J* 5:A1394, 1991.

123. Kubalak SW, Webb JG: Angiotensin II enhancement of hormone-stimulated cAMP formation in cultured vascular smooth muscle cells. *Am J Physiol* 264:H86-H96, 1993.

124. Lincoln TM, Cornwell TL, Taylor AE: cGMP-dependent protein kinase mediates the reduction of Ca^{2+} by cAMP in vascular smooth muscle cells. *Am J Physiol* 258:C399-C407, 1990.

125. Slakey LL, Gordon EL, Pearson JD: A comparison of ectonucleotidase activities on vascular endothelial and smooth muscle cells. *Ann NY Acad Sci* 603:366–378, 1990.

126. Malam-Souley R, Campan M, Gadeau A-P, Desgranges C: Exogenous ATP induces a limited cell cycle progression of arterial smooth muscle cells. *Am J Physiol* 264:C783-C788, 1993.

127. Wang D, Huang N, Heppel LA: Extracellular ATP and ADP stimulate proliferation of porcine aortic smooth muscle cells. *J Cell Physiol* 153:221–233, 1992.

128. Hillis LD, Lange RA: Serotonin and acute ischemic heart disease. *N Engl J Med* 324:688–690, 1991.

129. Nemecek GM, Coughlin SR, Handley DA, Moskowitz MA: Stimulation of aortic smooth muscle cell mitogenesis by serotonin. *Proc Natl Acad Sci USA* 83:674–678, 1986.

130. Kavanaugh WM, Williams LT, Ives HE, Coughlin SR: Serotonin-induced deoxyribonucleic acid synthesis in vascular smooth muscle cells involves a novel, pertussis toxin-sensitive pathway. *Mol Endocrinol* 2:599–605, 1988.

131. Lee SL, Wang WW, Moore BJ, Fanburg BL: Dual effect of serotonin on growth of bovine pulmonary artery smooth muscle cells in culture. *Circ Res* 68:1362–1368, 1991.

132. Lee SL, Dunn J, Yu FS, Fanburg BL: Serotonin uptake and configurational change of bovine pulmonary artery smooth muscle cells in culture. *J Cell Physiol* 138:145–153, 1989.

133. Re R, Fallon JT, Dzau V, Quay SC, Haber E: Renin synthesis by canine aortic smooth muscle cells in culture. *Life Sci* 30:99–106, 1982.

134. Lilly LS, Pratt RE, Alexander RW, et al: Renin expression by vascular endothelial cells in culture. *Circ Res* 57:312–318, 1985.

135. Anderson KM, Murahashi T, Dostal DE, Peach MJ: Morphological and biochemical analysis of angiotensin II internalization in cultured rat aortic smooth muscle cells. *Am J Physiol* 264:C179-C188, 1993.

136. Dubey RK, Roy A, Overbeck HW: Culture of renal arteriolar smooth muscle cells: mitogenic responses to angiotensin II. *Circ Res* 71:1143–1152, 1992.

137. Gunther S, Gimbrone MA Jr, Alexander RW: Identification and characterization of the high affinity vascular angiotensin II receptor in rat mesenteric artery. *Circ Res* 47:278–286, 1980.

138. Brock TA, Alexander RW, Ekstein LS, Atkinson WJ, Gimbrone MA: Angiotensin increases cytosolic free calcium in cultured vascular smooth muscle cells. *Hypertension* (suppl I)7:I-105-I-109, 1985.

139. Nabika T, Velletri PA, Lovenberg W, Beaven MA: Increase in cytosolic calcium and phosphoinositide metabolism induced by angiotensin II and [Arg]vasopressin in vascular smooth muscle cells. *J Biol Chem* 260:4661–4670, 1985.

140. Lang U, Vallotton MB: Effects of angiotensin II and of phorbol ester on protein kinase C activity and on prostacyclin production in cultured rat aortic smooth-muscle cells. *Biochem J* 259:477–484, 1989.

141. Hatori N, Fine BP, Nakamura A, Cragoe E, Aviv A: Angiotensin II effect on cytosolic rat vascular smooth muscle cells. *J Biol Chem* 262:5073–5078, 1987.

142. Pfeilschifter J, Ochsner M, Whitebread S, De Gasparo M: Down-regulation of protein kinase C potentiates angiotensin II-stimulated phosphoinositide hydrolysis in vascular smooth-muscle cells. *Biochem J* 26:285–291, 1989.

143. Tsuda T, Alexander RW: Angiotensin II stimulates phosphorylation of nuclear lamins via a protein kinase C-dependent mechanism in cultured vascular smooth muscle cells. *J Biol Chem* 265:1165–1170, 1990.

144. Pirola CJ, Wang H, Kamyar A, et al: Angiotensin II regulates parathyroid hormone-related protein expression in cultured rat aortic smooth muscle cells through transcriptional and post-translational mechanisms. *J Biol Chem* 268:1987–1994, 1993.

145. Takeuchi K, Nakamura N, Cook NS, Pratt RE, Dzau VJ: Angiotensin II can regulate gene expression by the AP-1 binding sequence via a protein kinase C-dependent pathway. *Biochem Biophys Res Comm* 172:1189–1194, 1990.

146. Griendling KK, Delafontaine P, Rittenhouse SE, Gimbrone MA Jr, Alexander RW: Correlation of receptor sequestration with sustained diacylglycerol accumulation in angiotensin II-stimulated cultured vascular smooth muscle cells. *J Biol Chem* 262:14555–14562, 1987.

147. Low BC, Ross IK, Grigor MR: Angiotensin II stimulates glucose transport activity in cultured vascular smooth muscle cells. *J Biol Chem* 267:20740–20745, 1993.

148. Berk BC, Vekshtein V, Gordon HM, Tsuda T: Angiotensin II-stimulated protein synthesis in cultured vascular smooth muscle cells. *Hypertension* 13:305–314, 1989.

149. Gibbons GH, Pratt RE, Dzau VJ: Vascular smooth muscle cell hypertrophy versus hyperplasia: autocrine

transforming growth factor-β_1 expression determines growth response to angiotensin II. *J Clin Inv* 90: 456–461, 1992.

150. Campbell-Boswell M, Robertson AL Jr: Effects of angiotensin II and vasopressin on human smooth muscle cells in vitro. *Exp Molec Pathol* 35:265–276, 1981.

151. Tseng H, Berk BC: The Na/K/2Cl cotransporter is increased in hypertrophied vascular smooth muscle cells. *J Biol Chem* 267:8161–8167, 1992.

152. Duff JL, Berk BC, Corson MA: Angiotensin II stimulates the pp44 and pp42 mitogen-activated protein kinases in cultured rat aortic smooth muscle cells. *Biochem Biophys Res Comm* 188:257–264, 1992.

153. Naftilan AJ, Pratt RE, Dzau VJ: Induction of platelet-derived growth factor A-chain and c-*myc* gene expressions by angiotensin II in cultured rat vascular smooth muscle cells. *J Clin Inv* 83:1419–1424, 1989.

154. Nakahara K, Nishimura H, Kuro-o M, et al: Identification of three types of PDGF-A chain gene transcripts in rabbit vascular smooth muscle and their regulated expression during development and by angiotensin II. *Biochem Biophys Res Comm* 184:811–818, 1992.

155. Gibbons GH, Pratt RE, Dzau VJ: Angiotensin II is a bifunctional vascular smooth muscle cell growth factor. *Hypertension* 14:358a, 1989.

156. Owens GK, Geisterfer AAT, Yang YW-H, Komoriya A: Transforming growth factor-beta-induced growth inhibition and cellular hypertrophy in cultured vascular smooth muscle cells. *J Cell Biol* 107:771–780, 1988.

157. Itoh H, Mukoyama M, Pratt RE, Gibbons GH, Dzau VJ: Multiple autocrine growth factors modulate vascular smooth muscle cell growth response to angiotensin II. *J Clin Inv* 91:2268–2274, 1993.

158. Luscher TF: Endothelin: systemic arterial and pulmonary effects of a new peptide with potent biologic properties. *Am Rev Respir Dis* 146:S56-S60, 1992.

159. Clozel M, Fischli W, Guilly C: Specific binding of endothelin on human vascular smooth muscle cells in culture. *J Clin Inv* 83:1758–1761, 1989.

160. Hirata Y, Yoshimi H, Takata S, et al: Cellular mechanism of action by a novel vasoconstrictor endothelin in cultured rat vascular smooth muscle cells. *Biochem Biophys Res Comm* 154:868–875, 1988.

161. Nishimura J, Chen X, Jahan H, Shikasho T, Kobayashi S, Kanaide H: cAMP induces up-regulation of ETA receptor mRNA and increases responsiveness to endothelin-1 of rat aortic smooth muscle cells in primary culture. *Biochem Biophys Res Comm* 188:719–726, 1992.

162. Gardner JP, Tokudome G, Tomonari H, Maher E, Hollander D, Aviv A: Endothelin-induced calcium responses in human vascular smooth muscle cells. *Am J Physiol* 262:C148-C155, 1992.

163. Araki S-I, Kawahara Y, Kariya K-I, Sunako M, Fukuzaki H, Takai Y: Stimulation of phospholipase C-mediated hydrolysis of phosphoinositides by endothelin in cultured rabbit aortic smooth muscle cells. *Biochem Biophys Res Comm* 159:1072–1079, 1989.

164. Jaiswal RK: Endothelin inhibits the atrial natriuretic factor stimulated cGMP production by activating the protein kinase C in rat aortic smooth muscle cells. *Biochem Biophys Res Comm* 182:395–402, 1992.

165. Little PJ, Neylon CB, Tkachuk VA, Bobik A: Endothelin-1 and endothelin-3 stimulate calcium mobilization by different mechanisms in vascular smooth muscle. *Biochem Biophys Res Comm* 183:694–700, 1992.

166. Muldoon LL, Rodland KD, Forsythe ML, Magun BE: Stimulation of phosphatidylinositol hydrolysis, diacylglycerol release, and gene expression in response to endothelin, a potent new agonist for fibroblasts and smooth muscle cells. *J Biol Chem* 264:8529–8536, 1989.

167. Miasiro N, Yamamoto H, Kanaide H, Nakamura M: Does endothelin mobilize calcium from intracellular store sites in rat aortic vascular smooth muscle cells in primary cultures? *Biochem Biophys Res Comm* 156: 312–317, 1988.

168. Komuro I, Kurihara H, Sugiyama T, Takaku F, Yazaki Y: Endothelin stimulates c-fos and c-myc expression and proliferation of vascular smooth muscle cells. *FEBS Lett* 238:249–252, 1988.

169. Han C, Li J, Minneman KP: Subtypes of α_1-adrenoceptors in rat blood vessels. *Eur J Pharmacol* 190:97–104, 1990.

170. Han C, Abel PW, Minneman KP: α_1-Adrenoceptor subtypes linked to different mechanisms for increasing intracellular Ca^{2+} in smooth muscle. *Nature* 329: 333–336, 1987.

171. Colucci WS, Black TA, Gimbrone MA, Alexander RW: Regulation of alpha-adrenergic receptor coupled calcium flux in cultured vascular smooth muscle cells. *Hypertension* 6:119–124, 1984.

172. Colucci WS, Gimbrone MA Jr, Alexander RW: Phorbol diester modulates α-adrenergic receptor-coupled calcium efflux and α-adrenergic receptor number in cultured vascular smooth muscle cells. *Circ Res* 58: 393–398, 1986.

173. Izzo NJ, Seidman CE, Collins S, Colucci WS: α_1-Adrenergic receptor mRNA level is regulated by norepinephrine in rabbit aortic smooth muscle cells. *Proc Natl Acad Sci USA* 87:6268–6271, 1990.

174. Mills DE, Buckman MT, Peake GT: Neonatal treatment with antiserum to prolactin lowers blood pressure in rats. *Science* 217:162–164, 1982.

175. Buckley AR, Putnam CW, Russell DH: Rapid elevation of plasminogen activator activity in rat tissues by prolactin. *Biochem Biophys Res Comm* 122:1005–1011, 1984.

176. Sauro MD, Zorn NE: Prolactin induces proliferation of vascular smooth muscle cells through a protein kinase C-dependent mechanism. *J Cell Physiol* 148:133–138, 1991.

177. Montgomery DW, Zukoski CF, Shah GN, et al: Concanavalin A-stimulated murine splenocytes produce a factor with prolactin-like bioactivity and immunoreactivity. *Biochem Biophys Res Comm* 145:692–698, 1987.

178. Inagami T: Atrial natriuretic factor. *J Biol Chem* 264: 3043–3046, 1989.

179. Itoh H, Pratt RE, Dzau VJ: Atrial natriuretic polypeptide inhibits hypertrophy of vascular smooth muscle cells. *J Clin Inv* 86:1690–1697, 1990.

180. Kawabe J-I, Ohsaki Y, Onodera S: Down-regulation of protein kinase C potentiates atrial natriuretic peptide-stimulated cGMP accumulation in vascular smooth muscle cells. *Biochim Biophys Acta* 1175:81–87, 1992.

181. Itoh H, Pratt RE, Ohno M, Dzau VJ: Atrial natriuretic polypeptide as a novel antigrowth factor of endothelial cells. *Hypertension* 19:758–761, 1992.

182. Guyton J, Rosenberg R, Clowes A, Karnovsky MJ: Inhibition of rat arterial smooth muscle cell proliferation by heparin. I. In vivo studies with anticoagulant and nonanticoagulant heparin. *Circ Res* 46:625–634, 1980.

183. Hoover RL, Rosenberg R, Haering W, Karnovsky MJ: Inhibition of rat arterial smooth muscle cell prolifera-

tion by heparin. II. In vitro studies. *Circ Res* 47: 578–583, 1980.

184. Majack RA, Clowes A: Inhibition of vascular smooth muscle cell migration by heparin-like glycosaminoglycans. *J Cell Physiol* 118:253–256, 1984.

185. Castellot JJ Jr, Addonizio ML, Rosenberg R, Karnovsky MJ: Cultured endothelial cells produce a heparinlike inhibitor of smooth muscle cell growth. *J Cell Biol* 90:372–379, 1981.

186. Fritze LMS, Reilly CF, Rosenberg RD: An antiproliferative heparan sulfate species produced by postconfluent smooth muscle cells. *J Cell Biol* 100:1041–1049, 1985.

187. Reilly CF, Kindy MS, Brown KE, Rosenberg RD, Sonenshein GE: Heparin prevents vascular smooth muscle cell progression through the G_1 phase of the cell cycle. *J Biol Chem* 264:6990–6995, 1989.

188. Pukac LA, Ottlinger ME, Karnovsky MJ: Heparin suppresses specific second messenger pathways for protooncogene expression in rat vascular smooth muscle cells. *J Biol Chem* 267:3707–3711, 1992.

189. Wright TC Jr, Pukac LA, Castellot JJ Jr, et al: Heparin suppresses the induction of c-fos and c-myc mRNA in murine fibroblasts by selective inhibition of a protein kinase C-dependent pathway. *Proc Natl Acad Sci USA* 86:3199–3203, 1989.

190. Au YPT, Kenagy RD, Clowes AW: Heparin selectively inhibits the transcription of tissue-type plasminogen activator in primate arterial smooth muscle cells during mitogenesis. *J Biol Chem* 267:3438–3444, 1992.

191. Coughlin SR, Vu TH, Hung DT, Wheaton VI: Characterization of a functional thrombin receptor. *J Clin Inv* 89:351–355, 1992.

192. Vu TH, Hung DT, Wheaton VI, Coughlin SR: Molecular cloning of a functional thrombin receptor reveals a novel proteolytic mechanism of receptor activation. *Cell* 64:1057–1068, 1991.

193. Berk BC, Taubman MB, Griendling KK, Cragoe EJ Jr, Fenton JW, Brock TA: Thrombin-stimulated events in cultured vascular smooth muscle cells. *Biochem J* 274: 799–805, 1991.

194. Noda-Heiny H, Fugii S, Sobel B: Induction of vascular smooth muscle cell expression of plasminogen activator inhibitor-1 by thrombin. *Circ Res* 72:36–43, 1993.

195. Hansson GK, Jonasson L, Holm J, Clowes MM, Clowes AW: τ-Interferon regulates vascular smooth muscle proliferation and Ia antigen expression in vivo and in vitro. *Circ Res* 63:712–719, 1988.

196. Garg UC, Hassid A: Nitric oxide-generating vasodilators and 8-bromo-cyclic guanosine monophosphate inhibit mitogenesis and proliferation of cultured rat vascular smooth muscle cells. *J Clin Inv* 1989;83:1774–1777, 1989.

197. Scott-Burden T, Schini VB, Elizondo E, Junquero DC, Vanhoutte PM: Platelet-derived growth factor suppresses and fibroblast growth factor enhances cytokine-induced production of nitric oxide by cultured smooth muscle cells: effects on cell proliferation. *Circ Res* 71: 1088–1100, 1992.

198. Nunokawa Y, Ishida N, Tanaka S: Cloning of inducible nitric oxide synthase in rat vascular smooth muscle cells. *Biochem Biophys Res Comm* 191:89–94, 1993.

199. Altura BM, Altura BT: Vascular smooth muscle and neurohypophyseal hormones. *Fed Proc* 36:1853–1860, 1977.

200. Penit J, Faure M, Jard S: Vasopressin and angiotensin

II receptors in rat aortic smooth muscle cells in culture. *Am J Physiol* 244:E72-E82, 1983.

201. Capponi AM, Lew PD, Vallotton MB: Cytosolic free calcium levels in monolayers of cultured rat aortic smooth muscle cells. *J Biol Chem* 260:7836–7842, 1985.

202. Aiyar N, Nambi P, Stassen FL, Crooke ST: Vascular vasopressin receptors mediate phosphatidylinositol turnover and calcium efflux in an established cell line. *Life Sci* 39:37–45, 1986.

203. Stassen FL, Heckman G, Schmidt D, Aiyar N, Nambi P, Crooke ST: Identification and characterization of vascular (V_1) vasopressin receptors of an established smooth muscle cell line. *Mol Pharm* 31:259–266, 1987.

204. Nambi P, Watt R, Whitman M, et al: Induction of c-fos by activation of vasopressin receptors in smooth muscle cells. *FEBS Lett* 245:61–64, 1989.

205. Sachinidis A, Wieczorek A, Weisser B, Locher R, Vetter W, Vetter H: Lipoproteins induce expression of the early growth response gene-1 in vascular smooth muscle cells from rat. *Biochem Biophys Res Comm* 192: 794–799, 1993.

206. Locher R, Weisser B, Mengden T, Brunner C, Vetter W: Lysolecithin actions on vascular smooth muscle cells. *Biochem Biophys Res Comm* 183:156–162, 1992.

207. Berk BC, Alexander RW, Brock TA, Gimbrone MA, Webb RC: Vasoconstriction: a new activity for platelet-derived growth factor. *Science* 232:87–90, 1986.

208. Huang CL, Ives HE: Guanosine 5'-O-(3-thiotrisphosphate) potentiates both thrombin- and platelet-derived growth factor-induced inositol phosphate release in permeabilized vascular smooth muscle cells: signaling mechanisms distinguished by sensitivity to pertussis toxin and phorbol esters. *J Biol Chem* 264:4391–4397, 1990.

209. Huang C-L, Takenawa T, Ives HE: Platelet-derived growth factor-mediated Ca^{2+} entry is blocked by antibodies to phosphatidylinositol 4,5-bisphosphate but does not involve heparin-sensitive inositol 1,4,5-trisphosphate receptors. *J Biol Chem* 266:4045–4048, 1991.

210. Berk BC, Brock TA, Webb RC, et al: Epidermal growth factor, a vascular smooth muscle mitogen, induces rat aortic contraction. *J Clin Inv* 75:1083–1086, 1985.

211. Homma Y, Sakamoto H, Tsunoda M, Aoki M, Takenawa T, Ooyama T: Evidence for involvement of phospholipase C-τ2 in signal transduction of platelet-derived growth factor in vascular smooth muscle cells. *Biochem J* 290:649–653, 1993.

212. Sharma RV, Bhalla RC: PDGF-induced mitogenic signaling is not mediated through protein kinase C and c-fos pathway in VSM cells. *Am J Physiol* 264:C71-C79, 1993.

213. Kihara M, Robinson PJ, Buck SH, Dage RC: Mitogenesis by serum and PDGF is independent of PI degradation and PKC in VSMC. *Am J Physiol* 256:C886-C892, 1989.

214. Kondo T, Konishi F, Inui H, Inagami T: Differing signal transductions elicited by three isoforms of platelet-derived growth factor in vascular smooth muscle cells. *J Biol Chem* 268:4458–4464, 1993.

215. Higashiyama S, Abraham JA, Miller J, Fiddes JC, Klagsbrun M: A heparin-binding growth factor secreted by macrophage-like cells that is related to EGF. *Science* 251:936–939, 1991.

216. Temizer DH, Yoshizumi M, Perrella MA, Susanni EE, Quertermous T, Lee ME: Induction of heparin-binding epidermal growth factor-like growth factor mRNA by

phorbol ester and angiotensin II in rat aortic smooth muscle cells. *J Biol Chem* 267:24892–24896, 1992.

217. Klagsbrun M, Edelman ER: Biological and biochemical properties of fibroblast growth factors: implications for the pathogenesis of atherosclerosis. *Arteriosclerosis* 9: 269–278, 1989.

218. Winkles JA, Friesel R, Burgess WH, et al: Human vascular smooth muscle cells both express and respond to heparin-binding growth factor I (endothelial cell growth factor). *Proc Natl Acad Sci* 84:7124–7128, 1987.

219. Folkman J, Klagsbrun M, Sasse J, Wadzinski M, Ingber D, Vlodavsky I: A heparin-binding angiogenic protein-basic fibroblast growth factor-is stored within basement membrane. *Am J Path* 130:393–400, 1988.

220. King GL, Goodman AD, Buzney S, Moses A, Kahn CR: Receptors and growth-promoting effects of insulin and insulinlike growth factors on cells from bovine retinal capillaries and aorta. *J Clin Inv* 75:1028–1036, 1985.

221. Pfeifle B, Ditschuneit H: Effect of insulin on growth of cultured human arterial smooth muscle cells. *Diabetologia* 20:155–158, 1981.

222. Clemmons DR: Exposure to platelet-derived growth factor modulates the porcine aortic smooth muscle cell response to somatomedin-C. *Endocrinology* 117:77–83, 1985.

223. Antonelli-Orlidge A, Saunders KB, Smith SR, D'Amore PA: An activated form of transforming growth factor β is produced by cocultures of endothelial cells and pericytes. *Proc Natl Acad Sci USA* 86: 4544–4548, 1989.

224. Saltis J, Agrotis A, Bobik A: TGF-β_1 potentiates growth factor-stimulated proliferation of vascular smooth muscle cells in genetic hypertension. *Am J Physiol* 263: C420–C428, 1992.

225. Bell L, Madri JA: Effect of platelet factors on migration of cultured bovine aortic endothelial and smooth muscle cells. *Circ Res* 65:1057–1065, 1989.

226. Majesky M, Lindner V, Twardzik DR, Schwartz SM, Reidy MA: Production of transforming growth factor β_1 during repair of arterial injury. *J Clin Inv* 88:904–910, 1991.

227. Basson CT, Kocher O, Basson MD, Asis A, Madri JA: Differential modulation of vascular cell integrin and extracellular matrix expression in vitro by TGF-β1 correlates with reciprocal effects on cell migration. *J Cell Physiol* 153:118–128, 1992.

228. Janat MF, Argraves WS, Liau G: Regulation of vascular smooth muscle integrin expression by transforming growth factor β1 and by platelet-derived growth factor-BB. *J Cell Physiol* 151:588–595, 1992.

229. Owens GK, Rabinovitch PS, Schwartz SM: Smooth muscle cell hypertrophy versus hyperplasia in hypertension. *Proc Natl Acad Sci USA* 78:7759–7763, 1981.

230. Goldberg ID, Rosen EM, Shapiro HM, et al: Isolation and culture of a tetraploid subpopulation of smooth muscle cells from the normal rat aorta. *Science* 226: 559–561, 1984.

231. Owens GK: Differential effects of antihypertensive drug therapy on vascular smooth muscle cell hypertrophy, hyperploidy, and hyperplasia in the spontaneously hypertensive rat. *Circ Res* 56:525–536, 1985.

232. Owens GK: Influence of blood pressure on development of aortic medial smooth muscle hypertrophy in spontaneously hypertensive rats. *Hypertension* 9: 178–187, 1987.

233. Lichtenstein AH, Brecher P, Chobanian AV: Effects of deoxycorticosterone-salt hypertension on cell ploidy in the rat aorta. *Hypertension* 8:II50–II54, 1986.

234. Sumpio BE, Banes AJ: Response of porcine aortic smooth muscle cells to cyclic tensional deformation in culture. *J Surg Res* 44(6):696–701, 1988.

235. Sumpio BE, Banes AJ, Link WG, Johnson GJ: Enhanced collagen production by smooth muscle cells during repetitive mechanical stretching. *Arch Surg* 123(10): 1233–1236, 1988.

236. Costa KA, Sumpio BE, Cerreta JM: Increased elastin synthesis by cultured bovine aortic smooth muscle cells subjected to repetitive mechanical stretching. *FASEB J* 5:A1609, 1991.

237. Leung DYM, Glagov S, Mathews MB: Cyclic stretching stimulates synthesis of matrix components by arterial smooth muscle cells in vitro. *Science* 191:475–477, 1976.

238. Kollros PR, Bates SR, Mathews MB, Horowitz AL, Glagov S: Cyclic AMP inhibits collagen production by cyclically stretched smooth muscle cells. *Lab Invest* 56: 410–417, 1987.

239. Berk BC, Elder E, Mitsuka M: Hypertrophy and hyperplasia cause differing effects on vascular smooth muscle cell Na^+/H^+ exchange and intracellular pH. *J Biol Chem* 265:19632–19637, 1990.

240. Ross R, Wight TN, Strandness E, Thiele B: Human atherosclerosis. I. Cell constitution and characteristics of advanced lesions of the superficial femoral artery. *Am J Pathol* 114:79–93, 1984.

241. Majesky MW, Giachelli CM, Reidy MA, Schwartz SM: Rat carotid neointimal smooth muscle cells reexpress a developmentally regulated mRNA phenotype during repair of arterial injury. *Circ Res* 71:759–768, 1992.

242. Walker LN, Bowen-Pope DF, Ross R, Reidy MA: Production of platelet-derived growth factor-like molecules by cultured arterial smooth muscle cells accompanies proliferation after arterial injury. *Proc Natl Acad Sci USA* 83:7311–7315, 1986.

243. Okazaki H, Majesky MW, Harker LA, Schwartz SM: Regulation of platelet-derived growth factor ligand and receptor gene expression by α-thrombin in vascular smooth muscle cells. *Circ Res* 71:1285–1293, 1992.

244. Simons M, Edelman ER, DeKeyser J, Langer R, Rosenberg RD: Antisense c-*myb* oligonucleotides inhibit intimal arterial smooth muscle cell accumulation in vivo. *Nature* 359:67–70, 1992.

245. Lynch CM, Clowes MM, Osborne WRA, Clowes AW, Miller AD: Long-term expression of human adenosine deaminase in vascular smooth muscle cells of rats: a model for gene therapy. *Proc Natl Acad Sci USA* 89: 1138–1142, 1992.

246. Plautz G, Nabel EG, Nabel GJ: Introduction of vascular smooth muscle cells expressing recombinant genes in vivo. *Circulation* 83:578–583, 1991.

247. Chapman GD, Lim CS, Gammon RS, et al: Gene transfer into coronary arteries of intact animals with a percutaneous balloon catheter. *Circ Res* 71:27–33, 1992.

248. Lim CS, Chapman GD, Gammon RS, et al: Direct in vivo gene transfer into the coronary and peripheral vasculatures of the intact dog. *Circulation* 83:2007–2011, 1991.

249. Flugelman MY, Jaklitsch MT, Newman KD, Casscells W, Bratthauer GL, Dichek DA: Low level in vivo gene transfer into the arterial wall through a perforated balloon catheter. *Circulation* 85:1110–1117, 1992.

250. Barbee RW, Stapleton DD, Perry BD, et al: Prior arterial injury enhances luciferase expression following in

vivo gene transfer. *Biochem Biophys Res Comm* 190: 70–78, 1993.

251. Bowers CW, Dahm LM: Maintenance of contractility in dissociated smooth muscle: low-density cultures in a defined medium. *Am J Physiol* 264:C229-C236, 1993.

252. Chamley JH, Campbell GR, McConnell JD, Groschel-Stewart U: Comparison of vascular smooth muscle cells from adult human, monkey and rabbit in primary culture and in subculture. *Cell Tiss Res* 177:503–522, 1977.

253. Gimbrone MA Jr, Cotran RS: Human vascular smooth muscle in culture. *Lab Invest* 33:16–27, 1975.

254. Ross R: The smooth muscle cell. II. Growth of smooth muscle in culture and formation of elastic fibers. *J Cell Biol* 50:172–186, 1971.

255. Travo P, Barrett G, Burnstock G: Differences in proliferation of primary cultures of vascular smooth muscle cells taken from male and female rats. *Blood Vessels* 17:110–116, 1980.

256. Gimbrone MA Jr, Cotran RS, Folkman J: Human vascular endothelial cells in culture: growth and DNA synthesis. *J Cell Biol* 60:673–684, 1973.

257. Aviv A, Migashino H, Hensten D, Bauman JW Jr, Lubit BW, Searle BM: Na⁺-K⁺ ATPase in rat vascular smooth muscle cells grown in vitro. *Am J Physiol* 251: C227-C233, 1983.

258. Chamley-Campbell J, Campbell GR, Ross R: The smooth muscle cell in culture. *Physiol Rev* 59:1–61, 1979.

259. Skalli O, Ropraz P, Trzeciak A, Benzonana G, Gillessen D, Gabbiani G: A monoclonal antibody against α-smooth muscle actin: a new probe for smooth muscle differentiation. *J Cell Biol* 103:2787–2796, 1986.

260. Chan P, Patel M, Betteridge L, et al: Abnormal growth regulation of vascular smooth muscle cells by heparin in patients with restenosis. *Lancet* 341:341–342, 1993.

261. Maurer HR: Towards chemically-defined, serum-free media for mammalian cell culture. In: Freshney RI (ed). *Animal Cell Culture*. Oxford, England: IRL Press; 13–32, 1986.

262. Libby P, O'Brien KV: Culture of quiescent arterial smooth muscle cells in a defined serum-free medium. *J Cell Physiol* 115:217–223, 1983.

263. Isales C, Rosales O, Sumpio BE: Mediators and mechanisms of cyclic strain and shear stress-induced vascular responses. In: Sumpio BE (ed). *Hemodynamic Forces and Vascular Cell Biology*. Austin, TX: RG Landes Co.; 1993.

264. Luscher TF, Boulanger CM, Dohi Y, Yang Z: Endothelium-derived contracting factors. *Hypertension* 19: 117–130, 1992.

CHAPTER 8

Macrophages

Howard P. Greisler, MD

The Macrophage and Vascular Disease

The macrophage is an extraordinarily versatile cell found in histologic sections of tissues representing a wide variety of pathologic conditions, including a large number of arteriopathies. By virtue of its roles in phagocytosis, antigen processing and presentation, production of a spectrum of secretory products including proteases, cytokines, and growth factors, and its role in lipid metabolism, the macrophage likely plays a central role in mediating the progression of these disease processes. A role for the macrophage has been speculated in the initiation and/or progression of atherogenesis, angiogenesis, aneurysmal dilatation, vasculitis, and the pathophysiologic reactions to many currently used interventional therapies including vascular graft implantation, angioplasty, and atherectomy. Many of these processes involve a coordinated interaction between the macrophage and B and T lymphocytes yielding inflammatory responses including local tissue destruction. The macrophage interacts with endothelial cells, smooth muscle cells (SMCs), and fibroblasts to mediate fibroplasia, angiogenesis, and intimal hyperplasia. The macrophage's activities in lipid metabolism, in concert with the release of a battery of monokines, may mediate atherogenesis and macrophage production of oxygen radicals, and a variety of proteases may modulate aneurysmal dilatation.

Isolated macrophage-derived foam cells have been found in the intima of infants in areas of fatty streaks, and this constitutes the earliest evidence of arterial wall lipid accumulation. Similarly, following balloon deendothelialization injuries in New Zealand White rabbits fed high cholesterol diets, macrophages occupy 85% of the neointimal area after 3 days. Inflammatory cytokines increase the adhesivity between endothelial cells and circulating monocytes in the area of vascular injury; these monocytes migrate into the subendothelial space, become activated, and synthesize and secrete numerous bioactive substances which likely modulate arterial disease processes. Activated monocytes initially respond with a respiratory burst and the release of products of oxygen metabolism as well as proteolytic enzymes, both of which induce cytotoxicity and matrix degradation of the local microenvironment. Acid hydrolases including proteases, lipases, ribonucleases, deoxyribonucleases, and others, and neutral proteases including collagenases, elastase, and plasminogen activator degrade the extracellular matrix (ECM) enabling SMCs to migrate into the intima. Released proteolytic enzymes may also release fibroblast growth factor type 2 (FGF-2) stored in the basement membrane, and thus, make it available to receptors on migrating SMCs. Activated macrophages similarly synthesize and secrete numerous cytokines which modulate the inflammatory reaction, to an undetermined extent, and myointimal hyperplasia. Among these cytokines are interleukins (IL) 1, 6, and 8, interferon (IFN), tumor necrosis factor (TNF), and colony stimulating factors (CSF). Growth factors released by these macrophages include platelet-derived growth factor (PDGF), FGFs, and transforming growth factor-β (TGF-β). The interactions among all of these cytokines and growth factors and the cells in the microenvironment of the arterial wall are complex, but a great deal of in vitro experimentation suggests conditions in which these effector molecules may induce SMC migration and proliferation consistent with the pathophysiology of atherogenesis and myointimal hyperplasia. Similarly, these monokines are potent stimuli for collagen and ECM production by SMCs and fibroblasts. Once in the subendothelial tissues, macrophages take up and metabolize oxidized low density lipoprotein (LDL). This results in the promotion of

From *The Basic Science of Vascular Disease*. Edited by Sidawy AN, Sumpio BE, and DePalma RG. Armonk, NY: Futura Publishing Company, Inc.; © 1997.

macrophage-derived foam cell formation as well as the generation of chemoattractants, inducing additional monocyte infiltration into the arterial wall.

Recent evidence strongly suggests the role for the macrophage in the pathogenesis of arterial aneurysms as well. Human aneurysm walls contain decreased elastic tissue and have been shown to possess increased elastolytic activity. Pancreatic elastase perfused into rat abdominal aortas induces aneurysmal dilatation secondary to loss of elastic tissue. Similar infusion of aortas with activated macrophages induces a similar loss of elastin and development of aneurysmal dilatation.

The Mononuclear Phagocyte System

Macrophages were first described by Metchnikoff in Messina[1] more than a century ago. However, a role for these cells in atherogenesis was first postulated in 1933 by Anitschow[2] who observed these cells in diet-induced lesions in rabbits. The presence of macrophages in human atherosclerosis was first described in 1961[3] using electron microscopy and in 1980[4] using immunohistochemical identification techniques. During this recent period, there has been an explosion in our understanding of macrophage biology leading to an increased understanding of the physiologic roles that macrophages within the atheromatous plaques may play in lipid metabolism, inflammatory processes, and modulation of mesenchymal cell proliferative activity.

Macrophages were assigned by Aschoff in 1924[5] to the reticulo-endothelial system (RES) which included not only monocytes, macrophages, and histocytes, but also fibroblasts, endothelial cells, and reticular cells. More recent studies have separated these cells based upon shared functional capacities and immunohistochemical identification, and in 1969 the present title, mononuclear phagocyte system (MPS), was defined.

The MPS consists of a variety of related tissue macrophage types (Figure) all stemming from monoblasts found in bone marrow. Monoblast division yields two promonocytes, which upon their division yields four monocytes. The monoblast itself is thought to derive within the bone marrow from a bipotent stem cell called either the granulocyte-monocyte progenitor cell or the colony-forming unit, granulocyte-macrophage (CFU-GM) which is able to give rise to both monocyte and neutrophil colonies in culture. Monocytes themselves are thought to remain in the bone marrow for less than 24 hours before entering the circulation, and are then distributed between circulating and marginating pools. In normal adult humans, the half-life in circulation of monocytes is estimated to be 70 hours,[6] and with a normal peripheral blood monocyte

count of 1% to 6% of the total leukocyte count, monocytes are present in the range of 300 to 700 cells/μL of blood. The marginating pool of monocytes includes those attached to the endothelium, many in the process of transendothelial migration to enter tissues and serous cavities and which then mature into resident macrophages. Monocyte-endothelial cell adherence involves a variety of high-molecular weight glycoprotein receptors in both cell types, the expression of many which can be upregulated by inflammatory cytokines resulting in an increased migration of mononuclear phagocytes to areas of inflammation. Once in the tissues, resident macrophages remain for many months, their ultimate fate dependent upon the persistence of inflammatory stimuli, foreign bodies, etc.

Monocytopoiesis

Monocytopoiesis in the bone marrow is regulated by a variety of growth factors including IL-3, granulocyte-macrophage colony stimulating factor (GM-CSF), and macrophage colony stimulating factor (M-CSF or CSF-1). The last two of these factors are products of macrophages themselves. Resident macrophages are found in large numbers within bone marrow and, thus may modulate their own numbers.[6] Macrophage production of M-CSF and GM-CSF is increased by exposure to endotoxin.[7] In addition, macrophages release IL-1 and TNF, which in turn can induce both endothelial cells and fibroblasts to produce M-CSF and GM-CSF and, thus modulate monocytopoiesis.[8-10] During active inflammation, the number of promonocytes and monocytes dramatically increases, induced by a humoral factor found in blood termed "factor increasing monocytopoiesis" (FIM).[11,12] FIM is monocyte specific and has not been reported to be detected in serum in the absence of active inflammation. FIM is an 18 to 25 kD glycoprotein released by macrophages themselves during phagocytosis.[11-14]

Among the growth factors listed above capable of stimulating proliferation of monocyte progenitor cells, the most potent is M-CSF. M-CSF is present in active concentrations in normal human serum and is required by both circulating monocytes and tissue macrophages for their survival. M-CSF may modulate macrophage physiologic functions including phagocytic activity and production of inflammatory cytokines including IL-1, TNF, and IFN.[15-17] Thus, the local production of M-CSF within arterial wall lesions may significantly impact on the atherogenesis process. Clinton et al[18] demonstrated that exposure of cultured endothelial cells or SMCs to bacterial liposaccharides (LPS), IL-1α, or TNF-α induced M-CSF mRNA accumulation in a dose-dependent fashion, correlating with increased staining for M-CSF protein using fluorescent antibod-

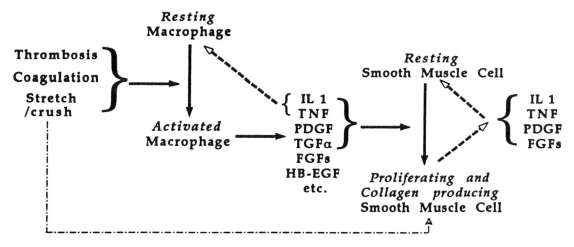

Figure. Cascade model of major pathways of signaling of smooth muscle proliferation and matrix accumulation. We hypothesize an intermediary role for cytokines and growth factors derived from macrophages as paracrine mediators of smooth muscle activation (**solid arrows**) and autocrine amplification loops from smooth muscle cells (SMCs) and macrophages (**dashed lines**). Our model does not exclude direct activation of SMCs by products of thrombosis and coagulation (**dot-dashed line**), but emphasizes the previously underemphasized contribution of macrophages, which could provide an important intermediary and amplification loop as schematized above. IL-1 = interleukin-1; TNF = tumor necrosis factor; PDGF = platelet-derived growth factor; TGFα = transforming growth factor-α; FGFs = fibroblast growth factors; HB-EGF = heparin-binding growth factor. (Reproduced with permission from Reference 28.)

ies. Plaques resected from diet-induced atherosclerosis in rabbit aortas showed elevated M-CSF mRNA compared with controls. Immunostaining of these tissues showed the M-CSF protein to be associated with both intimal SMCs and macrophages. Human atherosclerotic plaques analyzed by polymerase chain reaction (PCR) techniques showed elevated M-CSF mRNA as compared to nonatherosclerotic arteries and veins. The M-CSF receptor, c-fms, was not found on cultured endothelial cells or SMCs, suggesting the macrophage as the likely target for the M-CSF within these plaques. When cultured human monocytes were exposed to recombinant M-CSF, Northern analysis demonstrated an upregulation of mRNA for the acetyl-LDL (scavenger) receptor and apolipoprotein E (apo E) species. M-CSF has also been reported to stimulate clearance of lipoproteins containing apolipoprotein B-100 via both LDL receptor-dependent and independent pathways in rabbits[19] to stimulate macrophage lipoprotein lipase secretion,[20] and to stimulate macrophage uptake and degradation of acetylated LDL.[21] Human umbilical artery SMCs exposed to PDGF-BB homodimer showed a dose-dependent down-regulation of M-CSF mRNA, along with a reduced M-CSF protein production.[22]

Monocyte Recruitment and Activation

Although circulating monocytes adhere to endothelium in normocholesterolemic animals, this adhe-sivity is dramatically increased in the presence of hypercholesterolemia.[23] Following balloon de-endo-thelialization injury in New Zealand white rabbits fed a 2% cholesterol diet, immunohistochemical staining showed RAM-11 (a rabbit macrophage specific marker) positive macrophages to occupy 85% of the neointimal area 3 days following injury. By contrast, HHF-35 immunostaining for SMCs did not show their appearance in the neointima until 7 days following injury.[24] Similar balloon injury studies in normocholest-erolemic rats demonstrated the early appearance of intimal macrophages, and with the addition of hyper-cholesterolemia these macrophages represented the only cell type in this model to develop into foam cells.[25] In an autopsy study of coronary arteries and aortas of 1160 human subjects who died between full-term birth and age 29, isolated macrophage foam cells were found in the intima of infants and this constituted the earliest evidence of lipid retention. While these cells were present in 45% of infants under 8 months of age, their numbers transiently decreased until puberty at which time larger accumulations of macrophage-derived foam cells in the area of intimal thickening opposite flow dividers was found in 73% of children between the ages of 12 and 14 years.[26] While macrophage-derived foam cell accumulation and SMC proliferation have long been considered the hallmarks of atherogenesis, Gordon et al applied cell cycle-related antibodies to study cell proliferation in human atherosclerotic lesions, and found that in advanced plaques, immunohistochemically identified macrophages themselves had high rates of proliferation.[27]

The evidence for the early appearance of monocyte-derived macrophages in arterial lesions, including those of atherosclerosis and postangioplasty restenosis, is thus substantial. The etiologic role of these cells in the pathophysiology that ensues is a matter of intense investigation. The role of these macrophages in modulating the SMC proliferation characteristic of these proliferative arteriopathies has been suggested by numerous investigators. In an excellent recent review of the pathophysiology of postangioplasty restenosis, Libby and colleagues[28] have suggested a primary role for macrophage-derived cytokines and growth factors as paracrine mediators of SMC activation and proliferation (Figure). Vein grafts implanted into hypercholesterolemic rabbit carotid arteries underwent increased intimal thickening, due largely to the accumulation of lipid laden macrophages.[29] Similarly, bioresorbable vascular grafts implanted into the aortas of diet-induced atherosclerotic rabbits resulted in large accumulations of lipid laden macrophages within the neointimas.[30] Rabbit peritoneal macrophages cultured in the presence of different vascular graft materials have also been shown to release growth factors including basic FGF,[31] TGF-β,[32] and IL-1.[33]

Chemoattractants

Monocyte adhesion to endothelial cells in lesion prone areas is the earliest identifiable evidence of the development of an atherosclerotic plaque. This adherence has been described in a wide variety of animal models of experimentally induced atherosclerosis, and immunohistochemical techniques have demonstrated the presence of monocytes in early atherosclerotic lesions in human necropsy and carotid endarterectomy specimens.[34-36] Similarly, monocyte adherence to injured areas occurs early following therapeutic interventions, including implantation of vascular grafts, endarterectomy, and angioplasty. These monocytes may then differentiate successively into inflammatory monocytes, macrophages, and finally activated macrophages which, when faced with a foreign body such as a vascular graft, may coalesce to form foreign body giant cells. The signals stimulating the recruitment of monocytes to lesion prone areas or areas of vascular wall injury are manifold, deriving from products found within plasma as well as products secreted by or membranes associated with ingrowing cells, and by the presence of a foreign body itself. Many of the known monocyte chemotactic factors are listed in Table 1.

Transendothelial monocyte migration into the subendothelial space occurs via cell junctions, likely a response to chemoattractants within the vessel wall.

Table 1
Monocyte Chemotactic Factors

Interleukin-1	Bevilaqua (1985)
Thrombin	Bar-Shavit (1983)
PDGF	Deuel (1982)
C5a	Snyderman (1971)
Collagen fragments	Postlewaite (1976)
Elastin	Hunninghake (1981)
Fibronectin	Norris (1982)
Kallikrein	Gallin (1974)
Plasminogen activator	Gallin (1974)
SMC Product	Jauchem (1982)
E.C. Product	Berliner (1986)
Fibrinopeptides	Kay (1973)
IgG Proteolytic fragments	Ishida (1978)
Leukotriene B$_4$	Ford-Hutchinson (1980)
Platelet factor 4	Deuel (1981)

(Modified with permission from Greisler HP: *New Biologic and Synthetic Vascular Prostheses*. Austin, TX: RG Landes Publishing Company; 1991.)

Extracts of aortic tissues from hypercholesterolemic swine[37] and pigeons[38] were shown to be chemotactic for monocytes. Baboon SMCs were shown to produce a potent chemoattractant for circulating monocytes originally termed SMC chemotactic factor (SMC-CF),[39] later termed monocyte chemotactic peptide (MCP-1).[40] MCP-1 is the major chemotactic substance generated by the vessel wall and is currently under intense investigation. Following vascular graft implantation, monocytes are also attracted to both the graft material and to the fibrin coagulum, which forms on its surface, as well as to substances released by injured adjacent endothelial cells and SMCs. PDGF is a potent monocyte chemoattractant released by platelets, endothelial cells, SMCs, and by macrophages. PDGF production by endothelial cells is increased in vitro following cell injury induced by endotoxin or phorbol esters.[41] Endothelial cells within the area of pannus ingrowth following vascular graft implantation have been shown to maintain a persistently elevated mitotic index,[42] suggesting persistent endothelial cell injury which may yield an elevated local concentration of PDGF-inducing monocyte recruitment into the area. Monocytes preferentially adhere to areas of injured or regenerating endothelium.[43] Cytokines, including IL-1, also increase monocyte adhesivity to endothelium[44] by altering expression of cell adhesion molecules. Other potent cell-derived monocyte recruitment factors include leukotriene B$_4$ (LTB$_4$) and platelet factor 4 (PF-4). Monocyte chemoattractants in plasma include the complement-derived peptides C5a and C5a *des arg*, fibrinopeptides, and thrombin. Vascular injury in general and vascular graft implantation in specific activate both classic and alternative complement pathways, and also lead to the generation of thrombin and fibrinopeptides following platelet activation and release. Thus, monocyte recruitment is stimulated by all such interventional modalities. ECM bound monocyte chemotactic factors include fragments of collagen, elastin, and fibronectin.

Monocytes harvested from the blood of hypercholesterolemic patients were reported to be more sensitive to chemoattractants than monocytes harvested from normal patients.[45] Quinn has shown that oxidized LDL is a potent chemotactic substance for monocytes due to the presence of lysophosphatidylcholine PC (lyso PC), a lipid both chemotactic to monocytes and inhibitory to motility of resident macrophages,[46–48] thus promoting influx and inhibiting efflux of monocyte-derived macrophages in the developing lesion. Minimally modified LDL (mm-LDL) treatment of endothelial cells yields secretion of a monocyte chemoattractant,[49] and mm-LDL exposure to SMCs results in their secretion of MCP-1.[50] Exposure of either endothelial cells or SMCs to LDL did not yield MCP-1 secretion, whereas LDL exposure to co-cultures of these two cell lines resulted in increased MCP-1 secretion and monocyte transmigration.[51] MCP-1 gene transcription in monocytes themselves is up-regulated by exposure to a number of cytokines including IL-1, TNF, IFN-γ, and GM-CSF.[52,53] MCP-1 secretion by both endothelial cells and SMCs is also increased by exposure to IL-1 and TNF.[54] In addition to secreting MCP-1, monocytes also possess high affinity MCP-1 receptors.[55] MCP-1 itself is a basic polypeptide of molecular weight 14 kD, with maximal biologic activity for monocyte chemotaxis at concentrations 1 to 10 ng/mL. Arteries resected from hypercholesterolemic cyamologous monkeys were shown to exhibit increased MCP-1 mRNA levels in vivo as compared to normocholesterolemic controls.[56] MCP-1 mRNA was detected in 16% of cells harvested from human carotid endarterectomy specimens using in situ hybridization, with the highest expression in the area of organizing thrombi (33%) and in macrophage rich areas bordering the necrotic lipid core (24%), compared to the fibrous cap (8%) and the necrotic lipid core (5%).[57] Immunohistochemical staining showed the MCP-1 mRNA expressing cells to be both SMCs and macrophages. Very few cells (<0.1%) from normal arteries expressed MCP-1 mRNA.[57]

Monocyte Endothelial Cell Adherence

Circulating monocytes migrating along concentration gradients of chemoattractant substances must first adhere to endothelial cells, followed by their transendothelial migration into the subendothelial space. Many of the chemoattractants listed above also upregulate the expression of cell adhesion molecules in either the endothelial cell or the monocyte. Monocyte surface glycoproteins are required for adhesion to the endothelial cell, the endothelial cells expressing counter receptors. Inflammatory cytokines including IL-1 and TNF upregulate the expression of endothelial cell adhesion molecules including intercellular adhesion molecule 1 (ICAM-1), endothelial cell leukocyte adhesion molecule 1 (ELAM-1), granule membranae protein-140 (GMP-140), platelet activation dependent granule external membrane protein (PADGEM), and vascular cell adhesion molecule 1 (VCAM-1), along with additional adhesion molecules on monocytes including the leukocyte cell adhesion molecules (leuCAM [CD11/CD18]).

Adhesion proteins expressed by endothelial cells can be categorized into two classes: selectins, structurally related to lectins; and adhesion proteins of the immunoglobulin gene superfamily (Table 2).[58] The selectins are a family of glycoproteins which are not expressed on unstimulated endothelial cells, but are rapidly and transiently expressed following exposure to IL-1, LPS, thrombin, phorbol esters, and TNF.[58] The two selectins identified on endothelial cell membranes include E-selectin (ELAM-1) whose expression is rapidly induced and returns to baseline levels by 24 hours, and P-selectin (PADGEM or GMP-140), whose expression is very rapidly induced, returning to basal levels within minutes.

The immunoglobulin gene superfamily expressed by endothelial cells includes VCAM-1 which is expressed at low levels, but its expression is rapidly induced by cytokines which produce a sustained elevated expression.[59,60] ATHERO-ELAM is a VCAM-1 homolog detected in rabbit endothelial cells in areas overlying atherosclerotic lesions.[61,62] ICAM-1 is a constitutively expressed ELAM also enhanced by endothelial cell exposure to IL-1, TNF, and LPS.[63] ICAM-2 is a structurally related protein, constitutively expressed by cultured human umbilical vein endothelial cells (HUVEC), but without cytokine altered expression.

ICAM-1 interacts with the monocyte via the β-2 integrins LFA-1 (CD11a/CD18) and MAC-1 (CD11b/CD18).[64–66] The integrin family of CD11/CD18 heterodimeric leukocyte surface molecules are important modulators of endothelial cell-leukocyte adherence. These integrins are membrane glycoprotein heterodimers, and evidence suggests that ICAM-1-CD11a/CD18 affinity is modulated by alterations in the β-2 subunit.[67] In addition, other monocyte surface integrins may also bind to matrix ligands found in fibronectin, vitronectin (for example the RGD sequence), etc. A third mode

Table 2
Endothelial-Leukocyte Adhesion Molecules

	Size (kD)	Ligand	Ligand Cell Type	Expression on Human ECs In Vitro Constitutive Expression	Expression on Activated ECs (Max)
1. Selectin family					
a. E-selectin (ELAM-1)	115	Sialyl-Lewis X	PMNL, Monocyte	None	3–4 hours (down by 24 hours)
b. P-selectin (GMP-140/ PADGEM)	140	LNF III	PMNL, Monocyte	None	10–30 minutes
2. Immunoglobulin family					
a. VCAM-1 (INCAM-110)	110	VLA-4 ($\alpha^4\beta_1$)	Lymphocyte, Monocyte	Low	4–10 hours
b. ICAM-1 (CD54)	100	LFA-1 (CD11a/CD18) MAC-1 (CD11b/CD18) p150,95 (CD11c/CD18	Lymphocyte, Monocyte, PMNL	Moderate	12–24 hours
c. ICAM-2	46	LFA-1 (CD11a/CD18)	Lymphocyte, Monocyte, PMNL	Moderate	Unchanged

of integrin binding is to platelet glycoproteins such as GPIIb/IIIa. The three members of the CD11/CD18 integrin family share a common β chain (CD18) with distinct α chains (CD11a, CD11b, CD11c).

Monocyte Migration

Monocytes attached to the endothelial monolayer migrate across that cell layer and through the subendothelial connective tissue. The regulation of this cell migration is poorly understood, but is thought to involve both density gradients of the chemotactic substances described above, as well as CD11a/CD18, CD11b/CD18, and ICAM-1.[68] Even in the absence of chemotactic gradients, neutrophil migration can be stimulated by endothelial cell pretreatment with IL-1, TNF, or LPS[69]; this migration is significantly inhibited by prior exposure of the endothelium to monoclonal antibodies against either CD11a, CD18, or ICAM-1.[69,70] As discussed above, IL-1 exposure to endothelial cells induces their production of MCP-1 as does exposure to mm-LDL. Endothelial cells migrating through the endothelial monolayer are found initially between the endothelium and the basement membrane. These cells then insinuate themselves through apertures in the basement membrane, thereby entering the connective tissue. This process is thought to involve the synthesis and release of proteolytic enzymes from the monocyte, including elastase, collagenase, and plasminogen activators. However, attempts to inhibit this cell migration using a variety of proteinase inhibitors have failed.

Macrophage Activation

Both monocytes and resident macrophages attracted to arterial wall lesions become activated by complex mechanisms. Macrophage activation may be defined as the acquisition of competence to complete a complex function. Macrophages can be activated in numerous ways, each representing the enhancement or suppression of specific functions. Thus, macrophages within developing atherosclerotic plaques may be activated resulting in the increased secretion of specific monokines, whereas macrophages activated by exposure to a tumor mass or invading microorganisms, may be activated to result in a different secretory response. Macrophage activation can be induced by microbial products such as lipopolysaccharides (LPS), or by cytokines including IL-1, TNF, IL-8, and GM-CSF,[71] by the presence of low oxygen tensions,[72] as well as by elevated lactate concentrations.[73] Macrophages activated by phagocytosis release preformed lysosomal and granule contents. When confronted with material it cannot phagocytize, such as a vascular graft, this lysosomal and granule discharge still occurs in the absence of phagocytosis; this situation is referred to as "frustrated phagocytosis."[74]

The numerous cell surface receptors on the macrophage may induce the state of activation and regulate the specific macrophage functions. The large variety

Table 3
Surface Receptors of Monocytes and Macrophages

Fc receptors
   IgG_{2a}, IgG_{2b}/IgG_1, IgG_3, IgA, IgE

Complement receptors
   C3b, C3b, C3bi, C5a, C1q

Cytokine receptors
   MIF, MAF, LIF, CF, MFF, IL-1, IL-2, IL-3, IL-4
   $IFN\alpha$, $IFN\beta$, $IFN\gamma$
   Colony-stimulating factors (GM-CSF, M-CSF/CSF-1)

Receptors for peptides and small molecules
   H_1, H_2, 5HT
   1,2,5-Dihydroxy vitamin D3
   N-Formulated peptides
   Enkephalins/endorphins
   Substance P
   Arg-vasopressin

Hormone receptors
   Insulin
   Glucocorticosteroids
   Angiotensin

Transferrin and lactoferrin receptors

lipoprotein lipid receptors
   Anionic low density lipoproteins
   PGE_2, LTB_4, LTC_4, LTD_4 PAG
   Apolipoproteins B and E (chylomicron remnants, VLDL)

Receptors for coagulants and anticoagulants
   Fibrinogen/fibrin
   Coagulation factor VII
   α_1-Antithrombin
   Heparin

Fibronectin receptors

Laminin receptors

Mannosyl, fucosyl, galactosyl residue, AGE receptors

α_2-Macroglobulin-proteinase complex receptors

Others
   Cholinergic agonists
   α_1-adrenergic agonists
   β_2-adrenergic agonists

AGE: advanced glycosylation end-products; GM: granulocyte macrophages; CSF: colony-stimulating factor; VLDL: very low density lipoprotein; PG: prostaglandin; LT: leucotriene; IG: immunoglobulin; C: complement; MIF: macrophage inhibitory factor; MAF: macrophage-activating factor; LIF: leucocyte migration inhibition factor; MFF: macrophage fusion factor; IL: interleukin; H: histamine; 5HT: 5-hydroxytryptamine.
(Reproduced with permission from Reference 81.)

of surface receptors have been identified and are outlined in Table 3.

Macrophage Secretory Products

Proteases and Local Tissue Destruction

Once activated by inflammatory cytokines and/or receptor-mediated phagocytosis, the activated monocyte/macrophage responds initially with a respiratory burst and release of products of oxygen metabolism and of proteolytic enzymes, which may lead to cell death and matrix degradation in the local microenvironment. Maturation of the monocyte into the mature macrophage attenuates the respiratory burst. A phagocytic challenge yields a respiratory burst from the activated monocyte within minutes, and these cells then progressively mature into activated macrophages over the ensuing several days, during which time the macro-

phages synthesize and release numerous proteolytic enzymes. Exposure of the activated macrophage to cytokines including TNF, GM-CSF, and INF-γ, increases the cells release of reactive oxygen intermediates such as superoxide, hydrogen peroxide, and hydroxyl groups.[75-79] The regulation of this respiratory burst is incompletely understood. External stimuli require the activation of a nicotinamide adenine dinucleotide phosphate (NADPH) oxidase to generate reactive oxygen intermediates; this enzyme activation occurs within seconds and, thus, likely does not require de novo enzyme synthesis.[80]

Macrophages are known to synthesize and secrete over 100 identified substances (Table 4),[81] with molecular weights ranging from 32 D (superoxide anions) to 440000 D (fibronectin). Some of these secretory products are constitutively expressed such as lysozyme, complement components, and apolipoprotein E, whereas others are synthesized only when the cell is stimulated. This stimulation results in alterations at the

Table 4
Secretory Products of Mononuclear Phagocytes

Enzymes

Lysozyme

Lysosomal acid hydrolases
    proteases
    lipases
    (deoxy)ribonuclease
    phosphatases
    blycosidases
    sulphatases

Neutral proteases
    collagenase
    elastase
    myelinase
    angiotensin convertase
    plasminogen activator
    cytolytic proteinase

Lipases
    lipoprotein lipase
    phospholipase A2

Arginase

Enzyme & cytokine inhibitors

Protease inhibitors
    α_2-macroglobulin
    α_1-antitrypsin inhibitor
    plasminogen activator inhibitor
    collagenase inhibitor

Phospholipase inhibitor

IL-1 inhibitors

Complement components

Classical pathway
    C1, C4, C2, C3, C5

Alternative pathway
    Factor B, factor D, properdin

Active fragments
    C3a, C3b, C5a, Bb

Inhibitors
    C3b inactivator, β-1H

Reactive oxygen intermediates

Superoxide

Hydrogen peroxide

Hydroxyl radical

Arachidonic acid intermediates

Cyclo-oxygenase products:
    PGD$_2$, prostacyclin, thromboxane

Lipo-oxygenase products
    hydroxyeicosotetranoic acids
    leucotrienes
    Platelet-activating factors

Coagulation factors

Tissue factor

Prothrombin activator

Coagulation factors II, VII, IX, X, XIII

Plasminogen activator

Plasminogen activator inhibitors

Cytokines

IL-1, IL-6, IL-8

TNFα

IFNα, IFNβ

Platelet-derived growth factors

Fibroblast growth factor

Transforming growth factor β

GM-CSF

M-CSF

Erythropoietin

Factor-inducing monocytopoiesis

Angiogenesis factor

Others

Thrombospondin

Fibronectin

Lipronectin

Lipocortin

Transcobalamin II

Transferrin

Ferritin

Haptoglobin

Glutathione

Uric acid

Apolipoprotein E

Neopterin

(Reproduced with permission from Reference 81.)

transcriptional, translational, and post-translational levels depending on the particular secretory product.

Lysosomal acid hydrolases are released early by macrophages following their activation by complement, cytokines, bacterial products, or occupancy of Fc receptors.[82,83] These acid hydrolases degrade basement membrane and collagen, and include a variety of proteases, lipases, ribonucleases, deoxyribonucleases, phosphatases, glycosidases, and sulphatases.

Activated macrophages are also induced to synthesize and release a variety of neutral proteases, including collagenase types I, II, III, and IV, elastase, plasminogen activator, angiotensin convertase, and cysteine protease. While lysosomal acid hydrolases are active at low pH, the family of neutral proteases are more active at neutral pH levels. These proteolytic enzymes produce local matrix degradation. In addition, the resulting fragments of elastin and collagen are themselves monocyte chemotactic agents which, thus, perpetuate the cycle of monocyte recruitment to the area of local injury. By contrast, protease secretion by resident macrophages is much lower. A complex and possibly important interaction among macrophage-derived proteins may in part modulate angiogenesis. Exposure of macrophages to TGF-β_1 (itself a macrophage-derived growth factor) leads to an up-regulated macrophage expression of urokinase-type plasminogen activator (uPA) which is released into the surrounding matrix. When TGF-β_1-primed macrophages were cultured on matrices containing bound ^{125}I basic fibroblast growth factor (bFGF), FGF release was increased tenfold in the presence of plasminogen.[84] Normal arterial walls contain bFGF bound to the basement membrane which may be released by uPA secreted by activated macrophages.

Recent evidence has suggested a role for macrophage-derived neutral proteases in the pathogenesis of arterial aneurysms. Clinical studies have shown a loss of elastic tissue, along with increased elastolytic activity, in the media of human aneurysms. Perfusion of rat abdominal aortas with pancreatic elastase results in loss of elastic tissue and aneurysmal dilatation.[85] Similarly, infusion into the rat aorta of activated macrophages also yielded a loss of elastin with the development of true aneurysmal dilatation.[85]

Activated macrophages also release protease inhibitors including α_1 antitrypsin inhibitor, plasminogen activator inhibitors, and collagenase inhibitor. The secretion of proteases is reduced following macrophage surface receptor binding by α_2 macroglobulin-protease complexes.[86]

Many components of both the classic and alternative pathways of the complement cascade are synthesized and secreted by activated macrophages. In addition, macrophage proteases result in the generation of active complement fragments including C3a, C3b, C5a, and Bb.

Secretory Products in Hemostasis and Thrombosis

Human monocytes have long been known to express high concentrations of tissue factor on the cell surface. Tissue factor in the presence of phospholipid augments Factor VII activation of the extrinsic coagulation cascade. Macrophage tissue factor secretion has been shown to be increased in a dose- and time-dependent manner by cell exposure to endotoxin, immune complexes, and the complement component C5a.[87] In addition, activated monocytes were also reported to synthesize procoagulants, including the prothrombin activator and coagulation Factors II, VII, IX, and XIII. The secretion by the macrophage of both plasminogen activators and plasminogen activator inhibitors has been discussed above.

Murine peritoneal macrophages cultured on disks of Dacron and ePTFE graft materials were assayed for release of procoagulant activity in the presence and absence of LPS. Exposure to Dacron yielded an increased procoagulant activity both with and without LPS; these levels increased by the presence of LPS.[88]

Macrophages also synthesize and secrete products of arachidonic acid metabolism including prostacyclin and thromboxane, thereby modulating platelet/vessel wall adhesivity and vascular tone as well as LTB$_4$, a potent monocyte recruitment factor.

In addition, monokines including IL-1 and TNF-α can induce tissue factor synthesis and expression by endothelial cells, and also can result in a downregulation of endothelial cell protein C activity; these activities all promote thrombogenesis.[89]

Cytokines

Activated macrophages synthesize and secrete a number of cytokines (Table 4) which may modulate the inflammatory response and myointimal hyperplasia. Many of these cytokines have potent antimicrobial and tumoricidal activities, and additionally are potent modulators of SMC proliferation. The conditioned media in which macrophages are cultured stimulates SMC proliferation suggesting release of soluble factors.[90] Cell contact between macrophages and SMCs is required to induce 6-keto-PGF$_{1\alpha}$ production by these SMCs.[90] Immunohistochemical and in situ hybridization techniques have demonstrated expression of gap junction connexin43 mRNA in macrophage foam cells isolated from human atherosclerotic carotid arteries,[91] suggesting the possibility of gap junction communication in atherogenesis between macrophages and SMCs, and transmission of lower molecular weight mediators via these junctions.

Interleukin-1

IL-1 is a product of activated monocytes and macrophages along with endothelial cells and several other cell types. Macrophages additionally release an IL-1 inhibitor.[92] Two structurally related isotypes, IL-1α and IL-1β, have been cloned. These isotopes are both derived from a 30 kD precursor polypeptide lacking a signal sequence. The two isotopes share 26% amino acid homology. Both IL-1α and IL-1β are 17.5 kD, and share many functional characteristics. Three IL-1 receptors have now been identified including a high affinity 80 kD receptor.

IL-1 is a potent immunoregulatory protein which influences the production of IL-2, IL-4, IL-6, TNF-α, and IL-1. Cellular immune response is augmented by IL-1 in T cells, B cells, and NK cells. IL-1 is involved in the acute phase protein response, playing a role in the generation of fever and hypotension.

IL-1 in an endothelial cell growth inhibitor in vitro.[93,94] The production of IL-1 by endothelial cells increases with time in culture, and this has been reported to promote endothelial cell senescence.[95] The introduction of an antisense IL-1α oligonucleotide into endothelial cells extends cell longevity in vitro. IL-1 induces a decrease in endothelial cell FGF receptor expression[94]; this effect is possibly involved in the endothelial cell growth inhibitory activity of IL-1.

By contrast, IL-1 stimulates proliferation of fibroblasts and vascular SMCs, an effect possibly mediated by the reported IL-1 induction of PDGF transcription and subsequent PDGF activity.[96,97] Macrophages exposed to vascular graft materials in the presence of LPS have been shown to synthesize IL-1, and this may partly mediate the subendothelial fibroblast and/or SMC proliferation as well as possibly inhibit endothelial cell growth in the region of graft to artery anastomoses.[98–100] In addition, IL-1 can induce an increase in endothelial cell procoagulant activity in vitro.[101]

IL-1 is also a chemoattractant for monocytes, neutrophils, and lymphocytes. The net effect of IL-1 on angiogenesis in vivo is poorly understood and has been reported to both promote angiogenesis[102] and to inhibit angiogenesis.[94]

Interleukin-6

IL-6 is a phosphoglycoprotein secreted predominantly by activated monocytes and macrophages, but additionally by T cells, B cells, endothelial cells, and fibroblasts. IL-6 production is reportedly up-regulated by other cytokines including IL-1 and TNF-α. By contrast, macrophages express IL-4 receptors, and IL-4 reportedly downregulates IL-6 production. IL-6 initiates the synthesis of acute phase proteins in the liver and also induces proliferation of both immature and mature T cells.[103] In vitro studies have suggested an antiproliferative effect of IL-6 on cultured endothelial cells.[104]

Interleukin-8

IL-8 secretion by human monocytes was first reported following monocyte exposure to endotoxin and phorbol esters.[105] IL-8 mRNA expression is up-regulated in macrophages exposed to IL-1α, IL-1β, and TNF-α, as well as following the process of phagocytosis. IL-8 is a single nonglycosylated peptide chain whose signal sequence is cleaved to allow secretion of a 72 amino acid residue 8.4 kD active protein. IL-8 selectively induces neutrophil accumulation, a long lasting effect following intradermal IL-8 injection, which is most likely due to IL-8's resistance to enzymatic degradation. IL-8 has been found in large quantities in synovial fluids of arthritic joints and in cirrhotic lesions. Its role in the inflammatory aspects of atherosclerosis and/or vasculitis is unknown.

Interferon

Macrophages have been shown to produce IFN-α, the rate of production being increased in response to viruses, bacteria, and tumor and foreign cells.[106] In addition, some investigators have suggested the capability of macrophages to synthesize IFN-γ.[107,108] Both IFN-α and IFN-γ inhibit endothelial cell proliferation in vitro. IFN-α also inhibits PDGF-stimulated bovine aortic smooth muscle proliferation and bovine cappillary endothelial cell migration.[109]

IFN-γ has also been reported to inhibit endothelial cell proliferation,[110] to inhibit capillary tube formation in vitro,[111] and to inhibit angiogenesis following bFGF exposure.[112] IFN-γ additionally stimulates endothelial cell glycosaminoglycan secretion.[113] Other potent effects of these interferons include antiviral activity, upregulation of major histocompatibility complex (MHC) class II antigen expression, and an increase in NK cell activity.

Tumor Necrosis Factor

TNF-α, also referred to as cachectin, was originally named for its reported tumoricidal activity. Its gene has been cloned, sequenced, and assigned to chromosome 6 near the MHC locus. This macrophage-derived cytokine shares many, but not all, functions with IL-1. The major source of TNF-α is the activated monocyte and macrophage. TNF-α production by macrophages is stimulated by LPS, IL-2, GM-CSF, and IL-1. This monokine was shown to be growth inhibitory to endothelial cells in vitro,[114,115] but capable of stimulating angiogenesis in vivo.[116,117] This paradox may be explained by the in vivo inflammatory response induced by TNF-α, which results in the generation of secondary mediators of angiogenesis.

TNF-α has been reported to stimulate collagenase production by fibroblasts[118] and, thus may induce basement membrane degradation with secondary neovascularization. Other reported activities of TNF-α have included inflammatory, immunoregulatory, and procoagulant effects.[119] TNF-α is most likely involved in tumor necrosis, endotoxic shock, fever, cachexia, and the acute phase protein response.

Colony Stimulating Factors (G-CSF, GM-CSF, M-CSF)

Monocytes and macrophages stimulated by LPS or IL-1 increase their production of M-CSF, GM-CSF, and G-CSF. These three glycoproteins induce proliferation of hemopoietic cells, and have been reported to increase migration and proliferation of cultured endothelial cells.[120] A physiologic in vivo action of these cytokines within the vascular wall, however, has not been documented. As discussed previously, M-CSF mRNA expression in human atherosclerotic plaques was reported by PCR techniques to be at higher levels as compared to normal arteries and veins, but these investigators found no c-fms M-CSF receptor in cultured endothelial cells or SMCs and, thus, concluded that the macrophages were the likely target cells.[27] These same investigators additionally showed that cultured human monocytes exposed to M-CSF increased their mRNA expression for the acetyl LDL (scavenger) receptor and apolipoprotein E.

M-CSF induces the formation of monocyte precursors and stimulates the production of PGE$_2$, plasminogen activator, IL-1, IFN-γ, and TNF-α.[81] GM-CSF induces granulocyte, and monocyte colony formation, and modulates IL-1 and TNF-α production.[81] G-CSF induces granulocyte colony formation and enhances neutrophil function.[81]

Growth Factors

Platelet-Derived Growth Factor

PDGF is a dimeric cationic (pI 9.5 to 10.4) protein consisting of an A chain (18 kD) and a B chain (16 kD) with potent mitogenic activity against fibroblasts and

SMCs in vitro at concentrations of 1 to 6 ng/mL. Three dimeric combinations of A and B chains are found, AA, AB, and BB; the relative proportions of each dimer is dependent upon species. Originally found in the α granules of platelets, PDGF is also secreted by macrophages, endothelial cells, and SMCs. PDGF binds to a high affinity (kD 10^{-11} M) receptor found on SMCs and fibroblasts, but not on endothelial cell surfaces; these cells generally do not respond to PDGF stimulation. PDGF also is a potent chemoattractant for SMCs, monocytes, and neutrophils. The cell surface receptor is a glycoprotein of molecular weight 164000 D, with 40000 to 50000 receptors/SMCs. The PDGF receptor consists of α and β receptor subunits, the β receptor subunit specific for the PDGF B chain, while the α receptor subunit recognizes both PDGF A and B chains.

Following receptor binding by PDGF, tyrosine phosphokinase activity increases. The phosphorylation of intracytoplasmic phosphoproteins following PDGF exposure suggests second messenger system activation, with phosphorylation of both membrane associated and cytoplasmic proteins on both serine and tyrosine moieties occurring within seconds of PDGF receptor binding.

A transient exposure of cultured cells to PDGF results in an induced competency to progress through G_0/G_1 into the S phase; this competency is maintained for up to 13 hours following removal of the PDGF.[121,122] This competence state can be transferred by cytoplast fusion[123] suggesting mRNA mediation, and the PDGF B chain amino acid sequence shares an 87% homology with a region of the transforming gene product of the Simian Sarcoma Virus, the oncogene v-sis. The second messenger systems transducing the PDGF signal likely include tyrosine kinase phosphorylation, phosphatidylinositol turnover, protein kinase C (PKC) activation, and mobilization of calcium.[124–126] C-fos and c-myc proto-oncogenes are induced by PDGF prior to cell division.

PDGF's half-life in circulation is less than 2 minutes,[127] suggesting that in vivo activity would likely occur locally. Circulating proteins including α_2 macroglobulin may inhibit PDGF receptor binding.[128,129]

Immunohistochemical staining has identified the PDGF B chain protein within macrophages in all stages of atherosclerotic lesion development in both humans and nonhuman primates[130]; this data is consistent with the previous report of elevated PDGF B chain mRNA found by Northern analysis of human carotid endarterectomy specimens.[131] Endothelial denudation studies, however, have suggested that PDGF alone is not sufficient to induce a myointimal proliferation.[132,133] Rat carotid artery balloon de-endothelialization injury studies by Reidy and his colleagues have suggested a role for PDGF in stimulating SMC migration rather than proliferation.[134–136]

Fibroblast Growth Factor

FGF-1 (acidic FGF) and FGF-2 (bFGF) are both members of the heparin-binding growth factor family. FGF-1 production by activated macrophages was shown in a radioimmunoassay by Baird,[137] and FGF-1 and FGF-2 mRNA transcripts were identified by Winkles and Greisler[138] in macrophages harvested from both rabbit peritoneal cavities and rabbit aortic plaques. FGF-1 and FGF-2 share a 55% sequence homology, and can be separated by isoelectric points (pI 5 versus pI 9 to 10), as well by heparin-binding affinities with maximal elution from heparin sepharose at 1.1 versus 1.6 M NaCl. Heparin synergizes with the mitogenic activity of both FGF species, as well as affords them protection from proteolytic degradation.[139,140] FGF-1 in the absence of heparin possesses significantly less SMC mitogenic activity, while both FGF species are potent endothelial cell mitogens stimulating angiogenesis in many bioassay models.

FGF's mechanism of action is poorly understood. The protein possesses no signal sequence to permit its secretion from intact cells. However, secretion may occur following either cell injury or as a response to heat shock. Nuclear translocation has been suggested as a possible autocrine mode of action. In addition, FGF-2 has been detected in the basement membrane of arteries, attached to heparan sulfate[141,142]; this matrix-bound FGF-2 is released by exposure to heparanase,[143] and plasmin,[144] both of which are macrophage products. As discussed earlier, macrophage-released TGF-β may similarly induce release of basement membrane stored FGF-2. Both high affinity (FGF Type I receptor [flg]) and low affinity (heparan sulfate) FGF receptors have been found on endothelial cells. Transmembrane signaling is thought to involve PKC activation.[145] FGF exposure induces a rapid transient c-fos proto-oncogene expression in bovine endothelial cells.[139]

Balloon de-endothelialization studies of rat carotid arteries have suggested a mediating role for FGF-2 released by injured SMCs in the arterial media in stimulation of the first wave of SMCs cell proliferation prior to cell migration into the intima.[146] This proliferative response was significantly inhibited by infusion of an anti-FGF-2 antibody.[147] Immobilization of FGF-1 onto vascular grafts induces a transient elevation of tritiated thymidine uptake by both endothelial cells and SMCs in the first month following graft implantation into canine arteries.[148] Both endothelial cells and SMCs respond to FGF's chemoattractant activity, and FGF added to endothelial cells in culture promotes tube formation.[149]

Transforming Growth Factor-β

TGF-β is a product of a variety of malignant and normal cells including the activated macrophage. Three TGF-β homologs have been isolated, with TGF-β1 the most prevalent and well characterized. TGF-β1 is a 25 kD homodimeric peptide secreted in latent form requiring proteolysis or acidification prior to receptor binding. Three TGF-β receptors have also been identified.[150]

The mitogenic activity of TGF-β on endothelial cells and SMCs is complex. Endothelial cell growth in vitro is inhibited by TGF-β,[151] endothelial cell entry into the S phase is delayed,[152] and c-myc expression decreased.[153] By contrast, however, endothelial cells cultured in three-dimensional collagen gels are not inhibited by TGF-β.[154] Angiogenesis is induced by TGF-β installation into newborn mice in vivo,[155] and TGF-β installation into chorioallantoic membranes induces capillary sprouting and endothelial cell proliferation.[156] Higher TGF-β concentrations, however, resulted in an inhibition of endothelial cell migration and proliferation.[157]

A similar dose-dependent effect on SMC proliferation has been shown for TGF-β. SMC proliferation in vitro is stimulated at low TGF-β concentrations, but conversely is inhibited at higher concentrations. This is likely explained by a TGF-β-induced up-regulation of fibroblast and SMC PDGF transcription,[158] whereas higher concentrations of TGF-β simultaneously induce a down-regulation of the PDGF-β receptor subunit. TGF-β may also modulate myointimal hyperplasia and angiogenesis by inducing a secondary up-regulation of TNF-α, IL-1 FGF-2, as well as PDGF B.[159–161]

TGF-β is a potent stimulator of ECM molecule synthesis in vitro and in vivo. In vitro studies have shown an increase synthesis of many ECM molecules, proteinase inhibitors, and inhibition of proteinase synthesis.[162] Subcutaneous injection of TGF-β induces collagen synthesis.[163] TGF-β also induces both gene expression and protein synthesis of types I and III collagen and fibronectin.[164–166] TGF-β additionally modulates the expression of integrins, and inhibits IL-2's effects including IL-2-R expression.[167] TGF at picomolar concentrations induces gene expression for TNF-α, IL-1, FGF-2, and PDGFB.[161,168–170]

Lipid Metabolism

Accumulation of lipid in the arterial intima is central to the development of atherosclerosis. LDL modification in arterial walls with subsequent scavenger receptor mediated uptake by intimal macrophages are thought to be central to the formation of atherosclerotic plaques. Macrophages take up and degrade cholesterol containing lipoproteins by two mechanisms: 1) phagocytosis of whole cells or fragments of membranes containing cholesterol; or 2) by receptor mediated endocytosis of plasma lipoproteins either in solution or complexed in insoluble form with other tissue constituents. The scavenger (acetyl LDL) receptor is a high affinity saturable receptor which facilitates rapid uptake of modified LDL (modifications that abolish positive lysine residue charges and enhance the net negative charge), the receptor not regulated by intracellular cholesterol content. The normal in vivo ligand for the acetyl LDL/scavenger receptor is unknown, but the incubation of LDL with cultured endothelial cells generates an oxidized LDL (resembling the oxidized LDL product generated by in vitro incubation of LDL with copper), the uptake and degradation of which is receptor mediated and competitive with the uptake and degradation of acetyl LDL.[171–173] Native LDL does not cause lipid accumulation within macrophages, but must first be modified by any of several processes. Oxidative modification occurs within endothelial cells, which themselves can bind and incorporate native LDL. LDL may be proteolytically modified by elastase, plasmin, kallikrein, or thrombin. LDL entry into the intimal space exposes it to pro-oxidant conditions resulting in mm-LDL. mm-LDL can induce expression and secretion of M-CSF, GM-CSF, and G-CSF by human aortic endothelial cells[174] and can stimulate monocyte specific chemoattractant secretion including MCP-1 by cultured human aortic endothelial and SMCs.[175] MCP-1 and M-CSF mRNA were identified by in situ hybridization in macrophage rich regions of human and rabbit aortas, but not in control aortic tissues.[176,177] Thus, LDL oxidation induces both LDL uptake by macrophages to result in the promotion of foam cell formation, as well as the generation of chemoattractants yielding a further influx of circulating monocytes to the developing lesion.

Oxidized LDL induces an immunologic response as well. Auto antibodies against oxidized LDL epitopes are present in human serum and the titer of an autoantibody to an epitope of oxidized LDL, MDA-lysine, was reportedly an effective predictor of human carotid atherosclerosis progression.[178] Oxidized LDL also stimulates tissue factor released by macrophages, which may promote a prothrombotic balance in the region of macrophage rich plaques. A considerable research activity in many laboratories is currently in progress to investigate the relationship between oxidized LDL uptake by macrophages and the subsequent release of macrophage-derived cytokines and growth factors relevant to SMC proliferation.

The generation of profound hyperlipidemia in animals fed high cholesterol diets yields an abnormal cholesterol-rich, VLDL (d < 1.006 g/mL) which has a β mobility on electrophoresis and is, thus, designated β-VLDL, in contrast to the pre-β mobility seen in normal triglyceride carrying VLDL. This β-VLDL binds directly to macrophage receptors; these receptors differ from the scavenger acetyl-LDL receptor. A third family of macrophage binding sites mediates uptake of cholesteryl ester/protein complexes which can be isolated from human aortic atherosclerotic plaques.[179] This uptake results in a marked stimulation of cholesteryl oleate synthesis and cellular accumulation of cholesteryl esters.[179] This uptake is via high affinity saturable sites competitively blocked by polyamines including polyinosinic acid, dextran sulfate, and fucoidin, but not by polycytidylic acid.

Intracellular lipoprotein metabolism by macrophages occurs by sequential reactions in two cellular compartments. Lipoprotein bound cholesteryl esters entering the cell by receptor-mediated endocytosis are delivered first to lysosomes where they are hydrolyzed by an acid lipase. The liberated cholesteryl crosses the lysosomal membrane and enters the cytoplasm where it is either re-esterified by a microsomal enzyme (acyl-Co-A:cholesterol acyltranferase) and stored within the cytoplasm as cholesteryl ester, or is excreted from the cell.

Lipoprotein uptake by macrophages is considered by many to be a protective mechanism to rid the interstitial space of excessive lipoproteins. When this protective mechanism is overwhelmed, however, foam cell formation results because of either an overabundance of intimal lipoproteins too large for macrophages to process, or because of the limited ability of macrophages to excrete the processed cholesterol.

References

1. Karnovsky ML: Metchinkoff in Messina: a century of studies on phagocytosis. *N Eng J Med* 304:1178–1180, 1981.
2. Antischow E: Experimental arteriosclerosis in animals. In: Cowdry EV (ed). *Arteriosclerosis* New York: MacMillan; 271–322, 1967.
3. Geer JC, McGill HC, Strong JP: The fine structure of human atherosclerotic lesions. *Am J Path* 34:1764–1769, 1961.
4. Scaffner T, et al: Arterila foam cells with distinctive immunomorphological and histochemical features of macrophages. *Am J Path* 100:57–80, 1980.
5. Aschoff L: Das reticulo-entheliale system. *Ergeb Inn Med Kinderheilkd* 26:1–118, 1924.
6. Whitelaw DM: The intravascular life span of monocytes. *Blood* 28:445–464, 1966.
7. Jones AL, Miller JL: Growth factors in haemopoiesis. In: Clinical haematology: *A plastic ANaemia* (ed. EC Gordon-Smith) London: Bailliere Tindall; 1989.
8. Thorens B, Mermod JJ, Vassalli P: Phagocytosis and inflammatory stimuli induce GM-CSF mRNA in macrophages through post-transcriptional regulation. *Cell* 48:671–679, 1987.
9. Broudy VC, Kaushansky K, Segal GM, Harlan JM, Ad-

amson JW: Tumour necrosis factor type alpha stimulates human endothelial cells to produce granulocyte/macrophage colony-stimulating factor. *Proc Natl Acad Sci USA* 83:7467–7471, 1986.

10. Munker R, Gasson J, Ogawa M, Koeffler HP: Recombinant human tumour necrosis factor induces production of granulocyte-monocyte colony stimulating factor. *Nature* 323:79–82, 1986.

11. Bagby GC Jr, Dinarello CA, Wallace P, Wagner C, Hefeneider S, McCall E: Interleukin 1 stimulates granulocyte macrophage colony-stimulating activity release by vascular endothelial cells. *J Clin Invest* 78:1316–1323, 1986.

12. van Waarde D, Hulsing-Hesselink E, van Furth R: Properties of a factor increasing monocytopoiesis (FIM) occurring in serum during the early phase of an inflammatory reaction. *Blood* 50:727–741, 1977.

13. Sluiter W, Elzenga-Claasen I, Hulsing-Hesselink E, van Furth R: Presence of the factor increasing monocyto-poiesis (FIM) in rabbit peripheral blood during an acute inflammation. *J Reticuloendothel Soc* 34:235–252, 1983.

14. van Furth R, Sluiter W: Macrophages as autoregulators of mononuclear phagocytes proliferation. In: *Progress in Leukocyte Biology*. Vol. 4 Reichard S, Kojima M (eds). Alan R. Liss Inc.; New York: 111–123, 1985.

15. Moore RN, Oppenheim JJ, Farrar JJ, Carter CS, Waheed A, Shadduck PK: Production of lymphocyte-activating factor (interleukin-1) by macrophages activated with colony stimulating factors. *J Immunol* 125:1302–1305, 1980.

16. Moore RN, Larsen HS, Horohov DW, Rouse BT: Endogenous regulation of macrophage proliferative expansion by colony-stimulating factor-induced interferon. *Science* 223:178–180, 1984.

17. Warren MK, Ralph P: Macrophage growth factor CSF-1 stimulated human monocyte production of interferon, tumor necrosis factor, and colony stimulating activity. *J Immuno* 137:2281–2285, 1986.

18. Clinton SK, Underwood R, Hayes L, Sherman ML, Kufe DW, Libby P: Macrophage colony-stimulating factor gene expression in vascular cells and in experimental and human atherosclerosis. *Am J Pathol* 140:301–316, 1992.

19. Shimano H, Yamada N, Ishibashi S, et al: Human monocyte colony-stimulating factor enhances the clearance of lipoproteins containing apolipoprotein B-100 via both low density lipoprotein receptor-dependent amd -independent pathways in rabbits. *J Biol Chem* 265:12869–12875, 1990.

20. Mori N, Gotoda T, Isibashi S, et al: Effects of human recombinant macrophage colony-stimulating factor on the secretion of lipoprotein lipase from macrophages. *Arterioscler Thromb* 11:1315–1321, 1991.

21. Ishibashi S, Inaba T, Shimano H, et al: Monocyte colony-stimulating factor enhances uptake and degradation of acetylated low density lipoproteins and cholesterol esterification in human monocyte-derived macrophages. *J Biol Chem* 265:14109–14117, 1990.

22. Shimada M, Inaba T, Shimano H, et al: Platelet-derived growth factor BB-dimer suppresses the expression of macrophage colony-stimulating factor in human vascular smooth muscle cells. *J Biol Chem* 267:15455–15458, 1992.

23. Gerrity RG, Naito HK, Richardson M, Schwartz CJ: Dietary-induced atherogenesis in swine. I. Morphology of the intima in prelesion stages. *Am J Pathol* 95:775–792, 1979.

24. Stadius ML, Rowan R, Fleischhauer JF, Kernoff R, Billingham M, Gown AM: Time course and cellular characteristics of the iliac artery response to acute balloon injury. *Arterioscler Thromb* 12:1267–1273, 1992.

25. Verheyen AK, Vlaminckx EM, Lauwers FM, Saint-Guillani ML, Borgers MJ: Identification of macrophages in intimal thickening of rat carotid arteries by cytochemical localization of purine nucleoside phosphorylase. *Arteriosclerosis* 8:759–767, 1988

26. Stary HC: Evolution and progression of atherosclerotic lesions in coronary arteries of children and young adults. Arteriosclerosis 9(suppl I):I19–I32, 1989.

27. Gordon D, Reidy MA, Benditt EP, Schwartz SM: Cell proliferation in human coronary arteries. *Proc Natl Acad Sci USA* 87:4600–4604, 1990.

28. Libby P, Schwartz D, Brogi E, Tanaka H, Clinton SK: A cascade model for restenosis. *Circulation* 86(suppl III):III47–III52, 1992.

29. Zwolak RM, Kirkman TR, Clowes AW: Atherosclerosis in rabbit vein grafts. *Arteriosclerosis* 9:374–379, 1989.

30. Greisler HP, Ellinger J, Henderson SC, et al: The effects of an atherogenic diet on macrophage/biomaterial interactions. *J Vasc Surg* 14:10–23, 1991.

31. Greisler HP, Henderson SC, Lam TM: Basic fibroblast growth factor production in vitro by macrophages exposed to Dacron and polyglactin 910. *J Biomater Sci Polymer Ed.* 4:415–430, 1993.

32. Petsikas D, Cziperle DJ, Lam TM, Murchan PM, Henderson SC, Greisler HP: Dacron-induced TGF-β release from macrophages: effects on graft healing. Surg *Forum* 42:326–328, 1991.

33. Miller K, Rose-Caprara V, Anderson JM: Generation of IL1-like activity in response to biomedical polymer implants: a comparison of in vitro and in vivo models. *J Biomed Mat Res* 23:1007–1026, 1989.

34. Aqel NM, Ball RY, Waldmann H, Mitchinson MJ: Identification of macrophages and smooth muscle cells in human atherosclerosis using monoclonal antibodies. *J Pathol* 146:197–204, 1985.

35. Klurfeld DM: Identification of foam cells in human atherosclerotic lesions as macrophages using monoclonal antibodies. *Arch Pathol Lab Med* 109:445–449, 1985.

36. Johasson L, Holm J, Skalli O, Bondjer G, Hansson GK: Regional accumulations of T cells, macrophages, and smooth muscle cells in the human atherosclerotic plaque. *Arteriosclerosis* 6:131–138, 1986.

37. Gerrity RG, Goss JA, Soby L: Control of monocyte recruitment by chemotactic factor(s) in lesion-prone areas of swine aorta. *Arteriosclerosis* 5:55–66, 1985.

38. Denholm EM: Monocyte chemoattractants in pigeon aortic atherosclerosis. *Am J Pathol* 126:464–475, 1987.

39. Valente AJ, Fowler SR, Sprague EA, Kelley JL, Suenram CA, Schwartz CJ: Initial characterisation of a peripheral blood mononuclear cell chemoattractant derived from cultured arterial smooth muscle cells. *Am J Pathol* 117:409–417, 1984.

40. Salvemini D, deNucci G, Gryglewski RJ: Monocyte chemotactic protein 1 in human endothelial cells and smooth muscle cells. *Proc Natl Acad Sci USA* 87:5134–5138, 1990.

41. Fox PL, DiCorleto PE: Regulation of production of a platelet-derived growth factor-like protein by cultured bovine aortic endothelial cells. *J Cell Physiol* 121:298–308, 1984.

42. Clowes AW, Kirkman TR, Clowes MM: Mechanisms of arterial graft failure. II. Chronic endothelial and smooth muscle cell proliferation in healing polytetrafluoroethylene prostheses. *J Vasc Surg* 3:877–884, 1986.

43. DiCorleto PE, De La Motte CA: Characterization of the adhesion of the human monocytic cell line U-937 to cultured endothelial cells. *J Clin Invest* 75:1153–1161, 1985.

44. Bevilacqua MP, Pober JS, Wheeller ME, Cotran RS, Gimbrone MA, Jr: Interleukin-1 acts on cultured human vascular endothelium to increase the adhesion of polymorphonuclear leukocytes, monocytes, and related leukocyte cell lines. *J Clin Invest* 76:2003–2011, 1985.

45. Bath PM, Gladwin AM, Martin JF: Human monocyte characteristics are altered in hypercholesterolaemia. *Atherosclerosis* 90:175–181, 1991.

46. Quinn MT, Parthasarathy S, Fong LG, Steinberg D: Oxidatively modified low density lipoproteins: a potential role in recruitment and retention of monocyte/macrophages during atherogenesis. *Proc Natl Acad Sci USA* 84:2995–2998, 1987.

47. Quinn MT, Parthasarathy S, Steinberg D: Endothelial cell-derived chemotactic activity for mouse peritoneal macrophages and the effects of modified forms of low density lipoprotein. *Proc Natl Acad Sci USA* 82:5949–5953, 1985.

48. Quinn MT, Parthasarathy S, Steinberg D: Lysophosphatidylcholine: a chemotactic factor for human monocytes and its potential role in atherogenesis. *Proc Natl Acad Sci USA* 85:2805–2809, 1988.

49. Berliner JA, Territo MC, Sevanian A, Ramin S, Kim JA, Bamshad B, et al: Minimally modified low density lipoprotein stimulates monocyte endothelial interactions. *J Clin Invest* 85:1260–1266, 1990.

50. Cushing SD, Berliner JA, Valente AJ, Territo MC, Navab M, Parhami F, et al: Minimally modified low density lipoprotein induces monocyte chemotactic protein cells. *Proc Natl Acad Sci USA* 87:5134–5138, 1990.

51. Navab M, Imes SS, Hama SY, Hough GP, Ros LA, Bork RW, et al: Monocyte transmigration induced by modification of low density lipoprotein in cocultures of human aortic wall cells is due to induction of monocyte chemotactic protein 1 synthesis and is abolished by high density lipoprotein. *J Clin Invest* 88:2039–2046, 1991.

52. Moore SK, Appella E, Lerman MJ, Leonard EJ: Human monocyte chemoattractant protein-1 (MCP1): full-length cDNA cloning, expression in mitogen-stimulated blood mononuclear leukocytes, and sequence similarity to mouse competence gene JE. *FEBS Letts* 244:487–493, 1989.

53. Colotta F, Borre A, Wang JM, Tarranelli M, Maddalena F, Polentarutti N, et al: Expression of a monocyte chemotactic cytokine by human mononuclear phagocytes. *J Immunol* 148:760–765, 1992.

54. Wang JM, Sica A, Giuseppe P, Walter S, Padura IM, Libby P, et al: Expression of monocyte chemotactic protein and interleukin-8 by cytokine-activated human vascular smooth muscle cells. *Arterioscler Thromb* 11:1166–1174, 1991.

55. Yoshimura T, Leonard EJ: Identification of high affinity receptors for human monocyte chemoattractant protein-1 on human monocytes. *J Immunol* 145:292–297, 1990.

56. Yu X, Dluz S, Graves DT, et al: Elevated expression of monocyte chemoattractant protein 1 by vascular smmoth muscle cells in hyperclolesterolemic primates. *Proc Natl Acad Sci USA* 89:6953–6957, 1992.

57. Nelken NA, Coughlin SR, Gordon D, Wilcox JN: Monocyte chemoattractant protein-1 in human atheromatous plaques. *J Clin Invest* 88:1121–1127, 1991.

58. Faruqi RM, DiCorleto PE: Mechanisms of monocyte recruitment and accumulation. *Br Heart J* 69(suppl):S19–S29, 1993.

59. Sluiter W, Hulsing-Hesselink E, Elzenga-Claasen I, et al: Macrophages as origin of factor increasing monocytopoiesis. *J Exp Med* 166:909–922, 1987.

60. Annema A, Sluiter W, van Furth R: Effect of interleukin I, macrophage colony-stimulating factor, and factor increasing monocytopoiesis on the production of leukocytes in mice. *Exp Hematol* 20:69–74, 1992.

61. Sluiter W, Elzenga-Claasen I, van der Voort van der Kley-van Andel A, and van Furth R: Differences in the response of inbred mouse strains to the factor increasing monocytopoiesis. *J Exp Med* 159:524–536, 1984.

62. van Furth R, Sluiter W: Distribution of blood monocytes between a marginating and circulating pool. *J Exp Med* 163:474–479, 1986.

63. Pober JS, Gimbrone MA Jr, LaPierre LA et al: Overlapping patterns of activation of human endothelial cells by interleukin 1, tumor necrosis factor, and immuno interferon. *J Immunol* 137:1893–1896, 1986.

64. Marlin SD, Springer TA: Purified intercellular adhesion molecule-1 (ICAM-1) is a ligand for lymphocyte function-associated antigen 1 (LFA-1). *Cell* 51:813–819, 1987.

65. Diamond MS, Stanuton DA, de Fougerolles AR, et al: ICAM-1 (CD54): a counter-receptor for Mac-1 (CD11b/CD18). *J Cell Biol* 111:3129–3139, 1990.

66. Smith CW, Marlin SD, Rothlein R, Toman C, Anderson DC: Cooperative interactions of LFA-1 and Mac-1 with intercellular adhesion molecule-1 in facilitating adherence and transendothelial migration of human neutrophils in vitro. *J Clin Invest* 83:2008–2017, 1989.

67. Hibbs ML, Xu H, Stacker SA, Springer TA: Regulation of adhesion to ICAM-1 by the cutoplasmic domain of LFA-1 integrin β subunit. *Science* 251:1611–1613, 1991.

68. Furie MB, Tancinco MCA, Smith CW: Monoclonal antibodies to leukocyte integrins CD11a/CD18 and CD11b/CD18 or intercellular adhesion molecule-1 (ICAM-1) inhibit chemoattractant-stimulated neutrophil transendothelial migration in vitro. *Blood* 78:2089–2097, 1991.

69. Geng JG, Bevilacqua MP, Moore KL, et al: Rapid neutrophil adhesion to activated endothelium mediated by GMP-140. *Nature* 343:757–760, 1990.

70. Smith CW, Rothlein R, Hughes BJ et al: Recognition of an endothelial determinant for CD18 dependent human neutrophil and transendothelial migration. *J Clin Invest* 82:1746–1756, 1988.

71. Pober JS, Cotran RS: Cytokines and endothelial cell biology. *Physiol Rev* 70:427–451, 1990.

72. Knighton DR, Hunt TK, Scheuenstuhl H, Halliday BJ, Werb Z, Banda MJ: Oxygen tension regulates the expression of angiogenesis factor by macrophages. *Science* 39:233–238, 1983.

73. Jensen JA, Hunt TK, Scheuenstuhl H, Banda MJ: Effect of lactate, pyruvate, and pH on secretion of angiogenesis and mitogenesis factors by macrophages. *Lab Invest* 54:574–578, 1986.

74. Henson PM, Henson JE, Fittschen C, Bratton DL, Riches DWH: Degranulation and Secretion by Phagocytic Cells. In: Gallin JI, Goldstein IM, Snyderman R (eds). *Inflammation: Basic Principles and Clinical Cor-*

relates, 2nd Ed. New York: Raven Press; 511–539, 1992.

75. Grabstein KH, Urdal DL, Tushinski RJ, et al: Induction of macrophages tumoricidal activity by granulocyte-macrophage colony-stimulating factor. *Science* 232: 506–508, 1986.

76. De Tito EH, Catterall JR, Remington JS: Activity of recombinant tumor necrosis factor on Toxoplasma gondii and Trypanosoma cruzi. *J Immunol* 137:1342–1345, 1986.

77. Nathan CF, Murray HW, Wiebe ME, Rubin BY: Identification of interferon-γ as the lymphokine that activates human macrophage oxidative metabolism and antimicrobial activity. *J Exp Med* 158:670–689, 1983.

78. Murray HW, Rubin BY, Rothermel CD: Killing of intracellular Leishmania donovani by lymphokine-stimulated human mononuclear phagocytes: evidence that interferon-γ is the activating lymphokine. *J Clin Invest* 72:1506–1510, 1983.

79. Cassatella MA, Della Bianca V, Berton G, Rossi F: Activation by gamma interferon of human macrophage capability to produce toxic oxygen molecules is accompanied by decreased Km of the superoxide-generating NADPH oxidase. *Biochem Biophys Res Commun* 132: 908–914, 1985.

80. McPhail LC, Snyderman R: Activation of the respiratory burst enzyme in human polymorphonuclear leucocytes by chemoattractants and other soluble stimuli: evidence that the same oxidase is activated by different transductional mechanisms. *J Clin Invest* 72:192–200, 1983.

81. Auger MJ, Ross JA: The biology of the macrophage. In: Lewis CE and McGee JO'D (eds). *The Natural Immune System: The Macrophage* New York: Oxford University Press; 1–74, 1992.

82. Pantalone RM, Page RC: Lymphokine-induced production and release of lysosomal enzymes by macrophages. *Proc Natl Acad Sci USA* 72:2091–2094, 1975.

83. Gabig TG, Babior BM: The killing of pathogens by phagocytes. *Ann Rev Med* 32:313–326, 1981.

84. Falcone DJ, McCaffrey TA, Haimovitz-Friedman A, Garcia M: Transforming growth factor-β1 stimulates macrophage urokinase expression and release of matrix-bound basic fibroblast growth factor. *J Cell Physiol* 155:595–605, 1993.

85. Anidjar S, Salzmann J-L, Gentric D, Lagneau P, Camilleri J-P, Michel J-B: Elastase-induced experimental aneurysms in rats. *Circulation* 82:973–981, 1990.

86. Johnson WJ, Pizzo SV, Imber MJ, Adams DO: Receptors for maleylated proteins regulate secretion of neutral proteases by murine macrophages. *Science* 218: 574–576, 1982.

87. Edwards RL, Rickles FR: Macrophage procoagulants. In: Spaet TH (ed). *Progress in Haemostasis and Thrombosis*. New York Grune and Stratton Inc; 1984.

88. Kalman PG, Rotstein OD, Niven J, Glynn MFX, Romaschin AD: Differential stimulation of macrophage procoagulant activity by vascular grafts. *J Vasc Surg* 17:531–537, 1993.

89. Nawroth PP, Stern DM: Modulation of endothelial cell haemostatic properties by tumour necrosis factor. *J Exp Med* 163:740–745, 1986.

90. Zhang H, Downs EC, Lindsey JA, Davis WB, Whisler RL, Cornwell DG: Interactions between the monocyte/macrophage and the vascular smooth muscle cell. *Arterioscler Thromb* 13:220–230, 1993.

91. Polacek D, Lal R, Volin MV, Davies PF: Gap junctional communication between vascular cells. *Am J Pathol* 142:593–606, 1993.

92. Roberts NJ Jr, Prill AH, Mann TN: Interleukin-1 and interleukin-1 inhibitor production by human macrophages exposed to influenza virus or respiratory syncytial virus, respiratory syncytial virus is a potent inducer of inhibitor activity. *J Exp Med* 163:511–519, 1986.

93. Saegusa Y, Ziff M, Welkovich L, Cavender D: Effect of inflammatory cytokines on human endothelial cell proliferation. *J Cell Physiol* 142:488–495, 1990.

94. Cozzolino F, Torcia M, Aldinucci D, et al: Interleukin-1 is an autocrine regulator of human endothelial cell growth. *Proc Natl Acad Sci USA* 6487–6491, 1990.

95. Maier JAM, Voulalas P, Roeder D, Maciag T: Extension of the life-span of human endothelial cells by an interleukin-1-alpha antisense oligomer. *Science* 249: 1570–1574, 1990.

96. Gay CG, Winkles JA: Interleukin-1 regulates heparin-binding growth factor-2 gene expression in vascular smooth muscle cells. *Proc Natl Acad Sci USA* 88: 296–300, 1991.

97. Raines EW, Dower SK, Ross R: Interleukin-1 mitogenic activity for fibroblasts and smooth muscle cells is due to PDGF-AA. *Science* 243:393–396, 1989.

98. Bonfield TL, Colton E, Anderson JM: Plasma protein adsorbed biomedical polymers: Activation of human monocytes and induction of interleukin 1. *J Biomed Mater Res* 23:535–548, 1989.

99. Miller KM, Anderson JM: In vitro stimulation of fibroblast activity by factors generated from human monocytes activated by biomedical polymers. *J Biomed Mater Res* 23:911–930, 1989.

100. Miller KM, Rose-Caprara V, Anderson JM: Generation of IL 1-like activity in response to biomedical polymer implants: a comparison of in vitro and in vivo models. *J Biomed Mater Res* 23:1007–1026, 1989.

101. Bevilacqua MP, Pober JS, Majeau GR, Cotran RS, Gimbrone Jr MA: Interleukin I (IL-1) induces biosynthesis and cell surface expression of procoagulant activity in human vascular endothelial cells. *J Exp Med* 160: 618–623, 1984.

102. BenEzra D: Neovasculogenic ability of prostaglandins, growth factors, and synthetic chemoattractants. *Am J Ophthal* 86:455–461, 1978.

103. Matsuda T, et al: IL-6/BSF2 in normal and abnormal regulation of immune responses. *Ann NY Acad Sci* 557: 466–476, 1989.

104. May LT, Torcia G, Cozzolino F, et al: Interleukin-6 gene expression in human endothelial cells: RNA start sites, multiple IL-6 proteins and inhibition of proliferation. *Biochem Biophys Res Commun* 159:991–998, 1989.

103. Baggiolini M, Walz A, Kunkel SL: Neutrophil-activating peptide-1/interleukin-8, a novel cytokine that activates neutrophils. *J Clin Invest* 84:1045–1050, 1989.

106. Pestka S, Langer JA, Zoon KC, Samuel CE: Interferons and their actions. *Ann Rev Biochem* 56:727–777, 1987.

107. Robinson BWS, McLemore TL, Crystal RG: Gamma interferon is spontaneously released by alveolar macrophages and lung T lymphocytes in patients with pulmonary sarcoidosis. *J Clin Invest* 75:1488–1495, 1985.

108. Nathan C, Yoshida R: Cytokines: Interferon-gamma. In: Gallin JI, Goldstein IM and Snyderman R (eds). Inflammation: Basic Principles and Clinical Correlates, New York: Raven Press; 229–251, 1988.

109. Brouty-Boye D, Zetter BR: Inhibition of cell motility by interferon. *Science* 208:516–518, 1980.

110. Friesel R, Komoriya A, Maciag T: Inhibition of endothelial cell proliferation by gamma-interferon. *J Cell Biol* 104:689–696, 1987.

111. Tsuruoka N, Sugiyama M, Tawaragi Y, et al: Inhibition of in vitro angiogenesis by lymphotoxin and interferon-gamma. *Biochem Biophys Res Commun* 155:429–435, 1988.

112. Sato N, Nariuchi H, Tsuruoka N, et al: Actions of TNF and IFN-gamma on angiogenesis in vitro. *J Invest Dermat* 95:85S–89S, 1990.

113. Montesano R, Mossaz A, Ryser J-E, Orci L, Vassalli P: Leukocyte interleukins induce cultured endothelial cells to produce a highly organized, glycosaminoglycan-rich pericellular matrix. *J Cell Biol* 99:1706–1715, 1984.

114. Sato N, Goto T, Haranaka K, et al: Actions of tumor necrosis factor on cultured vascular endothelial cell: morphologic modulation, growth inhibition, and cytotoxicity. *JNCI* 76:1113–1121, 1986.

115. Robaye B, Mosselmans R, Fiers W, Dumont JE, Galand P: Tumor necrosis factor induces apoptosis (programmed cell death) in normal endothelial cells in vitro. *Am J Path* 138:447–453, 1991.

116. Frater-Schroder M, Risau W, Hallmann R, Gautschi P, Bohlen P: Tumor necrosis factor type α, a potent inhibitor of endothelial cell growth in vitro, is angiogenic in vivo. *Proc Natl Acad Sci USA* 84:5277–5281, 1987.

117. Rosenbaum JT, Howes EL Jr, Rubin RM, Samples JR: Ocular inflammatory effects of intravitreally-injected tumor necrosis factor. *Am J Path* 133:47–53, 1988.

118. Dayer J-M, Beutler B, Cerami A: Cachectin/tumor necrosis factor stimulates collagenase and PGE₂ production by human synovial cells and dermal fibroblasts. *J Exp Med* 162:2163–2168, 1985.

119. Pober JS, Cotran SR: The role of endothelial cells in inflammation. *Transplantation* 50:537–544, 1990.

120. Bussolino F, Wang JM, Defilippi P, et al: Granulocyte-and granulocyte-macrophage-colony-stimulating factors induce human endothelial cells to migrate and proliferate. *Nature* 337:471–473, 1989.

121. Pledger WJ, Stiles CD, Antoniades HN, Scher CD: Induction of DNA synthesis in BALB/c 3T3 cells by serum components: reevaluation of the commitment process. *Proc Natl Acad Sci USA* 74:4481–4485, 1977.

122. Pledger WJ, Stiles CD, Antoniades HN, Scher CD: An ordered sequence of events is required before BALB/c 3T3 cells become committed to DNA synthesis. *Proc Natl Acad Sci USA* 75:2839–2843, 1978.

123. Smith JC, Stiles CD: Cytoplasmic transfer of the mitogenic response to platelet-derived growth factor. *Proc Natl Acad Sci USA* 78:4363–4367, 1981.

124. Habenicht AJR, Glomset JA, King WC, Nist C, Mitchell CD, Ross R: Early changes in phosphatidylinositol and arachidonic acid metabolism in quiescent Swiss 3T3 cells stimulated to divide by platelet-derived growth factor. *J Biol Chem* 256:12329–12335, 1981.

125. Nishizuka Y: The role of protein kinase C in cell surface signal transduction and tumour promotion. *Nature* 308:693–698, 1984.

126. Sunderkotter C, Goebeler M, Schulze-Osthoff K, Bhardwaj R, Sorg C: Macrophage-derived angiogenesis factors. *Pharmac Ther* 51:195–216, 1991.

127. Bowen-Pope DF, Malpass TW, Foster DM, Ross R: Platelet-derived growth factor in vivo: levels, activity, and rate of clearance. *Blood* 64z;458–469, 1984.

128. Raines EW, Bowen-Pope DF, Ross R: Plasma binding proteins for platelet-derived growth factor that inhibit its binding to cell-surface receptors. *Proc Natl Acad Sci USA* 81:3424–3428, 1984.

129. Huang JS, Huang SS, Deuel TF: Specific covalent binding of platelet-derived growth factor to human plasma α₂-macroglobulin. *Proc Natl Acad Sci USA* 81:342–346, 1984.

130. Ross R, Masuda J, Raines EW, et al: Localization of PDGF-B protein in macrophages in all phases of atherogenesis. *Science* 1009–1012, 1990.

131. Barrett TB, Benditt EP: Platelet-derived growth factor gene expression in human atherosclerotic plaques and normal artery wall. *Proc Natl Acad Sci USA* 85:2810–2814, 1988.

132. Groves HM, Kinlough-Rathbone RL, Richardson M, Moore S, Mustard F: Platelet interaction with damaged rabbit aorta. *Lab Invest* 40:194–200, 1979.

133. Goldberg ID, Stemerman MB, Handin RI: Vascular permeation of platelet factor 4 after endothelial injury. *Science* 209:611–612, 1980.

134. Fingerle J, Johnson R, Clowes AW, Majesky MW, Reidy MA: Role of platelets in smooth muscle cell proliferation and migration after vascular injury in rat carotid arery. *Proc Natl Acad Sci USA* 86:8412–8416, 1989.

135. Jawien A, Bowen-Pope DF, Lindner V, Schwartz SM, Clowes AW: Platelet-derived growth factor promotes smooth muscle migration and intimal thickening in a rat model of balloon angioplasty. *J Clin Invest* 89:507–511, 1992.

136. Ferns GAA, Raines EW, Sprugel KH, Motani AS, Reidy MA, Ross R: Inhibition of neointimal smooth muscle accumulation after angioplasty by an antibody to PDGF. *Science* 253:1129–1132, 1991.

137. Baird A, Mormede P, Bohlen P: Immunoreactive fibroblast growth factor in cells of peritoneal exudate suggests its identity with macrophage-derived growth factor. *Biochem Biophys Res Commun* 126:358–364, 1985.

138. Winkles J, Greisler HP: Unpublished observations.

139. Burgess WH, Maciag T: The heparin-binding (fibroblast) growth factor family of proteins. *A Rev Biochem* 58:575–606, 1989.

140. Sommer A, Rifkin DB: Interaction of heparin with human basic fibroblast growth factor: protection of the angiogenic protein from proteolytic degradation by a glycosaminoglycan. *J Cell Physiol* 138:215–220, 1989.

141. Ingber DE: Fibronectin controls capillary endothelial cell growth by modulating cell shape. *Proc Natl Acad Sci USA* 87:3579–3583, 1990.

142. Saksela O, Moscatelli D, Sommer A, Rifkin DB: Endothelial cell-derived heparan sulfate binds basic fibroblast growth factor and protects it from proteolytic degradation. *J Cell Biol* 107:743–751, 1988.

143. Vlodavsky I, Folkman J, Sullivan R, et al: Endothelial cell-derived basic fibroblast growth factor. Synthesis and deposition into subendothelial extracellular matrix. *Proc Natl Acad Sci USA* 84:2292–2296, 1987.

144. Saksela O, Rifkin DB: Release of basic fibroblast growth factor-heparan sulfate complexes from endothelial cells by plasminogen activator-mediated proteolytic activity. *J Cell Biol* 110:767–775, 1990.

145. Daviet I, Herbert JM, Maffrand JP: Involvement of protein kinase C in the mitogenic and chemotaxis effects of basic fibroblast growth factor on bovine cerebral cortex capillary endothelial cells. *FEBS Lett* 259:315–317, 1990.

146. Lindner V, Lappi DA, Baird A, Majack RA, Reidy MA: Role of basic fibroblast growth factor in vascular lesion formation. *Circ Res* 68:106–113, 1991.

147. Lindner V, Reidy, MA: Proliferation of smooth muscle cells after vascular injury is inhibited by an antibody

basic fibroblast growth factor (bFGF). *Proc Natl Acad Sci USA* 88:3739–3743, 1991.

148. Greisler HP: Unpublished observations.

149. Montesano R, Vassalli J-D, Baird A, Guillemin R, Orci L: Basic fibroblast growth factor induces angiogenesis in vitro. *Proc Natl Acad Sci USA* 83:7297–7301, 1986.

150. Barnard JA, Lyons RM, Moses HL: The cell biology of transforming growth factor β. *Biochim Biophys Acta* 1032:79–87, 1990.

151. Frater-Schroder M, Risau W, Hallmann R, Gautschi P, Bohlen P: Tumor necrosis factor type α, a potent inhibitor of endothelial cell growth in vitro, is angiogenic in vivo. *Proc Natl Acad Sci USA* 84:5277–5281, 1987.

152. Heimark RL, Twardzik DR, Schwartz SM: Inhibition of endothelial regeneration by type-beta transforming growth factor from platelets. *Science* 233:1078–1080, 1986.

153. Takehara K, LeRoy EC, Grotendorst GR: TGF-β inhibition of endothelial cell proliferation: alteration of EGF binding and EGF-induced growth regulatory (competence) gene expression. *Cell* 49:415–422, 1987.

154. Madri JA, Pratt BM, Tucker AM: Phenotypic modulation of endothelial cells by transforming growth factor-beta depends upon the composition and organization of the extracellular matrix. *J Cell Biol* 106:1375–1384, 1988.

155. Roberts AB, Sporn MB, Assoian RK, et al: Transforming growth factor type β: rapid induction of fibrosis and angiogenesis in vivo and stimulation of collagen formation in vitro. *Proc Natl Acad Sci USA* 83:4167–4171, 1986.

156. Yang EY, Moses HL: Transforming growth factor beta 1-induced changes in cell migration, proliferation, and angiogenesis in the chicken chorioallantoic membrane. *J Cell Biol* 111:731–741, 1990.

157. Moses HL, Yang EY, Pietenpol JA: TGF-β stimulation and inhibition of cell proliferation: new mechanistic insights. *Cell* 63:245–247, 1990.

158. Leof EB, Proper JA, Goustin AS, Shipley GD, DiCorleto PE, Moses HL: Induction of c-sis mRNA and activity similar to platelet-derived growth factor by transforming growth factor beta: a proposed model for indirect mitogenesis involving autocrine activity. *Proc Natl Acad Sci USA* 83:2453–2457, 1986.

159. Wahl SM, Hunt DA, Wakefield IM, et al: Transforming growth factor type β induces monocyte chemotaxis and growth factor production. *Proc Natl Acad Sci USA* 84:5788–5792, 1987.

160. McCartney-Francis N, Mizel D, Wong H, Wahl LM, Washl SM: Transforming growth factor-beta (TGF-β) as an immunoregulatory molecule. *FASEB J* 2:A875, 1988.

161. Wiseman DM, Polverini PJ, Kamp DW, Leibovich SJ: Transforming growth factor-beta (TGFβ) is chemotactic for human monocytes and induces their expression of angiogenic activity. *Biochem Biophys Res Commun* 157:793–800, 1988.

162. Barnard JA, Lyons RM, Moses HL: The cell biology of transforming growth factor β. *Biochim Biophys Acta* 1032:79–87, 1990.

163. Roberts AB, Sporn MB, Assoian RK et al: Transforming growth factor type β: rapid induction of fibrosis and angiogenesis in vivo and stimulation of collagen formation in vitro. *Proc Natl Acad Sci USA* 83:4167–4171, 1986.

164. Ignotz RA, Endo T, Massague J: Regulation of fibronectin and type I collagen mRNA levels by transforming growth factor-β. *J Biol Chem* 262:6443–6446, 1987.

165. Varga J, Rosenbloom J, and Jimenez SA: Transforming growth factor-β (TGF-β) causes a persistent increase in steady-state amounts of type I and type III collagen and fibronectin mRNAs in normal human dermal fibroblasts. *Biochem* 247:597–604, 1987.

166. Rossi P, Karsenty G, Roberts AB, Roche NS, Sporn MB, DeCrombrugghe B: A nuclear factor 1 binding site mediates the transcriptional activation of a type I collagen promoter by transforming growth factor-β. *Cell* 52:405–414, 1988.

167. Chieftez S, et al: The transforming growth factor-beta system, a complex pattern of cross-reactive ligands and receptors. *Cell* 48:409–415, 1987.

168. Wahl SM, McCartney-Francis N, Allen JB, Dougherty EB, Dougherty SF: Macrophage production of TGF-β and regulation by TGF-β. *Ann NY Acad Sci* 593:188–196, 1990.

169. Wahl SM, Hunt DA, Wakefield IM, et al: Transforming growth factor type β induces monocyte chemotaxis and growth factor production. *Proc Natl Acad Sci USA* 84:5788–5792, 1987.

170. McCartney-Francis N, Mizel D, Wong H, Wahl LM, Wahl SM: Transforming growth factor-beta (TGF-β) as an immunoregulatory molecule. *FASEB J* 2:A875, 1988.

171. Brown MS, Basu SK, Falck JR, Ho YK, Goldstein JL: The scavenger cell pathway for lipoprotein degradation: specificity of the binding site that mediates the uptake of negatively-charged low density lipoprotein by macrophages. *J Supramol Struct* 13:67–81, 1980.

172. Henriksen T, Mahoney EM, Steinberg D: Enhanced macrophage degradation of low density lipoprotein previously incubated with cultured endothelial cells: recognition by receptors for acetylated low density lipoproteins. *Proc Natl Acad Sci USA* 78(10):6499–6503, 1981.

173. Steinbrecher UP, Parthasarathy S, Leake DS, Witzum JL, Steinberg D: Modification of low density lipoprotein by endothelial cells involves lipid peroxidation and degradation of low density lipoprotein phospholipids. *Proc Natl Acad Sci USA* 81:3883–3887, 1984.

174. Rajavashisth TB, Andalibi A, Territo MC, et al: Induction of endothelial cell expression of granulocyte and macrophage colony-stimulating factors by modified low density lipoproteins. *Nature* 344:254–257, 1990.

175. Cushing SD, Berliner JA, Valente AJ, et al: Minimally modified low density lipoprotein induces monocyte chemotactic protein 1 in human endothelial cells and smooth muscle cells. *Proc Natl Acad Sci USA* 87:5134–5138, 1990.

176. Yla-Herttuala S, Lipton BA, Rosenfeld ME, et al: Macrophages express monocyte chemotactic protein (MCP-1) in human and rabbit atherosclerotic lesions. *Proc Natl Acad Sci USA* 88:5252–5256, 1991.

177. Rosenfeld ME, Ula-Herttuala S, Lipton VA, Ord VA, Witztum JL, Steinberg D: Macrophage colony-stimulating factor mRNA and protein in atherosclerotic lesions of rabbits and man. *Am J Pathol* 140:291–300, 1992.

178. Salonen JT, Yla-Herttuala S, Yamamoto R, et al: Autoantibody against oxidised LDL and progression of carotid atherosclerosis. *Lancet* 339:883–887, 1992.

179. Goldstein JL, Hoff HF, Ho YK, Basu SL, Brown MS: Stimulation of cholesteryl ester synthesis in macrophages by extracts of atherosclerotic human aortas and complexes of albumin/cholesteryl esters. *Arteriosclerosis* 1:210–226, 1991.

CHAPTER 9

Platelets

William C. Krupski, MD

Historical Perspective

On March 7, 1842, at a session of the Académie des Sciences in Paris, Alfred Donné[1] described little globules ("globulins") in blood, now known as blood platelets. He distinctly differentiated them from other blood elements, although he erroneously attributed their origin to lymph, derived from the fatty particles in chyle. Also in 1842, Addison,[2] Gerber,[3] and Simon[4] independently demonstrated platelets, hypothesizing that they were precipitates from plasma or fragments of endothelium. At about the same time as Donné, Gustav Zimmermann, a German military physician, declared that platelets were precursors of red blood cells, calling them "elementarblächen." He remarked on their tendency to gather in clumps, even though he was among the first to use anticoagulants (potassium ferrocyanide) for the cytologic study of blood.[5] Zimmermann noted that anticoagulated blood contained "billions" of these small, colorless elementary bodies. Of interest, Rudolph Virchow, renowned for his contributions to pathology including his concept of thrombosis, wrote a scathing attack on Zimmermann's work in *Die Cellular-pathologie*[6]; Zimmermann replied with a similarly caustic article published in Virchow's own journal, *Virchow's Archiv*.

Max Schultze,[7] of Bonn, was among the first to attribute the origin of platelets to other blood elements. He corroborated Zimmermann's observation about clumping and called the subsequent granular masses "kugelchen," which he thought resulted from destruction of white blood cells. Others postulated that during anemias and cachectic states, white blood cells fragmented and gave rise to smaller corpuscles, which they termed "zerfallskoperchen" (disintegration bodies), analogous to Schultze's "kugelchen."

The next significant advance occurred in 1873. A young Canadian, recently graduated from McGill University, Dr. William Osler,[8] working in Professor Schaefer's laboratory in Oxford, demonstrated by observing his own blood that the "granular masses" of Schultze originated from the agglutination of small bodies; these occurred as single units in the circulation, coming together when blood was shed. Although he shared the erroneous opinion of other scientists of his era who thought platelets were related to bacteria, Osler's experiments in recently killed rats established platelets as normal constituents of circulating blood, not simply artifacts or byproducts of shed blood.[9] Georges Hayem,[10] a contemporary of Osler, held that platelets represented primitive red blood cells that had arrested in their evolution, coining the term "hematoblasts." According to Hayem, hematoblasts served to accelerate coagulation and regenerate blood after hemorrhage. He based these conclusions on changes in platelet shape after blood loss or severe illness in conjunction with fibrin formation. Hayem was both gifted and prolific; he became a full professor at the age of 38 at the Hôpital St. Antoine, retired from his clinic at 70, but continued to write until age 84, ten years before his death at 94.

In 1882, Giulio Bizzozero,[11] Professor of General Pathology at Turin, wrote a classic treatise that firmly established the platelet as a distinct element of circulating blood that promotes thrombosis. In this era, so-called "white thrombi" were thought to consist primarily of leukocytes. Bizzozero performed a number of imaginative experiments proving that the white portion of thrombi were composed almost exclusively of platelets, and accumulated at an area of vessel injury or obstructed blood flow. Bizzozero experimentally damaged blood vessel walls and observed that the first effect was adhesion of platelets to the point of injury; these platelet masses broke off into circulation and a

From *The Basic Science of Vascular Disease.* Edited by Sidawy AN, Sumpio BE, and DePalma RG. Armonk, NY: Futura Publishing Company, Inc.; © 1997.

new accumulation formed. He wrote "during a quarter of an hour one can see this game repeated three or four times, and this can last for hours. . ." When they formed a mass, platelets underwent changes in appearance and became sticky. His description was remarkably accurate: "[Platelets] become granular within the lumen of an injured vessel, and this change produces a substance which activates the coagulation system to form fibrin." Bizzozero referred to these bodies as "petites plaques" and Osler translated his expression "blut plättchen" as "blood plates." (Osler actually preferred the term "blood plaques.") The English word "platelet" did not appear until later in the nineteenth century, and "thrombocyte" did not appear until Dekhuyzen introduced the term in 1901.[12]

However, much disagreement and contradiction of Bizzozero's theories appeared in subsequent papers. Many investigators attributed the findings of the Italian scientist to remnants from vessel compression, circulatory disturbances, and anesthetic effects. Wooldridge[13] believed that platelets were a precipitate of the globulin portion of the plasma rather than a distinct component of blood, and Lowit[14] presented evidence against the existence of the platelet. In vitro experiments produced a confusing array of morphologic shapes and arrangements of platelets that presented many questions.

In a career than spanned over 50 years, the renowned American physiologist William Henry Howell, who at age 33 was appointed chairman of the Department of Physiology at the newly-opened Johns Hopkins Medical School, wrote several articles on platelets. The first confirmed Bizzozero's observations and appeared in *Science* in 1884.[15] One of the last was published in 1937, proposing the lungs instead of the bone marrow as the principal source of platelets, a concept still popular (see below).[16] Howell became dean of the Johns Hopkins Medical School at age 39, and at 45 he was elected to the first of his six consecutive terms as president of the American Physiological Association.[17]

In 1885, Professor J. C. Eberth and his assistant, the young German surgeon Curt Schimmelbusch, wrote an excellent paper on the relationship of blood-platelets and clotting, which supported Bizzozero's hypotheses.[18] Eberth and Schimmelbusch described the morphologic changes that occur when platelets come in contact with a foreign surface or a damaged vessel. They reported that these changes were associated with enhanced stickiness, so that platelets adhered to one another as well as to the abnormal surface, and introduced the term "viscous metamorphosis" to distinguish the process of platelet deposition and fibrin formation. These scientists also observed that platelets travel in the center of the blood stream with plasma on the periphery. Stasis of the circulation is accompanied by migration of leukocytes and platelets to the periphery of the stream, whereas red cells remain in the center. Laker[19] examined the behavior of platelets in vivo in dogs and other mammals, substantiating these concepts.

Counting platelets was hindered by technical difficulties, by Hayem[10] accurately reported platelet counts per cmm of blood. Hayem also concluded that because platelets play a central role in thrombus formation, a decrease or diminution in the number of circulating platelets should be associated with reduced hemostasis. He counted only 62,000 platelets per cmm of blood in a young patient with purpura, and he reported abnormally large platelets in patients with this disorder in conjunction with soft quality and poor retractility of formed thrombus.[20]

At the end of the nineteenth century, debate was raging over the origin of platelets, with most affirming that they arose from disintegrated erythrocytes. Confusion originated from the unavailability of stains to differentiate elements in the blood. Dominici,[21] using polychrome Romanowsky stains and azure dyes, introduced the concept that platelets were "organites," formed elements liberated by cells and lacking a nucleus. He described mononuclear "mother cells" of platelets with protoplasm distributed in long pedicles, which, when broken off, produced platelets. This notion influenced James Homer Wright,[22] who in 1906 showed that platelets were actually fragments of megakaryocytes, which Bizzozero[23] first described in 1869 and Howell[24] named in 1890. Examining blood smears with "improved Romanowsky stain" (later designated as Wright stain), Wright described intracytoplasmic blue hyaline material that surrounds central violet granules in both megakaryocytes and circulating platelet. In addition, he observed that both platelets and megakaryocytes formed pseudopods, suggesting a structural and functional relationship. These promising conjectures were largely ignored until the development of the electron microscope much later in the century.

Encouraged by Wright, who was his mentor when he was a house officer at Massachusetts General Hospital, W. W. Duke became interested in platelets and their role in bleeding disorders. The participation of platelets in spontaneous thrombosis, first suggested by Hayem, was convincingly shown by Duke. Duke developed the "bleeding time" test that bears his name. He correlated duration of bleeding time and platelet count, established the importance of platelets in hemostasis, and launched twentieth-century investigation of platelet function.

In 1918, Glannzmann[25] reported a patient with a bleeding disorder characterized by inability of clot to retract even in the presence of normal numbers of platelets. Glanzmann postulated that an internal platelet constituent was necessary for clot retraction—a contractile protein called thrombosthenin. The malady was called Glanzmann's *thrombasthenia* and was the first account of a qualitative platelet disorder.

The introduction of the electron microscope in the 1940s allowed investigators to study platelets at the molecular level. In 1947, Brinkhous[26] described platelet factors that participate in thrombin formation. In 1951, Harrington and associates[27] reported an antibody that attacked both platelets and the cytoplasm of megakaryocytes that gives rise to platelets.

Braunsteiner and Pakesch[28] discovered an abnormality in platelet function due to inadequate production of platelet factor 3 (PF3) in 1956, thus heralding the biochemical era of platelet research. That same year, Born[29] reported that adenosine triphosphate (ATP) was consumed in platelet aggregation. Discoveries of the significance of PF3 and ATP were crucial for elucidation of platelet behavior. Soon, introduction of sophisticated histochemical, immunologic, and molecular biologic techniques led to an abundance of research concerning the mechanisms of platelet function.

Platelet Production and Structure

Megakaryocytes

Megakaryocytes are the hematopoietic precursor cells that give rise to platelets.[22] Bizzozero first described the megakaryocyte in 1882, identifying it and the osteoclast as the two largest cells in bone marrow.[11] Megakaryocytes reach 150 μm (averaging 35 μm) in diameter and contain a single multilobulated nucleus, a feature that distinguishes them from the multinucleate osteoclasts. Osteoclasts are nonmyelogenous marrow cells that break down calcified bone and release ionic calcium into plasma. Megakaryocytes are relatively rare, comprising about 0.02% to 0.05% of the bone marrow nucleated cell population, with total numbers averaging $\sim 4 \times 10^7$.[30] Their large size and abundant cytoplasm allow them to produce several thousand platelets per cell. Their large *(mega)* nucleus *(karyon)* prompted their name. The mean ploidy of the normal human megakaryocyte is ~16N, in contrast to the normal 2N complement of DNA.

Although bone marrow is the principal location of megakaryocytes, they are found sporadically in all major organ tissues and are frequently present in the lung. This wide distribution has led some investigators to conclude that megakaryocytes do not shed platelets in the marrow, but are released into the circulation toward the end of the cell life cycle. They eventually reach the lung where, under the rigors of the voyage through the pulmonary vasculature, they ultimately discharge platelets.[31]

The rarity and fragility of megakaryocytes presented considerable obstacles to their study, especially at the molecular level. In the past decade, techniques were developed allowing isolation and enrichment of relatively pure populations of mature megakaryocytes and cloning of megakaryocyte progenitor cells in tissue culture. Several methods for isolating megakaryocytes are available, all of which take advantage of their large size, low density, or unique surface protein phenotype. These techniques include velocity sedimentation, isopycnic or density gradient sedimentation, counterflow centrifugal elutriation, immunologic separation using antibodies that recognize platelet glycoproteins, and combinations of these.[32,36]

Control of Megakaryocyte Production

The hematopoietic stem cell can differentiate into myelocytic, erythrocytic, and megakaryocytic cell lines. Determination of a cell line is controlled by plasma-soluble or *humoral* proteins called *poietins*, cell-derived regulators (elaborated by nonhematopoietic cells), and cytokines. The most well-known example of a humoral regulator is *erythropoietin*, which is secreted by the juxtaglomerular apparatus in the kidney nephron and regulates production of red blood cells by inducing proliferation of erythrocyte precursors via attachment to a receptor site on the stem cell membrane. Several regulators are responsible for control of megakaryocyte production, which act early in development at the level of the progenitor cell and late on terminally differentiating cells.

Megakaryocyte colony stimulating factor (Meg-CSF; also designated Meg-CSA [activity]) recruits stem cells for megakaryocytic differentiation, but does not influence growth or proliferation of committed megakaryocytes. Meg-CSF production depends primarily on the mass of bone marrow megakaryocytes.[37] Ancillary bone marrow cells, macrophages or lymphocytes, are probably the sources of Meg-CSF, and decreases in total numbers of megakaryocytes stimulate production of Meg-CSF by these cells. Meg-CSF is present in the blood and urine of patients recovering from cytotoxic chemotherapy, irradiation, and bone marrow transplantation, as well as those with aplastic anemia and thrombocytopenic purpura.[38] The exact amino acid structure or a cloned version of Meg-CSF remains to be developed. Absence of purified Meg-CSF illustrates the great technical difficulties of this endeavor. Available evidence suggests that Meg-CSF is a low-molecular weight glycoprotein immunologically distinct from erythropoietin, thrombopoietin, interleuken 3 (IL-3), and granulocyte macrophage colony stimulating factor (GM-CSF).[39]

Thrombopoietin (TPO), which like Meg-CSF is

difficult to separate from plasma, is known to be a glycoprotein with a molecular weight ranging between 15 and 30 kDa. TPO activity measurements are based on the ability of the factor to increase platelet size, platelet count, and incorporation of radiolabeled ^{35}S-selenomethionine or ^{35}S-sodium sulfate into newly-synthesized platelet proteins. The principal variables studied are the size of new platelets and megakaryocyte protein synthesis, which do not directly correlate with actual platelet production and, thus, only indirectly reflect TPO activity. In addition, these tests are performed in live animals, and are time-consuming and costly. The specific site of TPO production and the physiologic mechanism responsible for modulating TPO synthesis are unknown. Indirect evidence from patients with abnormalities of the long arm of chromosome 3 in whom megakaryocyte hyperplasia and thrombocytosis occur implicates this genetic locus as a control point. Cytokines, such as interleuken 1 (IL-1), play a role in regulation of production.[40] Ancillary marrow cells, stromal cells, and even endothelial cells are potential sources of IL-1, partially explaining the reactive thrombocytosis that accompanies inflammatory processes.[41] Because patients on dialysis rarely become thrombocytopenic, it is unlikely that the kidney is the major manufacturer of TPO, even though animal nephrectomy experiments have suggested this.[42,43]

Megakaryocyte colony simulating factor and thrombopoietin work together with respect to platelet production (Figure 1). Meg-CSF induces differentiation of the stem cell to the progenitor stage, whereas TPO regulates the number of mitotic divisions, the size, and the cytoplasmic content of the maturing megakaryocyte. When the action of Meg-CSF stops and the control of TPO begins, and how the two regulators influence each other are unknown. Likewise, the mechanisms by which Meg-CSF and TPO levels respond to decreased megakaryocyte mass and platelet availability are unknown.

Cell-derived regulators of megakaryocytopoiesis have been studied in various experimental models, largely based on ex vivo cell culture systems. T lymphocytes, monocytes, and natural killer (NK) cells have been shown to influence megakaryocyte progenitor cell proliferation with variable findings.[44-46] It has been hypothesized that these cells produce a Meg-CSF-like substance, but no such compound has been isolated. At present, there is no definitive in vivo evidence that these various ancillary cells play a major role in regulating normal megakaryocytopoiesis or in the reactive thrombocytosis that accompanies neoplastic or chronic inflammatory conditions.

Cytokines and growth factors also affect megakaryocyte cell development at both the progenitor cell and more mature cell levels. Most work has been performed with recombinant cytokines and factors, partic-

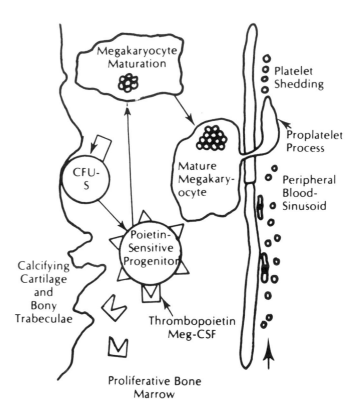

Figure 1. Platelet production from megakaryocytes. Megakaryocytes are recruited in the proliferative bone marrow from colony-forming units (CFUs). Megakaryocyte colony-stimulating factor (Meg-CSF) and thrombopoietin work together to initiate megakaryocyte differentiation. Meg-CSF recruits stem cells for megakaryocyte differentiation, but does not influence growth or proliferation of committed megakaryocytes. Thrombopoietin regulates the number of mitotic divisions, the size, and the cytoplasmic content of the maturing megakaryocyte. Early maturation of the megakaryoblasts (stage I megakaryocytes) and promegakaryocytes (stage II megakaryocytes) occurs in quiescent bone marrow. The mature megakaryocytes (stages III and IV) migrate to the margin of the sinusoid to initiate platelet dispersal. (Reproduced with permission from Reference 12.)

ularly IL-3 and GM-CSF.[47-49] IL-3 is more potent than GM-CSF, as measured by increased colony formation and proliferative capacity of progenitor cells.[50] In addition, there appears to be synergism between these agents.[51] Numerous other cytokines have been implicated in regulating megakaryocytopoiesis (Table 1).[52] Of these, interleukin 6 (IL-6) holds the most promise. It is synthesized by T cells, macrophages, and marrow stromal cells, and was originally defined by its ability to stimulate B-lymphocyte growth. Recently, it has been shown to increase megakaryocyte size and to augment the development of polyploidy.[53,54]

Inhibitors of megakaryocytopoiesis have not been as carefully studied as stimulatory factors. The concept of inhibitors arose from the discovery that megakaryo-

Table 1
Effects of Cytokines on Megakaryocytopoiesis

Cytokine	Cloning Efficiency
IL-1	No independent stimulatory activity, but synergizes with other cytokines to promote megakaryocyte colony formation
IL-3	Enhances
IL-4	No independent stimulatory activity, but synergizes with other cytokines to promote megakaryocyte colony formation
IL-6	Enhances
GM-CSF	No effect
CSF-1	No independent stimulatory activity, but synergizes with other cytokines to promote megakaryotyte colony formation
Erythropoietin	Conflicting results in the literature
G-CSF	No independent stimulatory activity, but synergizes with other cytokines to promote megakaryocyte colony formation
MK-CSF	Enhances
KIT ligand	No independent stimulatory activity, but synergizes with other cytokines to promote megakaryocyte colony formation
TGF-β	Inhibitory
Interferons	Inhibitory
Platelet factor 4	Inhibitory
Platelet released glycoprotein	Inhibitory

(Adapted with permission from Reference 52.)

cyte colony growth in serum is poorer than growth in platelet-poor plasma, suggesting that platelet constituents (released in serum) could inhibit megakaryocytopoiesis in vitro and raising the possibility of negative autocrine feedback.[55] Transforming growth factor β (TGF-β), a cytokine present in relatively high concentrations in platelets and widely distributed in other cells (not megakaryocytes), inhibits megakaryocytopoiesis at the progenitor cell level.[56] TGF-β inhibits the growth of many other hematopoietic and nonhematopoietic cell lineages; it most likely inhibits progenitor cells at a similar stage of differentiation or inhibits growth of stem cells. In addition, several platelet-specific proteins contained in α granules, including platelet factor 4 (PF4), β thromboglobulin, and platelet basic protein (PBP) inhibit megakaryocytopoiesis.[57,58] The mechanisms of inhibition are not completely understood.

There are several other known blood cells that inhibit megakaryocytopoiesis. T Lymphocytes and macrophages contain proteins that substantially suppress megakaryocyte production, resulting in subsequent thrombocytopenia.[45,59,60] Both cell lines generate interferon that inhibits megakaryocyte production.[61] The purpose of such cellular regulation of megakaryocyte development and platelet release is obscure.

Megakaryocyte response to changes in platelet counts has been studied in numerous animal models. Some investigators have reported that the pool of progenitor cells is dynamic and responds almost immediately to experimentally-induced thrombocytopenia,[62] whereas others have contended that they remain stable for up to 2 weeks after induction of thrombocytopenia.[63] Severity of thrombocytopenia may be important in the hematopoietic response. Severely thrombocytopenic rodents develop increased numbers of megakaryocytes in direct relation to the degree of platelet reduction.[64] In general, a bone marrow examination from an animal with acute thrombocytopenia shows normal numbers of megakaryocytes with increased size and DNA content. In chronic thrombocytopenia, size and DNA content are normal, but the number of megakaryocytes is increased.[65]

Megakaryocyte Differentiation and Developmental Biology

Like other myeloid cells, megakaryocytes have an undifferentiated pluripotent hematopoietic stem cell precursor. A stem cell can differentiate into one of several independent and disparate cell lines (Figure 2). The stem cell maintains itself by asymmetric mitosis,

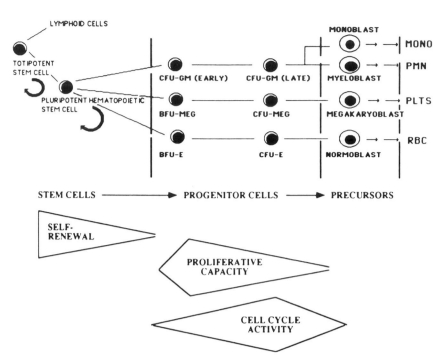

Figure 2. Diagram of hematopoietic cell development. Cells are arbitrarily divided into compartments of stem cells, progenitor cells, and precursor cells, giving rise to various cell types. The ability for self-renewal, proliferative capacity, and cell cycle activity is indicated at the bottom of the diagram. Precursor cells are morphologically distinct. CFU-GM = colony forming units-granulocyte, macrophage; BFU-MEG = burst forming unit-megakaryocyte; BFU-E = burst forming unit-erythrocyte; CFU-MEG = colony forming unit-megakaryocyte; MONO = monocyte; PMN = polymorphonuclear leukocyte; PLTS = platelets; RBC = red blood cell. (Reproduced with permission from Reference 52.)

in which one daughter cell remains pluripotential, whereas the other enters a pathway of differentiation under a variety of different stimuli. The differentiating daughter cells associated with megakaryocytopoiesis undergo maturation as 1) progenitor cells, and 2) morphologically recognizable megakaryocytes.

Progenitor Cells (Endomitosis)

The principal function of progenitor cells in the marrow is to enlarge the number of megakaryocyte-producing cells, because there are few stem cells that produce the lineage-committed progenitor cells. Three types of megakaryocyte progenitor cells have been described based on: 1) how long they require to develop in culture; 2) the types of colonies the produce; and 3) physical properties. The least mature progenitor cell type is the burst-forming unit-megakaryocyte (BFU-Meg) (Figure 2). BFU-Meg-derived colonies are comprised of multiple clusters of megakaryocytes (up to hundreds) and take approximately 21 days to develop in culture. A more mature progenitor cell type is the colony-forming unit-megakaryocyte (CFU-Meg), which gives rise to smaller cluster colonies (3 to 10

cells) of megakaryocytes in 10 to 12 days. The most mature progenitor is the light-density CFU-Meg (LD-CFU-Meg), which gives rise to small colonies because it has little proliferative capacity.[52] Both velocity sedimentation gradients and centrifugal elutriation can separate BFU-Megs and CFU-Megs. Megakaryocyte progenitor cells contain only the normal 2N level of DNA and cannot be distinguished morphologically form stem cells or other committed progenitor cells.[66] However, analysis of cell membrane epitopes can be used for identification.[67]

In the earliest stage of megakaryocyte development, the lineage-committed daughter cells undergo endomitosis (also called endoreduplication). Endomitosis is the process of nuclear division without formation of separate daughter cells. It is unique to megakaryocyte in human bone marrow.[68] Early endomitosis is not associated with the production of cytoplasm, which accounts for the undistinguished appearance of young megakaryocyte cells from other bone marrow cells. Duplication of nuclear material to 4N or 8N accompanies cytoplasmic changes that morphologically distinguish megakaryocyte progenitors. Mitosis does not continue beyond the progenitor stage; instead, the nucleus of a given cell increases in size and lobulation.

Cytoplasmic volume correlates with DNA concentration, but there is no relationship between the degree of lobulation and amount of DNA. When the DNA level reaches the 4N or 8N stage, the progenitor cells enter the maturation phase of development, and this first stage cell is called a *megakaryoblast*. Endomitosis continues as the cell grows and stops at 16N, 32N, or 66N.

Maturation

Major proliferative activity ceases as cells enter the maturation phase of development. These cells mature according to three or four well-defined stages (Table 2).[69]. When studied by immunohistochemistry, even the earliest cells in this developmental chain express platelet markers, such as PF4, factor VIII: Ag (vWF:Ag), and platelet glycoproteins Ib and IIb–IIIa. These very immature megakaryocyte cells represent a transitional developmental stage between the progenitor cells and morphologically identifiable megakaryocytes.[70] It has been estimated that transitional cells make up 5% of marrow megakaryocytes.[71]

Stage I megakaryocytes, called megakaryoblasts, have lobed and compact nuclei with the highest nuclear:cytoplasmic ratio (Figure 3A). Megakaryoblast cytoplasm is very basophilic owing to high RNA content; dense bodies, α granules, and beginnings of the demarcation membrane system are already present. The demarcation membrane system (DMS) is plasma membrane generated throughout the cytoplasm that ultimately results in complete compartmentalization. There is invagination and internal proliferation of the membrane structure that eventually results in formation of individual platelets. As noted above, megakaryoblasts still actively synthesize DNA and undergo endomitosis.

Stage II megakaryocytes, called *promegakaryocytes*, have horseshoe-shaped nuclei with a 1:1 nuclear: cytoplasmic ratio (Figure 3B). Their cytoplasm is more plentiful and contains more platelet organelles and a better developed membrane system.[72] Somewhere in the middle of the promegakaryocyte stage, endomitosis stops.[73]

Stage III megakaryocytes are the most abundant megakaryocytes in the bone marrow, constituting 85% of the cell line in normal human marrow. They are large ($\sim$40 to 150 μm) with copious eosinophilic cytoplasm (Figure 3B). The nuclei are multilobed and resemble bunches of balloons. Platelet organelles are extensive,

Table 2
Morphology of Megakaryocyte Maturation

Characteristic	Stage I	Stage II	Stage III†
Nomenclature	Megakaryoblast	Promegakaryocyte	Megakaryocyte
Shape	Oval or round	Irregular	Irregular
Size	15–50 μm	20–80 μm	40–150 μm
Nucleus	Nonsegmented round to oval; nucleoli present; dispersed chromatin and light staining	Lobulated; vestigial nucleoli; condensed chromatin and medium staining	Highly lobulated (bunch of balloons); dense chromatin; dark staining
Cytoplasm	Nongranular and basophilic; clear Golgi apparatus; brilliant blue stain owing to rough endoplasmic reticulum; mitochondria	Demarcation membrane system; lightly granular with azuroophilic granules owing to platelet organelles	Highly granular because of lysosomes, alpha granules, and dense bodies; demarcation membrane system complete; pseudopods may be present because of thrombosthenin
Nucleus/ Cytoplasm Ratio	5:1 or greater	$\sim$1:1	<1 mostly cytoplasm
Approximate percent of Population	$\sim$20	$\sim$25	$\sim$55
Mitoses	Present	Variable	Absent

† Stage IV megakaryocytes are called postmature and have very similar morphology to Stage III (see text).

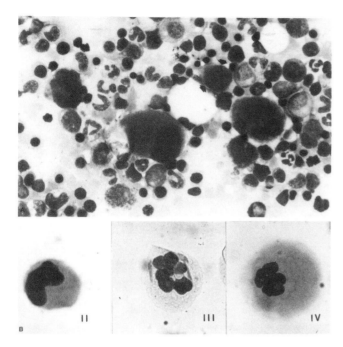

Figure 3. Megakaryocyte maturation. **Panel A (above):** Marrow smear showing megakaryocytes in various stages of maturation in vivo. The **arrow** points to a stage I megakaryoblast, which has a compact nucleus and a high nuclear: cytoplasmic ratio. The cytoplasm is basophilic owing to high RNA content. **Panel B (below):** Stage II megakaryocytes, called promegakaryocytes, have horseshoe-shaped nuclei with a 1:1 nuclear:cytoplasmic ratio. Stage III megakaryocytes constitute 85% of the cell line in the bone marrow. The nuclei are multilobed and the demarcation membrane system is fully developed. Stage IV megakaryocytes are called postmature and have the lowest nuclear:cytoplasmic ratio. Their nuclei are more compact and denser than stage III cells, suggesting that involution is occurring. (Reproduced with permission from Reference 52.)

and the demarcation membrane system is fully developed. Dense bodies and alpha granules that characterize platelets are readily identified in stage III megakaryocytes and account for the azure staining quality of the cytoplasm. Also visible are the microfilamentous molecules, collectively called *actomyosin,* that are identical to the molecules that constitute the myofilaments of skeletal muscle. By means of its contractile nature, actomyosin is responsible for locomotion and reorganization of the cell. The actomyosin found in megakaryocytes and platelets is also known as *thrombosthenin.*

Stage IV megakaryocytes are included in some classification systems.[74] They are called *postmature* and are morphologically similar to stage III megakaryocytes. Their nuclei are more compact and denser than stage III cells, suggesting that involution is occurring (Figure 3B). The eosinophilic cytoplasm of postmature megakaryocytes is most brilliantly and evenly stained. They also tend to be slightly smaller than stage III cells.

Both stage III and IV cells, in which granule content and development of the DMS are maximal, are thought to be responsible for actual platelet release.[52]

Megakaryocyte Proteins

With maturation of megakaryocytes, lineage-specific organelles (i.e., dense bodies, α granules, DMS) have been shown to contain a variety of proteins, most (but not all) of which are also contained in platelets. The proteins have a wide spectrum of activities. Although the megakaryocytic synthesis of some platelet granule proteins (e.g., PF4 von Willebrand factor [vWF], beta-thromboglobulin) is well accepted, others (e.g., albumin, IgG, fibrinogen) may be taken in by endocytosis.[75–77] A prodigious research effort has been aimed at elucidating the mechanisms of production and elaboration of megakaryocyte proteins. A list of some of these molecules is given in Table 3.

Fragmentation and Platelet Dispersal

There are two major postulated mechanisms for thrombopoiesis. The first is based on the formation from proplatelets. According to this hypothesis, parallel DMS channels fuse leading to fenestrated sheets of membrane. The sheets cleave along their perpendicular axes and form scalloped membranes that become the membranes of platelets.[78] Pseudopods form from megakaryocytes and extend into the sinuses of the bone marrow; the pseudopods fracture along the cleavage planes established by the DMS, releasing variably-sized pieces of megakaryocyte cytoplasm called *proplatelets.* Additional fragmentation along the DMS produces individual platelets.

The second theory is called the *flow model.* According to this hypothesis, the DMS is not organized into discrete domains, but is simply extruded into pseudopods as redundant membrane. Shear forces from flow in the capillary sinus constrict the pseudopods and weaken them enough to cause a break, thereby releasing platelets. It has been shown that DMS decreases as pseudopods form.[79]

Additional controversy exists over the exact site of platelet release. Most investigators think that proplatelets are formed in the bone marrow and released into the peripheral blood through the sinus endothelial cells. Once all the platelets have been shed, a bare or naked nucleus remains. The finding of naked nuclei in the marrow and proplatelets in the central venous blood support this hypothesis.[80,81] Alternatively, as previously noted, some scientists have suggested that platelet formation and dispersal occur in the lungs.[82] Megakaryocytes do circulate and, if mature, probably undergo fragmentation in whatever capillary bed they

Table 3
Megakaryocyte Proteins

Enzymes	Contractile Proteins	Coagulant Proteins	Miscellaneous
Acetylcholinesterase†	Actin	Fibrinogen	Platelet-derived growth Factor (PDGF)
Peroxidase	Myosin	Factor V	Transforming growth factor-β
Acid phosphatase	α-Actin	Factor XIII	Glycogen
α-Naphthyl acetate esterase	Filamin	Factor VIII antigen	Adenine nucleotides
5′Nucleotidase	Tubulin	Platelet Factor 4	Proteoglycans
		Platelet glycoproteins (Ib, IIb-IIIa, thrombospondin)	Arachidonic acid metabolites
		Fibronectin	Serotonin
		β-thromboglobulin	Thrombomodulin

† Present in rat, but no human megakaryocytes.

nest. Whether all megakaryocytes must obligatorily reside in the pulmonary vasculature remains speculative.

Platelet Structure

Morphology

Platelets are discoid structures averaging 2 μm to 4 μm in diameter that, when quiescent, spend about 7 to 10 days in the circulation before they are removed by the spleen. The range of sizes of normal platelets is wide: 1.5 μm to 6.5 μm. The range of size results from the random manner in which platelets fragment during production. There is some evidence that large platelets are young cells that have most recently come from megakaryocytes, whereas small platelets are older.[68] Large platelets must be differentiated from giant platelets, which are almost as large as red blood cells and indicate an underlying hematologic disorder, such as thrombocythemia, chronic myelocytic leukemia, gray platelet syndrome, Bernard-Soulier syndrome, and others.[83,84] Platelets in patients with these diseases can reach 20 μm in diameter.[85] Giant platelets are not seen in smears of normal individuals and indicate abnormal or uncontrolled maturation.

On light microscopy, Wright-stained platelets have a characteristic translucent purple-blue cytoplasm. A few centrally located granules may be faintly visible. Spiny processes may be present due to activation and contraction induced by contact with the glass slide. Organelles become concentrated together centrally when platelets spread on glass or aggregate; they

are surrounded by relatively clear cytoplasm. Wright referred to these regions as *granulomere* (organelles) and *hyalomere* (cytoplasm), an overly simplistic distinction.[22]

Ultrastructure

Electron microscopy has elucidated the complicated ultrastructure of platelets (Figures 4 and 5). Although platelets in the quiescent state appear to have a smooth convex surface, much like the biconcave erythrocyte, rigorous examination shows multiple random indentations (pores) on the platelet surface that represent communications between channels of the surface connecting system (SCS), which is also called the open canalicular system (OCS), and the cell exterior.[86] No other human cells are so porous.

It is useful to subdivide the platelet into four major regions, listed in Table 4 and illustrated in Figures 4 and 5. The *peripheral zone* consists of the membranes and associated structures that make up the surface of the platelet and the walls of the OCS. Three domains comprise the peripheral zone: 1) the exterior coat; 2) the unit membrane; and 3) the submembrane region. The OCS is made up of invaginations of the cell wall, thus, producing a far greater surface area than would be predicted by standard measurements of cell size and volume. In essence, the platelet resembles a sponge although it does not function like one.[87] The OCS has special intracellular and extracellular relationships, and these details are discussed later in the section concerning platelet membrane systems. Structurally, how-

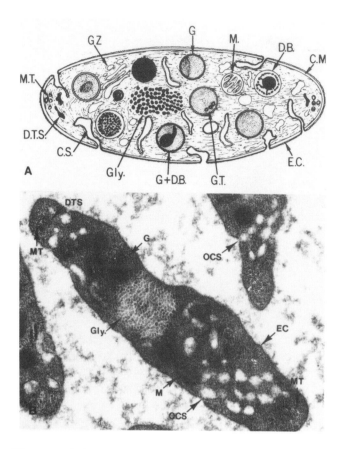

Figure 4. Quiescent discoid platelet. (**A**) The diagram indicates ultrastructural features of the platelet cross-sectioned in the coronal plane. The **peripheral zone** (see Table 4) consists of: the exterior coat (E.C.), the unit cell membrane (C.M.), and the submembrane region containing thrombosthenin filaments (S.M.F.). The **solid gel zone** (sometimes called the platelet cytoskeleton) consists of microtubules (M.T.). The **organelle zone** consists of mitochondria (M.), dense bodies (D.B.), α granules and lysosomes (G.), which are indistinguishable from one another in standard TEM preparations, and glycogen particles (Gly.) The **membranous zone** consists of platelet membrane systems: the surface-connected open canalicular system (C.S. or OCS, **below**) and the dense tubular system (D.T.S.). (**B**) TEM of platelet cross sectioned in the coronal plane, showing the ultrastructures in the **above diagram**. (magnification ×28,000). Reproduced with permission from Reference 90.)

Table 4
Major Platelet Regions

Peripheral zone	Cell Surface
	Exterior coat (glycocalyx)
	Submembrane region
Solid-Gel Zone	Microtubules
	Microfilaments
Organelle Zone	Mitochondria
	Dense bodies
	α granules
	Lysosomes
	Glycogen particles
Membrane Systems	Surface-connected, open canalicular system (OCS)
	Dense tubular system
	Membrane complexes

described, each of which shares a common beta subunit. Platelets contain several receptors in the β_1 family. The β_1 family of integrins interacts with many different cells and extracellular matrix, including collagen, laminin, and fibronectin. β_2 receptors are present in platelets and leukocytes, functioning in immune and inflammatory reactions. The β_3 family, designated as cytoadhesins, includes the megakaryocyte- and platelet-specific glycoprotein GPIIb–IIIa complex and the vitronectin receptor present on platelets and endothelial cells.

Platelet membrane glycoproteins that function as receptors assist in adhesion of platelets to surfaces. An exception is the GPIIb–IIIa receptor (fibrinogen, vitronectin, fibronectin, vWF, and thrombospondin), which is exclusively responsible for platelet aggregation. Unlike other integrins, GPIIb–IIIa is found *only* on platelets and is not functional on quiescent platelets. The other major integrins associated with platelets, which are functional on both resting and inactivated platelets, include: GPIa/IIa (collagen), GPIc/IIa (laminin), GPIc–IIa (fibronectin), Av/IIIa (vitronectin, fibrinogen, vWF, and thrombospondin), GPIV (thrombospondin, and collagen), and GPIb-IX (vWF and thrombospondin).

The middle layer of the peripheral zone consists of the unit membrane, which contains phospholids that serve as a surface for interactions with coagulation serine proteases. Because of these interactions, the unit membrane is of critical importance in hemostasis by accelerating the coagulation process.[91] The physical make up of the unit membrane provides a lipoprotein-rich catalytic surface for the occurrence of coagulation, a function referred to in older literature as PF3.[92] The mechanisms by which the constituents of the unit

ever, the OCS shares the same characteristics as the more exposed portions of the cell membrane.

The exterior coat or glycocalyx covers the outermost portion of the platelet; it differs substantially from the coverings of erythrocytes or leukocytes. The glycocalyx is rich in glycoproteins that serve as receptors for a variety of specific and nonspecific stimuli.[88,89] Several membrane glycoproteins are *integrins*, a large "superfamily" of receptors common to many cells.[90] Integrin receptors are characterized by the presence of alpha and beta subunits, joined by noncovalent bonds. Three families of integrins (β_1, β_2, and β_3) have been

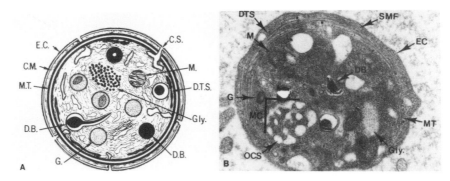

Figure 5. Quiescent discoid platelets. **(A)** The diagram indicates ultrastructural features of the platelet cross-sectioned in the equatorial plane. Abbreviations are the same as in Figure 4. **(B)** TEM of platelet cross-sectioned in the equatorial plane, showing the ultrastructures in the above diagram. (magnification ×28,000). (Reproduced with permission from reference 90.)

membrane are reorganized and exposed during this process are unknown. In some way, anionic phospholipids of the membrane that promote clotting move from the inside to the outside layer after thrombin activation.

The submembrane region is the third structural domain of the peripheral zone. It serves as a barrier to organelles inside the platelet matrix. There is a distinct system of filaments in the submembrane region that is associated with the platelet cytoplasmic cytoskeleton.[93] The submembrane filaments are composed of thrombosthenin (short-actin) and are most heavily concentrated just beneath the plasma membrane, where they articulate with proteins of the inner leaflet.[94]

Microfilaments in the submembrane region are randomly arranged, but when platelets become activated they line up in parallel bundles and participate in shape change. This parallel arrangement remains intact within pseudopodic processes in which filaments are particularly concentrated during platelet activation. The process of extrusion of cytoplasm into spiky extensions (pseudopods), whereas organelles move the opposite direction toward the center of the cell during platelet activation, has been the focus of much research.[95] A special regulatory system exists that permits the extrusion of pseudopods while the rest of the cytoplasm is contracting toward the platelet center.

The solid-gel zone is sometimes referred to as the platelet cytoskeleton. The matrix within a platelet more closely resembles a gel than a fluid. Microtubules and microfilaments constitute the solid-gel zone. Microtubules are hollow, nonbranching cylinders that measure 25 nm in diameter and many micrometers in length. In cross-sections of fixed platelets, they appear as a group of 8 to 24 circular profiles. The bundle lies close to the cell wall, but is separated from it by submembrane filaments. Microtubules are composed of

tubulin protein dimers that polymerize to form the wall of the microtubule.[96] Tubulin is dissociated by cold temperature, which causes platelets to lose their discoid shape, suggesting that microtubules are essential for cytoskeletal support. Rewarming to 37°C restores normal shape.[97] Drugs that inhibit mitosis, including colchicine, vincristine, and vinblastine, disassemble or hinder formation of microtubules and also cause platelets to lose lentiform appearance.[98]

In addition to maintaining resting platelet shape, microtubules participate in platelet contraction during activation. Platelets exposed to thrombin, adenosine diphosphate (ADP), or other activating agents lose discoid appearance and become irregular with bulky and spike-like pseudopods. The organelles become concentrated into the center of the cell and are encircled by circumferential microtubules.[99] This process is called reorganization and accounts for the appearance of the granulomere and hyalomere seen in light microscopic preparations; it is essential for the secretion of granular contents. Destroying the microtubule with the alkylating agents discussed above inhibits central migration of organelles. However, microtubules do not provide the direct contractile force, because treatment with these agents do not prevent platelet contraction. Thus, intact microtubules influence the wave of contraction, although the individual tubules are not the contractile elements.

Microfilaments comprise the second fiber system in the gel-zone.[90] Thrombosthenin microfilaments are dispersed throughout the platelet cytoplasm. Between 15% to 35% of the total platelet protein is actin.[100] The actin may exist in monomeric (globular) or multimeric (filamentous) form. The assembly of actin filaments is one of the earliest occurrences when the surface of platelets is activated. First, there is formation of a haphazard network of actin, soon followed by creation of

Table 5
Contents of Platelets

Cytoplasm	Lysosomes	α Granules	Dense Bodies
Factor XIII	α-arabinoside	**Enzymes**	ATP
PDECGF	β-galactosidase	α_1-antitrypsin	ADP
	β-glucuronidase	α_2-macroglobulin	Ionic calcium
	β-glycerophosphatase	α_2-antiplasmin	Serotonin
	N-acetylglucosaminidase	C1-esterase inhibitor	Phosphate
	Elastase	**Adhesive Proteins**	Guanine nucleotides
	Collagenase	Fibrinogen	
	Cathepsins	Fibronectin	
		vWF	
		Thrombospondin	
		Vitronectin	
		Growth Factors	
		PDGF	
		TGF Beta	
		EGF	
		ECGF	
		Platelet Specific Proteins	
		Platelet Factor 4	
		β-thromboglobulin	
		Coagulation Factors	
		HMWK	
		Plasminogen	
		Factor V	
		Factor XI	
		Fibrinogen	
		Protein S	
		PAI-1	

PDECGF = platelet-derived endothelial cell growth factor; vWF = von Willebrand Factor; PDGF = platelet-derived growth factor; TGF = transforming growth factor; EGF = epidermal growth factor; ECGF = endothelial cell growth factor; HMWK = high-molecular weight kininogen; PAI-1 = plasminogen activator inhibitor 1; ATP = adenosine triphosphate; ADP = adenosine diphosphate.

close parallel segregations that constitute lattice arrangement within pseudopods.

The organelle zone consists of structures listed in Table 4. A platelet does not contain a nucleus, rough endoplasmic reticulum (RER), or a Golgi apparatus and, thus, cannot synthesize proteins. Platelets do have mitochondria, glycogen granules, and three types of storage organelles: lysosomes, alpha granules, and dense bodies.[94] Lysosomes are indistinguishable from the azurophilic granules in human granulocytes, containing neutral proteinases, microbe-killing enzymes, and acid hydrolases (Table 5). Some granules are rich in peroxidase, some in acid β-galactosidase, and others in acid β-glycerophosphatase. The function of lysosomes in hemostasis remains unclear. They respond to activating agents for the release of their contents, but the activating stimulus must be greater than for secretion of substances from alpha granules or dense bodies.

Lysosomes and alpha granules are indistinguishable in standard TEM preparations. Both are filled with a dark gray homogeneous substance. Alpha granules tend to be slightly larger than lysosomes and sometimes have a denser central area, resembling a bull's eye.[101]

Alpha granules contain a host of proteins that participate in coagulation. Most are found in plasma, but are nonetheless probably of primary platelet origin. These proteins include plasma protease inhibitors (α_1 antitrypsin, α_2 macroglobulin, α_2 antiplasmin, C1 esterase inhibitor), and coagulation cofactors (high-molecular-weight kininogen, vWF, fibrinogen, fibronectin, Factor V). In addition, there are platelet-specific markers within alpha granules (β-thromboglobulin, PF4). These proteins can be measured to determine platelet activation.

Patients with gray platelet syndrome have giant platelets with almost no alpha granules.[102] Investigation of platelets from these patients has allowed characterization of the substances normally contained in alpha granules. For example, gray platelet syndrome platelets are markedly deficient in thrombospondin, β-thromboglobulin, PF4, and mitogenic activity.[103] In contrast, levels of serotonin and adenine nucleotides are normal, as would be expected because dense body content is normal. Likewise, lysosomal enzyme content is normal.

Dense bodies are smaller than lysosomes and alpha granules and are more electron-dense in TEM preparations. They are the storage sites for the nonmetabolic pool of adenine nucleotides (ATP, ADP), serotonin, pyrophosphate, and ionic calcium.[104] These substances are secreted by platelets during the release reaction, and participate in the recruitment and activation of additional platelets in clot formation. Patients with storage pool disease and Hermansky-Pudlak syndrome have diminished or absent dense bodies, which is associated with defective aggregation and hemorrhagic episodes.[105]

The membranous zone consists of platelet membrane systems—the surface connected OCS and the dense tubular system (DTS). The platelet is the only blood cell with an OCS, which is a patent internal tortuous invagination of the cell wall that tunnels throughout the cytoplasm in a serpentine fashion. This system gives the cell its vacuolar appearance on cross-section. The OCS is patent in activated, aggregated, and resting platelets, suggesting that the channels serve as conduits for substances extruded by platelets during the release reaction.[106] In fact, the OCS connects with platelet granules and communicates with the outside, providing a route for secretion as granules are squeezed during shape change and their contents pass outside the cell.

In addition, the OCS participates in the contractile process. When agonists bind to the cell wall, the OCS transmits chemical messages inward. Contraction of actomyosin in the platelet is regulated by calcium flux through the OCS, which functions like the tubules of the T-system of muscle cells that transport free calcium.

The DTS originates from the RER in the parent megakaryocyte. Channels of the dense tubular system have an amorphous material within them, similar in appearance to surrounding cytoplasm that differentiates this tubular system from the OCS.[107] Like the OCS, the DTS is randomly dispersed in the platelet cytoplasm, and because it derived from RER, it is considered residual smooth endoplasmic reticulum (SER), analogous to the sarcoplasmic reticulum of muscle cells.[108] The DTS is the main site for sequestration of internally functional calcium, whose release is necessary for cell activation. In addition, adenyl cyclase is present in the DTS. Adenyl cyclase converts ATP to cyclic adenosine monophosphate (cAMP), which promotes uptake of free calcium by the DTS, preventing platelet activation. Many inhibitors of platelet function (adenosine, prostaglandin E_1, and prostacyclin) act by stimulating platelet adenyl cyclase to produce increased cAMP.[109] The prostaglandin-related enzymes, cyclooxygenase and thromboxane synthetase, are also present in large amounts in the DTS, suggesting that the DTS is the principal location for platelet prostaglandin synthesis.[110]

Thus, when a platelet is activated the stimulus is transmitted by the OCS to the DTS, which releases free calcium. In turn, the free calcium initiates contraction of thrombosthenin microfilaments, controlling platelet reorganization.

Platelet Kinetics and Life Span

In normal human bone marrow there are about 6000000 megakaryocytes, which produce about 35000 platelets/μL of blood per day. In acute thrombocytopenia or stress, megakaryocytes can increase platelet production six- to eightfold. Two thirds of platelets circulate, whereas one third is sequestered by sinusoids within the red pulp of the spleen (near the endothelial surface in splenic sinusoids).[111] After splenectomy, all platelets reside in the bloodstream. In contrast, in splenomegaly vast numbers (up to 90%) of platelets become sequestered.

Both ^{51}Cr and ^{111}In are effective agents for labeling platelets. Both agents bind firmly and have little effect on clearance. Experiments using these radiolabels have shown that the average life span to human platelets is about 6.9 to 9.9 days, with a turnover rate of 10% per day.[112] However, in pathologic conditions such as immune thrombocytopenia, the life span may decrease to less than 1 day.

Most old platelets are destroyed in the bone marrow, liver, and spleen, although some are lost in peripheral vessels repairing sites of vascular injury. Cell destruction is based on senescence, but the exact features of older platelets responsible for their recognition and clearance is unknown. In disorders such as idiopathic thrombocytopenia purpura (ITP), thrombotic thrombocytopenic purpura (TTP), and hemoytic-uremic syndrome, the clearance curve is exponential, suggesting that the destruction is unrelated to platelet age.

Platelet Membrane Glycoproteins

Platelet membrane glycoproteins mediate many crucial processes involved in platelet function. Whereas some of the glycoproteins of platelets are unique, others share immunologic identity with glyco-

Table 6
Platelet Gene Families

Gene Family	Glycoprotein Receptor
Integrins	Glycoprotein IIb-IIIa (GP IIb-IIIa)
	Glycoprotein Ia-IIa (GP Ia-IIa)
	Fibronectin receptor
	Vitronectin receptor
	Laminin receptor
Leucine-rich Glycoprotein (LRG)	Glycoprotein Ib-IX (GP Ib-IX)
	Glycoprotein V (GPV)
Quadraspanin	p24/CD9
	ME491
Immunoglobulin Supergene	Platelet-endothelial cell adhesion molecule-1 (PECAM-1)
Selectins	GMP-140
	ELAM-1
	MEL-14

proteins of erythrocytes and leukocytes. Surface glycoproteins are often antigenic and may participate in autoimmune disorders such as ITP. Radiolabeling glycoproteins on the platelet surface with I^{125} or H^3 was the principal method by which the receptor sites were initially characterized. Many of these glycoproteins have now been produced using recombinant DNA technology, which has permitted sequencing of the amino acids comprising the receptor and cataloging several gene families.[113] An explosion of knowledge about receptor sites has resulted in antiplatelet therapy targeted to particular receptors and platelet functions.

Originally, glycoproteins on the platelet surface were separated into five electrophoretic fractions designated by roman numerals I through V. With the advent of genetic cloning experiments and more sophisticated molecular biologic techniques, additional receptors were discovered that made older classification schemes outmoded. Currently, platelet membrane glycoproteins are classified into five gene families (Table 6). In-depth discussion of all of these gene families and receptors is beyond the scope of this chapter, but two receptors, GPIb-IX and GPIIb-IIIa, warrant special attention.

GPIb-IX, a member of the leucine-rich-gene family, mediates platelet adhesion to the subendothelium. Approximately 25000 copies of GPIb-IX exist on the platelet surface. The glycoprotein complex is sialoglycoprotein (containing sialic acid) and contributes to the net negative charge of the platelet surface.[114] GPIb consists of two subunits that are liked by disulfide bonds: GPIbα (MW = 145 kDa, 610 amino acids in length) and GPIbβ (MW = 24 kDa, 122 amino acids in length), and is tightly complexed to GPIX (MW = 17,000, 134 amino acids in length) (115–117).

Patients with Bernard-Soulier syndrome have a bleeding disorder due to absence of the GPIb-IX on their platelets. They have provided much information about this glycoprotein receptor, along with monoclonal antibodies specifically targeted at the receptor.[118] For normal platelet adhesion to occur, vWF must bind to both the platelet and the subendothelium. The subendothelial vWF binding site is located on collagen, whereas the platelet binding site is GPIb-IX. We have shown that monoclonal antibodies directed against vWF effectively prevent platelet-dependent arterial thrombosis in a nonhuman primate model.[119] Circulating unactivated platelets do not bind to soluble vWF in the plasma, but they adhere to immobilized vWF in the subendothelium.[120] When vWF binds to collagen, it undergoes a conformational change that permits binding to the GPIb-IX receptor, even in the absence of platelet activation. This can be observed in vitro by adding to platelet-rich plasma the antibiotic ristocetin, which binds to vWF and changes it conformation to one similar to immobilized vWF. The inducement of binding of vWF to GPIb-IX is called *ristocetin cofactor activity* and results in platelet *agglutination*, not true aggregation.[121] Absence of ristocetin-induced aggregation that is corrected by the addition of vWF indicates von Willebrand disease, whereas lack of correction indicates Bernard-Soulier syndrome.

GP-Ib functions in platelet aggregation as well as adhesion. It recently has been shown that the binding of vWF to GPIb-IX, in addition to GPIIb-IIIa, plays an important role in thrombosis under conditions of high blood shear.[122,123] High shear induces platelet aggregation in the absence of platelet agonists. Aurin tricarboxylic acid (ATA) blocks the binding of vWF to GPIb, but does not block the binding of vWF to GPIIb-IIIa; ATA effectively inhibits shear-induced aggregation, indicating that the GPIb receptor is essential to this process.

The GPIIb-IIIa complex serves as a platelet receptor for fibrinogen, fibronectin, vitronectin, and vWF on activated platelets (Figure 6).[124] It is necessary for platelet aggregation, and more research has been focused on GPIIb-IIIa than any other platelet receptor. The GPIIb-IIIa complex is a member of widely disseminated family of receptors that mediate many cellular functions designated as integrins.[125] Integrins are transmembrane heterodimeric molecules. Each heterodimer contains an alpha and beta chain that are noncovalently linked. Platelets, endothelial cells, smooth muscle cells, fibroblasts, and leukocytes express one

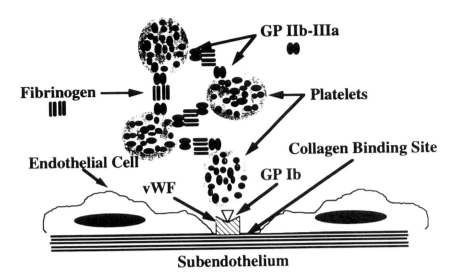

Figure 6. Illustration of the two most important receptors in platelet adhesion and aggregation. GPIb interacts with vWF which binds to its collagen binding site in the subendothelium. There are about 25000 copies of GPIb on the platelet surface. The GPIIb-IIIa complex serves as a platelet receptor for fibrinogen, fibronectin, vitronectin, and vWF on activated platelets. GPIIb-IIIa is the most numerous integrin on the platelet surface and is found exclusively on platelets. It is the most abundant glycoprotein on platelets with approximately 50000 copies per platelet.

or more receptor proteins in the integrin family, which cause adherence of adhesive proteins to the cell that in turn cause cell to cell, or cell to substratum, interactions.

GPIIb-IIIa is the most numerous integrin on the platelet surface and, in contrast to other integrins, is found exclusively on platelets an other cells that originate in megakaryoblasts. In fact, this integrin is the most abundant glycoprotein on platelets with approximately 50000 copies per platelet.[126] GPIIb consists of two disulfide-like subunits of MW 132kDa and 23 kDa.[127] GPIIIa consists of a single polypeptide chain with extensive intrachain disulfide bonds (MW = 114 kDa).[128] Both GPIIb and GPIIIa contain 15% carbohydrate by weight. GPIIb and GPIIIa form a 1:1 complex on the membrane surface in the presence of calcium, and the complex dissociates when the Ca^{++} concentration is very low.[129]

As is true of so many hematologic disorders, Glanzmann's thrombasthenia, a bleeding diathesis characterized by absence of platelet aggregation and fibrinogen binding of platelets, provided much information about the GPIIb-IIIa receptor.[130] Patients with Glanzmann's thrombasthenia have platelets that do not aggregate or bind to fibrinogen because they have either abnormal or low levels of GPIIb-IIIa receptors. Although the synthesis of GPIIb and GPIIIa are encoded by different genes on the long arm of chromosome 17, a defect in either gene can lead to the thrombasthenic phenotype and absence of GPIIb-IIIa on the platelet

surface.[131] Clinically, patients with this disorder typically present with hemorrhagic problems such as purpura or mucous membrane bleeding in early childhood.

The GPIIb-IIIa complex binds to fibrinogen, vWF, fibronectin, vitronectin, and other serum proteins.[128,132] The principal functional domain of GPIIb-IIIa with respect to its binding to extracellular adhesive plasma proteins is related to the argininine-glycine-aspartic acid (*Arg-Gly-Asp*, which is designated *RGD*) amino acid sequence that is present on each of the above listed ligands.[133] Of note, the RGD sequence is also present on several peptides found in snake venoms, including echistatin from *Echis carinatus* and applagrin from *Agkistrodon piscivorus*.[134] These low-molecular weight RGD-containing peptides, which have also been produced synthetically, are collectively called *disintegrins*. Adhesive plasma proteins such as fibrinogen do not bind to resting platelet; the binding sites must be exposed by platelet activation.[135,136]

In addition to investigation of platelets from patients with Glanzmann's thrombasthenia and experiments with disintegrins, monoclonal antibodies directed against the GPIIb-IIIa complex have provided much information about this receptor. We have shown that the monoclonal antibody LJ-CP8 is an effective agent to prevent vascular graft thrombosis in baboons by preventing GPIIb-IIIa-related platelet aggregation[137] (Figure 7). Other such antibodies, such as 7E3, prevents coronary and carotid artery thrombosis in the Folts model of thrombosis in dogs.[138] The 7E3 anti-

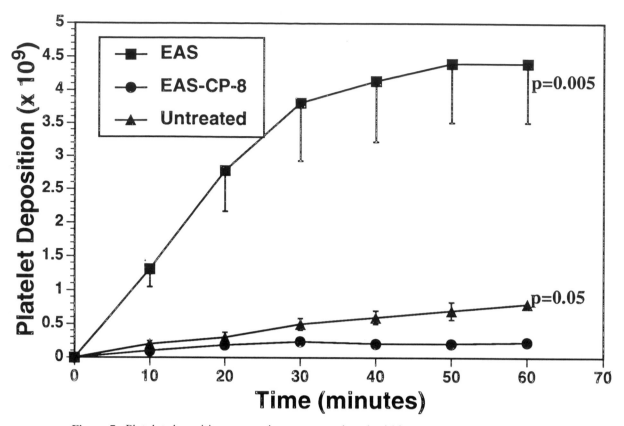

Figure 7. Platelet deposition on aortic segments placed within an externalized arteriovenous shunt in baboons and imaged with a gamma camera. [111]Indium-labeled platelet deposition on endarterectomized aortic segments (EAS, ■ n-6) was marked after 1 hour (4.40 ± 0.89 × 10^9 platelets/cm). Treatment of animals with LJ-CP8, a monoclonal antibody directed against GPIIb-IIIa, (EAS-CP8, ● n = 4) reduced platelet deposition to 0.23 ± 0.01 × 10^9 platelets/cm (p = 0.005 compared with EAS results). LJ-CP8 treatment permitted even less platelet deposition than on uninjured, nonendarterectomized aortic segments (Untreated, ▲ n = 6) which accumulated 0.89 ± 0.26 × 10^9 platelets/cm at 60 minutes. (p = 0.05 compared with EAS-CP8 results). (Reproduced with permission from Krupski WC, Bass A, Kelly AB, Ruggeri ZM, Harker LA, Hanson SR: Interruption of vascular thrombosis by bolus anti-platelet glycoprotein IIb/IIIa monoclonal antibodies in baboons. *J Vasc Surg* 17:294, 1993.)

body also shortens the time to reperfusion and prevents reocclusion in canine models of thrombosis.[139] These and other such studies have established the importance of GP IIb-IIIa in platelet thrombus formation, and may help explain why thrombolytic therapy is unsuccessful in one-fifth of acute coronary artery thromboses.[113]

Successful ablation of the GPIIb-IIIa complex in animal models by monoclonal antibodies soon led to their use in humans. After a pilot study of 7E3 showed efficacy in patients with unstable angina pectoris,[140] a larger multicenter trial of this anti-GPIIb-IIIa antibody was instituted in patients undergoing percutaneous transluminal coronary angioplasty.[141] In this 1994 study, a bolus infusion of placebo or monoclonal antibody (c7E3) directed against the platelet glycoprotein IIb-IIIa receptor was given to 2099 patients undergoing

high-risk coronary angioplasty in 56 centers. c7E3 produced a 35% reduction in the rate of the primary end point (death, nonfatal myocardial infarction, unplanned surgical revascularization, unplanned repeat percutaneous procedure, unplanned implantation of a coronary stent, or insertion of an intra-aortic balloon pump for refractory ischemia), but not surprisingly the risk of bleeding was increased.

Although monoclonal antibodies have increased our understanding of the GPIIb-IIIa complex, and they have been therapeutically effective, their antigenicity, expense, and irreversibility (with consequent effects on bleeding time and potential for clinical hemorrhage) have motivated a quest for more practical agents to block this receptor. To some extent, the disintegrins, i.e., RGD-containing peptides, have favorable pharmacologic characteristics. RGD peptides from snake venoms (trigramin, echistatin, bitistatin, and kistrin) are quickly cleared from plasma and have antiplatelet effect shorter-lived than those of monoclonal antibodies.[134,142,143] In addition, synthetic cyclic peptides containing the RGD sequence have been produced. However, both snake venom peptides and cyclic RGD peptides react with several integrins and are not specific for GPIIb-IIIa; they theoretically could have deleterious effects on other cell functions, such as adhesion of endothelial cells to matrix proteins.

Platelet Physiology

Platelets play a central role in hemostasis, which consists of the interaction of the vascular endothelium, vascular wall, platelets, and chemical coagulation. Platelets interact with the blood vessel wall, other platelets, and the coagulation proteins. The process of hemostasis begins with platelet adhesion, when platelets attach to nonendothelial surfaces, but not to one another. They then undergo a complex series of morphologic and biochemical changes termed shape change, aggregation, and secretion. A defect in any of these functions results in a bleeding disorder of some sort.

Adhesion

One-trillion circulating platelets survey 1000 m² of vascular endothelial surface area.[144] Adhesion is the platelet's first response to vessel injury, in which platelets attach to nonendothelial surfaces, but not to one another. The continuous endothelial surface is not thrombogenic, but when the subendothelial surface is exposed, as in vascular injury, platelets adhere to elements therein, especially collagen. The degree of platelet adhesion is directly dependent on the degree of vascular injury. Even small amounts of injury instigate this process. For example, dilatation of veins during general anesthesia results in separation of endothelial cells and exposes collagen; platelet adherence to the basement membrane may then play a role in initiation of deep venous thrombosis in this setting.

When the magnitude of vascular injury is small, such as when platelets bridge the gap between separated endothelial cells, adherent platelets do not change morphology and may detach and reenter the circulation. Platelets firmly adhere to larger areas of exposed collagen within seconds and generally undergo shape change, aggregation, and the release reaction; they do not reenter circulating blood. As this process repeats itself, a hemostatic plug is formed within minutes.

Adherent of platelets to the basement membrane

is dependent on a "bridging" plasma protein, the most important of which is vWF. As previously noted, vWF is a multimeric glycoprotein synthesized exclusively in megakaryocytes and endothelial cells.[145,146] vWF multimers are stored in endothelial cell secretory granules termed *Weibel-Palade bodies*.[147] Weibel-Palade bodies are unique to endothelial cells and are used to identify these cells by electron microscopy. In platelets, vWF is stored in and secreted from α granules.

In vivo, the vasopressin derivative desmopressin (1-Desamino-8-D-Arginine Vasopressin or DDAVP induces release of vWF by endothelial cells into the area of the basement membrane and surrounding area,[148,149] evidenced by loss of Weibel-Palade body-vWF on immunostained tissue sections obtained after DDAVP administration.[150]

All other plasma proteins involved in hemostasis are synthesized in the liver except for vWF, which in addition to its bridging function serves as the macromolecular weight portion of the factor VIII molecules (VIII:vWF). When combined with the procoagulant portion of factor VIII (VIII:C and VIII:vWF), Factor VIII$_a$ can be generated that is a cofactor for factor X activation. The exact site of production of VIII:C is uncertain.

Circulating vWF consists of a series of multimers ranging in size from about 800 kDa to 1200 kDa. Larger vWF multimers more effectively bind platelets to subendothelium than smaller multimers.[151] von Willebrand Disease (vWD), described by von Willebrand in 1927,[146] results from quantitative and qualitative deficiencies in vWF. Because it is involved both in platelet adhesion/aggregation and stabilization of factor VIII, clinical and laboratory findings may reflect impaired platelet function, impaired coagulation, or both.

There are three major types (and several subtypes) of vWD, defined by specific qualitative and/or quantitative abnormalities in vWF.[152] The production of vWF is controlled by genes on chromosome 5. All types of vWD are inherited as autosomal traits with variable genetic penetrance. Types I, IIA, and IIB, the commonest forms, are inherited as dominant traits transmitted by either parent. The most severe variety of vWD (type III) is inherited from both parents and may be either a homozygous recessive inheritance of a distinct defect or more severe expression of the other types of vWD in a homozygous or doubly heterozygous inheritance of two dominant genes.[153] In contrast, deficiency of the second portion of the factor VIII molecule, VIII:C, results in classic hemophilia A, which occurs almost exclusively in males as an X-linked recessive trait.

vWF is present in circulating blood, is deposited in the subendothelium by endothelial cells, and is stored within platelet alpha granules.[154–156] Neither circulating vWF, nor subendothelial vWF, normally binds to circulating platelets unless there is disruption of vascular endothelium. In vivo investigation of the mechanisms by which binding occurs is difficult. From in vitro experiments, however, it is clear that the nonintegrin receptor GPIb-IX is the site for this process. Of note, GPIb does not bind human vWF in plasma, whereas it does interact with vWF deposited in the subendothelial extracellular matrix. Only when ristocetin or certain snake venoms, such as botrocetin, are added will vWF interact with platelets in a plasma milieu.[157] As previously noted (see section on Platelet Membrane Glycoproteins), ristocetin is antibiotic; it has a marked positive charge that decreases the negative charge of the platelet, thereby unmasking the plasma vWF site for GPIb.[158] The electrostatic repulsion between vWF and the platelet surface plays an important role in preventing undue interactions in the circulation.[146]

About 20% of total circulating vWF is stored within the alpha granules of platelets. Of note, this storage pool is comprised mostly of the larger molecular-weight multimers of vWF that are more hemostatically active.[159,160] However, this source of vWF is not available for the initial interaction of platelets with the vessel wall. Alpha granule vWF is liberated only during the secretion (release reaction), when platelets are activated subsequent to adhesion (see below).

In addition to its interaction with GPIb-IX, vWF binds to platelets by a second mechanism distinct from ristocetin-induced binding. vWF competes with fibrinogen and other adhesive molecules (fibronectin and thrombospondin) for the GPIIb-IIIa binding site when platelets become activated in the presence of thrombin or ADP.[161,162] Because fribrinogen is present in far greater quantities than vWF, it usually "wins the battle" for the GPIIb-IIIa receptor site.[163,164] Hence, when platelets are activated, most of the GPIIb-IIIa receptor sites bind fibrinogen, not vWF. Thrombin-induced binding of vWF to platelets is calcium-dependent, requires activated platelets, and is prevented and *reversed* by prostacyclin, which produces increased intracellular cAMP. In essence, the two functional binding domains to which vWF attaches to platelets produces a "zipper effect" through multiple interactions between platelets and the subendothelium.[144]

The second mechanism of vWF binding has clinical relevance. Activated platelets from patients with Glanzmann's thrombasthenia (deficient in the GPIIb-IIIa receptor) do not bind to plasma vWF when stimulated by thrombin.[165] In addition, as previously discussed, the GPIIb-IIIa receptor is crucial for platelet aggregation; because vWF can bind to this site, it can substitute for fibrinogen in this process. This may explain why some patients with afibrinogenemia have

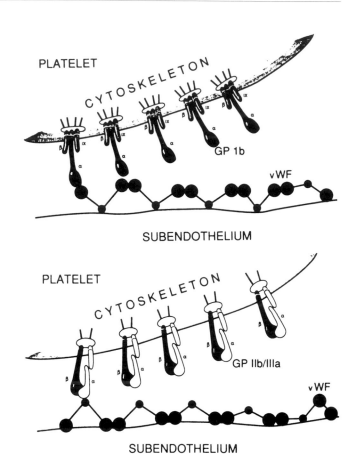

Figure 8. Cartoon of zippering mechanisms of platelet membrane receptors with vWF and the subendothelium. **(top)** Platelet GPIb forms multiple bond with the amino-terminal domain of vWF subunits attached in linear multimers. **(bottom)** Platelet GPIIb-IIIa forms multiple bonds with the carboxy-terminal domain of vWF subunits arranged in linear multimers. Zippering occurs because multiple bonds are formed adjacent to one another. (Reproduced with permission from Reference 144.)

less severe bleeding episodes.[166] Of importance, when platelets aggregate in conditions of high shear stress (e.g., turbulent arterial flow), large vWF multimers are released from stressed endothelial cells.[167,168] These exceptionally large vWF multimers may contribute to occlusive platelet thrombi in small arteries and arterioles that are affected by atherosclerosis or vasospasm.[144]

Figure 8 shows the interaction between platelet membrane receptors with vWF in the extracellular matrix, producing the zippering effect. Exposure of subendothelial collagen and other matrix proteins results in absorption of circulating high-molecular weight multimers of vWF, as well as binding of vWF released from nearby endothelial cells. Both plasma vWF and subendothelial-bound vWF are important in the subsequent optimal adhesion of platelets to this surface.[196]

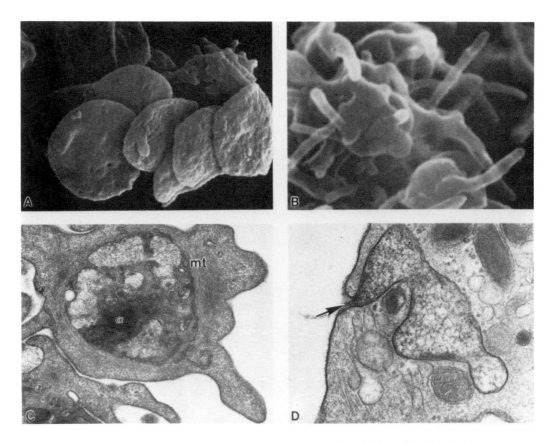

Figure 9. Scanning and transmission electron micrographs of alterations in platelets after activation. **(A)** SEM of quiescent platelet. The indentations and rough-appearing surface are caused by communication of the surface-connected open canalicular system with the cell exterior. (magnification ×7,000). **(B)** SEM of platelet activated with ADP showing long spiky pseudopod formation. (magnification ×21,000). **(C)** TEM of platelet activated with thrombin showing pseudopods, centralization of organelles, and the constricting microtubules [Mt] (magnification ×32,000). **(D)** TEM of actively secreting platelet showing fusion of granules with the surface open canalicular system (stained with tannic acid), which connects through the cell exterior through narrow pores **(arrow).** Alpha granules are secreted through these openings. (Reproduced with permission from References 196 and 197.)

Shape Change

After adhesion occurs, if platelets are exposed to a sufficiently strong stimulus (agonist), they soon undergo a shape change from discoid to irregular spheres with long pseudopods (Figures 9A and 9B). At the same time, organelles move to the central area of the cell and become enclosed within a close-fitting ring of microtubules and microfilaments (Figure 9C). This process has been likened to a sort of internal contraction. Agonists for platelet shape change and subsequent aggregation include collagen, ADP, thromboxane A_2, prostaglandin H_2, chymotrypsin, thrombin, platelet activating factor (PAF), and epinephrine.[170]

Platelet agonists are commonly classified as strong and weak, but the distinctions between these categories are often blurred (Table 7). Strong agonists are those that can elicit granule secretion even when aggregation is blocked (such as by removing extracellular Ca^{++} required for fibrinogen binding to GPIIb-IIIa.) Thrombin and collagen are examples of strong agonists, whereas ADP and epinephrine are weak agonists that require aggregation for secretion to occur. Theoretically, the strong agonists are primarily responsible for platelet aggregation in vivo, while the weak agonists play a supporting role, particularly ADP which is stored in dense granules and released during early stages of aggregation. The role of epinephrine is less straightforward. Most agonists cause internal redistribution of calcium from membrane-bound stores (e.g., in the DTS into the cytoplasm.[171] Free cytosolic calcium is then available for initiation of shape change and other platelet activation processes (see subsequent

Table 7
Platelet Agonists Relative Strengths

Strength	Agonist
Weak	ADP
	Epinephrine
	Platelet Activating Factor (PAF)
	vasopressin
	serotonin
Intermediate	Thromboxane A_2
Strong	Thrombin
	Trypsin
	Collagen
Unknown	Ristocetin
	Bovine factor VIII
	Antiplatelet antibodies

ADP = adenosine diphosphate.

section on Importance of Thromboxane. In contrast, epinephrine's interaction with its receptor allows calcium to enter the cell "from outside in."[172] When calcium levels are sufficiently high, additional calcium is released from internal stores, a phenomenon called "calcium-stimulated calcium release."[173] Although epinephrine can activate platelets on its own, its standard function may be to sensitize platelets to other agonists.[174] Curiously, epinephrine does *not* induce platelet shape change.

As previously noted, microtubules immediately beneath the plasma membrane maintain the normal discoid shape of platelets in their resting state. During shape change, by means of rising cytosolic calcium levels, the microtubules transiently disassemble. They reassemble in the spiky pseudopods, where they provide structural support. High cytosolic calcium levels also promote contraction of thrombosthenin (which, like thrombosthenin in megakaryocytes is identical to naturally occurring muscle actomyosin). The band of microfilaments that centralizes the platelet organelles is separate from the circumferential microtubules and is composed principally of thrombosthenin. The purpose of centralization of granules and the function of contraction of the microfilaments are incompletely understood. If cytosolic calcium levels rise to a sufficient level in response to the agonist, aggregation and secretion will ensue; if not, the process of shape change can reverse, and the platelet will return to its normal discoid shape.

Aggregation

Platelets circulating in blood, in plasma, or even as an isolated cell population in vitro do not interact with one another. If stimulated by an appropriate agonist, however, they stick to one another, the process known as aggregation (Figure 10).[175] The development of a simple technique for continuous monitoring of agonist-induced platelet aggregation in plasma greatly increased our understanding of this reaction.[176] Platelet aggregometers are special instruments designed for measuring changes in light transmission through suspensions of platelets.[177] At concentrations of 1 to 3 × 10^8/mL, platelet suspensions are opalescent. After an agonist is added, a stirred suspension of normal platelets will aggregate producing a visible decrease in turbidity and optical density.

Interaction of the agonist with its specific receptor initiates aggregation. Aggregation is energy-dependent, requiring ATP derived from glycolysis, and to some extent from oxidative phosphorylation in the mitochondria.[178] When oxidative phosphorylation is inhibited, ATP produced by glycolysis alone is inadequate to produce aggregation. Information about the structure of the receptors for agonists is limited. With the exception of epinephrine, whose receptor site has been identified with certainty, not much is known about specific binding sites. The numbers of binding sites for various agonists have been determined by binding studies (Table 8).

Fibrinogen and calcium are essential for platelet-platelet interaction.[179] Plasma fibrinogen is adequate to facilitate aggregation, but platelets contain additional fibrinogen that can be released and, under certain circumstances, support aggregation in the absence of plasma fibrinogen.[180] Fibrinogen plays a dual role in the formation of thrombus by virtue of its ability to aggregate platelets and form fibrin in the coagulation cascade. Calcium is also necessary for platelet-platelet interactions, although magnesium can support aggregation as long as a trace amount of calcium is also present.

As previously discussed, the glycoprotein IIb-IIIa complex is the fibrinogen binding site. In the resting platelet, IIb and IIIa exist as separate proteins.[181] When cytoplasmic calcium levels rise, however, the GPIIb-IIIa complex forms as a consequence of intracellular calcium flux and fibrinogen binds to the platelet surface.[182,183] After fibrinogen binds to its receptor, extracellular calcium facilitates formation of fibrinogen/fibrin bridges between platelets and development of platelet aggregates.[173] Fibrinogen contains two RGD sequences, one near the N-terminus and a second near the C-terminus.[184] Recent data suggests that it is the C-terminal RGD sequence that binds to GPIIb-IIIa.[185] The dimeric nature of fibrinogen permits each molecule to interact with two platelets, serving as a platelet-platelet "bridge." In certain circumstances, other adhesive proteins, such as vitronectin, fibronectin, thrombospondin, and vWF, may substitute for fi-

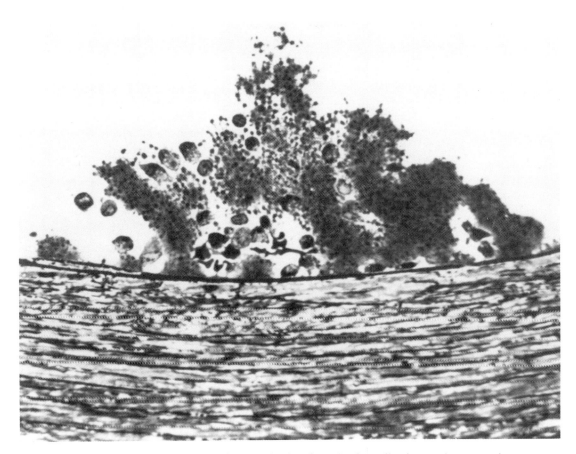

Figure 10. Scanning electron micrograph showing platelet adhesion and aggregation to denuded rabbit aorta in vivo. (magnification ×820). (Reproduced with permission from Reference 175.)

Table 8
Receptors for Platelet Agonists

Agonist	Approximate Number of Binding Sites	Antagonist
ADP	10^4–10^5	ATP, FSBA
Thrombin	10^2–10^3	PPACK-thrombin
Thromboxane	10^3	PTA-0H
Platelet activating factor	10^2	Multiple
Epinephrine	10^2	Yohimbine
Collagen	Unknown	Unknown

ADP = adenosine diphosphate; ATP = adenosine triphosphate; FSBA = 5′-p-fluoro-sulfonylbenzoyl adenosine; PPACK = L-prolyl-d-phenylalanyl-chloromethylketone; PTA-OH = $\alpha\beta$-gw-tetranor-TxA$_2$.

(Adapted with permission from References 266 and 275.)

brinogen in this process.[186] It has been postulated that under conditions of high shear, vWF may be dominant in producing aggregation.[187]

Four clinical examples illustrate the importance of calcium, fibrinogen, and GPIIb-IIIa in platelet aggregation. First, if blood is collected using EDTA, which tightly binds calcium, platelets will not aggregate. In contrast, the other commonly used anticoagulant, citrate, only weakly binds calcium and platelet aggregation can occur.[173] Second, when fibrinogen is removed from plasma and release of platelet alpha-granule-fibrinogen is inhibited, platelet aggregation cannot proceed. Third, patients with Glanzmann's thrombasthenia, whose platelets are deficient in the GPIIb-IIIa receptor, demonstrate abnormal platelet aggregation.[130] Fourth, monoclonal antibodies directed against GPIIb-IIIa profoundly block aggregation.[137,188]

Aggregation may proceed in two waves or phases, depending on the concentration of agonist. These phases are called *primary* and *secondary aggregation*. During primary aggregation small platelet aggregates form. If the concentration or relative strength of the agonist is low (e.g., low concentrations of ADP), the aggregates can break up and secondary aggregation does not occur. Eventually, all the small aggregates dissociate into individual platelets. Thus, primary aggregation is reversible. With higher doses of agonists, secondary aggregation proceeds after a variable lag period of time. The onset of secondary aggregation marks the beginning of platelet secretion. Secondary aggregation and secretion are intimately associated. In fact, secondary aggregation is dependent on molecules released from platelet granules, particularly ADP from dense bodies. Similarly, secretion is dependent on thromboxane A_2 (TXA_2) formed within the platelet (except when thrombin is used as an agonist). Blocking production of TXA_2 by agents such as aspirin usually prevents the second wave of platelet aggregation.

Secondary aggregation is often called irreversible. However, prostacyclin (PGI_2) and other TXA_2-inhibitors, such as PTA-OH, can reverse platelet aggregation even after the secondary phase has begun (Table 7).[189,190] However, after several minutes of secondary aggregation, the addition of even large amounts of PGI_2 will not reverse aggregation. Thus, there is a time-dependent stabilization of the platelet-platelet bridges.

Secretion (Release Reaction)

Platelet secretion or the release reaction is defined as extrusion of the contents of the storage organelles to the cells' environment without loss of constituents from other subcellular compartments (Figure 9C). Platelet secretion marks the final phase of platelet acti-

vation and accompanies secondary aggregation. Some authors describe secretion preceding aggregation in the process of platelet plug formation. The process takes 10 to 120 seconds, depending on the strength of the stimulus and which secreted substance is measured.[101,191] Secretion proceeds in an orderly fashion; contents of the dense granules are released first, followed by the contents of alpha granules and then lysosomes. The secreted molecules have effects on other cells, the platelets themselves, or they are converted to physiologically active substances in plasma or on cell surfaces.[101] In order for secretion to start, cytosolic calcium concentration must rise to a sufficient level, which generally occurs owing to thromboxane formation. Thrombin is a unique agonist in this regard; it can induce secretion independent of thromboxane, and it is classified as a *direct secretagogue,* causing secretion independent of aggregation.

Dense Bodies

Contents of platelet granules are listed in Table 5. There is a high metal ion (calcium, phosphate) content in dense bodies; in fact, they drive their name from their electron dense appearance on transmission electron micrographs.[101] As noted earlier, the ADP and calcium released from dense bodies are important for secondary aggregation and additional platelet activation. Serotonin (5 HT) derived from dense bodies serves several functions. Serotonin by itself is a weak platelet activating agent, but it promotes activation by other agonists, including ADP.[192] Serotonin also contributes to hemostasis by its potent vasoconstrictor effects. Although ATP inhibits ADP in vitro, the concentration is insufficient to produce this effect in vivo. Thus, the overall effect of dense granule release is to promote vasoconstriction and potentiate platelet aggregation and activation.

Alpha Granules

There are more alpha granules than dense bodies in platelets. Both structures are released by exocytosis, a process involving fusion of the secretory granule membrane with the plasma membrane.[193,194] This is not a simple process because most alpha granules move centripetally during secretion and, thus, are not in a position that easily allows fusion with the peripheral plasma membrane.[195-197] The mechanisms for exocytosis are still unsettled and the subject of controversy and ongoing research.[198]

Secretion of alpha granules begins with fusion of the granule membrane with the surface-connected open canalicular system (see above). The next step involves surface expression of GPIIb and GPIIIa and some alpha granule proteins (e.g., high-molecular-weight kininogen and platelet fibrinogen).[196,199] The 20 or more proteins in alpha granules can be grouped in several ways. One classification scheme is to divide them into two groups: 1) proteins that are platelet-specific (e.g., PF4, β-thromboglobulin) and 2) proteins that are similar or homologues of plasma proteins (e.g., fibrinogen vWF, high-molecular-weight kininogen). Another classification system is mostly based on the functions of various platelet proteins (Table 5).

Platelet Specific Proteins

Most textbooks include four proteins in this group: PF4, β-thromboglobulin, platelet-derived growth factor (PDGF) and thrombospondin. In fact, only the first two are found exclusively in platelets. Macrophages and other cells produce PDGF and endothelial cells also produce thrombospondin.[200]

Platelet Factor 4

PF4, a 70-amino acid monomer with a molecular weight of 7.8 kDa, is secreted from the platelet alpha granules complexed with a high-molecular-weight proteoglycan carrier.[201] It has many actions, including: 1) chemotaxis of neutrophils and monocytes[202]; 2) chemotaxis of fibroblasts[203]; 3) stimulation of histamine release by basophils[204]; 4) inhibition of contact activation of the coagulation cascade[205]; and 5) promotion of platelet aggregation owing to a high affinity PF4 binding site.[200] Thus, PF4 may play a role in the inflammatory process, wound healing, hypersensitivity reactions, and modulation of thrombosis.

The most important function of PF4, however, is its ability to bind and neutralize heparin. PF4 has a very high affinity for heparin; when the PF4-proteoglycan complex is exposed to heparin, the carrier is released, and PF4 binds to heparin and neutralizes its activity.[206] This action has been one proposed explanation for the resistance of high-flow, high-shear arterial thrombosis to heparin.[137]

Recombinant human PF4 is currently available and may have important clinical applications. For example, PF4 may be a useful substitute for protamine sulfate to reverse anticoagulant activity of heparin. Protamine can cause thrombocytopenia, leukopenia, hypotension, and pulmonary edema, whereas recombinant human rPF4 effectively reverses heparin without any adverse effects.[207] In addition, rPF4 suppresses angiogenesis, mitigates immunosuppression, and inhibits tumor growth in mice, suggesting a possible role for this substance in the treatment of malignant tumors.[208]

β-Thromboglobulin

β-Thromboglobulin (βTG) is a degradation product of two other compounds that are immunologically identical using polyclonal antibodies: PBP and low-affinity platelet factor 4 (LA-PF4), which is also called connective tissue activating peptide III (CTAP-III).[209] Thus, β-thromboglobulin is one of a group of βTG-like proteins (PBP, LA-PF4, [CTAP-III], βTG, and βTG-F).[210] The βTG-like proteins have a molecular weight ranging from 7 to 11 kDa, and all have a high degree of homology with PF4. Although βTG does neutralize heparin, it has a low affinity for it.[211] The biologic activities of PF4 and the βTG-like proteins differ substantially. For example, the major route of clearance of βTG is renal, whereas PF4 is metabolized in the liver (probably related to heparin-binding sites). The major biologic activities of the βTG-like proteins include chemotaxis of neutrophils and both chemotaxis and mitogenesis of fibroblasts, suggesting a role in inflammation and wound healing.[210,212]

Platelet-Derived Growth Factor

Serum, not plasma, is required in the medium for cultured cells to divide. This observation suggested the presence of cell growth factors in platelets. A polypeptide growth factor is defined as an agent that promotes cell proliferation by interacting with specific receptors that promote DNA synthesis and cell division.[213] At least four potent growth factors are present in platelet granules (see Table 5): platelet-derived growth factor (PDGF), platelet transforming growth factor β1 (platelet TGF-β), epidermal growth factor (EGF), and—most recently described—platelet-derived endothelial cell growth factor (PD-ECGF).[214-218] PDGF is one of the best characterized growth factors. PDGF purified from human platelets has a molecular weight of approximately 30,000 (ranging from 28000 to 35000, due to different levels of glycosylation and partial proteolytic cleavage in outdated plasma).[219] Each molecule consists of an alpha peptide chain (M_r: 14000) and a beta peptide chain (M_r: 17000) with multiple disulfide bonds, which are responsible for mitogenic activity. When it binds to its specific cell surface, high-affinity receptor (M_r: 170000–180000),[220] highly-purified PDGF is active in the picomolar range.[221]

PDGF is a potent mitogen for mesenchymally-derived connective tissue cells such as fibroblasts, smooth muscle cells, and glial cells, inducing cell doubling within 30 to 36 hours.[219] Chapter 5 discusses these properties in detail. Unlike some other growth factors, it is chemotactic for the same cells for which it is mitogenic.[222] Cells without PDGF-receptors, including epithelial cells, lymphocytes, and vascular endothelium, do not grow in response to the mitogen.

Exposure to PDGF induces a host of intracellular events in susceptible cells, including: calcium mobilization, increased DNA synthesis, expression of several genes (c-fos and c-myc), increased cholesterol synthesis, increased binding of low-density lipoprotein (LDL) to its receptor, increased prostaglandin formation, increased synthesis of RNA and protein, and changes in cell shape with reorganization of actin cables.[219,223,224] This last feature may have relevance to the recent finding that PDGF is an extremely potent vasoconstrictive agent, even more effective than angiotensin II (AII) in inducing smooth muscle contraction.[225]

PDGF is produced by megakaryoctes and carried in platelet α granules. As the first cell to appear at sites of vascular injury and the largest source of PDGF in the body, release of PDGF by activated platelets initiates and directs tissue repair.[226] Tissue macrophages, derived from circulating monocytes, are of equal importance in PDGF production. Unlike platelets, monocytes contain little or no preformed PDGF, and they are incapable of manufacturing the mitogen in cell culture unless they are activated. Once the monocyte departs the blood, enters the tissue, and is activated to become a macrophage, it can synthesize and secrete PDGF. Because PDGF-secreting macrophages, fibroblasts, and smooth muscle cells can be activated by PDGF, a positive autocrine feedback within the wound amplifies the initial platelet-derived signals and triggers release of a cascade of molecules that effects healing. Endothelial cells, which constitute a significant portion of proliferating wounds, secrete PDGF as well providing a paracrine stimulus for nearby smooth muscle cells. Interestingly, the concentrations of PDGF required for chemotaxis vary between neutrophils, monocytes, and fibroblasts, resulting in an orderly sequence of cellular infiltration into a wound according to concentration gradients.[227]

Thrombospondin

Thrombospondin is a high-molecular weight glycoprotein (approximately 450 kDa) originally described in 1971 as thrombin-sensitive protein.[228] Ultrastructural studies reveal that it exists as a trimer with three identical disulfide-bonded peptide chains. In addition to platelets, endothelial cells, macrophages, smooth muscle cells, and fibroblasts, synthesize and secrete thrombospondin.[229–232]

Thrombospondin is a multifunctional glycoprotein that binds to the surface of activated platelets on several binding sites including GPIIb, fibrinogen, the complex of GPIIIa and the alpha-chain vitronectin receptor, and others. It is a calcium-binding protein whose conformation is altered by chelation of calcium.[233]

Antibodies to thrombospondin inhibit platelet aggregation. Thrombospondin interacts with both fibrin and fibrinogen, forming a reversible, noncovalent complex, and is incorporated into the fibrin clot network.[231] Thus, it may play a major role in platelet aggregation by stabilizing the initially reversible platelet: fibrinogen interaction.[234]

Inhibition of Secretion

Substances that elevate the intracellular concentration of cAMP strongly inhibit platelet secretion. These agents include adenosine, papaverine, dipyridamole, methylxanthines, and several prostaglandins (E_2, D_2, and especially I_2 [prostacyclin]). The mechanism of inhibition is most likely related to removal of cytoplasmic Ca^{++} by means of sequestration in the DTS. Aspirin, indomethacin, and imidazole, and many of the nonsteroidal anti-inflammatory drugs prevent secretion by inhibition of aracidonate liberation, cyclooxygenase, and thromboxane synthetase. Calmodulin inhibitors also stop platelet secretion, indicating that minimal, submicromolar concentrations of Ca^{++} are required for signal processing. When the availability of ATP is decreased by increased consumption or inhibited production, platelet secretion ceases. Finally, platelet secretion may be stopped or decreased by interference with the Ca^{++} pump by Ca^{++} pump inhibitors, local anesthetics, and calcium antagonists.

Biochemistry of Platelet Activation

Importance of Thromboxane

Elevation of cytosolic calcium is the cornerstone of platelet activation and secretion. Only small amounts of free Ca^{++} are present in the cytoplasm of resting platelets, estimated to be in the range of 10^{-7} M.[173] How does Ca^{++} bring about platelet activation? In part, elevated cytosolic Ca^{++} activates enzymes that are not optimally functional in the quiescent platelet, which include phospholipases A_2 and C.[235] Arachidonate, a major 20-carbon fatty acid in platelets and endothelial cells, is liberated from phospholipids by hydrolysis (the actions of phospholipases A_2 and C) and by receptor-controlled G-proteins.[236,237] The arachidonate released from membrane phospholipids is first converted to Prostaglandin-G_2 (PGG_2) via the aspirin-sensitive cyclooxygenase pathway. PGG_2 is rapidly converted to PGH_2. Prostaglandin-H_2 (PGH_2) is acted on by thromboxane synthetase to form thromboxane A_2 (TXA_2). TXA_2 is the most potent platelet activator known.[238] TXA_2 interacts with an as yet uncharacterized platelet receptor to further raise cytosolic calcium levels and platelet activation and release; ADP appears to be important in the ability to TXA$_2$ to produce platelet aggregation, although this is somewhat controversial.[239]

Once formed, TXA$_2$ diffuses across the platelet membrane and activates other platelets, which amplifies the initial stimulus for platelet activation.[240] This phenomenon is largely confined to the specific area of injury owing to the short (about 30 seconds) half-life of TXA$_2$. Thromboxane spontaneously degrades to a stable metabolic end product designated thromboxane B$_2$ (TXB$_2$), which can be measured by radioimmunoassay using labeled antibodies. Under most circumstances, almost all PGH$_2$ is converted to TXA$_2$, but PGH$_2$ is itself a potent platelet activator that produces internal Ca^{++} mobilization.[170,171]

Of note, the enzymes involved in TXA$_2$ formation from arachidonate are located on the DTS. Thus, the DTS is very important in platelet aggregation. The DTS is close to the plasma membrane, which releases arachidonate (see section on *Ultrastructure*). The enzymes responsible for production of thromboxane, cyclooxygenase, and thromboxane synthetase are localized on the DTS.[241] Thromboxane production stimulates release of calcium from the DTS, raising cytosolic Ca^{++}. It is likely, though as yet unproven, that the thromboxane receptor is located on the DTS. In addition to its ability to release Ca^{++}, the DTS actively stores calcium. Thus, the DTS functions efficiently in platelet activation; it has been likened to the sarcoplasmic reticulum of muscle.[173]

Other Agonists of Platelet Activation

Although thromboxane plays a major role in platelet aggregation, inhibition of TXA$_2$ production does not lead to clinically important hemorrhagic episodes, because only one pathway of platelet activation is blocked. In contrast, severely thrombocytopenic patients do have bleeding problems. The following discussion describes other important agonists of platelet activation.

Thrombin

Thrombin, an important serine protease in the coagulation cascade whose substrates include fibrinogen, factor V, factor VIII, and protein C, is a potent platelet-aggregating agent that does *not* require TXA$_2$ generation for its action. Platelets promote thrombin generation because negatively charged phospholipids on the surface of activated platelets accelerate coagulation factor activation. Thrombin, in turn, causes platelet activation, thereby acting synchronously to foster hemostasis. Extremely small amounts of thrombin are required to produce platelet aggregation (about 0.1 nM). In addition, platelet-bound factor V-X$_a$ complex

catalyzes the prothrombin-thrombin conversion up to 30000 times faster than when the factors are acting freely in solution (see subsequent section on *Platelet Interactions with Coagulation Proteins*.[242] Therefore, the concentration of thrombin at the platelet surface is sufficient to produce activation long before fibrin formation occurs in the extracellular phase.[101,191]

As previously noted, thrombin is a direct secretagogue, producing secretion without antecedent platelet aggregation. It activates platelets by several mechanisms. Unlike most other agonists (collagen, TXA$_2$, epinephrine), thrombin stimulates platelets by an ADP-independent mechanism.[243] Thrombin 1) releases arachidonate from the platelet membrane by provoking enzymatic hydrolysis; 2) increases cytosolic free Ca^{++}; 3) causes fibrinogen receptor expression; and 4) suppresses cAMP synthesis.[244–246] Blocking thromboxane synthesis by cyclooxygenase or thromboxane synthetase inhibitors does not substantially interfere with thrombin-induced platelet activation, as the effects can easily be overcome by increasing the concentration of thrombin.

The thrombin receptor on platelets has only recently been identified. It is a 425 amino-acid transmembrane molecule with a large amino-terminal extracellular extension.[247] A novel proteolytic mechanism is responsible for platelet activation when thrombin binds to this receptor. The receptor undergoes proteolysis at arginine 41, giving rise to a new N-terminal. The new N-terminal peptide created by this cleavage functions as a ligand that activates an additional receptor that causes signal transduction across the platelet membrane. The identical thrombin receptor is present on endothelium and smooth muscle cells. Importantly, interaction of thrombin with endothelial cells is important in maintaining the equilibrium between hemostasis and normal blood flow, because thrombin stimulates endothelial cell release of PGI$_2$, a potent vasodilator and inhibitor of platelet activation (by increasing cAMP formation).

Because 1) thrombin is such a powerful agonist for platelet activation; and 2) thromboocclusive events remain a significant complication of mechanical interventional procedures for treating atherosclerotic disease (including endarterectomy, bypass grafting, and percutaneous transluminal angioplasty); and 3) thrombin-mediated, platelet-dependent thrombus formation is often resistant to conventional antithrombotic therapies (including aspirin and heparin),[248,249] we have studied novel antithrombins in several clinically-relevant models of thrombosis. The peptide D-Phe-Pro-ArgCH$_2$Cl (PPACK), a synthetic antithrombin, effectively interrupted heparin-resistant platelet deposition and thrombosis of thrombogenic metal vascular stents in baboons.[250] Whereas blood loss after systemically-administered PPACK was substantial when the agent was given before a carotid endarterectomy in baboons, we found that transiently infused PPACK *after* the endarterectomy had been performed produced lasting and safe interruption of endarterectomy thrombosis.[251] We have also shown that hirudin, a polypeptide produced by the leech *Hirudo medicinalis* (available as a recombinant product, desulfatohirudin), effectively interrupts heparin-resistant arterial thrombus formation in both endarterectomized arterial segments and synthetic vascular grafts in baboons.[252] Thus, both synthetic and biologic antithrombins may be useful substitutes for heparin.

Collagen

Collagen causes platelets to adhere to vessel walls, change shape, secrete, and aggregate.[253] Platelet activation by collagen requires ADP and the synthesis of prostaglandins.[254] Evidence for dependency on ADP comes from development of an ADP affinity analogue, 5'-p-fluorosulfonylbenzoyl adenosine (FSBA). When platelets were incubated with FSBA, the rate of aggregation induced by collagen decreased with time; also, fibrinogen binding to platelets is inhibited by FSBA.[255] FSBA prevents shape change induced by collagen, indicating that the arachidonate liberated by collagen is insufficient to produce shape change in the absence of ADP.

There are multiple genetically distinct types of collagen. Both connective tissue collagen (types I and III) and basement membrane collagen (types IV and V) can activate platelets.[256,257] Types I and III are more potent platelet activators than IV and V, which may explain why vessel damage that penetrates the subendothelium produces a greater thrombotic response than more superficial injuries.[257,258] In general, collagen monomers polymerize and form covalent cross-links by means of enzymes in the connective matrix. Although platelets can adhere to some forms of monomeric collagen, they require the quaternary structure of polymeric collagen for aggregation and secretion.[259,260]

Several potential collagen receptors on platelets have been suggested. The interaction of vWF with the GPIb receptor site on platelets has been discussed extensively in previous sections. GPIb is very important in the binding of platelets to collagen with vWF acting as a bridge.[115–118] In addition to vWF-mediated platelet:collagen interaction, platelets express specific collagen receptors to interact directly with collagen. Candidates for this role include glycosyl transferases, factor XIII, fibronectin, glycoprotein IV (also known as CD36 and previously identified as a receptor for thrombospondin), the glycoprotein Ia-IIa complex.[261–264]

The action of collagen on platelets proceeds in the classic biphasic fashion indicative of shape change followed by aggregation. This can be observed using platelet aggregometry (Figure 11). Upon addition of collagen, there is a rapid rise towards 100% light transmission which plateaus at a point halfway between baseline and full aggregation. After a short pause, a second rise ascends until full aggregation occurs. The first deflection is the primary curve, the latter is secondary. The primary curve represents the direct response of platelets to the agonist: shape change and formation of small aggregates. The second curve represents complete aggregation after release of intrinsic ADP and thromboxane. Platelet granule contents are secreted during the latter portion of primary aggregation during the plateau phase. If the agonist concentration is too low, primary aggregation may be followed by disaggregation.

ADP

In contrast to thrombin and collagen, ADP can come from within as well as from outside platelets, because ADP is stored in dense granules. Secretion of ADP in conjunction with thromboxane recruits additional platelets into a growing platelet plug. When added to platelets in vitro, ADP causes arachidonate formation, fibrinogen receptor formation, and an increase in cytosolic Ca^{++}. The increase in Ca^{++} is mostly due to increased Ca^{++} flux across the plasma membrane rather than to Ca^{++} released from the DTS by the phosphoinositide pathway.[235,265]

Low concentrations of ADP (0.1 to 0.5 μM) produce shape change only. At ADP concentrations of 0.5 to 1.5 μM), reversible aggregation follows shape change.[176] Secondary aggregation occurs at concentrations from 2 to 5 μM. Exogenous Ca^{++} is not required for shape change to occur, and aggregation and secretion can occur even at low calcium concentrations (50 to 100 μM), suggesting that released ADP and platelet collisions in the aggregometer are responsible for irreversible aggregation.[266] Like collagen, ADP produces biphasic aggregation in vitro (see above). Secondary aggregation is dependent on production of thromboxane. If thromboxane production is prevented (e.g., by inhibition of cyclooxygenase), secondary aggregation does not occur at moderate concentrations of ADP. If additional ADP is added, however, secondary aggregation can occur, because the ADP normally supplied by secretion is replaced by added ADP.

Numerous investigators have attempted to identify the platelet ADP receptor. Coleman and colleagues have described the many difficulties in studying the ADP receptor.[266] In brief, development of FSBA has been very useful in this regard. FSBA treatment

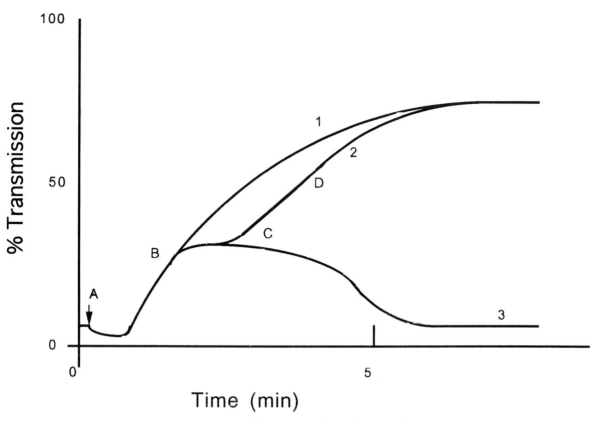

Figure 11. Aggregation response of human platelets. In order for aggregation to occur, divalent ions (Ca^{++}), an agonist (collagen) and an adhesive protein (fibrinogen) are required. Agonist (collagen) is added at **A.** Shape change is observed as a brief downward deflection (decrease in light transmission) induced by the agonist, followed by an increase in transmission (**B**) as the platelets undergo primary aggregation, forming a plateau (**C**). If sufficient agonist has been added, secondary aggregation-secretion then occurs, forming a biphasic curve (**D**). The biphasic nature of the curve is due to secondary aggregation (**2**). If sufficient agonist has been added, the platelets disaggregate after primary aggregation, curve (**3**). When the stimulus is strong (e.g., a high concentration of thrombin), there is rapid platelet aggregation with brisk rise in percent light transmission, as in the monophasic curve (**1**).

of platelets inhibits ADP-induced aggregation and prevents the exposure of fibrinogen receptors, effects that correlate with binding of FSBA to the cell.[267] At high concentrations, FSBA can behave as a weak agonist, an effect that is inhibited by ATP (a competitive antagonist of ADP).[268] There is strong evidence that ADP binds to a 100 kDa protein on the cell membrane, called aggregin, that bears superficial similarities to GP IIIa (the smaller component of the fibrinogen receptor [GP IIb-IIIa]).[266–268] However, several experiments have indicated that the two proteins are distinct.[269]

The ADP receptor is closely linked to the enzyme adenylate cyclase located on the inner surface of the plasma membrane. Adenylate cyclase converts ATP to cAMP. Increased cAMP results in decreased cytosolic free Ca^{++}, thereby inhibiting platelet activation. It has been proposed that free Ca^{++} is pumped into the DTS by a cAMP-driven pump.[270] When ADP interacts with its receptor, negative coupling with underlying adenylate cyclase *prevents* increase in intracellular cAMP; thus, the mechanism for *lowering* Ca^{++} is inhibited. The increase in cytosolic Ca^{++} generated by ADP also inhibits cAMP production.

Epinephrine

There are distinct differences between epinephrine and other agonists of platelet activation. Interestingly, epinephrine causes aggregation and secretion, but not shape change. Although many human cells have been shown to have at least three surface receptors for epinephrine (α_1, α_2, and β), platelets have only α_2 receptors, which—like ADP receptors—are negatively coupled to adenylate cyclase.[173] Binding of epinephrine to the α_2 receptor stops production of cAMP by inhibition of adenylate cyclase. Yohimbine is a specific antagonist for the α_2 receptors; binding of [^{3}H]-labelled yohimbine has been used to measure the number of α_2 receptors (Table 8).[271] There are about 200 to 300 α_2 binding sites per platelet.[272]

The activation of platelets by epinephrine is dependent on thromboxane production and can be suppressed by preincubating platelets with aspirin.[273] Unlike ADP, addition of excess epinephrine will not overcome thromboxane-blockade. In addition, the action of epinephrine is completely dependent on extracellular calcium.[274] Also unlike ADP, epinephrine does not cause release of intracellular calcium stores. Chelation of extracellular calcium by EDTA suppresses epinephrine-induced platelet activation. Platelet activation by epinephrine can also be prevented by phentolamine, which blocks the α_2 receptor, and verapamil, which blocks calcium channels.[274]

Platelet activation by epinephrine varies from individual to individual.[275] Depressed responsiveness to epinephrine in platelets from apparently normal human donors has been reported as a familial trait.[276] The etiology of this is uncertain. Two reports have described families in which mild bleeding was caused by impaired epinephrine-induced aggregation and decreased numbers of α_2 receptors.[277,278]

Epinephrine is approximately 10 times more potent than norepinephrine in activating platelets, although both substances act on α_2 receptors. At physiologic concentrations in plasma, epinephrine does not act as an independent platelet activator. In vitro concentrations tenfold higher are required for activation.[279] However, epinephrine potentiates the effects of other agonists such as thrombin, ADP, and collagen at concentrations of 0.01 to 0.1 M, which are present in vivo.[280]

Platelet Activating Factor

A substance released from leukocytes that produced platelet aggregation and secretion was discovered in the early 1970s.[173,281] PAF was found to be a choline-containing phospholipid contained in neutrophils, macrophages, eosinophils, and endothelial cells, but usually not in human platelets.[282,283] Under certain circumstances, platelets may produce PAF, but the importance of this is unknown.[284] In addition to platelet activation, PAF participates in acute allergic reactions, inflammation, and anaphylaxis.

The in vivo role of PAF in undetermined. It causes platelet aggregation in concentrations from 10 to 100 nM.[285] There are about 100 high-affinity PAF-binding sites per platelet, but the receptor has not yet been

characterized (Table 8).[286] It has been suggested that PAF causes platelet activation by a third pathway independent of thromboxane and secreted ADP;[287] however, this hypothesis is controversial. Studies are complicated by the ability of platelets and other cells to take up and metabolize PAF.[283,286] PAF-induced platelet aggregation and release are suppressed by aspirin (cyclooxygenase inhibition), ATP (ADP inhibition), FSBA (ADP receptor antagonism), and α_2 receptor blockade (the epinephrine receptor).[288]

Ristocetin

The structure and antimicrobial mechanism of action of the antibiotic ristocetin is similar to vancomycin. Ristocetin was introduced into clinical practice in the late 1950s, but it was soon withdrawn from the market because it produced thrombocytopenia. In 1971, Howard and Firkin recognized that ristocetin aggregated normal platelets, but had little or no effect on platelets from patients with vWD.[289] Aggregation is normalized by addition of normal plasma and is blocked by specific monoclonal antibodies directed against vWF.[140,290]

Ristocetin appears to bind to both platelet glycoprotein Ib and vWF. It apparently induces a change in surface charge or structure that permits bridging between ligand and receptor. Even after fixation with paraformaldehyde, which metabolically inactivates platelets, platelets will agglutinate in response to ristocetin in the presence of vWF.[291] Agglutination is contrasted with aggregation, which occurs when ristocetin is used with metabolically active platelets, because once vWF binds to GP Ib it induces GPIIb-IIIa activation, which in turn permits fibrinogen binding. vWD and Bernard-Soulier syndrome (congenital absence of GP Ib) are the only disorders in which ristocetin-induced agglutination is abnormal.[173]

Interaction of Agonists in Vivo

Although for discussion purposes platelet activating agents have been described individually, in vivo they work in concert with one another. After vascular injury, platelets are simultaneously exposed to a variety of platelet agonists. Vessel damage exposes collagen and releases tissue factor to initiate the extrinsic component of the coagulation cascade, forming thrombin. ADP and serotonin are released from the dense granules of those platelets attracted to the site of injury, recruiting additional platelets. Circulating epinephrine plays a supporting role, along with PAF released from leukocytes or even platelets themselves. Hence, numerous platelet activation pathways begin simultaneously that reinforce one another. Concentrations of agonists that in themselves might be insufficient to induce aggregation can activate platelets when added together.[173] Moreover, certain platelet granule contents, such as thromboxane and serotonin, are potent vasoconstrictors, further limiting blood loss after vascular injury.

Pathologic agonists of platelet activation also exist. The prototype condition resulting in unwanted platelet aggregation ironically is caused by heparin, the most commonly used antithrombin to produce anticoagulation. Heparin treatment can result in platelet-antibody formation, leading to activation, aggregation, and both arterial and venous thromboembolism.[292-295] Antigen-antibody complexes can also be generated by certain bacterial endotoxins, some antibiotics, and serotonin (which is a weak agonist by itself).

Platelet Interactions with Coagulant Proteins

Preceding sections have described the importance of platelet interactions with the vessel wall and with other platelets. Of equal importance in hemostasis is the interaction of platelets with the coagulation mechanism. The platelet membrane serves as the normal physiologic site of coagulation enzyme-cofactor-substrate assembly of the intrinsic pathway of fibrin clot formation. The tissue factor-extrinsic pathway of coagulation does not require the participation of platelets.

Walsh[296] has proposed at least seven major functions of platelets with respect to fibrin formation: 1) exposure of specific, high-affinity binding sites for coagulation enzymes and cofactors; 2) delivery of activated clotting factors to sites of vascular injury; 3) protection of coagulation enzymes from naturally occurring inhibitors; 4) amplification of small stimuli to promote the speedy formation of fibrin; 5) assembly of enzyme-substrate-cofactor complexes that profoundly accelerate the enzymatic reactions of the coagulation cascade; 6) provision of coagulant and inhibitory proteins (also present in plasma) from platelet granules; and 7) regulation of coagulation reactions to prevent generalized intravascular thrombosis.

Coagulation Proteins In Platelets

Fibrinogen

Fibrinogen comprises 3% to 10% of total platelet protein.[297] It is secreted from platelets by an energy-dependent process after activation by a variety of agonists, including ADP, thrombin, and collagen.[298,299] Controversy exists regarding the biochemical nature of platelet fibrinogen; some investigators have suggested

that it is qualitatively similar to plasma fibrinogen (immunologically, electrophoretically, physiochemically, and structurally), whereas others have found dissimilarities with respect to these parameters.[297,300,301] Platelet fibrinogen is processed intracellularly by a calcium-dependent mechanism, secreted from α granules, and expressed on the surface membranes of activated platelets.[302] However, the exact function of platelet fibrinogen is unclear, because afibrinogenemic platelets aggregate normally when exogenous fibrinogen is available.[303]

Factor V

Although it was originally thought that factor V was bound to the platelet surface, recent studies have shown that it is present within platelets rather than surface-associated.[304] Human platelets contain 18% to 25% of the factor V present in whole blood, and 80% of this is located in platelet α granules.[305,306] Platelet factor V is secreted in response to ADP, epinephrine, and collagen; secretion is thromboxane dependent, because aspirin is inhibitory.[306,307] Platelet factor V is a platelet receptor site for factor X_a binding to platelets, and the binding of factor X_a to factor V on the platelet surface is important in the activation of prothrombin.[308] Platelet factor V is more important than circulating levels of factor V. Patients with <1% *plasma* factor V activity, but *normal platelet* factor V do not have bleeding complications, whereas patients with *normal plasma* factor V activity, but markedly decreased platelet factor V have a severe bleeding diathesis (called Factor V Quebec).[309]

von Willebrand Factor

Platelet α-granules contain vWF in amounts equivalent to 10% to 25% of that present in plasma.[310] Platelet vWF is secreted in response to ADP, collagen, and thrombin, and it is immunochemically identical to plasma vWF.[311] Although the physiological function of platelet vWF is still undetermined, it may assist in platelet adherence to subendothelium; platelet vWF binds more tightly than exogenous vWF to thrombin-stimulated platelets.[312] In addition, platelet vWF along with plasma vWF mediates platelet-collagen interaction at high shear rates, and bleeding time and platelet vWF activity correlate closely, suggesting that platelet vWF plays an important role in hemostasis.[313]

High-Molecular-Weight Kininogen (HMWK)

When platelets are stimulated, HMWK contained in α granules is secreted and expressed on the activated platelet surface.[314] HMWK is important in contact activation. The activated form of Factor XII (XII$_a$) [Hageman Factor] is the first coagulant protein-factor in the intrinsic pathway (see Chapter 20). It is generated through proteolytic cleavage by kallikrein, and the active component is released into the fluid phase.[315] Factor XII$_a$ is an active enzyme capable of cleaving and activating prekallikrein and factor XI. Prekallikrein is associated with HMWK in plasma, and this complex binds to the platelet surface.[316] Moreover, HMWK binds factor XI. Thus, the necessary elements for contact activation are concentrated on the platelet surface or subendothelial structures bound to HMWK.[317] Platelet HMWK is thought to act in concert with plasma HMWK in this process.

Factor XI

Numerous immunologic studies have demonstrated that factor XI is present (albeit in relatively small amounts) within platelets.[318] The physiologic significance of factor XI in platelets is unknown. It may substitute for plasma factor XI in certain settings.[319] Of importance, patients with no detectable plasma factor XI, but with normal amounts of platelet factor XI (platelets contain only 0.4% of factor XI in normal plasma), have no history of abnormal bleeding.[318,319] In contrast, patients with the hereditary giant platelet syndrome who have normal *plasma* factor XI, but no detectable platelet factor XI have serious hemorrhagic complications, suggesting an important role in hemostasis for platelet factor XI.[320]

Factor XIII

Platelets contain factor XIII in a form that is enzymatically similar to plasma factor XIII, but consist only of dimerized a-subunits (in contrast to active a-chains linked to inactive b-subunits, as in plasma).[321] The a-subunits of factor XIII in platelets constitute 50% of the total factor XIII in the blood.[322] Platelet factor XIII is present within the cytoplasm rather than within granules. Thus, platelets do not secrete factor XIII and its functional significance is unclear. It has been postulated that the a-subunit of platelet factor XIII may be a source of the a-subunit for plasma factor XIII.[321]

Plasma Protease Inhibitors

In addition to delivering procoagulant proteins in high localized concentrations, platelets play a role in regulating plasma proteolysis. Numerous plasma protease inhibitors have been identified in human platelets. A complete discourse on each of these substances is beyond the scope of this chapter, but Walsh[323] has thoroughly discussed them. Platelet plasma protease inhibitors are listed in Table 9.

Platelet Contribution to the Coagulation Mechanism

Contact Activation

As previously noted, platelets serve to localize the coagulation cascade because they contain specific re-

Table 9
Plasma Protease Inhibitors in Platelets

Protein	Molecular Weight	Enzymes Inhibited
α_1-Protease Inhibitor	53,000	Thrombin, Kallikrein, Factor XI$_a$ Plasmin, urokinase, activated protein C
α_2-Macroglobulin	725,000	Thrombin, kallikrein, Factor XII$_a$ plasmin
C1 inhibitor	105,000	Kallekrein, Factor XII$_a$, Factor XI$_a$ plasmin
α_2-Antiplasmin	67,000	Thrombin, kallikrein, Factor XII$_a$ Factor XI$_a$, Factor X$_a$, plasmin, urokinase tissue plasminogen activator
Plasminogen activator Inhibitor-1 (PAI-1)	47,000	Kallikrein, Factor XII$_a$, Factor XI$_a$ tissue plasminogen activator, urokinase activated protein C
Extrinsic pathway inhibitor	46,000	Factor X$_a$/Factor VII$_a$/tissue factor complex
Protease nexin I	50,000	Thrombin, urokinase
Protease nexin II	120,000	Factor XI$_a$, plasmin
Platelet inhibitor of factor XI$_a$	8,500	Factor XI$_a$

(Adapted with permission from Reference 323.)

ceptors on their surfaces for procoagulant proteins. As discussed, contact activation (the intrinsic pathway) requires platelet participation owing to the platelet HMWK receptor. Factor XII, once activated to factor XII$_a$, cleaves prekallikrein to kallikrein. Active kallikrein can remain bound to the platelet surface or be released into plasma. Both bound and free kallikrein then convert additional factor XII to factor XII$_a$; this reaction takes place on the platelet surface.[324] Kallikrein not only activates factor XII, it also cleaves free and surface-bound HMWK, releasing bradykinin. Bradykinin is a potent vasoconstrictor that promotes hemostasis.

Fragments of factor XII are capable of activating plasminogen proactivator to plasminogen activator; plasminogen activator then converts plasminogen to plasmin. Whereas plasmin is usually thought of as beginning the process of clot lysis, in fact, it can also *promote* thrombosis by activating factor XII in the same manner as kallikrein.[325] This entire process is enhanced when platelets are activated.[326]

Factor XII$_a$ in turn activates factor XI bound to HMWK on the platelet surface to form Factor XI$_a$ and cleavage products. Factor XI$_a$ is bound to specific receptors on the platelet surface where it is protected from inactivation by plasma protease inhibitors (see Table 9).[323,326] Factor XII$_a$ and its fragments also activate factor VII in the extrinsic pathway of coagulation, thereby connecting the two pathways.[326] Factor XI$_a$ bound to the platelet surface converts Factor IX to IX$_a$, a process that requires Ca^{++}.

Activated platelets can activate factor XI independent of factor XII$_a$. The mechanism of this activation is unknown. Interestingly, because of this factor XII$_a$-independent pathway, the coagulation cascade can proceed even in the absence of Factor XII (Hageman Factor). Thus, patients with a deficiency of Hageman factor do not have a bleeding disorder. In fact, instead of bleeding they suffer thromboembolic complications, and Mr. Hageman in whom factor XII deficiency was originally described, died of complications from thromboembolism.[173] Thromboembolic complications are thought to arise from ineffective clot lysis because factor XII fragments are required to activate plasminogen proactivator.

Factor X

Factor X is the substrate for Factor IX$_a$. Activation of factor X begins the so-called *common pathway* of the coagulation cascade. Again, this process occurs at a specific receptor site for factor X on the platelet surface. Factor VIII, which is modified by thrombin, serves as a cofactor for the activation of factor X, and it too has a specific receptor on the platelet surface

adjacent to the factor X binding site. Although factor IX$_a$ can activate factor X independent of factor VIII, the reaction proceeds 300000 times faster when thrombin-modified factor VIII is present (designated VIII$_m$ or VIII$_a$).[327] Like factor XI$_a$, factor X$_a$ is protected from plasma protease inhibitors by its position on the platelet membrane.

Once activated, in the presence of calcium factor X$_a$ binds to a high affinity site on the platelet that is actually activated factor V.[328] Like factor VIII, factor V is modified by thrombin to V$_a$ (also designated V$_m$); also like factor VIII$_a$, factor V$_a$ functions as a cofactor for factor X$_a$.

Once factor X$_a$ binds to V$_a$, in the presence of calcium prothrombin (bound to the platelet surface) it is rapidly converted to thrombin. Phospholipid is required for this reaction. Prothrombin is converted to thrombin 300000 times faster when factor X$_a$ is bound to V$_a$-phospholipid, than when factor X$_a$ is unbound.[173] The thrombin formed in this process is released to plasma where it converts fibrinogen to fibrin.

Activated protein C serves to modulate activation of prothrombin in two ways: it is capable of degrading factor V (after it is bound to platelets) and factor VIII$_a$.[329] However, it cannot inactivate unbound factor V or V$_a$. Patients with protein C deficiency suffer thromboembolic complications.[330]

Summary

Platelets have specific receptors for: 1) the prekallikrein-HMWK complex; 2) the factor XI$_a$-HMWK complex; 3) factor XI$_a$; 4) the factor X$_a$-V$_a$ complex; and 5) prothrombin. Thus, platelets participate in activation of prekallikrein, and factors XII, XI, IX, X, and II. The adherence of platelets to sites of vascular injury focuses and localizes the coagulation mechanism to where it is needed.[173]

Platelet Inhibitors

Repair of vascular injury by platelets may also play a role in untoward events. For example, platelet-related thromboemboli contribute to transient ischemic attacks, strokes, angina pectoris, cardiac arrhythmias, myocardial infarctions, sudden death due to cardiac disease, failure of interventional procedures (vascular grafts, percutaneous transluminal angioplasty, etc.), and other intravascular adverse outcomes,[119,137,140,173,248] Antiplatelet agents, therefore, are important for preventing unwanted consequences of platelet activation.

Inhibition of Thromboxane

Because thromboxane plays a central role in platelet activation and aggregation, inhibition of its production is a principal strategy for interruption of unwanted thrombosis. Platelets rendered unresponsive by thromboxane-antagonists theoretically maintain ability to adhere to endothelium and respond normally to other agonists for aggregation, but no longer contribute to unfavorable intravascular occurrences.

Cyclooxygenase Inhibitors

Aspirin

In 1899, the Bayer Company introduced aspirin, a salicylate that rapidly became the most widely used drug ever developed.[331] Aspirin has been shown to reduce morbidity and mortality in patients with unstable angina[332,333] and myocardial infarction[334,335] and to be useful in secondary prevention of myocardial infarction,[336,337] presumably because of its effects on platelet function. A recent meta-analysis involving over 29000 patients with vascular disease from 31 trials of prophylactic antiplatelet therapy indicated a 15% (p < 0.0003) reduction in cardiovascular mortality with treatment.[338] Aspirin has also been shown to be of some benefit in maintaining patency of small vessel bypasses, particularly aortocoronary bypasses[339–341] and lower extremity prosthetic bypasses.[342] Likewise, antiplatelet therapy may improve the results of percutaneous transluminal angioplasty.[343,344]

Aspirin irreversibly inhibits platelet cyclooxygenase (CO) and, thereby, prevents conversion of arachidonate to thromboxane.[345] Importantly, aspirin also inhibits production of prostacyclin by CO in endothelial cells. Acetylsalicylic acid provides the acetyl group to CO, forming salicylic acid and irreversibly acetylated CO. After it is acetylated, CO cannot convert arachidonate to PGG_2, a thromboxane precursor. Because platelets cannot synthesize CO, the TXA_2 pathway is inhibited for the life of the platelet. New platelets will contain thromboxane because megakaryocytes do synthesize CO. Thus, about 7 to 10 days (the life span of the platelet) are required for normal reactivity to arachidonic acid. It is well to remember that more than 200 nonprescription preparations contain aspirin.[173]

The optimal antithrombotic dose of aspirin remains controversial. Theoretically, the lowest effective dose should be chosen because gastric side effects of aspirin are dose dependent, and lower doses are thought to block thromboxane A_2 production without permanently inhibiting prostacyclin synthesis.[346] Recent studies of low-dose aspirin have yielded conflicting data with respect to this hypothesis. Kyrle and coworkers[347] studied the effects of low-dose aspirin on the formation of thromboxane A_2 and prostacyclin in blood from a standardized skin incision and found greater than 80% inhibition of both prostaglandins. Aspirin may exert effects by mechanisms not limited to the inhibition of platelet function and thromboxane biosynthesis. For example, aspirin reduces catecholamine-induced vasoconstriction and lipolysis.[348] Aspirin also reduces arrhythmias in platelet-depleted animals.[349] Larger doses of aspirin may produce greater anti-inflammatory effects, and it has long been known that aspirin nonspecifically acetylates other plasma proteins such as albumin and hemoglobin in a dose-dependent fashion.[350] Conflicting data exist regarding dose-dependent antithrombotic effects of aspirin in animals,[351,352] and in humans given aspirin once daily; 10% of platelets remain normal, thus partially normalizing platelet function.[353]

Several trials have compared the effect of different doses of aspirin on thrombotic events with mixed results. In patients undergoing knee replacement operations, McKenna et al[354] found significant protection against deep venous thrombosis by a dose of aspirin of 3900 mg daily, but none from a dose of 975 mg daily. The design of the UK-TIA study[355] also allows separate comparisons of different aspirin doses. The risk of vascular events (nonfatal stroke, nonfatal myocardial infarction, vascular death) was reduced more by aspirin administered at a dose of 1200 mg per day than 300 mg per day, although the difference was not statistically significant. The Subcommittee on Cerebrovascular Disease of the 2nd ACCP Conference on Antithrombotic Therapy recently considered it premature to recommend a lower dose (325 mg) of aspirin in patients with transient cerebral ischemia, and instead suggested 1000 mg per day.[356] In contrast, in the ISIS-2 study of 17,187 patients with suspected acute myocardial infarction, low-dose aspirin (160 mg daily) reduced nonfatal reinfarction by 51% and nonfatal stroke by 47%.[357] Likewise, Lorenz and colleagues[358] showed improved patency of aortocoronary bypass grafts in patients taking 100 mg of aspirin daily. Finally, the Dutch TIA Trial Study Group recently reported that low-dose aspirin was equally effective as higher-dose aspirin for prevention of vascular events.[359]

Indomethecin and Sulindac

These agents, also anti-inflammatory and anti-pyretic, are similar in effect to aspirin. However, they are competitive inhibitors of CO, and they do not permanently inhibit the enzyme. Platelets recover ability to metabolize arachidonate within 1 to 2 days after discontinuation of drug intake.

Phenylbutazone and Sulfinpyrazone

Although both of these drugs have toxic side effects, both have uricosuric effects, making them useful in the treatment of gout. Of interest, sulfinpyrazone *(Anturane)* prolongs the survival of platelets in patients with various thromboembolic disorders. However, it is probably no more effective than aspirin alone in preventing platelet-related thrombosis.[360]

Nonsteroidal Antiinflammatory Drugs (NSAIDS)

Many of these agents have recently been approved the United States. NSAIDS are derivatives of propionic acid. They are aspirin-like drugs with similar antipyretic and anti-inflammatory effects, but with improved analgesia and generally fewer gastrointestinal side effects. All drugs in this class inhibit cyclooxygenase. Ibuprofen *(Motrin, Advil)* is the most widely prescribed of the many NSAIDS, and its use as a non-prescription medication has recently been approved. Other commonly used NSAIDS are naproxen and fenoprofen.

Dipyridamole

Dipyridamole *(Persantine)* alone or in conjunction with aspirin has been used to prevent arterial thromboembolic complications in several clinical settings, including treatment[343] of patients with cerebral transient ischemic attacks, coronary artery disease, and myocardial infarctions.[361,362] Dipyridamole has two important actions. It inhibits myocardial cellular reuptake and transport of endogenously produced adenosine, a potent coronary dilator. As adenosine accumulates in the interstitium, coronary vasodilation ensues. The administration of dipyridamole, through its adenosine effect, results in an increase in coronary flow by two- to threefold.[363] In addition, dipyridamole inhibits the enzyme responsible for cAMP metabolism, cAMP phosphodiesterase. The drug by itself produces little, if any, effect on platelets. Dipyridamole-treated platelets aggregate normally in response to standard agonists. However, the drug potentiates effects of other platelet inhibitors, with which it is usually combined.[361–362] When cAMP is stimulated and phosphodiesterase is inhibited, cytosolic cAMP levels remain high and platelet aggregation is inhibited.

Prostacyclin

PGI_2 is the most potent known inhibitor of platelet activation. It is also a powerful vasodilator. As noted previously, endothelial cells synthesize PGI_2 from ara-chidonic acid using cyclooxygenase. The half-life of PGI_2 is only 1 minute; thus, its effect on platelets is transient. PGI_2 reacts with a specific receptor on platelet membranes coupled to adenylate cyclase. Adenylate cyclase converts intracellular ATP to cAMP, which in turn results in a shift of cytosolic Ca^{++} to the DTS, thereby decreasing cytosolic free Ca^{++}. Aspirin blocks cyclooxygenase both in platelets and endothelial cells. However, vascular endothelium can regenerate PGI_2 within a few hours of a small dose of aspirin, whereas thromboxane production by platelets is permanently inhibited leading to interest in low-dose aspirin therapy (see above).

The clinical use of PGI_2 has been limited by its short half-life, expense, and profound vasodilating effects causing hypotension. These limitations have led to development of several prostacyclin analogues (e.g., iloprost) that are currently under investigation.

Thromboxane Synthetase Inhibitors

Selective inhibition of thromboxane formation can be achieved with specific inhibitors of thromboxane synthetase.[364] Theoretically, these are attractive agents because they might increase prostacyclin synthesis by donating accumulated PGH_2 to endothelial cells for conversion to PGI_2. Dazoxiben is the prototype drug in this class.[365] Unfortunately, for several reasons, most importantly the short half life of the drug, clinical studies of efficacy were largely negative. A theoretical limitation of thromboxane synthetase inhibition is that accumulated PGH_2 might substitute for TXA_2 and serve as a platelet agonist. A new drug with antagonism to both TXA_2 and PGH_2 ridogel has been developed and is currently being evaluated in large-scale clinical trials.

Thromboxane Receptor Antagonists

Thromboxane receptor antagonists are the newest agents for antiplatelet therapy. Most of these agents are analogues of prostaglandins or prostaglandin precursors, such as 13-APA (13-azaprotanoic acid). The drugs hold theoretical promise because they would not effect prostaglandins as does aspirin. A number of pilot studies have shown that TXA_2-receptor antagonists are well tolerated in doses that block platelet responses to agonists ex vivo, but the efficacy and safety of these compounds in clinical medicine remains to be defined.[366,367] Like thromboxane synthetase inhibitors, thromboxane receptor antagonists have not yet been approved for clinical use.

Ticlopidine

Ticlopidine, a thienopyridine derivative, recently received FDA approval for use in the prevention of strokes in patients with aspirin-intolerance. Its mode of action is obscure, but it has been postulated to selectively suppress expression of GP IIb-IIIa by ADP.[368] However, ADP is not the only agonist blocked by ticlopidine; it also inhibits platelet activation by thrombin, collagen, and PAF.[369] It does not affect cyclooxygenase, phosphodiesterase, adenylate cyclase, thromboxane synthetase, or platelet-dependent thrombin generation. Interestingly, it does not affect platelet function when tested in vitro. The onset of action of ticlopidine is delayed, requiring several days of oral administration to achieve maximum effect.[370]

Three large clinical studies of ticlopidine have recently been published. The first two established efficacy for prevention of stroke. The Canadian American Ticlopidine Study (CATS) randomized 1072 patients to ticlopidine (250 mg twice daily) or placebo within 1 week to 4 months of a completed stroke.[371] The incidence of combined end point (stroke, myocardial infarction, or vascular death) was reduced by about 30%. In the Ticlopidine Aspirin Stroke Study (TASS) 3069 patients with transient ischemic attacks, a reversible neurologic deficit, or minor stroke within the previous 3 months were randomized to ticlopidine (250 mg twice daily) or aspirin (650 mg daily).[372] Fatal and nonfatal stroke decreased by 21% at 3 years in the ticlopidine group, but the 3-year cumulative event rates for fatal and nonfatal myocardial infarction rates were similar between groups.

The third major study consisted of comparison of ticlopidine with placebo in 687 patients with intermittent claudication the Swedish Ticlopidine Multicenter Study (STIMS).[373] Although the study end points, myocardial infarction, stroke, and transient ischemic attack occurred with equal frequency between groups, the overall mortality was 30% lower in the ticlopidine group. Other studies of ticlopidine for diabetic retinopathy, unstable angina, and during cardiopulmonary bypass produced positive but less impressive results.[374-376]

Ticlopidine is the most widely prescribed antiplatelet drug in Japan, but it is unlikely to replace aspirin in the United States for several reasons. First, it is far more expensive than aspirin. Second, it causes more gastrointestinal side effects than low-dose aspirin. Third, it is associated with neutropenia in about 1% of patients, which is usually reversible, but occasionally profound. Fourth, in TASS, a significant (9%) increase in serum cholesterol was noted.

Glycoprotein IIb-IIIa Inhibitors

The importance of GP IIb-IIIa in platelet aggregation has been extensively discussed. The recently published large multicenter trial of monoclonal antibodies directed against this receptor in 2099 patients undergoing high-risk coronary artery angioplasty showed impressive results, but bleeding complications were substantial.[141] In addition, the expense, antigenicity, and irreversibility of monoclonal antibodies are problematic. To address these issues, pharmaceutical companies have developed several synthetic RGD peptides that may have clinical utility. For example, Rubin and coworkers have recently described efficacy of an RGD analogue (SC-49992) that effectively inhibited platelet adhesion and aggregation and eliminated platelet deposition on canine vascular grafts.[377] Human studies of these agents are currently underway.

References

1. Donné AD: L'origine des globules der san, de leur mode de formation et de leur fin. *CK Acad Sci* 14:366, 1842.
2. Addison W: On the colorless corpuscles and on the molecules and cytoblasts in the blood. *London Med Gaz (NS):* 30:144, 1842.
3. Gerber F: *Elements of General and Minute Anatomy of Man and Mammals.* London: G. Gulliver Co; 1842.
4. Simon JF: *Physiologische und pathologische antropochemie mit Berucksichtigung der eigentlichen Zoochemie. Handbuch der angewandten medizinischen chemie nach dem neuesten Standpunkte der wissenschaft und nach zahlreichen eigenen untersuchungen. Theil II.* Berlin: A Forstner; 1842.
5. Zimmerman G: Ueber die Formegebilde des menschlichen Blutes in ihrem nähern Verhältniss Zum Process der Entzundung und Eiterung. *Rust's Magazin f d Gesammte Heilk* unde 65:410, 1846.
6. Virchow R: *Die cellularpathologie.* In: *Begründung auf Physiologische und Pathologische. Gewebelehre.* Berlin A: Hirschwald; 1858.
7. Schultze M: Ein Heizbarer Objekttisch und seine Verwendung bei Untersuchungen des Blutes. *Arch f Mikr Anat* 1:36, 1865.
8. Osler W, Schaefer EA: Ueber einige im Blute vorhandene bakterienbildende Massen. *Centralb f ur Med Wissenschaft* 2:577, 1873.
9. Osler W: An account of certain organisms occurring in liquor sanguinis. *Proc Roy Soc* 22:391, 1874.
10. Hayem G: Recherches sur l'evolution des hematies dans le sang de l'homme et des vertebres. *Arch Physiol Norm Pathol* 5:692, 1878.
11. Bizzozero G: Uber eine neuen Formbestand there des blutes und desen Rolle bei der Thrrombose und der Blutgerinnung. *Virchows Arch Pathol Anat* 90:261, 1882.
12. Robb-Smith AHT: Why the platelets were discovered. *Brit J Haemat* 13:618, 1967.
13. Wooldridge LC: Note on a new constituent of blood serum. *Proc Roy Soc Lond* 42:230, 1887.
14. Lowit M: Die Blutplättchen und die Blutgerinnung. *Fortschr d Med, Berl* 3:173, 1885.
15. Howell WH: The new morphological element of the blood. *Science* 3:46, 1884.
16. Howell WH, Donahue DD: Production of blood platelets in lungs. *J Exp Med* 65:177, 1937.
17. Harvey AM: Fountainhead of American physiology: H.

Newell Martin and his pupil, William Henry Howell. *Bull Johns Hopkins Hosp* 136:38, 1975.

18. Eberth JC, Schimmelbusch C: Experimentalle untersuchungen uber thrombose. *Arch Path Anat u Physiol* 103:39, 1886.

19. Laker C: Die Blutscheibchen sind constante Formelemente des normal circuliren den Säugethierblutes. *Arch f Path Anat, Berl* 116:28, 1889.

20. Hayem G: Sur un cas de diathèse hémorrhagique. *Bull et Mem Soc Med Hop, Paris.* 8:389, 1891.

21. Dominici H: Le processus hisologique de la leucémie myélogène. *Presse Med Paris* 2:35, 1900.

22. Wright JH: The origin and nature of the blood platelet. *Boston Med Surg J* 154:643, 1906.

23. Tocantins LM: Historical notes on blood platelets. *Blood* 3:1073, 1948.

24. Howell WH: Observations upon the occurrence, structure, and function of the giant cells of the marrow. *J Morphol* 4:117, 1890.

25. Glanzmann E: Hereditare hamorrhagische thrombasthenie: ein beitrag zur pathologie der blutpattchen. *Jahrb Kinderheilkd* 88:113, 1918.

26. Brinkhous KM: Clotting defect in hemophilia: deficiency in a plasma factor required for platelet utilization. *Proc Soc Exp Biol Med* 66:117, 1947.

27. Harrington WJ, Minnick V, Hollingswirth JW, et al: Demonstration of a thrombocytopenic factor in the blood of patients with thrombocytopenic purpura. *J Lab Clin Med* 38:1, 1951.

28. Braunsteiner H, Pakesch F: Thrombocytasthenia and thrombocytopathia—old names and new diseases. *Blood* 11:965, 1956.

29. Born GR: The breakdown of adenosine triphosphate in platelets during clotting. *J Physiol* 133:61, 1956.

30. Harker LA, Finch CA: Thrombokinetics in man. *J Clin Invest* 47:452, 1968.

31. Stenberg PE, Levin J: Mechanisms of platelet production. *Blood Cells* 15:23, 1989.

32. Nakeff A, Maat B: Separation of megakaryoctes from mouse bone marrow by velocity sedimentation. *Blood* 43:591, 1974.

33. Shoff PK, Levine RF: Elutriation for isolation of megakaryocytes. *Blood Cells* 15:285, 1989.

34. Leven R: Elutriation for isolation of megakaryocytes. *Blood Cells* 15:306, 1989.

35. Tomer A, Harker LA, Burstein SA: Purification of human megakaryocytes by fluorescence-activated cell sorting. *Blood* 70:1735, 1987.

36. Van Pampus EC, Van Geel BJ, Huijgens PC, et al: Combining counter-flow centrifugal elutriation and glycoprotein Ib-dependent purification of human megakaryocytes: efficacy and selectivity. *Eur J Haematol* 47:299, 1991.

37. Miura M, Jackson CW, Steward SA: Increase in circulating megakaryocyte growth-promoting activity (Meg-GPA) following sublethal irradiation is not related to decreased platelets. *Exp Hematol* 16:139, 1988.

38. Hoffman R, Mazur E, Bruno E, Floyd V: Assay of an activity in the serum of patients with disorders of thrombogenesis that stimulates formation of megakaryocytic colonies. *N Engl J Med* 305:533, 1975.

39. Hoffman JR, Yang HH, Bruno E, Straneva JE: Purification and partial characterization of a megakaryocyte colony-stimulating factor from human plasma. *J Clin Invest* 75:1174, 1985.

40. Naki S, Aihara K, Hirai Y: Interleukin-1 potentiates granulopoiesis and thrombopoiesis by producing hematopoietic growth factors in vivo. *Life Sciences* 45:585, 1989.

41. Frenkel EP: The clinical spectrum of thrombocytosis and thrombocythemia. *Am J Med Sci* 301:69, 1991.

42. Jenkins RB, Tefferi A, Solberg LA Jr, Dewald GW: Acute leukemia with abnormal thrombopoiesis and inversions of chromosome 3. *Cancer Genet Cytogenet* 39:167, 1989.

43. McDonald TP: Thrombopoietin: its biology, clinical aspects, and possibilities. *Am J Pediatr Hematol Oncol* 14:8, 1992.

44. Geissler D, Konwalinka G, Peschel C, Braunsteiner H: The role of erythropoietin, megakaryocyte colony-stimulating factor, and T-cell-derived factors on human megakaryocyte colony formation: evidence for T-cell mediated and T-cell independent stem cell proliferation. *Exp Hematol* 15:485, 1987.

45. Gewirtz AM, Xu WY, Mangan KF: Role of natural killer cells in comparison with T lymphoscytes and monocytes, in the regulation of normal human megakaryocytopoiesis in vitro. *J Immunol* 139:2915, 1987.

46. Kelso A, Owens T: Production of two hemopoietic growth factors is differentially regulated in single T Lymphocytes activated with and anti T cell receptor antibody. *J Immunol* 140:1159, 1988.

47. Bruno E, Cooper RJ, Briddell RA, Hoffman R: Further examination of the effects of recombinant cytokines on the proliferation of human megakaryocyte progenitor cells. *Blood* 77:2339, 1991.

48. Mazur EM, Cohen JL, Newton J, et al: Human serum megakaryocyte colony-stimulating activity appears to be distinct from interleukin-3, granulocyte-macrophage conony-stimulating factor, and lymphocyte-conditioned medium. *Blood* 76:290, 1990.

49. Geissler K, Valent P, Bettelheim P, et al: In vivo synergism of recombinant human interleukin-3 and recombinant human interleukin-6 on thrombopoiesis in primates. *Blood* 79:1155, 1992.

50. Quesenberry PJ, Ihle JN, McGrath E: The effect of interleukin-3 and GM-CSA-2 on megakaryocyte and meyloid clonal colony formation. *Blood* 65:214, 1985.

51. Donahue RE, Seehra J, Metzger M, et al: Human IL-3 and GM-CSF act synergistically on stimulating hematopoiesis in primates. *Science* 241:1820, 1988.

52. Gewirtz AM, Schick B: Megakaryocytopoiesis. In: Colman RW, Hirsh J, Marder VJ, Salzman EW (eds). *Hemostasis and Thrombosis: Basic Principles and Clinical Practice*. 3rd Ed. Philadelphia: JB Lippincott Co; 1994.

53. Mei RL, Burstein SA: Megakaryocytic maturation in murine long-term bone marrow culture: role of interleukin-6. *Blood* 78:1438, 1991.

54. Ishida Y, Yano S, Yoshida T, et al: Biological effects of recombinant erythropoietin, granulocyte-macrophage colony-stimulating factor, interleukin-3, and interleukin-6 on purified ratmegakaryocytes. *Exp Hematol* 19:608, 1991.

55. Solbert LA Jr: Stimulators and inhibitors of megakaryocytopoiesis in human plasma. *Blood Cells* 15:186, 1989.

56. Ishibashi T, Miller SL, Burstein SA: Type β transforming growth factor is a potent inhibitor of murine megakaryocytopoiesis in vitro. *Blood* 69:1737, 1987.

57. Han ZC, Sensebe L, Abgrall JF, Briere J: Platelet factor 4 inhibitis human megakaryocytopoiesis in vitro. *Blood* 75:1234, 1990.

58. Han ZC, Bellucci S, Tenza D, Caen JP: Negative regulation of human megakaryocytopoiesis by human platelet factor 4 and beta thromboglobulin: comparative

analysis in bone marrow cultures from normal individuals and patients with essential thrombocythaemia and immune thrombocytopenic purpura. *Br J Haematol* 74: 395, 1990.

59. Evans DI: Immune amegakaryocytic thrombocytopenia of the newborn: association with anti-HLA-A2. *J Clin Pathol* 40:258, 1987.

60. Hoffman R, Briddel RA, van Besien K, et al: Acquired cyclic amegakaryocytic thrombocytopenia associated with an immunoglobulin blocking the action of granulocyte-macrophage colony-stimulating factor. *N Engl J Med* 321:97, 1989.

61. Ganser A, Carlo-Sella C, Greher J, Volkers B, Hoelzer D: Effect of recombinant interferons alpha and gamma on human bone marrow-derived megakaryocyte progenitor cells. *Blood* 70:1173, 1987.

62. Nakeff A, Bryan JE: Megakaryocyte proliferation and its regulation as revealed by CFU-M analysis. In: Golde DW, Cline MJ, Metcalf DJ (eds). *Hematopoietic Cell Differentiation.* Orlando: Academic Press Inc.; 1978.

63. Levin MJ, Levin FC, Penington DG, et al: Measurement of ploidy distribution in megakaryocyte colonies obtained from culture: with studies of the effects of thrombocytopenia. *Blood* 57:287, 1981.

64. Jackson CW: Cholinesterase as a possible marker for early cells in the megakaryocytic series. *Blood* 42:413, 1973.

65. Penington DG, Olsen TE: Megakaryocytes in states of altered platelet production: cell numbers, size, and DNA content. *Br J Haematol* 18:447, 1970.

66. Gewirtz AM: Human megakaryocytopoiesis. *Semin Hematol* 23:27, 1986.

67. Briddell RA, Brandt JE, Staneva JE, Srour EF, Hoffman R: Characterization of the human burst-forming unit megakaryocyte. *Blood* 74:145, 1989.

68. Long MW: Current concepts in the development and regulation of the bone marrow megakaryocyte. *J Med Technol* 1:681, 1984.

69. Williams N, Levine RF: The origin, development, and regulation of megakaryocytes. *Br J Haematol* 52:173, 1982.

70. Long MW, Williams N: Immature megakaryocytes in mouse: morphology and quantitation by acetylcholinesterase staining. *Blood* 58:1032, 1981.

71. Rabellino EM, Levene RB, Leung LLK, Nachman RL: Human megakaryocytes: II. Expression of platelet proteins in early marrow megakaryocytes. *J Exp Med* 154: 88, 1981.

72. Breton-Gorius J, Reyes R: Ultrastructure of human bone marrow cell maturation. *Int Rev Cytol* 46:251, 1976.

73. Ebbe S: Experimental and clinical megakaryocytopoiesis. *Clin Hematol* 8:371, 1979.

74. Levine RF: Isolation and characterization of normal human megakaryocytes. *Br J Haematol* 45:487, 1980.

75. McLauren ML, Pepper DS: Immunological localization of beta-thromboglobulin and platelet factor 4 in human megakaryocytes and platelets. *J Clin Pathol* 35:1227, 1982.

76. Sporn LA, Chavin SI, Marker VJ, et al: Biosynthesis of von Willebrand factor by human megakaryocytes. *J Clin Invest* 76:1102, 1985.

77. Handagama PJ, Shuman MA, Bainton DF: Incorporation of intravenously injected albumin, immunoglobulin G, and fibrinogen in guinea pig megakaryocyte granules. *J Clin Invest* 84:73, 1989.

78. Shakli M, Tavassoli: Demarcatio membrane system in rat megakaryocyte and the mechansim of platelet formation: a membrane reorganization process. *J Ultrastruct Res* 62:270, 1978.

79. White JG: Mechanisms of platelet production. *Blood Cells* 15:48, 1989.

80. Radley JM, Haller CJ: Fate of senescent megakaryocytes in the bone marrow. *Br J Haematol* 53:277, 1983.

81. Tong M, Seth P, Penington DG: Proplatelets and stress platelets. *Blood* 69:522, 1987.

82. Martin JF, Slater DN, Trowbridge EA: Platelet production in the lungs. *Agents Actions* (suppl) 21:37, 1987.

83. White JG: Ultrastructural studies of the gray platelet syndrome. *Am J Pathol* 95:445, 1979.

84. McGill M, Jamieson GA, Drouin J, Cho MS, Rock GA: Morphometric analysis of platelets in Bernard-Soulier syndrome: size and configurations in patients and carriers. *Thromb Haemost* 52:37, 1984.

85. Alagille D, Josso F, Binet JL, Blin ML: La dystrophie thrombocytaire hemorragipare: discussion nosologique. *Nouv Rev Fr Hematol* 4:755, 1964.

86. Behnke O: Electron microscopic observations on the membrane systems of the rat blood platelet. *Anat Rec* 158:121, 1967.

87. Adelson E, Rheingold JJ, Crosby WH: The platelet as a sponge: A review. *Blood* 17:767, 1961.

88. Phillips DR, Poh Agin P: Platelet plasma membrane glycoproteins. *J Biol Chem* 252:2121, 1977.

89. Coller BS: Platelets and thrombolytic therapy. *N Engl J Med* 322:33, 1990.

90. White JG: Anatomy and structural organization of the platelet. In: Colman RW, Hirsh J, Marder VJ, Salzman EW (eds). *Hemostasis and Thrombosis: Basic Principles and Clinical Practice.* 3rd Ed. Philadelphia: JB Lippincott, 1994.

91. Fantl P, Ward HA: The thromboplastic component of intact blood platelets is present in masked form. *Aust J Exp Biol* 36:499, 1955.

92. Marcus AJ, Zucker-Franklin D: Studies on subcellular platelet particles. *Blood* 23:389, 1964.

93. White JG: The submembrane filaments of blood platelets. *Am J Pathol* 56:267, 1969.

94. Gerrard JM, White JG: The structure and function of platelets with emphasis on their contractile nature. *Pathobiol Annu* 6:31, 1979.

95. White JG, Leistikow EL, Escolar G: Platelet membrane responses to surface and suspension activation. *Blood Cells* 16:43, 1990.

96. Pipeleers DG, Pipeleers-Marichal MH, Kipnis KM: Physiological regulation of total tubulin and polymerized tubulin in tissues. *J Cell Biol* 74:351, 1977.

97. White JG, Krivit W: An ultrastructural basis for the shape changes induced in platelets by chilling. *Blood* 30:638, 1968.

98. White JG: Effects of colchicine and vinca alkaloids on human platelets. I. Influence on platelet microtubules and contractile function. *Am J Pathol* 53:281, 1968.

99. White JG: Fine structural alterations induced in platelets by adenosine diphosphate. *Blood* 31:604, 1968.

100. Adelstein RS, Pollard TD: Platelet contractile proteins. *Prog Hemost Thromb* 4:37, 1978.

101. Holmsen H: Platelet metabolism and activation. *Semin Hematol* 22:219, 1985.

102. Raccuglia G: Gray platelet syndrome: a variety of qualitative platelet disorders. *Am J Med* 51:818, 1971.

103. Gerrard JM, Phillips DR, White JG: Severe deficiency of thrombin-sensitive protein (TSP) in the gray platelet syndrome. *Clin Res* 26:503A, 1978.

104. Martin JH, Carson FL, Race GH: Calcium containing platelet granules. *J Cell Biol* 60:775, 1974.

105. White JG, Gerrard JM: Ultrastructural features of abnormal blood platelets. *Am J Pathol* 83:590, 1976.

106. White JG: Identification of platelet secretion in the electron microscope. *Sem Hematol* 6:429, 1973.

107. Behnke O: The morphology of blood platelet membrane systems. *Sem Hematol* 3:3, 1970.

108. White JG: Is the canalicular system the equivalent of the muscle sarcoplasmic reticulum? *Hemostasis* 4:185, 1975.

109. Gerrard JM, Townsend D, Stoddard S, Witkop CJ Jr, White JG: The influence of prostaglandin G2 on the platelet ultrastructure and platelet secretion. *Am J Pathol* 86:99, 1977.

110. Gerrard JM, White JG, Rao GHJR, Townsend D: Localization of platelet prostaglandin production in the platelet dense tubular system. *Am J Pathol* 83:283, 1976.

111. Aster RH: Pooling of platelets in the spleen: role in the pathogenesis of "hypersplenic" syndrome. *J Clin Invest* 45:645, 1966.

112. Fritsma GA: Platelet production and structure. In: Corriveau DM, Fritsma GA (eds). *Hemostasis and Thrombosis in the Clinical Laboratory*. New York: JB Lippincott; 1988.

113. Charo IF, Kieffer N, Phillips DR: Platelet membrane glycoproteins. In: Colman RW, Hirsh J, Marder VJ, Salzman EW (eds). *Hemostasis and Thrombosis: Basic Principles and Clinical Practice*. 3rd ed. Philadelphia: JB Lippincott; 1994.

114. Clemetson KJ, McGregor JL, McEver RP, et al: Absence of platelet membrane glycoproteins IIb/IIIa from monocytes. *J Exp Med* 161:972, 1985.

115. Fox EB, Aggerbeck LA, Berndt MC: Structure of the glycoprotein Ib-IX complex from platelet membranes. *J Biol Chem* 263:4882, 1988.

116. Lopez JA, Chung DW, Fujikawa K, et al: The α and β chains of human platelet glycoprotein Ib are both transmembrane proteins containing a leucine-rich amino acid sequence. *Proc Natl Acad Sci USA* 85:2135, 1988.

117. Hickey MJ, Williams SA, Roth GJ: Human platelet glycoprotein IX: an adhesive prototype of leucine-rich glycoproteins with flank-center-flank structures. *Proc Natl Acad Sci USA* 86:6773, 1989.

118. Olson JD, Moake JL, Collins MF, et al: Adhesion of human platelets to purified solid-phase von Willebrand factor: studies of normal and Bernard-Soulier platelets. *Thromb Res* 32:115, 1983.

119. Krupski WC, Bass A, Cadroy Y, Kelly AB, Harker LA, Hanson SR: Antihemostatic and anti-thrombotic effects of monoclonal antibodies against von Willebrand factor (vWF) in the nonhuman primate. *Surgery* 112:433, 1992.

120. Weiss HJ, Turitto VJ, Baumgartner HR: Platelet adhesion and thrombus formation on subendothelium in platelets deficient in glycoproteins IIb-IIIa, Ib, and storage granules. *Blood* 67:322, 1986.

121. MacFarlane DE, Stibbe J, Kirby EP, et al: A method for assaying von Willebrand Factor (ristocetin cofactor). *Thromb Diath Haemorrh* 4:306, 1975.

122. Weiss HJ, Hawiger J, Ruggeri ZM, Turitto VT: Fibrinogen-independent platelet adhesion and thrombus formation on subendothelium mediated by glycoprotein IIb-IIIa complex at high shear rate. *J Clin Invest* 83:288, 1989.

123. Phillips MD, Moake JL, Nalasco L, Tuner N: Aurin

124. Phillips DR, Charo IF, Parise LV, Fitzgerald LA: The platelet membrane glycoprotein IIb-IIIa complex. *Blood* 71:831, 1988.

125. Hynes RO; Integrins: a family of cell surface receptors. *Cell* 48:549, 1987.

126. Fitzgerald LA, Leung B, Phillips DR: A method for purifying the platelet membrane glycoprotein IIb-IIIa complex. *Anal Biochem* 151:169, 1985.

127. Nachman RL, Ferris B: Studies on the proteins of human platelet membranes. *J Biol Chem* 247:4468, 1972.

128. Shattil SJ, Brass LF: Induction of the fibrinogen receptor on human platelets by intracellular mediators. *J Biol Chem* 262:992, 1987.

129. Fitzgerald LA, Phillips DR: Calcium regulation of the platelet membrane glycoprotein IIb-IIIa complex. *J Biol Chem* 260:11366, 1985.

130. George JN, Caen JP, Nurden AT: Glanzmann's thrombasthenia: the spectrum of clinical disease. *Blood* 75:1383, 1990.

131. Bray PF, Barsh G, Rosa JP, et al: Physical linkage of the genes for platelet membrane glycoproteins IIb and IIIa. *Proc Natl Acad Sci USA* 85:8683, 1988.

132. Niewiarowski S, Kornecki E, Budzynski AZ, Morinelli TA, Tuszynski G: Fibrinogen interaction with platelet receptors. *Ann NY Acad Sci* 408:536, 1983.

133. Pytela R, Pierschbacher MD, Ginsberg EF, Plow EF, Ruoslahti E: Platelet membrane glycoprotein IIb/IIIa: member of a family of arg-gly-asp-specific adhesion receptors. *Science* 231:1559, 1986.

134. Savage B, Marzec UM, Chao BH, Harker LA, Maraganore JM, Ruggeri ZM: Binding of the snake venom derived proteins applagin and echistatin to the arginine-glycine-aspartic acid recognition site(s) on platelet glycoprotein IIb/IIIa complex inhibits platelet function. *J Biol Chem* 265:211766, 1990.

135. Gachet C, Cazenave JP: ADP-induced blood platelet aggregation: a review. *Nouv Rev Fr Hematol* 33:347, 1991.

136. Handagama P, Bainton DF, Jacques Y, Conn MT, Lazarus RA, Shuman MA: Kistrin, an integrin antagonist, blocks endocytosis of fibrinogen into guinea pig megakaryocyte and platelet alpha-granules. *J Clin Invest* 91:193, 1993.

137. Krupski WC, Bass A, Kelly AB, Ruggeri ZM, Hanson SR, Harker LA: Interruption of vascular thrombosis by bolus anti-platelet glycoprotein IIb/IIIa monoclonal antibodies in baboons. *J Vasc Surg* 17:294, 1993.

138. Coller Bs, Folts JD, Scudder LE, Smith SR: Antithrombotic effect of a monoclonal antibody to the platelet glycoprotein IIb/IIIa receptor in an experimental animal model. *Blood* 68:783, 1986.

139. Yasuda T, Gold HK, Fallon JT, et al: Monoclonal antibody against the platelet glycoprotein (GP) IIb/IIIa receptor prevents coronary artery reocclusion following reperfusion with recombinant tissue-type plasminogen activator in dogs. *J Clin Invest* 81:1284, 1988.

140. Krupski WC, Bass A, Cadroy Y, Kelly AB, Harker LA, Hanson SR: Antihemostatic and anti-thrombotic effects of monoclonal antibodies against von Willebrand factor (vWF) in the non-human primate. *Surgery* 112:433, 1992.

141. EPIC Investigators: Use of a monoclonal antibody directed against the platelet glycoprotein IIb/IIIa receptor

in high-risk coronary angioplasty. *N Engl J Med* 330: 956, 1994.

142. Huang TF, Holt JC, Lukasiewicz H, Niewiarowski S: Tigramin. *J Biol Chem* 262:16157, 1987.

143. Shebuski RJ, Ramjit DR, Bencen GH, Polokoff MA: Characterization and platelet inhibitory activity of bitistatin, a potent arginine-glycine-aspartic acid-containing peptide from the venom of the viper *Bitis arietans*. *J Biol Chem* 264:21550, 1989.

144. Hawiger J: Adhesive interactions of blood cells and the vascular wall. In: Colman RW, Hirsh J, Marder VJ, Salzman EW (eds). *Hemostasis and Thrombosis: Basic Principles and Clinical Practice*. Philadelphia: JB Lippincott; 1994.

145. Hoyer LW, de los Santos RP, Hoyer JR: Antihemophilic factor antigen: localization in endothelial cells by immunofluorescent microscopy. *J Clin Invest* 52:2737, 1973.

146. Ruggeri ZM, Zimmerman TS: Platelets and von Willebrand disease. *Semin Hematol* 22:203, 1985.

147. Wagner DD, Olmstead JB, Marder VJ: Immunolocalization of von Willebrand protein in Weibel-Palade bodies of human endothelial cells. *J Cell Biol* 95:355, 1982.

148. Menon C, Berry EW, Ockelford P: Beneficial effect of DDAVP on bleeding time in vWD. *Lancet*: 743, 1978.

149. Moffat EH, Giddings JC, Bloom AL: The effect of desamino-D-arginine vasopressin (DDAVP) and naloxone infusions on factor VIII and possible endothelial cell related activities. *Br J Haematol* 57:651, 1984.

150. Takeuchi M, Nagura H, Kaneda T: DDAVP and epinephrine-induced changes in the localization of vWF antigen in endothelial cells of human oral mucosa. *Blood* 72:850, 1988.

151. Zimmerman TS, Ruggeri ZM: Von Willebrand's Disease. *Prog Hemost Thromb* VI:203, 1982.

152. Zimmerman TS, Ratnoff OD, Powell AE: Immunologic differentiation of classic hemophilia (factor VIII deficiency) and von Willebrand's disease. *J Clin Invest* 50: 244, 1971.

153. Weiss AE: The hemophilias. In: Corriveau DM, Fritsma GA (eds). *Hemostasis and Thrombosis in the Clinical Laboratory*. Philadelphia: JB Lippincott; 1988.

154. Zucker MB, Mosesson MW, Broekman MJ, et al: Release of fibronectin (cold-insoluble globulin) from alpha granules induced by thrombin and collagen: lack of requirement for plasma fibronectin in ADP-induced platelet aggregation. *Blood* 54:8, 1979.

155. Sussman II, Rand JH: Subendothelial deposition of von Willebrand's factor requires the presence of endothelial cells. *J Lab Clin Med* 100:526, 1982.

156. Fulcher CA, Zimmerman TS: Characterization of the human Factor VIII procoagulant protein with a heterologous precipitation antibody. *Proc Natl Acad Sci* 79: 1648, 1982.

157. Brinkhous KM, Read MS: Fixation of platelets and platelet agglutination/aggregation tests. *Methods Enzymol* 169:149, 1989.

158. Coller BS, Gralnick HR: Studies on the mechanism of ristocetin-induced platelet agglutination: Effects of structural modification of ristocetin and vancomycin. *J Clin Invest* 60:302, 1977.

159. Lopez-Fernandez MF, Ginsberg MH, Ruggeri ZM, et al: Multimeric structure of platelet Factor VII/von Willebrand factor: the presence of larger multimers and their reassociation with thrombin stimulated platelets. *Blood* 60:1132, 1982.

160. Ruggeri ZM, Mannucci PM, Federici AB, et al: Mul-

timeric composition of factor VII/von Willebrand factor following administration of DDAVP: implications for pathophysiology and therapy of von Willebrand's disease subtypes. *Blood* 59:1272, 1982.

161. Fujimoto T, Ohara S, Hawiger J: Thrombin-induced exposure and prostacyclin inhibition of the receptor for Factor VIII/von Willebrand factor on human platelets. *J Clin Invest* 69:1212, 1982.

162. Ruggeri ZM, DeMarco L, Gatti L, et al: Platelets have more than one binding site for von Willebrand factor. *J Clin Invest* 72:1, 1983.

163. Pietu G, Cherel G, Marguerie G, et al: Inhibition of von Willebrand factor-platelet interaction by fibrinogen. *Nature* 308:648–649.

164. Plow EF, Srouji AH, Meyer D, et al: Evidence that three adhesive proteins interact with a common recognition site on activated platelets. *J Biol Chem* 259:5388, 1984.

165. Ruggeri ZM, Bader R, DeMarco L: Glanzmann thrombasthenia: deficient binding of von Willebrand factor to thrombin-stimulated platelets. *Proc Natl Acad Sci USA* 79:6083, 1982.

166. DeMarco L, Girolami A, Zimmerman TS, Ruggeri ZM: von Willebrand factor interaction with the glycoprotein IIb-IIIa complex: its role in platelet function as demonstrated in patients with congenital afibrinogenemia. *J Clin Invest* 77:1272, 1986.

167. Moake JL, Turner NA, Stathopoulos NA, et al: Involvement of large plasma von Willebrand factor multimers and unusually large vWF forms derived from endothelial cells in shear stress-induced platelet aggregation. *J Clin Invest* 78:1456, 1986.

168. Peterson DM, Stathopouls NA, Giorgio TD, et al: Shear-induced platelet aggregation requires von Willebrand factor and platelet membrane glycoprotein Ib and IIb-IIIa. *Blood* 69:625, 1987.

169. Stel HV, Sakariassen KS, de Groot PG, et al: von Willebrand factor in the vessel wall mediates platelet adherence. *Blood* 65:85, 1985.

170. Brace LD, Venton DL, LeBreton GC: Thromboxane A_2/prostaglandin H_2 mobilizes calcium in human blood platelets. *Am J Physiol* 249:H1, 1985.

171. Brace LD, Venton DL, Le Breton GC: Reversal of thromboxane A_2/ prostaglandin H_2 and ADP-induced calcium release in intact platelets. *Am J Physiol* 249: H8, 1985.

172. Owen NE, Feinberg H, Le Breton GC: Epinephrine induces calcium uptake in human blood platelets. *Am J Physiol* 249:H483, 1980.

173. Brace LD: Platelet Physiology. In: Corriveau DM, Fritsma GA (eds). *Hemostasis and Thrombosis in the Clinical Laboratory*. Philadelphia: JB Lippincott; 1988.

174. Ware JA, Smith M, Salzman EW: Synergism of platelet-aggregating agents: role of elevation of cytoplasmic calcium. *J Clin Invest* 80:267, 1987.

175. Baumgartner HR: The role of blood flow in platelet adhesion, fibrin deposition, and formation of mural thrombi. *Microvasc Res* 5:167, 1973.

176. Born GV: Aggregation of blood platelets by adenosine diphosphate and its reversal. *Nature* 194:927, 1962.

177. Born GVR, Cross M: The aggregation of blood platelets. *J Physiol (Lond)* 168:178, 1963.

178. Holmsen H: Platelet metabolism and activation. *Semin Hematol* 22:219, 1985.

179. Marguerie GA, Plow EF: Interaction of fibrinogen with its platelet receptor: kinetics and effect of pH and temperature. *Biochemistry* 20:1074, 1981.

180. Keenan JP, Solum NO: Quantitative studies on the release of platelet fibrinogen by thrombin. *Br J Haematol* 23:461, 1972.

181. Bennett JS, Vilaire G, Cines DB: Identification of the fibrinogen receptor on human platelets by photoaffinity labelling. *J Biol Chem* 257:8048, 1982.

182. Fujimura K, Phillips DR: Calcium cation regulation of GPIIb-IIIa complex formation in platelet cell membranes. *J Biol Chem* 258:10247, 1983.

183. Phillips DR, Baughan AK: Fibrinogen binding to human platelet plasma membranes: clarification of two steps requiring divalent cations. *J Biol Chem* 258:10240, 1983.

184. Doolittle RF, Watt KWK, Cottrell BA, et al: The amino acid sequence of the alpha chain of human fibrinogen. *Nature* 280:464, 1979.

185. Cheresh DA, Berliner SA, J Vincente V, Ruggeri ZM: Recognition of distinct adhesive sites on fibrinogen by related integrins on platelets and endothelial cells. *Cell* 58:945, 1989.

186. Plow EF, Srouji AH, Meyer D, et al: Evidence that three adhesive proteins interact with a common recognition site on activated platelets. *J Biol Chem* 259:5388, 1984.

187. Weiss HJ, Hawiger J, Ruggeri ZM, et al: Fibrinogen-independent platelet adhesion and thrombus formation mediated by glycoprotein IIb-IIIa at high shear rate. *J Clin Invest* 83:288, 1989.

188. Coller BS, Peerscchke EI, Scudder LE, et al. A murine monoclonal antibody that completely blocks the binding of fibrinogen to platelets produces a thrombasthenic like state in normal platelets and binds GPIIb and/or IIIa. *J Clin Invest* 72:325, 1983.

189. Parise LV, Venton DL, LeBreton GC: Prostacyclin potentiates 13-azaprostanoic acid-induced platelet deaggregation. *Throm Res* 28:721, 1982.

190. Saussy DL Jr, Mais DE, Burch RM, Halushka PV: Identification of a putative thromboxane A2: prostaglandin H2 receptor antagonist binding site in human platelet membranes. *J Biol Chem* 261:3025, 1986.

191. Holmsen H: Platelet secretion and energy metabolism. In: Colman RW, Hirsh J, Marder VJ, Salzman EW (eds). *Hemostasis and Thrombosis: Basic Principles and Clinical Practice*. 3rd Ed. Philadelphia: JB Lippincott; 1994.

192. DeClerk F, Van Gorp L: Induction of circulating platelet aggregates by release of endogenous 5-hydroxytryptamine in the rat (abst). *Throm Haemost* 46:29, 1981.

193. Palade G: Intracellular aspects of the process of protein synthesis. *Science* 189:347, 1975.

194. Wencel-Drake JD, Plow EF, Kunicki TJ, et al: Localization of internal pools of membrane glycoproteins involved in platelet adhesive responses. 124:324, 1986.

195. Painter RG, Ginsberg MH: Centripetal myosin redistribution in thrombin-stimulated platelets. Relationship to platelet factor 4 secretion. *Exp Cell Res* 155:198, 1984.

196. Stenberg PE, Shuman MA, Levine SP, Bainton DF: Redistribution of alpha granules and their contents in thrombin-stimulated platelets. *J Cell Biol* 98:741, 1984.

197. Stenberg RE, Shuman MA, Levine SP, et al: Optimal techniques for the immunocytochemical demonstration of β-thromboglobulin, platelet factor 4, and fibrinogen in the qlpha granules of unstimulated platelets. *Histochem J* 16:983, 1984.

198. White JG, Krumwiede M: Further studies of the secretory pathway in thrombin-stimulated platelets. *Blood* 69:1196, 1987.

199. Gogstad GO, Brosstak F, Krutnes MB, et al: Fibrino-gen-binding properties of the human platelet glycoprotein IIb-IIIa complex: a study using crossed-radioimmunoelectrophoresis. *Blood* 60:663, 1982.

200. Holt JC, Niewiarowski S: Biochemistry of alpha granule proteins. *Semin Hematol* 22:151, 1985.

201. Deuel TF, Senior RM, Chang D, et al: Platelet factor 4: complete amino acid sequence. *Proc Natl Acad Sci USA* 74:2256, 1977.

202. Deuel TF, Senior RM, Chang D, et al: Platelet factor 4 is chemotactic for neutrophils and monocytes. *Proc Natl Acad Sci USA* 78:4584, 1981.

203. Senior RM, Criffin GL, Huang JS, et al: Chemotactic activity of platelet alpha granule proteins for fibroblasts. *J Cell Biol* 96:382, 1983.

204. Brindley LL, Sweet JM, Goetzl EJ: Stimulation of histamine release from human basophils by human platelet factor 4. *J Clin Invest* 72:1218, 1983.

205. Weerasinghe KM, Scully MF, Kakkar VV: Inhibition of the cerebroside sulphate (sulfatide)-induced contact activation reactions by platelet factor four. *Throm Res* 33:625, 1984.

206. Bock PE, Luscombe M, Marshall SE, Pepper DS, Holbrook JJ: The multiple complexes formed by the interaction of platelet factor 4 with heparin. *Biochem J* 191: 769, 1980.

207. Cook JJ, Niewiarowski S, Yan Z, et al: Platelet factor 4 efficiently reverses heparin anticoagulation in the rat without adverse effects of heparin-protamine complexes. *Circulation* 85:1102, 1992.

208. Zucker MB, Katz IR: Platelet factor 4: production, structure and physiologic and immunological action. *Proc Soc Exp Biol Med* 197:693, 1991.

209. Holt JC, Harris ME, Holt AM, et al: Characterization of human platelet basic protein, a precursor form of low-affinity platelet factor 4 and β-thromboglobulin. *Biochemistry* 25:1988, 1986.

210. Holt JC, Niewiarowski S: Platelet basic protein, low-affinity platelet factor 4, and beta-thromboglobulin: purification and identification. *Methods Enzymol* 169:224, 1989.

211. Moore S, Pepper DS, Cash JD: The isolation and characterization of a platelet-specific beta-globulin and the detection of anti-urokinase and anti-plasmin released from thrombin-aggregated washed human platelets. *Biochim Biophys Acta* 379:360, 1975.

212. Walz A, Baggiolini M: A novel cleavage product of beta-thromboglobulin formed in cultures of stimulated mononuclear cells activates human neutrophils. *Biochem Biophys Res Commun* 159:969, 1989.

213. McGrath MH: Peptide growth factors and wound healing. *Clin Plastic Surg* 17:421, 1990.

214. Antoniades HN, Scher CD, Stiles CD: Purification of the human platelet-derived growth factor. *Proc Natl Acad Sci USA* 76:1809, 1979.

215. Assoian RK, Komoriya AK, Meyers CA, et al: Transforming growth factor-β in human platelets: identification of a major storage site, purification, and characterization. *J Biol Chem* 258:7155, 1983.

216. Oka Y, Orth DN: Human plasma epidermal growth factor β urogastrone is associated with blood platelets. *J Clin Invest* 72:249, 1983.

217. Krupski WC. Growth factors and wound healing. *Semin Vasc Surg* 5:249, 1992.

218. Ishikawa F, Miyazono K, Hellman U, et al: Identification of angiogenic activity and the cloning and expression of platelet-derived endothelial cell growth factor. *Nature* 338:557, 1989.

219. Ross R: Platelet-derived growth factor. *Ann Rev Med* 38:71, 1987.
220. Bowen-Pope DF, Seifert RA, Ross R: The platelet-derived growth factor receptor. In: *Control of Animal Cell Proliferation*. Boynton AL, Leffert HL (eds). New York: Academic Press Inc.; 1985.
221. Ross R, Raines EW, Bowen-Pope DF: The biology of platelet-derived growth factor. *Cell* 37:9, 1986.
222. Grotendorst GR, Chang T, Seppa HE, et al: Platelet-derived growth factor is a chemoattractant for vascular smooth muscle cells. *J Cell Physiol* 113:261, 1982.
223. Zullo JN, Cochran BH, Huang A, Stiles CD: Platelet-derived growth factor and double-stranded ribonucleic acids stimulate expression of the same genes in 3T3 cells. *Cell* 43:793, 1985.
224. Habenicht AJR, Dresel HA, Goerig M, et al: Low-density lipoprotein receptor-dependent prostaglandin synthesis in Swiss 3T3 cells stimulated by platelet-derived growth factor. *Proc Natl Acad Sci USA* 83:1344, 1986.
225. Berk BC, Alexander RW, Brock TA, et al: Vasoconstriction: A new activity for platelet-derived growth factor. *Science* 232:87, 1986.
226. Deuel TF: Polypeptide growth factors: roles in normal and abnormal cell growth. *Ann Rev Cell Biol* 3:443–492, 1987.
227. Deuel TF, Huang JS: Platelet-derived growth factor: structure, function, and roles in normal and transformed cells. *J Clin Invest* 74:669–676, 1984.
228. Baenziger NL, Brodie GN, Majerus PW: A thrombin-sensitive protein of human platelet membranes. *Proc Natl Acad Sci USA* 68:240, 1971.
229. Mosher DF, Doyle MJ, Jaffe EA: Synthesis and secretion of thrombospondin by cultured human endothelial cells. *J Cell Biol* 93:343, 1982.
230. Schwatz BS: Monocyte synthesis of thrombospondin. *J Biol Chem* 264:7512, 1989.
231. Mosher DF: Physiology of thrombospondin. *Ann Rev Med* 41:85, 1990.
232. Lyons-Giordano B, Conaway H, Kefalides NA: The effect of heparin on fibronectin and thrombospondin synthesis by human smooth muscle cells. *Biochem Biophys Res Commun* 148:1264, 1987.
233. Lawler W, Simmons ER: Cooperative binding of calcium to thrombospondin. *J Biol Chem* 258:12098, 1983.
234. Leung LL: The role of thrombospondin in platelet aggregation. *J Clin Invest* 74:1764, 1984.
235. Majerus PW, Connolly TM, Bansal VS, et al: Inositol phosphates: synthesis and degradation. *J Biol Chem* 263:3051, 1988.
236. Bills TK, Smith JB, Silver MJ: Selective release of arachidonic acid from the phospholipids of human platelets in response to thrombin. *J Clin Invest* 60:1, 1977.
237. Silk ST, Clejan S, Witkom K: Evidence of GTP-binding protein regulation of phospholipase A_2 in isolated human platelet membranes. *J Biol Chem* 264:21466, 1989.
238. Hamberg M, Svensson J, Wakabayashi T, Samuelsson B: Isolation and structure of two prostaglandin endoperoxides that cause platelet aggregation. *Proc Natl Acad Sci USA* 71:435, 1974.
239. Rao AK, Willis J, Holmsen H: A major role of ADP in thromboxane transfer experiments: studies in patients with platelet secretion defects. *J Lab Clin Med* 104:116, 1984.
240. Brass LF, Shaller CC, Belmonte EJ: Inositol 1,4,5-triphosphate-induced granule secretion in platelets. Evidence that the activation of phospholipase C mediated

by platelet thromboxane receptors involves a guanine nucleotide binding protein-dependent mechanism distinct from that of thrombin. *J Clin Invest* 79:1269, 1987.
241. Carey F, Menashi S, Crawford N: Localization of cyclo-oxygenase and thromboxane synthetase in human platelet intracellular membranes. *Biochem J* 204:847, 1982.
242. Majerus PW, Miletich JP: Relationships between platelets and coagulation factors. *Ann Rev Med* 29:41, 1978.
243. Figures WR, Colman RF, Niewiarowski S, Colman RW: New evidence for an ADP-independent mechanism of thrombin-induced platelet activation. *Thromb Haemost* 46:94a, 1981.
244. Bell RL, Majerus PW: Thrombin-induced hydrolysis of phosphatidylinositol in human platelets. *J Biol Chem* 255:1790, 1980.
245. Broekman MJ, Ward JW, Marcus AJ: Phospholipid metabolism in stimulated human platelets. *J Clin Invest* 66:275, 1980.
246. Aktories K, Jokobs KH: Ni-mediated inhibition of human platelet adenylate cyclase by thrombin. *Eur J Biochem* 145:333, 1984.
247. Vu T-K H, Hung DT, Wheaton VI, Cough SR: Molecular cloning of a functional thrombin receptor reveals a novel proteolytic mechanism of receptor activation. *Cell* 64:1057, 1991.
248. Harker LA: Clinical trials evaluating platelet-modifying drugs in patients with atherosclerotic cardiovascular disease and thrombosis. *Circulation* 73:206, 1986.
249. Bock Pe, Luscombe M, Marshall et al: The multiple complexes formed by the interaction of platelet factor 4 with heparin. *Biochem J* 191:769, 1980.
250. Krupski WC, Bass A, Kelly AB, Marzec UM, Hanson Sr, Harker LA: Heparin-resistant thrombus formation by endovascular stents in baboons: interruption by a synthetic antithrombin. *Circulation* 81:570, 1990.
251. Lumsden AB, Kelly AB, Schneider PA, Krupski WC, et al: Lasting safe interruption of endarterectomy thrombosis by transiently infused antithrombin peptide D-Phe-Pro-ArgCH₂Cl in Baboons. *Blood* 81:1762, 1993.
252. Kelly AB, Marzec UM, Krupski WC, et al: Hirudin interruption of heparin-resistant arterial thrombus formation in baboons. *Blood* 77:1006, 1991.
253. Packham MA, Guccione MA, Greenberg JP, et al: Release of ¹⁴C-serotonin during initial platelet changes induced by thrombin, collagen, or A23187. *Blood* 50:915, 1977.
254. Kinlough-Rathbone RL, Packham MA, Mustard JF: Synergism between platelet-aggregating agents: the role of the arachidonate pathway. *Thromb Res* 11:567, 1977.
255. Colman RW, Figures WR, Scearce LM, et al: Inhibition of collagen-induced platelet activation by 5'-p-fluorosulfonylbenzoyl adenosine: evidence for an ADP requirement and synergistic influence of prostaglandin endoperoxidases. *Blood* 68:563, 1986.
256. Barnes MJ, Gordon JL, MacIntyre DE: Platelet aggregating activity of type I and III collagens from human aorta and chicken skin. *Biochem J* 160:647, 1976.
257. Barnes MJ, Gordon JL, MacIntyre DE: Platelet aggregation by basement membrane-associated collagens. *Thromb Res* 18:375, 1980.
258. Wester J, Sixma JJ, Geuze JJ, Heijnes HFG: Morphology of the hemostatic plug in human skin wounds: transformation of the plug. *Lab Invest* 41:182, 1979.
259. Brass LF, Bensusan HB: The role of collagen quaternary structure in the platelet: collagen interaction. *J Clin Invest* 54:1480, 1974.

260. Santoro SA: Identification of a 160,000 dalton platelet membrane protein that mediates the initial divalent cation-dependent adhesion of platelets to collagen. *Cell* 46: 913, 1986.

261. Jamieson GA, Urban CL, Barber AJ: Enzymatic basis for platelet: collagen adhesion as the primary step in hemostasis. *Nature* 234:5, 1971.

262. Chiang TM, Kang AK: Isolation and purification of collagen alpha 1 receptor from human platelet membrane. *J Biol Chem* 257:7581, 1982.

263. Sarto Y, Imada T, Tagkagi J, et al: Platelet factor XIII: the collagen receptor? *J Biol Chem* 261:1355, 1986.

264. Tandon NN, Kralisz U, Jamieson GA: Identification of glycopotein IV (CD36) as a primary receptor for platelet-collagen adhesion. *J Biol Chem* 264:7576, 1989.

265. Hallam TJ, Snchez A, Rink TJ: ADP increases cytoplasmic free Ca^{2+} in quin-2-loaded human platelets mainly by influx across the plasma membrane. *Thromb Haemost* 50:76, 1983.

266. Coleman RW, Cook JJ, Niewiarowski S: Mechanisms of platelet aggregation. In: Colman RW, Hirsh J, Marder VJ, Salzman EW (eds). *Hemostasis and Thrombosis: Basic Principles and Clinical Practice*. 3rd Ed. Philadelphia: JB Lippincott; 1994.

267. Bennett JS, Vilaire G, Colman RF, Colman RW: Localization of the human platelet membrane associated actomyosin using the affinity label 5′-p-fluorosulfonylbenzoyl adenosine. *J Biol Chem* 256:1185, 1981.

268. Figures WR, Scearce LM, Defeo P, et al: Direct evidence for the interaction of the nucleotide affinity analog 5′-p-fluorosulfonylbenzoyl adenosine with a platelet ADP receptor. *Blood* 70:796, 1987.

269. Colman RW, Figures WR, Wu Q-X, et al: Distinction between glycoprotein IIIa and the 100-kDa membrane protein (aggregin) mediating ADP-induced platelet activation. *Arch Biochem Biophys* 262:298, 1988.

270. Owen NE, LeBreton GC: Ca^{2+} mobilization in blood platelets as visualized by chlortetracycline fluorescence. *Am J Physiol* 241:H613, 1981.

271. Lefkowitz RJ, Caron MC, Stiles GL: Mechanims of membrane-receptor regulation. Biochemical, physiological, and clinical insights derived from studies of the adrenergic receptors. *N Engl J Med* 310:1570, 1984.

272. Motulsky HJ, Insel PA: [^{3}H]Dihydroergocryptine binding to alpha-adrenergic receptors in human platelets: a reassessment using the selective radioligands [^{3}H]prazosin, [^{3}H]yohimbine, and [^{3}H]rauwolscine. *Biochem Pharmacol* 31:2591, 1982.

273. Siess W, Eber PC, Lapetina EG: Activation of phospholipase C is dissociated from arachidonate metabolism during platelet shape change induced by thrombin or platelet-activating factor: epinephrine does not induce phospholipase C activation or platelet shape change. *J Biol Chem* 259:8286, 1984.

274. Owen NE, Feinberg H, LeBreton GC: Epinephrine induces calcium uptake in human blood platelets. *Am J Physiol* 239:H483, 1980.

275. Brass LF: The biochemistry of platelet activation. In: Hoffman R, Benz EJ Jr, Shattil SJ, Furie B, Cohen HJ (eds). *Hematology: Basic Principles and Practice*. New York: Churchill-Livingston, Inc.; 1991.

276. Scrutton MC, Clare KC, Hutton RA, Bruckdorfer KR: Depressed responsiveness to adrenalin in platelets from apparently normal human donors: a familial trait. *Br J Haematol* 49:303, 1981.

277. Rao AK, Willis J, Kowalska MA, et al: Differential requirements for platelet aggregation and inhibition of adenylate cyclase by epinephrine: studies of a familial platelet alpha 2-adrenergic defect. *Blood* 71:494, 1988.

278. Tamponi G, Pannocchia A, Arduino C, et al: Congenital deficiency of α_2-adrenoreceptors on human platelets: description of two cases. *Thromb Haemost* 58:1012, 1987.

279. Siess W: Molecular mechanisms of platelet activation. *Physiol Rev* 69:58, 1989.

280. Steen VM, Holmsen H: The platelet-stimulating effect of adrenaline through alpha-2-adrenergic receptors requires simultaneous activation by a true stimulatory platelet agonist: evidence that adrenaline per se does not induce human platelet activation in vitro. *Thromb Haemost* 70:506, 1993.

281. Beneveniste J, Henson PM, Cochrane CG: Leukocyte-dependent histamine release from rabbitt platelets: the role of IgE, basophils, and a platelet-activating factor. *J Exp Med* 13:56, 1972.

282. Clark PO, Hanahan DJ, Pinckard RN: Physical and chemical properties of platelet-activating factor obtained from human neutrophils and monocytes and rabbit neutrophils and basophils. *Biochim Biophya Acta* 628:69, 1980.

283. Braquet P, Touqui L, Shen JTY, Vargaftig BB: Perspectives in platelet-activating factor research. *Pharmacol Rev* 39:97, 1987.

284. Alam I, Smith JB, Silver MJ: Human and rabbit platelets form platelet-activating factor in response to calcium ionophore. *Thromb Res* 30:71, 1983.

285. MacIntyre DE, Pollock WK: Platelet-activating factor stimulates phosphatidylinositol turnover in platelets. *Biochem J* 212:433, 1983.

286. Kloprogge E, Akkerman JWN: Binding kinetics of PAF-acether to intact human platelets. *Biochem J* 223: 901, 1984.

287. Vargaftig BB, Chignard M, LeCouedic JP, Beneveniste J: One, two, three, or more pathways for platelet aggregation. *Acta Med Scand* 642:23, 1980.

288. Rao AK, Willis J, Hassel B, et al: Platelet-activating factor is a weak platelet agonist: evidence from normal human platelets and platelets with congenital secretion defects. *Am J Hematol* 17:153, 1984.

289. Howard MA, Firkin BG: Ristocetin—a new tool in the investigation of platelets. *Thromb Diath Haemorrh* 26: 362, 1971.

290. Kawai Y, Montgomery RR: Endothelial cell processing of von Willebrand proteins. *Ann NY Acad Sci* 509:60, 1987.

291. Allain JP, Cooper HA, Wagner RH, Brinkhous: Platelets fixed with paraformaldehyde: a new reagent for assay of vWf and platelet aggregating factor. *J Lab Clin Med* 85:318, 1975.

292. Kelton JG, Sheridan D, Santos A, et al: Heparin-associated thrombocytopenia: laboratory studies. *Blood* 72: 925, 1988.

293. Makhoul RG, Greenberg CS, McCann RL: Heparin-associated thrombocytopenia and thrombosis: a serious clinical problem and potential solution. *J Vasc Surg* 4: 522, 1986.

294. Sobel M, Adelman B, Szentpetery S, et al: Surgical management of heparin-associated thrombocytopenia: strategies in the treatment of venous and arterial thromboembolism. *J Vasc Surg* 8:395, 1988.

295. Becker PS, Miller VT: Heparin-induced thrombocytopenia. *Stroke* 20:1449, 1989.

296. Walsh PN: Platelet coagulant activities and hemostatasis: an hypothesis. *Blood* 43:597, 1974.

297. Nachman RL, Marcus AJ, Sucker-Franklin D: Immunologic studies of proteins associated with subcellular fraction of normal human platelets. *J Lab Clin Med* 69: 651, 1967.

298. Kaplan KL, Broekman J, Chernoff A, et al: Platelet alpha granule proteins: studies on release and subcellular localization. *Blood* 53:604, 1979.

299. Keenan JP, Solum NO: Quantitative studies on the release of platelet fibrinogen by thrombin. *Br J Haematol* 23:461, 1972.

300. Kunicki TJ, Newman PJ, Amrani DL, Mosesson MW: Human platelet fibrinogen: purification and hemostatic properties. *Blood* 66:808, 1985.

301. James HL, Ganguly P, Jackson CW: Characterization and origin of fibrinogen in blood platelets: a review with recent data. *Thromb Haemost* 38:939, 1977.

302. Legrand C, Dubernard V, Nurden AT: Studies on the mechanism of expression of secreted fibrinogen on the surface of activated human platelets. *Blood* 73:1226, 1989.

303. Inceman S, Caen J, Bernard J: Aggregation, adhesion, and viscous metamorphosis of platelets in congenital fibrinogen deficiencies. *J Lab Clin Med* 68:21, 1966.

304. Giddings JC, Shearn SAM, Bloom AL: Platelet-associated coagulation factors: Immunological detection and the effects of calcium. *Br J Haematol* 39:569, 1978.

305. Chiu HC, Schick P, Colman RW: Biosynthesis of coagulation factor V by megakaryocytes. *J Clin Invest* 75: 339, 1985.

306. Chesney CM, Pifer D, Cjolman JRW: Subcellular localization and secretion of factor V from human platelets. *Proc Natl Acad J Sci UJSA* 78:5180, 1981.

307. Vivic WJ, Lages B, Weiss HJ: Release of human platelet factor V activity is induced by both collagen and ADP and is inhibited by aspirin. *Blood* 56:448, 1980.

308. Kane WH, Lindhout MJ, Jackson CW, Majerus PW: Factor V_a dependent binding of factor X_a to human platelets. *J Biol Chem* 255:11170, 1980.

309. Tracy PB, Giles AR, Mann KG, et al: Factor 5 (Quebec): a bleeding diathesis associated with a qualitative platelet factor 5, deficiency. *J Clin Invest* 74:1221, 1984.

310. Zucker MB, Broekman MJ, Kaplan KL: Factor 8-related antigen in human blood platelets: localization and release by thrombin and collagen. *J Lab Clin Med* 94: 675, 1979.

311. Koutts J, Walsh PN, Plow JEF, et al: Active release of human platelet factor 8-related antigen by adenosine diphosphate, collagen, and thrombin. *J Clin Invest* 62: 1255, 1978.

312. Ruggeri ZM, Bader R, Zimmerman TS: High affinity interaction of platelet von Willebrand factor with distinct platelet membrane sites. *Clin Res* 31:322A, 1983.

313. Gralnick HR, Rick ME, McKeown LP, et al: Platelet von Willebrand factor: an important determinant of the bleeding time in type I von Willebrand's disease. Blood 68:58, 1986.

314. Gustafson E, Schutsky D, Schmaier AH: High molecular weight kininogen binds to the unstimulated platelet. *J Clin Invest* 78:310, 1986.

315. Revak SD, Cochrane CG: The relationship of structure and function in human Hageman factor: the association of enzymatic and binding activities with separate regions of the molecule. *J Clin Invest* 57:852, 1976.

316. Mandle R, Colman RW, Kaplan AP: Identification of prekallekrein and high molecular weight kininogen as a complex in human plasma. *Proc Natl Acad Sci USA* 11:4179, 1976.

317. Wiggins RC, Bouma BN, Cochrane CG, Griffin JH: Role of high molecular weight kininogen in surface-binding and activation of coagulation factor XI and prekallilrein. (Hageman factor, contact activation, fibrinolysis). *Proc Natl Acad Sci UJSA* 74:4636, 1977.

318. Lipscomb MS, Walsh PN: Human platelets and factor XI: localization in platelet membranes of factor-XI-like activity and its functional distinction from plasma factor XI. *J Clin Invest* 63:1006, 1979.

319. Tuszynski GP, Bevaqua SJ, Schmaier AH, et al: Factor XI antigen in the coagulant activity in human platelets. *Blood* 59:1148, 1982.

320. Walsh PN, Mills DCB, Pareti FI, et al: Hereditary giant platelet syndrome: absence of collagen-induced coagulant activity and deficiency of factor XI binding to platelets. *Br J Haematol* 29:639, 1975.

321. Schwartz ML, Pizzo V, Hill RL, McKee PA: Human factor XIII from plasma and platelets: Molecular weights, subunit structures, proteolytic activation, and cross-linking of fibrinogen and fibrin. *J Biol Chem* 248: 1395, 1973.

322. McDonagh J, Kiesselbach TH, Wagner RH: Factor XIII and antiplamin activity in human platelets. *Am J Physiol* 216:508, 1969.

323. Walsh PN: Platelet-Coagulant Protein Interactions. In: *Hemostasis and Thrombosis: Basic Principles and Clinical Practice*. 3rd Ed. Colman RW, Hirsh J, Marder VJ, Salzman EW (eds). Philadelphia: JB Lippincott; 1994.

324. Cochrane CG, Griffin JH: Molecular assembly in the contact phase of the Hageman factor system. *Am J Med* 67:657, 1979.

325. Burrowes CE, Morat HZ, Soltay MJ: The kinin system of human plasma. VI. The action of plasmin. *Proc Soc Exp Biol* 138:959, 1971.

326. Walsh PN, Griffin JH: Contributions of human platelets to the proteolytic activation of blood coagulation factors XII and XI. *Blood* 57:106, 1981.

327. Hultin MB: Role of human Factor VIII in Factor X activation. *J Clin Invest* 69:950, 1982.

328. Tracy PB, Nesheim ME, Mann KG: Coordinate binding of Va and factor Xa to the unstimulated platelet. *J Biol Chem* 256:743, 1981.

329. Comp PC, Esmon CT: Activated protein C inhibits platelet prothrombin-converting activity. *Blood* 54: 1271, 1979.

330. Griffin JH, Evatt B, Zimmerman JS, et al: Deficiency of protein C in congenital thrombocytic disease. *J Clin Invest* 68:1370, 1981.

331. Graham DY, Smith JL: Aspirin and the stomach. *Ann Int Med* 104:39, 1986.

332. Lewis HD Jr, Davis JW, Archibald DG, et al: Protective effects of aspirin against acute myocardial infarction and death in men with unstable angina: results of a Veterans Administration cooperative study. *N Engl J Med* 309:396, 1983.

333. Carins JA, Gent M, Singer J, et al: Aspirin, sulfinpyrazone, or both in unstable angina: results of a Canadian multicenter trial. *N Engl J Med* 313:1369, 1985.

334. Elwood PC, Cochrane AL, Burr ML: A randomized controlled trial of acetylsalicylic acid in the secondary prevention of mortality from myocardial infarction: comparison of acetylsalicylic acid, phenprocoumon, and placebo. A multicenter two-year prospective study. *Thromb Haemost* 4:225, 1979.

335. Elwood PC, Sweethorn PM: Aspirin and secondary mortality after myocardial infarction. *Lancet* 2:1313, 1979.

336. The Persantine-Aspirin Reinfarction Research Group: Persantine and aspirin in coronary heart disease. *Circulation* 62:449, 1980.

337. Steering Committee of the Physician's Health Study Research Group: Preliminary report: findings from the aspirin component of the ongoing Physicians's Health Study. *N Engl J Med* 318:262, 1988.

338. Antiplatelet trialists collaboration: Secondary prevention of vascular disease by prolonged antiplatelet treatment. *Br J Med* 296:320, 1988.

339. Lorenz RL, Weber M, Kotzar J, et al: Improved aortocoronary bypass patency by low dose aspirin (100 mg daily): effects on platelet aggregation and thromboxane formation. *Lancet* 1:1261, 1984.

340. Chesebro JH, Fuster V, Elveback LR, et al: Effect of dipyridamole and aspirin on late vein-graft patency after coronary bypass operations. *N Engl J Med* 310:209, 1984.

341. Fuster V, Chesbro JH: Role of platelets and platelet inhibitors in aortocoronary vein-graft disease. *Circulation* 73:227, 1986.

342. Clyne CAC, Archer TJ, Atuhaire LK, Chant ADB, Webster JHH: Random control trial of a short course of aspirin and dipyridamole (Persantin) for femorodistal grafts. *Br J Surg* 74:246, 1987.

343. Barnathan ES, Schwartz JS, Taylor L, et al: Aspirin and dipyridamole in the prevention of acute coronary thrombosis, complicating coronary angioplasty. *Circulation* 76:125, 1987.

344. Schwartz L, Bourassa MG, Lesperance J, et al: Aspirin and dipyridamole in the prevention of restenosis after percutaneous transluminal angioplasty. *N Engl J Med* 318:1714, 1988.

345. Smith JB, Willis AL: Aspirin selectively inhibits prostaglandin production in human platelets. *Naturenew Biol* 231:235, 1971.

346. Jaffe EA, Weksler BB: Recovery of endothelial cell prostacyclin production after inhibition by low doses of aspirin. *J Clin Invest* 63:532, 1979.

347. Kyrle PA, Eichler HG, Jager U, Lechner K: Inhibition of prostaglandin and thromboxane A$_2$ generation by low-dose aspirin at the site of plug formation in man in vivo. *Circulation* 75:1025, 1987.

348. Strom EA, Coffman JD: Effect of aspirin on circulatory responses to catecholamines. *Arth Rheum* 6:689, 1963.

349. Moschos CB, Haier B, DeLaCrux C Jr, Lyons MM, Regan TJ: Antiarrhythmic effects of aspirin during nonthrombotic coronary occlusion. *Circulation* 57:681, 1978.

350. Roth GJ, Majerus PW: The mechanism of the effect of aspirin on human platelets. I. Acetylation of a particulate fraction protein. *J Clin Invest* 56:624, 1975.

351. Peterson J, Zucker MB: The effect of adenosine monophosphate, arcaine, and anti-inflammatory agents on thrombosis and platelet function in rabbits. *Thrombosis et Diathesis Haemorrhagica* 23:148, 1970.

352. Kelton JG, Hirsh J, Carter CJ, Buchanan MR: Thrombogenic effect of highdose aspirin in rabbits. Relationship to inhibition of vessel was synthesis of prostaglandin I$_2$-like activity. *J Clin Invest* 62:892, 1978.

353. Cerskus AL, Ali M, McDonald JWD: Possible significance of functional platelets circulating between doses of aspirin. *Blood* (suppl 1)52:160, 1978.

354. McKenna R, Galante J, Bachmann F, Wallace DL, Kaushal SP, Meredith P: Prevention of venous thromboembolism after total knee replacement by high-dose aspirin or intermittent calf and thigh compression. *BMJ* 280:514, 1980.

355. UK-TIA Study Group: The United Kingdom transient ischaemic attack (UK-TIA) aspirin trial: interim results. *BMJ* 296:316, 1988.

356. Hirsh J, Salzman EW, Harker LA, et al: Aspirin and other platelet active drugs: relationship among dose, effectiveness, and side effects. *Chest* (suppl)95:12S–18S, 1989.

357. ISIS-2 (Second International Study of Infarct Survival) Collaborative Group: Randomized trial of intravenous streptokinase, oral aspirin, both or neither among 17,189 cases of suspected acute myocardial infarction: ISIS-2. *Lancet* 2:34, 1988.

358. Lorenz RL, Weber M, Kotzar J, et al: Improved aortocoronary bypass patency by low dose aspirin (100 mg daily): effects on platelet aggregation and thromboxane formation. *Lancet* 1:1261, 1984.

359. The Dutch TIA Study Group: A comparison of two doses of aspirin (30 mg vs. 283 mg a day) in patients after a transient ischemic attack or minor ischemic stroke. *N Engl J Med* 325:1261, 1991.

360. The Anturane Reinfarction Trial Research Group: Sulfinpyrazone in the prevention of sudden death after myocardial infarction. *N Engl J Med* 302:250, 1980.

361. Bousser MG, Eschwege E, Haguenau M, et al: "AICLA" controlled trial of aspirin and dipyridamole in the secondary prevention of atheroemolic cerebral ischemia. *Stroke* 14:5, 1983.

362. American-Canadian Cooperative Study Group: Persantine aspirin trial in cerebral ischemia. Part II. End point results. *Stroke* 16:406, 1985.

363. Mays AE, Cobb FR: Relationship between regional myocardial blood flow and thallium 201 redistribution in the presence of coronary artery stenosis and dipyridamole-induced vasodilation. *J Clin Invest* 73:1359, 1984.

364. Fitzgerald GA, Brash AK, Oates JA, Pedersen AK: Endogenous prostacyclin biosynthesis and platelet function during selective inhibition of thromboxane synthesis in man. *J Clin Invest* 72:1336, 1983.

365. Vermylen J, Defreyn NG, Carreras AS, et al: Thromboxane synthetase inhibition as an antithrombotic strategy. *Lancet* 1:1073, 1981.

366. Darius H, Lefer AM: Antiaggregatory effects of thromboxanes receptor antagonists in vivo. *Thromb Res* 40:663, 1985.

367. Pierucci A, Simonetti BM, Pecci G, et al: Improvement in renal function with selective thromboxane antagonism in lupus nephritis. *N Engl J Med* 320:421, 1989.

368. Hardisty RM, Powling MJ, Nokes TC: The action of ticlopidine on human platelets: studies on aggregation, secretion, calcium mobilization, and membrane glycoproteins. *Thromb Haemost* 64:150, 1990.

369. Defreyn G, Bernat A, Delebassee D, Maffrand JP: Pharmacology of ticlopidine: A review. *Semin Thromb Hemost* 15:159, 1989.

370. DiMinno G, Cerbone AM, Mattioli PL, et al: Functionally thrombasthenic state in normal platelets following administration of ticlopidine. *J Clin Invest* 75:328, 1985.

371. Gent M, Easton JD, Hachinski VC, et al., and the CATS Group: The Canadian American Ticlopidine Study (CATS) in thromboembolic stroke. *Lancet* 1:1215, 1989.

372. Hass WK, Easton JD, Adams HP, et al. for the Ticlopidine Aspirin Stroke Study Group: A randomized trial

comparing ticlopidine hydrochloride with aspirin for the prevention of stroke in high-risk patients. *N Engl J Med* 321:501, 1989.

373. Janzon L, Bergquist D, Boberg J, et al: Prevention of myocardial infarction and stroke in patients with intermittent claudication: effects of ticlopidine. Results from STIMS, the Swedish Ticlopidine Multicenter Struy. *J Intern Med* 227:301, 1990.

374. The TIMAD Study Group: Ticlopidine treatment reduces the progression of nonproliferative diabetic retinopathy. *Arch Ophthalmol* 108:1577, 1990.

375. Balsano F, Rizzon R, Violai F, et al., and the STAI Group: Antiplatelet treatment with ticlopidine in unstable angina: a controlled multicenter clinical trial. *Circulation* 82:17, 1990.

376. Renner C, Guilmot D, Curtet JM: Ticlopidine in cardiac surgery with extracorporeal circulation. *Nouv Presse Med* 1487, 1991.

377. Rubin BG, McGraw DJ, Sicard GA, Santoro SA: New RGD analogue inhibits human platelet adhesion and aggregation and eliminates platelet deposition on canine vascular grafts. *J Vasc Surg* 15:683, 1992.

CHAPTER 10

Response of the Arterial Wall to Injury and Intimal Hyperplasia

Larry W. Kraiss, MD; Alexander W. Clowes, MD

Introduction

The management of the exuberant intimal hyperplastic response to injury in blood vessels is one of the most important and difficult therapeutic challenges facing cardiovascular specialists today. This process dooms a large proportion (10% to 50%) of all vascular interventions to clinical failure, whether they are in the coronary[1-4] or peripheral circulations.[5-8]

This chapter reviews the histology and pathophysiology of clinical and experimental intimal hyperplasia, as well as the usefulness and limitations of various animal models of arterial injury. A paradigm depicting intimal hyperplasia as the end-product of three distinct pathophysiologic processes is presented. The final section of the chapter discusses various strategies designed to control intimal hyperplasia.

The topic of transplant-related arteriosclerosis will not be addressed in any detail.

Degrees of Vascular Injury

There are many forms of "injury" that ultimately result in an intimal hyperplastic lesion. These injuries can differ dramatically in the type or degree of insult applied to the vessel wall. A means of classifying vascular injury (or at least the immediate histologic effect of injury; see Table 1) is useful since it is likely that different pathophysiologic processes are initiated with different degrees of injury.[9]

Type I is known as nondenuding endothelial injury. In this type of injury, there is no loss of endothelium and, therefore, no thrombus formation. Platelet adherence is minimal. That endothelial injury is present is indicated by clear increases in endothelial cell turnover and, often, changes in endothelial morphology. The "response to injury" theory of atherosclerosis[10] currently invokes this type of vascular injury as the inciting event.

In type II injury, there is endothelial denudation, but the internal elastic lamina (IEL) remains intact and the media incurs little if any trauma. This type of injury can result from adherent cytotoxic leukocytes, air desiccation, various techniques of vein graft preparation[11] or "routine" vascular instrumentation such as arterial catheterization. Where endothelium is missing, platelets adhere and a small, transient amount of thrombus may form. One widely used model of type II injury is filament (gentle) denudation of the rat carotid artery.[12]

The most severe injury is type III—a transmural injury that results in medial or even adventitial damage. This injury is imparted by many vascular interventional techniques designed to rupture or remove atherosclerotic plaque including balloon angioplasty, atherectomy, and surgical endarterectomy. Histologically, these injuries are characterized by extensive platelet

From *The Basic Science of Vascular Disease*. Edited by Sidawy AN, Sumpio BE, and DePalma RG. Armonk, NY: Futura Publishing Company, Inc.; © 1997.

Table 1
Types of Vascular Injury

Injury Type	Description	Histologic Findings	Examples
I	Nondenuding endothelial injury	No endothelial loss; possible morphologic changes or leukocyte adhesion	?Atherosclerosis ?Homocystinemia ?Hyperlipidemia ?Altered hemodynamics
II	Denuding endothelial injury	Loss of endothelium; internal elastic lamina remains intact; variable platelet adhesion and thrombus formation	Simple vascular instrumentation, ie, valvulotomy, arterial catheterization
III	Combined endothelial and medial injury	Loss of endothelium; internal elastic lamina disrupted; SMC necrosis; thrombus formation	Balloon dilatation Atherectomy Endarterectomy Stenting

deposition and even occlusive mural thrombus formation. Hence, anticoagulants, usually heparin, are frequently used during these procedures.

How are these forms of injury different and how are they alike? One of the main differences between the various forms of injury is the degree to which the coagulation cascade is activated and the likelihood of thrombus formation. This observation may have pathophysiologic and, therefore, therapeutic significance in humans. However, it should also be noted that intimal thickening can occur after any type of injury; the absence of thrombus formation is not an indication that injury is not occurring, nor is thrombus necessary for the ultimate development of intimal hyperplasia. The feature common to all forms of injury is dysfunction or loss of endothelium. Thus, intimal hyperplasia may be considered the final common pathway of a variety of vascular injuries that always involve some endothelial damage.

A useful classification scheme should also roughly predict the degree of intimal hyperplasia that will result from a vascular injury. Evidence exists from animal models that more severely injured arteries develop more significant intimal lesions.[12-14]

General Characteristics of Intimal Hyperplasia

The lesions that arise from vascular injuries are remarkably similar in ultimate histologic appearance despite the diverse nature of the injuries: laser or electrical stimulation,[15] air desiccation,[16] balloon dilatation,[17] atherectomy,[18,19] endarterectomy,[20] and vascular grafting with autogenous or prosthetic material.[8,21] There are, however, some notable differences in the

way these histologically similar lesions develop in various settings.[22] These differences will be highlighted throughout this discussion.

The smooth muscle cell (SMC) is the primary cellular component of intimal thickening, but ultimately comprises only ~20% of the total intimal volume; the remainder of the intima is filled with extracellular matrix (ECM).[23-26] Macrophages and lymphocytes can also be found within the lesion.[27-29] Depending upon when the injury occurred and its extent, the luminal surface may or may not be endothelialized.[12,30]

Intimal hyperplasia develops fairly rapidly after injury. In most experimental models, the process is well under way within 1 week and is often complete by 2 to 3 months.[22] A similarly accelerated course of events occurs clinically. Most complications attributed to restenosis because of intimal hyperplasia occur within 1 or 2 years of intervention.[1,2,5,7]

Intimal Hyperplasia Distinguished From Restenosis

It is critical to make a clear distinction between restenosis and intimal hyperplasia. Restenosis is the term applied to the loss of luminal diameter after a vascular intervention, for whatever reason. Intimal hyperplasia is only one possible mechanism contributing to restenosis: others are vasospasm and mural thrombus accumulation.

Most clinical studies of vascular injury use restenosis as an end point. It is important to note the particular definition of restenosis used in a study, since there is little uniformity and the definition used may greatly affect the reported incidence of restenosis. Restenosis is commonly defined as recurrence of luminal narrowing of ≥ 50%, especially in the peripheral vascular surgery literature. However, coronary angiographers often define restenosis as the loss of 50% of original gain in luminal diameter. Consider a 90% lesion dilated to a 40% stenosis by balloon angioplasty. During follow-up, the loss of an additional 20% of luminal diameter (now a 60% lesion) would qualify as restenosis, according to one definition but not the other.

Since the focus of this chapter is intimal hyperplasia, the other possible mechanisms of restenosis will not be addressed in any great detail. Yet, it is important to remember these other processes for several reasons. The occurrence of restenosis does not automatically mean the existence of severe intimal hyperplasia. Similarly, the persistent occurrence of restenosis in clinical trials testing drugs designed to limit intimal hyperplasia does not mean that these drugs failed to inhibit intimal hyperplasia; restenosis may be present because other mechanisms were at work. Articles describing risk factors for restenosis are not necessarily describing risk factors for exuberant intimal hyperplasia. Finally, animal models of vascular injury developed to assess intimal hyperplasia may not adequately represent other processes contributing to restenosis.

Types of Injury Resulting in Intimal Hyperplasia

The clinical interventions that most commonly result in intimal hyperplasia are balloon angioplasty, atherectomy, stenting, endarterectomy, and vein or prosthetic grafting. For our purposes, we will consider angioplasty, atherectomy, stenting and endarterectomy together since all involve the destruction of vascular tissue, and the events leading to intimal hyperplasia after these interventions may be very similar. The primary model for these injuries is the rat carotid injury model. Vein and prosthetic grafting will be addressed individually (along with appropriate models), since the mechanisms of lesion development in grafts may be quite different from balloon angioplasty.

Angioplasty and Similar Injuries

Balloon angioplasty is a technique that uses a catheter-borne balloon to dilate arterial narrowings, usually due to atherosclerosis. Much of the gain in luminal diameter is accomplished by fracture of the atherosclerotic plaque, often with significant degrees of medial disruption and dissection.[31,32] Plaque compression also occurs and may account for up to half of the gain in luminal cross-sectional area. The overall vessel cross-sectional area is often slightly increased, indicating that the entire vessel has been significantly stretched.[32] It is obvious that this technique often produces significant

vessel wall injury (type III), especially since one of the most feared and deadly complications of this procedure is vessel rupture. Even when significant medial injury does not occur, endothelial denudation (type II injury) is probable.

The Rat Carotid Injury Model

Probably the most widely used experimental model of arterial injury and intimal hyperplasia is the rat carotid artery injury preparation, originally utilized by Baumgartner[17] and extensively characterized by Clowes and Reidy.[23,30,33,34] There are two basic variants (Table 2): 1) a type III injury in which an inflated 2F embolectomy balloon is pulled through the artery, denuding the endothelial lining and injuring the media, and 2) a type II injury in which only the endothelium is deleted by passing a fine nylon loop through the vessel without causing significant medial injury.[12] The second variant allows the effects of endothelial denudation to be separated from the effects of medial distention. A large number of experiments studying the expression of various growth factor systems, matrix production, and pharmacologic approaches to control of intimal hyperplasia are based on variations of this model.

With balloon dilatation, the endothelial lining is completely denuded, the IEL is frequently disrupted or destroyed, and a significant fraction (20% to 30%) of medial SMC are killed.[12,30] Platelet adherence to the raw surface is almost immediate, followed very shortly thereafter by macrophage attachment. Around 24 hours later, 20% to 40% of the surviving medial SMC enter the cell cycle as a cohort and begin to proliferate.[33] The remainder of the medial SMC do not appear to divide. By 4 days, SMC begin to migrate from the media to the intima. Roughly half of the migrating SMC are cells that did not proliferate in the media.[33]

The intimal compartment then expands as some SMC continue to divide and produce ECM. Simultaneously, endothelial coverage of the damaged vessel occurs via ingrowth from either end of the denuded segment. As the endothelium covers the intima, the proliferative activity of the underlying intimal SMC declines, implying a growth inhibitory function for endothelium. SMC proliferative rates return to baseline (from a peak of 46% in the media and 73% in the intima) in areas covered with endothelium, but remain elevated in regions lacking endothelium.[30] The capacity for endothelial regrowth is limited. If the denuded segment is longer than 1 or 2 cm, regeneration will be incomplete even 1 year later, and the luminal cells in the central portion of the injured artery are still SMC. These SMC morphologically resemble endothelium, but do not stain with anti-Factor VIII antibodies; rather, they stain with anti-actin markers. Luminal

Table 2
Comparison of Events in Various Models of Vascular Injury

	Balloon–Injured Artery	Gently-Denuded Artery	Vein Graft	Prosthetic Graft
Thrombus formation	Present	Present	Variable	Present
Endothelial Regeneration	Variable (depends on distance between sources of endothelium)	Complete	Complete	Variable (incomplete in nonporous grafts; complete in porous grafts)
Chronic endothelial proliferation	No	No	Yes (fivefold over baseline)	Yes (20- to 30-fold over adjacent native endothelium)
Speculated effect of endothelium on SMC activation	Inhibitory	Inhibitory	Permissive or stimulatory	Permissive or stimulatory
Basal SMC proliferation (per day)	0.06%	0.06%	<0.05%	<0.01% (in adjacent vessel)
Peak medial SMC proliferation	20–50% (48 hours)	<2% (48 hours)	Not reported	Not applicable
Peak intimal SMC proliferation	~73% (4 days)	~48% (7 days)	~10% (7 days)	8% (1 month at growing edge in nonporous grafts); 0.8% (1 month in porous grafts)
Chronic intimal SMC proliferation	Yes (~8% in nonendothelialized region)	No	Yes (fourfold over basal level)	Yes (15- to 40-fold over adjacent arterial endothelium in nonporous; fivefold higher in porous)
Intimal thickening	Significant (two- to threefold increase in total wall area)	Modest (one- to twofold increase in total wall area)	Significant (tenfold increase in total wall area)	Significant
Hemodynamic regulation of intimal structure	Possibly	No	Yes	Yes

SMC: smooth muscle cells.

SMC proliferation remains above baseline, but is matched by cell loss, and the intimal thickness does not change after 3 months. The denuded luminal surface remains mildly thrombogenic, with detectable platelet adherence.[35] The final composition of the intima is approximately 20% SMC volume and 80% ECM,[24] em-phasizing the important role of matrix production in producing the intimal lesion.

Vasospasm is at least partly responsible for luminal narrowing in the rat carotid balloon injury model. Two weeks after injury, luminal narrowing is partly reversible by papaverine while at 12 weeks it is not.[22]

It is worth noting that at 12 weeks, when a large amount of intimal hyperplasia is present, the lumen is only narrowed by 35%. Thus, while the rat carotid balloon injury model generates a significant intimal lesion, it is not a very good model of luminal stenosis (or restenosis).

The filament denudation model causes less medial injury than the balloon angioplasty model. There is also much less medial SMC proliferation (2% versus 40%), but platelets adhere to the denuded surface to at least the same degree, if not greater.[12] SMC migration to the intima occurs, but the intimal lesion is only 50% as thick as that in the balloon model. The differences in cellular injury noted between the balloon dilatation and the filament denudation models led Reidy and Lindner to pursue the hypothesis that growth factors released from the damaged cells (e.g., basic fibroblast growth factor [bFGF]) stimulate the remaining medial SMC to proliferate.[36-38]

The rat carotid injury model has limitations. It is an unfounded assumption that the response to injury of a normal rat carotid artery is the same as in stiff, calcific, atherosclerotic human vessels. Furthermore, many of the drugs that inhibit intimal hyperplasia in the rat do not work in higher animal models or in humans. There is also much less thrombus in injured rat arteries compared to larger animals such as the pig or humans. This difference may prove to be very important if thrombin or other coagulation products help to regulate intimal lesion formation in humans.

Other Balloon Injury Models

Balloon injury of rabbit arteries induces a similar sequence of events and produces an intimal lesion that is similar to the rat.[39-43] Balloon injury of an already diseased vessel might be expected to more closely mirror the clinical situation. Thus, hypercholesterolemic rabbits are frequently used to model vascular injury.[13,44,45] The effects of hypercholesterolemia and balloon injury appear to be synergistic in the production of intimal hyperplasia, suggesting that diseased vessels may be predisposed to restenosis following balloon injury.[45-47] However, even with this enhanced lesion formation, mean luminal narrowing barely reaches 50%.[44]

The pig is often used as a model of balloon injury because it is large, and atherosclerotic changes can be induced in its vessels by cholesterol feeding.[14,48,49] Balloon angioplasty of the porcine carotid artery typically produces complete endothelial denudation and platelet deposition at 1 hour.[49] Mural thrombus accumulates in arteries with medial tearing, but not in less injured vessels. Detectable losses of SMC in the media are present by 24 hours. The degree of platelet deposition begins to decline by 4 days, as endothelium begins to regenerate. Endothelial regeneration is complete by 7 days and platelet deposition is then absent. However, intimal thickening continues through 14 days and is stable at 30 and 60 days. Unless acute thrombotic occlusion occurs, mere balloon injury of porcine vessels does not reliably cause luminal stenosis, even though a significant intimal lesion forms.[48,49]

Our laboratory and others have used baboons to study vascular injury because of this animal's hematologic similarities to humans.[50] Balloon injury of the femoral artery results in intimal hyperplasia, but the lesion is relatively small and thin.[51] The major cellular component is the SMC.[52] The kinetics of lesion development and endothelial regeneration in this model have yet to be described, although it seems clear, at this point, that at least normal primate arteries will not develop significant stenosis after balloon injury.

Atherectomy

Atherectomy restores luminal diameter by cutting or resecting the plaque.[1,2,53,54] Tissue may be retrieved for histologic or other forms of analysis. At times, recognizable fragments of adventitia have been retrieved, thus documenting transmural (type III) injury.[19] The deeper the resection, the more likely restenosis is to occur.[53] These restenotic lesions resemble other forms of intimal hyperplasia, containing SMC and ECM.[18,19,55,56]

Intravascular Stenting

Expandable stents are often placed within the lumen of a narrowed artery when the outcome of angioplasty or atherectomy is uncertain, such as in long stenoses, recanalized occlusions, or after obvious vessel wall dissection.[57-59] Most stents are metallic and fabricated into a mesh-like configuration and are either balloon-expandable or self-expandable. When deployed, the stent applies a constant outward force on the vessel, maintaining the desired dimensions of the lumen by preventing stenosis due to spasm or progressive dissection.

Intimal hyperplasia after stent placement is probably the primary process narrowing the lumen at late times, although thrombus accumulation is another possibility. Restenosis as a result of stent compression does not appear to occur.[60] Whether the restenosis is primarily a result of the adjunctive intervention or the stent itself is unclear. The addition of a stent to an angioplasty or atherectomy most likely increases the degree of injury because a chronic irritant and outward force are now constantly present.[48]

Stents removed from human arteries at various

times after placement show platelet and leukocyte adherence to the stent wires in the first few days.[61,62] At 3 months, the stent wires are embedded in the intimal lesion. By 6 months, extracellular lipid and cholesterol crystals are present. Endothelialization occurs, but is discontinuous; platelet and leukocyte adherence persists at 10 months. At all times, SMC and ECM comprise the dominant portion of the lesion, although cell density decreases at later times indicating an accumulation of ECM. A foreign body response has not been documented in clinical specimens.[60,63]

Stented arteries often have initially greater gains in luminal diameter compared to ballooned arteries. However, the later loss of luminal diameter is also accelerated in the stented patients, suggesting increased or more virulent intimal hyperplasia.[64] Most of the luminal narrowing occurs in the first 3 months,[58] consistent with the time course of intimal hyperplasia. The durability of stent intervention in the femoropopliteal location is particularly poor, with 30% to 50% failure rates 20 months after placement.[65,66]

Animal models of intravascular stenting have been developed using the rabbit,[67] dog,[68] and pig.[69,70] Histologic examination of the stents within hours of placement reveals endothelial destruction (at a minimum a type II injury) and platelet deposition on the stent material.[70] In all of these models, an SMC-rich intimal lesion covers the wires so that the stent becomes embedded within the artery. In the dog and pig models, endothelialization occurs between 1 to 2 weeks, with maximal intimal thickening at 4 to 8 weeks. The degree of thickening then stabilizes or even regresses from this point, such that luminal diameter is preserved.[68,70] Stents can induce a significant inflammatory response in the pig[69]—a finding that differs from the general lack of inflammation observed to date in human stented arteries.[60,63]

In rabbits[67] and pigs,[69] stenting results in more significant hyperplasia than balloon angioplasty, and is more resistant to inhibition by heparin than the balloon-injury lesion.[67] These studies suggest that placement of a stent increases the amount of injury sustained by the vessel wall above and beyond the balloon dilatation. This concept is buttressed by Schwartz's observation that stenting balloon-injured pig coronary arteries more commonly resulted in luminal stenosis than balloon injury alone.[48]

Endarterectomy

Surgical endarterectomy is defined as the removal of the intimal (usually atherosclerotic) lesion, as well as a significant portion of the vessel media. By definition, this is a type III injury.

After carotid endarterectomy, restenosis is a fairly common occurrence, with a 30% cumulative incidence in the University of Washington experience.[5] The restenotic lesion generally has the histologic appearance of intimal hyperplasia, especially when examined within 2 years of the endarterectomy. Lesions that become clinically significant more than 2 years after the original procedure generally represent recurrence of atherosclerosis, not intimal hyperplasia.[71]

Endarterectomies of normal carotid arteries have been experimentally performed in the dog[20] and baboon.[51] Significant thrombus forms on the injured surface and is replaced by intimal hyperplasia. The relevance of these models to human endarterectomy is unknown.

Vein Grafting

Coronary saphenous vein grafts develop two fairly distinct lesions. Early after grafting, intimal hyperplasia is often present.[28] Later, atheromatous lesions appear superimposed upon the intimal thickening and contain large concentrations of T-cells and macrophages in the subendothelial space, as well as foam cells, calcification, and regions of necrosis.[28,55]

Both manifestations of vein graft injury—the early hyperplastic response and the later atherosclerotic degeneration—may reflect failure of a type I or type II injury to resolve. In a study of harvested saphenous coronary grafts, focal intimal proliferative lesions were the sites of least responsiveness to endothelium-dependent vasodilators, indicating that these sites were either still de-endothelialized or were covered with dysfunctional endothelium.[72]

Lipid uptake by veins placed in a simulated arterial environment is increased and associated with changes in endothelial morphology.[73] This may reflect a type I injury and account for later atherosclerotic degeneration.

Peripheral saphenous vein grafts display the same pathologic and physiologic alteration as coronary grafts.[8,74,75] Overall, the mechanisms producing these changes are probably the same in peripheral and coronary vein grafts.

A number of animal models have been used to study the response of veins grafted into the arterial circulation. These include the rat,[76] rabbit,[77] dog,[78,79] pig,[80] and nonhuman primate.[81]

Zwolak[77] studied the development of intimal hyperplasia in rabbit vein grafts (Table 2). Immediately after grafting, there is loss of endothelium, especially near the anastomoses, with platelets and leukocytes adhering to the denuded regions. Re-endothelialization occurs in association with an increase in endothelial proliferation at 1 week (8% versus 0.02% at quiescence). Although regeneration of an endothelial lining is complete at 2 weeks, endothelial proliferation remains higher than baseline at 24 weeks (0.1%). SMC proliferation peaks at 1 week (10% versus 0.05% at quiescence) and declines to 0.22% at 24 weeks, still about fourfold higher than baseline. Absolute SMC mass is maximal at 4 weeks and does not change at later times despite the elevated proliferative rate. Vein graft thickening lags behind the cellular proliferative response, not reaching a maximum until 12 weeks. Thus, the increase in wall thickness and cross-sectional area after 4 weeks is primarily a result of ECM production. The lumen of the thickened vein graft is lined with cells staining for Factor VIII-related antigen (endothelium), and the intima and media are dominated by actin-positive cells (SMC). Macrophages account for less than 1% of stained cells. The overall thickening of the vein wall is accounted for by equal increases in the medial and intimal compartments.

The process of intimal thickening in experimental vein grafts appears to differ from that in models of arterial injury in several important respects. First, re-endothelialization in vein grafts is rapid and complete, whereas in injured arteries, it is delayed[42] and may be incomplete.[35] In injured arteries, SMC proliferation appears to be inhibited once re-endothelialization has occurred,[30] yet it remains significantly elevated even after endothelial coverage in vein grafts. Wall thickening in vein grafts occurs over a more protracted period of time (12 weeks), compared to injured arteries where the peak wall thickness occurs at 2 weeks.[42] Medial thickening contributes proportionally more to total wall thickness in vein grafts than injured arteries. These differences suggest several possibilities: 1) the fundamental response to vascular injury is different in veins and arteries; 2) regenerated endothelium in vein grafts has an altered physiology, allowing underlying SMC to proliferate; 3) the injury to vein grafts persists beyond the perioperative period and is not completely mitigated by re-endothelialization.

The concept of altered endothelial function in vein grafts has considerable experimental support. Acetylcholine-induced (endothelium-dependent) relaxation in rabbit vein grafts explanted from the arterial circulation is impaired.[82] If the grafts are returned to the venous environment, relaxation in response to acetylcholine returns. Qualitatively, similar findings were reported by Fann in a dog model.[78] The endothelial lining of 1-year-old arterialized vein grafts in normocholesterolemic rabbits fails to exclude macromolecules, despite a morphologically intact endothelial lining.[83] Overall wall thickness is the same as at 12 weeks, but significant structural degeneration is present, with subendothelial hemorrhage along with cholesterol and foam cell accumulation.

Despite the important information gained from them, the available animal models of vein grafting are not clearly relevant to humans. The veins used are often valveless, undergo different preparation and, therefore, may not reflect the unique adaptation of the human saphenous vein to arterial conditions. The animal models also do not mimic the pattern of intimal hyperplasia that in humans occurs primarily near anastomoses or valves.[7]

Mechanisms of Vein Graft Injury

Interventions such as balloon angioplasty or atherectomy destroy tissue and often result in intimal hyperplasia. Why, after careful and delicate preparation, does intimal hyperplasia occur in a previously normal vessel such as a saphenous vein when it is used as an arterial graft? There may be no single cause of intimal hyperplasia in vein grafts. We will review three possibilities: mechanical trauma, ischemia-reperfusion, and hemodynamic adaptation, or "arterialization." Blaming all of the intimal hyperplasia in veins to the process of grafting may be inaccurate since over 90% of "normal" saphenous veins contain some degree of intimal hyperplasia.[74]

Even in the best hands, the vein is mechanically injured to some degree during harvest, preparation, and implantation. Depending upon the amount of trauma, this injury is a type II or type III insult.[9,11,84,85] Vein grafts can incur type III transmural injury during preparation. A study of human saphenous veins, prepared as in situ or reversed peripheral grafts, found evidence of medial injury (SMC necrosis) more often after passage of a valvulotome than after fluid distention alone.[11] Another study concluded that the in situ technique was less traumatic to canine vein grafts than the reversed technique.[86]

The evidence for type II mechanical injury comes from histologic studies showing loss of endothelium without medial injury in grafts distended with saline,[11,86] and from studies demonstrating lack of normal endothelial function after graft preparation.[75,82,85,87] These latter studies frequently focus on impaired endothelium-dependent vasorelaxation in vein grafts, without always demonstrating actual loss of endothelium. Thus, they might only represent a type I injury in which the endothelium, although still present, is dysfunctional.

Veins that are completely removed from the leg undergo a period of ischemia, then "reperfusion" when grafted. The ischemic insult is probably more significant if the vein wall is thickened—a feature common to many distal saphenous veins.[74] Ischemia induced by disruption of the vasa vasorum causes medial SMC proliferation in rabbit arteries and increases expression of platelet-derived growth factor (PDGF),[88] a growth factor thought to be important in vascular

SMC growth control. Ischemia might also result in generation of toxic free radicals, which then cause endothelial or SMC damage. If this hypothesis is true, antioxidant treatment should prevent free radical-induced injury to excised veins and subsequent intimal hyperplasia. This protective effect has been demonstrated for one antioxidant molecule, desferrioxamine manganese. Ex vivo treatment of rabbit vein grafts with this agent after harvest, but before grafting, results in significantly less intimal hyperplasia than untreated veins. The treated veins also retain normal, endothelium-dependent function after grafting.[89]

The arterial environment, with its increased wall tension and shear stress relative to the venous side, may be injurious to the vein graft. Intimal thickening may be an adaptive response by the vein to these new hemodynamic conditions—a process of "arterialization." This process might be construed as a transmural or type III injury, even though endothelial loss might only be patchy.

The arterial circulation has a significantly higher intraluminal pressure than the venous circulation. The law of Laplace states that tangential wall tension (T), the circumferential distending force, is directly proportional to intraluminal pressure (P) and radius (R):

$$T = PR.$$

Wall thickness (h) tends to reduce this distending force. Inclusion of this term yields the equation for wall stress (S):

$$S = PR/h$$

which has the dimensions force per unit area (dynes/cm^2).[90]

Differences in wall tension may account for developmental differences in wall thickness between vessels with different intraluminal pressures (arteries and veins), as well as vessels with different radii (elastic versus muscular arteries).[91] The same principle can be invoked to partially explain the increase in medial thickness in the arteries of hypertensive animals.[92] These differences in wall thickness tend to equalize wall stress for many vessels of different size or intraluminal pressure. The thin-walled vein graft is often of larger diameter than the recipient artery. Thus, the vein experiences a significant increase in tangential wall stress when placed in the arterial circulation because of its large diameter, thin wall, and the higher pressure.[93]

Assuming a constant intraluminal pressure, the radius to wall thickness ratio is a surrogate parameter for wall stress. Rabbit vein grafts cease to thicken when the radius to wall thickness ratio of the graft approximates that of the carotid artery (Figure 1).[77] This finding suggests that increased wall stress is a significant factor in promoting vein graft wall thickening, and could explain why thickening and SMC proliferation persist even after re-endothelialization occurs. The results of another study using rigid external support to reduce vein graft wall tension were consistent with this notion. Wall thickening was reduced in the segments of vein with external support.[94]

Shear stress can be thought of as the frictional force applied to the luminal surface of the vein by the flowing blood. By the Hagen-Poiseuille relationship,

$$\tau \; \alpha \; Q/_{\pi r^3}$$

shear stress, τ, is directly proportional to blood volume flow, Q, (which is directly proportional to mean velocity) and inversely proportional to the cube of vessel radius, r.[90] It is difficult to exactly estimate the changes in shear that a vein experiences when it is transplanted into the arterial circuit. Arterial blood flow velocity is higher than venous velocity, but acute increases in venous diameter after grafting have also been documented.[77,94] These changes would tend to cancel each other, or even result in reduced shear (since shear varies with the cube of the radius). Berceli[93] calculated that the canine jugular vein experienced a sixfold reduction in shear stress relative to the carotid artery after grafting, mainly due to the increased diameter of the vein. However, the change in shear stress that the vein experienced as a result of being transplanted from the venous circulation to the arterial circulation was not modeled.

Intimal thickening in vein grafts varies inversely with blood velocity (or shear stress).[95–97] However, overall wall thickening is just as much a result of medial as intimal thickening.[77] These two processes may very well be different.[42,79] In a study designed to separate the influences of wall stress and shear stress on overall vein graft wall thickening, wall tension was found to primarily influence medial thickening and shear stress regulates intimal thickening.[97] It seems clear that the vein graft is exposed to significantly higher wall tension in the arterial position. The graft may also experience a net reduction in shear stress, although this is less certain. Increased wall tension and decreased shear would be a potent combination favoring overall thickening of the vein graft.

Prosthetic Grafting

The host response to insertion of a prosthetic graft has many histologic similarities to other forms of vascular injury, especially at the anastomoses. Yet, no convincing evidence exists that grafts inserted into the

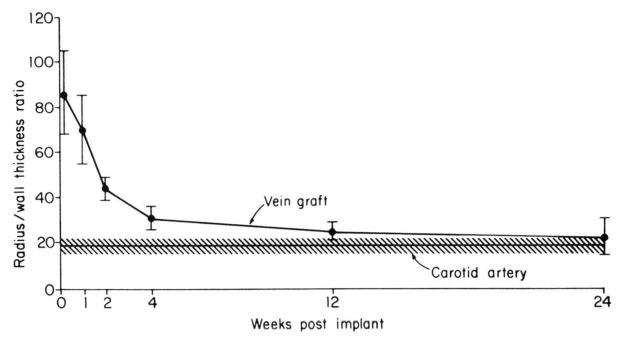

Figure 1. Graph of vein graft luminal radius/wall thickness ratio plotted against weeks after implantation. **Time 0** represents grafts excised 1 hour after implant. Values expressed as mean + standard deviation. Carotid artery value did not change during the course of the experiment and represents nine animals. (Reproduced with permission from Reference 77.)

human circulation develop an endothelialized neointima that completely lines the flow surface. Obviously, systematic studies of graft incorporation in humans are difficult if not impossible to perform. The available specimens usually come from grafts that have thrombosed and are removed during reconstruction, or from cadavers with inconsistent preparation for histologic study.[98-101] By necessity then, much of what is known about prosthetic graft incorporation comes from animal models.

The striking difference between most animal models and humans is the regularity of neointimal development in animals, regardless of species. Dogs have been a favorite host for years, and many reports are available detailing the healing pattern of various prosthetic materials. In hopes of developing a model more relevant to humans, our laboratory has characterized the healing response to prosthetic grafting (mainly polytetrafluoroethylene [PTFE]) that occurs in nonhuman primates.[102-107] A fundamental observation from this series of experiments is that the mechanism of graft healing is porosity-dependent.[105,106] The low-porosity PTFE grafts (30 μm internodal distance) currently in clinical use heal only to the extent that SMC and endothelium can migrate over the prosthetic surface from the cut arterial edge,[102,103,105,106] whereas more porous grafts (PTFE 60 or 90 μm internodal distance and knitted Dacron) heal by transmural ingrowth of vascular cells.[104-106] The capacity for longitudinal migration

from the cut arterial edge is limited to only a few centimeters; long low-porosity grafts are not completely endothelialized even 1 year later.[103] Healing in higher porosity grafts occurs relatively rapidly, although the more porous Dacron grafts lag behind the PTFE, perhaps reflecting a material-dependent healing mechanism as well.[104-106,108] In the high porosity grafts, the neointimal cells migrate through the substance of the graft from the perivascular tissue to reach the luminal surface.[104]

The neointima of the baboon PTFE grafts is consistently endothelialized and composed of SMC, ECM, and occasional macrophages.[27,102-104] During the healing phase of the high-porosity PTFE grafts, an intriguing sequence of cell appearance occurs.[104] Endothelial cells appear first on the luminal surface of the graft followed by SMC. Thickening then occurs as SMC migrate into the neointima and proliferate beneath an intact endothelial lining. This sequence is the opposite of what is observed in injured arteries, where SMC proliferation occurs in unendothelialized regions and quiescence is reestablished by endothelial coverage. Additionally, endothelial cells in completely covered grafts maintain a high proliferative rate,[107] a feature that distinguishes them from the quiescent endothelial cells lining regenerated regions of injured arteries. This pattern of cell proliferation and healing resembles the events that occur in vein grafts more than they resemble the healing response in injured arteries (Table 2).

Thus, even though the cellular constituents of the hyperplastic lesions in injured arteries, vein grafts, and prosthetic grafts are the same (endothelium, SMC, and occasional macrophages), the biology of these cells and, therefore, the mechanisms of (neo)intimal thickening, differs significantly.

If the mechanism of (neo)intimal thickening is different for injured arteries and grafts, perhaps the stimulus or its source is also different. The pattern of healing in injured arteries is consistent with the notion that blood-borne substances are involved in intimal growth regulation; when the normal barrier function of endothelium is restored, intimal proliferation subsides. (Of course, this does not rule out other possibilities or mechanisms; it is just one possible explanation.) However, in the baboon prosthetic graft model, neointimal proliferation is initiated and continues under an apparently intact endothelium that excludes macromolecules and prevents platelet adherence.[107]

In this situation, we have hypothesized that the neointimal cells are themselves the source of the growth stimulus. In support of this hypothesis are the findings of our lab and others that PTFE grafts in baboons[27,109–111] and dogs[112,113] are capable of SMC growth factor production. In fact, work by Kaufman[112,113] suggests that growth factor production by endothelialized grafts is actually greater than nonendothelialized grafts.

How might prosthetic arterial grafts activate endothelial cells and SMC to cause intimal hyperplasia? The possibilities include a foreign body response to the prosthetic material, compliance mismatch, and hemodynamic flow disturbances at the anastomoses.

Prosthetic grafts explanted from humans and animals contain multinucleated macrophages resembling foreign body giant cells.[27,99,102] The prosthetic material may, through a foreign body response, activate macrophages resulting in polyploidy and elaboration of growth factors and cytokines that then promote neointimal thickening.[114–118] In this regard, Dacron appears more stimulating to macrophages than PTFE, at least in vitro.[114,117,118]

Prosthetic material may also activate blood-borne elements, primarily platelets, to release growth factors that would then act upon peri-anastomotic tissues to cause neointimal hyperplasia.[119] This theory was developed to explain the more severe hyperplasia at distal compared to proximal anastomoses and should only apply as long as grafts are not completely endothelialized. This explanation may be very relevant clinically, since prosthetic grafts in humans do not reliably endothelialize, and platelets accumulate on prosthetic grafts (especially Dacron) in humans for years after implantation.[120,121]

No prosthetic graft is as compliant as the artery to which it is sewn. This mismatch in compliance produces a region of significantly enhanced compliance just a few millimeters to the arterial side of the anastomosis. Here, SMC in the wall of the artery are subjected to abnormally increased amounts of strain.[122] SMC exposed to cyclic strain in vitro respond in ways that might promote neointimal hyperplasia with increased cell turnover and ECM production.[123–125]

The peri-anastomotic region, especially with a distal end-to-side anastomosis, contains closely apposed regions of widely varying shear and flow separation.[126] Depending upon the velocity of blood flow and the degree of any stenosis, true turbulence may also exist in the peri-anastomotic region. These hemodynamic factors have been implicated in the development of anastomotic neointimal hyperplasia.

Bassiouny[127] has shown that anastomotic neointimal thickening occurs typically in two distinct regions: at the suture line and at the floor of the recipient vessel of an end-side anastomosis (Figure 2). The degree and location of anastomotic hyperplasia were shown to correlate with regions of low shear stress and flow separation. The propensity of vascular lesions to occur in regions of low shear and flow separation is known.[127]

Conversely, high shear stress seems to reduce intimal or neointimal growth, both at the anastomosis and in the body of the graft.[25,95,96,128,129]

Cell Biology of Intimal Hyperplasia

Biology of Normal Arterial Cells

Endothelium

For the most part, the endothelium is the only cell occupying the undiseased intima, although in certain cases, intimal accumulations of SMC may be normal.[74,130] Endothelium is identified ultrastructurally by the presence of tight junctions and Weibel-Palade bodies,[131] and immunochemically by the presence of Factor VIII.[132] The normal endothelium, with its tight junctions, isolates the blood from the subendothelial space,[133] but is also very metabolically active.

Differentiated endothelium produces prostacyclin,[134] nitric oxide (NO),[135] tissue plasmin activator (tPA),[136] and heparan sulfate,[137] making it intensely thromboresistant.

The observation that SMC proliferation subsides after endothelium has regenerated over injured segments of artery led to the concept that the endothelium imposes an antiproliferative effect on the underlying SMC.[30] Many endothelial products are growth inhibitory for SMC, at least in vitro. These include prostacyclin[138] and heparan sulfate.[139] Which of these products, if any, actually maintains SMC in quiescence in vivo is not known.

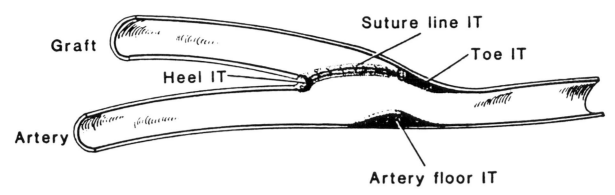

Figure 2. Illustration of sagittal section of end-to-side anastomosis depicts sites of localization of intimal thickening (**IT**) at suture line and artery floor. Intimal thickening on the artery floor is located in regions of flow separation and low shear stress. (Reproduced with permission from Reference 127).

The endothelium modulates vessel wall tone by producing both vasodilators and vasoconstrictors. The prominent vasodilators are prostacyclin[140] and NO,[135] while endothelin is a very potent vasoconstrictor.[141] Endothelial cells sense and metabolically respond to changes in the hemodynamic environment,[142] particularly changes in shear stress.[143] The expression of many endothelial genes are influenced by shear stress including prostacyclin,[134] NO,[135] tPA,[144] endothelin,[145] and PDGF.[146] Resnick[146] has demonstrated the existence of a specific shear-responsive element in the promoter region of the PDGF-B gene and reports similar sequences in the promoter regions of other genes known to be shear-sensitive.

Many endothelial products have more than one physiologic function. Molecules with antiplatelet effects, like NO and prostacyclin, are also SMC growth inhibitors and vasodilators. It is important to stress that vasodilation in response to increased shear stress, thromboresistance, and SMC growth inhibition are the functional properties of normal, unperturbed, differentiated endothelium; the corollary is that endothelium can exist in a dysfunctional or undifferentiated state with vasoconstrictive, procoagulant, and mitogenic effects. This line of reasoning implies that the traditional vascular surgical goal of preserving or promoting the mere existence of endothelium may be insufficient. Endothelium must not only be present for normal vessel function, it must also exist in its normally differentiated state.

Smooth Muscle Cells

The IEL is the endothelial basement membrane and forms the histologic boundary between the intima and media. The media is primarily composed of SMC and ECM. SMC do the work of vasoconstriction or

vasodilation and are the pivotal cells in the development of intimal hyperplasia, since they form the bulk of the cellular volume of the lesion and elaborate the ECM that ultimately comprises most of the (neo)intimal volume.[24,25]

Cell culture studies have demonstrated that SMC are of two basic phenotypes: the contractile state (differentiated) or the synthetic (dedifferentiated) state.[147] The contractile phenotype is the quiescent, nonproliferative, vasoactive state of normal adult vascular SMC. These cells contain large amounts of actin and myosin and contract in response to angiotensin II (AII), norepinephrine, and mechanical stimulation. Daily replicative rates of contractile SMC in normal, uninjured vessels are very low, less than 0.1%.[30,77] On the other hand, the synthetic phenotype proliferates readily in response to mitogens, and resembles fibroblasts with abundant cytoplasmic organelles and rough endoplasmic reticulum. Synthetic SMC have little or no detectable myosin. There are several actin isoforms (α, β, and γ), and SMC of different phenotypes differ in the isoforms they express.[148] Contractile SMC mainly express the α-isoform, whereas synthetic SMC in culture, intimal hyperplasia, and atherosclerosis express mostly β-actin. SMC in lesions of intimal hyperplasia appear to be of the synthetic phenotype and are characterized by abundant rough endoplasmic reticulum, loss of myosin, and a shift in actin expression to the β-isoform.[149] During fetal development, vascular SMC more closely resemble the synthetic than contractile phenotype.[133,150]

The phenotypic state of the SMC profoundly affects the amount of ECM in the intimal lesion. Synthetic SMC produce four- to fivefold more matrix than contractile cells, which may explain the relative hypocellularity of mature intimal lesions compared to the normal arterial media.[150]

Adventitial Elements

The outermost layer of the artery, the adventitia, is a loose investment of connective tissue through which nutrient vasa vasora and autonomic nerve fibers travel. Fibroblasts, pericytes, microvascular endothelial cells, and mast cells are the main cell types. The autonomic nervous system helps to coordinate vascular tone throughout the entire organism, but may also help to maintain the SMC of the media in the quiescent, contractile phenotype.[151] Extensive surgical exposure and dissection of blood vessels can deprive the media of nutrient blood flow by removing vasa vasorum[88] and also induce SMC to switch phenotypes by removing autonomic nerve fibers which had kept them in a contractile phenotype.

Thrombogenesis

Arterial injury activates thrombosis through the extrinsic pathway by disrupting arterial wall elements and unmasking tissue factor which binds Factor VII and leads to the activation of Factor X.[152] Fibrinogen and other coagulation proteins of the intrinsic pathway coat the luminal surface of prosthetic grafts immediately upon restoration of blood flow, forming thrombin and fibrin on the graft surface.[153] Thrombin may help regulate early events in intimal hyperplasia formation.[154]

Platelet adhesion, activation, and aggregation are integral to clot formation and occur at sites of vascular injury along with activation of the coagulation cascade. Platelets carry a variety of molecules potentially important in intimal hyperplasia including PDGF, transforming growth factor-β (TGF-β), and serotonin.

The importance of thrombosis for intimal hyperplasia is not always evident. Hyperplasia can occur throughout vein grafts, yet thrombus formation is often minimal and localized to areas that have been de-endothelialized during graft preparation.[77]

Thrombus formation is also less prominent in balloon-injured rat carotid arteries than after simple endothelial deletion without medial injury.[155] Yet, intimal hyperplasia is more severe after balloon injury than with gentle denudation.[12] In the pig, however, platelet deposition is directly related to the depth of medial injury which is also proportional to the amount of intimal hyperplasia in this model.[14,84] This situation may more closely reflect the human response.

The Three-Wave Model of Intimal Hyperplasia

The development of intimal hyperplasia after injury of normal artery (especially balloon angioplasty) involves three processes (Table 3).[156,157] First, SMC in the media of the vessel proliferate to replace the cells lost as a consequence of the injury. Second, SMC must migrate into the intima from the media. Third, SMC that migrate to the intima proliferate and produce the ECM that ultimately comprises most of the intimal volume.

It might not be necessary for all three processes to occur in some forms of injury. An atherosclerotic lesion is already an intimal lesion. After injury, restenosis might only involve further proliferation of intimal cells already in place with little additional contribution from the media. Injuries that result primarily in endothelial denudation (simple endovascular instrumentation) without medial distention may mostly represent migration and subsequent intimal proliferation.

Table 3
Three-Wave Model of Intimal Hyperplasia

Wave	Major Events	Possible Mediators*
First Wave	Medial SMC proliferation	Basic fibroblast growth factor (bFGF) Angiotensin II ?catecholamines ?thrombin
Second Wave	Medial SMC migration into the intima	Platelet-derived growth factor (PDGF) ?Transforming growth factor β (TGF-β)
Third Wave	Intimal SMC proliferation Extracellular matrix production	Angiotensin II ?TGF-β PDGF ?TGF-β

* Roles for factors wtihout "?" are supported by more than one type of experiment, i.e., an infusion and a blocking experiment (either pharmacologic or antibody).
SMC: smooth muscle cells.

We will now consider the cellular and molecular regulation of SMC behavior following arterial injury and how these processes might result in intimal hyperplasia, using the three-wave theory as a paradigm. A complete categorization of all known SMC growth regulators is beyond the scope of this chapter and the reader is referred to several excellent reviews.[133,157]

First Wave: Medial Smooth Muscle Cell Proliferation

Endothelial damage or destruction results in thrombus formation. Approximately 24 hours later, if there has been enough damage to the vessel wall, a proportion of medial SMC begin to proliferate. These cells enter the cell cycle together as a wave; the remaining cells do not proliferate later.

The process(es) that determine which SMC in the media will proliferate are not known. The artery wall becomes permeable to macromolecules once the endothelium is gone,[158] giving serum or platelet-borne mitogens access to medial SMC. Alternatively, growth factors released by injured or dying SMC might stimulate adjacent SMC to proliferate (see next section).

Another theory is that some SMC in the normal vessel are phenotypically different than others, and this intrinsic cellular difference is what determines whether a cell will proliferate or not in response to an injury.[150] Indirect evidence supporting this "stem cell" hypothesis comes from Chan's work[159] showing that apparently normal venous SMC from patients with clinical restenosis are refractory to the growth inhibitory effects of heparin in culture, while SMC grown from saphenous veins of patients without restenosis are more likely to be inhibited by heparin. Thus, a subset of SMC within apparently normal vessels may be more predisposed to the synthetic, proliferative phenotype than others and may be more easily recruited to divide. This theory is also consistent with observations that coronary angioplasty patients who have developed restenosis in one artery are more likely to do so when another artery is dilated.[160] Perhaps SMC proliferate when an inhibitory influence normally present in the vessel wall is removed.[133,150] The obvious source for this inhibitory influence is the endothelium, since its removal, damage, or dysfunction seem to be necessary for intimal hyperplasia to occur. Endothelium produces heparan sulfate proteoglycan (HSPG), a large molecule that is incorporated in the cell membrane as well as the ECM.[137,139,161] SMC in culture that are post-confluent, i.e., growth-arrested, also make HSPG.[162] Heparan sulfate, which can be released from HSPG, and its close relative, heparin, have profound growth inhibitory effects on vascular SMC in vitro and in vivo.[16,34,137,139,161–166] Arterial injury could impair heparan sulfate's growth inhibitory function by removing

its source (endothelial destruction), or by giving heparinolytic enzymes access to the ECM of the media. Platelets contain an endoglycosidase that can degrade heparin[139]; when platelets adhere to the site of an injury, release of this enzyme could destroy matrix-incorporated HSPG and release the SMC from growth inhibition.[150]

TGF-β released from endothelium might also inhibit SMC growth. TGF-β is a peptide growth regulator that usually inhibits growth, although there are circumstances in which it stimulates SMC growth.[138,167–169] When endothelium and SMC are grown in co-culture, the latent form of TGF-β is activated.[167] Heparin may facilitate this activation of TGF-β.[170]

Other endothelium-derived substances that may maintain SMC quiescence are NO,[171] formerly known as endothelium-derived relaxing factor (EDRF),[135] and various natriuretic peptides (NP).[172] These two substances are similar in that they both increase intracellular cyclic guanosine monophosphate (cGMP) content, and thus may share certain intracellular pathways involved in growth control.[173]

Platelet-Derived Growth Factor

One of the first growth factors for cultured SMC to be isolated and defined was PDGF.[174] Since its original description, the story of PDGF has become quite complex (see review by Raines).[175] PDGF exists as a dimer of two different peptide subunits, PDGF-A or PDGF-B. These ligand subunits can associate to form three different types of dimers: -AA, -AB, or -BB. These dimers then interact with specific receptors on the cell membrane (PDGFR), which are also dimers composed of two different subunits: PDGFR-α or PDGFR-β.[176] Similar to the ligands, the receptor subunits associate to form three different dimers: -$\alpha\alpha$, -$\alpha\beta$, or -$\beta\beta$. The ligand and receptor subunits do not universally interact with one another. The PDGF-A ligand can only interact with PDGFR-α, while PDGF-B can interact with both PDGFR-α and -β. Thus, PDGF-BB can be regarded as the "universal ligand" capable of binding to any PDGF receptor, and the PDGFR-α receptor is the "universal receptor" capable of binding any PDGF ligand. Knowledge of these ligand-receptor relationships is critical, not just for PDGF, but for any growth factor that interacts with cell-membrane receptors, since the presence of both the ligand and receptor is necessary for a biologic response to occur. In other words, it is not enough to show that a particular growth factor is present—the presence of the relevant receptor should also be demonstrated before a role for the growth factor in the genesis of SMC proliferation can be proposed.

Is PDGF involved in first-wave medial SMC proliferation? Three different types of experiments suggest it is probably not the major mitogen controlling this process. First, intimal lesion formation after balloon injury is decreased in platelet-deficient animals compared to controls, but medial SMC proliferation is not affected.[177] Thus, while platelet-borne products (i.e., PDGF) are involved in intimal lesion formation, they are not necessary for medial SMC proliferation. However, PDGF might not have to come from platelets; both endothelial cells[27,178–180] and SMC[27,179,181–183] can synthesize PDGF. Second, anti-PDGF antibodies which block the action of PDGF (from whatever source) reduce the amount of intimal thickening compared to control, but do not affect medial SMC proliferation.[184] Third, pharmacologic infusions of PDGF-BB (the universal PDGF ligand) have only a weak mitogenic effect for medial SMC in rats with type II carotid injury.[185] If PDGF is not the major mitogen, what is?

Basic Fibroblast Growth Factor

Lindner and Reidy[36–38] have provided convincing evidence that bFGF is primarily responsible for the first wave of SMC proliferation in the media, at least in the rat. SMC proliferation is significantly reduced by administration of anti-bFGF antibodies,[37] is enhanced by administration of bFGF,[36] and the relevant receptor for bFGF is expressed by the proliferating SMC.[38]

Basic FGF lacks the putative signal sequence that allows proteins to be secreted outside the cell,[186] yet it is known to induce SMC proliferation by a receptor-mediated process. It is also deposited in the ECM, from where it can be released into the circulation by intravenous heparinization.[187] How does bFGF get outside the cell? Recently, it has been shown that bFGF can be released by an exocytotic mechanism independent of the endoplasmic reticulum-Golgi complex.[188] This mechanism may explain the existence of small amounts of bFGF in the ECM of previously untraumatized vessels. bFGF is also released by dying or damaged cells[186,189] and it is probably this mechanism that explains the bFGF-mediated wave of proliferation after arterial injury. Up to 30% of medial SMC are killed by balloon dilatation of the rat carotid artery,[30,34] indicating that a significant amount of growth factor can suddenly become available to the surviving medial SMC. Release of bFGF through cell lysis is also consistent with observations that more severe injury results in greater degrees of intimal hyperplasia.[12–14,53,190]

Angiotensin II

The renin-angiotensin system consists of five basic components: 1) the precursor molecule, angiotensinogen; 2) renin, an enzyme that catalyzes the formation of angiotensin I from angiotensinogen; 3) angiotensin-converting enzyme (ACE) which converts angiotensin I to 4) AII, the primary effector molecule in the system, and 5) receptors for AII.

In the last decade, much has been learned about the biochemistry and molecular biology of this system; the development of techniques to analyze gene expression for each of the system's components has led to a major revision in the proposed physiologic role of the system.[191] Historically, the renin-angiotensin system was thought to function in the circulating blood with its components synthesized in separate organs (angiotensinogen in the liver, renin in the kidney, ACE in the lung, and the receptors in the vasculature or the adrenals). It is now apparent that these component genes are expressed in many different tissues; also, many individual tissues simultaneously express several of the genes, including vascular tissue.[191] These findings suggest that there may be tissue-localized renin-angiotensin systems, as well as the more generalized circulating system.[192]

In vitro, AII can stimulate SMC to proliferate.[193] Treatment with AII also induces expression of PDGF-A, bFGF, TGF-β, and the proto-oncogenes, c-myc and c-fos.[169,194,195] Proto-oncogene expression accompanies cell division, and these proteins may participate in intracellular events related to mitogenesis.[196]

The in vivo evidence for a mitogenic effect of AII on medial SMC is also fairly strong.[157] Arterial injury results in increased angiotensinogen gene expression in the media[197] as well as enhanced angiotensin receptor (AT-1) expression,[198] suggesting that injured arteries may have enhanced production of, as well as sensitivity to, AII. Antagonists to these receptors reduce medial SMC proliferation and subsequent intimal hyperplasia in injury models,[199–202] and direct infusion of AII increases medial and intimal SMC proliferation and subsequent intimal hyperplasia.[201–204]

The proliferative effects of AII may also be mediated by the adrenergic nervous system since α-adrenergic antagonists block the mitogenic effect of AII on SMC.[204]

Other Potential Smooth Muscle Cell Mitogens

A few other mitogens, although not as extensively studied as PDGF, bFGF, or AII, deserve some mention. Given the inevitable interaction of the exposed media with the coagulation cascade, the possible role of thrombin must be considered. However, while thrombin has been shown to be mitogenic for SMC in vitro and to interact with other SMC mitogens such as PDGF,[123,154] demonstration of a clear-cut mitogenic effect in vivo has been more difficult. Rabbits treated with hirudin, a direct inhibitor of thrombin, after balloon angioplasty of the femoral arteries develop less intimal hyperplasia than heparin-treated animals.[205] However, whether hirudin affects SMC proliferation or other processes involved in intimal hyperplasia is unknown.

Catecholamines have mitogenic effects on cultured SMC[157] at physiologically relevant concentrations. This finding is consistent with the trophic effects for SMC exerted by autonomic fibers.[151,206] The involvement of catecholamines in SMC growth after injury is suggested by reduced SMC proliferation and intimal hyperplasia after treatment with adrenergic blockers such as prazosin.[40,43,204,207] Catecholamines also appear to interact with other known mitogens such as PDGF[208] and AII.[204]

Mitogenic effects on SMC by the potent vasoconstrictor endothelin have been described,[209] but there is no evidence for its role in vivo.

In summary, the first wave of proliferation after vascular injury is unlikely to be mediated by PDGF, but strong evidence exists for a primary role by bFGF and possibly AII. Catecholamines may also participate, but the current evidence is not as strong as for bFGF or AII. SMC may also proliferate because of removal of the growth inhibitory influences of heparan sulfate, TGF-β, NO, and the NPs.

Second Wave: Smooth Muscle Cell Migration

Human vessels requiring intervention usually have established vascular lesions, such as an atherosclerotic plaque or a restenotic lesion from a previous intervention. As such, there is already a significant amount of intimal tissue that may absorb the damage of the dilatation or atherectomy. There are no well-characterized models of injury superimposed upon preexisting disease, so it is unclear how much of a role additional SMC migration plays in the development of a restenotic lesion, especially after simple balloon angioplasty. Furthermore, it is difficult to measure migration when SMC are already present in the intima. After endarterectomy or atherectomy, some migration must occur from the remaining media, but the relative proportions of migration or proliferation (medial or intimal) are not known. A recent study of atherectomy specimens suggests that SMC proliferation in restenotic tissue is rare; the implication is that the intimal lesion is largely populated by migrating cells.[56]

The rat carotid artery intima contains only endothelial cells. For intimal thickening to occur, SMC must migrate from the media. SMC begin to appear in the intima 4 days after injury, and intimal cell mass accumulates for approximately 1 month.[30,33]

Clowes and Schwartz[33] have deduced that only 50% of all cells that migrate from media to intima after balloon injury are committed to proliferate. This finding suggests that the cohort of SMC selected to migrate after injury is substantially different from that selected to proliferate. Even less is known about the selection process for migration than for proliferation. Is there a migratory phenotype? Are these cells selected all at once, as the proliferating population seems to be, or is migration a more continuous process occurring over a longer period of time? The answers to these questions are unknown.

The Extracellular Matrix

A more detailed consideration of the ECM is necessary at this point. SMC can be thought of as being "suspended" in the ECM they produce. Endothelial cells also make ECM. The ECM consists of two basic domains: the basement membrane (IEL) produced by endothelial cells and the interstitial matrix made by SMC. Basement membrane is rich in laminin, type IV collagen, and heparan sulfate proteoglycans, while the interstitial matrix is rich in fibronectin, thrombospondin, collagen I and III, chondroitin and dermatan sulfate proteoglycans, and elastin.[210] These substances help determine SMC phenotype since changing the composition of the ECM can cause SMC to change phenotypes.[211] SMC interact with the ECM via specialized transmembrane proteins (mainly integrins and proteoglycans) that link the ECM moieties with the cytoskeleton. The ECM is continuously remodeled, not only by altered patterns of synthesis, but also by matrix metalloproteinases.[212]

What must SMC do to migrate? Most simply, they must break their attachments to the ECM and then form new attachments with matrix components[213] or degrade the ECM in the path of migration. It is likely that migration is a combination of the two processes. Arterial injury induces expression of plasminogen activators (tPA and uPA) within the vessel which are capable of stimulating ECM degradation and, by extension, disrupting existing cell-matrix attachments.[214] Plasmin, derived from plasminogen through the action of tPA or uPA, degrades most matrix components and activates matrix metalloproteinases.[212] Plasmin probably participates in SMC migration since tranexamic acid, a plasmin inhibitor, reduces the number of SMC appearing in the intima of the ballooned rat carotid artery.[215]

The effects of heparin and heparan sulfate provide more evidence for the role of proteases in SMC migration. Heparin, both in vivo and in vitro, inhibits the induction of genes encoding for tissue plasminogen activator and collagenase,[216–218] and decreases intimal hyperplasia and SMC migration.[16,34,163,219] In culture, the ECM of postconfluent, nonmigrating SMC contains a species of heparan sulfate that is potently inhibitory for SMC.[162] Arterial injury might induce protease expression by removing the constitutive inhibition of heparan sulfate. Endothelial destruction, platelet deposition, or both, could alter the composition of the ECM to one more conducive to protease expression[139] and subsequent SMC migration.

The Role of Platelets and Migratory Factors

Many of the growth regulators involved in SMC proliferation also affect SMC migration.[220] These include bFGF,[221] PDGF,[185,222] TGF-β,[221] and AII.[200,223] All can affect plasminogen activator expression and, therefore, matrix metalloproteinase activation and ECM degradation.[215,223,224]

There is strong evidence that PDGF stimulates SMC migration from the media to intima, but in a complicated way. The dimers PDGF-BB and -AB enhance SMC migration in vitro. PDGF-AA has no effect when added alone, but *inhibits* -AB- and -BB-induced migration. PDGF-AA also inhibits SMC migration in response to fibronectin, a prominent ECM component.[222] These findings suggest that the PDGFR-α and -β receptor subunits have different functions in the cell. Specifically, it appears that PDGF-induced migration is mediated by the PDGFR-β subunit, and that migratory stimuli are significantly inhibited by the activation of PDGFR-α.[225]

Other growth factors interact with PDGF to influence SMC migration. Added alone, TGF-β stimulates SMC migration in vitro. However, when combined with PDGF at less than 1/10 dose that stimulates migration, TGF-β inhibits PDGF-induced migration.[226] These findings illustrate the multifunctional character of TGF-β as a growth factor, and hint at the complexity of growth factor interactions that might exist in vivo.

The Role of Endothelium

Endothelium (or at least differentiated endothelium) appears to inhibit SMC migration in much the same way that it controls SMC proliferation. In the gentle denudation model of rat carotid injury, no intimal thickening occurs in regions that re-endothelialize within 7 days.[12] The reappearance of endothelium apparently inhibits SMC migration from the media to the intima. Medial distention alone is also insufficient to produce intimal thickening; some form of endothelial denudation has to occur.[190] The endothelium may func-

tion merely as a barrier, preventing the influx of blood-borne factors that stimulate medial SMC to migrate, but it may prevent SMC migration by other mechanisms as well. Perhaps the endothelium maintains or, after injury, reestablishes the type of ECM that holds SMC in check. Recall that the endothelium-derived IEL is rich in heparan sulfate proteoglycan, relative to the SMC-derived interstitial matrix.[210] Thus normal, uninjured endothelium with an intact IEL might stand as a barrier to SMC migration. Removal of the endothelium or disruption of the heparan-enriched IEL may, thus, remove a tonic inhibitory influence on SMC migration.

However, the mere existence of endothelium may not be sufficient to prevent SMC migration. The endothelial layer in arteries seems to inhibit SMC growth, while in synthetic and vein grafts it fails to do so. When vein grafts are placed into the arterial circulation, they are thought to retain much of their endothelium.[77] Yet these vein grafts develop intimal hyperplasia, with migration from media being the only apparent explanation for the appearance of SMC in the intima. Porous PTFE grafts also appear to endothelialize first, and *then* develop an SMC-rich neointima.[104] Also, certain areas of the apparently normal arterial tree develop intimal accumulations of SMC, particularly at branch points where there is low shear stress or a high degree of shear variation throughout the cardiac cycle.[127,130] These areas are endothelialized, yet SMC migration occurred at some point. Endothelium can, thus, be dysfunctional (or become less differentiated) at certain times or under certain conditions, and fail to exert its expected inhibitory influence on SMC behavior. We can speculate that in these situations the endothelium fails to elaborate the same type of ECM or some other endothelium-dependent factor (such as heparan or NO) found in normal arteries.

Undifferentiated endothelium may not just allow SMC migration to occur—it might even *promote* intimal hyperplasia. Cultured endothelial cells produce SMC mitogens and promigratory factors such as PDGF; this production and release is increased when endothelial cells are stressed, damaged, or killed.[178,180] Endothelial cells in atherosclerotic plaque[179,227] and prosthetic PTFE grafts[27,110,111] express the genes for PDGF. In PTFE grafts, mitogenically active PDGF is present, indicating that not only are PDGF genes transcribed, but PDGF protein is produced as well.[27,110] This work, as well as the demonstration of increased endothelial cell turnover in these grafts, at late times suggestive of ongoing nondenuding endothelial cell injury,[107] has led our group to postulate that the signals for SMC proliferation and migration arise from the endothelium. This concept was further reinforced by a study[26] showing that endothelialized PTFE grafts undergo a dramatic and sudden burst of intimal thickening when shear stress is abruptly lowered. The relative importance of SMC migration and proliferation in this process has not been determined. Our working hypothesis is that endothelial cells, when suddenly exposed to a low-shear environment (or other possible perturbations), communicate to the underlying SMC a growth-promoting or promigratory signal. Graham and coworkers, using a canine model of endothelial cell-seeding in prosthetic grafts, have shown that PDGF production and subsequent anastomotic neointimal thickening is actually enhanced in grafts seeded with endothelium compared to unseeded grafts, and that PDGF production correlates positively with graft area covered by endothelium and inversely with platelet deposition.[112,113] These findings implicate the endothelium as the source of the growth factor.

Third Wave: Intimal Expansion

The third major process in the development of intimal hyperplasia is intimal expansion, often at the expense of luminal area. An increase in intimal area might occur in three ways: ongoing SMC migration, proliferation of SMC within the intima after migration, and production of ECM. It is difficult to know precisely the contribution made by ongoing SMC migration from the media, but pulse thymidine labeling studies indicate that SMC in the intima (or neointima) proliferate.[30,77,102] These SMC also produce a great deal of ECM, since the mature intimal lesion is approximately 60% to 80% ECM by volume.[24-26]

Intimal Smooth Muscle Cell as a Separate Phenotype

Intimal SMC exhibit the characteristics of a secretory, proliferative phenotype while medial SMC are of the contractile, quiescent phenotype.[148-150,228] This difference is important since SMC of different phenotypes have different patterns of growth responsiveness and function.

Intimal SMC can be distinguished morphologically from medial SMC in culture.[111,183] Intimal SMC secrete significantly (approximately fivefold) higher amounts of PDGF into culture media than do medial SMC.[183] However, intimal cells have fewer PDGF receptors and respond poorly to purified PDGF, casting doubt on the role PDGF might play in stimulating intimal SMC to proliferate. Conversely, these results showed that intimal SMC are capable of PDGF-independent (more autonomous?) growth. Cells cultured from human hyperplastic lesions also produce PDGF.[182,229]

Intimal and fetal SMC have many similarities, suggesting that intimal SMC may reactivate the program of gene expression characteristic of the developing or-

ganism. Expression of the PDGFR-α is significantly depressed in intimal SMC, as it is in fetal or neonatal SMC.[181,230,231] Injury-induced intimal tissue expresses an angiotensin receptor subtype (subtype 2) usually seen only during development.[199] A number of other genes appear to be expressed differently by intimal and fetal SMC compared to medial SMC.[228,230]

Intimal Smooth Muscle Cell Growth Control

All of the peptide growth factors involved in medial SMC proliferation (first wave) are candidates for promoting intimal SMC proliferation. Interestingly, bFGF may not participate significantly in intimal SMC growth control. Infusions of bFGF begun at the time of injury result in a doubling of the amount of intimal hyperplasia,[36] but the relative effects of bFGF on medial SMC proliferation, SMC migration, or intimal SMC proliferation are not known. Administration of anti-bFGF antibodies has no effect on intimal SMC proliferation in a rat carotid artery injured 5 days previously. The initial peak in bFGF production has subsided by this time, suggesting that endogenous bFGF may have little to do with perpetuating the proliferation of intimal SMC.[232]

Pharmacologic infusions of PDGF-BB produce a modest, but real growth response in rat carotid intimal SMC weeks after injury.[185] This result shows that intimal SMC can respond to PDGF-BB, but it does not mean that endogenous PDGF-BB regulates intimal SMC proliferation in vivo. One is obligated to show that endogenous PDGF-BB exists in the wall and that selective blockade of PDGF-BB decreases proliferation. However, in the injured rat carotid artery, PDGF-A and PDGFR-β predominate in the intima at late times.[181] A similar pattern is seen in the mature neointima of prosthetic PTFE grafts.[27] This particular combination of ligand and receptor expression does not support a role for PDGF in sustaining intimal proliferation since, according to the currently accepted model, PDGF-A can only interact with PDGFR-α.[176]

AII may be an important growth factor for intimal SMC. When infused into rats with a well-developed carotid lesion 2 weeks after injury, AII produces a fourfold increase in intimal SMC proliferation and a 60% increase in intimal cross-sectional area. These rats also have significantly higher blood pressures, so it is not clear whether AII directly causes SMC to proliferate, or whether the mitogenic response is indirectly mediated by a mechanical effect of hypertension.

TGF-β usually inhibits SMC proliferation,[170] but it can induce SMC growth under certain circumstances.[168,233] The net effect of TGF-β on SMC growth in vitro is dependent upon the per cell concentration of TGF-β.[168,233] When a given amount of TGF-β is added to a sparse culture, the per cell concentration of TGF-β is high and SMC growth is inhibited. When TGF-β is added to a confluent culture, the per cell concentration is lower, and SMC are stimulated. The onset of DNA synthesis after addition of TGF-β is delayed by about 4 hours, compared to other SMC mitogens such as PDGF. This delay suggests that the effect of TGF-β is mediated by another growth factor. TGF-β induces PDGF-A expression, and anti-PDGF antibodies neutralize much of TGF-β's mitogenic effect.[233] Release of PDGF-A into the conditioned media of cultured SMC and transcription of the PDGFR-α gene is increased by TGF-β.[168] However, as the per cell concentration of TGF-β increases, PDGFR-α transcription goes down and the mitogenic effect of PDGF-A disappears. The TGF-β gene is induced within 6 hours of rat carotid balloon injury and remains elevated for at least 2 weeks,[234] easily long enough to influence the development of an intimal lesion. Immunocytochemical studies show that intimal SMC stain positively for TGF-β protein, and intimal SMC proliferation increases when this growth factor is infused into rats with an established lesion.[234] Restenotic lesions from human coronary arteries obtained by atherectomy express the TGF-β1 gene and protein to a greater extent than primary atherosclerotic lesions.[235] Thus, the particular conditions of intimal hyperplasia after arterial injury may favor the expression of TGF-β's growth-stimulating effects over its growth-inhibitory properties. Until specific TGF-β antagonists are available for in vivo use, the exact role of TGF-β in intimal lesion development will remain unclear.

There are several other, less well-studied peptides that may regulate intimal SMC growth including insulin-like growth factor (IGF),[236] gamma interferon (γ-IFN),[237] and interleukin-1 (IL-1).[238] An in-depth consideration of their roles is not possible here.

Extracellular Matrix Production

Intimal expansion depends not only upon SMC proliferation, but perhaps most upon deposition of ECM. Currently, it appears that the amount of matrix ultimately produced is closely tied to the number of SMC that exist in the intima, regardless of the size of the intimal lesion. Studies of the hemodynamic regulation of SMC growth in the neointima of PTFE grafts[25,26,129] have shown that the proportional contribution of SMC and ECM volumes to the overall intimal volume remains constant over a range of shear stresses and intimal volumes. However, this is only true when SMC proliferation has subsided. Near the lumen, where most of the SMC proliferation occurs in this model,[25,110] the relative proportion of SMC to ECM is much higher.[25] Thus, the bulk of matrix production and the continued increase in intimal cross-sectional area

in injured arteries,[30] vein grafts,[77] and prosthetic PTFE grafts[26] occur when SMC proliferation has waned.

Not much is known about the control of matrix production in the intima. Intimal hyperplastic lesions contain proportionally more ECM than the quiescent media. This difference probably reflects the predominant SMC phenotype in each of these areas. In culture, the intimal secretory phenotype synthesizes much more ECM than medial contractile SMC.[150] If the amount of matrix production is tightly linked to cellular phenotype, the degree of intimal hyperplasia due to ECM may not be independently regulated apart from controlling the number or the phenotype of SMC that accumulate within the intima.

Growth factors such as TGF-β and PDGF are also fibroplastic, i.e., they stimulate ECM production by SMC.[239] Thus, the same factors that might stimulate SMC proliferation could simultaneously increase ECM production, a potent combination favoring enlargement of the intimal lesion.

In summary, third-wave intimal expansion probably occurs as a result of SMC accumulation through proliferation, continued migration, or both, as well as relatively exuberant ECM synthesis. The processes of SMC accumulation and volume of ECM production appear to be tightly linked, with fairly constant proportions of SMC to ECM volumes characterizing the intimal lesions that arise after a variety of vascular injuries.

What Regulates the Extent of Intimal Hyperplasia?

In most models and probably most clinical situations, the process of intimal hyperplasia is self-limited: medial SMC proliferation, migration from media to intima, intimal SMC proliferation, and ECM production spontaneously subside and a new equilibrium is established. Even when endothelial regeneration is incomplete in injured arteries, the accumulation of intimal tissue usually reaches a limit.[35] Why does this occur?

Balloon injury induces TGF-β expression in the intima of the rat carotid artery.[234] TGF-β induces PDGF-A expression and, perhaps even more importantly, seems to inhibit SMC proliferation by suppressing expression of PDGFR-α.[168,233] This is the pattern of PDGF ligand and receptor expression in the mature (neo)intima of several models.[27,181] We can speculate that, many weeks after injury, TGF-β expression increases to the point that it becomes growth inhibitory and intimal accumulation eventually ceases. However, this scenario is difficult to reconcile with the increase in SMC proliferation that occurs in the intima after TGF-β infusion.[234]

Another possibility is that the size of the intimal lesion is hemodynamically regulated. Vein grafts carrying blood at higher velocity develop less intimal hyperplasia than vein grafts carrying blood at lower velocity.[95–97] The same regulatory phenomenon has been observed in healing prosthetic grafts,[25,26,128,129] and blood flow specifically regulates SMC proliferation in the neointima of baboon PTFE grafts.[25,26] Acute reductions in flow also appear to induce expression of PDGF-A in baboon PTFE grafts.[240]

Shear stress is the physical parameter most likely to regulate the extent of intimal hyperplasia. Shear stress is directly proportional to volume flow (which is directly proportional to mean velocity) and inversely proportional to the cube of the radius. The luminal cells of a blood vessel that experience a given shear stress, τ, at a certain flow, Q, before injury will experience an eightfold increase in shear stress at the same flow rate if intimal hyperplasia narrows the lumen by one half. Obviously, intimal hyperplasia can greatly affect shear stress. In fact, arteries appear to respond initially to the growth of intimal lesions by enlarging or vasodilating, which tends to keep shear stress at or near normal levels for as long as the vessel can compensate.[241]

Endothelial cells in culture respond to alterations in shear stress with a variety of biologic responses, including changes in morphology,[143] proliferative rate,[241] and augmented prostacyclin,[134] tPA,[144] and PDGF-B production.[146]

It is not known how the influences of shear stress are transduced through or by endothelial cells to the underlying SMC. SMC, themselves, are also sensitive to changes in shear stress,[242] and differences in flow affect the development of intimal hyperplasia in injured rat carotid arteries that do not re-endothelialize.[243]

Therefore, whether or not an intimal lesion is endothelialized, the luminal cells appear to be capable of responding to increases in shear stress. The balance of the experimental evidence implies that high shear stress would be inhibitory to intimal growth. Conclusive evidence that shear stress governs the upper limit of intimal hyperplasia would likely consist of a strong inverse correlation between shear stress and intimal hyperplasia, or a positive correlation between final luminal diameter and shear stress. Also, the demonstration of a threshold level of shear stress above which no further intimal thickening occurred would be persuasive. At this point, the evidence that shear stress actually limits the amount of intimal hyperplasia is minimal; however, the concept is theoretically sound and consistent with the available evidence.

A synthesis of the biologic events leading to intimal hyperplasia in injured arteries, vein grafts, and prosthetic grafts is presented in Figures 3 through 5.

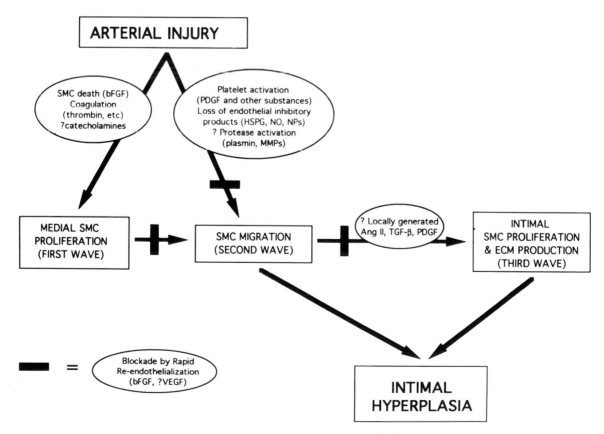

Figure 3. Possible events leading to intimal hyperplasia after arterial injury.

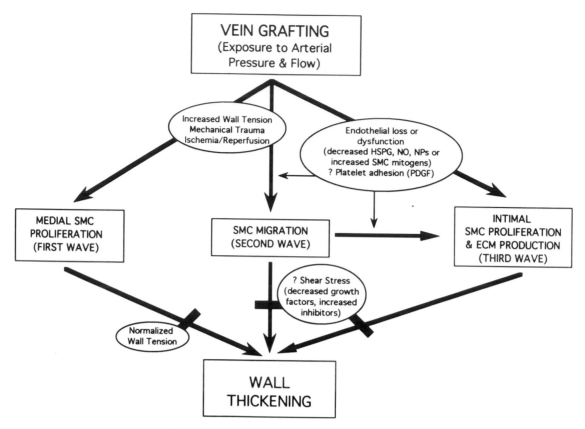

Figure 4. Possible events leading to intimal hyperplasia after vein grafting.

Prospects for Control of Intimal Hyperplasia

This section must be prefaced with the statement that there is no agent, substance, or technique clinically proven to prevent or reduce restenosis in humans.

Surgical Technique

For surgeons, it is axiomatic that adherence to Halsted's principles is important in obtaining a good clinical outcome. Vascular surgeons are especially cognizant of these principles, placing great emphasis on gentle, minimal handling of tissue, and developing less traumatic ways of preparing vein grafts and controlling vessels in preparation for an anastomosis. Yet, despite virtual universal acceptance and observance of these principles, intimal hyperplasia remains a significant problem. No study has shown a difference in incidence of intimal hyperplasia according to technique. Surgeons should still strive to minimize injury to blood vessels since these precautions do no harm and might still be beneficial in ways that are not easily measured.

Promoting Endothelialization

Intimal hyperplasia almost always follows some kind of injury or damage to the endothelium. Thus, measures that enhance endothelial regeneration and coverage of the denuded region might minimize intimal hyperplasia. This goal can be accomplished in basically two ways: 1) increasing the rate at which native endothelial cells regenerate; or 2) covering the unendothelialized surface with exogenously supplied endothelium (endothelial cell seeding).

The endothelial layer should be restored most rapidly when vessels have been minimally traumatized. The theoretical basis for this concept comes from the rat carotid injury model. When a type III injury of the artery is induced by balloon distention, complete regrowth of endothelium does not occur.[30,35] However, when only a type II injury is inflicted, complete endothelial regeneration is seen.[155]

Providing an endothelial mitogen at the time of injury could also enhance the regrowth of endothelium. The prototypical endothelial mitogens are the FGFs,[244] and exogenously administered bFGF increases the rate and extent of re-endothelialization after balloon injury in the rat carotid artery.[245] However, bFGF is also a potent SMC mitogen, and systemic administration increases SMC proliferation and intimal hyperplasia in injured rat carotid arteries.[36] This latter effect might neutralize the positive effects of enhanced re-endothelialization. Another endothelial mitogen is vascular endothelial growth factor (VEGF) which differs from bFGF in that it has no effect on SMC.[246] There are as yet no reports of the effects of VEGF administration in models of vascular injury.

Endothelial cell seeding is another way to rapidly reestablish an endothelial covering.[247,248] This technique may be most applicable to prosthetic grafting, since humans seem unable to re-endothelialize prosthetic grafts, as well as other interventions that injure long segments of arteries. Endothelial seeding improves patency and reduces intimal hyperplasia in a canine model of carotid endarterectomy.[20] Clinical experience with endothelial seeding has produced mixed results. When measured by radiolabeled platelet imaging techniques, platelet uptake by seeded grafts is significantly reduced compared to unseeded grafts.[249] However, another study observed no difference in serum markers of platelet activation between seeded and nonseeded PTFE femoropopliteal grafts at 1 year.[120] All prosthetic grafts, seeded or not, activate platelets to a greater extent than saphenous vein grafts. To date, no clinical study has shown that endothelial seeding has a beneficial effect on neointimal hyperpla-

sia or even patency; rather, when seeded grafts fail, they do so because of neointimal hyperplasia.[250]

These clinical observations reinforce the point that the mere presence of endothelium is probably insufficient to prevent intimal hyperplasia. The endothelium may be present, but dysfunctional or undifferentiated, i.e., experiencing a chronic type I injury. Such endothelium could conceivably promote SMC proliferation, or at least fail to exert the expected inhibitory influences of normal endothelium on nearby SMC.

Pharmacologic Control of Smooth Muscle Cell Activity

Clinical studies evaluating therapies for intimal hyperplasia can be difficult to interpret because the end points are clinical or based on imaging techniques, such as quantitative angiography or duplex scanning. These end points cannot distinguish between restenosis due to intimal hyperplasia, vasospasm, or thrombus. Newer techniques, such as high resolution duplex scanning and examination of tissue retrieved by ather-

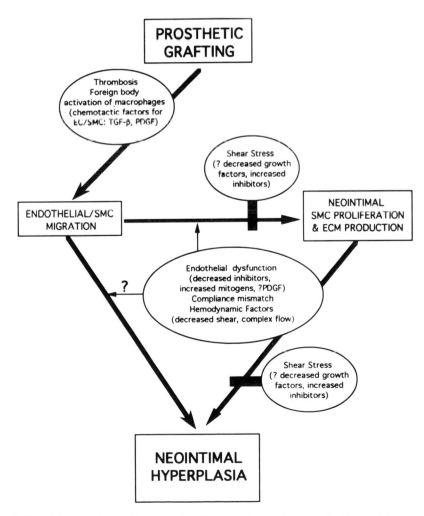

Figure 5. Possible events leading to intimal hyperplasia after prosthetic grafting.

ectomy, may permit such conclusions in the future; however, the series now available for analysis have not used these newer techniques.

While experimental evidence has suggested that a wide variety of agents (warfarin, hirudin, heparin, antiplatelet drugs, angiotensin-converting enzyme inhibitors, calcium antagonists, steroids, cyclosporine, angiopeptin, lipid-lowering drugs, fish oils, anti-oxidants, etc.) hold promise as inhibitors of intimal hyperplasia, none has consistently been shown to produce clinically significant results. This topic has been the subject of a number of comprehensive reviews[157,251,252] and the reader is referred to them for details regarding any individual agent.

The Problem With Animal Models

The fact that so many agents have shown promise in animals, but have failed to show similar results clinically, indicates that the current animal models do not accurately model the problem of clinical restenosis in humans. A better model of arterial injury is clearly needed. The more we learn about restenosis in humans through examination of atherectomy specimens and intravascular imaging techniques, the more apparent it is that the existing animal models are inadequate.

The three-wave paradigm of intimal hyperplasia is founded primarily on the injury of normal rat carotid arteries. While this paradigm is useful for discussion, it may be completely irrelevant to the injury of human atherosclerotic vessels that already have clinically significant intimal pathology. The histologic appearance of atherosclerotic arteries after balloon dilatation differs greatly from normal vessels. Diseased vessels frequently show fracturing of the vessel wall into the tunica media or adventitia.[31,32] Actual fracture or disruption of normal vessel wall architecture is seldom seen when normal vessels are ballooned. Intimal SMC proliferation may not occur to any significant degree after clinical balloon angioplasty or atherectomy.[56] SMC migration may not be that important either, since atherosclerotic vessels already have SMC in the plaque. Exuberant ECM production by existing SMC might be more important clinically than is suggested by animal models which are more focused on SMC proliferation and migration. Animal models, apart from the pig or baboon, may also not adequately reflect the importance of thrombus formation after injury, a process thought to be very important in humans.[50,84]

The clinical problem is restenosis, not necessarily intimal hyperplasia. Animal models reproduce intimal hyperplasia that is histologically very similar to human intimal hyperplasia, but very few animal models reliably produce restenosis or luminal compromise. The pig model of coronary stenting[48] seems to produce restenosis more reliably than most other models, but at the expense of stent placement. The response of an artery to the chronic presence of a stent may not be relevant to other injuries that occur at discrete points in time.

The current and best models for clinical restenosis are humans, themselves. Hopefully, as more techniques become available that permit study of the human lesion as it evolves, we will learn as much about arterial injury in humans as we know now about arterial injury in animals. Based on this knowledge, therapies can be devised that may be more likely to work in humans.

Strategies for the Future

For the most part, the attempts to prevent restenosis and intimal hyperplasia after vascular injury have involved only one agent or a single class of agents. However, it is almost certain that myriad factors, molecules, and pathways interact and cooperate to produce the intimal hyperplastic lesion. Similarly, there is no reason to expect that a single drug or substance will successfully overcome the cascade of cellular events that accompanies vascular injury. In animal models, combinations of several agents have proven to be more potent in reducing the degree of intimal hyperplasia than any single agent.[253,254]

Local drug delivery techniques such as stents[67] or perivascular controlled-release devices[255] may bring higher concentrations of therapeutic agents to bear at sites of injury than could be achieved by systemic administration.

There may be some promise in a more biologic and less pharmacologic approach to intimal hyperplasia. Some of the tools that have been used experimentally to dissect the pathophysiologic mechanisms of intimal hyperplasia may also be useful in treating it. Among these tools are specific antibodies to the growth factors PDGF[184] and bFGF,[37] antisense nucleotides to key mRNA transcripts involved in SMC proliferation,[256] and transferred genes that are expressed focally in the vessel wall.[257,260]

Conclusion

The development of intimal hyperplasia and luminal restenosis will occur in a large proportion of all vascular interventions, often dooming them to clinical failure and the need for reintervention. The mechanisms underlying the development of the restenotic lesion in various forms of injury may be rather distinct (Figures 3 through 5); the factors contributing to the accumulation of intimal tissue in the de-endothelialized, balloon-injured artery may be largely different from those that cause restenosis in vein or prosthetic grafts. The search for a clinical solution to restenosis has mainly focused on coronary angioplasty. The largely negative results in these studies should not automatically be extrapolated to the peripheral vascular surgical patient whose intimal hyperplastic lesion might arise through different mechanisms and, therefore, be more (or less) amenable to therapy.

References

1. Adelman AG, Cohen EA, Kimball BP, et al: A comparison of directional atherectomy with balloon angioplasty for lesions of the left anterior descending coronary artery. *New Engl J Med* 329:228, 1993.

2. Topol EJ, Leya F, Pinkerton CA, et al: A comparison of directional atherectomy with coronary angioplasty in patients with coronary artery disease. *New Engl J Med* 329:221, 1993.

3. Lytle BW, Loop FD, Cosgrove DM, et al: Long-term (5 to 12 years) serial studies of internal mammary artery and saphenous vein coronary bypass grafts. *J Thorac Cardiovasc Surg* 89:248, 1985.

4. Platko WP, Hollman J, Whitlow PL, et al: Percutaneous transluminal angioplasty of saphenous vein graft stenosis: long-term follow-up. *J Am Coll Cardiol* 14:1645, 1989.

5. Healy DA, Zierler RE, Nicholls SC, et al: Long-term follow up and clinical outcome of carotid stenosis. *J Vasc Surg* 10:662, 1989.

6. Johnston KW: Femoral and popliteal arteries: reanalysis of results of balloon angioplasty. *Radiology* 183:767, 1992.

7. Mills JL, Fujitani RM, Taylor SM: The characteristics and anatomic distribution of lesions that cause reversed vein graft failure: a five-year prospective study. *J Vasc Surg* 17:195, 1993.

8. Szilagyi DE, Elliott JP, Hagemann JH, et al: Biologic fate of autogenous vein implants as arterial substitutes: clinical, angiographic, and histopathologic observations in femoro-popliteal operations for atherosclerosis. *Ann Surg* 178:232, 1973.

9. Ip JH, Fuster V, Badimon L, et al: Syndromes of accelerated atherosclerosis: role of vascular injury and smooth muscle proliferation. *J Am Coll Cardiol* 15:1667, 1990.

10. Ross R: The pathogenesis of atherosclerosis: a perspective for the 1990s. *Nature* 362:801, 1993.

11. Sayers RD, Watt PA, Muller S, et al: Structural and functional smooth muscle injury after surgical preparation of reversed and nonreversed (in situ) saphenous vein bypass grafts. *Br J Surg* 78:1256, 1991.

12. Fingerle J, Au YPT, Clowes AW, et al: Intimal lesion formation in rat carotid arteries after endothelial denudation in absence of medial injury. *Arteriosclerosis* 10:1082, 1990.

13. Sarembock IJ, LaVeau PJ, Sigal SL, et al: Influence of inflation pressure and balloon size on the development of intimal hyperplasia after balloon angioplasty: a study in the atherosclerotic rabbit. *Circulation* 80:1029, 1989.

14. Schwartz RS, Huber KC, Murphy JG, et al: Restenosis and the proportional neointimal response to coronary artery injury: results in a porcine model. *J Am Coll Cardiol* 19:267, 1992.

15. Hassenstein S, Hanke H, Kamenz J, et al: Vascular injury and time course of smooth muscle cell prolifera-

tion after experimental holmium laser angioplasty. *Circulation* 86:1575, 1992.

16. Clowes AW, Karnovsky MJ: Suppression by heparin of smooth muscle cell proliferation in injured arteries. *Nature* 265:625, 1977.

17. Baumgartner HR: Eine neue methode zur erzeugung von thromben durch gezeilte uberduhnung der gefasswand. *Z Gesellschaft Exp Med* 137:227, 1963.

18. Johnson DE, Hinohara T, Selmon MR, et al: Primary peripheral arterial stenoses and restenoses excised by transluminal atherectomy: a histopathologic study. *J Am Coll Cardiol* 15:419, 1990.

19. Schnitt SJ, Safian RD, Kuntz RE, et al: Histologic findings in specimens obtained by percutaneous directional coronary atherectomy. *Hum Pathol* 23:415, 1992.

20. Bush HL, Jakubowski JA, Sentissi JM, et al: Neointimal hyperplasia occurring after carotid endarterectomy in a canine model: effect of endothelial cell seeding vs perioperative aspirin. *J Vasc Surg* 5:118, 1987.

21. Szilagyi DE, Smith RF, Elliot JP, et al: Long-term behavior of a dacron arterial substitute: clinical, roentgenologic, and histologic correlations. *Ann Surg* 162:453, 1965.

22. Clowes AW: Intimal hyperplasia and graft failure. *Cardiovasc Pathol* 2:179, 1993.

23. Clowes AW, Reidy MA, Clowes MM: Mechanisms of stenosis after arterial injury. *Lab Invest* 49:208, 1983.

24. Snow AD, Bolender RP, Wight TN, et al: Heparin modulates the composition of the extracellular matrix domain surrounding arterial smooth muscle cells. *Am J Pathol* 137:313, 1990.

25. Kraiss LW, Kirkman TR, Kohler TR, et al: Shear stress regulates smooth muscle proliferation and neointimal thickening in porous polytetrafluoroethylene grafts. *Arteriosclerosis Thromb* 11:1844, 1991.

26. Geary RL, Kohler TR, Vergel S, et al: Time course of flow-induced smooth muscle cell proliferation and intimal thickening in endothelialized baboon vascular grafts. *Circ Res* 74:14, 1994.

27. Kraiss LW, Raines EW, Wilcox JN, et al: Regional expression of the platelet-derived growth factor and its receptors in a primate graft model of vessel wall assembly. *J Clin Invest* 92:338, 1993.

28. van der Wal AC, Becker AE, Elbers JR, et al: An immunocytochemical analysis of rapidly progressive atherosclerosis in human vein grafts. *Eur J Cardiothorac Surg* 6:469, 1992.

29. Holm J, Hansson GK: Cellular and immunologic features of carotid artery disease in man and experimental animal models. *Eur J Vasc Surg* 4:49, 1990.

30. Clowes AW, Reidy MA, Clowes MM: Kinetics of cellular proliferation after arterial injury. I. Smooth muscle growth in the absence of endothelium. *Lab Invest* 49:327, 1983.

31. Castaneda-Zuniga WR, Sibley R, Amplatz K: The pathologic basis of angioplasty. *Angiology* 35:195, 1984.

32. Losordo DW, Rosenfield K, Pieczek A, et al: How does angioplasty work? Serial analysis of human iliac arteries using intravascular ultrasound. *Circulation* 86:1845, 1992.

33. Clowes AW, Schwartz SM: Significance of quiescent smooth muscle migration in the injured rat carotid artery. *Circ Res* 56:139, 1985.

34. Clowes AW, Clowes MM: Kinetics of cellular proliferation after arterial injury. IV. Heparin inhibits rat smooth muscle mitogenesis and migration. *Circ Res* 58:839, 1986.

35. Clowes AW, Clowes MM, Reidy MA: Kinetics of cellular proliferation after arterial injury. III. Endothelial and smooth muscle growth in chronically denuded vessels. *Lab Invest* 54:295, 1986.

36. Lindner V, Lappi DA, Baird A, et al: Role of basic fibroblast growth factor in vascular lesion formation. *Circ Res* 68:106, 1991.

37. Lindner V, Reidy MA: Proliferation of smooth muscle cells after vascular injury is inhibited by an antibody against basic fibroblast growth factor. *Proc Natl Acad Sci USA* 88:3739, 1991.

38. Lindner V, Reidy MA: Expression of basic fibroblast growth factor and its receptor by smooth muscle cells and endothelium in injured rat arteries: an en face study. *Circ Res* 73:589, 1993.

39. Friedman RJ, Stemerman MB, Wenz B, et al: The effect of thrombocytopenia on experimental arteriosclerotic lesion formation in rabbits: smooth muscle cell proliferation and re-endothelialization. *J Clin Invest* 60:1191, 1977.

40. Vashisht R, Sian M, Franks PJ, et al: Long-term reduction of intimal hyperplasia by the selective alpha-1 adrenergic antagonist doxazosin. *Br J Surg* 1992:1285, 1992.

41. Chervu A, Moore WS, Quinones-Baldrich WJ, et al: Efficacy of corticosteroids in suppression of intimal hyperplasia. *J Vasc Surg* 10:129, 1989.

42. Kohler TR, Kirkman TR, Clowes AW: Effect of heparin on adaptation of vein grafts to arterial circulation. *Arteriosclerosis* 9:523, 1989.

43. O'Malley MK, McDermott EW, Mehigan D, et al: Role for prazosin in reducing the development of rabbit intimal hyperplasia after endothelial denudation. *Br J Surg* 76:936, 1989.

44. Gellman J, Ezekowitz MD, Sarembock IJ, et al: Effect of lovastatin on intimal hyperplasia after balloon angioplasty: a study in an atherosclerotic hypercholesterolemic rabbit. *J Am Coll Cardiol* 17:251, 1991.

45. Stevens SL, Hilgarth K, Ryan US, et al: The synergistic effect of hypercholesterolemia and mechanical injury on intimal hyperplasia. *Ann Vasc Surg* 6:55, 1992.

46. Shinomiya M, Shirai K, Saito Y, et al: Inhibition of intimal thickening of the carotid artery of rabbits and of outgrowth of explants of aorta by probucol. *Atherosclerosis* 97:143, 1992.

47. Kisanuki A, Asada Y, Hatakeyama K, et al: Contribution of the endothelium to intimal thickening in normocholesterolemic and hypercholesterolemic rabbits. *Arteriosclerosis Thromb* 12:1198, 1992.

48. Schwartz RS, Murphy JG, Edwards WD, et al: Restenosis after balloon angioplasty: a practical proliferative model in porcine coronary arteries. *Circulation* 82:2190, 1990.

49. Steele PM, Chesebro JH, Stanson AW, et al: Balloon angioplasty: natural history of the pathophysiological response to injury in a pig model. *Circ Res* 57:105, 1985.

50. Harker LA, Kelly AB, Hanson SR: Experimental arterial thrombosis in nonhuman primates. *Circulation* 83:IV41, 1991.

51. Hanson SR, Powell JS, Dodson T, et al: Effects of angiotensin converting enzyme inhibition with cilazapril on intimal hyperplasia in injured arteries and vascular grafts in the baboon. *Hypertension* 18:II 70, 1991.

52. Geary RL, Koyama N, Wang TW, Vergel S, Clowes AW: Failure of heparin to inhibit intimal hyperplasia in injured baboon arteries: the role of heparin-sensitive and -insensitive pathways in the stimulation of smooth muscle cell migration and proliferation. *Circulation* 91:2972–2981, 1995.

53. Simpson JB, Selmon MR, Robertson GC, et al: Transluminal atherectomy for occlusive peripheral vascular disease. *Am J Cardiol* 61:96, 1988.

54. Garratt KN, Holmes DR Jr, Bell MR, et al: Restenosis after directional coronary atherectomy: differences between primary atheromatous and restenosis lesions and influence of subintimal tissue resection. *J Am Coll Cardiol* 16:1665, 1990.

55. Popma JJ, De Cesare NB, Pinkerton CA, et al: Quantitative analysis of factors influencing late lumen loss and restenosis after directional coronary atherectomy. *Am J Cardiol* 71:552, 1993.

56. Garratt KN, Edwards WD, Kaufmann UP, et al: Differential histopathology of primary atherosclerotic and restenotic lesions in coronary arteries and saphenous vein bypass grafts: analysis of tissue obtained from 73 patients by directional atherectomy. *J Am Coll Cardiol* 17:442, 1991.

57. O'Brien ER, Alpers CE, Stewart DK, et al: Proliferation in primary and restenotic coronary atherectomy tissue: implications for antiproliferative therapy. *Circ Res* 73:223, 1993.

58. George BS, Voorhees WD III, Roubin GS, et al: Multicenter investigation of coronary stenting to treat acute or threatened closure after percutaneous transluminal coronary angioplasty: clinical and angiographic outcomes. *J Am Coll Cardiol* 22:135, 1993.

59. Kastrati A, Schomig A, Dietz R, et al: Time course of restenosis during the first year after emergency coronary stenting. *Circulation* 87:1498, 1993.

60. Becker GJ: Intravascular stents: general principles and status of lower-extremity arterial applications. *Circulation* 83:I122, 1991.

61. Anderson PG, Bajaj RK, Baxley WA, et al: Vascular pathology of balloon-expandable flexible coil stents in humans. *J Am Coll Cardiol* 19:372, 1992.

62. van Beusekom HM, van der Giessen WJ, van Suylen R, et al: Histology after stenting of human saphenous vein bypass grafts: observations from surgically excised grafts 3 to 320 days after stent implantation. *J Am Coll Cardiol* 21:45, 1993.

63. Strauss BH, Umans VA, van Suylen RJ, et al: Directional atherectomy for treatment of restenosis within coronary stents: clinical, angiographic, and histologic results. *J Am Coll Cardiol* 20:1465, 1992.

64. Serruys PW, Strauss BH, van Beusekom HM, et al: Stenting of coronary arteries: has a modern Pandora's box been opened? *J Am Coll Cardiol* 17:143, 1991.

65. Kimura T, Nosaka H, Yokoi H, et al: Serial angiographic follow-up after Palmaz-Schatz stent implantation: comparison with conventional balloon angioplasty. *J Am Coll Cardiol* 21:1557, 1993.

66. Zollikofer CL, Antonucci F, Pfyffer M, et al: Arterial stent placement with use of the Wallstent: midterm results of clinical experience. *Radiology* 179:449, 1991.

67. Sapoval MR, Long AL, Raynaud AC, et al: Femoropopliteal stent placement: long-term results. *Radiology* 184:833, 1992.

68. Rogers C, Karnovsky MJ, Edelman ER: Inhibition of experimental neointimal hyperplasia and thrombosis depends on the type of vascular injury and the site of drug administration. *Circulation* 88:1215, 1993.

69. Schatz RA, Palmaz JC, Tio FO, et al: Balloon-expandable intracoronary stents in the adult dog. *Circulation* 76:450, 1987.

70. Karas SP, Gravanis MB, Santoian EC, et al: Coronary intimal proliferation after balloon injury and stenting in swine: an animal model of restenosis. *J Am Coll Cardiol* 20:467, 1992.

71. Rodgers GP, Minor ST, Robinson K, et al: The coronary artery response to implantation of a balloon-expandable flexible stent in the aspirin- and nonaspirin-treated swine model. *Am Heart J* 122:640, 1991.

72. Das MB, Hertzer NR, Ratliff NB, et al: Recurrent carotid stenosis: a five-year series of 65 reoperations. *Ann Surg* 202:28, 1985.

73. Ku DD, Caulfield JB, Kirklin JK: Endothelium-dependent responses in long-term human coronary artery bypass grafts. *Circulation* 83:402, 1991.

74. Berceli SA, Borovetz HS, Sheppeck RA, et al: Mechanisms of vein graft atherosclerosis: LDL metabolism and endothelial actin reorganization. *J Vasc Surg* 13:336, 1991.

75. Sayers RD, Jones L, Varty K, et al: The histopathology of infrainguinal vein graft stenoses. *Eur J Vasc Surg* 7:16, 1993.

76. Park TC, Harker CT, Edwards JM, et al: Human saphenous vein grafts explanted from the arterial circulation demonstrate altered smooth muscle and endothelial responses. *J Vasc Surg* 18:61, 1993.

77. Dilley RJ, McGeachie JK, Prendergast FJ: A review of the histologic changes in vein-to-artery grafts, with particular reference to intimal hyperplasia. *Arch Surg* 123:691, 1988.

78. Zwolak RM, Adams MC, Clowes AW: Kinetics of vein graft hyperplasia: association with tangential stress. *J Vasc Surg* 5:126, 1987.

79. Fann JI, Sokoloff MH, Sarris GE, et al: The reversibility of canine vein-graft arterialization. *Circulation* 82:IV 9, 1990.

80. Dobrin PB, Littooy FN, Golan J, et al: Mechanical and histologic changes in canine vein grafts. *J Surg Res* 44:259, 1988.

81. Violaris AG, Newby AC, Angelini GD: Effects of external stenting on wall thickening in arteriovenous bypass grafts. *Ann Thorac Surg* 55:667, 1993.

82. McCann RL, Hagen P-O, Fuchs JCA: Aspirin and dipyridamole decrease intimal hyperplasia in experimental vein grafts. *Ann Surg* 191:238, 1980.

83. Davies MG, Klyachkin ML, Dalen H, et al: Regression of intimal hyperplasia with restoration of endothelium-dependent relaxing factor-mediated relaxation in experimental vein grafts. *Surgery* 114:258, 1993.

84. Kohler TR, Kirkman TR, Gordon D, et al: Mechanism of long-term degeneration of arterialized vein grafts. *Am J Surg* 160:257, 1990.

85. Fuster V, Badimon L, Badimon JJ, et al: The porcine model for the understanding of thrombogenesis and atherogenesis. *Mayo Clin Proc* 66:818, 1991.

86. Sayers RD, Watt PA, Muller S, et al: Endothelial cell injury secondary to surgical preparation of reversed and in situ saphenous vein bypass grafts. *Eur J Vasc Surg* 6:354, 1992.

87. Cambria RP, Megerman J, Abbott WM: Endothelial preservation in reversed and in situ autogenous vein grafts: a quantitative experimental study. *Ann Surg* 202:50, 1985.

88. Yang Z, Luscher TF: Endothelium-dependent regulatory mechanisms in human coronary bypass grafts: possible clinical implications. *Z Kardiol* 78:80, 1989.

89. Martin JF, Booth RF, Moncada S: Arterial wall hypoxia following thrombosis of the vasa vasorum is an initial lesion in atherosclerosis. *Eur J Clin Invest* 21:355, 1991.

90. Hagen PO, Davies MG, Schuman RW, et al: Reduction of vein graft intimal hyperplasia by ex vivo treatment with desferrioxamine manganese. *J Vasc Res* 29:405, 1992.

91. Milnor WR: *Hemodynamics*. 2nd ed. Baltimore: Williams & Wilkins; 419, 1989.

92. Wolinsky H, Glagov S: A lamellar unit of aortic medial structure and function in mammals. *Circ Res* XX:99, 1967.

93. Owens GK: Influence of blood pressure on development of aortic medial smooth muscle hypertrophy in spontaneously hypertensive rats. *Hypertension* 9:178, 1987.

94. Berceli SA, Showalter DP, Sheppeck RA, et al: Biomechanics of the venous wall under simulated arterial conditions. *J Biomech* 23:985, 1990.

95. Kohler TR, Kirkman TR, Clowes AW: The effect of rigid external support on vein graft adaptation to the arterial circulation. *J Vasc Surg* 9:277, 1989.

96. Rittgers SE, Karayannacos PE, Guy JF, et al: Velocity distribution and intimal proliferation in autologous vein grafts in dogs. *Circ Res* 42:792, 1978.

97. Berguer R, Higgins RF, Reddy DJ: Intimal hyperplasia: an experimental study. *Arch Surg* 115:332, 1980.

98. Dobrin PB, Littooy FN, Endean ED: Mechanical factors predisposing to intimal hyperplasia and medial thickening in autogenous vein grafts. *Surgery* 105:393, 1989.

99. Berger K, Sauvage LR, Rao AM, et al: Healing of arterial prostheses in man: its incompleteness. *Ann Surg* 175:118, 1972.

100. Kohler TR, Stratton JR, Kirkman TR, et al: Conventional versus high-porosity polytetrafluoroethylene grafts: clinical evaluation. *Surgery* 112:901, 1992.

101. Sottiurai VS, Yao JST, Flinn WR, et al: Intimal hyperplasia and neointima: an ultrastructural analysis of thrombosed grafts in humans. *Surgery* 93:809, 1983.

102. Guidoin R, Chakf'e N, Maurel S, et al: Expanded polytetrafluoroethylene arterial prostheses in humans: histopathological study of 298 surgically excised grafts. *Biomaterials* 14:678, 1993.

103. Clowes AW, Gown AM, Hanson SR, et al: Mechanisms of arterial graft failure. I. Role of cellular proliferation in early healing of PTFE prostheses. *Am J Pathol* 118:43, 1985.

104. Clowes AW, Kirkman TR, Clowes MM: Mechanisms of arterial graft failure. II. Chronic endothelial and smooth muscle cell proliferation in healing polytetrafluoroethylene prostheses. *J Vasc Surg* 3:877, 1986.

105. Clowes AW, Kirkman TR, Reidy MA: Mechanisms of arterial graft healing: rapid transmural capillary ingrowth provides a source of intimal endothelium and smooth muscle in porous PTFE prostheses. *Am J Pathol* 123:220, 1986.

106. Golden MA, Hanson SR, Kirkman TR, et al: Healing of polytetrafluoroethylene arterial grafts is influenced by graft porosity. *J Vasc Surg* 11:838, 1990.

107. Clowes AW, Zacharias RK, Kirkman TR: Early endothelial coverage of synthetic arterial grafts: porosity revisited. *Am J Surg* 153:501, 1987.

108. Reidy MA, Chao SS, Kirkman TR, et al: Endothelial regeneration VI. Chronic nondenuding injury in baboon vascular grafts. *Am J Pathol* 123:432, 1986.

109. Zacharias RK, Kirkman TR, Clowes AW: Mechanisms of healing in synthetic grafts. *J Vasc Surg* 6:429, 1987.

110. Zacharias RK, Kirkman TR, Kenagy RD, et al: Growth factor production by polytetrafluoroethylene vascular grafts. *J Vasc Surg* 7:606, 1988.

111. Golden MA, Au YPT, Kirkman TR, et al: Platelet-derived growth factor activity and mRNA expression in healing vascular grafts in baboons: association in vivo of platelet-derived growth factor mRNA and protein with cellular proliferation. *J Clin Invest* 87:406, 1991.

112. Golden MA, Au YPT, Kenagy RD, et al: Growth factor gene expression by intimal cells in healing polytetrafluoroethylene grafts. *J Vasc Surg* 11:580, 1990.

113. Kaufman BR, Fox PL, Graham LM: Platelet-derived growth factor production by canine aortic grafts seeded with endothelial cells. *J Vasc Surg* 15:699, 1992.

114. Kaufman BR, DeLuca DJ, Folsom DL, et al: Elevated platelet-derived growth factor production by aortic grafts implanted on a long-term basis in a canine model. *J Vasc Surg* 15:806, 1992.

115. Bonfield TL, Colton E, Marchant RE, et al: Cytokine and growth factor production by monocytes/macrophages on protein preadsorbed polymers. *J Biomed Mater Res* 26:837, 1992.

116. Miller KM, Anderson JM: In vitro stimulation of fibroblast activity by factors generated from human monocytes activated by biomedical polymers. *J Biomed Mater Res* 23:911, 1989.

117. Greisler HP, Dennis JW, Endean ED, et al: Macrophage/biomaterial interactions: the stimulation of endothelialization. *J Vasc Surg* 9:588, 1989.

118. Miller KM, Huskey RA, Bigby LF, et al: Characterization of biomedical polymer-adherent macrophages: interleukin-1 generation and scanning electron microscopy studies. *Biomaterials* 10:187, 1989.

119. Miller KM, Anderson JM: Human monocyte/macrophage activation and interleukin-1 generation by biomedical polymers. *J Biomed Mater Res* 22:713, 1988.

120. Cantelmo NL, Quist WC, LoGerfo FW: Quantitative analysis of anastomotic intimal hyperplasia in paired Dacron and PTFE grafts. *J Cardiovasc Surg* 30:910, 1989.

121. Fasol R, Zilla P, Deutsch M, et al: Human endothelial cell seeding: evaluation of its effectiveness by platelet parameters after one year. *J Vasc Surg* 9:432, 1989.

122. Stratton JR, Thiele BL, Ritchie JL: Platelet deposition on Dacron aortic bifurcation grafts in man: quantitation with indium-111 platelet imaging. *Circulation* 66:1287, 1982.

123. Hasson JE, Megerman J, Abbott WM: Increased compliance near vascular anastomoses. *J Vasc Surg* 2:419, 1985.

124. Wilson E, Mai Q, Sudhir K, et al: Mechanical strain induces growth of vascular smooth muscle cells via autocrine action of PDGF. *J Cell Biol* 123:741, 1993.

125. Iba T, Maitz S, Furbert T, et al: Effect of cyclic stretch on endothelial cells from different vascular beds. *Circ Shock* 35:193, 1991.

126. Sumpio BE, Banes AJ, Link WG, et al: Enhanced collagen production by smooth muscle cells during repetitive mechanical stretching. *Arch Surg* 123:1233, 1988.

127. Bassiouny HS, White S, Glagov S, et al: Anastomotic intimal hyperplasia: mechanical injury or flow induced. *J Vasc Surg* 15:708, 1992.

128. Zarins CK, Giddens DP, Bharadvaj BK, et al: Carotid bifurcation atherosclerosis: quantitative correlation of plaque localization with flow velocity profiles and wall shear stress. *Circ Res* 53:502, 1983.

129. Binns RL, Ku DN, Stewart MT, et al: Optimal graft diameter: effect of wall shear stress on vascular healing. *J Vasc Surg* 10:326, 1989.

130. Kohler TR, Kirkman TR, Kraiss LW, et al: Increased blood flow inhibits neointimal hyperplasia in endothelialized vascular grafts. *Circ Res* 69:1557, 1991.

131. Friedman MH, Bargeron CB, Deters OJ, et al: Correlation between wall shear and intimal thickness at a coronary artery branch. *Atherosclerosis* 68:27, 1987.

132. Wagner DD, Bonfanti R: von Willebrand factor and the endothelium. *Mayo Clin Proc* 66:621, 1991.

133. Ruiter DJ, Schlingemann RO, Rietveld FJ, et al: Monoclonal antibody-defined human endothelial antigens as vascular markers. *J Invest Dermatol* 93:25, 1989.

134. Schwartz SM, Heimark RL, Majesky MW: Developmental mechanisms underlying pathology of arteries. *Physiol Rev* 70:1177, 1990.

135. Frangos JA, Eskin SG, McIntire LV, et al: Flow effects on prostacyclin production by cultured human endothelial cells. *Science* 227:1477, 1985.

136. Moncada S, Palmer RMJ, Higgs EA: Nitric oxide: physiology, pathophysiology, and pharmacology. *Pharmacol Rev* 43:109, 1991.

137. van Hinsbergh VW: Regulation of the synthesis and secretion of plasminogen activators by endothelial cells. *Haemost* 18:307, 1988.

138. Marcum JA, Atha DH, Fritze LM, et al: Cloned bovine aortic endothelial cells synthesize anticoagulantly active heparan sulfate proteoglycan. *J Biol Chem* 361:7507, 1986.

139. De Mey JGR, Schiffers PM: Effects of the endothelium on growth responses in arteries. *J Cardiovasc Pharmacol* 21:S22, 1993.

140. Castellot JJ Jr, Favreau LV, Karnovsky MJ, et al: Inhibition of vascular smooth muscle cell growth by endothelial cell-derived heparin: possible role of a platelet endoglycosidase. *J Biol Chem* 257:11256, 1982.

141. Shepherd JT, Katusi'c ZS: Endothelium-derived vasoactive factors: I. Endothelium-dependent relaxation. *Hypertension* 18:III76, 1991.

142. Yanagisawa M, Kurihara H, Kimura S, et al: A novel potent vasoconstrictor peptide produced by vascular endothelial cells. *Nature* 332:411, 1988.

143. Langille BL, O'Donnell F: Reductions in arterial diameter produced by chronic decreases in blood flow are endothelium-dependent. *Science* 231:405, 1986.

144. Davies PF, Dewey CF Jr, Bussolari SR, et al: Influence of hemodynamic forces on vascular endothelial function: in vitro studies of shear stress and pinocytosis in bovine aortic cells. *J Clin Invest* 73:1121, 1984.

145. Diamond SL, Eskin SG, McIntire LV: Fluid flow stimulates tissue plasminogen activator secretion by cultured human endothelial cells. *Science* 243:1483, 1989.

146. Sharefkin JB, Diamond SL, Eskin SG, et al: Fluid flow decreases preproendothelin mRNA levels and suppresses endothelin-1 peptide release in cultured human endothelial cells. *J Vasc Surg* 14:1, 1991.

147. Resnick N, Collins T, Atkinson W, et al: Platelet-derived growth factor B chain promoter contains a cis-acting fluid shear-stress-responsive element. *Proc Natl Acad Sci USA* 90:4591, 1993.

148. Chamley JH, Campbell GR, McConnell JD, et al: Comparison of vascular smooth muscle cells from adult human, monkey, and rabbit in primary culture and in subculture. *Cell Tissue Res* 177:503, 1977.

149. Gabbiani G, Kocher O, Bloom WS, et al: Actin expression in smooth muscle cells of rat aortic intimal thicken-

ing, human atheromatous plaque, and cultured rat aortic media. *J Clin Invest* 73:148, 1984.

150. Kocher O, Skalli O, Bloom WS, et al: Cytoskeleton of rat aortic smooth muscle cells: normal conditions and experimental intimal thickening. *Lab Invest* 50:645, 1984.

151. Schwartz SM, Campbell GR, Campbell JH: Replication of smooth muscle cells in vascular disease. *Circ Res* 58:427, 1986.

152. Chamley JH, Campbell GR: Trophic influences of sympathetic nerves and cyclic AMP on differentiation and proliferation of isolated smooth muscle cells in culture. *Cell Tiss Res* 161:497, 1975.

153. Furie B, Furie BC: Molecular and cellular biology of blood coagulation. *New Engl J Med* 326:800, 1992.

154. Pankowsky DA, Ziats NP, Topham NS, et al: Morphologic characteristics of adsorbed human plasma proteins on vascular grafts and biomaterials. *J Vasc Surg* 11:599, 1990.

155. Okazaki H, Majesky MW, Harker LA, et al: Regulation of platelet-derived growth factor ligand and receptor gene expression by alpha-thrombin in vascular smooth muscle cells. *Circ Res* 71:1285, 1992.

156. Lindner V, Reidy MA, Fingerle J: Regrowth of arterial endothelium: denudation with minimal trauma leads to complete endothelial cell regrowth. *Lab Invest* 61:556, 1989.

157. Clowes AW, Clowes MM, Fingerle J, et al: Regulation of smooth muscle cell growth in injured artery. *J Cardiovasc Pharmacol* 14:S12, 1989.

158. Jackson CL, Schwartz SM: Pharmacology of smooth muscle cell replication. *Hypertension* 20:713, 1992.

159. Goldberg ID, Stemerman MB, Handin RI: Vascular permeation of platelet factor 4 after endothelial injury. *Science* 209:611, 1980.

160. Chan P, Munro E, Patel M, et al: Cellular biology of human intimal hyperplastic stenosis. *Eur J Vasc Surg* 7:129, 1993.

161. Weintraub WS, Brown CL, Liberman HA, et al: Effect of restenosis at one previously dilated coronary site on the probability of restenosis at another previously dilated coronary site. *Am J Cardiol* 72:1107, 1993.

162. Castellot JJ Jr, Addonizio ML, Rosenberg R, et al: Cultured endothelial cells produce a heparinlike inhibitor of smooth muscle cell growth. *J Cell Biol* 90:372, 1981.

163. Fritze LM, Reilly CF, Rosenberg RD: An antiproliferative heparan sulfate species produced by postconfluent smooth muscle cells. *J Cell Biol* 100:1041, 1985.

164. Clowes AW, Clowes MM: Kinetics of cellular proliferation after arterial injury. II. Inhibition of smooth muscle growth by heparin. *Lab Invest* 52:611, 1985.

165. Reilly CF, Kindy MS, Brown KE, et al: Heparin prevents vascular smooth muscle cell progression through the G1 phase of the cell cycle. *Biol Chem* 264:6990, 1989.

166. Reilly CF, Fritze LM, Rosenberg RD: Antiproliferative effects of heparin on vascular smooth muscle cells are reversed by epidermal growth factor. *J Cell Physiol* 131:149, 1987.

167. Reilly CF, Fritze LM, Rosenberg RD: Heparin inhibition of smooth muscle cell proliferation: a cellular site of action. *J Cell Physiol* 129:11, 1986.

168. Antonelli-Orlidge A, Saunders KB, Smith SR, et al: An activated form of transforming growth factor beta is produced by cocultures of endothelial cells and pericytes. *Proc Nat'l Acad Sci USA* 86:4544, 1989.

169. Battegay EJ, Raines EW, Seifert RA, et al: TGF-β induces bimodal proliferation of connective tissue cells via complex control of an autocrine PDGF loop. *Cell* 63:515, 1990.

170. Itoh H, Mukoyama M, Pratt RE, et al: Multiple autocrine growth factors modulate vascular smooth muscle cell growth response to angiotensin II. *J Clin Invest* 91:2268, 1993.

171. McCaffrey TA, Falcone DJ, Brayton CF, et al: Transforming growth factor-beta activity is potentiated by heparin via dissociation of the transforming growth factor-beta/alpha 2-macroglobulin inactive complex. *J Cell Biol* 109:441, 1989.

172. Garg UC, Hassid A: Nitric oxide-generating vasodilators and 8-bromo-cyclic guanosine monophosphate inhibit mitogenesis and proliferation of cultured rat vascular smooth muscle cells. *J Clin Invest* 83:1774, 1989.

173. Porter JG, Catalano R, McEnroe G, et al: C-type natriuretic peptide inhibits growth factor-dependent DNA synthesis in smooth muscle cells. *Am J Physiol* 263:C1001, 1992.

174. Kariya K, Kawahara Y, Araki S, et al: Antiproliferative action of cyclic GMP-elevating vasodilators in cultured rabbit aortic smooth muscle cells. *Atherosclerosis* 80:143, 1989.

175. Ross R, Glomset J, Kariya B, et al: A platelet-dependent serum factor that stimulates the proliferation of arterial smooth muscle cells in vitro. *Proc Natl Acad Sci USA* 71:1207, 1974.

176. Raines EW, Bowen-Pope DF, Ross R: Platelet-derived growth factor. In: Sporn MB, Roberts AB(eds). *Handbook of Experimental Pharmacology: Peptide Growth Factors.* New York: Springer-Verlag, Inc; 173, 1990.

177. Seifert RA, Hart CE, Phillips PE, et al: Two different subunits associate to create isoform-specific platelet-derived growth factor receptors. *J Biol Chem* 264:8771, 1989.

178. Fingerle J, Johnson R, Clowes AW, et al: Role of platelets in smooth muscle cell proliferation and migration after vascular injury in rat carotid artery. *Proc Natl Acad Sci USA* 86:8412, 1989.

179. Fox PL, DiCorleto PE: Regulation of production of a platelet-derived growth factor-like protein by cultured bovine aortic endothelial cells. *J Cell Physiol* 121:298, 1984.

180. Barrett TB, Benditt EP: Platelet-derived growth factor gene expression in human atherosclerotic plaques and normal artery wall. *Proc Natl Acad Sci USA* 85:2810, 1988.

181. DiCorleto PE, Bowen-Pope DF: Cultured endothelial cells produce a platelet-derived growth factor-like protein. *Proc Natl Acad Sci USA* 80:1919, 1983.

182. Majesky MW, Reidy MA, Bowen-Pope DF, et al: PDGF ligand and receptor gene expression during repair of arterial injury. *J Cell Biol* 111:2149, 1990.

183. Libby P, Warner SJ, Salomon RN, et al: Production of platelet-derived growth factor-like mitogen by smooth-muscle cells from human atheroma. *New Engl J Med* 318:1493, 1988.

184. Walker LN, Bowen-Pope DF, Ross R, et al: Production of platelet-derived growth factor-like molecules by cultured arterial smooth muscle cells accompanies proliferation after arterial injury. *Proc Natl Acad Sci USA* 83:7311, 1986.

185. Ferns GA, Raines EW, Sprugel KH, et al: Inhibition of neointimal smooth muscle accumulation after angioplasty by an antibody to PDGF. *Science* 253:1129, 1991.

186. Jawien A, Bowen-Pope DF, Lindner V, et al: Platelet-

derived growth factor promotes smooth muscle migration and intimal thickening in a rat model of balloon angioplasty. *J Clin Invest* 89:507, 1992.

187. D'Amore PA: Modes of FGF release in vivo and in vitro. *Canc Metastasis Rev* 9:227, 1990.

188. Thompson RW, Whalen GF, Saunders KB, et al: Heparin-mediated release of fibroblast growth factor-like activity into the circulation of rabbits. *Growth Factors* 3:221, 1990.

189. Mignatti P, Morimoto T, Rifkin DB: Basic fibroblast growth factor, a protein devoid of secretory signal sequence, is released by cells via a pathway independent of the endoplasmic reticulum-Golgi complex. *J Cell Physiol* 151:81, 1992.

190. McNeil PL, Muthukrishnan L, Warder E, et al: Growth factors are released by mechanically wounded endothelial cells. *J Cell Biol* 109:811, 1989.

191. Jamal A, Bendeck M, Langille BL: Structural changes and recovery of function after arterial injury. *Arteriosclerosis Thromb* 12:307, 1992.

192. Griendling KK, Murphy TJ, Alexander RW: Molecular biology of the renin-angiotensin system. *Circulation* 87:1816, 1993.

193. Campbell DJ: Circulating and tissue angiotensin systems. *J Clin Invest* 79:1, 1987.

194. Cambell-Boswell M, Robertson AL Jr: Effects of angiotensin II and vasopressin on human smooth muscle cells in vitro. *Exp Mol Pathol* 35:265, 1981.

195. Naftilan AJ, Pratt RE, Eldridge CS, et al: Angiotensin II induces c-fos expression in smooth muscle via transcriptional control. *Hypertension* 13:706, 1989.

196. Naftilan AJ, Pratt RE, Dzau VJ: Induction of platelet-derived growth factor A-chain and c-myc gene expressions by angiotensin II in cultured rat vascular smooth muscle cells. *J Clin Invest* 83:1419, 1989.

197. Bos TJ: Oncogenes and cell growth. *Adv Exp Med Biol* 321:45, 1992.

198. Rakugi H, Jacob HJ, Krieger JE, et al: Vascular injury induces angiotensinogen gene expression in the media and neointima. *Circulation* 87:283, 1993.

199. Viswanathan M, Stromberg C, Seltzer A, et al: Balloon angioplasty enhances expression of angiotensin II AT1 receptors in neointima of rat aorta. *J Clin Invest* 90:1707, 1992.

200. Janiak P, Pillon A, Prost J-F, et al: Role of angiotensin subtype 2 receptor in neointima formation after vascular injury. *Hypertension* 20:737, 1992.

201. Prescott MF, Webb RL, Reidy MA: Angiotensin-converting enzyme inhibitor versus angiotensin II, AT1 receptor antagonist: effects on smooth muscle cell migration and proliferation after balloon catheter injury. *Am J Pathol* 139:1291, 1991.

202. Osterrieder W, Muller RK, Powell JS, et al: Role of angiotensin II in injury-induced neointimal formation in rats. *Hypertension* 18:II60, 1991.

203. Laporte S, Escher E: Neointima formation after vascular injury is angiotensin II mediated. *Biochem Biophys Res Comm* 187:1510, 1992.

204. Daemen MJAP, Lombardi DM, Bosman FT, et al: Angiotensin II induces smooth muscle cell proliferation in the normal and injured rat arterial wall. *Circ Res* 68:450, 1991.

205. van Kleef EM, Smits JFM, De Mey JGR, et al: alpha-1-adrenoreceptor blockade reduces the angiotensin II-induced vascular smooth muscle cell DNA synthesis in the rat thoracic aorta and carotid artery. *Circ Res* 70:1122, 1992.

206. Sarembock IJ, Gertz SD, Gimple LW, et al: Effectiveness of recombinant desulphatohirudin in reducing restenosis after balloon angioplasty of atherosclerotic femoral arteries in rabbits. *Circulation* 84:232, 1991.

207. Bevan RD: Effect of sympathetic denervation on smooth muscle cell proliferation in the growing rabbit ear artery. *Circ Res* 37:14, 1975.

208. Jackson CL, Bush RC, Bowyer DE: Inhibitory effect of calcium antagonists on balloon catheter-induced arterial smooth muscle cell proliferation and lesion size. *Atherosclerosis* 69:115, 1988.

209. Majesky MW, Daemen MJ, Schwartz SM: Alpha 1-adrenergic stimulation of platelet-derived growth factor A-chain gene expression in rat aorta. *J Biol Chem* 265:1082, 1990.

210. Takuwa Y, Yanagisawa M, Takuwa N, et al: Endothelin, its diverse biological activities and mechanisms of action. *Prog Growth Factor Res* 1:195, 1989.

211. Carey DJ: Control of growth and differentiation of vascular cells by extracellular matrix proteins. *Annu Rev Physiol* 53:161, 1991.

212. Pauly RR, Passaniti A, Crow M, et al: Experimental models that mimic the differentiation and dedifferentiation of vascular cells. *Circulation* 86:III68, 1992.

213. Murphy G, Doherty AJ: The matrix metalloproteinases and their inhibitors. *Am J Respir Cell Mol Biol* 7:120, 1992.

214. Tooney PA, Agrez MV, Burns GF: A re-examination of the molecular basis of cell movement. *Immunol Cell Biol* 71:131, 1993.

215. Clowes AW, Clowes MM, Au YPT, et al: Smooth muscle cells express urokinase during mitogenesis and tissue-type plasminogen activator during migration in injured rat carotid artery. *Circ Res* 67:61, 1990.

216. Jackson CL, Raines EW, Ross R, et al: Role of endogenous platelet-derived growth factor in arterial smooth muscle cell migration after balloon catheter injury. *Arteriosclerosis Thromb* 13:1218, 1993.

217. Au YPT, Kenagy RD, Clowes AW: Heparin selectively inhibits the transcription of tissue-type plasminogen activator in primate arterial smooth muscle cells during mitogenesis. *J Biol Chem* 267:3438, 1992.

218. Au YP, Montgomery KF, Clowes AW: Heparin inhibits collagenase gene expression mediated by phorbol ester-responsive element in primate arterial smooth muscle cells. *Circ Res* 70:1062, 1992.

219. Clowes AW, Clowes MM, Kirkman TR, et al: Heparin inhibits the expression of tissue-type plasminogen activator by smooth muscle cells in injured rat carotid artery. *Circ Res* 70:1128, 1992.

220. Majack RA, Clowes AW: Inhibition of vascular smooth muscle cell migration by heparin-like glycosaminoglycans. *J Cell Physiol* 118:253, 1984.

221. Madri JA, Bell L, Marx M, et al: Effects of soluble factors and extracellular matrix components on vascular cell behavior in vitro and in vivo: models of de-endothelialization and repair. *J Cell Biochem* 45:123, 1991.

222. Sprugel KH, McPherson JM, Clowes AW, et al: Effects of growth factors in vivo. I. Cell ingrowth into porous subcutaneous chambers. *Am J Pathol* 129:601, 1987.

223. Koyama N, Morisaki N, Saito Y, et al: Regulatory effects of platelet-derived growth factor-AA homodimer on migration of vascular smooth muscle cells. *J Biol Chem* 267:22806, 1992.

224. Bell L, Madri JA: Influence of the angiotensin system

on endothelial and smooth muscle cell migration. *Am J Pathol* 137:7, 1990.

225. Rifkin DB, Moscatelli D, Bizik J, et al: Growth factor control of extracellular proteolysis. *Cell Differ Dev* 32: 313, 1990.

226. Koyama N, Hart CE, Clowes AW: Different functions of alpha- and beta-receptors for platelet-derived growth factor (PDGF) in the migration and proliferation of cultured primate smooth muscle cells. *Circulation* 88:I-468, 1993.

227. Koyama N, Koshikawa T, Morisaki N, et al: Bifunctional effects of transforming growth factor-beta on migration of cultured rat aortic smooth muscle cells. *Biochem Biophys Res Comm* 169:725, 1990.

228. Wilcox JN, Smith KM, Williams LT, et al: Platelet-derived growth factor mRNA detection in human atherosclerotic plaques by in situ hybridization. *J Clin Invest* 82:1134, 1988.

229. O'Brien ER, Schwartz SM: Update on the biology and clinical study of restenosis. *Trends Cardiovasc Med* 4:169–178, 1994.

230. Birinyi LK, Warner SJC, Salomon RN, et al: Observations on human smooth muscle cell cultures from hyperplastic lesions of prosthetic bypass grafts: production of a platelet-derived growth factor-like mitogen and expression of a gene for a platelet-derived growth factor receptor—a preliminary study. *J Vasc Surg* 10:157, 1989.

231. Majesky MW, Giachelli CM, Reidy MA, et al: Rat carotid neointimal smooth muscle cells reexpress a developmentally regulated mRNA phenotype during repair of arterial injury. *Circ Res* 71:759, 1992.

232. Majesky MW, Benditt EP, Schwartz SM: Expression and developmental control of platelet-derived growth factor A-chain and B-chain/Sis genes in rat aortic smooth muscle cells. *Proc Natl Acad Sci USA* 85:1524, 1988.

233. Olson NE, Chao S, Lindner V, et al: Intimal smooth muscle cell proliferation after balloon catheter injury: the role of basic fibroblast growth factor. *Am J Pathol* 140:1017, 1992.

234. Majack RA, Majesky MW, Goodman LV: Role of PDGF-A expression in the control of vascular smooth muscle cell growth by transforming growth factor-β. *J Cell Biol* 111:239, 1990.

235. Majesky MW, Lindner V, Twardzik DR, et al: Production of transforming growth factor beta 1 during repair of arterial injury. *J Clin Invest* 88:904, 1991.

236. Nikol S, Isner JM, Pickering JG, et al: Expression of transforming growth factor-beta 1 is increased in human vascular restenosis lesions. *J Clin Invest* 90:1582, 1992.

237. Ferns GA, Motani AS, Anggard EE: The insulin-like growth factors: their putative role in atherogenesis. *Artery* 18:197, 1991.

238. Hansson GK, Jonasson L, Holm J, et al: Gamma-interferon regulates vascular smooth muscle proliferation and Ia antigen expression in vivo and in vitro. *Circ Res* 63:712, 1988.

239. Raines EW, Dower SK, Ross R: Interleukin-1 mitogenic activity for fibroblasts and smooth muscle cells is due to PDGF-AA. *Science* 243:393, 1989.

240. Kraiss LW, Geary RL, Mattsson EJR, Vergel S, Au YPT, Clowes AW: Acute reductions in blood flow and shear stress induce PDGF-A expresssion in baboon prosthetic grafts. *Circ Res* 70:45–53, 1996.

241. Pierce GF, Vande Berg J, Rudolph R, et al: Platelet-derived growth factor-BB and transforming growth factor beta 1 selectively modulate glycosaminoglycans, collagen, and myofibroblasts in excisional wounds. *Am J Pathol* 138:629, 1991.

242. Glagov S, Weisenberg E, Zarins CK, et al: Compensatory enlargement of human atherosclerotic coronary arteries. *New Engl J Med* 316:1371, 1987.

243. Davies PF, Remuzzi A, Gordon EJ, et al: Turbulent fluid shear stress induces vascular endothelial turnover in vitro. *Proc Natl Acad Sci USA* 83:2114, 1986.

244. Sterpetti AV, Cucina A, D'Angelo LS, et al: Response of arterial smooth muscle cells to laminar flow. *J Cardiovasc Surg* 33:619, 1992.

245. Kohler TR, Jawien A: Flow affects development of intimal hyperplasia after arterial injury in rats. *Arteriosclerosis Thromb* 12:963, 1992.

246. Burgess WH, Maciag T: The heparin-binding (fibroblast) growth factor family of proteins. *Annu Rev Biochem* 58:575, 1989.

247. Lindner V, Majack RA, Reidy MA: Basic fibroblast growth factor stimulates endothelial regrowth and proliferation in denuded arteries. *J Clin Invest* 85:2004, 1990.

248. Ferrara N, Houck KA, Jakeman LB, et al: The vascular endothelial growth factor family of polypeptides. *J Cell Biochem* 47:211, 1991.

249. Herring MB: Endothelial cell seeding. *J Vasc Surg* 13: 731, 1991.

250. Herring MB: The use of endothelial seeding of prosthetic arterial bypass grafts. *Surg Annu* 23 Pt 2:157, 1991.

251. Ortenwall P, Wadenvik H, Risberg B: Reduced platelet deposition on seeded versus unseeded segments of expanded polytetrafluoroethylene grafts: clinical observations after a 6-month follow-up. *J Vasc Surg* 10:374, 1989.

252. Herring MB, LeGrand DR: The histology of seeded PTFE grafts in humans. *Ann Vasc Surg* 3:96, 1989.

253. Herrman J-PR, Hermans WRM, Vos J, et al: Pharmacological approaches to the prevention of restenosis following angioplasty: the search for the Holy Grail? (Part 1). *Drugs* 46:18, 1993.

254. Herrman J-PR, Hermans WRM, Vos J, et al: Pharmacological approaches to the prevention of restenosis following angioplasty: the search for the Holy Grail? (Part II). *Drugs* 46:249, 1993.

255. Clowes AW, Clowes MM, Vergel SC, et al: Heparin and cilazapril together inhibit injury-induced intimal hyperplasia. *Hypertension* 18:II-65, 1991.

256. Berk BC, Gordon JB, Alexander RW: Pharmacologic roles of heparin and glucocorticoids to prevent restenosis after coronary angioplasty. *J Am Coll Cardiol* 17: 111, 1991.

257. Edelman ER, Nugent MA, Karnovsky MJ: Perivascular and intravenous administration of basic fibroblast growth factor: vascular and solid organ deposition. *Proc Natl Acad Sci USA* 90:1513, 1993.

258. Simons M, Edelman ER, DeKeyser JL, et al: Antisense c-myb oligonucleotides inhibit intimal arterial smooth muscle cell accumulation in vivo. *Nature* 359:67, 1992.

259. Lynch CM, Clowes MM, Osborne WRA, et al: Long-term expression of human adenosine deaminase in vascular smooth muscle cells of rats: a model for gene therapy. *Proc Natl Acad Sci USA* 89:1138, 1992.

260. Plautz G, Nabel EG, Nabel GJ: Introduction of vascular smooth muscle cells expressing recombinant genes in vivo. *Circulation* 83:578, 1991.

CHAPTER 11

Atherosclerosis:
Theories of Etiology and Pathogenesis
Ralph G. DePalma, MD

In the previous text, this chapter[1] considered atherosclerosis and reactions of the injured arterial wall together. The reasons for this were evident particularly to vascular surgeons who recognized that arterial trauma, such as clamping or balloon injury, can produce stenoses and that vascular injuries, ranging from minor to severe, might initiate myointimal hyperplasia or atheroma. One of the theories of atherogenesis at that time was that this process was most often a response to injury. In that scenario, physical or chemical agents caused endothelial denudation leading to platelet adherence and subsequent release of platelet-derived growth factor (PDGF)[2] which then triggered smooth muscle cell migration from the media to the intima, smooth muscle cell proliferation, and lipid accumulation. This sequence applies in specific situations with injury of the arterial wall when the internal elastic lamina is disrupted by a deep longitudinal injury.[3]

However, the injury hypothesis initially proposed by Ross and Glomset[4] was not completely supported by subsequent investigations. These showed that arterial denudation is a rare event in early atherogenesis in humans and animals, although endothelial cells can be injured and remain in place.[5,6] Virtually all of the cells of the arterial wall are capable of secreting growth factors which, if not identical to PDGF and its derivatives, are quite similar to it. Thus, the role of autocrine or local cell-derived growth factors were later emphasized in the development of the atherosclerotic plaque as a useful working concept in considering mechanisms of atherogenesis.[5]

The responses of the arterial wall after injury remain of interest both in atherogenesis and intimal hyperplasia. In the last 7 years, considerable conceptual change has occurred. Chapter 10 of this volume details a ''three-wave model'' of intimal hyperplasia in response to injury. Here, early medial smooth muscle proliferation is the first step, influenced primarily by basic fibroblast growth factor (bFGF).[7] Migration and production of extracellular matrix comprise the second and third stages of injury. These mechanisms are relevant in trauma-provoked atheromas which occur as a result of clamping or balloon injuries even with modestly elevated levels of low density lipoprotein (LDL) cholesterol.[8] Other mitogens include angiotensin II which causes smooth muscle to proliferate as well as to induce expression of other growth factors (see Chapter 10),[9,10] one of which is TGF-β, which exhibits dual stimulatory or inhibitory effects in different circumstances. Injury also induces medial angiotensinogen gene expression along with angiotensin receptor expression.[11] Other smooth muscle antigens include thrombin, catecholamine, and possibly endothelin. Thus, atheromas developing in a setting of injury—mechanical, immunologic, or infectious, such as viral—are probably influenced by these trauma-induced growth factors in varying degrees and sequences. In turn, plasma LDL elevation accentuates the formation of neointimal hyperplasia[12,13] without actual atheroma formation in the classic sense.

Atherosclerosis cannot be considered as comprehensively as one might wish in this chapter. References to classic lesions, pathogenesis,[14] and late complica-

From *The Basic Science of Vascular Disease*. Edited by Sidawy AN, Sumpio BE, and DePalma RG. Armonk, NY: Futura Publishing Company, Inc.; © 1997.

tions should guide the reader to comprehensive recent reviews. Another caveat is a willingness to address atherosclerosis as if it were a single disease. Some view this entity or process as a polypathogenic family of closely related vascular disorders rather than as a single disease.[15,16] Moreover, were multiple "risk factors" considered as "etiologic" factors, a single disease view would not be logically valid.

Many lines of evidence suggest that, in a variety of circumstances, low density lipoprotein cholesterol (LDLC) entry into the arterial wall is an initiating step in early plaque inception. Subsequent plaque and clinical complications might be exacerbated or accelerated by associated risk factors from cigarette smoking, diabetes, and hypertension. These risk factors are not singular or univariate, but multiple and interactive. Presumably, these might influence early or moderately advanced lipid-based lesions. The fact that in certain areas of the world, populations free of coronary disease exhibit total cholesterol levels below 150 mg/dL and LDL cholesterol levels below 100 mg/dL led Roberts[17] to question the primacy of other "atherosclerotic risk factors" which are not uncommon in these populations.

This chapter considers atherosclerosis as a single disease; however, this process encompasses a spectrum of pathologic lesions, probably with different modes of pathogenesis, patterns of distribution,[18] and progression rates.[16] A critique of the usefulness of etiologic theories accounting for lesion variability is provided along with classic and more recent concepts of pathogenesis.

Atherosclerotic Lesions

Atheroma is derived from the Greek word *athere* meaning porridge or gruel. Sclerosis means induration or hardening; these differing characteristics exist in varying degrees in different plaques, different disease stages, and in different individuals. Von Haller, in 1755 as noted by Haimovici,[19] first applied the term atheroma to a common type of plaque, which, on sectioning, exuded a yellow, pultaceous content from its core. Figure 1 illustrates a typical fibrous plaque containing a central atheromatous core with a fibrous or fibromuscular cap, macrophage accumulation, and round cell adventitial infiltration. Although a classic definition of atherosclerotic plaque characterized the lesion as "a variable combination of changes in the intima of arteries consisting of focal accumulation of lipids, complex carbohydrates, blood and blood products, fibrous tissue and calcium deposits,"[20] this description does not encompass adequately the spectrum of advanced lesions encountered. Advanced plaques invade the media; atheromas at certain stages produce bulging, even enlargement of arteries, while round cell infiltration, medial changes, and neovascularization of the ad-

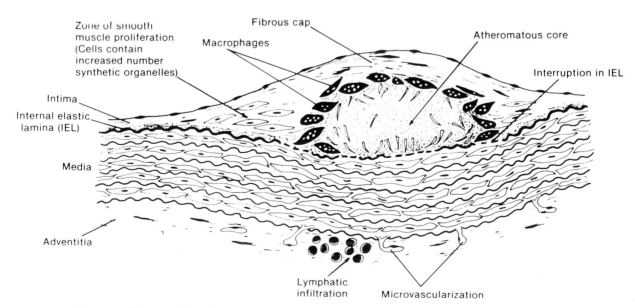

Figure 1. Schema of typical atheroma. Note central lipid core, fibrous cap, macrophage accumulation, and zone of synthetically active smooth muscle at the "shoulders" of the core. Note tendency of the lesion to bulge outward, neovascularization, and adventitial lymphocyte infiltration. (Modified with permission from DePalma RG: Pathology of atheromas. In: Bell PRF, Jamieson CW, Buckley CV (eds). *Surgical Management of Vascular Disease*. London: WB Saunders Co., Ltd.; 21–34, 1992.)

ventitia are characteristic of many advanced atherosclerotic lesions. This process involves the entire
arterial wall. The descriptions that follow consider progressively severe types of plaques which are accepted
under the rubric of atheromas. Certain lesions, however, might not always evolve in the same way.

Fatty Streaks

Fatty streaks are gross and minimally raised yellow lesions found frequently in the aorta of infants and
children (Figure 2). These lesions contain lipids deposited intracellularly in macrophages and in smooth muscle cells. A recent special report[21] defined initial fatty
streaks and intermediate lesions of atherosclerosis as
follows: type I lesions, found in children, are the very
earliest microscopic lesions consisting of increased intimal macrophages with the appearance of foam cells;
type II lesions are grossly visible. In contrast to type
I lesions, type II lesions stain with Sudan III or IV.

Fatty streaks are characterized by foam cells, lipid
droplets also in intimal smooth muscle cells, and heterogeneous droplets of extracellular lipids. Type III
lesions are considered intermediate lesions; these are
possibly the bridge between the fatty streaks (Figure
3) and the prototypical atheromatous fibrous plaque
illustrated in Figure 1. Type III lesions occur in plaque
expression-prone localities in the arterial tree,[22] i.e.,
those sites exposed to forces that cause increased LDL
influx, particularly low shear stress (Figures 4A and
4B).[23]

The fatty streak type II lipids are chemically similar to those of the plasma,[24] although the manner in
which the plasma lipids enter the arterial wall might
occur in several ways. The plasma threshold level for
LDL entry into the arterial wall is unknown.[21] The
earliest hypotheses suggested that lipids simply infiltrated from the plasma into the arterial wall. However,
even in these early theories, intimal changes before
lipid entry were postulated.[25] There are various itera-
tions of the lipid hypothesis.

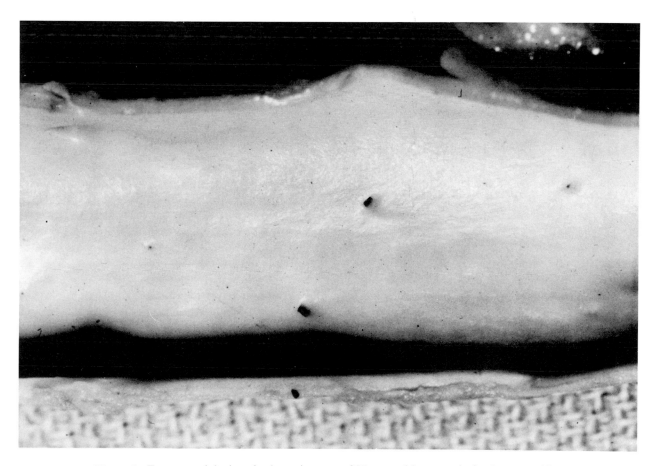

Figure 2. Fatty streak lesions in thoracic aorta of 20-year-old woman in fatal auto accident.
(Courtesy of Dr. Pacita Maralo, Professor of Pathology, University of Nevada School of
Medicine.)

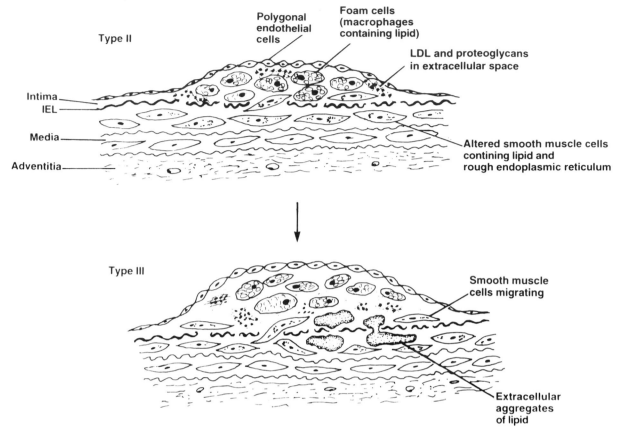

Figure 3. Diagrammatic representation of type IIa fatty streak lesions with foam cells, low density lipoprotein (LDL) particles in matrix, altered smooth muscle cells with developed rough endoplasmic reticulum also containing lipid particles. Type III: possible evolution to intermediate more advanced lesion now containing extracellular aggregates or pools of lipid deep in the intima and extending into the media.

As described in a recent review of pathogenesis,[14] LDL accumulation may occur because of 1) alterations in the permeability of the intima; 2) increases in the interstitial space in the intima; 3) poor metabolism of LDL by vascular cells; 4) impeded transport of LDL from the intima to the media; 5) increased plasma/LDL concentrations; or 6) specific binding of LDL to connective tissue components, particularly proteoglycans in the arterial intima. Experimental studies show that LDL cholesterol accumulates in the intima even before lesions develop and in the presence of intact endothelium. These observations are quite similar to those of early lesion formation described by Aschoff[25] at the beginning of this century, and Virchow[26] in the nineteenth century.

A second event in early atherogenesis has been shown in animal experiments to be the binding of monocytes to the endothelial lining with their subsequent diapedesis into the subintimal layer to become tissue macrophages.[27-29] Experimentally, fatty streaks are populated mainly by monocyte-derived macrophages. These lipid-engorged scavenger cells mainly become the foam cells characterizing fatty streaks and

other lesions. An interesting recent development is the observation that LDL must be altered in some manner,[30] as by oxidation or acetylation, to be taken up by the macrophages to form foam cells. Furthermore, oxidized LDL (OxLDL) is a powerful chemoattractant for monocytes. Another aspect of this theory suggests that endothelium modifies LDL to promote foam cell formation.

The interactions of plasma LDL levels with the arterial wall are the subject of intense interest. LDL traverses the endothelium mostly through receptor-independent transport though some does occur through cell breaks.[31] Endothelial cells,[32] smooth muscle cells,[33] and macrophages[34] are all capable of promoting oxidation of LDL, and OxLDL, in turn, further attracts monocytes into the intima and promotes their transformation into macrophages. Macrophages produce cytokines including PDGF, TGFβ, and interleukin 1 (IL-1). OxLDL also induces gene products ordinarily unexpressed in normal vascular tissue. A notable example is tissue factor (TF), the cellular initiator of the coagulation cascade expressed by atheroma monocytes and foam cells.[35] TF expression requires the presence of

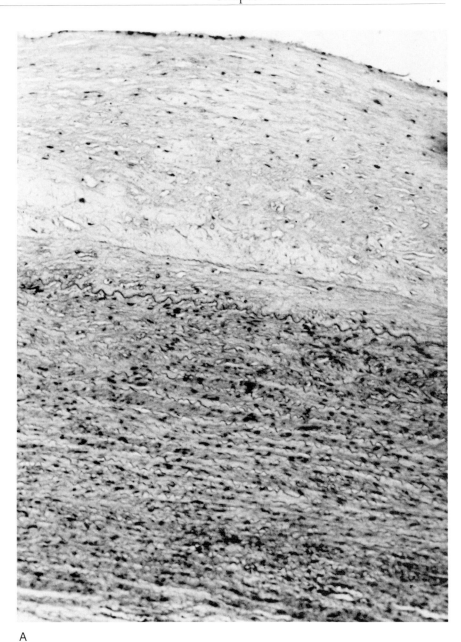

Figure 4A. Hematoxylin and éosin stain showing fatty streak lesion. Note medial cellular proliferation and lipid accumulation deep in lesion.

A

bacterial lipopolysaccharides, suggesting that hypercoagulability in atherosclerosis can be enhanced by endotoxemia.

Altered Characteristics of Arterial Cells

Initial Fatty Streak

Stary et al[21] have provided a comprehensive summary of cellular alterations in early lesions which will be briefly outlined for each layer of the arterial wall.

Endothelium

Animal studies show that endothelial cells tend to be oriented away from the direction of flow; these cells show increased stigmata or stomata, increased proliferation, and a decrease in microfilament bundles. In humans and animals, endothelial cells become polyhedral or rounded; in humans, there is increased formation of multinucleated cells and cilia. Animal studies show increased proliferation and cell death with retraction and exposure of subendothelial foam cells. The endothelium becomes more permeable to macromolecules in experimental models; in humans, it exhibits increased mural thrombus formation and tissue factor expression. Leukocyte adherence increases with the expression of a monocyte adhesion molecule (VCAM-1). Endothelial-derived relaxing factor and prostacyline release are decreased with enhanced vasoconstriction.

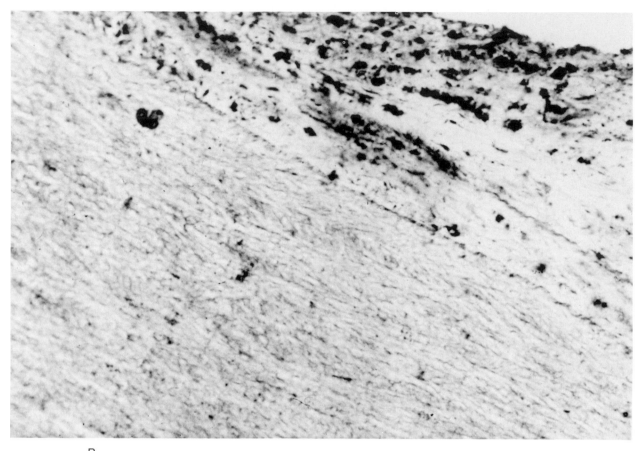

B

Figure 4B. Fat stain of fatty streak lesion. Note lipid deposits in macrophages and in media. (Courtesy of Dr. Pacita Maralo, Professor of Pathology, University of Nevada School of Medicine.)

Media

Experimentally, the smooth muscle shows increased proliferation with increased rough endoplasmic reticulum, phenotypic change, and increased production of altered intracellular and extracellular matrices. These in humans include increased expression of type I and type III collagen, dermatan sulfate, proteoglycan, and stromolysens. The smooth muscle cells produce cytokines including macrophage colony stimulating colony factor (MCSF), tumor necrosis factor (TNF), and monocyte chemotactic protein-I (MCP). The myocytes accumulate native and modified lipoproteins both by native receptor pathways and by nonspecific phagocytosis; these cells also express increased lipoprotein lipase activity and experimentally display a scavenger receptor similar to that of foam cells.

Macrophages

These cells proliferate and express: MCP1, MCSF, TNF, IL-1, PDGF, immune antigen, and tissue factor[35] as previously mentioned. Macrophages contain increased free and esterified cholesterol, increased acetyl CoA:cholesterol acyl transferase, and acid cholesterol ester hydrolase, while neutral cholesterol ester hydrolase decreases. The altered cells also express the scavenger receptor, 15-lipoxygenase, and exhibit increased lipoprotein oxidation products in humans and in animal models.

The extensive changes outlined indicate the complexity of morphologic, functional, biochemical, and genetic expressions of the arterial wall in early atherosclerosis. The reader is referred to the original report for comprehensive details with references to each of the cellular alterations described.[21]

Gelatinous Plaques

Another type of early atheroma precursors are intimal gelatinous lesions. These were also first described by Virchow in 1856[26] and later cited by Haust[36] as important progenitors of advanced atherosclerosis.

The methodical study of these lesions has been relatively neglected, but their identification has been recently stressed by Smith.[37,38] A variety of data show that virtually all the plasma proteins, particularly hemostatic components, are capable of entering the arterial intima. Gelatinous lesions appear translucent and neutral in color with central areas which are grayish or opaque. Certain lesions are characterized by finely dispersed, perifibrous lipids, along with collagen strands around the lesions. As described, gelatinous lesions feel soft, and with gentle lateral pressure, will seem to "wobble." Gelatinous plaques are often observed during arterial surgery (the author is struck by the frequency with which these occur in heavy smokers.) The gelatinous material separates easily from the underlying arterial wall without entering the usual endarterectomy plane. Gelatinous plaques are most commonly seen in the aorta. According to Smith,[37] gelatinous plaques occur as extensive areas of flat, translucent thickenings, particularly in the lower abdominal segment. These lesions are characterized by low lipid and high fluid content. Protein content is variable, but in some plaques, numerous smooth muscle cells occur and the lesions contain substantial amounts of cross-linked fibrin.

Fibrous Plaques

Figure 1 typifies the more advanced atherosclerotic lesion, the fibrous plaque. The atheroma is composed of a large number of smooth muscle cells and connective tissue, which form a fibrous cap over an inner yellow (atheromatous) core. This soft core contains cholesterol esters, mainly cholesteryloleate, believed to be derived from disrupted foam cells. A second type of particle contains both free cholesterol and cholesterol linoleates. The particle is thought to be derived directly from LDL, possibly by modification of LDL by specific lipolytic enzymes capable of hydrolyzing LDL cholesterol esters.[14] Fibrous plaques are also composed of large numbers of smooth muscle cells, connective tissue, and macrophages. There has been a recent emphasis[39] on the composition and integrity of the cap. This structure is probably important in stabilizing the atheroma and preventing intraluminal rupture of the soft core.

Fibrous plaques appear chronologically later and often in similar locations as fatty streaks. Some, but not all, fibrous plaques are believed to be derived from fatty streaks; other precursors such as the gelatinous plaques or injured arterial areas might also lead to fibrous plaque formation. It is important to note that conversion of a mural thrombus into an atheroma can occur, as demonstrated by chronic intra-arterial catheter implantation.[40]

Fibrous plaques protrude into the arterial lumen in fixed cut sections; however, when arteries are fixed at arterial pressure, they produce an abluminal or external bulge. For example, coronary plaques in vivo must occupy at least 40% of the arterial wall before angiographic detection,[41] and atheroma compression can be compensated for by arterial enlargement.[42] Remodelling of coronary arteries in subhuman primates and humans has been recently stressed.[43] However, ultimately, due to lesion growth, ulceration, rupture, or overlying thrombosis with advancing disease, the arterial lumen is compromised; when this occurs, distal ischemia develops. It is possible that a unique adaptive response involving dilation, with atheromatous involvement of the entire arterial wall and participation of inflammatory cells and immunologically active T-lymphocytes, might predispose to aneurysm formation.

During the evolution from fatty streak to fibrous plaque, cholesterol esters appear in the form of ordered crystalline arrays of intracellular lipid crystals in early states, while in intermediate type III and fibrous plaques, the lipids assume isotropic forms and occur extracellularly.[44] These cholesterol esters and oxysterols are quite irritating and cause severe inflammatory reactions in the connective tissue[45] they probably behave similarly within the arterial wall. Thus, striking periarterial inflammation, fibrosis, and lymphocytic infiltration occur. Advancing neovascularization from the adventitia characterizes intermediate fibrofatty and fibrous plaque lesions. Atherosclerotic lesions contain immune globulin gamma (IgG) in large quantities and complement components. The IgG recognizes epitopes characteristic of OxLDL indicating that immunologic processes also characterize more advanced atherosclerotic plaques.[46]

Complicated Plaques

Fibrous plaques are complicated by calcification, ulceration, intraplaque hemorrhage, or extensive necrosis. These are late developments in atherosclerosis; such changes relate to the clinical complications of stroke, gangrene, and myocardial infarction. Aneurysm formation in certain cases might represent a unique genetic interaction with atherosclerosis. Alternatively, aneurysms can also be viewed as nonspecific or inflammatory, degenerative, or purely mechanical arterial responses. We have reported a high prevalence of risk factors for atherosclerosis in subjects with abdominal aortic aneurysms along with concurrent atherosclerotic involvement of other arteries.[47] As indicated by Ernst,[48] no unified concept of pathogenesis of aneurysms has yet evolved.

Theories of Atherogenesis

The Lipid Hypothesis

Virchow's[26] original concept was that the cellular changes in atherosclerosis were reactive events in response to lipid infiltration; later Aschoff[25] remarked, "From plasma of low cholesterin content no deposition of lipids will occur even though mechanical conditions are favorable." As can be seen from fatty streak and fibrous plaque evolution, lipids, particularly LDL cholesterol, play a pivotal role in lesion morphology, composition, and evolution. Early experiments by Anitschkow,[49] where cholesterol was fed to rabbits to produce atherosclerosis, appeared to validate a simple "lipid filtration hypothesis." However, the situation is much more complex. Atherosclerosis develops in various species in proportion to the ease with which an experimental regimen will displace the normal lipid pattern toward hypercholesterolemia, particularly hyperbetalipoproteinemia; at the same time, arterial susceptibility varies between location, species, and individuals.

The author's experience with canine and subhuman primate models (rhesus and cynomolgus) of atherosclerosis demonstrates progression in response to dietary manipulation[50-58] as well as plaque regression in response to serum cholesterol lowering. It is important to understand that lesion progression is not simple dietary cholesterol overloading. Any diet which causes hypercholesterolemia will induce experimental atherosclerosis. It is not necessary to have excess, or even any cholesterol in atherogenic diets. In our early subhuman primate feeding experiments, reduction of cholesterol content to .5% combined with sugar and eggs produced lesions when high cholesterol addition up to 7% by weight did not.[53,54] In rabbits, a variety of semipure, purified cholesterol-free diets and various interactions of amino acid induced hypercholesterolemia and atherosclerosis.[59]

Epidemiologic observations provide important circumstantial evidence linking hyperlipidemia to atheromas.[60] Additionally, compelling evidence for the view that elevated LDL cholesterol is an etiologic factor in atherosclerosis is demonstrated by genetic hyperlipidemias, in spite of objections[61] that highly cellular lipid-laden atheromas might be a different lesion in these patients. These metabolic disorders are most often due to a lack or abnormality of LDL receptors on hepatocytes, which cause an ability to internalize and metabolize LDL.[62] The resulting serum cholesterol levels are markedly elevated early in life; individuals with this homozygous condition die prematurely from atherosclerosis; it is rare for them to live beyond the age of 26.

Unfortunately, the heterozygous condition is not uncommon; with total cholesterol levels ranging up to 350 mg/dL, these individuals account for 1 in 500 live births,[63] and will suffer from premature atherosclerosis, generally in middle age. Having had the opportunity to operate on some of these individuals, the atheromas to this observer are similar in morphology and effect to those seen in individuals with acquired hyperlipidemias or with premature atherosclerosis associated with heavy smoking.

This unfortunate natural experiment is powerful evidence that elevated LDL cholesterol is a relentless factor in plaque inception and rapid progression of atherosclerosis to lethal consequences. Recent experience with liver transplantation has been favorable[64] in retarding the progress of this type of atherosclerosis. Familial hypercholesterolemias are characterized by autosomal dominant disorders produced by at least 12 different molecular defects of the LDL receptors; familial abnormalities of high density lipoprotein (HDL), a negative risk factor for atherosclerosis, also exists. Not only is the status of LDL and HDL metabolism important in pathogenesis, surface proteins of the lipoprotein complex or apoproteins are also relevant. These are discussed by LaRosa in Chapter 19, "Plasma Lipoproteins in Vascular Disease."

Thrombogenic Hypothesis

In the mid-nineteenth century, Rokitansky[65] postulated that fibrinous substances deposited on the arterial intimal surface as a result of abnormal hemostatic elements in the blood could undergo metamorphosis into atheromatous masses containing cholesterol crystals and globules. The Rokitansky theory held that typical atheromatous lesions resulted mainly from degeneration of blood proteins, i.e., fibrin essentially deposited in the arterial intima. Duguid[66] repopularized this theory in 1946. It is interesting to note that in particular experimental models, usually rabbits, indwelling arterial catheters[40] or arterial injury[3] will result in cholesterol accumulation in lesions, without the necessity of added dietary cholesterol. In addition, the gelatinous plaques, described by Haust[36] and Smith,[37,38] might, under certain circumstances, evolve in a manner in which accumulation of blood proteins tend to dominate lesion development.

Mesenchymal Hypothesis

Hemodynamic Effects

The proliferation of smooth cells in the intima and subsequent production by these cells of connective tissue elements are considered, by some, to be primary and crucial steps in atherogenesis.[67,68] An important arterial wall element is proteoglycan, which might be responsible for trapping of infiltrated LDL, even if LDL were not elevated in the blood. Collagen represents the other space-filling component of advanced atherosclerotic lesions. Hauss et al[69] proposed that the migration of smooth muscle cells from the media to the intima, with proliferation and production of connective tissue, comprise a nonspecific reaction of the artery to any injury and that pathogenesis of atherosclerosis simply reflects this. Chisolm et al[14] termed this the "nonspecific" mesenchymal hypothesis. These scenarios are thought to be similar to wound healing in response to injury. In part, this type of theory attempts to explain why physical factors, such as shear stress, vasoactive agents, and different types of injuries, induce similar sequences of events in the vessel wall.

Stehbens,[61] who is highly skeptical of the lipid hypothesis, believes that "atherosclerosis constitutes the degenerative and reparative process consequent upon the hemodynamically-induced engineering fatigue of the blood vessel wall." He postulates that "the vibrations consisting of the pulsations associated with cardiac contractions and the vortex shedding generated in the blood vessels at branchings, unions, curvatures, and fusiform dilatations (carotid sinus) over a lifetime are responsible for fatigue failure after a certain, but individually variable, number of vibrations." In this view, atherosclerosis, a process of wear and tear, becomes an inexorable process associated with aging. It has been shown that hypertension and tachycardia induced in experimental animals[70] on atherogenic feeding caused accelerated plaque development, while bradycardia induced by sinoatrial node ablation in monkeys reduced coronary and carotid atherosclerosis.[71,72]

Monoclonal Hypothesis

Smooth Muscle Proliferation

The morphologic similarity of smooth muscle proliferation in some atherosclerotic lesions to uterine smooth muscle myomas led Benditt and Benditt[67] to suggest that atherosclerotic lesions are derived from a singular or, at most, a few mutated smooth muscle cells, that, like tumor cells, proliferate in an unregulated fashion. This evidence is based on the finding of only one allele for glucose-6 phosphate dehydrogenase in lesions from heterozygotes. A homology exists between the B-chain of human PDGF and the protein product of the V-SIS oncogene, which is a tumor-causing gene derived from Simian sarcoma virus. Tumor-forming cells in culture have been observed to express the genes for one or both of the PDGF chains and secrete PDGF into the medium.[14] This hypothesis assigns importance to events causing smooth muscle cell

proliferation as critical in atherogenesis. Other growth factors include fibroblast growth factor and transforming growth factors, which might stimulate or inhibit cell proliferation, depending on the circumstances, as well as macrophage-derived cytokines. These all influence smooth muscle proliferation, transformation, and collagen secretion. The reader again should note that all of the cells within arteries, endothelium, macrophages, and smooth muscle elaborate chemotactic and growth factors previously described.

Response to Injury Hypothesis

As a result of experimental data and deductive reasoning, Ross[4] initially postulated two pathways for the promotion of atheroma formation. In the first, as for example in hypercholesterolemia, monocytes and macrophage migration occurred without endothelial denudation. In some instances, there might also be endothelial loss with platelet carpeting of bare areas, and in this event, platelets would stimulate proliferation of smooth muscle by PDGF release. In a second pathway, endothelium was postulated to release growth factors stimulating smooth muscle proliferation. Experimental rabbit arterial balloon injury shows that regrowing endothelium induces myointimal proliferation beneath its advancing edges with the accumulation of collagen[73] and glycosaminoglycans.[74] As previously mentioned, stimulated smooth muscle cell releases growth factors leading to a continued autocrine proliferative response. In the initial iteration, the second pathway was postulated to be relevant in atheromas stimulated by diabetes, possibly due to insulin, cigarette smoking, or hypertension. Although hypertension causes endothelial injury, there are striking differences between the behavior of smooth muscle cells in atherosclerosis and hypertension. Atherosclerosis stimulates an overt smooth muscle proliferative response, while in pure hypertension, thickening of the arterial wall occurs in most instances by virtue of increased protein synthesis, without an increase in cell number.[75]

Lesion Arrest and Regression

Regression of atherosclerosis in response to lowered serum cholesterol has been demonstrated in autopsy studies of starved humans,[25] in animal models,[76] and in recent clinical angiographic trials.[77] Complete exposition of these extensive observations is beyond the scope of this chapter. However, in experimental models and humans, subject to some degree of controversy, plaque arrest and regression are known to occur.

As atherosclerotic plaques in experimental animals regress, plaque bulk is reduced mainly by lipid egress, as shown in plaque regression experiments using hypercholesterolemic dogs[50,51] and monkeys.[54,55] The exact mechanisms of atherogenesis, as well as lesion regression or atheroexodus, as it were, are as yet incompletely understood. However, this author and his coworkers demonstrated regression using serial observations of lessened bulk of individual plaques, lessened luminal encroachment as shown by edge defects on sequential angiography, and lessened plaque lipid and altered fibrous protein content measured histologically and chemically.[55] An important technical aspect of this research was the confirmation of regressive changes by immediate autopsy or surgical observation and biopsy, which closely followed the angiographic change.[52,53]

This type of correlative observation is not readily obtained in humans. Lessening of luminal intrusion on sequential angiography does, experimentally, coincide with decreased plaque size and lessened lipid content, though in some instances of regression, fibrous protein increased, and in other circumstances it was seen to decrease. Potentially, fibrosis limits regression, but this process also might convert a soft atheromatous plaque into a more stable, fibrotic plaque. In order to produce regression consistently, serum cholesterol had to be reduced generally below 200 mg/dL; conversely, serum cholesterol levels were shown above which lesions inevitably progressed.[55,58] This threshold in humans might approximate a total serum cholesterol of 150 to 170 mg/dL or an LDL level of 100 mg/dL, the levels Roberts[17] cited in populations where atherosclerosis is virtually absent.

In an attempt to modify platelet activity, and based on the initial PDGF stimulatory theory of atherogenesis, we performed long-term experiments to test this hypothesis. We observed that therapeutic doses of aspirin and dipyridamole administered to rhesus monkeys fed sucrose, egg yolk, and .5% cholesterol caused rapid anatomic and angiographic progression as compared to controls on atherogenic diet alone.[58] Hollander had similar results in cynomolgus monkeys.[78] These antiplatelet agents in combination clearly did not arrest disease progression; treated individuals as compared to controls exhibited more severe atherosclerosis with medial calcification and arterial thrombosis with complicated plaque formation. In the rhesus monkey, this is a distinctly unusual progression. Clinically, combinations of these two drugs are now seldom used.

As mentioned earlier, the lesion complications and deleterious clinical events associated with atherosclerosis are not singular and univariate, but multiple and interactive. It must be understood that the late pathogenesis of atheromas and the resulting instability of fibrous plaques involve more than simple continued lipid accumulation. In understanding possible concepts

of etiology, Holman et al,[79] in 1960, indicated that one must make "a sharp line of distinction between atherogenesis and the subsequent evolution of lesions that may or may not precipitate the disease, for the factors involved in the evolution of lesions beyond the stage of fatty streaks may be entirely different from the factors that initiate fatty streaks." Among these factors are altered fibrous proteins and the accumulation of blood elements within the atheroma.

Hypotheses of pathogenesis and etiology are constantly tested by manipulating risk factors that are associated with atherosclerosis. Among all the interventions so far tried to produce plaque stabilization or regression, only lipid manipulation, i.e., factors which decrease LDL cholesterol or increase HDL cholesterol, have been found to promote favorable changes in the atheroma itself. Generally, these lipid reductions also require cessation of smoking as well. Presently, about 2000 individuals have been studied by serial coronary angiography and regression trials which use mostly lipid reduction.[60] Overall, with the most lipid reduction, most favorable plaque changes in terms of arrest or regression occur. Blankenhorn and Hodis[77] reviewed these data noting that regression and stabilization are 1.5 to 2 times more common in treated subjects as compared to those on placebos. While the angiographic studies do show plaque regression trends, these changes are usually small as compared to lesion stabilization. Ornish et al[80] reported highly favorable results using serial coronary angiography among patients randomly assigned to an experimental group consuming 10% fat, 12 mg. cholesterol diet, smoking cessation, stress management training, and exercise. After one year, 82% of the treated group was said to show regressive changes in the coronary arteries, which depended somewhat upon the amount of initial lesion encroachment.

In spite of the limitations of angiography in assessing plaques, angiography provides a measure of lesion size by delineating the arterial lumen; computer-enhanced techniques can be used to quantify wall changes. Furthermore, with care, arteriography can be repeated for sequential studies. While, because of arterial remodeling, angiography might not be an absolute measure of plaque severity, it is a measure. Most would agree that more plaque intrusion is worse and less is better. Undoubtedly, magnetic resonance imaging and further development of ultrasound techniques will continue to develop as important quantifiable methods of serial assessment of arterial wall change.

Another treatment approach might be modification of the plaque itself, so that smooth muscle transformation with increased fibrous protein synthesis would produce a stable, fibrotic plaque as opposed to a soft, friable plaque containing an unstable, atheromatous core covered by a thin cap. In evaluating hypotheses with a view toward better prediction and control of this process, it is obviously necessary to treat or ameliorate atherosclerotic plaques and to provide quantifiable evidence of favorable changes. Desirable changes include more fibrotic and smaller plaques, which not only permit enhanced blood flow, but also are more stable than soft friable lesions.

Atherosclerosis is often segmental and the disease can be effectively treated by bypassing or removing arterial lesions. These observations were, over 3 decades ago, uniquely surgical insights.[16] Such interventions, now including endovascular approaches, are the most important means of treatment for advanced atheromas, including particular patterns of coronary involvement, high-grade carotid lesions, and limb occlusive disease. It is recognized, of course, that strictly surgical approaches to treatment do not prevent disease progression; with certain disease patterns, life expectancy remains shortened. Prevention of superimposed embolic phenomena and clotting can be influenced by aspirin and anticoagulants. Modification of inflammatory responses by intervening in the cytokine-derived or immunologic modulating factors might be fruitful, but requires the ability to influence in the enormously complex interactions occurring even in early lesions.[21]

Another productive approach might be decreasing arterial spasm which is provoked by relatively minor plaques, particularly in coronary or cerebral arteries. Atherosclerotic plaques impair the normal effect of endothelial-derived relaxing factor[81,82] and cause failure of vasodilator responses in coronary and cerebral arteries.[83] Dietary treatment of experimental atherosclerosis restores endothelium-dependent relaxation responses within certain limits,[84] while long-term inhibition of nitric oxide synthesis by feeding promotes atherosclerosis experimentally.[85]

The Cholesterol Controversy

Unanswered Questions

Dock[86] stated in 1974 that, regarding the etiology of atherosclerosis, the cholesterol controversy was over. Steinberg[87] in 1989 asked why this took so long. Nonetheless, controversy continued. The lipid hypothesis of atherogenesis elicits strong contending views. Not among the least of these are intense emotions stimulated by public health dietary recommendations aimed at reduction of serum cholesterol.[61,88] In some minds, this effort has been elevated to a "cholesterol conspiracy."[89] Clinicians testify to the difficulties of altering lifelong dietary traditions and deleterious lifestyle habits such as smoking. However, based on available science, national and international scientific leadership is dedicated to these goals, particularly serum cholesterol reduction and smoking cessation.

One of the specifics called into question is the possibility of lesion arrest or regression in humans based on drug or dietary therapy. This author believes regression is possible for certain types and stages of disease, having observed clear-cut regression of intrusive intermediate fibrofatty atheromas confirmed directly *in seriatim* in atherosclerotic animals, as well as regressive change in human peripheral arteries. Lesions capable of regression in animals appear similar to those observed in human arteries, and probably comprise type II and type III lesions, and some fibrous plaques. Current angiographic trials support evidence mainly for plaque arrest with some evidence of regression. Regressive changes must be qualified by the technical limitations of current imaging methods and further, should not be awaited when surgical or endovascular interventions are needed. In one trial, sequential angiography accurately presaged individual coronary events.[90] More outcome data such as these are urgently needed.

Stimuli for continued controversy include valid scientific skepticism; a focus on more rational delineation of pathogenic mechanisms, and quite importantly, the anomalous results of trials showing no decreased mortality or increased life span in primary lipid interventions. Increased noncardiovascular mortality in treated groups in some primary trials compounded this problem.[60]

The use of surrogate end points, i.e., "coronary heart disease (CHD) events" or CHD mortality in lieu of atheroma quantification, is a serious scientific limitation of human trials. The hypocholesterolemia associated with morbid conditions such as cancer, hepatic diseases, and pulmonary disease further confuses cardiovascular trial issues, as these high mortality patients become randomized. Documentation of a favorable effect on lesions demands quantitative morphologic, and ideally, biochemical measurements of the process itself.

Controversy and Unanswered Questions

We now practice in an era when deaths from cardiovascular disease have declined by more than one third in the past 3 decades. While this decline has been, in part, attributed to changing risk factors, the real reasons for this decrease are unknown. The mortality decrement probably relates not only to changing risk factors in the population, but also to effective therapy for hypertension, as well as surgical treatment for coronary, carotid, and aneurysmal disease. Recently, average cholesterol levels in the United States have fallen to levels which support the possibility of plaque arrest or even regression. The current average adult serum cholesterol in the United States is now estimated to be

205 mg/dL with almost half the adult population having levels below 200 mg/dL.[90] However, some[68] now question the importance of screening for lipids, given the failure of cholesterol reduction alone to dramatically influence results in the primary dietary trials.[60] At the same time, drug therapy and secondary regression trials have demonstrated clear-cut reductions in CHD events. Based on the most current data,[91] about 40% of all adults over the age of 20 might require lipoprotein analysis if treatment were to be considered and 29% of all adults would be candidates for dietary therapy. The cost of screening and drug therapy for dietary nonresponders continues to be controversial.

New treatment vistas include expanded roles for antioxidants such as vitamin C, vitamin E, and the drug probucol. One of the scientific bases for antioxidant therapy is the demonstration[30] that LDL uptake by macrophages to form foam cells requires LDL alteration by oxidation, glycosylation, or some other form of degradation. The atherogenic potentiating cellular effects of oxidized LDL have been considered in detail. This phenomenon might also be relevant in diabetes where glycosylation and oxidation of LDL account for enhanced LDL atherogenicity. Further research on the efficacy and mode of action of antioxidents could yield practical results based on known mechanisms of atherogenesis.

One of the most important risks or pathogenic factors promoting atherosclerosis is diabetes. This has not been the subject of controlled clinical trials as have lipid interventions. Diabetes is associated with an increased prevalence of severe infracrural and coronary atherosclerosis. Unfortunately, as indicated by Bierman,[92] the current diabetes control and complications trial,[93] showing favorable reduction in microvascular complications with tight control, has not been designed to study atherosclerosis end points. Further, diabetes as it affects atherogenesis has not been modeled extensively in animal models of atherosclerosis. Causes of enhanced atherogenesis in diabetes include abnormalities in apoprotein and lipoprotein particle distributions, particularly elevated levels of lipoprotein (a),[94] which is now believed to be an independent thromboatherosclerotic risk factor. In poorly controlled diabetes, a procoagulant state exists; insulin resistance and hyperinsulinemia might also contribute to smooth muscle proliferation. Not only do glyco-oxidation and oxidation contribute to LDL entry into macrophages, but glycation of proteins and plasma in the arterial wall could contribute further to accelerated atherosclerosis in diabetics. Finally, hormones, growth factors, and cytokine enhanced smooth muscle cell proliferation and increased foam cell formation are also postulated to be unique aspects of atherogenesis in diabetes mellitus. However, which of these factors dominates atherogenesis in diabetes and why the distal vessels are more severely affected are unanswered questions.

Ultimately, the usefulness of theories of etiology and pathogenesis of atherosclerosis depends upon their ability to provide for effective prevention or intervention. These two *might not* be identical. It is possible that elaboration of events in early atherogenesis and better understanding of the cellular factors controlling arterial injury and cytokine-induced changes would lead to prevention or modification of initial lesions. At the same time, public health measures, such as lipid reduction in the general population and risk factor control, provide clear benefits in the form of decreased disease prevalence. With the exception of diabetes, the prevalence trends of risk factors for atherosclerosis in the United States continue to improve. With current efforts directed at lipid modification, cessation of smoking, and control of hypertension, the next few decades should witness a further decrease in the prevalence and severity of atherosclerosis and its clinical complications.

References

1. DePalma RG: Atherosclerosis and reactions of the injured arterial wall. In: Giordano JM, Trout HH III, DePalma RG (eds). *The Basic Science of Vascular Surgery*. Armonk, NY: Futura Publishing Company, Inc.; 235–272, 1988.
2. Ross R, Glomset F, Kariya B, et al: A platelet dependent factor that stimulates the proliferation of arterial smooth muscle cells in vitro. *Proc Nat'l Acad Sci USA* 71:1207, 1974.
3. Bjorkerud JS, Bondjers G: Arterial repair and atherosclerosis after mechanical injury: 2 tissue response after induction of a total necrosis (deep longitudinal injury). *Atherosclerosis* 14:259, 1971.
4. Ross R, Glomset JA: The pathogenesis of atherosclerosis. *N Engl J Med* 295:369, 1976.
5. Ross R: The pathogenesis of atherosclerosis: an update. *N Eng J Med* 314:488, 1986.
6. Ross R: The pathogenesis of atherosclerosis: a perspective for the 1990s. *Nature* 362:801, 1993.
7. Lindner V, Lappi DA, Baird A, et al: Role of basic fibroblast growth factor in vascular lesion formation. *Circ Res* 68:106, 1991.
8. DePalma RG, Chidi CC, Sternfeld WC, Koletsky S: Pathogenesis and prevention of trauma provoked atheromas. *Surgery* 82:429, 1977.
9. Campbell-Bodwell M, Robertson AL Jr: Effects of angiotensin II and vasopressin on human smooth muscle cells in vitro. *Exp Med Pathol* 35:265, 1981.
10. Itoh H, Mukuyawa M, Pratt RE, et al: Multiple autocrine growth factors modulate vascular smooth muscle in response to angiotensin II. *J Clin Invest* 91:2268, 1993.
11. Viswanathan M, Stromberg C, Seltzer A, et al: Balloon angioplasty enhances expression of angiotensin II, ATI receptors in neointima of rat aorta. *J Clin Invest* 90:1707, 1992.
12. Stevens SL, Hilgarth K, Ryan US, et al: The synergistic effect of hypercholesterolemia and mechanical injury on intimal hyperplasia. *Ann Vasc Surg* 6:55, 1992.

13. Baumann DS, Doblas M, Dougherty A, et al: The role of cholesterol accumulation in prosthetic vascular graft anastomotic intimal hyperplasia. *J Vasc Surg* 19:435, 1994.

14. Chisolm GM, DiCarleto PE, Erhart LA, et al: Pathogenesis of atherosclerosis in peripheral vascular diseases. In: Young JR, Graor RA, Olin JW, Bartholomew JR (eds). St. Louis: Mosby Year Book; 137–160, 1991.

15. McMillan GC: Development of atherosclerosis. *Am J Cardiol* 31:542, 1973.

16. DeBakey ME: Atherosclerosis: patterns and rates of progression. In: Gotto AM, South LL, Allen B (eds). *Atherosclerosis*. New York: Springer-Verlag; 3, 1980.

17. Roberts WC: Atherosclerotic risk factors: are there ten or is there only one? *Am J Cardiol* 64:552, 1989.

18. DePalma RG: Patterns of peripheral atherosclerosis: implications for treatment. In: Shepherd J (ed). *Atherosclerosis Developments, Complications, and Treatment*. Amsterdam: Elsevier Science; 161, 1987.

19. Haimovici H, DePalma RG: Atherosclerosis: biologic and surgical considerations. In: Haimovici H, DePalma RG, Ernst CB, Hollier LH (eds). *Vascular Surgery Principles and Techniques*. 3rd ed. Norwalk, CT: Appleton and Lange; 161–187, 1989.

20. Report of a Study Group: Classification of Atherosclerotic Lesions. WHO Technical Report Series 1958, No. 143, Geneva, 1620.

21. Stary, HC (Chair), Chandler AB, Glagov S, et al: A definition of initial fatty streak and intermediate lesions of atherosclerosis: a report from the Committee on Vascular Lesions of the Council on Atherosclerosis, American Heart Association. *Arterioscler Thromb* 14:840, 1994.

22. Cornhill JF, Hederick EE, Stary HC: Topography of human aortic sudanophilic lesions. *Monogr Atheroscler* 15:13, 1990.

23. Glagov S, Zarins C, Giddens DP, et al: Hemodynamics and atherosclerosis: insights and perspectives gained from studies of human arteries. *Arch Pathol Lab Med* 112:1018, 1988.

24. Insull W Jr, Bartch GE: Cholesterol, triglyceride, and phospholipid content of intima, media, and atherosclerotic fatty streak in human thoracic aorta. *J Clin Invest* 45:513, 1966.

25. Aschoff L: Atherosclerosis. In: *Lectures on Pathology*. New York: Hoeber, Inc.; 131:153, 1924.

26. Virchow R: *Gesammelt Abhandungen zur Wissenschaftlichen Medicin*. Frankfurt: Meidinger John & Co.; 496, 1856.

27. Fagiotto A, Ross R, Harker L: Studies of hypercholesterolemia in the nonhuman primate I: changes that lead to fatty streak formation. *Arteriosclerosis* 4:323, 1984.

28. Fagiotto A, Ross R: Studies of hypercholesterolemia in the nonhuman primate II: fatty streak conversion to fibrous plaque. *Arteriosclerosis* 4:341, 1984.

29. Gerrity RG: The role of the monocyte in atherogenesis I: transition of blood borne monocytes into foam cells in fatty lesions. *Am J Pathol* 103:181, 1981.

30. Steinberg D, Parthasarathy S, Carew TE, et al: Beyond cholesterol: modifications of low density lipoprotein that increase its atherogenicity. *N Engl J Med* 320:915, 1989.

31. Wiklund O, Carew TF, Steinberg D: Role of the low density lipoprotein receptor in the penetration of low density lipoprotein into the rabbit aortic wall. *Arteriosclerosis* 5:135, 1985.

32. Steinbrecher UP: Role of superoxide in endothelial-cell modification of low density lipoprotein. *Biochem Biophys Acta* 959:20, 1988.

33. Heinecke JW, Baker L, Rosen L, Chait A: Superoxide mediates modification of low density lipoprotein by arterial smooth muscle cells. *J Clin Invest* 77:757, 1986.

34. Parthasarathy S, Printz DJ, Boyd D, et al: Macrophage oxidation of low density lipoproteins generates a form recognized by the scavenger receptor. *Arteriosclerosis* 6:505, 1986.

35. Brand K, Banka CL, Mackman N, et al: Oxidized LDL enhances lipopolysaccharide induced tissue factor expression in human adherent monocytes. *Arterioscler Thromb* 14:790, 1994.

36. Haust MD: The morphogenesis and fate of potential and early atherosclerotic lesions in man. *Human Pathol* 2:1, 1971.

37. Smith EB: Identification of the gelatinous lesion. In: Schettler G, Gott AM (eds). *Atherosclerosis VI*. New York: Springer-Verlag; 170, 1983.

38. Smith EB: Fibrin in the arterial wall. *Atherosclerosis* 70:186, 1988.

39. Davies MJ, Thomas A: Thrombosis and acute coronary artery lesions in sudden cardiac ischemic death. *N Engl J Med* 310:1137, 1984.

40. Moore S: Thromboatherosclerosis in normolipemic rabbits: a result of continued endothelial damage. *Lab Invest* 29:478, 1973.

41. Stiel GN, Stiel LSG, Schofer J, et al: Impact of compensatory enlargement of atherosclerotic arteries on angiographic assessment. *Circulation* 80:1603, 1989.

42. Glagov S, Weisenberd E, Zarins C, et al: Compensatory enlargement of human atherosclerotic coronary arteries. *New Engl J Med* 316:1371, 1987.

43. Clarkson TB, Prichard RW, Morgan TM, et al: Remodeling of coronary arteries in human and nonhuman primates. *JAMA* 271:289, 1994.

44. Hata Y, Hower J, Insull W, Jr: Cholesterol ester-rich inclusions from human aortic fatty streak and fibrous plaque lesions of atherosclerosis. *Am J Pathol* 75:423, 1974.

45. Baranowski A, Adams CWM, Bayliss-High OB, et al: Connective tissue responses to oxysterols. *Atherosclerosis* 41:255, 1982.

46. Yla-Herttuala S, Palinski W, Butler S, et al: Rabbit and human atherosclerotic lesions contain IgG that recognizes epitopes of oxidized LDL. *Atheroscler Thromb* 13:32, 1993.

47. DePalma RG, Sidawy AN, Giordano JM: Associated etiological and atherosclerotic risk factors in abdominal aneurysms. In: Greenhalgh RM, Mannick JA (eds). *The Cause and Management of Aneurysm*. London: WB Saunders Co.; 37–46, 1990.

48. Ernst CB: Abdominal aortic aneurysm. *N Engl J Med* 328:1167, 1993.

49. Anitschkow R: Experimental atherosclerosis in animals. In: Cowdry V (ed). *Arteriosclerosis: Review of Problem*. New York: MacMillan Co.; 1933.

50. DePalma RG, Hubay CA, Insull W Jr, Robinson AV, Hartman PH: Progression and regression of experimental atherosclerosis. *Surg Gynecol Obst* 131:633, 1970.

51. DePalma RG, Insull W Jr, Bellon EM, et al: Animal models for study of progression and regression of atherosclerosis. *Surgery* 72:268, 1972.

52. DePalma RG, Bellon EM, Insull W Jr, et al: Studies on progression and regression of experimental atherosclerosis: techniques and application to the rhesus monkey. *Med Primatol* III:313, 1972.

53. DePalma RG, Bellon EM, Klein L, et al: Approaches to evaluating regression of experimental atherosclerosis.

In: Manning GM, Haust MD (eds). *Atherosclerosis: Metabolic, Morphologic, and Clinical Aspects.* New York: Plenum Publishing; 459, 1977.

54. DePalma RG, Bellon EM, Koletsky S, et al: Atherosclerotic plaque regression in rhesus monkeys induced by bile acid sequestrant. *Exp Mol Pathol* 31:423, 1979.

55. DePalma RG, Klein L, Bellon EM, et al: Regression of atherosclerotic plaques in rhesus monkeys. *Arch Surg* 115:1268, 1980.

56. DePalma RG: Angiography in experimental atherosclerosis: advantages and limitations. In: Bond JG, Insull W Jr, Glagov S, Cornhill JF, Chandler AB (eds). *Clinical Diagnosis of Atherosclerotic Lesions: Quantitative Methods of Evaluation.* New York: Springer-Verlag; 99, 1983.

57. DePalma RG, Koletsky S, Bellon EM, et al: Failure of regression of atherosclerosis in dogs with moderate cholesterolemia. *Atherosclerosis* 27:297, 1977.

58. DePalma RG, Bellon EM, Manalo PM, Bomberger RA: Failure of antiplatelet treatment in dietary atherosclerosis: a serial intervention study. In: Gallo LL, Vahouny GV (eds). *Cardiovascular Disease: Molecular and Cellular Mechanisms Prevention and Treatment.* New York: Plenum Press; 407, 1987.

59. Kritchevsky D: Atherosclerosis and nutrition. *Nutr Int* 2:290, 1986.

60. LaRosa JC: Cholesterol lowering, low cholesterol and mortality. *Am J Cardiol* 72:776, 1993.

61. Stehbens WE: *The Lipid Hypothesis of Atherosclerosis.* Austin, TX: RG Landes; 1993.

62. Brown MS, Goldstein JL: Lipoprotein receptors in the liver: control signals for plasma cholesterol traffic. *J Clin Invest* 72:743, 1983.

63. Schonfeld G: Inherited disorders of lipid transport. In: LaRosa JC (ed). *Endocrinology and Metabolism Clinics of North America.* Vol. 19, No. 2. Philadelphia: WB Saunders Co.; 211, 1990.

64. Hoeg JM: Familial hypercholesterolemia: what the zebra can teach us about the horse. *JAMA* 271:543, 1994.

65. Rokitansky C von: *A Manual of Pathological Anatomy*, translated by Dan GE. London: The Sydenhams Society, 1852.

66. Duguid JB: Thrombosis as a factor in the pathogenesis of coronary atherosclerosis. *J Pathol* 58:207, 1946.

67. Benditt EP, Benditt JM: Evidence for a monoclonal origin of human atherosclerotic plaques. *Proc Natl Acad Sci USA* 70:1753, 1973.

68. Schwartz SM: Cellular proliferation in atherosclerosis and hypertension. *Proc Soc Exp Biol Med* 173:1, 1983.

69. Hauss WH, Junge-Hulsing G, Hollanden HJ: Changes in metabolism of connective tissue associated with aging and arterio or atherosclerosis. *J Atheroscler Res* 6:50, 1962.

70. Koletsky S, Roland C, Rivera-Velez JM: Rapid acceleration of atherosclerosis in hypertensive rats on a high fat diet. *Exp Mol Pathol* 9:322, 1968.

71. Beere PA, Glagov S, Zarins CK: Retarding effects of a lowered heart rate on coronary atherosclerosis. *Science* 226:180, 1984.

72. Beere PA, Glagov S, Zarins CK: Experimental atherosclerosis at the carotid bifurcation of the cynomolgus monkey: localization, compensatory enlargement and the sparing effect of lowered heart rate. *Atheroscler Thromb* 12:1245, 1992.

73. Chidi CC, DePalma RG: Collagen formation by transformed smooth muscle after arterial injury. *Surg Gynecol Obstet* 152:8, 1981.

74. Wight TV, Curwen KD, Litrenta MM, et al: Effect of endothelium on glycosaminoglycan accumulation in the injured rabbit aorta. *Am J Pathol* 113:156, 1983.

75. Schwartz SM, Ross R: Cellular proliferation in atherosclerosis and hypertension. *Proc Cardiovasc Dis* 26:355, 1984.

76. St. Clair RSW: Atherosclerosis regression in animal models: current concepts of cellular and biochemical mechanisms. *Prog Cardiovasc Dis* 26:109, 1983.

77. Blankenhorn DH, Hodis HN: Arterial imaging and atherosclerosis reversal. *Arterioscler Thromb* 14:177, 1994.

78. Hollander W, Kirkpatrick B, Paddock J, et al: Studies on the progression and regression of coronary and peripheral atherosclerosis in the cynomolgus monkey. I. Effects of dipyridamole and aspirin. *Exp Mol Pathol* 30:55, 1979.

79. Holman RLH, McGill HC Jr, Strong JP, Geer JC: Atherosclerosis: the lesion. *Am J Clin Nutr* 8:84, 1960.

80. Ornish D, Brown SE, Shewritz LW, et al: Can lifestyle changes reverse coronary heart disease: The Lifestyle Heart Trial. *Lancet* 336:129, 1990.

81. Chester AH, O'Neill GS, Moncada S, et al: Low basal and stimulated release of nitric oxide in atherosclerotic epicardial coronary arteries. *Lancet* 336:897, 1990.

82. Forstermann U, Mugge A, Alheid U, et al: Selective attenuation of endothelium-mediated vasodilation in atherosclerotic human coronary arteries. *Circ Res* 62:185, 1988.

83. Heistad DD, Breese K, Armstrong ML: Cerebral vasoconstrictor responses to serotonin after dietary treatment of atherosclerosis: implications for transient ischemic attacks. *Stroke* 18:1068, 1987.

84. Harrison DG, Armstrong ML, Freiman DC, Heistad DD: Restoration of endothelium dependent relaxation by dietary treatment of atherosclerosis. *J Clin Invest* 80:1808, 1987.

85. Naruse K, Shimizu K, Muramatsu M, et al: Long-term inhibition of NO synthesis promotes atherosclerosis in the hypercholesterolemic rabbit thoracic aorta. *Arterioscler Thromb* 14:746, 1994.

86. Dock W: Atherosclerosis: why do we pretend the pathogenesis is mysterious? *Circulation* 50:647, 1974.

87. Steinberg D: The cholesterol controversy is over: why did it take so long? *Circulation* 80:1070, 1989.

88. Holley SB, Walsh JMR, Newman TB: Health policy on blood cholesterol: time to change directions. *Circulation* 80:1026, 1992.

89. South RL, Pickney ER: *The Cholesterol Conspiracy.* St. Louis: Warren H. Green Inc.; 1991.

90. Johnson CL, Rifkind BM, Sempos CT, et al: Declining total serum cholesterol levels among US adults. *JAMA* 269:3002, 1993.

91. Sempos CT, Cleeman JI, Carrol MD, et al: Prevalence of high blood cholesterol among US adults. *JAMA* 269:3009, 1993.

92. Bierman EI: Atherogenesis in diabetes. *Arterioscler Thromb* 12:647, 1992.

93. The Diabetes Control and Complications Trial Research Group: The effect of intensive treatment of diabetes on the development and progression of long-term complications in insulin-dependent diabetes mellitus. *N Engl J Med* 329:977, 1993.

94. Loscalzo J: Lipoprotein (a): a unique risk factor for atherothrombotic disease. *Arteriosclerosis* 10:672, 1990.

CHAPTER 12

Histopathologic Features of Nonarteriosclerotic Diseases of the Aorta and Arteries

Max Robinowitz, MD

Clinical Pathologic Approach

This chapter describes morphologic aspects of nonarteriosclerotic diseases of the aorta, and medium-sized and small-sized arteries >300 μm in external diameter; vessels within the range of direct surgical repair or involved in diseases frequently diagnosed with the aid of a surgical biopsy. Many exogenous and endogenous agents may act directly or indirectly on vessels, but the vascular system responds to a diversity of injuries in a limited number of ways. Identification of the specific agents or pathogenetic processes usually requires close coordination between clinicians and pathologists to ensure optimal therapeutic results.

The initial question is whether a biopsy would be diagnostically useful. If the answer is yes, then the answer to how, where, and what should be biopsied is based on the clinical presentation of the patient. Although a strictly morphologic approach can identify etiologic agents such as microorganisms, the usual pathologic diagnosis of vascular disease requires pattern recognition of microscopic findings and the synthesis of all available clinical, radiological, and other imaging information, immunologic, and laboratory test information. The additional information a biopsy yields ranges from a negative diagnosis, i.e., no recognizable morphologic variation from normal, to a positive, pathognomonic diagnosis. The degree of certitude of a biopsy diagnosis, positive or negative, ranges between possible, probable, and definitive. False-negative diagnoses may occur with sampling errors, especially when a disease is focal in distribution or if the area selected for sampling is not a likely target tissue for the disease process under study. A possible or equivocal biopsy diagnosis occurs when a disease elicits nonspecific histologic pattern that mimic variants of normal, aging, degenerative processes, or other disease.

Usually, performance of a biopsy early in the course of a vascular disease yields more productive diagnostic information than one taken after progression of a disease to its end stage. At this time, the identifiable etiologic agent or pathogenetic processes might no longer be present, or secondary scarring and degeneration can obscure characteristic morphologic features. This timing problem is analogous to the biopsy diagnosis of liver disease that has progressed to cirrhosis, kidney disease at the stage of chronic glomer-

From *The Basic Science of Vascular Disease*. Edited by Sidawy AN, Sumpio BE, and DePalma RG. Armonk, NY: Futura Publishing Company, Inc.; © 1997.

ulonephritis, or lung disease that has terminated in emphysema.[1]

Influence of Structure and Function on Development of Disease

Regional structural and functional differences of the circulatory system influence the types of injury and repair that are likely to occur. The aorta and arterial system serve as conduits to transport blood, but also serve to modulate the pulsatile flow. The relative thickness and composition of each of the three layers of the aorta and arteries, i.e., intima, media, and adventitia, vary in proportion to the intensity and oscillations of the systolic pressure wave.[2] The wall of the ascending aorta is predominantly comprised of a media consisting of approximately 56 elastic lamellar units. Each lamellar unit is a composite of overlapping smooth muscle cells (SMCs) and elastic fiber fascicles lying parallel to the longitudinal plane of the vessel. Interposed between the elastin systems are wavy collagen fiber bundles and a pericellular ground substance composed of proteoglycans (acid mucopolysaccharides).[3] Vascular elastic tissue stores kinetic energy of systole, and releases the energy in diastole with a net energy balance that is essentially zero.[2,4] The systolic pulse wave in the abdominal aorta has less oscillation than in the ascending aorta, due to losses as the wave distends the wall of the aorta. In addition, waves reflected off the bifurcation of the aorta and various branches of the aorta dampen the forward-directed systolic aortic pulse wave.

Developmentally, in humans and animals, the number of elastic lamellae in the aorta is proportional to the pressure distending the wall. At the aortic bifurcation, the forward pulse wave decreases in intensity and only about 28 elastic lamellar units are present in the media. In the aortic areas, 28 or more elastic lamellar units thick, the outer one third of the media is perfused by nutrient arteries, the vasa vasorum, that enter the adventitia and outer media with increasing frequency in direct proportion to the thickness of the wall. The ascending aorta has the greatest concentration of vasa vasorum. The aortas of small animals with less than 28 elastic lamellar units in the wall have fewer vasa vasorum because their thinner walls are perfused adequately from the aortic lumen via the aortic intima.[1–3,5–7] The tensile strength of the aorta is derived principally from the collagen in the media and adventitia. Collagen has tensile strength several orders of magnitude greater than elastin, and serves as a check on overdistention of the elastic fibers.[3,8]

The medias of major branch arteries are also composed of musculoelastic fascicles, but the encompassing elastic fiber systems are less prominent than in the aorta. The size and orientation of the fascicles in arteries are in the direction and intensity of tensile stress.[3]

Degenerative Changes in the Aorta and Arteries

Age-Related Changes in the Aorta

Repetitive stress and strain in the aorta and arteries lead to degenerative changes that are probably universal with aging and senescence. The aging aorta tends to be less elastic and more stiff. This is probably secondary to degenerative changes resulting in more fibrosis, fewer SMCs in the media, and fragmentation of elastic lamellae in the aortic wall. There is also decreased water content in the aortic wall with aging. These morphologic and biochemical changes are reflected clinically in a widened arterial pulse pressure and elevation of the systolic blood pressure.[9,10]

Some changes similar to aging of the normal aorta can be seen when the aortic tissue has inherently decreased elastic and/or collagen structure or function, i.e., Marfan's syndrome, Ehlers-Danlos syndrome, or when there are abnormally increased hemodynamic forces on the vascular wall, i.e., systemic hypertension and coarctation of the aorta.[10,11] The elastic lamellar unit structure of the aorta becomes altered by wear and tear in a manner similar to aging. In aging and in degenerative conditions, pools of mucoid proteoglycan material appear in the media where there is focal loss of SMCs. These foci are termed cystic medial necrosis, cystic medial degeneration, or cystic medionecrosis. Originally, these terms were based on the theory that the spaces were due to SMC necrosis and replacement by collections of basophilic mucoid substance. It is now believed that these are nonspecific collections of ground substance.[10,13] Actual cysts do not develop, but rather areas filled with ground substance exist between fragmented elastic lamellae.

The smooth muscle of the media is probably replaced by fibrosis because of aging and hypertension.[10] The diameter of the aorta increases and the wall thickness stays the same or even thickens with age. Thus, the total amount of aortic elastic fibers may not decrease, but the relative amount of elastin decreases as the other components increase in amount per unit thickness of the aortic and arterial wall.[9] Degenerative aging changes are most striking in the proximal aorta, and cause decreased elasticity and decreased ability to transmit the recoil of the pulse wave in diastole. The aorta gradually dilates and increases diameter with age and increases in length, causing an unwinding or tortuosity characteristic of the aging aorta. This process is independent of superimposed atherosclerosis, which is basically an intimal process.[10–13]

Compliance and elasticity of the aortas of elderly patients can also be impaired by amyloid deposition. This material has the microscopic appearance of amyloid, i.e., stains with Congo red and is birefringent with polarized light; but this material is different chemically from the material found in senile cardiac amyloid.[1]

Aortic Dissection

Aortic dissection, formerly known as dissecting aneurysm of the aorta, refers to the longitudinal splitting of the outer media in a plane parallel to the course of the blood flow in the lumen of the aorta, and consequent development of an intramural hematoma that does not necessarily increase the external dimension of the involved aorta.[13] The peak presentation of aortic dissection is in later middle age (about age 60) and is two to three times more common in men than in women. Ninety percent of male patients with aortic dissection have left ventricular hypertrophy, and 70% have known systemic hypertension. The frequency of occurrence of aortic dissection increases with increasing severity of hypertension. In women, more than 25% of aortic dissections occur during pregnancy. People with Marfan's syndrome are susceptible to aortic dissection. The greater incidence of aortic dissection in black men probably relates to their increased incidence of systemic hypertension. No geographic risk for increased incidence of aortic dissection has been identified. The major etiologic factors are systemic hypertension and Marfan's syndrome. Risk increases directly with the age of the patient.[13,14]

An aortic dissection begins with a structural weakness in the media of the aorta that leads to decreased support of the overlying intima. An intimal tear develops, usually a transverse tear in the proximal ascending aorta, and blood from the lumen then dissects into the media. Once within the media, the dissection becomes an intramural hematoma extending longitudinally within the outer media in a course parallel to the flow of blood in the lumen. The dissection plane extends distally or proximally. Secondary ischemic necrosis of the media follows the dissection plane as the process disrupts the vasa vasorum of the aorta, further weakening the aortic wall. Impairment of the aorta can be severe as the dissection splits the aorta, often within seconds. Major branch vessels anywhere from the aortic arch to the distal bifurcation of the aorta can be sheared off. The vascular beds previously served by the sheared off branch arteries develop ischemia, which leads to infarcts and organ failure.[1,5,10,13,15]

Gross examination of an aortic dissection reveals a transverse primary intimal tear in the aorta in about 95% of cases (Figure 1). About two thirds of the tears occur in the proximal ascending aorta about 2 cm above the aortic valve annulus. The next most frequent site is in the distal aortic arch or upper descending thoracic aorta. In both sites, the tears are usually less than one half to one third of the circumference of the aorta.

The course of the dissection may extend into the aortic root for varying distances from the ascending aorta or towards the bifurcation. The dissection plane is usually along the greater curvature of the aorta and comprises less than the total circumference of the aorta. Beyond the aortic isthmus, the dissection plane usually pursues a spiral course and may extend outward into the orifices of branch vessels. When the dissection is in the ascending aorta, the most frequent route is into the aortic root. This can compromise the right coronary ostium. Distal extension of an aortic dissection may be limited by medial scarring or atrophy associated with severe arteriosclerosis, especially in the area of the isthmus of the aorta near the ligamentum arteriosum and in the abdominal aorta below the renal arteries. Dissection of the aorta is also limited by congenital isthmic coarctation of the aorta.[13,15]

Microscopically, an aortic dissection is found usually between the inner two thirds and outer one third of the media (Figure 2). Cystic medial necrosis (cystic medial degeneration) usually is found, along with disruption of the elastic lamella (Figure 3). The dissection plane actually can form a false channel for blood to course along the aortic wall. The outer wall may rupture externally with resultant hemorrhage.[13,15] The false channel of an aortic dissection can remain as a blind pouch, and extend and rupture into the lumen to create a patent false channel and true lumen. The false channel contents may expand to push the inner media into the true lumen and obliterate the true lumen, or the outer portion of the media and adventitia may rupture with massive blood loss or exsanguination.[13,15]

When the ischemic changes as a consequence of medial aortic dissection are limited and the patient survives, the surface of the false channel within the media becomes covered by fibrin and platelets. This coagulum forms a matrix for the ingrowth of SMCs and endothelial cells. Eventually, a nonthrombogenic neointima may form.[13] Approximately 90% of untreated cases of aortic dissection die. The prognosis is better if reentry occurs. The most frequent cause of death in aortic dissection is external rupture of the right anterolateral wall of the proximal aorta, near the site of the intimal tear in the ascending aorta.[13,14,16]

Classification of aortic dissection depends on whether it involves the ascending aorta, the descending aorta, or both segments. The DeBakey classification type I involves the ascending and descending aortas; type II involves only the ascending aorta; and type III involves only the descending aorta. The Daily classification type A combines DeBakey's type I and II. Daily type B is equivalent to DeBakey's type III. Involvement of the ascending aorta is associated with a poorer prognosis than those dissections limited to the descending aorta, and requires different medical and surgical therapy.[14,16]

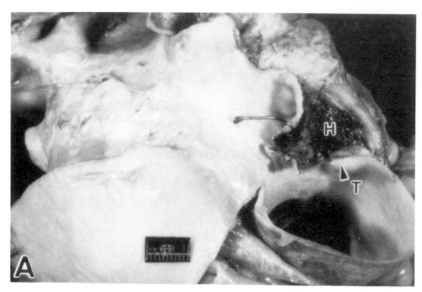

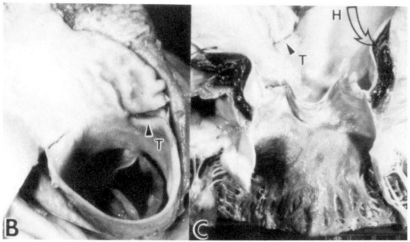

Figure 1. **A.** and **B.** Aortic dissection with transverse intimal tear (**T**) in the first portion of the ascending aorta. **C.** A hematoma (**H**) dissects into the media (**open arrow**) distally and proximally. The patient was a middle-aged man with systemic hypertension and no clinical stigmata of Marfan's syndrome. There is no dilatation of the sinuses of Valsalva.

Aortic dissection due to medial degeneration differs from rupture of atherosclerotic aneurysm. Atherosclerosis is primarily an intimal process that leads to secondary atrophy and thinning of the media. One view of atherosclerotic aneurysm pathogenesis is that severe diffuse atherosclerotic intimal involvement, especially in the abdominal aorta below the renal arteries, leads to decreased diffusion to the inner media, decreased tensile strength, and aneurysmal dilatation. The probability of rupture of an aortic aneurysm and direct communication into the periaortic space increases in direct relation to the increased diameter of an aneurysm. However, dissection into the aortic wall is not a likely consequence of atherosclerosis.[13,15]

Heritable Disorders of Connective Tissue

Heritable disorders of connective tissue include disorders of the structural fibers collagen, elastin, and fibrillin and the nonfibrous components of the ground substance, i.e., glycosaminoglycans and proteins. Disorders of the structural fibers include Marfan's syndrome, Ehlers-Danlos syndrome, congenital contractural arachnodactyly, cutis laxa, osteogenesis imperfecta, pseudoxanthoma elasticum, Weill-Marchesani syndrome, and various coalition syndromes. Disorders of the ground substance include the mucopolysaccharidoses, mucolipidoses, glycoproteinoses, and lipidoses.[17] In the future, it may be possible to identify the genetic defects responsible for the biochemical defects underlying the heritable connective disorders by nucleic acid probes. Some of these conditions can be identified by the presence or absence of certain metabolic products, others by enzyme deficiencies. All of these conditions originally were defined from the clinical appearance of the patient. Detailed family studies have demonstrated dominant and recessive inheritance and varying degrees of impairment by what is probably the same basic defect. Most of these

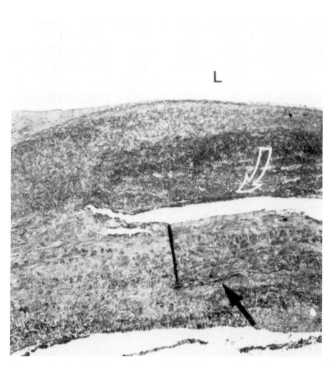

L

Figure 2. Aortic dissection within the media of the aorta of a middle-age man with systemic hypertension. **L** = lumen; **open white arrow** = dissection plane within muscularis; **black arrow** = junction of media with adventitia. (×30, Movat pentachrome stain.)

conditions are rare, and details about involvement of the cardiovascular system are not complete.[13,17,18]

Although collagen is the locus of disease in certain heritable connective disease, these conditions are not the same as those immunologic conditions labeled collagen disease by Klemperer et al in 1942.[19] They found that patients with scleroderma and systemic lupus erythematosus had eosinophilic deposition of fibrin-like material in the interstitial fibrous tissue of various organs. They applied the term "collagen disease" as a unifying concept to explain the pathogenesis of these diseases. Rich[20] later expanded their concept and changed the original terminology to collagen vascular disease.

Marfan's Syndrome

Marfan's syndrome is the most commonly encountered cardiovascular complication of heritable connective tissue disease. This is an autosomal dominant, pleiotropic, heritable disorder of connective tissue of unclear, yet probably heterogeneous causes. It afflicts an estimated 23000 people in the United States, or 1 American in 10000. The syndrome is characterized by abnormalities of the connective tissues, leading to structural weakness in the skeletal, cutaneous, ocular, and cardiovascular systems. Structural weakness of the blood vessels usually causes dilatation of the sinuses of Valsalva of the aorta (sinotubular portion of the aorta), and may result in aortic dissection and death in the teens or early adult life.[1,13,17,21,22]

No pathognomonic light or electron microscopic morphologic findings have been described for Marfan's syndrome. The cardiovascular diagnosis of Marfan's syndrome is based on the clinical recognition of abnormalities that occur with high frequency in Marfan's syndrome patients and family members exhibiting clinical manifestations of Marfan's syndrome. M-mode echocardiography demonstrates an egg-shaped dilatation of the sinuses of Valsalva, i.e., >3.5 to 3.8 cm diameter in women and >3.8 to 4.0 cm in men. Other cardiovascular findings include mitral valve prolapse, aortic regurgitation, and sometimes mitral regurgitation. The musculoskeletal abnormalities include a stature taller than comparable people of the same age and sex; disproportionately long limbs; an arm span that exceeds the patient's height; reduced upper/lower body ratio; arachnodactyly; hyperflexibility of the joints; lax hands; pectus excavatum or carinatum; scoliosis; genu recurvatum (abnormal hyperextensibility of the knees); long narrow and flat feet; high arched palate; downward slanting palpebral fissures; and malocclusion of the teeth. Superior dislocation of the lenses is an important diagnostic feature in Marfan's syndrome. A less specific ocular finding is myopia. Cutaneous striae are also seen with increased frequency. Not all of these abnormalities occur in each patients.[21–23]

The marfinoid habitus can be diagnosed at birth. In addition, linear longitudinal growth curves based on the ratio of upper to lower body length can aid in the diagnosis of Marfan's syndrome early in life, but the major cardiovascular morbidity usually is not seen until the late teens and peaks in the third decade. Marfan's syndrome occurs in all racial, geographic, and ethnic groups.[17,23]

Decreased aortic medial tensile strength in patients with Marfan's syndrome leads to disruption of elastic medial lamellar structural units, particularly in the area between the outer and midportion of the media. Trauma or sudden deceleration forces such as occur in an automobile accident may trigger an aortic dissection in an individual with Marfan's syndrome. Within the areas of disrupted elastic lamellae, proteoglycans or ground substance collects, resulting in the histologic appearance of cystic medial necrosis. This change is qualitatively similar to that described in aging and hypertension. Support of the overlying intima becomes impaired and may lead to aortic dissection. Usually, however, dilatation of the sinuses of Valsalva pre-

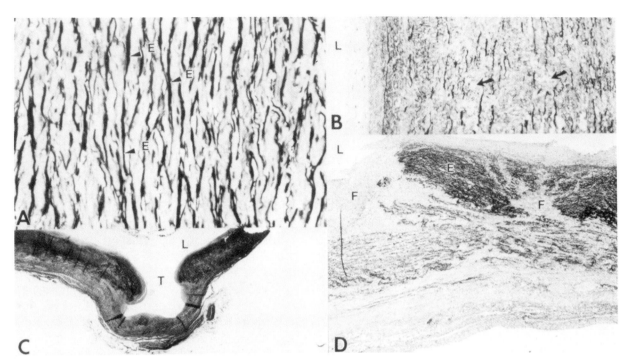

Figure 3. Comparison of normal aorta with aorta showing cystic medial necrosis. **A.** Media of normal aorta from 22-year-old male traffic victim. Note the elastic lamellae (**E**), which alternate with collagen fibers and smooth muscle cells (SMCs), (×300; Movat pentachrome stain). **B.** Fragmented elastic lamellae and areas showing absent elastin and SMCs consistent with cystic medial necrosis (**arrows**) (×75; Movat pentachrome stain). **C.** Marfan's syndrome patient with partial aortic dissection and formation of false aneurysm formation at tear (**T**) (×7.5; Movat pentachrome stain). **D.** Border of aortic tear showing disruption elastic lamellae (**E**) and partial healing by fibrous tissue (**F**). (×30; Movat pentachrome stain.)

cedes development of an aortic dissection in Marfan's syndrome.[8,10,12,13,15,17]

The gross pathology of aortic dissection is similar to that of patients without Marfan's syndrome, except that the aortic wall is usually very thin and may be translucent. The aortic annulus is typically dilated. Aortic root dilatation is less common in aortic dissection in patients without Marfan's syndrome.[8,10,12,13,15,17] Cystic medial necrosis is the microscopic hallmark of Marfan's syndrome, but is also found in other conditions. There is fragmentation and loss of elastic fibers in the media of the aorta, and secondary loss of SMCs and filling of the defect with increased mucoid proteoglycan ground substance. In patients over age 40, cystic medial change is more likely due to diseases other than Marfan's syndrome.[8,10,12,13,15,17]

Healing of an aortic dissection in Marfan's syndrome is less likely than in hypertension-related aortic dissection, because the wall is inherently more fragile in Marfan's syndrome. Incomplete tears also may be seen in the aorta in Marfan's syndrome (Figure 3). Untreated aortic dissection in Marfan's syndrome has a

fatality of greater than 95% and mortality, overall, in Marfan's syndrome principally is due to aortic dissection.[17]

Ehlers-Danlos syndrome, osteogenesis imperfecta, or cutis laxis syndrome are characterized by degeneration of elastic tissue. Individuals with these syndromes lack the Marfan's habitus and show other characteristic features. Ehlers-Danlos syndrome comprises at least 10 distinct disorders. Originally, the syndromes shared one or more phenotypic features that include hyperextensibility of skin, increased joint mobility, and abnormal tissue fragility. Later additions to the group are based on biochemical defects in structural fibers of the connective tissues. The most notable cardiovascular disorder is found in the Ehlers-Danlos syndrome type IV. There is a defect in type III collagen, the component that constitutes about 50% of the collagen in the wall of the aorta and arteries. The arteries may be extremely friable, and any elastic or muscular artery may rupture spontaneously. Aortic dissection or dilatation is not usually found. Direct surgical repair may not be possible because of the inability of the arterial wall to retain sutures. Cystic medial necrosis is absent. The affected vessel wall may be thinned, and internal elastic lamina may be irregular or fragmented. No pathognomonic microscopic features of Ehlers-Danlos syndrome are described in the literature or in the several cases examined at the Armed Forces Institute of Pathology.[1,13,17]

Annulo-aortic ectasia, defined as dilatation of the ascending aorta, dilatation of the aortic annulus, and progressive insufficiency of the aortic valve, may occur in classic Marfan's syndrome patients with skeletal, ocular, and cardiovascular abnormalities, or the annulo-aortic ectasia may be an isolated finding. Aortic dissection can occur. This entity is associated with microscopic features similar to Marfan's syndrome, and degenerative changes associated with cystic medial necrosis in patients over age 40. Until a definitive biochemical test of the structural disorders in the vessels is developed, or a laboratory test becomes available to identify the gene(s) responsible for Marfan's syndrome and related disorders, it may not be possible to separate subgroups of patients with structural disorders of the aorta without clinical features of the classic Marfan's syndrome.[17,27,28]

Acquired Structural Defects

Cystic Adventitial Disease

Cystic adventitial disease refers to the presence of an intramural cyst that narrows or occludes the lumen of the affected artery. The most typical example is the popliteal artery cyst.[18,29] Cystic advential disease is a rare, treatable cause of claudication of the leg and may present as a surgical emergency. Males outnumber females 6:1 in the incidence, and there is usually a history of manual labor. The peak onset of symptoms is in the fourth to fifth decade, in males and the sixth decade in females. The typical presentation is calf pain on flexion of the leg in an individual, without any generalized arterial insufficiency. Popliteal aneurysm should be suspected in patients with a prominent popliteal pulse who present with intermittent claudication and in patients developing acute ischemia of the leg due to thrombosis or distal embolization. Urgent surgery may be needed, and failure to recognize these diagnoses may result in limb loss.[18,29]

Intramural cysts are most frequently located at or just above the upper level of femoral condyles in the popliteal artery, but may also be found in the external iliac, common femoral, radial, and ulnar arteries. Least common is the finding of intramural cysts in veins. Bilateral aneurysms may be present in about 50% of patients (Figure 4).[18,29]

The cause of intramural cysts of arteries has not been identified. Trauma is suggested by the history of

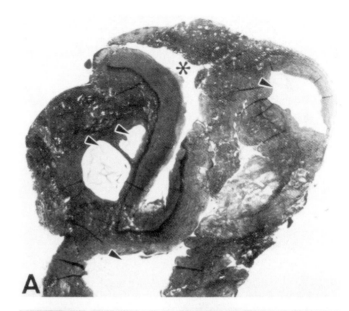

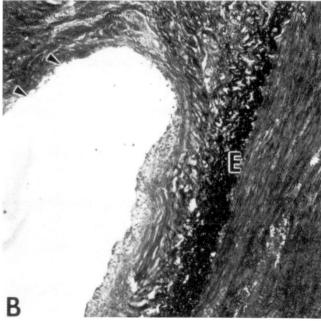

Figure 4. Popliteal artery with cystic adventitial disease. Note cystic spaces filled with mucoid material **(arrowheads).** The cysts compress the arterial lumen (*). (**A.** ×7.5, **B.** ×75; Movat pentachrome stain.)

manual labor in many individuals and the presence of hemorrhage or hemosiderin within the walls of some cysts. The mucin-like material within the cysts is similar to ganglion cysts of tendon sheath and is derived from the adjacent connective tissue; no lining cells are present in the cysts. Intramural cysts filled with clear fluid or gelatinous contents may be uniloculated or multiloculated. If completely excised, an intramural cyst does not usually recur.[18,29]

Developmental or Acquired Structural Abnormalities of Arteries

Fibromuscular Dysplasia

Fibromuscular dysplasia is a generic term for a group of structural abnormalities of one or more layers of medium-sized and large arteries. These abnormalities can result in luminal narrowing by fibrous, smooth muscle or fibromuscular tissue with or without associated aneurysms. The process usually is due to congenital malformation of the arterial structure. Its classification is based on the angiographic appearance and histopathologic localization and pattern of the structural abnormalities. Numerous and sometimes confusing synonyms have been applied to the overall group and each of its subdivisions.[1,18,30–32] All of these lesions may cause ischemia, particularly those involving the renal arteries. They may also be associated with dissection of the media.

Fibromuscular dysplasia located predominantly in the intima is called intimal fibroplasia and comprises about 5% of all cases of fibromuscular dysplasia. It may occur in all age groups including children, but is most commonly found in females of child-bearing age. Corkscrew or irregular, long tubular luminal stenoses are seen angiographically. These stenoses lead to is-

chemia in the organ served by the involved artery. The most frequent clinical presentation of intimal fibroplasia is renovascular hypertension secondary to stenosis of the renal arteries. Other sites of involvement include the carotid, vertebral, and splanchnic arteries; all of these arteries may be involved by obstruction, dissecting aneurysm, or emboli from mural thrombi within aneurysms. In disseminated cases, veins can also be affected. Microscopically, there is circumferential or eccentric intimal thickening by fibrous tissue without lipid deposition or inflammatory cell infiltrate (Figure 5). The process spares the internal elastic lamina, media, and adventitia. Endarteritis, secondary to inflammatory conditions within organs or trauma, may be associated with intimal fibroplasia in muscular arteries. These might mimic the histologic picture of intimal fibroplasia-type fibromuscular dysplasia. In addition, the morphologic picture may be virtually indistinguishable from that of secondary or reactive intimal fibroplasia seen after endarterectomy or in the initial proliferative stage of atherosclerosis. Intimal fibroplasia may be isolated or occur concomitantly with medial fibromuscular dysplasia.[1,18,30–32]

The second type of fibromuscular dysplasia, medial fibromuscular dysplasia, is subdivided into three variants: medial fibroplasia comprised of fibrous and muscular ridges (Figures 6A and 6B), medial hyperpla-

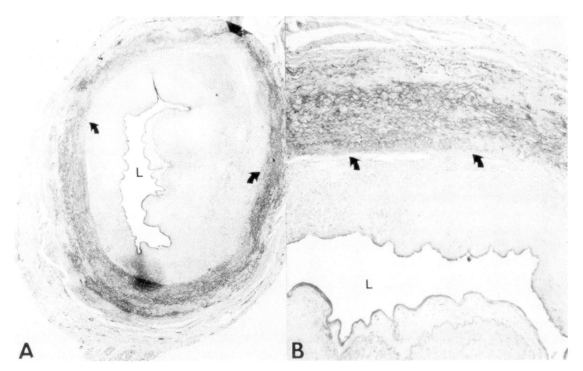

Figure 5. Medium-sized artery involved by fibromuscular dysplasia of the intimal fibroplasia type. The process spares the internal elastic lamina (**arrows**), media, and adventitia. L = lumen. (**A.** ×10, **B.** ×75; Movat pentachrome stain.)

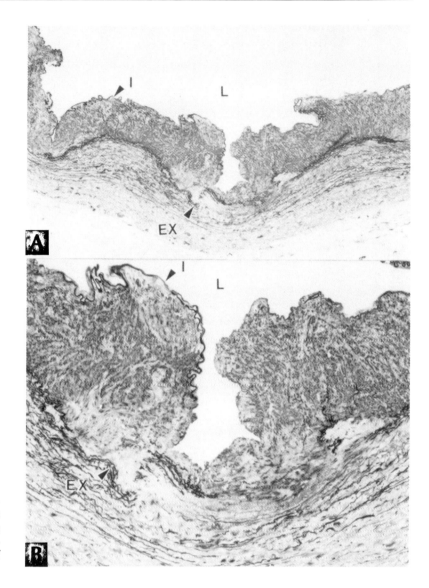

Figure 6. Medium-sized arteries involved by fibromuscular dysplasia. **A** and **B** represent the medial fibroplasia type represented by fibrous and muscular ridges, which produce the string-of-beads appearance in clinical angiograms of such arteries.

sia comprised of excessive proliferation of SMCs (Figures 6C and 6D), and perimedial fibroplasia characterized by the presence of dense fibrous tissue in the outer media. Each of these conditions is idiopathic. The major clinical presentation is arterial stenosis with or without aneurysms.[1,18,30–32] Medial fibroplasia comprises 60% to 85% of idiopathic renal arterial stenosis and is found in the distal two thirds of the renal artery and its main branches, and carotid, mesenteric, hepatic, and iliac arteries. It may angiographically present a string-of-beads appearance of stenosis alternating with aneurysms. This appearance is due to fibrous and SMC ridges alternating with aneurysms, where there has been collagenous replacement of smooth muscle and internal elastic lamina. Tubular stenoses or a single stenotic focus may also be seen.[1,18,30–32]

The next most common variant of medial fibromuscular dysplasia is perimedial fibroplasia. This condition is responsible for 10% to 25% of idiopathic renal stenosis. Angiographically, the appearance of perimedial fibroplasia is nonaneurysmal beading. This appearance is due to irregular severe luminal stenosis localized in the midportion of the renal artery. Microscopically, there is deposition of dense collagenous and elastic fibrous tissue in the outer media or even throughout the thickness of the media, with or without replacement of the external elastic lamina and development of small vessels in the media by neovascularization. The inner portion of the media usually is normal in appearance. Arterial dissection can occur at the interface of fibrous layer and muscle in the area of the neovascularization. Aneurysms rarely occur.[1,18,30–32]

The third and least common variant of fibromuscular dysplasia is medial hyperplasia, comprising only 1% to 15% of nonatheromatous renal artery stenosis. Angiographically and grossly, the appearance is that of

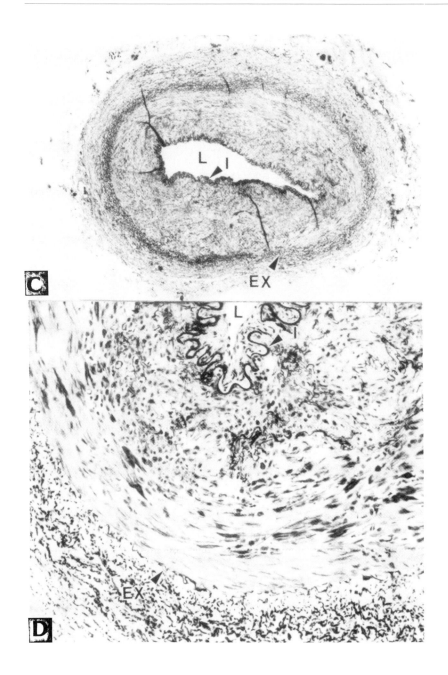

Figure 6. **C** and **D** show the medial hyperplasia variant with marked thickening of the media. Some disarray of smooth muscle cells is present. EX = external elastic lamina; I = internal elastic lamina; L = lumen. (**A** and **B**, ×30, **C** and **D**, ×150; Movat pentachrome stain.)

stenosis with aneurysms. The microscopic picture consists of a normal appearance of the arterial wall, but there is marked thickening of media by increased numbers of SMCs, which are normally arranged in the media and cause luminal narrowing. The intima, internal and external elastic laminae, and adventitia are spared. A condition related to fibromuscular dysplasia is periarterial fibroplasia, a thickening of a muscular artery due to dense collagenous replacement in the loose fibrous tissue of the arterial adventitia. This process can extend into the surrounding adipose and connective tissues. The media and intima are normal.[1,18,30–32]

Hormonal irregularities, physical stresses, arterial wall ischemia, viral infection, and congenital malformation all have been proposed as the possible etiologies for fibromuscular dysplasia. Currently, there is no animal model or definite explanation of this process. Because fibromuscular dysplasia has been found in cases of chronic ergotamine or methysergide intoxication, it has been suggested that fibromuscular dysplasia may be a consequence of chronic, repeated, discontinuous, and sub-obstructing spasms.[1,18,30–33]

The natural history of fibromuscular dysplasia depends on whether the process is localized to one vessel or multivessel sites, what organs are involved, and if an aneurysm develops, whether there is dissection and potentially fatal exsanguination.[1,18,30–32]

Inflammatory Conditions of the Aorta and Arteries

Vasculitis

Vasculitis, or angiitis, is the generic term for inflammation of the media of arteries and veins with or without involvement of the intima and the adventitia. Vasculitis may be primary or secondary to localized or generalized inflammatory conditions. Most examples of primary vasculitis are idiopathic and are classified on the basis of the size of blood vessels involved, type of vascular injury, predominant cellular component of the inflammatory reaction, and gross and microscopic localization and patterns of involvement of the tissue injury and repair. If there is morphologic evidence of tissue necrosis, especially with deposition of fibrin (fibrinoid necrosis), the condition is often called *necrotizing vasculitis*. Some types of vasculitis appear to be more prevalent in particular geographic areas or racial groups.[34,35]

Inflammation is a fundamental host defense mechanism that is mediated by the selective extravasation of certain cellular and noncellular blood components into perturbed tissues. The inflammatory response delivers complement antibodies and leukocytes to areas of microbial invasion and cell injury. As a result, the provoking agent is neutralized and healing begins. In certain instances, inflammation may be harmful to the host; a seemingly benign disturbance misdirects a similar outpouring of inflammatory elements, which initiates an autoimmune reaction against the host.[36–38]

The recognition of distinctive clinicopathologic vasculitis syndromes may help in identifying the underlying process. However, the same etiologic agent may cause different vasculitis syndromes that may progress and lead to the demise of the patient, or cause a syndrome that follows a chronic indolent course. These variations in the inflammatory response are influenced by the individual biologic variations of each patient's genetic makeup and immune system, the age and sex of the patient, and risk factors such as nutritional status, and coexisting disease or medications, i.e., corticosteroids. Also, differences in vascular response may be due to variations in the route of exposure of the etiologic agent, the form and amount of the inciting dose, and the presence of excitatory or inhibitory cofactors.[34,35]

Aortitis is vasculitis involving the aorta. The etiologic agent usually is presumed to be a microorganism, particularly a virus, or foreign antigens, particularly drugs. In the early inflammatory stage, evidence of tissue necrosis and active inflammation are typical. There often are varying amounts of lymphocytic and plasma cell infiltrates. Giant cells may be seen in many types of vasculitis, especially aortitis. Giant cells are multinucleated tissue macrophages that are associated with cell-mediated immunity and granulomatous reactions (Figure 7). Abundant quantities of giant cells characterize giant cell aortitis, a condition with a distinctive clinicopathologic constellation.[1,13,34,35]

In most forms of aortitis, the inflammation weakens the aortic media and can lead to aneurysmal dilatation. Takayasu's aortitis may be unique in its potential to also cause luminal narrowing and even occlusion of the aorta and its major branch arteries.[1,39]

Figure 7. Typical multinucleated giant cell derived from tissue macrophages or blood monocytes. It is found in a variety of inflammatory conditions in the aorta and arteries. (×750; hematoxylin and eosin.)

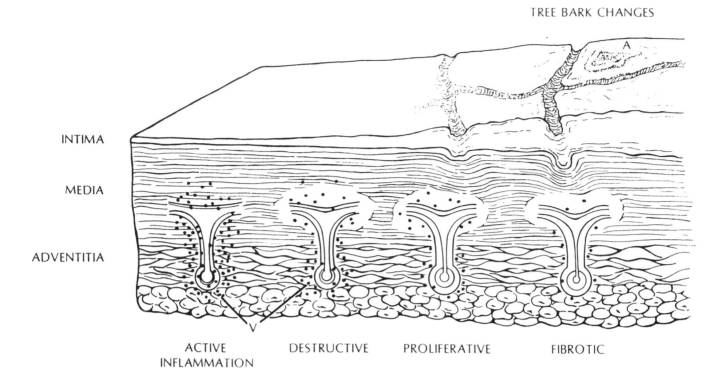

TREE BARK CHANGES

INTIMA

MEDIA

ADVENTITIA

ACTIVE   DESTRUCTIVE   PROLIFERATIVE   FIBROTIC
INFLAMMATION

Figure 8. Early to late stages in aortitis beginning with active inflammation involving the vasa vasorum followed by destructive changes in these vessels and the surrounding aortic wall. The proliferative response by intimal and medial smooth muscle cells leads to thickening of the vasa vasorum, luminal compromise, and ischemia in the aortic wall. Fibrosis follows in addition to retraction of the scar tissue, tree-bark intimal change, and superimposed atherosclerosis. These changes are nonspecific, but are typical of syphilitic aortitis. **A** = atherosclerotic plaque; **V** = vasa vasorum.

Intimal scarring and/or retraction of medial scars are found in almost any form of aortitis. The process may lead to wrinkling of the intimal surface by depressed scars that alternate with raised islands of intima. The resultant appearance of the intima is commonly called "tree-barking." Although tree-barking of the intima is frequent in syphilitic aortitis, it is not specific for syphilitic aortitis (Figures 8 and 9).[1,13]

In general, the vascular reaction to intimal injury of an artery or vein is migration of cells from the media

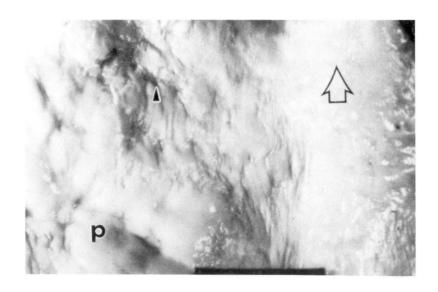

Figure 9. Gross appearance of aortic intima involved by aortitis. The **arrowhead** points to depressed scars surrounded by raised islands of intima leading to a tree-bark appearance. **P** = atherosclerotic plaque; **arrow** = direction of blood flow; **marker** = 2 cm.

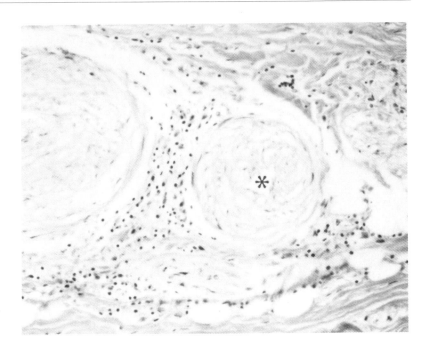

Figure 10. Two vasa vasorum (nutrient arteries of aorta) involved by proliferative endarteritis. Smooth muscle cells, fibrous tissue, and ground substance narrow the arterial lumen (*). Plasma cells and lymphocytes surround the arteries. (×250, hematoxylin and eosin.)

into the intima and proliferation of SMCs and modified SMCs or myofibroblasts within the intima. These SMCs and myofibroblasts produce collagen, elastin, and proteoglycans. The deposition of fibrous proteins and fibromuscular proliferation causes varying degrees of luminal narrowing that are often devoid of inflammatory infiltrate (Figure 10).[1,40]

Syphilitic Aortitis

Syphilitic or luetic aortitis is one of the characteristic cardiovascular manifestations of untreated syphilis. The process usually is clinically silent after the primary chancre and secondary stages until late into the teritary stage of syphilis. Syphilitic aortitis was seen in about 7.0% of the autopsies performed in 1939 (the preantibiotic era), but in only 0.7% of autopsies from 1950–1965. Since 1965, syphilitic aortitis has become extremely rare and is now found almost exclusively in elderly patients who contracted syphilis many years ago.[1,13]

Cardiovascular syphilis presents as one or more of the following clinicopathologic entities: aortitis, aortic aneurysm, aortic valvulitis with or without aortic root dilatation and aortic regurgitation, coronary artery ostial stenosis, and gumma formation within the wall of the aorta or myocardium. The first clinical manifestation of cardiovascular syphilis might be rupture of a syphilitic aortic aneurysm, chronic aortic regurgitation, or myocardial ischemia from coronary ostial stenosis. Pressure atrophy and necrosis can occur in bones and organs adjacent to a syphilitic aortic aneurysm. The definitive diagnosis of cardiovascular syphilis requires a positive history of syphilis, positive serologic test for syphilis, and/or tissue demonstration of *Treponema pallidum*. All three findings are preferable for a definitive diagnosis (Table 1).[1,13,41,42]

Treponema pallidum is the organism that causes syphilis. There is no identified risk factor, geographic, or familial susceptibility. The reported increased incidence in males in the past probably reflected past social customs more than a difference in gender susceptibility.[13]

The basic involvement in any bodily organ of congenital syphilis and syphilis acquired later in life is a small artery endarteritis, particularly the vasa vasorum—the nutrient arteries of the aorta (Figure 10). The endarteritis is characterized by inflammation of small muscular arteries and a reactive proliferation of SMCs. Collagen fibers and ground substance both deposit, which, in aggregate, narrow the lumen of the nutrient artery and cause ischemic damage and weakening of the aortic wall, aortic aneurysmal dilatation, and rupture. The frequency of distribution of the lesions of syphilitic aortitis follows the distribution pattern of the vasa vasorum. Syphilitic aortic aneurysms are almost always found in the ascending aorta with a variable extension distally. Only about 10% of syphilitic aortic aneurysms are limited to the abdominal aorta. It is rare for the process to extend beyond the upper abdominal aorta.[1,13,41,42]

The term *endarteritis* is also used as part of the generic diagnostic term "endarteritis obliterans," a nonspecific descriptive term for luminal narrowing of arteries in reaction to an injury. In a computerized search of the National Medical Library files from 1983 to 1986, only non-English medical articles used the

Table 1
Clinical Features of Aortitis

	Syphilitic	Rheumatoid	Ankylosing Spondylitis	Reiter's	Takayasu's	Giant Cell	Infective
Mean age	>50	>40	<40	<30	15	Elderly	Any age
Sex	M > F	F > M	M > F	M ≫ F	F ≫ M	F > M	Prob. M = F
Etiology	T. palidum	Viral?		Shigella + +	Unknown	Unknown	Bacteria, fungi, etc.
Association			HLA-B27	HLA-B27		Polymyalgia rheumatica	Vascular injury/sepsis
Pathologic features of aortitis:							
Typical involvement	ASC Ao	ASC Ao	AVA, Tub Ao LVOT Ridge	AVA, TUB Ao	ASC Ao + +	Variable	Anywhere
Stenosis of arteries	Coronary ostia		Coronary ostia		+ +/+ + +		
Aneurysm	+ +/+ + +		AVA DIL	AVA DIL			
Aneurysm location	ASC Ao*	Variable					
Vasa vasorum endarteritis & tree-barking	+ + +	+ +	+ +	+ +	±	±	±
Fibrinoid	No; but GUMMA 20%	No; but RA granuloma + +	Granuloma ±	−	±	±	±
Inflammatory reaction	P, L	L	L, P	L, P	L	L, G C	PMN, L, MAC
Giant cells	±	±	−	−	+	+ +/+ + +	Depends on ETX
Eosinophils	−	+/±	−	−	−	+	Depends on ETX

−: absent; ±: present occasionally; +: usually present; + +: frequently present; + + +: almost always present; *Ao: aorta; ASC: ascending; AVA: aortic valve annulus; DIL: dilatation; ETX: etiology; F: female; GC: giant cells; L: lymphocytes; LVOT: left ventricular outflow tract; M: male; MAC: macrophages; P: plasma cells; PMN: polymorphonuclear leukocytes; RA: rheumatoid arthritis; TUB: tubular portion.

term endarteritis as a diagnostic term in the title. More specific etiologic and morphologic diagnostic terms have supplanted the term *endarteritis obliterans*. In the past, endarteritis obliterans referred to the changes in a small artery that may follow inflammatory injury from infection or chemical injury. Examples are arteries at the base of a peptic ulcer, traumatic injury, involutional regressive changes as seen in the postpuerperal uterine arteries or in the stump of an amputated limb, and pressure-related arterial changes found in the intrarenal arteries in hypertension. The narrowing of the lumen may not have much clinical significance if the organ (e.g., the uterus) served has involuted and has a decreased demand for blood. Endarteritis obliterans has also been misused as a synonym for thromboangiitis obliterans or Buerger's disease.[18]

Grossly, syphilitic aortitis produces a thickened, wrinkled tree-bark intimal surface that usually becomes covered by secondary, superimposed atherosclerosis that is greater in the thoracic than in the ab-

dominal aorta (Figure 9). Gross or microscopic aortic calcification is identifiable radiographically in more than 50% of cases. Syphilitic aneurysm may be fusiform or saccular and may enlarge to 10 cm or more in diameter prior to rupture.[1,13,41,42]

Microscopically, endarteritis of the vasa vasorum of the aorta is an obliterative, proliferative inflammation of the small nutrient arteries of the aorta. Lymphocytes and plasma cells infiltrate in a perivascular cuffing pattern around and within the vasa vasorum (Figure 10). Decreased blood flow through the affected small arteries leads to destruction of the smooth muscle and elastic tissue of the media. Healing occurs by formation of scars in the media. Retraction of the scars results in the gross picture of tree-barking of the intima.[1,13,41,42]

About 20% of serologically proved syphilitic aortitis show gummas usually in the ascending aorta. Gummas are foci of tissue necrosis. Microscopically, a gumma is an area of deeply eosinophilic amorphous material in the media that is surrounded by a few lymphocytes and plasma cells and rarely by a few giant cells. Treponema pallidum organisms may be identified in these necrotic areas with special, silver impregnation stains (Levaditi's stain). This stain is available in consultation laboratories.[1,13,41,42] Severe coronary artery ostial narrowing, secondary to aortic intimal thickening or inflammatory endarteritis, can cause myocardial ischemia.[13]

Syphilis has been called the great imitator in clinical medicine because its widespread involvement in the vascular system results in symptoms that overlap with many other diseases. Pathologically, cardiovascular syphilis also is a great imitator. A previously positive serologic test for syphilis in a patient with untreated syphilis may decrease to low undetectable titers over many years. While special stains for Treponema pallidum demonstrate the organisms's characteristic morphology, tissue stains have low sensitivity and the organisms are usually found only in areas of active necrosis. A tentative diagnosis of syphilitic aortitis may be made in the absence of positive serology and history if the patient is over 50 years of age; aortitis and aortic aneurysm are maximal in the ascending thoracic aorta, and there is a plasma cell and lymphocytic cuffing and obliterative endarteritis involving the vasa va-

sorum. Superimposed intimal atherosclerotic plaques and medial degenerative changes from hypertension might obscure aortic changes due to syphilis.[1,13,41,42]

The most frequent cause of aortic aneurysms in middle-age and older patients is atherosclerosis. These aortic aneurysms are more common in the abdominal aorta and usually show less severe inflammatory infiltrates than syphilitic aneurysms. Obliterative endarteritis of the vasa vasorum is not a feature of atherosclerosis. Hypertension accelerates the development of atherosclerosis with and without syphilis.[1,13]

Inflammatory Aortic Aneurysms and Retroperitoneal Fibrosis

Some atherosclerotic aneurysms in the abdominal aorta are accompanied by intense inflammation. These have been termed inflammatory abdominal aortic aneurysms. Typically, inflammatory abdominal aortic aneurysms show excessive thickening of the aortic wall and perianeurysmal adhesions to adjacent structures. Lymphocytes and plasma cells comprise the inflammatory infiltrate, which possibly is triggered by some constituent of the atherosclerotic plaque (Figures 11 and 12.)[43-46]

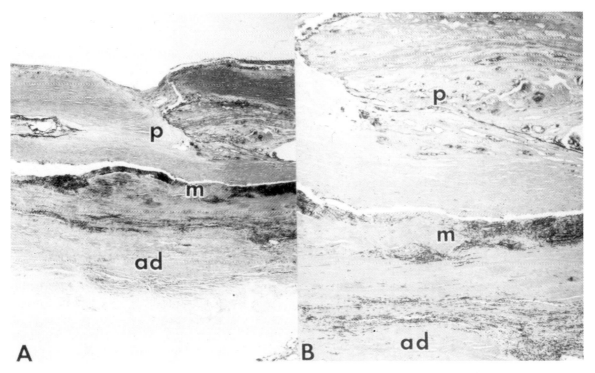

Figure 11. Atherosclerotic aortic aneurysm showing thinning of the wall, particularly the media underlying the atherosclerotic plaque. A small amount of lymphocytic inflammation is present beneath the plaque, but there is minimal extension of the infiltrate and no adventitial fibrosis. **Ad** = adventitia; **M** = media; **P** = atherosclerotic plaque. (**A.** ×30, **B.** × 75; Movat pentachrome stain.)

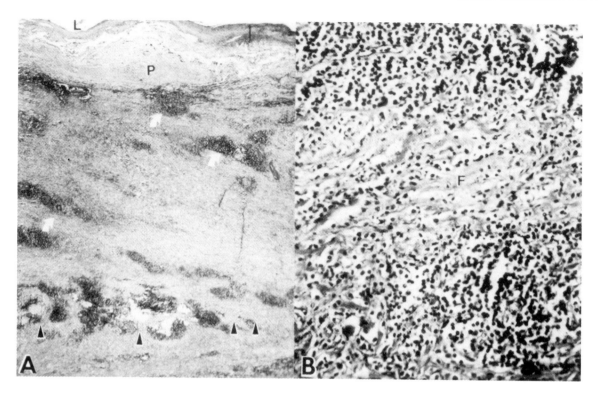

Figure 12. Inflammatory aortic aneurysm showing extensive lymphocytic inflammation (**white arrows**) and fibrosis (**F**) in the media underlying the atherosclerotic plaque. The inflammation and fibrosis extend past the medial-adventitial border (**black arrowheads**). (**A.** ×15, **B.** × 300; hematoxylin and eosin.)

Some inflammatory abdominal aortic aneurysms with extensive adventitial and periaortic inflammation and fibrosis are indistinguishable from the condition known as idiopathic retroperitoneal fibrosis, Ormand's disease (Figure 13).[47–49] Also, idiopathic retroperitoneal fibrosis encompasses other inflammatory diffuse fibrosis conditions known as idiopathic mediastinal fibrosis, Riedel's thyroiditis, sclerosing cholangitis, and pseudotumors of the orbit. Idiopathic retroperitoneal fibrosis rarely is associated with involvement of the coronary arteries.[50] Retroperitoneal fibrosis may present without aortic aneurysm formation. All of the clinical-pathologic variations seem to have an immunologic pathogenesis and are usually sensitive to corticosteroid therapy.[51–53] An experimental model of retroperitoneal fibrosis and periaortitis has been described in simian-acquired immunodeficiency syndrome (SAIDS).[54]

Rheumatoid Panaortitis

The panaortitis associated with rheumatoid arthritis has a nonspecific morphologic pattern (Figure 14) (Table 1). Recognition of the rheumatic or rheumatoid etiology of the panaortitis requires clinical, radiologic, and laboratory confirmations. At the core of the diagnostic problem is the fact that rheumatoid arthritis is a heterogeneous, chronic inflammatory disorder that combines nonsuppurative inflammation of the diarthrodial joints with a variety of extra-articular manifestations. The inflammation probably is related to the presence of circulating rheumatoid factors. Syndromes such as aortitis associated with rheumatoid arthritis are termed *seropositive aortitis*. The presence of rheumatoid factors often parallels the clinical course of the rheumatoid arthritis disease manifestations. The overall course of the disease is frequently characterized by exacerbations and remissions. Rheumatoid arthritis may be found in 2% to 3% of the adult population and afflicts all racial groups. Its peak incidence occurs in the fourth and fifth decades of life, and the disease is two to three times more frequent in females than in males.[55–56]

The pathogenetic mechanisms of rheumatoid arthritis are multifactorial. A genetic predisposition, probably involving the human leukocyte antigen (HLA) system, may render an individual susceptible to the action of an undefined microbial agent, which is most likely viral. This mechanism initiates an inflammatory reaction in the various organs affected in rheumatoid arthritis.[55–56] Rheumatoid aortitis principally involves the proximal aorta in a manner similar to syphilitic aortitis. Rheumatoid aortitis of the proximal

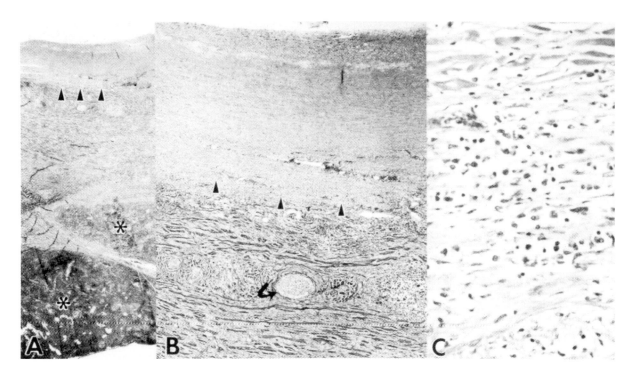

Figure 13. Section of aorta involved by retroperitoneal fibrosis. Note there is minimal atherosclerotic intimal change, but extreme fibrosis extending from and within the aortic media. **Arrowheads** mark the medial-adventitial border. **A. *** = periaortic lymph nodes enveloped by fibrous tissue; **B. Curved black arrow** = entrapped periaortic nerve; **C.** Plasma cells and lymphocytes within infiltrate in media. (**A.** × 7.5, **B.** × 30, **C.** × 300; Movat pentachrome stain.)

aorta may lead to aortic valvular insufficiency by dilation of the aortic valve annulus.[1,13]

Seronegative Spondyloarthritides

Seronegative spondyloarthritides constitute a group of arthritic syndromes that have been separated from rheumatoid arthritis on the basis of an absence of rheumatoid factor in the blood. Some of these conditions have cardiovascular involvement in addition to articular disease. Seronegative spondyloarthritides include ankylosing spondylitis, Reiter's disease, psoriatic arthropathy, and other interrelated conditions such as enteropathic sacroiliitis due to Crohn's disease or ulcerative colitis, uveitis, Behcet's disease, Whipple's disease, and pustulotic arthroosteitis. Based on newer diagnostic criteria, the incidence of ankylosing spondylitis may be as frequent as rheumatoid arthritis. The subclassification of seronegative spondyloarthritides is based on the pattern of joint involvement, associated clinical features, pattern of remissions or relapses, and the extra-articular manifestations (Table 1).[58]

Ankylosing spondylitis is the most common of the seronegative spondyloarthritides (Table 1). There is a tendency toward familial aggregation and the presence of haplotype HLA-B27. The incidence of HLA-B27 in patients with ankylosing spondylitis is 95%. About 6% to 14% of the white population in the United States has HLA-B27 and approximately 2% to 20% of these individuals have ankylosing spondylitis, i.e., 0.4% to 1.6% of the white population has ankylosing spondylitis. The clinical diagnostic criteria of ankylosing spondylitis include insidious onset of musculoskeletal discomfort, age less than 40 years, persistence of symptoms for more than 3 months, and morning stiffness that improves with exercise. The radiologic criteria are confirmatory and include squaring of the superior and inferior margins of the vertebral body due to inflammatory disease at the site of insertion of the outer fibers of the annulus fibrosus, leading ultimately to the characteristic bamboo spine picture.[59]

The incidence of cardiovascular involvement in ankylosing spondylitis is 3.5% to 10%, including aortic incompetence, cardiomegaly, and persistent conduction defects. These cardiovascular conditions may be clinically silent, or the patient may present with cardiovascular symptoms before the arthritic condition is clinically apparent. The grossly apparent involvement of the aorta involved by ankylosing spondylitis is limited to the aortic valve, aortic valve annulus, the si-

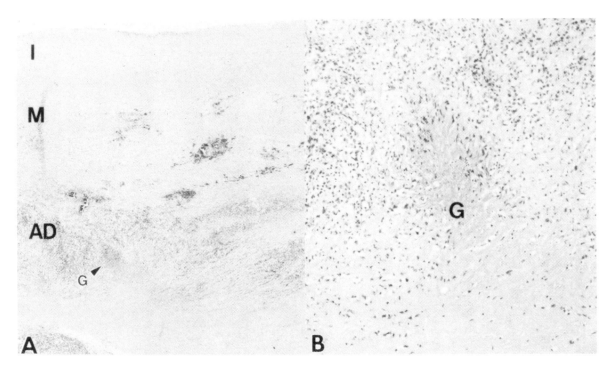

Figure 14. Rheumatoid panaortitis involving the full thickness of aorta. The focal granulomas **(G)** with palisading histiocytes that are seen within the media are characteristic of rheumatoid arthritis, but may occur in other conditions. **AD** = adventitia; **I** = intima; **M** = media. (**A.** × 30, **B.** × 150; hematoxylin and eosin.)

nuses of Valsalva, and the first portion of the ascending aorta (tubular portion). Typically, the aortic valve leaflets are fibrotic, shortened, and bow into the left ventricular outflow tract. Aortic valve involvement is maximal at the base of the leaflets and the distal margins. The fibrous thickening of the valve leaflets extends into the left ventricular outflow tract as a subaortic ridge.[60]

Microscopically, the aortic valve leaflets are infiltrated by lymphocytes and macrophages. The sinuses of Valsalva show destruction of the elastic and SMCs of the media and replacement with fibrous scar and lymphocytic inflammatory infiltrate (Figures 15 to 17). In the active phase, there is endarteritis of the vasa vasorum, and perivascular lymphocytic and plasma cell inflammation (Figure 16). This inflammatory phase is followed by destruction of all layers of the aortic wall and replacement with fibrous scar that may calcify. When this process extends into the coronary ostia, ostial stenosis results. Fibrous involvement of the left ventricular outflow tract can interrupt the atrioventricular bundle of the conduction system (Figure 17).[1,61–66]

The most common cause of an inflammatory oligoarthropathy in a young male is Reiter's syndrome, a seronegative spondyloarthritis. The disease is less common in females. The common clinical presentation is a triad of nongonococcal urethritis, conjunctivitis,

and arthritis, especially of the sacroiliac joint. Also, ulceration of balanitis is common. Most patients test positive for HLA-B27 and have a specific infection, usually due to *Shigella* or possibly a venereal infection such as *Chlamydia* or *Mycoplasma*. One percent of patients with nonspecific urethritis may develop Reiter's syndrome. Shigella dysentery is followed by Reiter's syndrome in 1% to 2% of cases, i.e., 20% of HLA-B27-positive patients. HLA-B27 acts potentially either as a receptor site for an infective agent, a marker for an immune-response gene, or it may induce tolerance to foreign antigens with which it cross-reacts.[58] Clinical cardiovascular involvement in Reiter's syndrome occurs about 17 months to 2 years after the onset of Reiter's syndrome. About 2% to 5% of patients with Reiter's syndrome develop aortitis with dilatation, aortic regurgitation, pericarditis, myocarditis, and various conduction delays, usually transient first-degree heart block. Grossly, there may be dilatation of the aortic annulus. Microscopically, there is an inflammatory infiltrate similar to that of ankylosing spondylitis, i.e., lymphocytes and plasma cells. There is a panaortitis, followed by scarring and fibrosis of the wall and loss of elastic fibers and SMCs in the ascending aorta. Reiter's syndrome usually does not involve the distal aorta.[1,67–76]

Some of the arthritic conditions of childhood, previously diagnosed as juvenile rheumatoid arthritis,

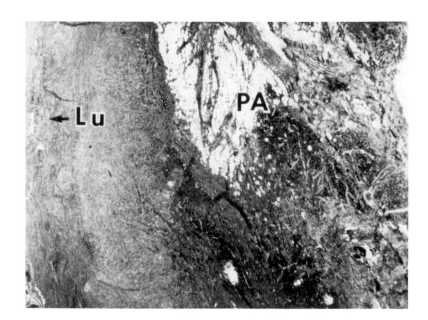

Figure 15. Ankylosing spondylitis involving the full thickness of the aorta near the root of the aorta. Periaortic adipose and fibrous tissue (PA) show dense lymphocytic and plasma cell infiltrate. Lu = direction of lumen. (×25, Movat pentachrome stain.)

now appear to be examples of seronegative spondyloarthritis, especially cases with psoriasis or inflammatory bowel disease. HLA-B27 and or rheumatoid factor may be present in these children. Because clinical, radiologic, and laboratory criteria are still evolving, the cardiovascular manifestations of childhood spondyloarthritis are not described.[58]

Enteropathic arthropathies, psoriatic arthropathy, Behcet's syndrome, and Whipple's disease have a lower frequency of vascular involvement than ankylosing spondylitis. Behcet's syndrome may manifest pericarditis and granulomas, similar to those found in rheumatoid arthritis, which have been noted in the heart.[77] Whipple's disease is an inflammation of the intestine caused by a PAS-positive bacillus and may manifest seronegative spondyloarthritis and cardiovascular involvement. The heart may show lesions that resemble rheumatic mitral stenosis.[78]

Aortitis following rheumatic fever may involve the entire length of the aorta and simultaneously may involve the pulmonary artery. The cardiovascular manifestations following rheumatic fever are mainly cardiac. Aortitis insufficiency is rare; mitral valve stenosis or aortic stenosis secondary to commissural fusion of the mitral and aortic valve leaflets are usual, whereas symptoms due to the aortitis per se are rare as a primary presentation.[1,13]

Microscopically, rheumatic panaortitis resembles rheumatoid panaortitis and syphilitic aortitis. There is endarteritis obliterans and fibrosis in the adventitia, mesaortitis with focal destruction of the media, and fibrous proliferation of the intima. Tree-barking and superimposed atherosclerosis are also seen. A mononuclear inflammatory infiltrate of lymphocytes and plasma cells usually occurs in the intima and adventitia. Patients with chronic rheumatic heart disease may show fibrotic, thickened aortas, with a paucity of inflammation consistent with a healed stage of panaortitis.[1,13] Although the incidence of rheumatic fever has fallen in the United States, rheumatic fever and cardiovascular sequelae are still common in developing countries, and a possible resurgence exists in some areas of the United States.[79,80]

Takayasu's Aortitis

Takayasu's aortitis is a chronic panaortitis that causes destruction of the aortic wall and extensive replacement of the wall with fibrous tissue. About 10% of patients may develop aneurysms, however, luminal constriction of the aorta and its branches is characteristic of Takayasu's aortitis. This luminal compromise has led to various synonyms for the condition, such as pulseless disease and aortic arch syndrome (Table 1).[81]

Although Takayasu's aortitis originally was described in Japan and is most commonly found in Asia, many cases have been described from other areas of the world and in all racial groups. Eighty percent to 90% of Takayasu's aortitis occurs in females from 10 to 50 years of age with 90% presenting before 30 years of age, with a mean age of 15. There is an increased occurrence in monozygotic twins and in individuals with haplotype HLA-B5. The principal clinical signs and symptoms present after a long prodrome of nonspecific malaise, low-grade fever, weight loss, polyarthralgia, muscle pains, and nausea. Later, there may be visual disturbances and markedly decreased pulses in the upper extremities due to fibrous thickening of

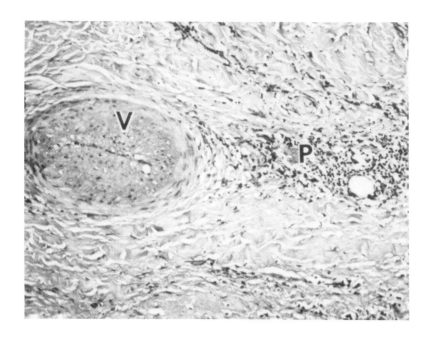

Figure 16. Ankylosing spondylitis aortitis with proliferative endarteritis and perivascular inflammation (**P**) involving the vasa vasorum (**V**) of the aorta, a feature not limited to syphilitic aortitis. (×160, Movat pentachrome stain.)

the aorta with narrowing or obliteration of the origins of the arteries arising from the aorta, especially from the aortic arch. Hypertension occurs when there is obstruction of the renal arteries. Coronary artery involvement leads to angina pectoris. When the process of Takayasu's aortitis extends into aortic branch arteries, it is called Takayasu's arteritis and may involve any of the arch branches, renal, subclavian, coronary, and mesenteric arteries.[1,13,82,83]

No etiologic factor has been identified. Because of the high incidence of tuberculin positivity in patients described in the early 1900s, tuberculosis or an allergic reaction to tuberculosis were suspected etiologies of Takayasu's aortitis, but no experimental, pharmacologic, or morphologic proof has developed to support this hypothesis.[84]

Four patterns of vascular involvement are found in Takayasu's aortitis. The most frequent one (about 33% of cases) is localization to the aortic arch and its major branches. Twelve percent of cases are limited to the descending thoracic and abdominal aorta, sparing the ascending aorta and aortic arch. The third most frequent pattern is involvement of the aortic arch, its branches, and the thoracic and abdominal aorta—a

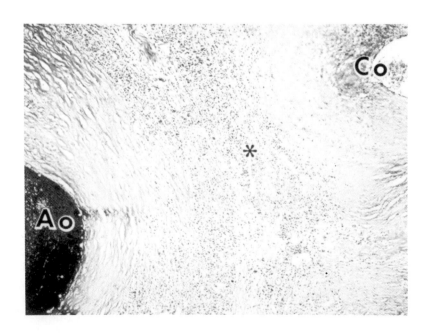

Figure 17. Ankylosing spondylitis aortitis showing extension of inflammation and fibrosis throughout the aortic wall and extension into a coronary artery ostium (**Co**). **Ao** = lumen of aorta. * = inflammatory infiltrate. (×60, hematoxylin and eosin.)

combination of the first and second patterns. The fourth pattern is the concomitant involvement of the pulmonary artery, as well as any portion of the aorta. Overall, 50% of Takayasu's aortitis cases show concomitant pulmonary artery involvement.[83]

Grossly, all layers of the affected aorta and involved branches are thickened. Typically, the intima is wrinkled and mildly thickened. The bulk of the severe thickening involves the media and adventitia. The aorta and its involved branches resemble stiff, rigid tubes with virtual obliteration of the lumen. Superimposed secondary thrombosis is a complication. Aneurysms associated with Takayasu's aortitis and arteritis are usually saccular, but may be fusiform and occur in the aorta or its branches.[1,13,84,85]

Early in the course of Takayasu's aortitis, there is an edematous mononuclear inflammatory infiltrate involving the vasa vasorum in the adventitia, similar to that seen in syphilitic aortitis; but unlike syphilitic aortitis, there is simultaneous mononuclear infiltration of the media and granulomatous changes within the media with Langhans' giant cells surrounding areas of necrosis. Involvement of the branch arteries is mainly narrowing of the ostium by thickening of the aorta. Unlike aortic involvement, the arterial media and adventitia of affected branch arteries are spared. An involved artery may show fibrinoid necrosis, giant cells, focal destruction of the internal elastic lamellae, and luminal thrombosis. Rarely, myocarditis is seen in cases of Takayasu's aortitis.[1,13,84,85]

The inflammation associated with Takayasu's aortitis and arteritis may regress spontaneously and allow fibrotic healing in areas of vascular destruction. This is the basis for the clinical quiescent-fibrotic stage. However, aneurysms and luminal stenoses once developed persist despite the cessation of inflammation (Figure 18).[1,13,84–86]

Mediastinal radiation therapy may induce arterial ostial stenosis, and thickening and fibrosis of the aorta and arteries that may mimic the fibrotic stage of Takayasu's disease. The initial injury of radiation is damage to endothelial cells in the lumen of large and small vessels, but the late reactions include accelerated atherosclerosis, atrophy due to loss of SMCs and fibrosis.[87]

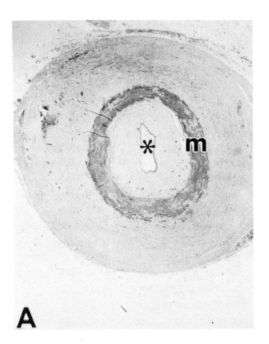

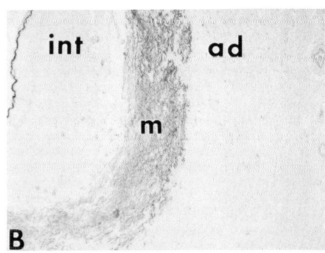

Figure 18. Fibrotic stage of Takayasu's aortitis extending into the common carotid artery. Note the severe thickening of the intima and adventitia by dense fibrous tissue. Although inflammation is sparse, there is persistent luminal compromise and increased wall stiffness. **ad** = adventitia; **int** = intima; **m** = media. (**A.** × 5; **B.** × 25; elastic van Gieson stain.)

Giant Cell Aortitis

Giant cell aortitis is an idiopathic panaortitis that may be part of the same disease as giant cell or temporal arteritis (Table 1). Like giant cell arteritis, giant cell aortitis usually is limited to elderly patients who often have the polymyalgia rheumatica syndrome. When the aorta is involved, the coronary ostia and aortic arch are spared. Superimposed mural thrombus is not common. The giant cell reaction, occurring in giant cell arteritis, is maximal around elastic tissue within the aortic media. Intramural thrombus may be present near the giant cells. The presence of giant cells is not fully diagnostic of giant cell arteritis, as giant cells may be plentiful in Takayasu's aortitis, occasionally present in syphilitic aortitis, and rarely appear in rheumatic and rheumatoid aortitis. Aneurysm formation, aortic insufficiency, aortic rupture, and aortic dissection are more frequent complications of giant cell aortitis than is Takayasu's aortitis. Both giant cell aortitis and Takayasu's aortitis show little inflammatory involvement of the intima.[1,13,88–91]

Infectious Aortitis

Infectious aortitis is an inflammation of the aorta from colonization of the aorta by microorganisms. An old term for infective aortitis is mycotic aneurysm. Although mycotic suggests fungal origin, mycotic aneurysms are most often due to bacterial agents (Table 1).[92] The aorta may become infected by various infectious agents by embolization of microorganisms from an intravascular site such an infective endocarditis, especially if the aorta is damaged from atherosclerotic plaques, syphilitic aortitis, or structural malformation.[93–95] Circulating microorganisms from a bacteremia or fungemia may gain access to the aorta via the vasa vasorum and produce infective aortitis. The aorta adjacent to synthetic vascular graft material may be especially susceptible to colonization by microorganisms, as well as the tissues lining and covering the vascular graft. *Salmonella* species are notable for their ability to colonize damaged areas of the aortic wall.[96,97] Spread of infection from contiguous osteomyelitis, abscesses, or direct inoculation from trauma, surgical, or other iatrogenic entry into the aorta can initiate infective aortitis.[1,13] Tuberculous infective aortitis may occur in the thoracic or abdominal aorta from hematogenous or direct extension.[98] Infective agents induce varying degrees of tissue necrosis and aneurysmal dilatation in the aorta. Rupture may be inevitable unless the affected area is sterilized by antibiotics or resected.[1,13]

The type of inflammatory reaction in infectious aortitis depends on the etiologic agents. Suppurative organisms such as *Staphylococcus* produce abscesses and marked destruction. *Mycobacterium tuberculosis* typically produces caseous necrosis with giant cells; polymorphonuclear leukocytes are seen only in the very earliest lesions. Cultures for detection of an etiologic agent should be performed at surgical exploration of any suspected inflammatory aortic lesions because special stains of resected tissue are not as sensitive or specific as cultures.[1,13,98]

Collagen Vascular Diseases

Collagen vascular diseases are a group of diseases that share a common morphologic lesion in the connective tissue. At some stage of collagen vascular disease, eosinophilic deposits of fibrin and related proteins are deposited in the collagen or ground substance in various parts of the body. The etiology, clinical course, severity, prognosis, morbidity, and mortality of the individual diseases within this large group vary in most other respects. Fibrinoid necrosis refers to collections of fibrin, increased ground substance, swollen fragmented collagen fibers, necrosis of parenchyma, and the histologic appearance of structureless eosinophilic deposits. This lesion can be seen in rheumatoid arthritis, systemic lupus erythematosus, scleroderma (progressive systemic sclerosis), dermatomyositis, polymyositis, polyarteritis nodosa, and thrombotic thrombocytopenic purpura. Fibrinoid necrosis occurs with lesser frequency and extent as part of Wegener's granulomatosis, ankylosing spondylitis, Reiter's syndrome, psoriatic arthritis, and relapsing polychondritis.[1,13,18–20]

Collagen vascular diseases are considered autoimmune diseases that are probably mediated through immunologic mechanisms directed against the host's own tissues. The older term, collagen disease,[19] refers to a concept that a chemical change in the collagen per se initiated the pathogenesis of the disease. This view is not accepted today.

Classification of collagen vascular disease is based on the clinical presentation and clinical course. The gross and microscopic pathologic features of the particular condition often are difficult to differentiate on morphology alone, particularly in the later stages. Collagen vascular diseases vary in their clinical features, time course, location of lesions, pathologic picture, and immune findings.

The pathologic findings in the various organs in collagen vascular disease are diverse and include one or more of the following: angiitis, glomerulonephritis, immunoglobulin abnormalities, and autoantibodies with differing specificity and reactivity. Most collagen vascular disease involves the smaller vessels, especially the venules. Impairment of the small arteries produces ischemic changes within organs. Disorders of large vessels, such as aneurysms, are usually not a major feature of collagen vascular disease. Biopsies are helpful in the diagnosis of these conditions, but direct surgical therapeutic interventions usually are not required for collagen vascular diseases.[1,13,18,99]

Scleroderma

Scleroderma is a systemic disease characterized by thickening of the arterioles and capillaries in various organs and large arteries including pulmonary, renal, and arteries in the hands and feet. The blood vessel is a major target organ. Microvascular abnormalities are the earliest detectable change in the patient destined to develop classic scleroderma. Characteristic diminished or absent capillary loops can be seen in the nailfold capillary bed. In the digital arteries, the thickening is due to severe fibromuscular intimal thickening, and medial hypertrophy may lead to total luminal occlusion. In small arteries, the intimal fibromuscular proliferation results in an onionskin pattern similar to that seen in malignant hypertension. Aortic involvement rarely produces clinical symptoms, but a nonspecific panaortitis has been reported in scleroderma.[100,101]

No etiologic agent has been identified, and the pathogenesis of scleroderma is not clear. Perivascular lymphocytic cuffing of small blood vessels is an early feature of scleroderma and suggests immunologic activity.[1,18,100-103]

Giant Cell Arteritis

Giant cell arteritis is a generalized inflammation of muscular arteries that sometimes presents with systemic signs and symptoms (Table 2). It is often most severe in the temporal artery. Its inflammatory infiltrate typically contains giant cells during its active stage (see *Giant Cell Aortitis*) (Figure 19). Giant cell arteritis is also known as temporal arteritis, polymyalgia rheumatica et arteritica, granulomatous arteritis, and cranial arteritis.[1,18,89-91,104]

Giant cell arteritis may simply present as isolated, painful nodules over the involved artery, or nodules associated with generalized symptoms of nonspecific headache, anorexia, fever, fatigue, weight loss, myalgia in the muscles of the neck, back, and proximal limbs, and arthralgia. The erythrocyte sedimentation usually is elevated. These generalized symptoms constitute the syndrome of polymyalgia rheumatica. The affected patient is usually over age 50 (average age, 70). It is the most common vasculitis over the

Table 2
Clinical Features of Arteritis

	Temporal Arteritis	Thromboangiitis Obliterans	Polyarteritis Nodosa	Allergic Granulomatosus	Overlap Syndrome
Mean age	70	35	50*	30	25
Sex	F	M	M	F	
Clinical features	Painful nodules Polymyalgia	Claudicacation, UE LE	Multisystem Symptoms and Signs	Asthma, Hypereosinophilia, Organ ischemia	Overlap with PAN and AG
Etiology	Unknown	Tobacco + +	Viruses + +	Unknown	Unknown
Pathologic features of arteritis:					
Size of vessels involved	MA (temporal) ± LA, SA	MA + SA MV + SV	MA + SA Not PA and spleen	SA, SV, PA, PV Spleen A + V	SA, SV, MA, MV, PA ± PV ±
Necrosis	+ +	+ +	+ + + Fibrinoid	+ + + Fibrinoid	+ + + Fibrinoid
Giant	+ +	±	±	+	±/+
Eosinophils	+	+	+ + +	+ + +	+ + +
Internal elastic lamina	Fragmented	Intact	Destruction (asymmetric)	Variable	Destruction ±
Luminal thrombus	+	+ + (Abscess)	+	±	±
Intimal inflammation	+ +	+	+ +	GR	±/+ +
Medial inflammation	+	±	+ +	GR	+/+ + GR ±
Healing	FIB	Recanalized TH	FIB	FIB	FIB
Aneurysm			Branch points		
Typical features	Giant cells + + +	Thrombi microabscess + + +/+ +	Multiple stages of inflammation + +	Granulomas asthma + +/+ + +	Cutaneous involvement + + to + + +

−: absent; ±: present occasionally; +: usually present; + +: frequently present; + + +: almost always present. A: artery; ABD: abdominal aorta; AG: allergic granulomatosis; AT: arterioles; F: females; FIB: fibrosis; GR: granulomas; LA: large arteries; M: males; MA: muscular arteries; MV: muscular veins; PA: pulmonary arteries; PAN: polyarteritis nodosa; SA: small arteries; SV: small veins; TH: thrombus; UE: upper extremities; V: veins.

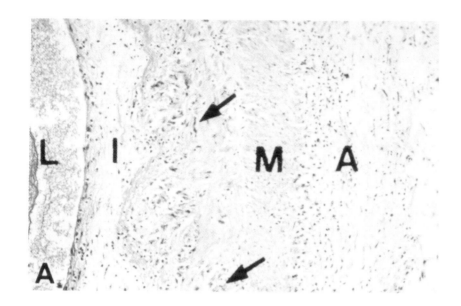

Figure 19. A. Temporal arteritis showing a panarteritis with dense inflammation in all layers of the arterial wall, but most marked in the area of the internal elastic lamina (**arrows**).

age of 80 years. Involvement of the ophthalmic artery can cause blindness and is a medical emergency.[1,18,89–91,104]

There is no definite geographic, genetic, familial, or racial predisposition. Females are more frequently involved than males. The cause and risk factors of giant cell arteritis are unknown. The initial injury probably elicits a granulomatous inflammation in the intima without giant cells. As this inflammation spreads to the area of the internal elastic lamella, giant cells form and are associated with destruction and phagocytosis of the elastin. This suggests cell-mediated immunity to arterial antigens. Rheumatoid factors and other serological tests are usually negative, and no infectious agents have been identified.[1,18,89–91,104]

In order of frequency of involvement, the principal

sites of involvement of giant cell arteritis are the medium-sized arteries such as the temporal, subclavian, coronary, renal, skeletal muscle arteries, limb arteries, and mesenteric arteries. Occasionally, large and small arteries also may be affected, but arteries within organs are usually spared. The impairment of involved arteries is one of luminal narrowing within the focus of inflammation. Saccular aneurysms of the aortic and aortic dissection have been associated with giant cell arteritis.

Giant cell arteritis involvement can localize to a very small segment of artery or multiple small segments of multiple arteries with "skip areas" of uninvolved vessel. In an otherwise normal temporal artery biopsied for the diagnosis of giant cell arteritis, lesions only 330 μm long have been found in an examination

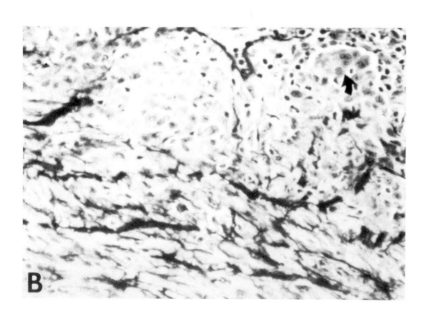

Figure 19. B. Abundant giant cells and disrupted elastic lamellae. **A** = adventitia; **I** = intima; **L** = lumen; **M** = media. (**A.** ×90, **B.** × 300; Movat pentachrome stain.)

of 6000 serial microscopic sections of arteritis in 60 patients studied for temporal arteritis.[105] The inflammation thickens the artery wall, which appears white and may contain luminal thrombus (Figure 19).[1,18,89–91,104]

In biopsies of temporal arteries in patients with giant cell arteritis, 50% show granulomatous inflammation with giant cells; 37.5% show only intimal proliferation by SMCs and fibrous tissue, and in 12.5%, there is granulomatous inflammation without giant cells. The intimal proliferation pattern actually may be a healing phase. The hallmark of this disease is focal destruction of the internal elastic lamella. Other findings include giant cells, fibrinoid necrosis, polymorphonuclear leukocytes, lymphocytes, and occasional eosinophils in the media and intima. Spontaneous healing or amelioration of the inflammation with corticosteroid therapy leads to regression of the inflammation and fibrosis of the areas of inflammation. Luminal narrowing may persist and even leave the involved artery as an obliterated fibrous cord.[1,18,89–91,104]

Untreated giant cell arteritis can progress to organ necrosis, i.e., blindness. Death from giant cell arteritis is rare, but may occur when a vital organ is affected, i.e., myocardial or cerebral infarction.[1,18,89–91,104]

The differential diagnosis of temporal artery nodules includes a number of conditions. Young adults may present with painless nodules in the area of the temporal arteries and ear and may be erroneously diagnosed as having giant cell arteritis. If the condition is painless and without accompanying systemic signs and symptoms, it is more likely that the diagnosis is juvenile temporal arteritis. This condition is probably a different disease than giant cell arteritis and giant cell aortitis. A biopsy is confirmatory. Microscopically, there is a granulomatous inflammation with varying amounts of giant cells, medial disruption and microaneurysm formation, and perivascular angiolymphoid hyperplasia. Usually, there is an absence of destruction of the internal elastic lamella, fibrinois necrosis, and luminal thrombosis.[18]

Angiolymphoid hyperplasia with eosinophilia, also known as subcutaneous angiolymphoid hyperplasia and Kimura's disease or intravascular atypical endothelial proliferation, is a condition that also present with thickening of the temporal artery or other arteries around the head and neck of young adults. There is usually an absence of systemic signs and symptoms. Microscopically, there is a proliferation of endothelial cells in sheets and nodules, and the arterial lumen may be obliterated. These conditions are probably benign, neoplastic proliferative processes involving histiocytoid endothelial cells forming hemangiomas that elaborate chemotactic factors for eosinophils and lymphoid

cells rather than a typical vasculitis. These lesions are quite indolent and are probably self-limited. Excisional biopsy probably is curative.[106–108]

Disseminated visceral giant cell arteritis is a widespread granulomatous inflammation of arteries and arterioles within organs including the heart, lung, kidney, liver, pancreas, and stomach. This condition is not accompanied with polymyalgia rheumatic symptoms. It is found in young individuals. Microscopically, there is widespread fibrinoid necrosis and giant cells.[109] The temporal artery also can be affected in polyarteritis nodosa, hypersensitivity angiitis, and nonspecific arteritis.[18]

A negative biopsy in a patient clinically suspected to have giant cell arteritis may represent a sampling error due to the often very focal nature of giant cell arteritis. If there is a risk of organ failure, particularly possible blindness, many authorities recommend institution of anti-inflammation based on clinical grounds alone.[110]

Polyarteritis Nodosa

Polyarteritis nodosa is the classic example of systemic necrotizing vasculitis involving systemic muscular arteries. Destruction of the artery and superimposed luminal thrombosis induce ischemia and organ failure. This condition has also been called macroscopic polyarteritis nodosa, periarteritis nodosa, and panarteritis nodosa (Table 2).[34,35,112–114]

The peak incidence of polyarteritis nodosa is about age 50. It occurs two to three times more commonly in males than in females. Polyarteritis nodosa can involve any systemic muscular artery, but spares the lungs and is rare in the spleen. Its clinical presentation is highly variable and depends upon the artery or arteries involved. Infarctions, ischemic atropy, and hemorrhages within the kidneys, heart, skeletal muscle, skin, mesentery, intestine, spleen, pancreas, lungs, liver, and peripheral nerves may present as renal failure, hypertension, abdominal pain, cramps, melena, muscular aches, and pains, or peripheral neuritis. There are usually three stages including acute, healing, and healed stages. All three stages often appear concurrently. This phenomenon contrasts with most other types of vasculitis in that the morphologic picture usually is synchronized, i.e., acute, healing, or healing, rather than the simultaneous mixture of stages seen in polyarteritis nodosa. This mixture of different stages of vasculitis suggests ongoing persistence of the inciting etiologic or pathogenetic agent in polyarteritis nodosa in contrast to some type of short-term exposure. The condition may undergo remission and recur. Low-grade fever, malaise, weakness, and leukocytosis are common. Polyarteritis nodosa is probably the result of the deposition of antigen-antibody complexes in the walls of muscular arteries. Hepatitis B may be responsible for as many as 40% of cases of polyarteritis nodosa. Immune complexes elicit an acute inflammatory response and fibrinoid necrosis, a general reaction characterized by destruction of the vessel wall and fibrin deposits within areas of necrosis.[18,34,35,112–114]

Grossly, small nodules up to 3 mm in diameter may be seen over the distribution of small- and medium-sized muscular arteries. These occur particularly at branch points in the hila of organs, striated skeletal muscle, and peripheral nerves. The microscopic feature of the acute stage is fibrinoid necrosis of the full thickness of the arterial wall. Polymorphonuclear leukocytes infiltrate within and around the arterial wall. Later eosinophils and mononuclear cells comprise more than 50% of the inflammatory cells. Necrosis may be focal or extend through the thickness of the arterial wall and lead to aneurysm formation, thrombosis of the lumen, and destruction of the elastica, especially the internal elastic lamina. The lesions may be eccentric or involve the entire circumference of the affected artery (Figure 20).[1,18,34,35,112–114]

The healing phase shows continuing necrosis and fibroblastic proliferation within the media and intima.

Concentrically arranged intimal SMCs proliferate and thicken the arterial wall and narrow the lumen. The large numbers of macrophages and plasma cells in the arterial wall and perivascular tissue form nodules. Polymorphonuclear leukocytes are absent. Luminal thrombus becomes organized and forms a fibrous cord within the lumen.[1,18,34,35,112–114] The healed lesion is characterized by fibrotic thickening of the affected arterial wall, scattered lymphocytes, plasma cells, occasional calcium deposits, and loss or fragmentation of the internal elastic lamella, which is replaced by fibrous tissue.[1,18,34,35,112–114]

Untreated polyarteritis nodosa has a poor prognosis; about two thirds of untreated patients die of renal failure and cerebral hemorrhage, or intestinal infarction may present within 1 year from the onset of symptoms. Corticosteroids and immunosuppressive drugs may be curative, but a definitive diagnosis is required prior to beginning treatment. Complications that occur as part of the natural history of polyarteritis nodosa can mimic the complications of corticosteroid therapy and vice versa. Because therapy is most effective early in the course of polyarteritis nodosa and clinical signs and symptoms are often vague, biopsy of an affected organ is the most expedient way to establish the diagnosis.[35] The most frequent sites for biopsy are

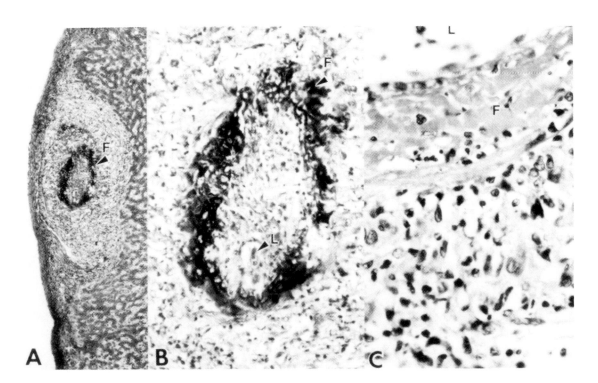

Figure 20. Small muscular artery involved by polyarteritis showing fibrinoid necrosis (**F**). The full thickness of the artery is necrotic. Lymphocytes and macrophages infiltrate the area of necrosis. The destroyed arterial wall is aneurysmally dilated and the lumen is almost obliterated. **L** = lumen. (**A.** ×75, **B.** × 150, **C.** × 300; Movat pentachrome stain.)

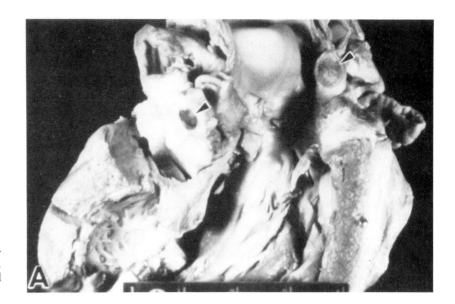

Figure 21. Fatal coronary arteritis in a 5-month-old child with Kawasaki's disease. **A. Arrowheads** point to thrombosed left and right coronary artery transverse sections.

skin and skeletal muscle followed by percutaneous liver biopsy, percutaneous kidney biopsy, temporal artery biopsy, testicular biopsy, and nerve biopsy. A positive biopsy is diagnostic, but a negative biopsy may be a false-negative due to sampling. Some patients even require laparotomy for evaluation of abdominal complaints that are suspicious for systemic necrotizing arteritis. Even if surgical exploration is grossly negative, however, liver and omental biopsies should be performed since liver and omental biopsies obtained at operation have been positive in 50% of macroscopically negative laparotomies.[35]

Infants and children at times present with a systemic necrotizing arteritis that has many features similar to polyarteritis in the adult. This childhood illness is called the mucocutaneous cutaneous lymph node syndrome or Kawasaki's disease. It probably represents an infantile form of polyarteritis nodosa. Clinically, it is an acute illness of young children and infants (rarely adults). It is often preceded by viral-like upper respiratory illness. The clinical diagnosis is based on the findings of fever unaffected by antibiotics, viral-like upper respiratory infection, conjunctival and oral erythema and erosions, skin rash, especially on the palms and soles with desquamation, and enlargement of lymph nodes. Although the disease is endemic in Japan, it has been found on all continents and in all racial groups.[115–120]

Like classic polyarteritis nodosa, Kawasaki's disease involves muscular arteries including coronary, iliac, and cerebral arteries, but it spares the pulmonary arteries. The inflammation leads to vessel wall necrosis, aneurysm formation, and thrombosis. Grossly and microscopically, the necrotizing arteritis of Kawasaki's disease resembles polyarteritis nodosa (Figure 21).[115–121] The etiology of Kawasaki's disease is thought to be infectious. The vascular injury and lesion pathogenesis are probably consequences of antigen-antibody complex deposition.[120]

Untreated Kawasaki's disease has a 1% to 2% mortality, usually from involvement of the coronary arteries and resultant acute myocardial infarction. Patients who survive the acute illness may present months to years later with aneurysms of a systemic muscular artery previously involved by the inflammatory process.[115–120]

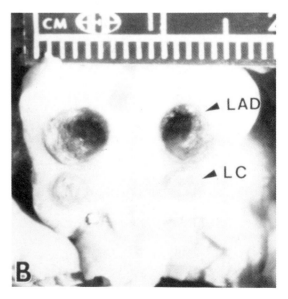

Figure 21. B. Left anterior descending **(LAD)** and left circumflex **(LC)** coronary arteries involved by arteritis and thrombosis.

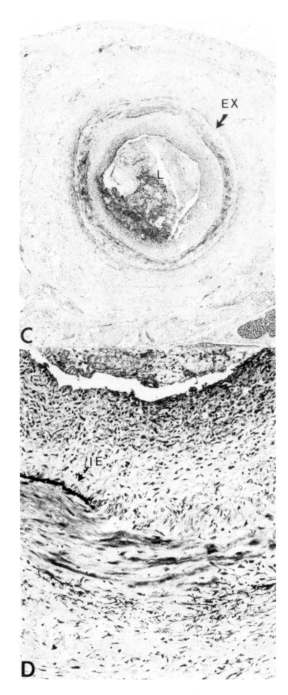

Figure 21. C. and **D.** Panarteritis with destruction of external (**EX**) and internal elastic (**IE**) laminas and fibromuscular proliferative reaction. (**C.** ×30, **D.** × 150; Movat pentachrome stain.)

Allergic Granulomatosis and Angiitis

Allergic granulomatosis and angiitis, or Churg-Strauss arteritis, is a necrotizing systemic angiitis of small- and medium-sized arteries and small- and medium-sized veins (Table 2). Its clinical presentation includes features of classic polyarteritis nodosa, plus a high incidence of bronchial asthma and peripheral eo-

sinophilia.[121,122] Unlike polyarteritis nodosa, allergic granulomatosis almost always involves the lungs. The peripheral nerves, skin, and spleen are the next most frequent areas of involvement. Microscopically, there are intra- and extravascular necrotizing granulomas with palisading histiocytes and prominent eosinophilic infiltrates. Immune complexes have been demonstrated suggesting an immunologic pathogenesis. Respiratory antigens are the suspected candidates for the etiologic agents.[121,123]

A biopsy is essential to establishing the diagnosis of this condition. The presence of infectious agents in the biopsy specimen should be searched for by culture and special stain. Once an infectious etiology is excluded, the diagnosis is specific. The 1-year survival rate of untreated allergic granulomatosis is only about 50%, but 90% 5-year survival may be possible with corticosteroids and cyclophosphamide therapy.[121]

Polyangiitis Overlap Syndrome

The polyangiitis overlap syndrome is a heterogeneous group of systemic necrotizing vasculitides with clinical and pathologic features of classic polyartcritis nodosa, and allergic angiitis and granulomatosis (Churg-Strauss arteritis), which do not fit precisely into either category (Table 2). It is a diagnosis of exclusion, after recognized collagen vascular disease syndromes and infectious disease have been ruled out. One third of cases previously classified as necrotizing arteritis by Fauci et al have now been reclassified as polyangiitis overlap syndrome.[124]

The overlap syndrome differs from classic polyarteritis nodosa in that the patients tend to be young, i.e., mean age at onset is 25 years, and none had hepatitis B antigenemia. The disease involves the pulmonary arteries, and systemic arterioles and venules. Cutaneous involvement often is found; cutaneous involvement is not typical of polyarteritis nodosa. The microscopic appearance of polyangiitis overlap syndrome may be indistinguishable from localized leukocytoclastic hypersensitivity vasculitis. The clinical history of systemic symptoms is mandatory in order to separate localized from systemic disease; a diagnosis cannot be made from histology alone.[122,124]

In some examples of the overlap syndrome, there may be a granulomatous component in the inflammatory reaction, but unlike allergic granulomatosis and angiitis, asthma and peripheral eosinophilia are absent. This condition may also be an overlap with aspects of temporal arteritis, Takayasu's arteritis, Henoch-Schonlein purpura, giant cell arteritis, or Wegener's granulomatosis.[124]

Thromboangiitis Obliterans

Thromboangiitis obliterans, Buerger's disease, is an inflammatory and thrombotic disease involving the distal portions of medium-sized arteries and veins and the adjacent nerves. It is characterized by ischemic episodes that may lead to gangrene and amputation of digits and ultimately one or both of the lower or upper limbs. The English language description of the condition was published by Buerger in 1908; however, the disease may be identical to the condition described by Winiwarter, endarteritis obliterans, in the German literature in 1879.[18]

Buerger's disease typically presents with relapsing waxing and waning symptoms similar to migratory phlebitis, but involves arteries as well as veins in the lower extremities principally. It also involves the upper extremities. The target population appears to be men, and it occurs with a peak around age 35, but its initial presentation can occur from the early 20s to the late 40s. Less than 1% of patients are women.[125]

Migratory thrombophlebitis may precede or coincide with arterial involvement. Claudication, the presenting complaint, is usually due to thrombosis of the arterial lumen.[126,127] The major risk factor for Buerger's disease is cigarette smoking. Buerger's disease occurs independently of organic heart disease, arterial aneurysms, diabetes mellitus, hypercholesterolemia, and radiographically recognizable calcification of the peripheral arteries.[127-129]

Although Buerger's disease was once thought to be found predominantly in Jewish people because Buerger first described the condition at Mt. Sinai Hospital in New York City, a major Jewish teaching hospital. It has been shown to occur in all races and in many countries. It has been described in Asia in populations with a low incidence of arteriosclerosis.[18,126]

The major presentation is gangrene of the lower extremity or upper extremity. The vessels most frequently involved are medium-sized arteries and veins, such as the popliteal artery down to the dorsalis pedis artery. The radial and ulnar arteries of the upper extremities can be involved. Less common involvement includes the coronary, cerebral, and iliac arteries. Buerger's disease can also affect the mesenteric arteries and, therefore, the intestinal tract (Figure 22).[18,128]

The etiology of Buerger's disease is unknown, but cell-mediated immunity directed against the vessel wall is suspected, possibly to a component in cigarette smoke. Abstinence from cigarette smoking is almost always beneficial, but no clear-cut benefit has been shown for immunosuppressive therapy, anticoagulants, antiplatelet agents, or vasodilating drugs.[129-131]

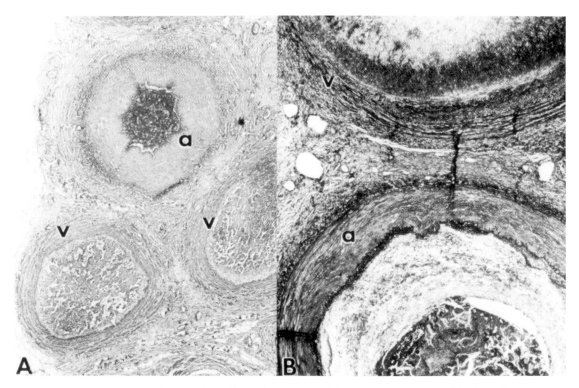

Figure 22. Amputation specimen from cigarette smoking 22-year-old man with thromboangiitis obliterans (Buerger's disease). There is cellular, organizing thrombus in both the artery and the vein, preservation of the arterial internal elastic lamina, thrombophlebitis, and early fibrosis surrounding the vessels. **a** = artery; **v** = vein. (**A.** ×10, **B.** ×30; Movat pentachrome stain.)

Few studies are available of biopsies early in the course of Buerger's disease, and certain cases of related conditions have been misdiagnosed as Buerger's disease. Its major feature of thrombosis is usually found in conjunction with inflammatory changes. Usually, there is an absence of intimal or medial disease in the affected vessel. Early in the disease, all layers of the affected vessel may be involved by an inflammatory infiltrate comprised of polymorphonuclear leukocytes without necrosis of the structures. The characteristic feature is the presence of microabscesses within the thrombosis in the lumen. The thrombosis may become organized by granulation tissue containing foreign body giant cells of the Langhans type. Recanalization may occur, and the internal elastic lamella and the media usually remain intact. Other characteristic features of Buerger's disease are the presence of highly cellular organizing thrombosis and panarteritis with concomitant panphlebitis. Vasculitis of the vasa vasorum in the arterial wall has been described. Late in the natural history is the development of dense adventitial fibrosis, which may involve the contiguous connective tissue and adjacent veins and nerves (Figure 22).[18,126–128]

Although thromboangiitis obliterans does not usually cause death, cigarette smokers with Buerger's disease have a high probability of limb loss if they continue to smoke. The diagnosis of thromboangiitis obliterans is a diagnosis of exclusion and should not be made in the presence of diabetes mellitus, a history of previous frostbite, embolic disease, proximal atherosclerosis, and hypercoagulability states. Thromboangiitis obliterans is distinct from atherosclerosis of the intima and media calcific arteriosclerosis of the Mönckeberg's type.[18,126]

Ergot-Alkaloid Associated Arterial Disease

Ergot alkaloids, especially methysergide maleate, can induce dose-related spasm and arterial occlusive disease especially in coronary, cerebral, and peripheral arteries that have been involved previously by atherosclerosis.[18,132–135] About 4% of patients with migraine headaches treated with methysergide maleate might develop peripheral artery ischemia and claudication.[133] Retroperitoneal fibrosis and endocardial sclerosis of the heart are also adverse effects of methysergide maleate. Similar changes have been observed in Europe in people who have eaten rye contaminated with ergot fungus, *Claviceps purpura*.[18,134]

Ergot alkaloids act directly on smooth muscle of arteries to induce vasoconstriction, which, if prolonged, can cause vascular stasis and vascular injury. Vascular SMCs do respond to vascular injury with intimal and medial fibromuscular proliferation, the general reaction of vessels to vascular injury. Acute thrombosis or late thrombosis may occlude the lumen totally and result in tissue death in the organ served by the affected artery. Fibromuscular intimal proliferative lesions may hyalinize and slightly shrink. Recanalization of organized thrombi may occur, but usually the reactive proliferative lesions persist, and permanent ischemia can result even though blood flow is partially restored. (Figure 23) Treatment requires abstinence from the inciting ergot preparation.[18,132–135]

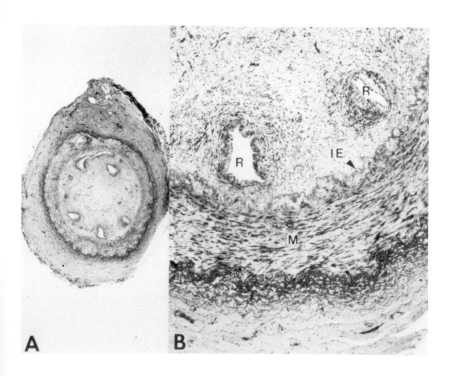

Figure 23. Transverse section of femoral artery of a teenaged girl with leg claudication. Patient had ergotamine for 2 months and headaches, and smoked cigarettes for 2 years. No other risk factors. No clinical or morphologic involvement of veins. The arterial lumen is occluded by fibromuscular tissue and is partially recanalized. Note the intact internal elastic lamina and muscularis and paucity of inflammation. **IE** = internal elastic lamina; **M** = media; **R** = recanalized lumens. (**A.** ×15, **B.** ×75; elastic Van Gieson stain.)

References

1. Virmani R, McAllister HA Jr: Pathology of the aorta and major arteries. In: Lande A, Berkmen YM, McAllister HA Jr (eds). *Aortitis: Clinical, Pathologic, and Radiographic Aspects.* New York: Raven Press; 1986.

2. O'Rourke MF, Yaginuma T: Wave reflections and the arterial pulse. *Arch Intern Med* 144:366, 1984.

3. Clark JM, Glagov S: Transmural organization of the arterial media: the lamellar unit revisited. *Arteriosclerosis* 5:19, 1985.

4. Sandberg LB, Soskel NT, Leslie JG: Elastin structure, biosynthesis, and relation to disease states. *N Engl J Med* 304:566, 1981.

5. Roberts WC: The aorta: its acquired disease and their consequences as viewed from a morphologic perspective. In: Lindsay J Jr (ed). *The Aorta.* Orlando: Grune & Stratton; 51, 1979.

6. Mulvany MJ: Determinants of vascular hemodynamic characteristics. *Hypertension* 6[suppl III]:13, 1984.

7. Lee RM, Smeda JS: Primary versus secondary structural changes of the blood vessels in hypertension. *Can J Physiol Pharmacol* 63:392, 1985.

8. Perejda AJ, Abraham PA, Carnes WH, et al: Marfan's syndrome: structural, biochemical, and mechanical studies of the aortic media. *J Lab Clin Med* 106:376, 1985.

9. Spina M, Garbisa S, Hinnie J, et al: Age-related changes in composition and mechanical properties of the tunica media of the upper thoracic human aorta. *Arteriosclerosis* 3:64, 1983.

10. Schlatmann TJM, Becker AE: Histologic changes in the normal aging aorta: implications for dissecting aortic aneurysm. *Am J Cardiol* 39:13, 1977.

11. Simon AC, Levenson J, Bouthier J, et al: Evidence of early degenerative changes in large arteries in human essential hypertension. *Hypertension* 7:675, 1985.

12. Klima T, Spjut HJ, Coelho A, et al: The morphology of ascending aortic aneurysms. *Hum Pathol* 14:810, 1983.

13. Heggtveit HA: Nonatherosclerotic disease of the aorta. In: Silver MD (ed). *Cardiovascular Pathology.* New York: Churchill Livingstone Inc; 707, 1983.

14. Slater EE, DeSanctis RW: The clinical recognition of dissecting aortic aneurysm. *Am J Med* 60:625, 1976.

15. Schlatmann TJ, Becker AE: Pathogenesis of dissecting aneurysms of aorta: comparison histopathologic study of significance of medial changes. *Am J Cardiol* 39:21, 1977.

16. Daily PO, Trueblood HW, Stinson EB, et al: Management of acute aortic dissection. *Ann Thorac Surg* 10:237, 1970.

17. Pyeritz RE: Cardiovascular manifestations of heritable disorders of connective tissue. *Prog Med Genet* 5:191, 1985.

18. Rose AG: Diseases of medium-sized arteries, including hypertension: diseases of peripheral arteries. In: Silver MD (ed). *Cardiovascular Pathology.* New York: Churchill Livingstone, Inc; 739, 1983.

19. Klemperer P, Pollack AD, Baehr G: Diffuse collagen disease: acute disseminated lupus erythematosus and diffuse scleroderma. *JAMA* 19:331, 1942.

20. Rich AR: Hypersensitivity in disease, with special reference to periarteritis nodosa, rheumatic fever, disseminated lupus erythematosus, and rheumatoid arthritis. *Harvey Lect* 42:106, 1947.

21. Pyeritz RE, McKusick VA: Marfan's syndrome: diagnosis and management. *N Engl J Med* 300:722, 1979.

22. Pyeritz RE: Marfan's syndrome. In: Emery AEH, Rimoin DL (eds). *Principles and Practice of Medical Genetics.* Edinburgh: Churchill Livingstone; 820, 1983.

23. Pyeritz RE, Murphy EA, Lin SJ, et al: Growth and anthropometrics in the Marfan's syndrome. *Prog Clin Biol Res* 200:355, 1985.

24. Uitto J, Murray LW, Blumberg B, et al: UCLA conference. Biochemistry of collagen in diseases. *Ann Intern Med* 105:740, 1986.

25. Ramirez F, Sangiorgi FO, Isipouras P: Human collagens: biochemical, molecular, and genetic features in normal and disease states. *Horiz Biochem Biophys* 8:341, 1986.

26. Judd KP: Hyperelasticity syndromes. *Cutis* 33:494, 1984.

27. Halme T, Peltonen J, Sims TJ, et al: Collagen in human aorta: changes in the type III/I ratio and concentration of the reducible crosslink, dehydrohydroxy-lysinonorleucine in ascending aorta from healthy subjects of different ages and patients with annuloaortic ectasia. *Biochim Biophys Acta* 881:222, 1986.

28. Savunen T, Aho HJ: Annulo-aortic ectasia: light and electron microscopic changes in aortic media. *Virchows Arch* [A] 407:279, 1985.

29. Downing R, Grimley RP, Ashton F, et al: Problems in diagnosis of popliteal aneurysms. *J R Soc Med* 78:440, 1985.

30. Harrison EG Jr, McCormack LJ: Pathologic classification of renal arterial disease in renovascular hypertension. *Mayo Clin Proc* 46:161, 1971.

31. Ratliff NB: Renal vascular disease: pathology of large blood vessel disease. *Am J Kidney Dis* 5:A93, 1985.

32. Dean RH: Renovascular hypertension. *Curr Probl Surg* 22:1, 1985.

33. Fievez ML: Fibromuscular dysplasia of arteries: a spastic phenomenon? *Med Hypotheses* 13:341, 1984.

34. Cupps TR, Fauci AS: The vasculitides. In: Smith LH Jr (ed). *Major Problems in Internal Medicine.* Philadelphia: WB Saunders, Co; 13:1, 1981.

35. McCauley RL, Johnston MR, Fauci AS: Surgical aspects of systemic necrotizing vasculitis. *Surgery* 97:104, 1985.

36. O'Flaherty JT: Age dependency of the inflammatory response (editorial). *Lab Invest* 56:600, 1986.

37. Fantone JC, Ward PA: Polymorphonuclear leukocyte-mediated cell and tissue injury: oxygen metabolites and their relations to human disease. *Hum Pathol* 16:973, 1985.

38. Reidy MA: A reassessment of endothelial injury and arterial lesion formation. *Lab Invest* 53:513, 1985.

39. Virmani R, Lande A, McAllister HA Jr: Pathological aspects of Takayasu's arteritis. In: Lande A, Berkmen YM, McAllister HA Jr (eds). *Aortitis: Clinical, Pathologic, and Radiographic Aspects.* New York: Raven Press; 55, 1986.

40. Schwartz SM, Campbell GR, Campbell JH: Replication of smooth muscle cells in vascular disease. *Cir Res* 58:427, 1986.

41. Pomerance A, Yacoub MH, Gula G: The surgical pathology of thoracic aortic aneurysms. *Histopathology* 1:257, 1977.

42. Gormsen H: Postmortem diagnosis of syphilitic aortitis, including serological verification on postmorten blood. *Forensic Sci Int* 24:51, 1984.

43. Pennell RC, Hollier LH, Lie JT, et al: Inflammatory

abdominal aortic aneurysms: a thirty-year review. *J Vasc Surg* 2:859, 1985.

44. Crawford JL, Sorwe CL, Safi HJ, et al: Inflammatory aneurysms of the aorta. *J Vasc Surg* 2:113, 1985.

45. Feiner HD, Raghavendra BN, Phelps R, et al: Inflammatory abdominal aortic aneurysm: report of six cases. *Hum Pathol* 15:454, 1984.

46. Parums DV, Chadwick DR, Mitchinson MJ: The localisation of immunoglobulin in chronic periaortitis. *Atherosclerosis* 61:117, 1986.

47. Mitchinson MJ: Chronic periaortitis and periarteritis. *Histopathology* 8:589, 1984.

48. Ormond JK: Idiopathic retroperitoneal fibrosis: an established clinical entity. *JAMA* 174:1561, 1960.

49. Mitchinson MJ: Retroperitoneal fibrosis revisited. *Arch Pathol Lab Med* 110:784, 1986.

50. Miro I, Bakir R, Chanu B, et al: Riedel's thyroiditis and retroperitoneal fibrosis: apropos of a case of multiple fibrosing disease. *Ann Med Interne* (Paris) 135:212, 1984.

51. Hershkowitz M, Fogari R, Chandra M: Idiopathic retroperitoneal fibrosis: implications for a systemic disorder. *Clin Exp Rheumatol* 1:157, 1983.

52. Stewart TW Jr, Friberg TR: Idiopathic retroperitoneal fibrosis with diffuse involvement: further evidence of systemic idiopathic fibrosis. *S Med J* 77:1185, 1984.

53. Sevenet F, Capron-Chivrac D, Delcenserie R, et al: Idiopathic retroperitoneal fibrosis and primary biliary cirrhosis: a new association? *Arch Intern Med* 145:2124, 1985.

54. Giddens WE Jr, Tsai CC, Morton WR, et al: Retroperitoneal fibromatosis and acquired immunodeficiency syndrome in macaques: pathologic observations and transmission studies. *Am J Pathol* 119:253, 1985.

55. Krane SM, Simon LS: Rheumatoid arthritis: clinical features and pathogenetic mechanisms. *Med Clin North AM* 70:263, 1986.

56. Espinoza LR: Rheumatoid arthritis: etiopathogenetic considerations. *Clin Lab Med* 6:27, 1986.

57. Kouri T: Etiology of rheumatoid arthritis. *Experientia* 41:434, 1985.

58. Calin A: Seronegative spondyloarthritides. *Med Clin N Amer* 70:323, 1986.

59. Wagener P, Mau W, Zeidler H, et al: HLA-B27 and clinical aspects of ankylosing spondylitis: result of prospective studies. *Immunol Rev* 86:93, 1985.

60. La Bresh KA, Lally EV, Sharma SC, et al: Two-dimensional echocardiographic detection of preclinical aortic root abnormalities in rheumatoid variant diseases. *Am J Med* 78:908, 1985.

61. Ansell BM, Bywaters EGL, Doniach I: The aortic lesion of ankylosing spondylitis. *Br Heart J* 20:507, 1958.

62. Graham DC, Smythe HA: The carditis and aortitis of ankylosing spondylitis. *Bull Rheum Dis* 9:171, 1958.

63. Davidson P, Baggenstoss AH, Slocum CH, et al: Cardiac and aortic lesions in rheumatoid spondylitis. *Mayo Clin Proc* 38:427, 1963.

64. Bulkley BH, Roberts WC: Ankylosing spondylitis and aortic regurgitation: description of the characteristic cardiovascular lesion from study of eight necropsy patients. *Circulation* 48:1014, 1973.

65. Kinsella TD, Johnson LG, Sutherland RI: Cardiovascular manifestations of ankylosing spondylitis. *Can Med Assoc J* 3:1309, 1974.

66. McGuigan LE, Geczy AF, Edmonds JP: The immunopathology of ankylosing spondylitis—a review. *Semin Arthritis Rheum* 15:81, 1985.

67. Paronen I: Reiter's disease—a study of 344 cases observed in Finland. *Acta Med Scand* 21 (suppl):1, 1948.

68. Csonka GW, Oates JK: Pericarditis and electrocardiographic changes in Reiter's syndrome. *Br Med J* 1:866, 1957.

69. Neu LT, Reider RA, Mack RE: Cardiac involvement in Reiter's disease: report of a case with review of the literature. *Ann Intern Med* 53:215, 1960.

70. Csonka GW, Litchfield JW, Oates JK: Cardiac lesions in Reiter's disease. *Br Med J* 1:243, 1961.

71. Weinberger HW, Ropes MW, Kulka JP, et al: Reiter's syndrome, clinical and pathological observations. *Medicine* 41:35, 1962.

72. Zvaifler NJ, Weintraub AM: Aortitis and aortic insufficiency in the chronic rheumatic disorders—a reappraisal. *Arthritis Rheum* 6:241, 1963.

73. Block SR: Reiter's syndrome and acute aortic insufficiency. *Arthritis Rheum* 15:218, 1972.

74. Good AE: Reiter's disease: a review with special attention to cardiovascular and neurologic sequelae. *Semin Arthritis Rheum* 3:253, 1974.

75. Wilkins RF, Arnett FC, Bitter T: Reiter's syndrome—evaluation of preliminary criteria for definite disease. *Bull Rheum Dis* 32:31, 1983.

76. Morgan SH, Asherson RA, Hughes GRV: Distal aortitis complicating Reiter's syndrome. *Br Heart J* 52:115, 1984.

77. Huycke EC, Robinowitz M, Cohen IS, et al: Rheumatoid granulomatous endocarditis with systemic embolism in Behcet's disease. *Ann Inter Med* 102:791, 1985.

78. McAllister HA Jr, Fenoglio JJ Jr: Cardiac involvement in Whipple's disease. *Circulation* 52:152, 1975.

79. Veasy LG, Wiedmeier SE, Orsmond GS, et al: Resurgence of acute rheumatic fever in the intermountain area of the United States. *N Engl J Med* 316:421, 1987.

80. Bisno AL: Acute rheumatic fever: forgotten but not gone. *N Engl J Med* 316:8, 1987.

81. Lande A, LaPorta A: Takayasu's arteritis: an arteriographic pathologic correlation. *Arch Pathol* 100:437, 1976.

82. Lande A, Bard R, Rossi P, et al: Takayasu's arteritis: a worldwide entity. *NY State J Med* 76:1477, 1976.

83. Lupi Herrera E, Sanchez-Torres G, Marchushamer J, et al: Takayasu's arteritis: clinical study of 197 cases. *Am Heart J* 93:94, 1977.

84. Rose AG, Halper J, Factor SM: Primary arteriopathy in Takayasu's disease. *Arch Pathol Lab Med* 108:644, 1984.

85. Rosen AG, Sinclair-Smith CC: Takayasu's arteritis: a study of 16 autopsy cases. *Arch Pathol Lab Med* 104:231, 1980.

86. Ishikawa K: Natural history and classification of occlusive thromboaortaopathy (Takayasu's disease). *Circulation* 57:27, 1978.

87. McGill CW, Holder TM, Smith TH, et al: Postradiation renovascular hypertension. *J Ped Surg* 14:831, 1979.

88. Huston KA, Hunder GG, Lie JT, et al: Temporal arteritis: a 25-year epidemiologic, clinical, and pathologic study. *Ann Intern Med* 88:162, 1978.

89. Lie JT, Failoni DD, Davis DC Jr: Temporal arteritis with giant cell aortitis, coronary arteritis, and myocardial infarction. *Arch Pathol Lab Med* 110:857, 1986.

90. Venna N, Goldman R, Tilak S, et al: Temporal arteritis-like presentation of carotid atherosclerosis. *Stroke* 17:325, 1986.

91. Allen NB, Studenski SA: Polymyalgia rheumatica and temporal arteritis. *Med Clin North Am* 70:369, 1986.

92. Osler W: The Gulstonian lectures on malignant endocarditis. *Br Med J* 1:467, 1885.

93. Bennet DE, Cherry JK: Bacterial infection of aortic aneurysms: a clinicopathologic study. *Am J Surg* 113:321, 1967.

94. Davies OG, Thornburg JD, Powell P: Cryptic mycotic abdominal aortic aneurysm: diagnosis and management. *Am J Surg* 136:96, 1978.

95. Bardin JA, Collins GM, Devin JB, et al: Nonaneurysmal suppurative aortitis. *Arch Surg* 116:954, 1981.

96. Silberman S, Greenblatt M: Primary mycotic aneurysm of the aorta: a complication of salmonellosis. *Angiology* 14:372, 1963.

97. Mendelowitz DA, Ramstedt R, Yao JST, et al: Abdominal aortic salmonellosis. *Surgery* 85:514, 1979.

98. Volini FI, Olfield RC Jr, Thompson JR, et al: Tuberculosis of the aorta. *JAMA* 181:78, 1962.

99. Ansari A, Larson PH, Bates HD: Cardiovascular manifestations of systemic lupus erythematosus: current perspective. *Prog Cardiovasc Dis* 27:421, 1985.

100. Rocco VK, Hurd ER: Scleroderma and scleroderma-like disorders. *Semin Arthritis Rheum* 16:22, 1986.

101. Haustein UF, Herrmann K, Bohme HJ: Pathogenesis of progressive systemic sclerosis. *Int J Dermatol* 25:286, 1986.

102. LeRoy EC: Pathogenesis of scleroderma (systemic sclerosis). *J Invest Dermat* 79(suppl 1):87s, 1982.

103. Jayson MIV: Systemic sclerosis: a collagen or microvascular disease? *Br Med J* 288:1855, 1984.

104. Greene GM, Lain D, Sherwin RM, et al: Giant cell arteritis of the legs: clinical isolation of severe disease with gangrene and amputations. *Am J Med* 81:727, 1986.

105. Klein RG, Campbell RJ, Hunder GG, et al: Skip lesions in temporal arteritis. *Mayo Clin Proc* 51:504, 1976.

106. Rosai J, Gold J, Landy R: Histiocytoid hemangioma. *Hum Pathol* 10:707, 1979.

107. Wechsler J, Clerici T, Capron F, et al: Angiolymphoid hyperplasia with eosinophilia: optical and histoimmunological study of five cases with an electron microscopy study of one of the cases. *Ann Pathol* 5:271, 1985.

108. Hirashima M, Sakata K, Tashiro K, et al: Spontaneous production of eosinophil chemotactic factors by lymphocytes from patients with subcutaneous angioblastic lymphoid hyperplasia with eosinophilia. *Clin Immunol Immunopathol* 39:231, 1986.

109. Lie JT: Disseminated visceral giant cell arteritis: histopathologic description and differentiation from other granulomatous vasculitides. *Am J Clin Pathol* 69:299, 1978.

110. Hall S, Hunder GG: Is temporal artery biopsy prudent? *Mayo Clin Proc* 59:793, 1984.

111. Fauci AS, Katz P, Haynes BF, et al: Cyclophosphamide therapy of severe systemic necrotizing vasculitis. *N Engl J Med* 301:235, 1979.

112. Lie JT: Coronary vasculitis: a review in the current scheme of classification of vasculitis. *Arch Pathol Lab Med* 111:224, 1987.

113. Mittal B, Kinare S, Mayekar K: Polyarteritis nodosa: an autopsy study. *J Postgrad Med* 31:206, 1985.

114. Savage CO, Winearls CG, Evans DJ, et al: Microscopic polyarteritis: presentation, pathology, and prognosis. *Q J Med* 56:467, 1985.

115. Kawasaki T, Kosaki F, Okawa S, et al: A new infantile acute febrile mucocutaneous lymph node syndrome (MLNS) prevailing in Japan. *Pediatrics* 54(3):271, 1974.

116. Landing BH, Larson EJ: Are infantile periarteritis nodosa with coronary artery involvement and mucocutaneous lymph node syndrome the same? Comparison of 20 patients from North America with patients from Hawaii and Japan. *Pediatrics* 59(5):651, 1977.

117. Everett ED: Mucocutaneous lymph node syndrome (Kawasaki disease) in adults. *JAMA* 242(6):542, 1979.

118. Resnick AH, Esterly NB: Vasculitis in children: *J Dermatol* 24:139, 1985.

119. Mead RH, Brandt L: Manifestation of Kawasaki disease in New England outbreak of 1980. *J Pediatr* 100:558, 1982.

120. Fujiwara H, Fujiwara T, Kao TC, et al: Pathology of Kawasaki disease in the healed stage: relationships between typical and atypical cases of Kawasaki disease. *Acta Pathol Jpn* 36:857, 1986.

121. Leavitt RY, Fauci AS: Pulmonary vasculitis. *Am Rev Respir Dis* 134:149, 1986.

122. Lie JT: The classification of vasculitis and a reappraisal of allergic granulomatosis and angiitis (Churg-Strauss syndrome). *Mt Sinai J Med* 53:429, 1986.

123. Kayes SG: Nonspecific allergic granulomatosis in the lungs of mice infected with large, but not small inocula of the canine ascarid, Toxocara canis. *Clin Immunol Immunopathol* 41:55, 1986.

124. Leavitt RY, Fauci AS: Polyangiitis overlap syndrome: classification and prospective clinical experience. *Am J Med* 81:79, 1986.

125. Leavitt RY, Bressler P, Fauci AS: Buerger's disease in a young woman. *Am J Med* 80:1003, 1986.

126. Nakata Y, Ban I, Hirai M: Onset and clinicopathological course in Buerger's disease. *Angiology* 27:509, 1976.

127. Chopra BS, Zakariah T, Sodhi JS, et al: Thromboangiitis obliterans: a clinical study with special emphasis on venous involvement. *Angiology* 27:126, 1976.

128. McAllister HA Jr, Ferrans VJ: Granulomas of the heart and major blood vessels. In: Ioachim HL (ed). *Pathology of Granulomas*. New York: Raven Press; 75, 1986.

129. Scharffetter K, Blasius S, Franke RP, Kohler M, Mittermayer C: Pathogenetic key position of thromboangiitis: the endothelial cell serum dependent proliferation studies of endothelial cells in obliterative angiopathies. *Vasa* 15:34, 1986.

130. Vermylen J, Blockmans D, Spitz B, et al: Thrombosis and immune disorders. *Clin Haematol* 15:393, 1986.

131. Simic L, Pirnat L: Immunological aspect of smoking in patients with thromboangiitis obliterans. *Vasa* 14:349, 1985.

132. Goldfischer JD: Acute myocardial infarction secondary to ergot therapy: report of a case and review of the literature. *N Engl J Med* 262:860, 1960.

133. Graham JR: Methysergide for prevention of headache: Experience in 500 patients over three years. *N Engl J Med* 270:67, 1964.

134. Whelan TJ, Baugh JH: Nonatherosclerotic arterial lesions and their management. *Curr Prob Surg Mar* 1, 1967.

135. Perrin VL: Clinical pharmokinetics of ergotamine in migraine and cluster headache. *Clin Parmacokinet* 10:334, 1985.

CHAPTER 13

Regulation of Vasomotor Tone and Vasospasm

Colleen M. Brophy, MD; Mark Awolesi, MD
Bauer E. Sumpio, MD, PhD

Introduction and Overview

Regulation of Vasomotor Tone

The important role of the endothelium in modulating vasomotor tone was highlighted in 1980 by Furchgott and Zawadzki with the discovery of the "endothelial-derived relaxation factor" (EDRF).[1] These investigators demonstrated that the administration of acetylcholine to blood vessel rings pre-contracted with norepinephrine resulted in an increase in the contractile response. However, if the endothelium was carefully preserved, the addition of acetylcholine to rings pre-contracted with norepinephrine resulted in a relaxation response. They postulated that an "endothelial-derived relaxing substance" caused this vasorelaxation response in the blood vessel rings in which the endothelium had been carefully preserved. Seven years later, the effects of EDRF were determined to be in large part due to the effects of nitric oxide (NO).[2] The discovery of NO provided the framework for much of the advancement in vascular biology.

A wide variety of factors including autocrine, paracrine, and endocrine vasoactive substances—the ionic milieu—and mechanical forces impact on vascular smooth muscle contraction and relaxation (Figure 1). The response of the vascular smooth muscle to vasoactive agents on the luminal aspect of the vessel depends on whether the endothelial layer is intact or damaged. In the presence of an intact endothelium, many substances interact with receptors on the endothelium which results in the subsequent release of vasoactive substances that influence the vascular smooth muscle in a paracrine fashion (Figure 2). These responses are "endothelial-dependent." For example, bradykinin, angiotensin II, histamine, norepinephrine, serotonin, and thrombin incite the endothelium to release NO which leads to vascular smooth muscle relaxation. Alternatively, if the endothelium is absent, these same pharmacologic substances interact with receptors on the vascular smooth muscle and generate a contractile response (Table 1). Thus, smooth muscle responses in the absence of an intact endothelium, "endothelial-independent," are often markedly different than "endothelial-dependent" responses. Injury to the endothelium in vivo has been implicated in vasospasm and in atherosclerosis.

Vascular smooth muscle cells are capable of producing substances which influence the responses of neighboring vascular smooth muscle cells in an autocrine fashion. In addition, it is likely that vascular smooth muscle cells are capable of producing substances which influence the response of endothelial cells. In particular, parathyroid hormone-related peptides (PTHrP) have been shown to be released by smooth muscle cells and cause vascular smooth muscle relaxation and inhibit endothelin release from endothelial cells.[3]

In addition to paracrine and autocrine substances,

From *The Basic Science of Vascular Disease.* Edited by Sidawy AN, Sumpio BE, and DePalma RG. Armonk, NY: Futura Publishing Company, Inc.; © 1997.

MODULATION OF VASOMOTOR TONE

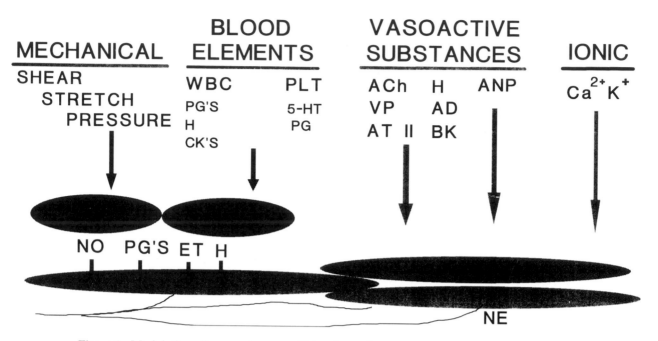

Figure 1. Modulation of vasomotor tone. This schematic oversimplifies some of the numerous factors and forces that modulate vasomotor tone. These signals originate from the lumen of the vessel, from cells in the vessel wall, and from the adventitial aspect of the vessel. The vasomotor response to many substances depends on whether the endothelium is present or absent. Endothelial cells respond to many intraluminal influences with the release of nitric oxide (**NO**), prostaglandins (**PGs**), endothelin (**ET**), and histamine (**H**). Mechanical forces, such as shear stress and pressure resulting from the pulsatility of blood flow, impact on vasomotor tone. Blood elements, such as white blood cells (**WBC**) and platelets (**PLT**) release PGs, H, cytokines (**CKs**), and serotonin (**5-HT**). Circulating vasoactive substances include acetylcholine (**ACh**), arginine vasopressin (**VP**), angiotensin II (**ATII**), H, adenosine (**AD**), bradykinin (**BK**), and atrial natriuretic peptides (**ANP**). The extracellular concentration of ions such as calcium (Ca^{2+}) and potassium (K^+) also influences vascular tone. Innervation of the smooth muscle impacts on tone via the release of neurotransmitters such as norepinephrine (**NE**). Thus, the regulation of vasomotor tone depends on multiple signals and responses to those signals.

vasomotor tone is regulated by circulating endocrine substances such as catecholamines, by substances released by blood components such as macrophages and platelets, and by the ionic milieu that bathes vascular cells (Figure 1). Other factors, such as mechanical forces, are also capable of modulating vasomotor tone (Figure 1). The physiologically relevant mechanical forces of cyclic strain and pressure have been shown to affect endothelial cells, and in some instances, smooth muscle cell responses (Figure 1). Vasomotor tone in blood vessels in the brain can be altered by substances that interact on the adventitial surface of the vessel. Subarachnoid hemorrhage results in blood in the cerebrospinal fluid, and it is thought that some component of blood, possibly oxyhemoglobin, leads to the intense vasospasm that occurs in association with subarachnoid hemorrhage.[4]

There is recent experimental evidence that vasoactive substances capable of inducing contraction in the vascular smooth muscle, such as endothelin, angiotensin II, catecholamines, and serotonin, are also mitogenic and induce smooth muscle proliferation.[5,6,7] Substances that are known to be potent vascular smooth muscle mitogens, such as platelet-derived growth factor (PDGF), and epidermal growth factor (EGF), are also capable of inducing vascular smooth muscle contraction.[8,9] The converse is also true in that substances that induce relaxation in the vascular smooth muscle, such as nitrosovasodilators and prostacyclin, prevent proliferation of vascular smooth muscle.[10] Thus, the signal for vascular smooth muscle contraction may ultimately incite fixed obliterative athero-occlusive lesions (Figure 3).

Vasomotor tone reflects a balance between con-

VASOACTIVE SUBSTANCES

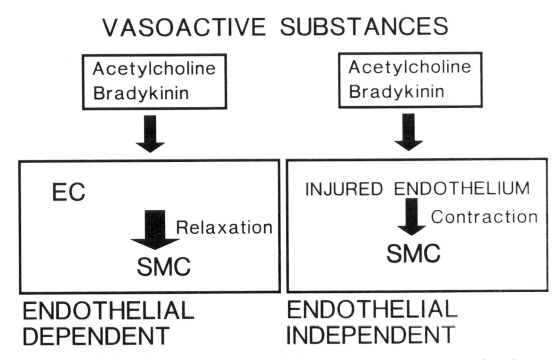

Figure 2. Endothelial-dependent and endothelial-independent responses to vasoactive substances. Vasoactive substances such as acetylcholine and bradykinin have differential effects on vasomotor tone depending on whether the endothelium is present or absent. In the presence of an intact endothelial layer, the endothelial cells (**EC**) respond to these substances by releasing diffusible substances such as nitric oxide (**NO**), that cause the vascular smooth muscle (**SMC**) to relax. In the absence of an intact endothelial layer, the direct effect of these substances on the smooth muscle is vasocontraction.

tracting and relaxing stimuli (Figure 1). Physiologic regulation of vasomotor tone is essential to meet the metabolic needs of the tissues supplied by the various vascular beds. Alterations in vasomotor tone can result in pathologic conditions such as hypertension, atherosclerosis, and vasospasm.

Table 1
Substances Capable of Inducing
"Endothelial-Independent" Vascular Smooth
Muscle Contraction and Relaxation

Vasocontraction	Vasorelaxation
Neuropeptide Y	Adenosine
Acetylcholine	Atrial naturetic peptides
Angiotensin II	Isoproteronol
Bradykinin	Nitrosovasodilators
Histamine	Prostacyclin
Serotonin	Calcium channel blockers
Thrombin	
Thromboxane	
Vasopressin	
Endothelin	

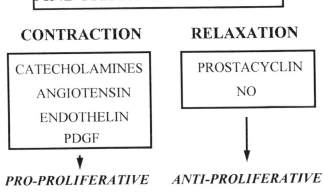

Figure 3. Vasomotor responses and atherogenesis. Substances which cause the vascular smooth muscle to contract are also mitogenic and induce smooth muscle proliferation and matrix production. This may lead to structural changes in the vessel wall. The converse is also true in that substances which cause the vascular smooth muscle to relax are antiproliferative and may prevent structural narrowing of blood vessels. Thus, the same forces that lead to physiologic narrowing of the blood vessel may predispose to fixed narrowing or atherosclerosis.

Vasospasm

Vasospasm is an alteration in vasomotor tone in which sustained contraction predominates.[11] This may be produced by a deficiency of vasorelaxing substances, or by an increase in vasocontracting substances. True vasospasm, however, represents a state of smooth muscle contraction refractory to relaxation by the addition of potent vasorelaxants (refractory to "active relaxation") and refractory to removal of vasoconstrictors (refractory to "passive relaxation").[12] Based on this more precise definition, vasospasm can be viewed as a state inherent to the vascular smooth muscle.[11] This implies that vasospasm may result from a primary alteration in smooth muscle cell signalling events that modulate the state of contraction and relaxation.

Vasospasm plays an important role in the pathogenesis of many clinical conditions. For example, vasospasm can occur in vessels in proximity to an extremity injury, as in long bone fractures and joint dislocations. The morbidity of subarachnoid hemorrhage is directly related to the extent of vasospasm that ensues after the hemorrhage. Vasospasm in the mesenteric vasculature contributes to both occlusive and nonocclusive mesenteric ischemia.[13] Spasm in autologous vein grafts may compromise peripheral vascular reconstructions.[14] Anginal pain not related to exercise associated with ST-segment elevation has been termed "Prinzmetal's angina," or variant angina. Prinzmetal's angina has been attributed to spasms in the main coronary vessels and can be induced by the administration of ergonovine.[15] In addition, vasospasm may occur in conjunction with coronary thrombosis and contribute to myocardial infarction. Raynaud's phenomenon, with characteristic triphasic color changes of the digits and associated pain and paresthesias, is caused by vasospasm in the digital vessels.

Vasospasm may play a role in both the initiation and maintenance of atherosclerosis. For instance, it has been demonstrated that atherosclerotic blood vessels display enhanced contractile responses to a variety of agonists.[16] Enhanced contractile responses to histamine have been observed in atherosclerotic pig coronary artery smooth muscle and to ergonovine in atherosclerotic dog coronary arteries.[17,18] Enhanced contractile responses have also been observed in response to serotonin in the hind limb of atherosclerotic monkeys and in the aorta of hereditary hyperlipidemic rabbits.[19,20] Thus, atherosclerotic vessels may be more prone to vasospasm.

Experimental Models

The biology and physiology of vascular smooth muscle can be examined in a variety of systems. Traditionally, vasomotor responses of arterial smooth muscle have been examined in muscle baths (Figure 4). Fresh whole vessels can be stored in sterile physiologic saline solution [such as Hepes buffered saline—140mM NaCl, 4.7mM KCl, 1.0mM $MgSO_4$, 1.0mM NaH_2PO_4, 1.5mM $CaCl_2$, 10mM glucose, and 10mM Hepes (pH 7.4)] at 4°C for 48 to 72 hours. A wide variety of animal tissues have been used as a source of vessels. A convenient, inexpensive source of vascular tissue is a local abattoir. In addition, fresh human tissue can be obtained from the operating room (as in extra segments of saphenous vein) or from organ donors.

For muscle bath experiments, the vessels are carefully dissected while bathed in the buffer solution. The adventitia is removed and either rings or strips of muscle are prepared. For strips of muscle, the vessels are opened lengthwise and transverse strips of muscle 1 to 2 mm wide are cut. If the purpose of the experiment is to examine endothelium-independent responses, the endothelium can be denuded with a cotton-tip applicator. Rings are often used to examine endothelial-dependent responses. The strip or ring of vascular smooth muscle is then fixed at one end and attached to a strain gauge transducer at the other end. The preparation is placed in a bath containing a physiologic saline solution [such as krebs bicarbonate buffer—120mM NaCl, 4.7mM KCl, 1.0mM $MgSO_4$, 1.0mM NaH_2PO_4, 10mM glucose, 1.5mM $CaCl_2$, and 25mM Na_2HCO_3 (pH 7.4) equilibrated with 95%O_2/5%CO_2] maintained at 37°C with a jacketed water bath. Pharmacologic agents can be added directly to the muscle bath preparation. Responses to these interventions can be recorded on a strip chart recorder or a computer (Figure 4). Concurrent intracellular biochemical events can be determined by homogenizing the strips and performing assays for specific pathways. This classic system has been widely employed to examine vascular smooth muscle physiology and pharmacology.

Whole vessel responses have been examined in ex vivo vasomotor perfusion devices.[21,22] These systems typically maintain constant flow through isolated perfused blood vessels and record changes in pressure with various interventions. A recently described apparatus utilizes a laser optical micrometer to measure changes in vessel wall diameter in response to pharmacologic manipulations.[22] Isolated perfused whole vessel models allow agents to be administered to either the external surface of the blood vessel or to the perfusate, thus differentiating between luminal and adventitial responses. In addition, if the endothelium is carefully preserved, this model allows evaluation of endothelial-dependent versus endothelial-independent responses. Endothelial-independent responses can be examined by denuding the endothelium with intraluminal passage of a balloon catheter.

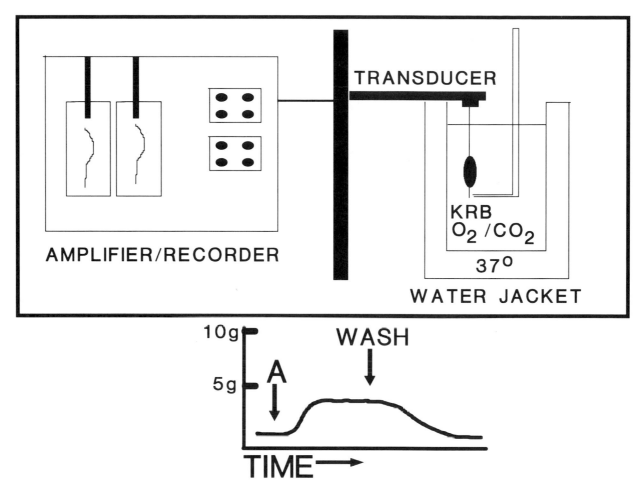

Figure 4. Muscle bath physiology. The classic system employed to examine muscle physiology is the muscle bath. Strips or rings of vascular smooth muscle are secured between a transducer and a fixed point. The strips are equilibrated in a physiologic saline solution and the temperature maintained at 37°C by a water jacket. Agonists can be added directly to the bath and the contractile response recorded on a strip chart or computer. The **tracing at the bottom** depicts a typical contractile response to an agonist (**A**) followed by relaxation when the agonist is washed out.

While no true model of vasospasm has been developed ex vivo, models of vasospasm have been developed in intact animals. Cerebral vasospasm can be produced in dogs by the injection of fresh autologous blood into the cisterna magna.[23] Vasospasm in the basilar arteries is then assessed angiographically. Using this model, investigators have determined that substances such as oxyhemoglobin, applied to the adventitial surface of cerebral vessels, can lead to vasospasm.[4]

The components of the blood vessel wall can also be examined in cell culture systems. Bovine aortic endothelial cells and human umbilical vein endothelial cells have both been well characterized in culture. Arterial smooth muscle cells can also be grown in cell culture systems. The advantage of cultured vascular cells is that the responses of large numbers of a single cell line can be readily determined. Vascular cells in culture, however, undergo phenotypic changes that

likely alter their physiologic response. For instance, vascular smooth muscle cells in culture characteristically modulate their phenotype from a spindle-shaped ''contractile'' phenotype to a more pleomorphic ''synthetic'' phenotype. Thus, when extrapolating data obtained from cells in culture to potential physiologic responses, it is important to recognize that significant phenotypic alterations may have occurred.

Fresh single vascular smooth muscle cells can be prepared by proteolytic digestion of the arterial wall. Contraction in these cells can be observed under the microscope.[24] The advantage of this system is that the individual cells can be manipulated with microtools, compounds can be injected in the cells, and the cells can be readily exposed to antibodies for immunocytochemical studies. In addition, these smooth muscle cells are phenotypically closer to smooth muscle cells in vivo than cultured smooth muscle cells.

Thus, the pharmacology and physiology of blood vessel contractile responses can be examined in a wide range of systems, from cultured vascular cells to whole vessels in vivo. It is important to recognize that data describing vasomotor tone are dependent on the presence or absence of an intact endothelium, the vascular bed involved, and the model used to assess tone. In order to elucidate some of the mechanisms underlying the regulation of vasomotor tone and vasospasm, this chapter will focus on the intracellular mechanisms which modulate these processes and highlight some of the physiologic agonists which incite vasoconstriction and relaxation.

Vasoconstriction

Molecular Mechanisms of Vasoconstriction

Physiologic substances which cause the vascular smooth muscle to contract include molecules which interact with specific cell surface receptors and extracellular ions which alter the polarization of the cell membrane (Table 1). The vascular muscle responds by initiating a cascade of events which culminate in contraction of the muscle. This cascade of events by which external stimuli are transduced into cellular responses are commonly referred to as intracellular signalling events.

Vascular smooth muscle contractions are different from cardiac or skeletal muscle contractions.[25] Vascular smooth muscle is especially unique in that sustained contractions can be maintained with minimal energy consumption. A common theme underlying the mechanism of vascular smooth muscle contraction is that an increase in intracellular Ca^{2+} concentration ($[Ca^{2+}]_i$) is important for the initiation of the contraction (Figure 5). This increase in $[Ca^{2+}]_i$ results in the formation of Ca^{2+}-calmodulin complexes that bind to and activate the myosin light chain kinase (MLCK). MLCK phosphorylates myosin light chains (MLC_{20}) which in turn activate the actinomycin ATPase resulting in cross bridge formation and contraction.

The plasma membrane forms a barrier for a ten-thousandfold concentration gradient between the extracellular (approximately 1 to 2.5 mM $[Ca^{2+}]$) and intracellular (approximately 80 to 200 nM $[Ca^{2+}]$) calcium domains. The cellular mechanisms that allow calcium to enter the smooth muscle cell include Ca^{2+} entrance into the cell via voltage-dependent Ca^{2+} channels (L-type channels), receptor operated Ca^{2+} channels, and Na^+/Ca^{2+} exchange. Ca^{2+} is extruded from the smooth muscle by a plasma membrane ATPase and by Na^+/Ca^{2+} exchange. Calcium channel blockers such as verapamil and nifedipine produce relaxation of vascular smooth muscle by blocking L-type channels, thus preventing the entrance of Ca^{2+} into the smooth muscle cell. The normal smooth muscle transmembrane potential is -40 to -55 mV. Depolarization of the smooth muscle membrane with high extracellular $[K^+]$ results in a rapid increase in ($[Ca^{2+}]_i$) and muscle contraction.

Agonists which interact with receptors on the cell surface, such as bradykinin, angiotensin, serotonin, and endothelin, lead to the hydrolysis of membrane-bound phosphoinositols. One of the breakdown products of phosphoinositol hydrolysis, inositol trisphosphate (IP^3), leads to increases in $[Ca^{2+}]_i$ through the release of Ca^{2+} from intracellular pools. The major intracellular calcium pool in the vascular smooth muscle is the sarcoplasmic reticulum. In addition, agonists can activate calcium influx from extracellular sources via direct activation of calcium channels and by indirectly inducing membrane depolarization.

Thus, both physiologic agonists and ionic influences can lead to increases in $[Ca^{2+}]_i$. These increases in $[Ca^{2+}]_i$ can be measured using a variety of Ca^{2+} indicators including calcium chelators such as fura-2 and the photoluminescent photoprotein, aequorin. Aequorin is a 21 kDa photoprotein that emits light when exposed to Ca^{2+}. Aequorin can be "loaded" into smooth muscle cells using reversible permeabilization.[26] Aequorin has been used to determine the temporal course of cytoplasmic $[Ca^{2+}]_i$ concurrently with vascular smooth muscle contraction. Carbachol-induced contractions in tracheal smooth muscle loaded with aequorin are associated with a rapid rise in $[Ca^{2+}]_i$ followed by a lower plateau phase that remains slightly but significantly higher than the unstimulated baseline value.[26] Experiments in which extracellular Ca^{2+} is removed suggest that the main source of mobilized Ca^{2+} for the initial Ca^{2+} transient is an intracellular pool (presumably the sarcoplasmic reticulum), and that the main source of Ca^{2+} during the plateau phase is an extracellular pool.[26]

Myosin light chain phosphorylation can be examined experimentally using two-dimensional gel electrophoresis.[27] With this technique, smooth muscles are pre-labeled with ^{32}P-orthophosphate and stimulated with various agonists. The muscles are then homogenized and the proteins separated by charge using isoelectric focusing (IEF). The proteins are then further resolved with SDS polyacrylamide electrophoresis (SDS-PAGE). The various isoforms of phosphorylated myosin light chain are present at 20 kDa. In addition to MLC_{20}, there are other low molecular weight phosphoproteins that are phosphorylated in a temporal manner concurrent with vascular smooth muscle contraction.[27] It is likely that many of these proteins are important mediators of vascular smooth muscle contraction, but the specific role of many of these phosphoproteins is only currently being characterized.

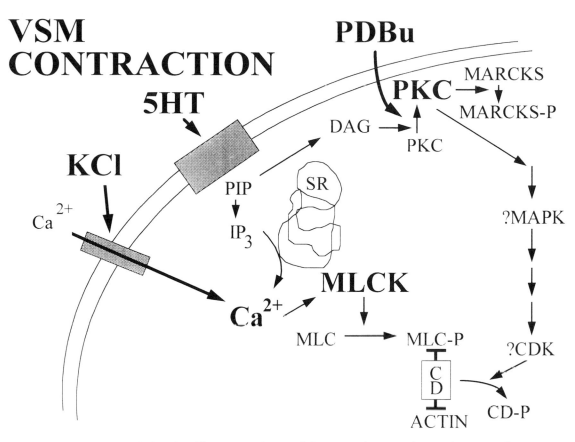

Figure 5. Intracellular signalling events that modulate vascular smooth muscle contraction. Agonists induce vascular smooth muscle contraction via phosphoinositol hydrolysis and the generation of the important intracellular signalling messengers inositol triphosphate (**IP$_3$**) and diacylglycerol (**DAG**). IP$_3$ causes release of Ca^{2+} from the sarcoplasmic reticulum (**SR**) and DAG activates protein kinase C (**PKC**). High extracellular KCl depolarizes the membrane allowing an influx of Ca^{2+}. Increases in Ca^{2+} activate the calcium-calmodulin-dependent enzyme, myosin light chain kinase (**MLCK**), which phosphorylates myosin light chains (**MLC**) and leads to activation of an ATPase and contraction. It is possible that PKC, acting through a kinase cascade that may involve mitogen-activated protein kinase (**MAPK**), is important for sustained vascular smooth muscle contractions. The phosphorylation of caldesmon (**CD**) by caldesmon kinase (**CDK**) reverses its inhibition of actinomyosin ATPase.

Much of the controversy surrounding the physiology of vascular smooth muscle contraction centers on the findings that: 1) maintenance of MLC$_{20}$ phosphorylation is not necessary for the maintenance of vascular smooth muscle contraction, and 2) sustained contraction can be maintained under circumstances when the [Ca^{2+}]$_i$ in the fully contracted muscle is nearly identical to the relaxed muscle.[28] To explain these data, Hai et al[29] have developed a model that describes a "latch state." In their model, rapidly cycling crossbridges, which form between myosin and actin, undergo dephosphorylation in such a way that kinetically stable bridges or "latch" crossbridges form. This new kinetic state is characterized by slow dissociation of the high affinity actinomyosin complex. These postulated latch bridges are thought to be essential to the tonic phase of contraction.

Rasmussen and other investigators have proposed that a second regulatory process may explain maintenance of sustained vascular smooth muscle contraction.[28] These investigators propose that activation of a separate pathway, the protein kinase C (PKC) pathway, is important for maintaining the sustained phase of smooth muscle contraction (Figure 5). PKC translocation, which coincides with activation, exhibits a temporal pattern similar to the contractile response observed after exposure to agonists such as histamine and endothelin.[30] Many agonists of smooth muscle contraction stimulate phosphatidylinositol hydrolysis resulting in a rapid and transient rise in IP$_3$ which mobilizes calcium from intracellular sources. In addition, phosphoinositol hydrolysis leads to increases in membrane diacylglycerol content (DAG). DAG activates PKC which results in translocation, or movement of the enzyme

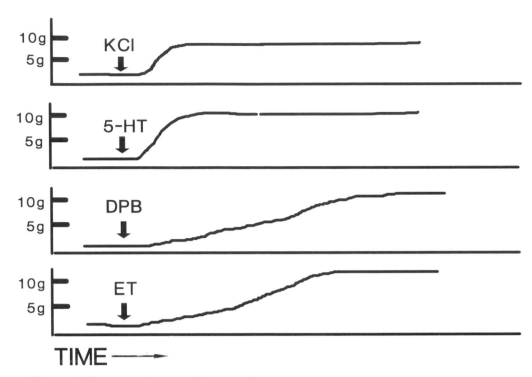

Figure 6. Representative vascular smooth muscle contractile responses. Depolarization of the muscle membrane with high extracellular potassium chloride (**KCl**) leads to an influx of Ca^{2+} and a rapidly induced contraction. Agonists such as serotonin (**5–HT**) also cause rapid contractions. Phorbol esters (**DPB**) induce slowly developing sustained contractions, possibly through the direct activation of protein kinase C. Endothelin (**ET**) the most potent vasoconstrictor known, induces slowly developing sustained contractions similar to those induced by phorbol esters.

from the cytosol to the membrane of the cell. Phorbol esters, which mimic DAG in activating PKC, have been shown to induce sustained contractions in a wide variety of smooth muscles.[30] Phorbol ester-induced contractions are slowly developing tonic contractions which mimic the development of the sustained phase of vascular smooth muscle contraction (Figure 6).

It is unlikely that direct phosphorylation of MLC_{20} by PKC modulates the regulation of smooth muscle contraction. PKC phosphorylates MLC_{20} at regions clearly distinct from the regions phosphorylated by MLCK. It has been proposed that PKC modulates sustained contraction through a kinase cascade which leads to the phosphorylation of several intermediate and thin filament proteins such as desmin, caldesmon, calponin, and other low-molecular weight cytosolic proteins.[30]

Mitogen-activated protein kinase (MAP kinase) may be an intermediate in PKC-modulated contraction. MAP kinase has been shown to phosphorylate the intermediate filament protein caldesmon. In a dephosphorylated state, caldesmon blocks the interaction of actin and myosin via inhibition of the actinomyosin ATPase. Once phosphorylated, caldesmon is no longer able to block this interaction and actinomyosin cross-links form.[31]

Thus, it is possible that increases in $[Ca^{2+}]_i$ and activation of MLCK are important for the rapid initial phase of vascular smooth muscle contraction. Maintenance of the tonic phase of contraction, however, may be regulated by a different cascade of signalling events activated by PKC.

PKC may also be important in mediating the tonic contractions that constitute vasospasm. There is evidence that under certain conditions of persistent high intracellular calcium, a Ca^{2+}-dependent neutral protease, calpain, becomes activated. Calpain catalyzes the hydrolysis of peptide bonds linking the regulatory and catalytic domains of PKC (Figure 7). This cleavage results in a constituitively activated catalytic domain, termed protein kinase M. Minami et al, using a canine basilar artery model of vasospasm and specific inhibitors of protein kinase C (calphostin) and calpain (calpeptin), suggested that the majority of the catalytic domain of protein kinase C is dissociated from the regulatory domain in vasospasm.[32] Thus, proteolysis of protein kinase C, resulting in a constituitively active enzyme, represents a tenable mechanism for the sustained vascular smooth muscle contraction in vasospasm.

Thus, the intracellular signalling mechanisms that modulate vascular smooth muscle contraction remain

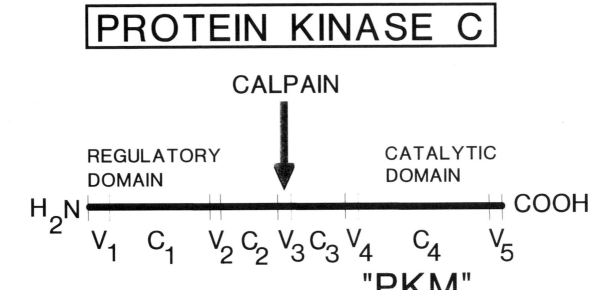

Figure 7. Cleavage of **PKC** by the enzyme calpain leads to the generation of constituitively active catalytic domain of protein kinase M (**PKM**). This is one hypothesis for a molecular mechanism of vasospasm.[44]

incompletely characterized. It is likely that multiple pathways modulate vascular smooth muscle contraction. It is possible that sequential activation of one or more of these signalling pathways leads to a persistent contractile state or vasospasm.

Mediators of Vascular Smooth Muscle Contraction

The endothelium produces several vasoactive compounds which act as autocrine and paracrine substances. A specific endothelial-derived contracting substance, endothelin, and an endothelial-derived relaxing factor, NO, have changed our understanding of the interaction between the endothelium and the underlying smooth muscle cell (SMC). Information has been recently accumulated regarding the role of these vasoactive paracrine and autocrine substances in regulating vasomotor tone, and in vasospasm.

Endothelin

Endothelin is the most potent vascular smooth muscle contracting factor known. Endothelin has only recently been identified and characterized.[33] In 1988, Yanagisawa and his colleagues reported the sequence and cloning of endothelin.[34] This resulted in an explosion of data regarding what is currently known as a family of vasoconstricting polypeptides. Four isotypes of endothelin have been described: endothelin-1 (ET-

1), endothelin-2 (ET-2), endothelin-3 (ET-3), and β-endothelin (β-ET), otherwise known as vasoactive intestinal peptide (VIP). ET-1 can be produced by both endothelial cells and vascular smooth muscle cells. However, vascular smooth muscle cells produce one-hundredfold less ET-1 than endothelial cells. Exogenously administered endothelins to whole organisms produce profound and sustained vasoconstriction; however, endothelin production does not account for all of the contracting activity generated by the endothelium. The identity of other endothelial-derived vasoactive substances is currently an active area of research.

The structure of the endothelins is highly conserved. All endothelins are 21 amino acid polypeptides with an estimated molecular weight of 2492 daltons. They contain two disulfide bonds and a carboxy terminal tryptophan molecule. The activity of the endothelins is dependent on the conservation of this structure. The endothelins have a hydrophilic N-terminal and a hydrophobic C-terminal. Nuclear magnetic resonance studies suggest that endothelin resembles a snail with a helical tail. The structure of ET-2, ET-3, and vasoactive intestinal peptide are very similar to that of ET-1. The structure of the endothelins is closely related to that of a toxic component in the venom of the burrowing asp, *Atractaspis engaddensis*, sarafotoxin S6. This toxin causes sustained coronary vasospasm leading to cardiac arrest.

ET-1 is encoded by a gene on the human chromosome 6, while ET-3 is located on the human chromosome 20. Thus, although the two compounds have very similar properties, they are not genetically linked. The 2026 nucleotide mRNA for ET-1 is encoded in five exons distributed over 6.8 kilobase pairs of the genome.[35] The 5' flanking region of ET-1 contains an octa-nucleotide sequence for the phorbol ester-responsive elements, the *fos-jun* complex, consensus motifs for the binding site of nuclear factor 1, and a hexa-nucleotide sequence for the acute phase reactant regulatory elements. The acute phase reactant regulatory elements may be involved in the induction of endothelin under acute physical stress in vivo.[35]

Two promoter regions, positions -148 to -117 and -117 to -98, appear to be necessary for the transcription of preproendothelin-1 in endothelial cells. The proximal 143 base pair 5' flanking sequence of the endothelin-1 gene appears to be sufficient for maximum transcription. Likewise, a consensus sequence for AP-1 at positions -109 to -102 is necessary for full transcriptional activity. This sequence may mediate responsiveness to phorbol esters and serve as binding sites for specific members of the *fos* and *jun* family of oncoproteins. The endothelin promoter also contains a TATC (GATA) motif that is critical for promoter function. Two alternative promoter regions have also recently been described which may be involved in the transcription of the endothelin gene.[36]

Translation of the ET mRNA results in the production of a large polypeptide, preproendothelin, which consists of 203 amino acid residues. Preproendothelin is an unstable protein with a half-life of about 15 minutes. Preproendothelin is cleaved to a 39 amino acid compound, proendothelin or big endothelin. The enzyme responsible for the conversion of proendothelin to ET-1, endothelin converting enzyme, is a membrane-bound neutral metalloprotease. The conversion of proendothelin to ET-1 is very rapid and efficient. Big endothelin has weak vasoconstrictor activity, one-hundredfold less than ET-1. Studies in rats have demonstrated a marked pressor effect upon intravenous injection of big endothelin, which can be effectively blocked by the administration of the metalloprotease inhibitor, phosphoramidon.

Although the mechanism of synthesis of the endothelins has been well studied, the mode of secretion is still not clearly defined. It is unlikely that there are significant intracellular stores of preformed endothelins, in that ultrastructural analysis of endothelial cells has not revealed secretory granules. It is more likely that endothelin secretion arises from de novo synthesis. Induction of ET-1 mRNA and peptide release in endothelial cells is enhanced by agents such as thrombin, transforming growth factor β, angiotensin II, vasopressin, interleukin-1, hypoxia, phorbol esters, and calcium ionophores. The stimulation of endothelin production by the calcium ionophore A23187 and phorbol

ester suggests a possible role for phospholipase C activation and increased intracellular calcium in the mechanism of endothelin release from endothelial cells.[37]

Endotoxin is a potent stimulus for endothelin production. Cultured endothelial cells exposed to endotoxin produce a dose-dependent increase in the secretion of immunoreactive endothelin. In several laboratory animals, a significant increase in the level of immunoreactive endothelin can be demonstrated after the infusion of endotoxin. Endothelin production has also been demonstrated in patients with sepsis.[38] TNF-α, a cytokine produced in septic shock, induces endothelin-1 production in bovine glomerular capillary cells, cultured bovine aortic endothelial cells, and bovine renal artery.

Several substances including prostacyclin, heparin, atrial natriuretic peptide, NO, and nitrovasodilator compounds inhibit the production of endothelin.[39,40,41] Co-culture of endothelial cells with vascular smooth muscle cells or fibroblasts results in significant reduction in the amount of endothelin in the media. Likewise, incubation of endothelial cells with conditioned media from smooth muscle or fibroblast cultures will down-regulate endothelin production. Thus, it appears that smooth muscle cells produce a yet unidentified substance which inhibits endothelin production by endothelial cells.

The release of the atrial natriuretic peptide (ANP) is augmented by endothelin. Since many of the observed actions of ANP oppose the actions of endothelin, ANP has been postulated as a negative feedback mechanism. ANP inhibits the vasoconstriction effect of ET-1. ANP induces natriuresis and increases renal blood flow whereas ET-1 has antinatriuretic effects and decreases renal blood flow.

Hemodynamic forces have also been demonstrated to regulate the synthesis of endothelin in cultured endothelial cells. There have been conflicting reports on the effect of shear stress on the production of endothelin. Exposure of cultured porcine endothelial cells to low (5 dynes/cm2) shear stress results in an increase in endothelin mRNA over 1 to 4 hours with a return to static levels over 12 to 24 hours and an increase in immunoreactive endothelin levels in the media.[41A] However, others have described a reduction in the level of preproendothelin mRNA in endothelial cells exposed to 24 hours of high laminar shear stress (25 dynes/cm2) accompanied by a concomitant decrease in ET-1 release into the culture media.[42] It is likely that the effect of shear stress on the endothelin regulation is dependent on the duration and level of shear stress. A short duration and low level of shear stress results in an increase in endothelin release while long duration and high shear stress levels inhibit endothelin release.

Cyclic strain, analogous to the pulsatile distension experienced by the vessel wall in vivo, has been demonstrated by our laboratory and other investigators to increase ET-1 immunoreactivity in bovine aortic endothelial cells.[43,44] This increase is mediated by an increase in endothelin mRNA.[45]

The endothelins mediate their effects by binding to specific receptors. After binding to a receptor, endothelin is internalized into the cell. Endothelin binding to receptors is nearly irreversible and is resistant to dissociation by acid treatment.[34] Long-term exposure of vascular smooth muscle cells to endothelin leads to a down-regulation of the receptor.[34] The ubiquitous distribution of ET receptors in cardiac muscle, central nervous system, the kidneys, lungs, adrenal medulla, spleen, corneal epithelium, intestine, and blood vessel walls has been documented by binding studies utilizing ^{125}I-endothelin.[46] Multiple subtypes of endothelin receptors have been described and have recently been classified into two major groups: endothelin-A (ET-A) and endothelin-B (ET-B). Both ET-A and ET-B receptors are present in blood vessels.[47] ET-A has a one-hundredfold higher affinity for ET-1 than ET-3, hence it is often referred to as the ET-1 specific receptor.[48] The affinity of ET-B for endothelin is similar for all of the isotypes. Endothelial cells express the ET-B receptor while vascular smooth muscle cells express the ET-A receptor.[48] The endothelin receptors have a transmembrane morphology similar to other G-protein coupled receptors.[47,48]

Several biologic functions have been ascribed to the endothelins. Intravenous administration of endothelins triggers a biphasic blood pressure response. There is an initial rapid fall in blood pressure followed by sustained increase in arterial blood pressure.[49] The initial vasodilatory effect of endothelin occurs by selective vasodilation of the musculocutaneous vascular beds, but not the visceral vasculature.[49] The initial vasodilatory response is due to the release of EDRF and prostacyclin from endothelial cells. The pressor effect of the endothelins is likely a direct effect of endothelin on the vascular smooth muscle.

In addition to a direct effect on vascular smooth muscle cells, stimulation of the sympathetic nervous system has been implicated in the vasoconstrictor response to exogenous ET-1. Chronic infusion of endothelin into the cerebral vessels of laboratory animals evokes a marked increase in arterial blood pressure which is accompanied by a systemic elevation of catecholamines and vasopressin.[50] Thus, endothelins produced in the central nervous system may affect tonic vascular responses. Endothelins may also affect tonic vascular responses through modulation of baroreflexes. Release of endothelin, in the region of the carotid sinus, aortic arch, heart, and lungs may modulate the baroreflex. For example, endothelins have been reported to decrease the activity of baroreceptors in isolated canine carotid sinus after the application of increased carotid sinus pressure.

In addition to the cardiovascular system, endothelin has major effects in other regional vascular beds including the kidneys. Intravenously administered endothelin leads to a dose-dependent reduction in glomerular filtration rate.[51] This may be the result of afferent arteriolar constriction. Endothelin also increases the activity of the angiotensin-converting enzyme which results in an increase in circulating angiotensin II levels. Endothelin also stimulates aldosterone synthesis in isolated zona glomerulosa cells. Water deprivation has been shown to result in production of endothelin from the hypothalamus. Thus, endothelin may be an important component of the fluid homeostatic system.

Endothelin appears to function as a paracrine and possibly an autocrine hormone. Baseline circulating levels of endothelin are 1 to 2 pg/mL.[52] Elevated endothelin levels have been reported in essential hypertension, angina, acute myocardial infarction, renal failure, shock, and endotoxemia.[52,53,54] Patients with hemangioendotheliomas, which are associated with hypertesion, have markedly elevated circulating levels of ET-1.[55] Resection of the tumor has been associated with a fall in blood pressure, and hypertension recurs in patients with recurrence of the tumor.[55] Plasma levels of endothelin increase with age in healthy patients.

Endothelin may be an important mediator of vasospasm. Vascular smooth muscle contractions induced by endothelin are slow to develop and relax very slowly when endothelin is removed (Figure 6). This unique property of endothelin suggests that endothelin may be important in generating the sustained vascular smooth muscle contractions that occur with vasospasm. In addition, after complete depletion of intracellular calcium, endothelin induces a contraction which can be inhibited by the protein kinase C inhibitor H7. Phorbol esters have also been shown to elicit calcium-independent vascular smooth muscle contraction.[56] Isoforms of PKC that require less calcium for activation, namely epsilon and zeta, are present in vascular smooth muscle. Thus, activation of calcium-independent isoforms of PKC by endothelin may represent a novel pathway for production of sustained, irreversible contractions as seen in vasospasm.

Vasorelaxation

Molecular Mechanisms of Vasorelaxation

The vascular smooth muscle responds to stimuli that elicit vasorelaxation via specific intracellular pathways. The actions of NO and nitrosovasodilators (such as sodium nitroprusside and nitroglycerine) appear to be mediated through activation of intracellular soluble

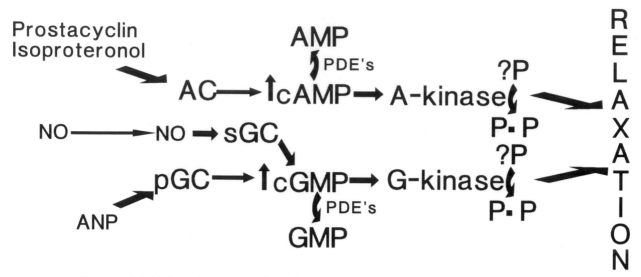

Figure 8. Multiple pathways have been implicated in modulating vascular smooth muscle relaxation. Prostacyclin and isoproteronol activate adenylate cyclase leading to the generation of **cAMP**. cAMP activates cAMP-dependent protein kinase (**A-kinase**). Nitric oxide (**NO**) diffuses across the plasma membrane and activates soluble guanylate cyclase in the cytoplasm leading to the generation of **cGMP**. Atrial natriuretic peptides (**ANP**) interact with cell surface receptors and activate an immunologically distinct guanylate cyclase (**pGC**) which also leads to the generation of cGMP. cGMP activates cGMP-dependent protein kinase (**G-kinase**). While multiple substrates have been described for A-kinase and G-kinase, the physiologically relevant late phase signalling events that modulate vascular smooth muscle relaxation remain incompletely understood.

guanylate cyclase and the production of guanosine 3',5'-cyclic monophosphate (cGMP) (Figure 8).[57] In addition, a family of low-molecular-weight, heat stable peptides, ANP, affect smooth muscle relaxation through receptor-mediated activation of an immunologically distinct, particulate guanylate cyclase with production of cGMP.[58]

Activation of a second pathway, the adenylate cyclase/cAMP pathway, also leads to vascular smooth muscle relaxation. Prostacyclin and β-adrenergic agonists activate adenylate cyclase through a receptor-mediated, GTP-binding protein mechanism, resulting in an increase in cAMP concentrations.[59] Forskolin, which directly activates adenylate cyclase, causes relaxation of smooth muscle from many sources including dog, bovine, and guinea pig coronary arteries, rat aorta, porcine brain arteries, and bovine renal and carotid arteries.[60]

Vasorelaxation can also be induced by agents which raise cyclic nucleotide concentrations via inhibition of phosphodiesterases (PDE), enzymes which catalyze the hydrolysis of cAMP and cGMP. At least four major types of PDEs exist in mammalian tissues. In vascular smooth muscle, the major PDEs are type I (Ca^{2+}-calmodulin regulated enzyme) and type IV (high affinity for cAMP).[61] Exogenous phosphodiesterase inhibitors (i.e., papaverine, 1-isobutyl-3 methylxan-

thine—IBMX), inhibit PDEs resulting in increases in intracellular cyclic nucleotide concentrations.

The specific mechanisms by which cyclic nucleotides induce smooth muscle relaxation are not completely understood. cAMP modulates many intracellular signalling processes through activation of cAMP-dependent protein kinase (A-kinase). Most tissues contain two forms of A-kinase designated types I and II based on their order of elution from DEAE-cellulose. Both types exist as an inactive holoenzyme composed of a regulatory subunit dimer and two monomeric catalytic subunits. The enzyme is activated by the binding of cAMP to the regulatory subunit and release of the free catalytic subunit. The different properties of type I and type II A-kinase are dependent on their distinct regulatory subunits.

The specific substrate proteins that A-kinase phosphorylates to initiate a physiologic relaxation response are not well characterized.[62] MLCK is phosphorylated in smooth muscle by A-kinase.[63] It has been proposed that this phosphorylation decreases the affinity of MLCK for the Ca^{2+}-calmodulin complex and hence induces vasorelaxation. Takuwa and Rasmussen, using bovine carotid artery smooth muscle, have demonstrated that forskolin stimulation results in changes in phosphorylation of other intracellular proteins.[27] In particular, an increase in the phosphorylation of two 20 kDa phosphoproteins (designated #3 and #8) occurs after forskolin treatment. We have recently shown that sodium nitroprusside treatment also increases the phosphorylation of phosphoproteins #3 and #8.[12] Potential candidates for these phosphoproteins include small GTP-binding proteins, phospholamban aggregates, phospholemman, or other uncharacterized regulatory proteins.

Although it is clear that activation of cyclic nucleotide-dependent protein kinases leads to vascular smooth muscle relaxation, further work is needed to define more clearly the mechanisms whereby these kinases modulate subsequent cellular processes leading to vasorelaxation. While a number of substrate proteins for cyclic nucleotide-dependent protein kinases have been described in vascular smooth muscle, the particular proteins that participate in physiologic vasorelaxation, and the specific biochemical events that lead to vasorelaxation, have not been well characterized. In addition, several lines of evidence suggest that cAMP may induce vasorelaxation via activation of cGMP-dependent protein kinase rather than cAMP-dependent protein kinase.[64,65,66]

An important effector for transducing cGMP signals into biologic responses is cGMP-dependent protein kinase or G-kinase.[57,67] G-kinase is a dimer of 80 kDa subunits with 2 cGMP binding sites per subunit. These sites exhibit cooperative binding.[67,68,69] Two isoforms of G-kinase have been identified and characterized.[70] While A-kinase is a ubiquitous enzyme found in most cells, high concentrations of G-kinase have been found only in vascular smooth muscle, cerebellar purkinje fibers, mesangial cells, and platelets.[67] The presence of high concentrations of G-kinase in vascular smooth muscle suggests an important physiologic role for this kinase in vascular smooth muscle.

The mechanisms through which G-kinase affects vascular smooth muscle relaxation are not well understood. While three in vitro substrates of G-kinase have been identified in rabbit aorta (M_r 240000, 130000, and 85000),[71] a physiologic role for these phosphoproteins has not yet been established. G-kinase phosphorylates itself as well as regulatory subunits of A-kinase.[72] We have recently found that activation of G-kinase with sodium nitroprusside in intact BCASM results in an increase in phosphorylation of the same 20 kDa phosphoproteins (#3 and #8) as seen after forskolin treatment.[12] Studies in intact platelets have identified a 50 kDa substrate for G-kinase.[73] Other putative substrates for G-kinase include the plasma membrane Ca^{2+} pump,[74] intermediate regulatory proteins such as phospholamban,[75] small GTP-binding proteins,[76] and cytoskeletal elements.[77]

Thus, the specific agonists which incite vasorelaxation and the early signalling responses of the smooth muscle have been well characterized. However, the late signalling events which modulate vascular smooth muscle relaxation remain to be elucidated. In addition, interactions between signalling pathways which modulate vasocontraction and pathways which modulate vasorelaxation have not been carefully examined. Significant investigative effort has recently focused on the endothelial-derived vasorelaxants, NO and prostacyclin.

Nitric Oxide

A diffusible substance released by the endothelium capable of inducing smooth muscle relaxation, EDRF was first described in 1980.[1] EDRF was subsequently identified as NO.[2] However, while several investigators have demonstrated a similarity between the diverse actions of NO and EDRF in vivo and in vitro, EDRF and NO are not identical. EDRF is more potent than NO and has a longer duration of action as a vasodilator.[78] EDRF cannot be evaporated from an aqueous medium, whereas NO is a volatile gas. EDRF is not as effective as NO in the relaxation of nonvascular smooth muscle cells.[79] Investigators have recently suggested that EDRF is a nitrosyl-non-heme-iron complex with thiol groups.[80]

NO is one of the most ubiquitous messenger molecules in mammals. Prior to the discovery of NO, only complex molecules were thought to regulate physiologic function. Currently, all mammals studied have been shown to utilize NO in the regulation of several biologic functions. Interestingly, NO exerts its biologic effect by diffusing across the plasma membrane instead of interacting with membrane receptors. Thus, NO represents a ubiquitous, simple, and ancient autocrine messenger. Medications that mimic the action of NO on the vascular system have been part of the armamentarium of physicians for more than 100 years. For example, the salutary effect of amyl nitrite on angina pectoris was first described by Bruton in 1863. It is now well recognized that the nitrovasodilators exact their effect by donating NO at their site of action.[81]

NO is a small, simple, paramagnetic molecule that reacts with iron-containing compounds to form paramagnetic iron-nitrosyl complexes. NO may exist in one of three redox forms, nitrosonium cation (NO^+), nitric oxide ($NO^·$), and nitrosyl anion ($NO^{·-}$), depending on the number of electrons in the 2p antibonding electron orbital. Thus, NO can exist as a reactive free radical and all three redox forms may play important roles in biologic processes.

Some of the actions of NO depend on reactions with transition metals such as those found in metalloproteins. The most widely studied NO interacting metalloproteins are the heme-containing proteins, guanylate cyclase and hemoglobin. The affinity of

Fe(II) for NO is several magnitudes greater than that of O_2. NO binds effectively to both Fe(II) heme and Fe(III) heme while O_2 and CO primarily bind to Fe(II). Upon binding, NO converts Fe(III) heme to Fe(II) heme. NO also reacts with non-heme transition metals such as the iron sulphur center of several proteins and complexes I and II of the mitochondrial electron transport chain. The formation of iron-nitrosyl complexes and the subsequent destruction of iron-sulphur centers may be responsible for some of the cytotoxic effects of NO.

NO reacts with oxygen to produce nitrate and nitrite ions very rapidly and thus has a very short biological half-life (2 to 5 seconds). NO produced in vivo circulates in plasma as S-nitrosoalbumin which has a relatively long half-life. S-nitrosoalbumin may be the circulating form or reservoir of endogenous NO.[82]

Interactions between NO and other free radicals may have significant biologic effects. Peroxynitrite anion (ONOO-), a product of NO and O^{2-}, is extremely reactive and vigorously oxidizes protein and nonprotein sulfhydryl groups.[83] This leads to a loss of free radical scavenging molecules such as cysteine and glutathione. In addition, oxidation leads to a diminished activity of sulfhydryl-containing proteins. O^{2-} and NO are by-products of metabolic reactions in EC, hence O^{2-} may contribute significantly to the cellular damage seen in conditions in which O^{2-} is increased, such as in hyperoxia, ischemia-reperfusion, and inflammation.

The first evidence for a mammalian metabolic pathway for nitrogen oxides was described in 1916.[84] It was determined that mammalian urine contained more nitrates than could be attributed to the intake of nitrate in the diet. It was not until 1981, however, that Green et al demonstrated conclusively that nitrogen oxides are metabolic by-products of nitrogen metabolism in mammals.[85]

In all cell types studied, NO is believed to be produced by NO synthase (NOS) from the terminal guanidino moiety of L-arginine.[86] The first step in the synthesis of NO is the mono-oxygenation of L-arginine to Nw-hydroxy-L-arginine.[87] The reaction is a five electron oxidation with N^G-hydroxy-L-arginine as a possible intermediate. Molecular oxygen is required for the reaction and L-citrulline is a by-product. The enzyme requires FAD, FMN, and tetrahydrobiopterin as cofactors, and NADPH is a cosubstrate. This reaction is stereospecific and the D isomer of arginine is not a substrate for the enzyme. NOS can be competitively inhibited by Nw-substituted L-arginine analogs.

NOS exists as multiple isotypes. The most widely accepted classification groups the enzymes into two major isotypes, a constitutive (cNOS) and an inducible (iNOS) form. The enzyme present in unstimulated endothelial cells is referred to as the constitutive enzyme, while the enzyme stimulated by lipopolysaccharide (LPS) is referred to as the inducible form. However, this classification does not accurately describe the biology of the NO syntheses. It has recently been shown that cNOS can be induced by the mechanical forces of shear stress and cyclic strain.[88] EC cNOS activity is dependent on calcium and the calcium-binding protein, calmodulin.

A number of agonists are known to activate endothelial cell cNOS including vasodilators such as histamine, bradykinin, adenosine, acetylcholine, leukotriene, and the calcium ionophore A23187. Intracellular arginine levels have not been shown to be important in the regulation of cNOS under physiologic conditions, and it appears endothelial cells can generate l-arginine from l-citrulline. However, the systemic administration of L-arginine magnifies hypotensive responses to acetylcholine, suggesting that extracellular sources of arginine may be important for the production of NO.

The activity of cNOS may be regulated by phosphorylation. It has been demonstrated that PKC, cAMP-dependent protein kinase, and calcium/calmodulin-dependent protein kinase can phosphorylate cNOS.[89] The PKC-directed phosphorylation is associated with a reduction in enzyme activity.[89] However, enzymatic activity is preserved after the phosphorylation of cNOS by cAMP-dependent protein kinase.

The human endothelial cNOS is encoded by a gene on chromosome 7. It contains 26 exons over 21 kilobases of DNA. The 5' flanking promoter region is "TATA-less" but contains a GATA and two Sp1 binding sites. The functional significance of these transcription factor binding sites has not yet been determined. The 5' flanking region also contains potential AP-1, AP-2, NF-1, acute phase response element, heavy metal, and sterol responsive element binding sites. In addition, both the bovine and human EC cNOS have been purified and the gene cloned.[88] The deduced molecular weight is 135 kDa, identical to the molecular weight of the native enzyme. EC cNOS is myristylated at the N-terminal and this regulates the localization of NOS to the particulate or membrane fraction of the cell.

iNOS was first described in inflammatory cells such as macrophages, neutrophils, and hepatocytes. iNOS has also been described in endothelial cells, vascular smooth muscle cells, fibroblasts, mesangial cells, and astrocytes. The gene for the rat macrophage and vascular smooth muscle cell iNOS has been cloned.[90] The mouse macrophage iNOS has been the most extensively studied enzyme and is cytosolic in location, has a Km of 3 μM, a molecular weight of about 130 kDa and has an activity of 1313 nmol of NO/min/mg prot. Calmodulin binds tightly and irreversibly to the macrophage iNOS and they readily copurify.[91] This association of calmodulin with iNOS might explain the calcium-independence of the enzyme.

iNOS is usually absent in target cells under basal conditions, but an appropriate stimulus such as bacterial lipopolysaccharide or tumor necrosis factor (TNF) induces the production of the enzyme.[92] The enzyme activity appears about 4 hours after exposure to the stimulus. Once expressed, the activity of iNOS is stable for hours. Induction of iNOS is inhibited by dexamethasone and other steroidal anti-inflammatory agents. This observation may explain the beneficial effects of glucocorticoid administration prior to the onset of shock and the apparent lack of an effect once the hypotension is manifested.

There is a tonic, basal level of NO production which is important for maintaining vasodilator tone in blood vessels. Infusion of inhibitors of NO synthesis abolishes this basal vasodilator tone leading to hypertension in experimental animals and human subjects. Decreased endothelial-mediated vasodilation has been demonstrated in hypertensive experimental animals and human hypertensive patients.[93] The finding that acetylcholine-induced vasodilation is impaired in normotensive subjects with a familial history of hypertension suggests that endothelial dysfunction may precede the development of hypertension.

In addition to its vasorelaxing properties, NO inhibits platelet aggregation and adhesion.[94,95] NO modulates leukocyte adhesion and migration.[96] Inactivation of NO by superoxide generated in acute inflammation may enhance sequestration of leukocytes.

Decreased NO production by an injured endothelium has been implicated in the pathogenesis of atherosclerosis. The interaction between reduced NO production as a consequence of endothelial dysfunction and inhibition of NO by oxidized low density lipoprotein (LDL) may be additive in atherosclerosis. Oxidized LDL has been shown to inhibit the actions of NO.[97] Animal models fed an atherogenic diet develop a substantial reduction in NO-mediated vasodilation in response to acetylcholine which is reversible by feeding a lipid reducing diet.[98] NO and nitrovasodilators inhibit smooth muscle proliferation.[10] NO depresses ^{3}H-thymidine incorporation, a measure of DNA synthesis, and inhibits the stimulation of DNA synthesis by 10% fetal calf serum and endothelin in smooth muscle cells.[99]

The NO pathway has been implicated in the regulation of renal arterial tone, renal plasma flow, renal cortical flow, renal medullary flow, papillary blood flow, electrolyte excretion, and the prevention of medullary hypoxic injury. Infusion of L-arginine, the NO precursor, in human subjects produces a diuresis and natriuresis as well as an increase in the urinary excretion of nitrite and nitrates.[100]

NO may be important in the development of diabetes mellitus. NO participates in the cytotoxicity of activated macrophages toward pancreatic islet cells.[101] Inhibition of NO production by L-monomethyl-arginine (L-NMMA) attenuates the development of diabetes in streptozocin-treated mice. The advanced glycosylation end products (AGES) produced in diabetics may quench NO.[102]

NO has also been implicated in the pathogenesis of the hypotension associated with liver cirrhosis. The administration of L-NMMA leads to a significant increase in systemic and portal pressures in cirrhotic animals.[103] It has been postulated that bacterial endotoxin from the gut bypasses the liver through porto-systemic shunts and enters the systemic vasculature and induces NO synthesis.

In summary, it appears that there is a basal secretion of NO, which maintains a state of basal vasodilation. Inhibition of NO production with L-arginine analogs such as L-NMMA is associated with an increase in peripheral resistance, decreased tissue perfusion and oxygen delivery, and an increase in blood pressure. It has also been postulated that impairment of NO production as a sequela of endothelial dysfunction contributes to an increase in platelet aggregation and platelet adhesion. This constellation of effects may have profound implications in the pathogenesis of atherosclerosis.

Summary and Conclusions

Blood vessels modulate the flow of intravascular contents via elaborate and intricate mechanisms. Intraluminal or blood-borne substances modulate vasomotor tone via vasoactive endocrine substances. Blood elements, such as platelets and white blood cells, are capable of releasing a variety of vasoactive substances. The vasomotor response of the vascular smooth muscle to these factors depends on whether an intact endoluminal endothelial layer is present or absent. When present, the endothelium responds to blood-borne substances and can subsequently influence vascular smooth muscle contractility by the production of paracrine mediators such as NO. If the endothelium is absent, the direct effect of many blood-borne hormones on the vascular smooth muscle is vasocontraction.

Most substances which induce functional vasoconstriction are mitogenic and theoretically could be involved in the production of structural narrowing of blood vessels as occurs in atherosclerosis. The converse is also true, in that substances which induce vasorelaxation are antimitogenic and may prevent fixed athero-obliterative lesions.

While no good ex vivo model of vasospasm currently exists, it is likely that vasospasm represents a state inherent to the vascular smooth muscle. An understanding of the molecular mechanisms of vasocontraction and vasorelaxation, as well as interactions between pathways that modulate vasomotor tone, will likely lead to a better understanding of mechanisms important to a variety of pathologic states, including vasospasm and atherogenesis.

References

1. Furchgott RF, Zawadzki JW: The obligatory role of endothelial cells in the relaxation of smooth muscle cells by acetylcholine. *Nature* 288:373, 1980.
2. Palmer RMJ, Ferrige AG, Moncada S: Nitric oxide release accounts for the biological activity of endothelium derived relaxing factor. *Nature* 327:524, 1987.
3. Mok L, Nickols G, Thompson JC, Cooper C: Parathyroid hormone as a smooth muscle relaxant. *Endocrine Rev* 10:420, 1989.
4. Steele JA, Stockbridge N, Maljovic G, Weir B: Free radicals mediate actions of oxyhemoglobin on cerebrovascular smooth muscle cells. *Circ Res* 68:416, 1991.
5. Blaes N, Boissel J: Growth stimulating effect of catecholamines on rat aortic smooth muscle cells in culture. *J Cell Phys* 116:16, 1983.
6. Bobik A, Grooms A, Millar JA, et al: Growth factor activity of endothelin on vascular smooth muscle. *Am J Physiol* 258:408, 1990.
7. Nemecek G, Coughlin S, Handley D: Stimulation of aortic smooth muscle cell mitogenesis by serotonin. *Proc Natl Acad Sci* 83:674, 1986.
8. Berk BC, Alexander RW, Brock TA, et al: Vasoconstriction: a new activity for platelet-derived growth factor. *Science* 232:78, 1986.
9. Berk BC, Brock TA, Webb RC, et al: Epidermal growth factor, vascular smooth muscle mitogen, induces rat aortic contraction. *Clin Invest* 75:1083, 1985.
10. Garg UC, Hassid A: Nitric oxide-generating vasodilators and 8-bromo-cGMP inhibit mitogenesis and proliferation of cultured rat vascular smooth muscle cells. *J Clin Invest* 83:1774, 1989.
11. Ganz P, Alexander W: New insights into the cellular mechanisms of vasospasm. *Am J Cardiol* 56:11E, 1985.
12. Berg C, Brophy CM, Dransfield D, Lincoln TM, Goldenring J, Rasmussen H: Impaired cyclic nucleotide-dependent relaxation in human umbilical artery smooth muscle. *Am J Physiol* 268:H202, 1995.
13. Brophy CM: Gastrointestinal vascular and ischemic syndromes. *Current Opinion in General Surgery* 224, 1993.
14. Komori K, Schini VB, Gloviczki P, et al: The impairment of endothelium-dependent relaxations in reversed vein grafts is associated with a reduced production of cyclic guanosine monophosphate. *J Vasc Surg* 14:67, 1991.
15. Maseri A: Variant angina: one aspect of a continuous spectrum of vasospastic myocardial ischemia. *Am J Cardiol* 42:1019, 1078.
16. Ginsberg R, Bristow MR, Davis K, et al: Quantitative pharmacologic responses of normal and atherosclerotic isolated human epicardial coronary arteries. *Circulation* 69:430, 1984.
17. Yamamoto Y, Tomoike H, Egashira K, et al: Attenuation of endothelium-related relaxation and enhanced responsiveness of vascular smooth muscle to histamine in spastic coronary arterial segments from miniature pigs. *Circ Res* 61:772, 1987.
18. Kawachi Y, Tomoike H, Maruoka Y, et al: Selective hypercontraction to ergonovine of the canine coronary artery under conditions of induced atherosclerosis. *Circulation* 69:441, 1984.
19. Heistad DD, Armstrong ML, Marcus ML, et al: Augmented responses to vasoconstrictor stimuli in hypercholesterolemic and atherosclerotic monkeys. *Circ Res* 54:711, 1984.
20. Yokoyama M, Akita H, Mizutani T, et al: Hyperreactivity of coronary arterial smooth muscles in response to ergonovine from rabbits with hereditary hyperlipidemia. *Circ Res* 53:63, 1983.
21. Bjoro K, Pedersen SS: In vitro perfusion studies on human umbilical arteries. *Acta Obstet Gynecol Scand* 65:351, 1986.
22. Ligush J, Labadie RF, Bercell SA, et al: Evaluation of endothelium-derived NO-mediated vasodilation utilizing ex vivo perfusion of an intact vessel. *J Surg Res* 52:416, 1992.
23. Varsos VG, Liszczak TM, Han DH, et al: Delayed cerebral vasospasm is not reversible by aminophylline, nifedipine, or papaverine in a "two-hemorrhage" canine model. *J Neurosurg* 58:11, 1983.
24. Collins EM, Walsh MP, Morgan KG: Contraction of single vascular smooth muscle cells by phenylephrine. *Am J Physiol* 262:H754, 1992.
25. Hathaway DR, March KL, Lash JA, et al: Vascular smooth muscle, a review of the molecular basis of contractility. *Circulation* 83:382, 1991.
26. Takuwa Y, Takuwa N, Rasmussen H: Measurement of cytoplasmic free Ca^{2+} concentration in bovine tracheal smooth muscle using aequorin. *Am J Physiol* 253:C817, 1987.
27. Takuwa Y, Kelley G, Takuwa N, et al: Protein phosphorylation changes in bovine carotid artery smooth muscle during contraction and relaxation. *Mol Cell Endo* 60:71, 1988.
28. Rasmussen H, Takuwa Y, Park S: Protein kinase C in the regulation of smooth muscle contraction. *FASEB J* 1:177, 1987.
29. Hai CM, Murphy RA: Crossbridge phosphorylation and regulation of the latch state in smooth muscle. *Am J Physiol* 254:C99, 1989.
30. Haller H, Smallwood JI, Rasmussen H: Protein kinase C translocation in intact vascular smooth muscle strips. *Biochem J* 270:375, 1990.
31. Katsuyama H, Wang CL, Morgan KG: Regulation of vascular smooth muscle tone by caldesmon. *J Biol Chem* 267:14555, 1992.
32. Minami N, Tani E, Maeda Y, Yamaura I, Fukami M: Effects of inhibitors of protein kinase C and calpain in experimental delayed cerebral vasospasm. *J Neurosurg* 76:111–118, 1992.
33. Yanigisawa M, Kurihara H, Kimura S, et al: A novel potent vasoconstrictor peptide produced by vascular endothelial cells. *Nature* 332:411, 1988.
34. Hirata Y, Yoshimi H, Takaichi S, Yanagisawa M, Masaki T: Binding and receptor down-regulation of a novel vasoconstrictor endothelin in cultured rat vascular smooth muscle cells. *FEBS Lett* 2391:13, 1988.
35. Inoue A, Yanagisawa M, Takuwa Y, Mitsui Y, Kobayashi M, Masaki T: The human preproendothelin-1 gene: complete nucleotide sequence and regulation of expression. *J Biol Chem* 26425:14954, 1989.
36. Benatti L, Bonecchi L, Cozzi L, Sarmientos P: Two

preproendothelin-1 mRNAs transcribed by alternative promoters. *J Clin Invest* 913:1149, 1993.

37. Yanagisawa M, Inoue A, Takuwa Y, Mitsui Y, Kobayashi M, Masaki T: The human preproendothelin-1 gene: possible regulation by endothelial phosphoinositide turnover signaling. *J Cardiovasc Pharm* (13 suppl)5:S13-S17, 1989.

38. Weitzberg E, Lundberg JM, Rudehill A: Elevated plasma levels of endothelin in patients with sepsis syndrome. *Circ Shock* 334:222, 1991.

39. Imai T, Hirata Y, Emori T, Marumo F: Heparin has an inhibitory effect on endothelin-1 synthesis and release by endothelial cells. *Hypertension* 213:353, 1993.

40. Boulanger CM, Luscher TF: Hirudin and nitrates inhibit the thrombin-induced release of endothelin from the intact porcine aorta. *Circ Res* 686:1768, 1991.

41. Boulanger C, Luscher TF: Release of endothelin from the porcine aorta: inhibition by endothelium-derived nitric oxide. *J Clin Invest* 852:587, 1990.

41A. Yoshizumi M, Kurihara H, Sugiyama T, et al: Hemodynamic shear stress stimulates endothelin production by cultured endothelial cells. *Biochem Biophys Res Comm* 1612:859, 1989.

42. Sharefkin JB, Diamond SL, Eskin SG, McIntire LV, Dieffenbach CW: Fluid flow decreases preproendothelin mRNA levels and suppresses endothelin-1 peptide release in cultured human endothelial cells. *J Vasc Surg* 141:1, 1991.

43. Sumpio BE, Widmann MD: Enhanced production of an endothelium-derived contracting factor by endothelial cells subjected to pulsatile stretch. *Surgery* 108:277, 1990.

44. Carosi JA, Eskin SG, McIntire LV: Cyclical strain effects on production of vasoactive materials in cultured endothelial cells. *J Cell Phys* 1511:29, 1992.

45. Wang DL, Tang CC, Wung BS, Chen HH, Hung MS, Wang JJ: Cyclic strain increases endothelin-1 secretion and gene expression in human endothelial cells. *Biochem Biophys Res Comm* 1952:1050, 1993.

46. Neuser D, Steinke W, Dellweg H, Kazda S, Stasch JP: 125I-endothelin-1 and 125I-big endothelin-1 in rat tissues: autoradiographic localization and receptor binding. *Histochemistry* 956:621, 1991.

47. Arai H, Hori S, Aramori I, Ohkubo H, Nakanishi S: Cloning and expression of a cDNA encoding an endothelin receptor. *Nature* 348:730, 1990.

48. Lin HY, Kaji EH, Winkel GK, Ives HE, Lodish HF: Cloning and functional expression of a vascular smooth muscle endothelin-1 receptor. *PNAS* 888:3185, 1991.

49. Hoffman A, Grossman E, Ohman KP, Marks E, Keiser HR: The initial vasodilation and the later vasoconstriction of endothelin-1 are selective to specific vascular beds. *Am J Hypertens* 310:789, 1990.

50. Makino S, Hashimoto K, Hirasawa R, Hattori T, Ota Z: Central interaction between endothelin and brain natriuretic peptide on vasopressin secretion. *J Hypertens* 101:25, 1992.

51. Goetz KL, Wang BC, Madwed JB, Zhu JL: Cardiovascular, renal, and endocrine responses to intravenous endothelin in conscious dogs. *Am J Physiol* 255:R1064, 1988.

52. Qiu S, Theroux P, Marcil M, Solymoss BC: Plasma endothelin-1 levels in stable and unstable angina. *Cardiology* 821:12, 1993.

53. Lechleitner P, Genser N, Mair J, et al: Endothelin-1 in patients with complicated and uncomplicated myocardial infarction. *Clin Investig* 7012:1070, 1992.

54. Pittet JF, Morel DR, Hemsen A, et al: Elevated plasma endothelin-1 concentrations are associated with the severity of illness in patients with sepsis. *Ann Surg* 2133:261, 1991.

55. Yokokawa K, Tahara H, Kohno M, et al: Hypertension associated with endothelin-secreting malignant hemangioendothelioma. *Ann Intern Med* 1143:213, 1991.

56. Whitney EG, Throckmorton D, Yeh J, Isales C, Rasmussen H, Brophy CM: Kinase activation and smooth muscle contraction in the presence and absence of calcium. *J Vasc Surg*. (In press.)

57. Lincoln TM: Cyclic GMP and mechanisms of vasodilatation. *Pharmac Ther* 41:479, 1989.

58. Tremblay J, Gerzer R, Vinay P, Pang SC, Beliveau R, Hamet P: The increase of cGMP by atrial naturetic factor correlates with the distribution of particulate guanylate cyclase. *FEBS Lett* 181:17, 1985.

59. Moncada S: Biological importance of prostacyclin. *Gr J Pharmacol* 76:3, 1982.

60. Seamon KB, Daly JW: Forskolin: its biological and chemical properties. *Adv Cycl Nucleotide Protein Phosphorylation Res* 20:1, 1986.

61. Silver P, Hamel L, Perrone M, et al: Differential pharmacologic sensitivity of cyclic nucleotide phosphodiesteras isozymes isolated from cardiac muscle, arterial and airway smooth muscle. *Eur J Pharm* 150:85, 1988.

62. Haynes J, Robinson J, Saunders L, et al: Role of cAMP-dependent protein kinase in cAMP-mediated vasodilation. *Am J Physiol* 262:H511, 1992.

63. DeLanerolle P, Nishikawa M, Yost DA, Adelstein RS: Increased phosphorylation of myosin light chain kinase after an increase in cAMP in intact smooth muscle. *Science* 223:1415, 1984.

64. Parks TP, Nairn AC, Greengard P, Jamieson JD: The cyclic nucleotide-dependent phosphorylation of aortic smooth muscle membrane proteins. *Arch Biochem Biophys* 255:361–371, 1987.

65. Lincoln TM, Cornwell TL: Towards an understanding of the mechanism of action of cyclic AMP and cyclic GMP in smooth muscle relaxation. *Blood Vessels* 28:129–137, 1991.

66. Jaing H, Colbran JL, Francis SH, Corbin JD: Direct evidence for cross-activation of cGMP-dependent protein kinase by cAMP in pig coronary arteries. *J Biol Chem* 267:1015–1019, 1992.

67. Walter U: Physiologic role of cGMP and cGMP-dependent protein kinase in the cardiovascular system. *Rev Physiol Biochem Pharmacol* 113:41, 1989.

68. Kuo JF, Greengard P: Cyclic nucleotide-dependent protein kinase VI: isolation and partial purification of a protein kinase activated by cGMP. *J Biol Chem* 245:2493, 1970.

69. Lincoln TM, Dills WL, Corbin JD: Purification and subunit composition of cGMP-dependent protein kinase from bovine lung. *J Biol Chem* 252:4269, 1977.

70. Lincoln T, Thompson M, Cornwell T: Purification and characterization of two forms of cGMP-dependent protein kinase from bovine aorta. *J Biol Chem* 263:17632, 1989.

71. Casnellie JE, Ives HE, Jamieson JD, Greengard P: Cyclic GMP-dependent protein phosphorylation in intact medial tissue and isolated cells from vascular smooth muscle. *J Biol Chem* 255:3770, 1980.

72. Landgraf W, Hullin R, Gobel C, Hofmann: Phosphorylation of cGMP-dependent protein kinase increases the affinity for cAMP. *Eur J Biochem* 154:113, 1986.

73. Reinhard M, Halbrugge, Scheer U, et al: The 46/50 kDa

phosphoprotein VASP purified from human platelets is a novel protein associated with actin filaments and focal contacts. *EMBP* 11:2063, 1992.

74. Furukawa K, Nakamura H: Cyclic GMP regulation of the plasma membrane (Ca^{2+}-Mg^{2+}) ATPase in vascular smooth muscle. *J Biochem* 101:287, 1987.

75. Raeymaekers L, Hofmann F, Casteels R: cGMP-dependent protein kinase phosphorylates phospholamban in isolated sarcoplasmic reticulum from cardiac and smooth muscle. *Biochem J* 252:269, 1988.

76. Miura Y, Kaibuchi K, Itoh T, et al: Phosphorylation of smg p21B/rap 1Bp21 by cGMP-dependent protein kinase. *FEBS Lett* 297:171, 1992.

77. Baltensperger K, Whiesi M, Carafoli E: Substrates of cGMP kinase in vascular smooth muscle and their role in the relaxation process. *Biochemistry* 29:9753–9760, 1990.

78. Myers PR, Minor RJ, Guerra RJ, Bates JN, Harrison DG: Vasorelaxant properties of the endothelium-derived relaxing factor more closely resemble S-nitroso-cysteine than nitric oxide. *Nature* 345:161, 1990.

79. Shikano K, Ohlstein EH, Berkowitz BA: Differential selectivity of endothelium-derived relaxing factor and nitric oxide in smooth muscle. *Br J Pharm* 923:483, 1987.

80. Vanin AF: Endothelium-derived relaxing factor is a nitrosyl iron complex with thiol ligands. *FEBS Lett* 289:1, 1991.

81. Marks GS, Mclaughlin BE, Nakatsu K, Brien JF: Direct evidence for nitric oxide formation from glyceryl trinitrate during incubation with intact bovine pulmonary artery. *Can J Phys Pharm* 70:308, 1992.

82. Stamler JS, Jaraki O, Osborne J, et al: Nitric oxide circulates in mammalian plasma primarily as an S-nitroso adduct of serum albumin. *PNAS* 8916:7674, 1992.

83. Radi R, Beckman JS, Bush KM, Freeman BA: Peroxynitrite oxidation of sulfhydryls: the cytotoxic potential of superoxide and nitric oxide. *J Biol Chem* 2667:4244, 1991.

84. Mitchell HH, Schonle HA, Grindly HS: The origin of the nitrates in the urine. *J Biol Chem* 24:461, 1916.

85. Green LC, Tannenbaum SR, Goldman P: Nitrate synthesis and reduction in the germ-free and conventional rat. *Science* 212:56, 1981.

86. Palmer RM, Rees DD, Ashton DS, Moncada S: L-arginine is the physiological precursor for the formation of nitric oxide in endothelium-dependent relaxation. *Biochem Biophys Res Comm* 1533:1251, 1988.

87. Stuehr DJ, Kwon NS, Nathan CF, Griffith OW, Feldman PL, Wiseman J: N-omega-hydroxy-L-arginine is an intermediate in the biosynthesis of nitric oxide from L-arginine. *J Biol Chem* 26610:6259, 1991.

88. Nishida K, Harrison DG, Navas JP, et al: Molecular cloning and characterization of the constitutive bovine endothelial cell nitric oxide synthase. *J Clin Invest* 90:2092, 1992.

89. Bredt DS, Ferris CD, Snyder SH: Nitric oxide synthase regulatory sites. *J Biol Chem* 2675:10976, 1992.

90. Lyons CR, Orloff GJ, Cunningham JM: Molecular cloning and functional expression of an inducible nitric oxide synthase from a murine macrophage cell line. *J Biol Chem* 2679:6370, 1992.

91. Cho HJ, Xie QW, Calaycay J, et al: Calmodulin is a subunit of nitric oxide synthase from macrophages. *J Experiment Med* 1762:599, 1992.

92. Lamas S, Michel T, Collins T, Brenner BM, Marsden PA: Effects of interferon-gamma on nitric oxide synthase activity and endothelin-1 production by vascular endothelial cells. *J Clin Invest* 903:879, 1992.

93. Calver A, Collier J, Moncada S, Vallance P: Effect of local intra-arterial NG-monomethyl-L-arginine in patients with hypertension: the nitric oxide dilator mechanism appears abnormal. *J Hypertension* 109:1025, 1992.

94. Radomski MW, Palmer RM, Moncada S: The role of nitric oxide and cGMP in platelet adhesion to vascular endothelium. *Biochem Biophys Res Comm* 1483:1482, 1987.

95. Radomski MW, Palmer RM, Moncada S: The anti-aggregating properties of vascular endothelium: interactions between prostacyclin and nitric oxide. *Br J Pharm* 923:639, 1987.

96. Kubes P, Suzuki M, Granger DN: Nitric oxide: an endogenous modulator of leukocyte adhesion. *PNAS* 8811:4651, 1991.

97. Chin JH, Azhar S, Hoffman BB: Inactivation of endothelial-derived relaxing factor by oxidized lipoproteins. *J Clin Invest* 891:10, 1992.

98. Harrison DG, Armstrong ML, Freiman PC, Heistad DD: Restoration of endothelium-dependent relaxation by dietary treatment of atherosclerosis. *J Clin Invest* 806:1808, 1987.

99. Nakaki T, Nakayama M, Kato R: Inhibition by nitric oxide and nitric oxide-producing vasodilators of DNA synthesis in vascular smooth muscle cells. *Eur J Pharm* 1896:347, 1990.

100. Kanno K, Hirata Y, Emori T, et al: L-arginine infusion induces hypotension and diuresis/natriuresis with concomitant increased urinary excretion of nitrite/nitrate and cyclic GMP in humans. *Clin Exp Pharm Physiol* 199:619, 1992.

101. Kroncke KD, Kolb BV, Berschick B, Burkart V, Kolb H: Activated macrophages kill pancreatic syngeneic islet cells via arginine-dependent nitric oxide generation. *Biochem Biophys Res Comm* 1753:752, 1991.

102. Bucala R, Tracey KJ, Cerami A: Advanced glycosylation products quench nitric oxide and mediate defective endothelium-dependent vasodilatation in experimental diabetes. *J Clin Invest* 872:432, 1991.

103. Pizcueta P, Pique JM, Fernandez M, et al: Modulation of the hyperdynamic circulation of cirrhotic rats by nitric oxide inhibition. *J Gastroenterol* 1036:1909, 1992.

CHAPTER 14

Venous System of the Lower Extremities:
Physiology and Pathophysiology

James O. Menzoian, MD; Elias J. Arbid, MD
Tania J. Phillips, MD; Jag Bhawan, MD
Wayne W. LaMorte, MD, PhD, MPH

Disorders of the venous system of the legs are common, but current treatment and preventive measures have limited effectiveness. As a result, patients all too frequently are forced to learn to live with these chronic recurrent problems. Our shortcomings in dealing with venous disease in the lower extremities reflect significant gaps in our knowledge of the pathophysiology of these disorders and underscore the importance of developing an understanding of the basic science of venous disease.

The view that the veins of the lower extremities are simply conduits through which blood returns to the heart is clearly an oversimplification. Even for this seemingly simple task, the upright posture that our species has adopted poses a significant hemodynamic problem. The solution which has evolved relies on the integrity of certain structural features (patency of the veins and normal function of the vein valves) and normal function of the musculoskeletal system (providing an adequately functioning calf muscle pump). When venous disease is present, one can usually find abnormalities in both structure and function, but it is not always clear whether these are causes or effects.

It is also increasingly clear that the cellular elements of blood frequently play an important role in these venous disorders. There is substantial evidence to indicate a dynamic interaction between the cellular and noncellular elements of blood, and the endothe-

lium of arteries and veins. Venous thrombosis is initiated by platelet adherence to the endothelium and subsequent activation and release of mediators. Other evidence suggests that monocyte entrapment and activation play an important role in the pathogenesis of lipodermatosclerosis and venous ulceration. These observations provide compelling reasons for studying the venous system of the lower extremities from a basic science perspective which simultaneously examines anatomy, hemodynamics, and cellular physiology.

Anatomy

The veins in the lower extremities consist of a superficial and a deep system that are connected by a communicating system of veins. The muscular plexus of veins constitutes a fourth component of the lower extremities' venous system.

The Superficial System of Veins

The venous system begins at the cutaneous microcirculation where it can be differentiated from the arterial system by the ultrastructure of its walls. A parallel network of arterioles and venules is present in the papillary dermis, from which capillary loops arise and connect to the postcapillary vessels in the deeper layers

From *The Basic Science of Vascular Disease*. Edited by Sidawy AN, Sumpio BE, and DePalma RG. Armonk, NY: Futura Publishing Company, Inc.; © 1997.

of the dermis and fat. Venules in the deep layer of the skin drain into the small veins of the foot and are the first vessels in which valves can be identified.[1] Digital veins drain individual toes to join the larger internal and external marginal veins on either side of the foot. A dorsal venous arch forms between the intermetatarsal and marginal veins. On the plantar aspect, a plexus of veins known as the "rete venosum plantare" drains the toes and skin and empties into the marginal veins.

In the leg, the superficial venous system consists of a large number of cutaneous and subcutaneous veins which drain into two main superficial veins. These veins run between the skin and deep fascia embedded in subcutaneous fat and are known as the saphenous veins. The *greater saphenous vein*, from the word "saphena" meaning "hidden,"[2] originates from the dorsal arch and medial marginal veins of the foot (Figure 1). It is quite superficial and can be easily palpated in adults 1 to 2 cm in front of the medial malleolus. The vein then curves medially and ascends in the leg 2 cm from the edge of the tibia accompanied by the saphenous nerve. It crosses the knee in a more superficial plane and continues in a straight course to enter the femoral canal at the fossa ovalis, 2 to 4 cm lateral to and 1 to 2 cm below the tubercle of the symphysis pubis. In the leg, it receives two main branches which join it below the knee, and in the distal thigh it has three main tributaries. Duplication of the greater saphenous vein is reported to occur in 10% to 37% of the population, with the two limbs often joining in the thigh within 10 cm

of the knee joint. Less commonly, a complete double system or a triple trunk may be encountered.[2,3,4] As the vein approaches the fossa ovalis, it receives 4 to 6 branches which can be quite variable, although the three most proximal ones are fairly constant (Figure 1). All of these branches have the potential for varicose formation.[2,3] Occasionally, the greater saphenous vein will not join the femoral vein but will continue beyond it, crossing the inguinal ligament to terminate in a cutaneous vein.[2]

The *lesser saphenous vein* originates from the lateral marginal vein and runs between the lateral malleolus and the Achilles tendon (Figure 1). It ascends in the leg in the subcutaneous tissues and enters the deep fascia at varying levels in the leg; its most distal portion is subcutaneous and subject to varicose formation. It travels in close proximity to the sural nerve, and enters the popliteal vein between the two heads of the gastrocnemius muscle, usually 3 cm above the popliteal space.[2,5] The lesser saphenous vein may join the superficial femoral vein in the thigh, or it may communicate with the greater saphenous vein, ending in mid-thigh or at the level of the knee.[6,7] A true duplication of the lesser saphenous vein is rarely reported, the more common variant being a low junction with the gastrocnemius vein giving the appearance of a double system.[2]

The Deep System of Veins

The deep system starts with the intermetatarsal veins which unite in the foot to form the deep plantar arch. Three separate veins emerge from the arch. The *anterior tibial vein* arises from the dorsal arch and runs medial to the hallicus longus extensor to enter the leg under the extensor retinaculum. The *posterior tibial vein* is formed by the junction of the medial and lateral plantar veins; it crosses the ankle inferior to the medial malleolus. The *peroneal vein* forms at the level of the lateral malleolus from the junction of the anterior and posterior lateral malleolar branches of the tibial veins. The deep veins of the foot communicate with the superficial veins through interdigital and interosseus branches as well as lateral and medial connecting branches.

The deep veins of the leg emerge from the foot as two or three vena commitantes with various ramifications embracing the arteries bearing the same name. They fuse proximally into single trunks which unite at different levels; a common tibioperoneal trunk is joined by the anterior tibial vein to form the *popliteal vein* which ascends behind the knee usually as a single vein. A double system draining into either one or two femoral veins, or even a triple popliteal vein may be encountered.[2] In the thigh, the popliteal vein becomes the *superficial femoral vein* at the adductor canal and travels

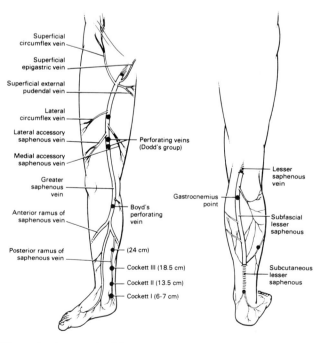

Figure 1. Anatomy of the venous system and location of perforators in the lower extremity.

Superficial circumflex vein
Superficial epigastric vein
Superficial external pudendal vein
Lateral circumflex vein
Lateral accessory saphenous vein
Medial accessory saphenous vein
Greater saphenous vein
Anterior ramus of saphenous vein
Posterior ramus of saphenous vein

Perforating veins (Dodd's group)

Boyd's perforating vein

(24 cm)
Cockett III (18.5 cm)
Cockett II (13.5 cm)
Cockett I (6-7 cm)

Lesser saphenous vein
Gastrocnemius point
Subfascial lesser saphenous
Subcutaneous lesser saphenous

posterior to the artery, commonly as a double system.[2,4,8] It is joined, 8 to 9 cm below the inguinal ligament, by the *deep femoral or profunda vein* which drains the muscles of the thigh. They form the *common femoral vein* which travels in the femoral sheath medial to the artery. As it crosses the ligament, the femoral vein becomes the *external iliac vein* and receives many branches from the deep iliac circumflex, the epigastric and the obturator veins. The *internal iliac vein* joins it after it receives a large number of tributaries from the internal pudendal, the uterine, the vesical, and the rectal plexuses of veins. Together they form the *common iliac vein* which joins its counterpart from the other side to form the inferior vena cava to the right of the midline. The left common iliac vein is, therefore, longer, and is compressed against the fifth lumbar vertebra by the right iliac artery. As a result of that compression, up to 20% of left iliac veins have been shown to have adhesive bands and spurs which may contribute to the higher incidence of thrombosis on the left side.[2,3]

The Perforating Veins

The perforating veins provide communications between the deep and superficial systems in the leg. Some connect the superficial veins directly with the posterior tibial vein on the medial aspect of the leg; others are indirect perforators connecting the superficial and deep systems via muscular veins (Figure 2).[7,9,10] To reach the deep veins, perforating veins have to pierce the deep fascia of the leg; after entering the superficial fibers of the fascia, perforators run intrafascially for a short distance surrounded by a thin sheath of fatty tissue before they bend sharply inwards to reach the deep veins. During their intrafascial course, perforating veins take a horizontal or slightly upward direction.[10] This anatomic relation between perforating veins and fascia may be important for normal emptying of perforating veins into the deep system; a reversal of this upward direction has been reported in extremities with varicose veins in which the majority of perforators seem to take an obliquely downward direction.[10]

The greater saphenous vein has one perforator (Boyd's perforator) in the proximal leg about 8 to 10 cm below the knee joint that drains into the posterior tibial vein (Figure 1). Three other perforators, known as the ankle perforators of Cockett, are present in the distal leg. An upper perforator is almost always located at the mid leg level on the posterior margin of the tibia; a middle perforator occurs about 7 to 10 cm above the medial malleolus; and a lower perforator can be found at the level of the malleolus.[11] The upper two perforators are joined by a venous arcade, and when the upper perforator is large, the middle one tends to be small.

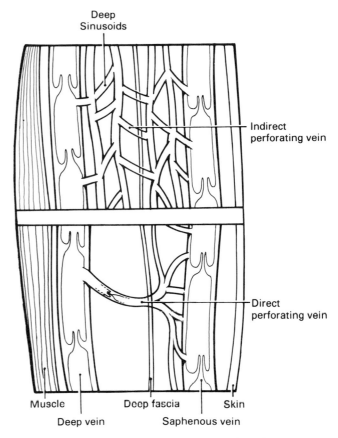

Figure 2. Direct and indirect types of perforators.

They both enter the posterior tibial vein at the same point as the soleus arcade of veins, creating a pathway through which a thrombus in the soleus vein can propagate into the perforator with the potential for valve destruction and venous insufficiency. Above the knee, two perforating veins are present between the greater saphenous and the superficial femoral veins in the distal third of the thigh; these perforators, also known as Dodd's perforators, are clinically important as they often are the first veins to become incompetent with varicose changes.[2]

In the lesser saphenous system, a constant perforator is found at the junction of the middle and lower thirds of the leg ending in the peroneal vein (Figure 1). Four indirect communicating veins of considerable size are also present between the lesser saphenous and the soleus-gastrocnemius sinusoids.[10] In addition, numerous communicating veins exist between the lesser and greater saphenous veins.[10]

Muscular Veins

The muscular veins of significance in the pathophysiology of venous insufficiency in the lower extremities are the venous plexuses of the soleus and gastrocnemius muscles. They consist of spindle-shaped intramuscular veins and venous sinusoids. An arcade of veins drains the soleus muscle and empties into the posterior tibial and peroneal veins, while the gastrocnemius veins usually drain into the popliteal vein. Soleus and gastrocnemius sinusoids are also present; they represent valveless dilatations of the venous arcades where blood pools before it is ejected by the calf muscle.

Vein Valves

Vein valves are bicuspid extensions of the intima into the lumen of the vessel. They are formed by a connective tissue core covered on either side by endothelium. Smooth muscle cells are present in the cusps.[12] The two leaflets have a free margin in the center of the vessel and attach to the vessel on either side. Unicuspid and tricuspid valves have been reported.[2,13] The space between the concave aspect of the leaflet and the wall takes the shape of a sinus that allows rapid closure of the valve when blood flow is reversed, but at the same time creates a cul-de-sac where stagnant flow and thrombosis will often start.

Valves tend to occur distal to major tributaries and seem to be more numerous below the knee.[2,4,11] They are absent from the soleus sinusoids and vena cava. The greater and lesser saphenous veins have an average of 10 to 12 valves about 40 mm apart.[4,11] At their junction with the femoral and popliteal veins, the superficial veins have a distinct valve referred to as the "sentinel" or "first" valve. It has strong, white cusps with a firm thickened attachment to the vessel wall and appears noticeably different from the other valves in the superficial veins.[2,4]

In the deep system, vein valves are approximately 22 mm apart. The anterior and posterior tibial veins have an average of nine valves each, while the peroneal vein has about six or seven.[4,11] Only one or two valves are found in the popliteal vein, but many are present in the perforating and muscular veins, and these seem to play a major role in preventing reflux into the superficial system.[2,4,11] The superficial femoral vein has four to six valves. Two of these, one at the adductor canal and another at the mid femoral level, are almost invariably present. The profunda vein has a constantly occurring valve just before it joins the common femoral vein and two to three valves more distally. In the common femoral and external iliac veins, one or two valves resist the transmission of intra-abdominal pressure. If these are absent or incompetent, intra-abdominal pressure will be transmitted directly to the first valve in the greater saphenous vein, potentially contributing to the development of varicosities.[2]

Structure of the Venous Wall

The walls of the veins, like those of arteries, are composed of three primary layers: intima, media, and adventitia. Although arteries and veins share some morphologic features, there are important structural and functional differences. Venous endothelial cells are thinner, but larger, and they form a more continuous barrier with minimal fenestrations. The intima of veins is more permeable than that of arteries, and its internal elastic lamina is much less defined. The media is thin with few elastic lamellae. Veins have a smaller number of smooth muscle cells, which tend to be longitudinally arranged and separated by few collagen fibers.

These structural characteristics correlate with important functional differences between arteries and veins. Veins are more compressible and much less elastic. As a result, the caliber of veins shows greater variability than that of arteries and is more prone to change under physiologic conditions. Veins are also more thrombogenic due to the presence of valves, a lower shear stress (resulting in less rapid clearance of thrombogenic substances), and an increased sensitivity to vasoconstrictors. Finally, lipolysis is slower, lipid uptake is more rapid, and lipid synthesis is more active in veins; these features may be related to the conspicuous absence of atherosclerosis in veins.[14]

Physiology

The venous system in the lower extremities has the difficult task of returning blood to the heart against gravity and serving as a capacitance reservoir which can store varying volumes of blood as dictated by posture and systemic hemodynamic considerations. The system does not function passively, and energy is required. Contraction of the calf muscles ejects blood into the thigh and pelvis, and propulsion of blood to the heart is further facilitated by the abdominal and thoracic muscles. Valves ensure forward flow and prevent reflux, while the endothelium actively contributes to maintenance of blood fluidity and venous tone.

Venous Hemodynamics

As in all hydraulic systems, blood flows in vessels because of a driving energy which is the net result of propulsive and resisting forces. The propulsive energy required for blood flow in the veins of the lower extremities is imparted by several muscular pumps: the heart, the muscles of the leg and foot, and the thoracoabdominal muscles. The pumping action of the heart generates the energy to deliver blood to all body organs, including the lower extremities. It also provides some of the energy required to return blood to the heart (referred to as "vis-a-tergo"). Contraction of foot and leg muscles also provides energy for venous return, and helps propel blood into the thigh and pelvis. In addition, excursion of the abdominal and thoracic walls during breathing creates pressure gradients between the chest and abdomen, and generates energy which further facilitates the flow of blood into the right side of the heart ("vis-a-fronte").

As blood circulates, it encounters a number of forces which resist flow. The primary one is friction, which is particularly important because of large molecules in blood and frequent branching of the vascular tree. In addition, stenotic or compressive lesions as well as alterations in vessel tone and diameter in response to temperature and hemodynamic changes are also important factors. In a cylindrical conduit, Poiseuille's law dictates that resistance increases directly with the length of the vessel and blood viscosity, and is inversely proportional to the fourth power of the radius.[15] Consequently, a small reduction in the size of a cylindrical conduit will cause a significant increase in its resistance. However, veins are not rigid cylindrical conduits. They have the ability to change shape in response to the circulating volume and are often elliptical conduits when partially collapsed. Because of the ability of veins to assume an elliptical shape, the resistance inside the conduit may vary although the total circumference may not change.[15] If the circumference of a vein remains constant, increasing ellipticity will rapidly result in a great increase in resistance and a low flow rate for a given pressure. When ellipticity is increased and there is a simultaneous decrease in circumference, such as when a vein collapses, total resistance is even higher. Conversely, as a vein fills to its capacity and its diameter increases, resistance to flow decreases.[15]

Viscosity is also a significant determinant of resistance. Blood flows in a laminar pattern with concentric layers of blood sliding past one another. As this occurs, a viscous drag is generated from friction between the layers, producing slower flow along the vessel wall compared to the center of the vessel. The force per unit area tending to impede this sliding movement is referred to as the shear stress and is proportional to the product of viscosity and shear rate (the relative velocity between two adjacent layers). Shear stress increases when either viscosity or shear rate is increased.[16] Among the various factors which have the potential to influence flow and shear stress through their effect on viscosity, hematocrit seems to play the predominant role; viscosity increases exponentially as hematocrit increases. Additional factors which increase viscosity include low temperature, stagnant flow, and increased concentrations of fibrinogen and other large molecules.[16]

Flow is impeded not only by high viscosity, but also by turbulence. Under certain conditions that produce high linear velocity, such as at branch sites and areas of stenosis, laminar flow breaks down into a turbulent pattern with swirls and eddies. Turbulence can be expressed as the Reynold's number, which is proportional to the product of blood density and flow rate divided by the vein diameter and blood viscosity; the lower the viscosity and the smaller the vessel lumen, the higher the turbulence.[16]

Venous Pressures

Venous pressures are influenced by several interacting factors, including the extent to which the vein is filled, vasomotor tone, posture, and muscle activity. When partially collapsed, veins are able to accommodate a relatively large volume of blood with minimal change in venous pressure. As intravenous volume increases, veins change from an elliptical to a more cylindrical shape (Figure 3). Higher pressures are needed at that point to stretch the vein wall which becomes stiffer and less compliant. If the veins are stretched to near maximum capacity, the addition of even a small volume will then markedly increase venous pressure. Clinically, the ability of the venous system to adjust its capacitance in response to changes in systemic hemodynamics or pharmacologic alterations in vascular tone provides an important buffer function during manipulation of cardiac preload and filling pressures.

In the supine position, the net driving energy generates a venous pressure that averages 10 to 15 mm Hg at the ankle and 0 to 5 mm Hg at the level of the right atrium. When one assumes the erect position, about 250 cc of blood shifts into each of the lower extremities, and calf volume increases by 2% to 3%.[15] Most of the blood is diverted from the heart and intra-

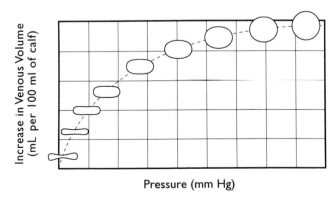

Figure 3. Relationship between venous volume and transmural venous pressure. Veins are able to accommodate a large volume of blood with a minimal change of pressure as they change from an elliptical to a cylindrical shape.

thoracic vasculature, and only a small amount comes from the arms. As blood fills the veins, the hydrostatic pressure generated by the weight of the column of blood rises, and venous pressure at the ankle increases, reaching 50 to 70 mm Hg in the sitting position and 90 to 110 mm Hg in the standing position.[15] Because hydrostatic pressure increases equally in the arterial system, an arteriovenous gradient of about 80 mm Hg is maintained, but mean capillary pressure rises from 25 mm Hg to about 125 mm Hg. As a result of the Starling forces that govern fluid exchange across capillaries, fluid will extravasate into the interstitial space until the pressure in the interstitial space rises sufficiently to prevent further extravasation.[15] Further increases in hydrostatic and capillary pressures can occur when either the valves are incompetent or there is significant obstruction to flow.

The Calf Muscle Pump

In the standing position, the energy required to return blood from the leg to the heart is substantial. When standing still, this energy is supplied solely by the dynamic pressure generated by the heart (vis-a-tergo) and thoracoabdominal muscles (vis-a-fronte). With ambulation, venous return is greatly facilitated by the pumping action of the muscles in the foot and calf.

Priming of the calf muscle pump begins in the plantar plexus of veins.[15] Contraction of the muscles in the calf exerts pressures up to 200 mm Hg on the intramuscular veins in that compartment.[15] This pressure squeezes blood out of the soleus-gastrocnemius sinusoids and deep veins, and propels it into the posterior tibial and popliteal veins. Pressure rises in the deep veins and is greater in the posterior tibial vein favoring rapid egress of blood into the thigh. Contraction of the leg muscles leads to deep fascia tightening in the leg; this exerts pressure on the superficial veins and forces blood flow toward the thigh where the intramuscular pressures are much lower. As this occurs, valves in the perforating veins and below the site of compression close, thereby preventing blood from flowing from the deep veins into superficial veins or into the foot (Figure 4). Valve closure occurs when reversal of the transval-

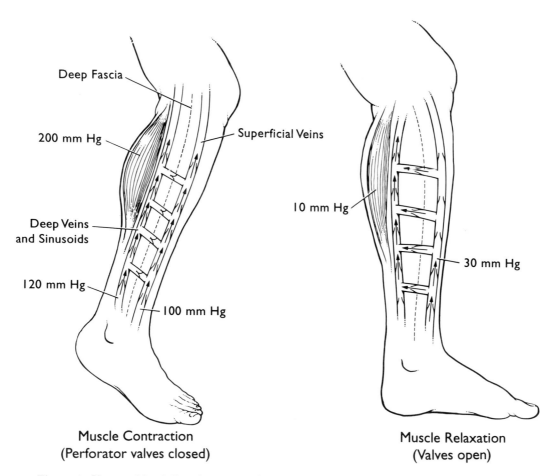

Figure 4. Venous blood flow in a normal leg. During muscle contraction, the perforator valves are closed. Blood is squeezed out of the deep veins into the thigh. When the muscles relax, the perforator valves are open and blood is decompressed from the superficial system into the deep system.

vular pressure gradient promotes retrograde flow; it begins within 100 msec after a reverse flow velocity of 30 cm/s or more is attained.[17] Additional factors which may play a role with valve closure include compliance of the venous wall and segmentation of blood between the valves.[15,18]

During muscle relaxation, pressure in the muscular compartments of the legs falls, allowing blood to flow from the capillaries and deep veins into the soleus sinusoids. Blood flows from the distal tibial veins into the muscular veins and proximal tibial veins. Valves in the perforating veins open and blood flows out of the superficial system where pressures are high, effectively decompressing it (Figure 4). It is still not clear whether or not the smooth muscle present in the vein wall plays any role in facilitating emptying of venous blood.

With a single step, pressure in the saphenous veins drops to about 45 mm Hg, and within 20 to 30 seconds there is return to the starting pressure of about 80 to 90 mm Hg.[15] After 8 to 10 contractions of the calf muscles, most of the venous blood is evacuated from the leg, and venous pressure at the ankle normally falls to about 20 mm Hg. This is referred to as the ambulatory venous pressure (AVP). As venous pressure drops, the gradient between the capillaries and venules decreases, and more blood flows into the venules and sinusoids where it pools until the next muscular contraction. Thus, the calf muscle pump performs two important functions: 1) it assists the heart during exercise by increasing venous return and facilitating flow through the muscles of the leg, and 2) it relieves venous congestion and decreases peripheral edema by decreasing hydrostatic and capillary pressures. Failure of the AVP to remain at a low level (yet undefined) is referred to as venous hypertension and is felt to be the underlying hemodynamic abnormality leading to chronic venous insufficiency.

The Thoracoabdominal Muscle Pump

Because of the collapsible nature of the venous wall and the compartmentalization of pressures between the abdominal and thoracic cavities, breathing has a significant effect on venous return. During inspiration, the diaphragm descends, and intra-abdominal pressure rises, while intrathoracic pressure falls. Blood flows out of the abdominal compartment into the right side of the heart, and flow from the thigh stops temporarily due to higher venous pressures in the abdominal compartment. With expiration the reverse takes place: intrathoracic pressure increases, and flow into the chest slows, while flow from the thigh into the abdominal compartment resumes. However, this seemingly simple mechanism is complicated by other factors. An increase in abdominal pressure can either increase or decrease venous return in the vena cava, depending on whether transmural pressure in the vena cava at the thoracic inlet significantly exceeds or is below the critical closing transmural pressure.[15,19] Clinically, these fluctuations in venous return during breathing have a significant effect on venous flow in the lower extremities which can be demonstrated using Doppler ultrasound (Figure 5).

Venous Tone

Venomotor tone is significantly influenced by the autonomic nervous system and by signal molecules released by the endothelium in reponse to local stimuli. Veins possess adrenergic receptors in the media, and their ability to act as a capacitance system is regulated to a large extent by sympathetic-mediated changes in venous tone. Venous volume may change passively, as occurs when one assumes the standing position, or actively, as a result of sympathetic control.[15] The increase in venomotor tone mediated by the sympathetic nervous system can shift large volumes of blood from the peripheral veins into the central circulation without significant changes in venous pressures. These shifts are essential to maintain cardiac output under a number of stressful conditions including exercise, shock, and hemorrhage.[15]

Stimulation of the alpha-adrenergic receptors by external changes in temperature and cold also results in venoconstriction. The highest density of alpha-receptors is present in the cutaneous and superficial veins, which play a significant role in heat conservation by actively diverting blood away from the skin into the deeper tissues. Deeper veins do not seem to be as responsive to sympathetic venoconstriction and therefore contribute very little to temperature regulation. The sympathetic control of the cutaneous veins is under the control of hypothalamic thermoregulatory centers, which will augment or diminish sympathetic outflow to the cutaneous veins as dictated by body temperature. Veins also vasoconstrict locally when exposed to cold temperatures, a response that can be abolished to a large extent by ganglionic blockade. Additional constricting factors include local trauma, pain, emotional stress, and heart failure. Venodilatation, on the other hand, occurs in response to a variety of drugs, smoking, anesthesia, and sympathetic blockade. The extent to which heat induces venodilatation, if any, is still unclear.

The Venous Endothelium

The endothelium is a monolayer of polygonal cells which lines all blood vessels. Previously thought to be inert and only serve a structural role, it is now clear

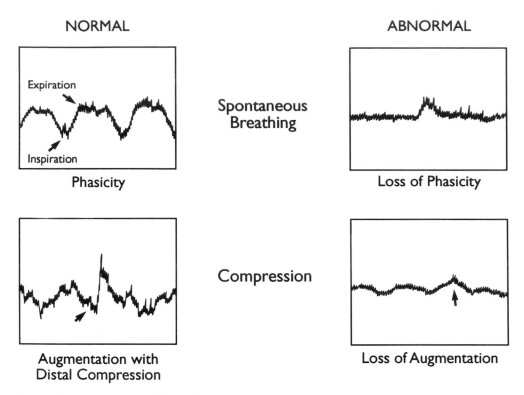

NORMAL

ABNORMAL

Spontaneous
Breathing

Expiration

Inspiration

Phasicity

Loss of Phasicity

Compression

Augmentation with
Distal Compression

Loss of Augmentation

Figure 5. Effects of breathing and manual compression on Doppler venous velocity signals in the lower extremity.

that endothelial cells are metabolically active and that they respond to a wide variety of stimuli. As the interface between the blood stream and the vessel wall, endothelial cells play a critical role in communication of biologic information. They constantly monitor alterations in the physiologic milieu and process biochemical signals from the vessel lumen. In response to these signals, the endothelium adjusts its synthesis of biomolecules which regulate hemostasis, vasomotor tone, and attachment of cellular elements of blood (Table 1). Consequently, the endothelium plays a key role in maintaining a delicate balance between growth promotion and inhibition, vasoconstriction and vasodilatation, and anticoagulation and procoagulation. In addition, the endothelium participates in inflammatory and immunologic responses.[20-22]

Endothelium plays a critical role in the regulation of vascular tone. A wide variety of intraluminal stimuli including endotoxin, hypoxia, humoral agents, and alterations in shear stress and pressure induce endothelial cells to increase or decrease their synthesis of a number of signal molecules.[23] These molecules can induce contraction (e.g., endothelins, endothelial-derived contracting factor [EDCF]), or relaxation (e.g., prostacyclin and nitric oxide) in the underlying vascular smooth muscle.[24] In many instances, these signal molecules influence cell proliferation as well. Thus, the endothelium not only serves a sensory function by con-

Table 1
Endothelial Cell Molecules Involved in Thrombosis, Inflammation, and Venous Tone

Prothrombotic	Antithrombotic
Platelet activating factor	Prostacyclin
Tissue factor	Antithrombin III
von Willebrand factor	Heparin like molecules
tPA inhibitor	tPA activator
Factor V	Thrombomodulin
Cytokines	EDRF
Growth factors	

Cell-Adhesion Molecules	Vasoregulators	
	Dilators	Constrictors
ICAMs:		
ICAM-1, ICAM-2	PGI$_2$	Endothelins
VCAM-1	EDRF	EDCF
	EDHP	
Selectins:		
ELAM-1, GMP-140	ADP	
Integrins:		
VLA, L-CAM,		
Cytoadhesins		

tinuously monitoring a host of intravascular factors, but also acts as a central processing unit which formulates and directs an appropriate contractile response. In addition, endothelial cells can influence vasomotor tone indirectly by clearing locally generated vasoactive substances.[24]

The endothelium also plays a vital role in maintaining the delicate balance of hemostasis. When intact, the endothelium acts as an effective barrier, preventing activation of platelets and coagulation. In addition, by orchestrating the synthesis of various procoagulants, and antithrombotic and fibrinolytic molecules, it plays a key role in regulating coagulation in both health and disease. Normally, the coagulation cascade is in a state of readiness, but not fully activated; it is held in check by molecules which neutralize the procoagulant activity. Examples of endothelial procoagulants include tissue factor, platelet activating factor, and von Willebrand factor. Typical antithrombotic molecules are prostacyclin, heparan sulfate, thrombomodulin, and plasminogen activators.

This delicate hemostatic balance is upset when the endothelium is injured, when a hypercoagulable state exists (e.g., malignancy, surgery, trauma), or when stasis is present. Denudation of the endothelium exposes the subendothelial matrix, triggering a sequence of biochemical reactions which result in thrombosis. Migration of platelets, neutrophils, monocytes, and lymphocytes to the injured area is directed by expression of specific cell adhesive molecules (CAMs) on endothelial cells (Table 1).[20-22] Platelet adhesion to the subendothelium is mediated by some members of the integrin family of molecules.[20,21] Adherence of platelets to the vessel wall is followed by aggregation of more platelets and enhancement of the coagulation cascade.

Leukocytes are also attracted to the site of injury and adhere to the vascular wall by binding to fibrinogen molecules.[20] The interaction with leukocytes and macrophages causes the endothelial cell to release a number of cytokines, including interleukins, chemotactic substances, platelet and fibroblast growth factors, and other mediators of inflammation.[20,21]

Clinical Tests of Physiologic Function of the Venous System

The ability to measure physiologic function is crucial to understanding the pathogenesis of venous diseases. In addition, tests of hemodynamic function provide a means of gauging the severity of disease and determining optimal management. Over the years, we have seen the introduction of a large number of tests of venous hemodynamic function. It is beyond the scope of this chapter to discuss each of these techniques at length, but several excellent publications describe them in detail.[25-31] The four methods commonly used to study venous hemodynamics are: 1) direct measurements of venous pressures, 2) contrast venography, 3) plethysmography, and 4) ultrasound evaluation. Each of these tests provides useful information about venous hemodynamics, but no single test completely characterizes the venous system of the lower extremity. As a result, several tests may provide complementary information.

Ambulatory Venous Pressure

This is probably the oldest quantitative diagnostic test for venous incompetence (Figure 6). Venous pressure is measured directly from a needle inserted into a dorsal foot vein, and pressures are recorded with the patient standing and during a variety of maneuvers. When the calf muscle is contracted to mimic walking, pressure drops as blood is propelled cephalad by the action of the calf muscle pump. When calf muscle contraction ceases, venous pressure slowly returns to its initial level. The pressure achieved after contracting the calf muscles is referred to as the AVP and is defined as the lowest pressure attained following exercise. The time required for intravenous pressure to return to its initial level is the venous refill time; with reflux, the venous refill time is markedly shortened. The application of a venous tourniquet to control reflux from the superficial system is sometimes useful in distinguishing superficial and deep venous incompetence. AVP is influenced by several factors: 1) the efficiency of the calf muscle pump, 2) the magnitude of venous reflux, and 3) the resistance to flow. Although AVP measurements are accurate and reliable, they have the disadvantage of being invasive and cumbersome to perform.[32,33]

Arm-Foot Pressure Differential

This technique, described by Raju,[34] involves the simultaneous recording of venous pressure in the foot

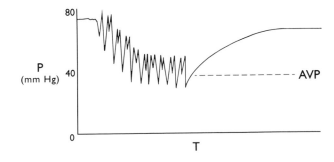

Figure 6. Typical recording of effect on venous pressure of 10 tiptoe movements. P = pressure; T = time; AVP = ambulatory venous pressure at the end of exercise. (Reproduced with permission from Reference 36.)

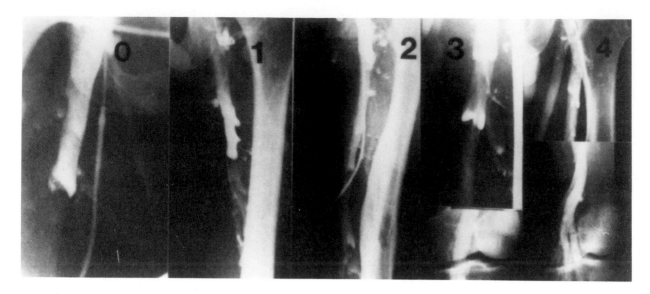

Figure 7. Descending venography demonstrating various grades of venous reflux (grade 0 to 4).

and hand with the patient in the supine position. In normal limbs, the arm-foot pressure differential is less than 5 mm Hg, while patients with venographic evidence of obstruction have marked increases in the arm-foot pressure differential. Using this technique, Raju was able to quantitate and define four grades of outflow obstruction.

Ascending and Descending Venography

Ascending venography has been used for many years to delineate the anatomic abnormalities associated with venous obstruction. Intravenous contrast is injected into a dorsal vein in the foot and is followed proximally. By tilting the table and applying a tourniquet at the ankle, one is able to divert blood to the deep veins. Both obstruction to flow (indicating vein thrombosis) or deep-to-superficial reflux can then be identified. This test has now been largely replaced by duplex ultrasound and air-plethysmography (APG).

Descending venography, on the other hand, continues to play a valuable role in the quantification of venous incompetence, especially when valve reconstruction is contemplated.[35] Contrast is injected in the femoral vein with the patient in a semi-upright position (Figure 7). Venous reflux can be detected if present, and quantitated to some extent. The degree of reflux is typically graded from grade 0 (no reflux below the confluence of the superficial and profunda femoris veins) to grade IV (reflux through all of the femoral popliteal and calf veins to the level of the ankle). While descending venography provides useful information and is still employed, it is likely to be replaced by newer, noninvasive techniques such as duplex ultrasound and APG.

Air-Plethysmography

APG, introduced by Christopoulos et al,[36] was developed to replace water and strain gauge plethysmographic techniques, which were cumbersome and did not reflect changes in the whole extremity. With this technique, changes in venous volume in the lower leg are sensed by an air-filled polyurethane cuff which surrounds the leg from the knee to the ankle. Changes in lower leg venous volume are monitored during a series of maneuvers which enable the investigator to test for proximal outflow obstruction, venous refilling time, and calf muscle pump ejection fraction (Figure 8). In addition, AVP can be estimated. Since its introduction, numerous reports have demonstrated the usefulness of APG in providing accurate measurements of venous reflux and venous obstruction.[36–40] More recently, APG has been used to assess the results of venous surgery.[41]

Photoplethysmography

Changes in the number of red cells in the skin affect the back scatter of light detected by a skin probe with a light source and a light-sensitive diode. Elevated venous pressure increases the number of capillary red cells and causes a decreased signal from the skin probe. As a result, alterations in venous pressure caused by changes in the position of the leg or by proximal venous

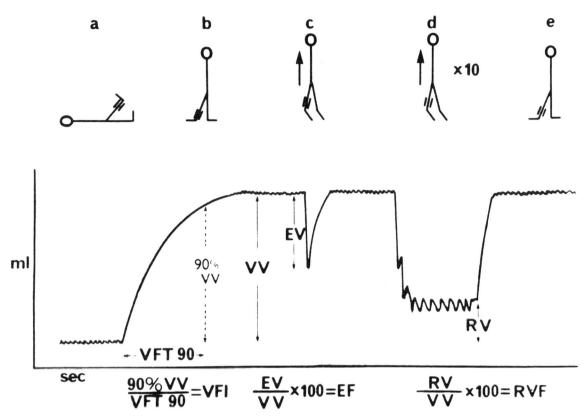

Figure 8. Volume changes in the lower extremity during standard sequence of postural changes and exercise. **a)** Patient in supine position with leg elevated 45 degrees; **b)** patient standing with weight on nonexamined leg; **c)** single tiptoe movement; **d)** ten tiptoe movements; **e)** same as in b. VV = functional venous volume; VFT = venous filling time; VFI = venous filling index; EV = ejected volume; RV = residual volume; EF = ejection fraction; RVF = residual volume fraction. (Reproduced with permission from Reference 40).

occlusion can be detected. Venous refill time can also be measured by photoplethysmography (PPG), and several studies have found these measurements to correlate well with direct measurements of AVP.[42-45] Although PPG is noninvasive and relatively easy to perform, it does not quantitate the degree of deep venous insufficiency, and only one area of the leg can be evaluated at a time.

Duplex Ultrasound

Duplex scanning first gained popularity as an extremely reliable noninvasive modality for diagnosis of deep venous thrombosis. More recently it has been found to be very helpful in the study of venous valve function and venous reflux.[46-49] Duplex scanning combines Doppler with B-mode ultrasound, making it possible to visualize veins and simultaneously assess their degree of reflux.[50,51]

Strandness and Van Bemmelen[52] have described several duplex scanning techniques using a combina-

tion of the Trendelenburg position, the Valsalva maneuver, and rapid inflation/deflation cuffs to more accurately quantitate venous reflux, and to determine velocity and direction of flow. The duration of reverse flow and the time to valve closure can be measured as well. More recent modifications by Araki,[53] using the effects of position and compression, have also contributed to a more precise and reliable evaluation of vein incompetence. A more detailed description of duplex scanning and its application in venous disease can be found elsewhere.[52]

Pathophysiology of the Venous System

Varicose Veins

Varicose veins are distended, elongated, tortuous superficial veins with incompetent valves.[54] They are referred to as primary varicose veins when they develop spontaneously without antecedent history of deep vein thrombosis. Primary varicose veins tend to be familial and involve predominantly the greater saphenous vein and its tributaries. Secondary varicose veins usually occur as a result of deep vein thrombosis and the postphlebitic syndrome.

Epidemiology of Varicose Veins

The prevalence of varicose veins is generally reported to range from 20% to 70% among adults in industrialized nations,[55–63] but varicose veins are distinctly less common in less technologically advanced populations.[64] The wide range of prevalence among industrialized countries probably results partly from differences in diagnostic criteria and partly from differences in the study populations. For example, prevalence is generally reported to be higher among women and prevalence increases with age. Most studies suggest that varicose veins are associated with parity,[55–57,59–63] family history of varicose veins,[57,59,61] obesity,[56,61–63,65] sedentary lifestyle,[62,65] and occupations requiring prolonged standing or sitting.[56,61–63] Increased intra-abdominal pressure may play an etiologic role as well, since varicose veins have been associated with inguinal hernia in men and wearing corsets in women.[56] Increased intra-abdominal pressure due to straining during defecation might explain the higher prevalence of varicose veins reported in patients with diverticular disease compared to age- and sex-matched controls.[66] Alternatively, dietary factors might play an important role.[67] Many of the retrospective case-control studies that have been performed may have been biased by the inability to select a control group which is truly comparable to the varicose vein cases; failure to control for confounding is also a common problem. One of the best studies to date is one from Brand et al using follow-up data from the Framingham Study.[65] These investigators found that, in women, development of varicose veins was associated with obesity, lower levels of physical activity, higher systolic blood pressure, and older age at menopause; among men, varicose veins were associated with low levels of physical activity and smoking.[65]

Pathology of Varicose Veins

Several histologic studies show that the collagen content of primary varicose veins is less than that of normal veins.[68,69] This results in disruption of the normal architecture of the vein wall[55] and produces disorganization of the smooth muscle layer. The muscle content of varicose veins is actually high,[69] but normal longitudinal and circular muscle fibers can no longer be distinguished, and areas of muscle are broken up by disorganized collagen.[55,68–70] These findings might

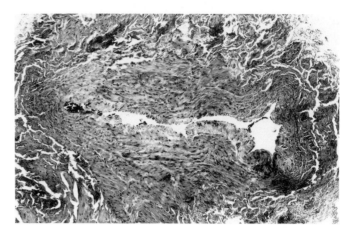

Figure 9. Deep vein with marked thickening of the wall and compromise of the lumen ($\times 45$).

account for the diminished elasticity found in varicose veins.[55]

A variety of metabolic changes have also been found in the walls of varicose veins. Histochemical studies by Haardt have shown a decrease in phosphatases in the muscle coats of the vein wall and an increase in collagen-splitting enzymes in the vein wall connective tissue resulting in decreased collagen content of varicose veins. Thus, the weakness of varicose vein walls may be related not only to anatomic disorganization of the vein structure, but also to deficiency of key enzymes.[69–71]

Primary varicose veins show no evidence of infection or signs of antecedent thrombophlebitis, but they do have noteworthy changes in the vein wall and in the valve cusps. The primary change in the commissure is dilatation of the wall, first seen as an evagination followed by widening with a consequent separation of the cusps' attachments. Secondary restorative changes are then superimposed later in the process.[72]

When secondary varicose veins occur following thrombosis, fibroblasts, mast cells, polymorphonuclear leukocytes, and histiocytes invade the vein wall, and the occluded lumen is usually restored by a combination of thrombus retraction and recanalization.[55] Instead of the vein wall becoming thin and weak as in primary varicose veins, the walls of previously thrombosed veins are thicker and less distensible than those of normal veins due to collagen deposition by fibroblasts in the process of recanalization (Figure 9).[55]

Pathophysiology of Varicose Veins

The critical factors involved in the development of varicose veins are still only partially understood. Over the years, several theories have been put forward to account for their occurrence, but despite extensive research, the etiology of primary varicose veins is still debated. Proponents of these theories argue that the critical factor(s) involved in varicose vein formation are: 1) arteriovenous communications in the microcirculation, 2) biochemical defects in the vein wall, 3) absence or incompetence of femoral valves, and 4) increased intra-abdominal pressure.

One of the oldest theories is that varicose veins result from arteriovenous communications (AVCs) through which arterial pressure is transmitted to venous tributaries which progressively dilate and eventually become incompetent. The presence of such AVCs was first suggested by Blalock in 1929,[73] when he demonstrated that oxygen saturation was greater in blood from varicose vein segments than that from nonvaricosed veins. Haimovici[74] later provided some anatomic and angiographic evidence that supported the existence of small (0.1–0.6 mm) AVCs which originate from subfascial arteries and terminate in venous tributaries. However, recent studies have not substantiated an increase in oxygen saturation in varicose vein segments, and this argues against AVCs as a significant factor in the development of varicose veins.

Biochemical defects in the vein wall have long been thought to play an essential role in the development of primary varicose veins.[68–71] Genetic enzymatic defects could be responsible for the morphologic and histologic changes previously decribed and could eventually lead to venous dilation, valve incompetence, and reflux.[71]

In addition to enzymatic or biochemical defects, hormonal influences may be important as well. The higher incidence of varicose veins in women compared to men suggests a hormonal effect on vein wall function.[60] It is possible that progesterone predisposes to varicose vein formation by inducing vein wall relaxation and dilation. To some extent, of course, the higher incidence of varicose veins in women probably reflects the effects of pregnancy, during which venous congestion increases as a result of increased pelvic blood flow, fluid retention, increased blood volume, and compression of the vena cava by an enlarged uterus. On the other hand, varicose veins are less prevalent among women in underdeveloped countries, even though they have a higher average parity than women in developed countries. Consequently, instead of being a primary cause of varicose veins, pregnancy may simply induce transient varicosities or exacerbate a predisposition to varicose vein formation.

Bergan recently suggested a unifying hypothesis in which an interaction between a "hereditary-hormonal substrate" and hemodynamic conditions causes the development of primary varicose veins.[75] This concept is supported by Lowell's findings of endothelial and smooth muscle abnormalities in vein segments taken from varicose vein patients who required coronary artery bypass grafting.[76] Biochemical and structural abnormalities were found not only in varicosed segments, but also in nonvaricosed veins, suggesting a generalized abnormality of the veins which was genetic.

Yet another theory is that reflux, vein distention, and venous hypertension are caused by absence or incompetence of valves. While there is agreement that valvular incompetence may be present, it is not clear whether this is a primary cause or a secondary result of vein distention and varicose formation. It seems clear, however, that there is no key valve and no particular combination of valves whose incompetence leads to varicose veins. Some authors had felt that saphenofemoral junction incompetence is a prerequisite for the development of varicose veins, but we have not found that to be the case (Table 2).[77] In our studies, saphenofemoral incompetence was not uniformly present, and furthermore, the greater saphenous vein was often normal, even in the presence of saphenofemoral incompetence. An additional piece of evidence suggesting that saphenofemoral incompetence is not a critical abnormality leading to varicose veins comes from anatomic studies which demonstrate that there are many individuals without saphenofemoral or common femoral valves who are clinically normal and do not have varicosities.[78,79]

For many years, varicosities were also believed

Table 2
Anatomic Distribution (%) of Incompetence in Extremities with Varicose Veins or Venous Ulcers

Location	Varicose Veins (n = 54)	Venous Ulcers (n = 95)
Superficial	100	79
Perforator	46	63
Deep	24	38
Superficial only	33	17
SFJ* only	9	—
Perforating only	7	8
Deep only	4	2
Superficial & deep	7	12
Superficial & perforating	9	19
Perforating & deep	9	4
Superficial, perforating, and deep (all 3)	20	30
No incompetence	—	6

* SFJ: saphenofemoral junction.
(Adapted with permission from References 77 and 113.)

to occur exclusively as a result of valve incompetence in superficial veins. It is now recognized that valve incompetence can occur anywhere in the lower extremity. Browse noted that incompetence could be found in any vein of the lower leg in patients with varicose veins.[80] Our studies using duplex scanning demonstrated that varicose formation and valve incompetence are more common in superficial veins and occur more frequently in tributaries rather than in the main trunk of the greater or lesser saphenous veins (Table 2).[77] The infrequency of incompetence in the main trunk of the greater saphenous vein may well be related to its well-developed media and investing fascia, in contrast to the distal venous branches which have much less smooth muscle and lie unsupported in the subcutaneous tissues. Varicosities are also much more common in the distal third of the lesser saphenous vein, which is in the subcutaneous layer, than in its proximal two thirds, which runs beneath the fascia. It has been suggested that the investing fascia of the proximal vein inhibits the development of varicosities.

In addition to superficial vein incompetence, many of these patients were noted to have deep and perforating vein incompetence as well. In fact, up to 20% of patients with primary varicose veins had combined superficial, deep, and perforating vein valve incompetence, yet only 7% of these patients showed clear evidence of deep vein thrombosis when examined by duplex.[77] Similar findings were reported by Mayberry, who found evidence of previous thrombosis in only 14% of patients with deep venous incompetence.[81] Ferris proposed that some of these individuals have a "primary" abnormality of the deep valves, such as a congenital absence or "floppy valves,"[82] a view that is not widely accepted. An alternative explanation is that these are secondary varicose veins which evolved after deep vein thrombosis destroyed valves in the deep system, but that thrombosis resolved without leaving telltale evidence.

When one considers the histologic, biochemical, and epidemiologic factors associated with the development of varicose veins, it seems plausible that pathogenesis may be multifactorial. Perhaps genetic factors establish the potential for developing varicose veins, while subsequent events and exposures to other factors dictate their occurrence and severity. Thus, primary biochemical or anatomic abnormalities in the vein wall may provide a necessary, but not solely sufficient condition for the evolution of varicosities. Subsequently, other factors, some of which are related to lifestyle, may trigger the formation of varicose veins and determine their severity. It is particularly easy to envision how certain risk factors related to lifestyle could contribute to varicose vein formation by their effects on venous hemodynamics. We have already noted that the pregnant uterus can cause venous congestion by

compressing the vena cava. Increased venous pressures might also result from suboptimal function of the calf muscle pump as a result of a sedentary lifestyle. A low-fiber diet might interfere with the thoracoabdominal pump as a result of straining during defecation or as a result of pressure on the external iliac veins from a feces-laden colon. Chronic obstructive lung disease might also have an adverse effect on the efficiency of the thoracoabdominal muscle pump, and this might account for the observed association between smoking and varicose veins. Each of these effects by itself might be quite small, but the sum of these effects over a period of many years may be sufficient to increase the probability of clinically overt disease and account for the greater incidence of varicose veins in developed countries.

Chronic Venous Insufficiency

There is no strictly uniform definition of chronic venous insufficiency (CVI), and this sometimes causes confusion. Here, we refer to CVI as a syndrome which results primarily from incompetence of valves and/or venous outflow obstruction in the lower extremity and evolves into a characteristic clinical picture. Initially, there is ankle swelling and discomfort. Edema and pain worsen as the disease progresses, and the skin in the so-called "gaiter" area of the leg becomes inflamed, hyperpigmented, and develops eczematoid changes. Eventually, there is subcutaneous fibrosis (lipodermatosclerosis), and skin ulcerations may develop. Recurring cycles of ulceration and healing are not unusual in the advanced stages and can cause significant distress and incapacitation.

Epidemiology of Chronic Venous Insufficiency

A large study in Australia identified 259 patients with chronic leg ulceration in a population of 238,000 (0.1%),[83] and a British study found a point prevalence of 0.18% in the adult population.[84] Not surprisingly, prevalence increases with age.[83–86] Interpretation of studies on the prevalence and epidemiology of venous ulceration is frequently complicated by a lack of clear evidence that the ulcers studied were venous in origin, although most studies conclude that venous disease is the primary cause of leg ulcerations. Several studies also note that, in patients with ulceration, venous disease not infrequently coexists with arterial disease, rheumatoid arthritis, or diabetes.[83–86] The significance of these coexisting conditions is unclear, however, since these diseases are more prevalent in older populations, and most studies to date have not been adjusted for age.

It is well established that CVI can occur following

deep vein thrombosis, and the conditions associated with venous thrombosis are well known. These include immobilization and convalescence; orthopedic, abdominal, and thoracic surgery; trauma, including fractures of the legs and pelvis; pregnancy; estrogen therapy; and hypercoagulable states. In each case, the association of these conditions with thrombosis can be directly linked to dysfunction of the normal venous physiology whereby the delicate hemostatic balance is tilted in the direction of thrombosis.

It is unclear, however, whether CVI is strictly a consequence of deep vein thrombosis, since many patients with CVI have no demonstrable evidence of previous thrombosis. In these patients, primary valve incompetence, leading to reflux and venous hyper tension, could be an alternative cause of CVI. One problem, however, is that some patients with varicose veins have significant reflux and venous hypertension without developing skin changes characteristic of CVI. In fact, several studies suggest that the pattern of venous incompetence and the extent of hemodynamic malfunction among patients with lipodermatosclerosis and/or venous ulceration is actually quite similar to that seen in patients with uncomplicated varicose veins.[77,87] Why, then, are some patients with venous insufficiency afflicted with skin changes and ulceration while others are not?

In a preliminary case-control study, we compared characteristics of patients with venous ulceration (N = 61) to patients with significant but uncomplicated varicose veins (N = 93). Patients with ulceration were older, more likely to be hypertensive, and more likely to be male than patients with varicosities. Even after adjusting for these differences, however, the ulcer patients were much more likely to have a past history of serious leg trauma (odds ratio = 7.7, p = .0002), even though a past history of phlebitis or thrombosis was only slightly more common in the ulcer patients. To our surprise, the ulcer patients are also more likely to be without health insurance (odds ratio = 5.0, p = .01). These findings raise the possibility that subclinical deep vein thrombosis may be an important predisposing factor and that ill-defined socioeconomic factors may also play a role.

Pathology of Chronic Venous Insufficiency

CVI is associated with a spectrum of characteristic skin changes which include edema, dermatitis, pigmentation, fibrosis of the skin (lipodermatosclerosis) with or without ulceration, and atrophie blanche.[88]

The dermatitis seen with venous insufficiency (so-called stasis dermatitis) may occur in subacute form or chronic form. Subacute stasis dermatitis is characterized by scaling, erythema, and weeping of the skin. Histologically, there is spongiosis, intracellular edema,

and vesicles at various levels of the epidermis. There is moderate acanthosis (thickening of the epidermis), and in the stratum corneum parakeratosis and crusting may be seen (Figure 10).[89] In chronic dermatitis, the skin is thickened, and acanthosis is more evident with elongation of the rete ridges. There is also hyperkeratosis with areas of parakeratosis. Slight spongiosis may be present, but vesicles are absent. An inflammatory infiltrate may be present in a perivascular distribution, but usually does not extend into the epidermis. Dermal fibrosis and vascular proliferation are commonly seen (Figure 11). They are usually accompanied by extravasation of red cells and hemosiderin deposits which are responsible for the characteristic hyperpigmentation (Figure 12).[89]

Lipodermatosclerosis is characterized not only by hyperpigmentation, but also by more advanced induration and inflammation (Figures 13A and 13B). Acute or early lesions show a lymphocytic infiltrate in the subcutaneous septa with areas of ischemic necrosis.[90,91] This progresses to fibroplastic thickening of the septa with a mixed inflammatory infiltrate, and areas of sclerosis within the fat. Advanced areas of lipodermatosclerosis occur in the more chronic states referred to by some as sclerosing panniculitis, and show marked sclerosis in the fat with little inflammatory infiltrate.[90,91] Within the dermis there is a superficial and deep mixed perivascular infiltrate.[90,91]

Atrophie blanche is a smooth, ivory-white plaque of sclerosis stippled with telangiectasia and surrounded by hyperpigmentation.[88] It is frequently seen in pa-

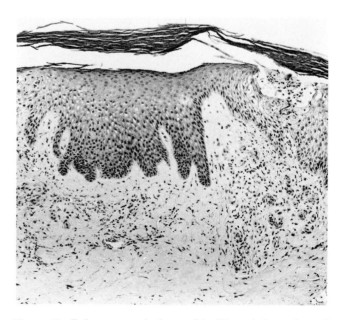

Figure 10. Subacute stasis dermatitis. There is irregular epidermal hyperplasia, with focal spongiosis and spongiotic vesicles. There is increased vascularity and mild perivascular inflammatory infiltrate ($\times 45$).

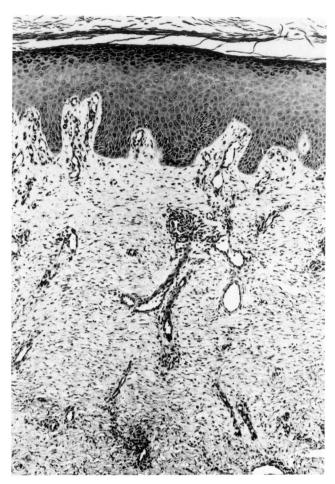

Figure 11. Chronic stasis dermatitis. Hypergranulosis and hyperkeratosis, epidermal hyperplasia, and marked dermal fibrosis with prominent vessels (×90).

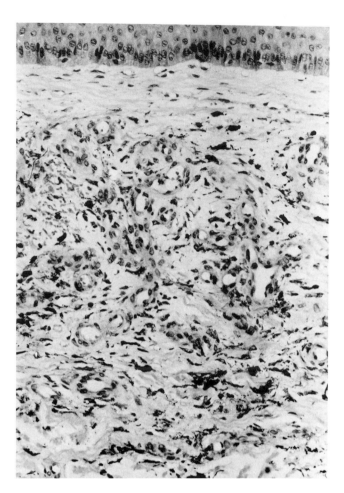

Figure 12. Hemosiderin deposits. There is vascular proliferation with extravasation of red cells and abundant hemosiderin deposition (×90).

tients with CVI. Histologically, this is characterized by an atrophic epidermis with scleroderma-like changes in the dermis with little or no inflammatory reaction. There is new vessel formation in the subpapillary layer with capillary tufting and dilation.[90]

In addition to the changes described above, biopsies from the margins of chronic venous ulcers show markedly irregular epidermal hyperplasia,[92,93] and increased mitotic activity.[93] Some authors have reported the skin surrounding the ulcer to appear normal, although in most specimens there was increased fibrosis and changes consistent with lipodermatosclerosis.[93] Histochemically, the epidermis in chronic venous ulcers demonstrates staining with hyperproliferative keratin markers, anti-involucrin staining throughout the epidermis, and staining with antibody to integrin 13 around the margins of epithelial cells.[94] These findings suggest that the epidermis at the edge of venous ulcers is hyperproliferative and demonstrates features of migration. The failure to re-epithelialize these wounds may be due to inability of the epidermis to undergo

keratinocytic maturation and terminal differentiation rather than its ability to proliferate.[93]

The underlying dermis at the ulcer margin contains numerous small and medium-sized blood vessels. The superficial dermis tends to contain numerous, tortuous capillaries which have a glomerulus-like appearance, narrow lumina, and cubic endothelial cells.[95,96] The basement membrane of these capillary loops is usually split up into multiple layers, and in contrast to normal skin capillaries, there is no clear separation between basement membranes and the surrounding connective tissue.[96] There is partial or complete destruction of the capillary pericyte envelope or "corset," possibly accounting for capillary dilation.[96] In the deep dermis, only a few dilated capillaries with a flattened endothelial layer are seen.[96] The remainder of the dermis consists of fibrous tissue in which chronic inflammatory cells and red cells are scattered and interstitial edema is present.

Most capillaries are surrounded by thick, organized fibrin cuffs with deposition of immunoglobulins, complement, fibrin, and neutrophils around vessels in

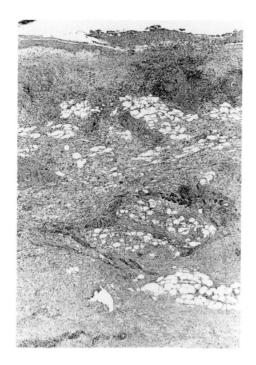

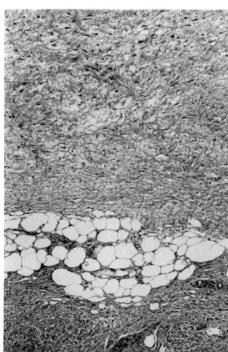

Figure 13. Lipodermatosclerosis. **A.** Low-power view with focal ulceration, underlying inflammatory infiltrate and sclerosis of underlying subcutis (×18). **B.** Close-up of subcutis with widened sclerotic septae with entrapment of fat (×45).

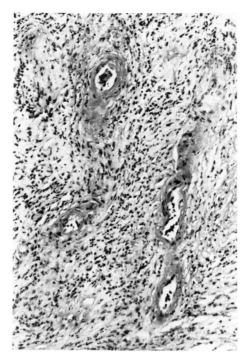

Figure 14. Pericapillary fibrin deposition and surrounding mixed inflammatory infiltrate of neutrophils and lymphoid cells.

lipodermatosclerotic non-ulcerated skin and at the edge of venous ulcers (Figure 14).[97–104] Histochemically, the fibrin cuffs around the capillaries contain fibrin, laminin, fibronectin, tenascin, collagens 1 and 3, and often trapped monocytes, macrophages, and polymorphonuclear leukocytes.[97] These findings suggest that so-called "fibrin cuffs" are not formed purely by the accumulation of blood-borne products extravasated through the vessel walls, but instead are actively synthesized and assembled by the endothelium and adjacent connective tissue cells.

The base of venous ulcers is often covered with a layer of fibrinous exudate of variable thickness which contains numerous polymorphonuclear leukocytes as well as bacteria and necrotic debris.[95,97] A layer of hyaline, apparently acellular collagen, is often observed sandwiched between the exudate and ulcer base together with a mild chronic inflammatory infiltrate. Granulation tissue can be seen beneath the ulcer, with fibrosis in the deep dermis or subcutis. Focally extravasated red blood cells, small perivascular deposits of hemosiderin, and macrophages are present in the ulcer base, along its edge and in the surrounding tissues.[94,97]

Pathogenesis of Chronic Venous Insufficiency

When all the components of the venous system including various muscle pumps and valves work properly, blood is returned to the heart against gravity. Under certain pathologic conditions resulting from improper valve function, venous obstruction, or calf muscle pump dysfunction, blood refluxes back down the legs and venous pressure rises. It is believed that when venous hypertension persists for prolonged periods of time, it initiates a sequence of events, at both the macro- and microcirculatory levels, that lead to the development of CVI syndrome with its characteristic skin changes.

For many years, chronic venous hypertension was thought to develop primarily as result of proximal deep vein thrombosis, and early investigators viewed CVI merely as a consequence of post-thrombotic abnormalities in the deep and perforating veins.[105–107] Virchow described a triad of physiologic changes associated with an increased incidence of thrombosis: 1) endothelial injury, 2) blood stasis, and 3) hypercoagulable states. These factors, alone or in combination, may initiate interaction between the vein wall and cellular elements of blood and trigger the coagulation cascade. Surgical and nonsurgical trauma may cause direct endothelial injury. Immobilization during surgery and convalescence interferes with the function of the calf muscle pump and the thoracoabdominal pump. As a result, venous flow in the lower extremities is impaired and the likelihood of thrombosis is increased. Perhaps of even greater significance is impaired function of the fibrinolytic system, which is known to occur after surgery or trauma and in patients with hypercoagulable states.

Over the last two decades, advances in radiologic and laboratory diagnostic methods have led to a better understanding of the natural history and pathophysiology of venous thrombosis in the lower extremities and its contribution to the development of CVI. It is now recognized that thrombus formation may begin in the soleus and calf muscles, and in up to 20% of cases progresses cephalad to cause more proximal occlusion.[108] The thrombus is believed to start mainly in the valve sinuses where flow is more stagnant; eventually, the thrombus becomes firmly attached to the wall by fibrin strands,[72] and there is progressive organization of the clot, which leads finally to malfunction or destruction of the valve and reflux.[72]

The process of valvular destruction and incompetence is believed to occur slowly, often requiring 3 to 6 months.[109] Once a thrombus forms on the valve, the fibrinolytic system is activated, and clot lysis begins. As the thrombus is reorganized and lysed by the fibrinolytic system, recanalization of the occluded segment takes place. This has been observed to occur as early as 1 week after thrombosis, but more than half of the occluded deep veins will not recanalize before 6 months, and it may take up to 1 year for the majority of occluded veins to recanalize.[110]

Despite a better understanding of the natural history of venous thrombosis, it is not clear that deep vein thrombosis is the sine qua non for CVI. A basic problem has been the inability to link the morphologic changes found in the veins following thrombosis to the development of hemodynamic abnormalities seen with CVI. Substantial evidence suggests that there is no direct correlation between the extent of lower extremity venous thrombosis or the presence of collaterals and the development of CVI and ulceration. In fact, only 35% to 45% of patients with CVI have evidence of previous deep vein thrombosis based on history or noninvasive testing.[111–113]

Since evidence for DVT is not always found in patients with CVI, primary valvular incompetence has been suggested as an alternative cause of venous hypertension. Dysfunction of certain valves as a result of an intrinsic defect in the vein wall or valves may be the primary abnormality responsible for reflux and venous hypertension. Even though it is believed that incompetence in the deep system of veins, particularly the popliteal vein, is an important component in the development of CVI, the location of valvular incompetence in patients with CVI seems to be very variable.

Despite a large number of studies, no specific pattern of incompetence has yet been identified. Using duplex scanning, patients with CVI have been shown to have valve dysfunction and reflux in the deep veins of the leg; furthermore, the presence of distal reflux in the popliteal segment has been demonstrated to correlate well with the severity of disease.[114] In fact, some have argued that this is an essential feature, in the absence of which, patients are unlikely to progress to an advanced stage of the disease. However, in our studies of patients with CVI, valvular incompetence was not limited to the deep system of veins (Table 2).[113] Some patients with CVI had abnormalities in the superficial veins only with no evidence of reflux in their deep veins,[113] a finding which seems to be in agreement with other reports.[115,116] Thus, it would appear that deep or perforating vein incompetence is not a prerequisite for CVI and, further, that some patients with deep or perforator incompetence will not necessarily progress to lipodermatosclerosis and ulceration.

Regardless of the primary abnormality, there is general agreement that venous hypertension is an important factor in the development of CVI. Shull[114] noted that venous ulceration was associated with elevated AVP and the presence of incompetent popliteal valves. Using light reflection rheography, Mac-Enroe[117] found that 79% of patients with venous ulcers had abnormal venous refill times; patients with less severe CVI had less abnormal venous refill times. Christopoulos[37] correlated the clinical severity of chronic venous disease with the severity of reflux, and in a more recent report by Nicolaides,[118] elevated ambulatory venous pressures appeared to be strongly associated with venous ulceration.

While hemodynamic abnormalities can be demonstrated in some patients with CVI, physiologic studies have generally failed to define clear parameters associated with development of CVI. Raju[119] was unable to document elevated venous pressures in a large proportion of patients with CVI and suggested that ambulatory venous hypertension may not be the only factor responsible for the generation of stasis ulcerations. We used APG to compare and contrast venous hemodynamics in normal subjects, patients with CVI, and patients with varicose veins but no evidence of CVI. Not surprisingly, both the patients with CVI and those with varicose veins differed substantially from the normal subjects (Table 3).[87] There were some differences between CVI patients and varicose vein patients as well. As a group, the CVI patients tended to have somewhat more evidence of outflow obstruction (decreased maximal venous outflow [MVO]), slightly worse reflux (higher venous filling index [VFI]), and significantly higher residual volume fractions (RVF), suggesting higher AVP. However, for each of these parameters there was an enormous amount of overlap between the CVI and varicose vein patients, and there was no abnormality or combination of abnormalities clearly associated with CVI. In fact, one was struck more by the remarkable degree of similarity between extremities with varicose veins and those with CVI than by any differences. Similar findings have since been reported by Van Bemmelen.[120]

Our inability to clearly identify the critical events or elements in CVI pathogenesis is related to several factors. First, it is unclear what proportion of CVI is a late sequela of venous thrombosis or how often thrombosis results in CVI. Venous thrombosis of the lower extremities appears to be extremely common, but it is often subclinical, so a past history of thrombosis is unlikely to be a sensitive indicator of its occurrence. In addition, the recognition that a given individual is developing CVI is likely to occur years after an episode of thrombosis that may have been responsible for initiating the process. Another problem is that the available diagnostic tests are relatively good at identifying abnormalities in large proximal veins, but the venous pathology which is responsible for triggering CVI may be limited to the smaller veins of the calf, which are beyond the limits of detection at present. Consequently, it is possible that important morphologic or physiologic differences between patients with CVI and those with varicose veins will eventually be discovered. Finally, there may be other factors in addition to hemodynamic abnormalities which contribute to the evolution of CVI. For example, it has been reported that patients with CVI tend to trap monocytes in their legs in the dependent position.[121] This phenomenon could be indicative of leukocyte activation and might be important in understanding what triggers the inflammatory reaction seen in these patients. If so, it would be important to determine whether leukocyte activation is a consequence of the hemodynamic abnormalities or whether activation is more likely in these individuals because of other factors (e.g., immunologic, dietary, or environmental factors) which have not yet come to our attention.

Future investigations correlating the anatomy, physiology, and epidemiology of venous insufficiency will undoubtedly improve our understanding of its pathophysiology. Further anatomic and radiologic studies of the muscular veins in the leg and their fascial coverings may identify specific abnormalities in patients with CVI. Additional studies looking at the effects of pregnancy, posture, occupation, and trauma on venous hemodynamics may help to better define patients at risk and identify clinically significant hemodynamic abnormalities at an early stage in order to interrupt the progression to end-stage disease. Finally, continued studies of cellular physiology and the interaction between the cellular elements of blood and the vessel wall will likely provide essential information regarding the pathogenesis of lipodermatosclerosis and venous ulceration.

Table 3
Characterization of Normal, Varicose Vein, and Venous Ulcer Patients by Air Plethysmography (mean ± SE)

	Normal (n = 59)	Varicose Vein (n = 39)	CVI (n = 83)
MVO	54.4 ± 1.4	54.4 ± 1.2	51.3 ± 1.6*
VFI	1.0 ± 0.1	5.4 ± 0.6	6.8 ± 0.6
VVol	108.8 ± 4.2	144.6 ± 7.1	141.1 ± 7.9
EF	58.6 ± 1.9	48.6 ± 1.8	51.9 ± 1.6
RVF	30.5 ± 1.9	39.8 ± 2.6	50.9 ± 2.0**

MVO: maximal venous outflow; VFI: venous filling index; VVol: total venous volume; EF: ejection fraction; RVF: residual volume fraction.

* Differs from varicose vein, $p < 0.05$ (age-adjusted).

** Differs from varicose vein, $p < 0.01$ (age-adjusted).

(Reproduced with permission from Reference 87.)

References

1. Braverman IM: Ultrastructure and organization of the cutaneous microvasculature in normal and pathologic states. *J Invest Dermat* 93:2S-9S, 1989.

2. Negus D: The surgical anatomy of the veins of the lower limb. In: Dodd H, Cockett FB, (eds). *The Pathology and Surgery of the Veins of the Lower Limb.* Edinburgh: Churchill Livingstone; 18, 1976.

3. Shah DM, Chang BB, Leopold PW: The anatomy of the greater saphenous system. *J Vasc Surg* 3:273–283, 1986.

4. May R: *Surgery of the Veins of the Leg and Pelvis.* Philadelphia: W.B. Saunders Company; 1–36, 1979.

5. Haeger K: The surgical anatomy of the sapheno-femoral and sapheno-popliteal junctions. *J Cardiovasc Surg* 6:420–427, 1962.

6. Kosinski C: Observations on the superficial venous system of the lower extremity. *J Anat* 60:131–141, 1926.

7. Van Limborgh J: L'anatomie du système veineux de l'extrémité inferieure en relation avec la pathologie variqueuse. *Folia Angiol* 8:3–12, 1961.

8. Kerr TM, Smith JM, McKenna P, et al: Venous and arterial anomalies of the lower extremities diagnosed by duplex scanning. *Surg Gynecol Obstet* 175(4):309–312, 1992.

9. Linton RR: The communicating veins of the lower leg and the operative technique for their ligation. *Ann Surg* 107:582–588, 1938.

10. Askar O: On the surgical anatomy of the communicating veins of the leg. *J Cardiovasc Surg* 4:138–151, 1963.

11. Cockett FB: The pathology and treatment of venous ulcers of the leg. *Br J Surg* 179:260–266, 1955.

12. Bouchet A: Anatomie morphologique des valvules des membres inferieures. *Phlebologie* 45(3):233–244, 1992.

13. Saphir O, Lev M: Venous valvulitis. *Arch Pathol Lab Med* 53:456–469, 1952.

14. Cox JL, Chiasson DA, Gotlieb A: Stranger in a strange land: the pathogenesis of saphenous vein graft stenosis with emphasis on structural and functional differences between veins and arteries. *Prog Cardiovasc Dis* 34(1): 45–68, 1991.

15. Sumner DS: Hemodynamics and pathophysiology of venous disease. In: Rutherford RB (ed). *Vascular Surgery*, 3rd ed. Philadelphia: WB Saunders Company; 1483, 1989.

16. Webster MW, Ramadan F: Vascular physiology. In: Simmons, Steed (eds). *Basic Science Review for Surgeons.* Philadelphia: WB Saunders Company; 203, 1992.

17. Van Bemmelen PS, Beach K, Bedford G: The mechanism of venous valve closure. *Arch Surg* 125:617–619, 1990.

18. Raju S, Fredericks R, Lishman P, et al: Observations on the calf venous pump mechanism: determinants of postexercise pressure. *J Vasc Surg* 17:459–469, 1993.

19. Takata M, Wise RA, Robotham JL: Effects of abdominal pressure on venous return: abdominal vascular zones conditions. *J Appl Physiol* 69(6):1961–1972, 1990.

20. Cotran RS: New roles for the endothelium in inflammation and immunity. *Am J Path* 129:407–411, 1987.

21. Wu KK: Endothelial cells in hemostasis, thrombosis, and inflammation. *Hosp Pract* 4:87–98, 1992.

22. Davies MG, Hagen PO: The vascular endothelium: a new horizon. *Ann Surg* 218(5):596–609, 1993.

23. Nerem RM, Girard PR: Hemodynamic influences on vascular endothelial biology. *Toxicol Path* 18:572–582, 1990.

24. Griendling KK: Control of vascular tone by the endothelium: new insights. *J Crit Illness* 8(3):355–370, 1993.

25. Bernstein EF (ed): *Noninvasive Diagnostic Techniques in Vascular Disease.* St. Louis: The CV Mosby Company; 1985.

26. Nicolaides AN, Sumner DS: *Investigation of Patients with Deep Vein Thrombosis and Chronic Venous Insufficiency.* London: Med-Orion Publishing Company; 1991.

27. Bergan JJ, Yao JST (eds). *Venous Disorders.* Philadelphia: WB Saunders Company; 1991.

28. Talbot SR: B-mode evaluation of peripheral arteries and veins. In: Zwiebel WJ (ed). *Introduction to Vascular Ultrasonography.* 2nd ed. Philadelphia: WB Saunders Company; 351, 1992.

29. Bergan JJ, Kistner RL (eds): *Atlas of Venous Surgery.* Philadelphia: WB Saunders Company; 1992.

30. Van Bemmelen PS, Bergan JJ: *Quantitative Measurement of Venous Incompetence.* RG Landes Company; 1992.

31. Bergan JJ: Historical highlights in healing venous insufficiency. In: Bergan JJ, Yao JST (eds). *Venous Disorders.* Philadelphia: WB Saunders Company; 1991.

32. Belcaro G, Labropoulos N, Christopoulos DC, et al: Noninvasive tests in venous insufficiency. *J Cardiovasc Surg* 34:3–11, 1993.

33. Belcaro G, Christopoulos DC, Nicolaides AN: Lower extremity venous hemodynamics. *Ann Vasc Surg* 5: 305–310, 1991.

34. Raju S: New approaches to the diagnosis and treatment of venous obstruction. *J Vasc Surg* 4:42–54,1986.

35. Kistner RL, Ferris EB, Randhawa G, et al: Method of performing descending venography. *J Vasc Surg* 4: 464–468, 1986.

36. Christopoulos DC, Nicolaides AN, Szendro G: Air-plethysmography and the effect of elastic compression on venous haemodynamics of the leg. *J Vasc Surg* 5: 148–159, 1987.

37. Christopoulos DC, Nicolaides AN, Szendro G: Venous reflux: quantification and correlation with the clinical severity of chronic venous disease. *Br J Surg* 75: 352–356, 1988.

38. Christopoulos DC, Nicolaides AN: Noninvasive diagnosis and quantification of popliteal reflux in the swollen and ulcerated leg. *J Cardiovasc Surg* 29:535–539, 1988.

39. Christopoulos DC, Nicolaides AN, Galloway JM, et al: Objective noninvasive evaluation of venous surgical results. *J Vasc Surg* 8:683–687, 1988.

40. Christopoulos DC, Nicolaides AN, Irvine A, et al: Pathogenesis of venous ulceration in relation to the calf muscle pump function. *Surgery* 106:829–835, 1989.

41. Gillespie DL, Cordts PR, Hartono C, et al: The role of air-plethysmography in monitoring results of venous surgery. *J Vasc Surg* 16:674–678, 1992.

42. Raju S, Fredericks R: Evaluation of methods for detecting venous reflux: perspectives in venous insufficiency. *Arch Surg* 125:1463–1467, 1990.

43. Pearce WH, Ricco JB, Queral LA, et al: Hemodynamic assessment of venous problems. *Surgery* 93:715–720, 1983.

44. Norris CS, Beyrau A, Barnes RW: Quantitative photoplethysmography in chronic venous insufficiency: a new method of noninvasive estimation of ambulatory venous pressure. *Surgery* 94:758–764, 1983.

45. Abramowitz HB, Queral LA, Flinn WR, et al: The use of photoplethysmography in the assessment of venous insufficiency: a comparison to venous pressure measurements. *Surgery* 86:434–441, 1979.

46. McEnroe CS, O'Donnell TF Jr: Noninvasive evaluation

of chronic venous insufficiency. *Seminars in Vascular Surgery* 1:73–85, 1988.

47. Hanrahan LM, Araki CT, Fisher JB, et al: Evaluation of the perforating veins in the lower extremity using high resolution duplex imaging. *J Cardiovasc Surg* 32:87–97, 1991.

48. Rollins DL, Semrow CM, Friedell ML, et al: Use of ultrasonic venography in the evaluation of venous valve function. *Am J Surg* 154:189–191, 1987.

49. Szendro G, Nicolaides AN, Zukowski AJ, et al: Duplex scanning in the assessment of deep venous incompetence. *J Vasc Surg* 4:237–242, 1986.

50. Weingarten MS, Branas CC, Czeredarczuk M, et al: Distribution and quantification of venous reflux in lower extremity chronic venous stasis disease with duplex scanning. *J Vasc Surg* 18:753–759, 1993.

51. Cranley JJ (ed): *Atlas of Duplex Scanning.* Philadelphia: WB Saunders Company; 1992.

52. Strandness DE, Van Bemmelen PS: Quantitations of venous duplex scanning. In: Bergan JJ, Yao JST (eds). *Venous Disorders.* Philadelphia: WB Saunders Company; 1991.

53. Araki CT, Back TL, Padberg FT Jr, et al: Refinements in the ultrasonic detection of popliteal vein reflux. *J Vasc Surg* 18:742–748, 1993.

54. Negus D: *Leg Ulcers: A Practical Approach to Management.* Oxford, UK: Butterworth-Heineman Ltd.; 1991.

55. Coon WW, Park WW, Keller JB: Venous thromboembolism and other venous diseases in the Tecumseh community health study. *Circulation* 158:839–846, 1973.

56. Abramson JH, Hopp C, Epstein LM: The epidemiology of varicose veins: a survey in western Jerusalem. *J Epidemiol Community Health* 35:213–217, 1981.

57. Hirai M, Aniki K, Nakayama R: Prevalence and risk factors of varicose veins in Japanese women. *Angiology* 41:228–232, 1990.

58. Franks PJ, Wright DD, Moffatt CJ, et al: Prevalence of venous disease: a community study in West London. *Eur J Surg* 158:143–147, 1992.

59. Dindelli M, Parazzini F, Basellini A, et al: Risk factors for varicose disease before and during pregnancy. *Angiology* 44:361–367, 1993.

60. Saddick NS: Predisposing factors of varicose veins and telangectatic veins. *J Dermatol Surg Oncol* 18:883–886, 1992.

61. Eberth-Willershausen W, Marshall M: Prevalence, risk factors, and complications of peripheral venous diseases in the Munich population. *Hautarzt* 35:68–77, 1984.

62. Stvrtinova V, Kolesar J, Wimmer G: Prevalence of varicose veins of the lower limbs in women working at a department store. *Int Angiol* 10:2–5, 1991.

63. Sun JM: Epidemiologic study on peripheral vascular diseases in Shanghai. *Chung Hua Wai Tsa Chih* 28:480–483, 1990.

64. Alexander CJ: The epidemiology of varicose veins. *Med J Aust* 1:215–218, 1972.

65. Brand FN, Dannenberg AL, Abbott RD, et al: The epidemiology of varicose veins: the Framingham study. *Am J Prev Med* 4:96–101, 1988.

66. Latto C, Wilkinson RW, Gilmore OJA: Diverticular disease and varicose veins. *Lancet* 19:1089–1090,1973.

67. Geelhoed GW, Burkitt DP: Varicose veins: a reappraisal from a global perspective. *South Med J* 84:1131–1134, 1991.

68. Rose SS: The aetiology of varicose veins. In: Negus D,

Jantet G (eds). *Phlebology 1985.* London: Libbey; 6, 1986.

69. Svejcar, Prerovsky I, Linhart J, et al: Content of collagen, elastin, and hexosamine in primary varicose veins. *Clin Sci* 24:325–330, 1963.

70. Haardt B: A comparison of the histochemical enzyme pattern in normal and varicose veins. *Phlebology* 2:135–158, 1987.

71. Gandhi RH, Irizarry E, Nackman GB, et al: Analysis of the connective tissue matrix and proteolytic activity of primary varicose veins. *J Vasc Surg* 18:814–820, 1993.

72. Edwards JE, Edwards EA: The saphenous valves in varicose veins. *Am Heart J* 19:338–340, 1940.

73. Blalock A: Oxygen content of blood in patients with varicose veins. *Arch Surg* 19:898–900, 1929.

74. Haimovici H, Steinman C, Caplan LH: Role of arteriovenous anastomoses in vascular diseases of the lower extremity. *Ann Surg* 164:990–992, 1966.

75. Bergan JJ: New developments in the surgical treatment of venous disease. *Cardiovasc Surg* 1:624–631, 1993.

76. Lowell RC, Gloviszki P, Miller VM: In vitro evaluation of endothelial cells and smooth muscle function of primary varicose veins. *J Vasc Surg* 16:679–686, 1992.

77. Hanrahan LM, Kechejian GJ, Cordts PR, et al: Patterns of venous insufficiency in patients with varicose veins. *Arch Surg* 126:687–691, 1988.

78. Basmajian JV: The distribution in the femoral, external iliac, and common iliac veins and their relationship to varicose veins. *Surg Gynecol Obstet* 95:537–542, 1952.

79. Egen SA, Casper SL: Etiology of varicose veins from an anatomic aspect based on dissection of 38 adult cadavers. *JAMA* 123:148–189, 1943.

80. Browse NL. Commentary. In: Eclof B, Gjores JE, Phulesius D, Berjquist D (eds). *Controversies in the Management of Venous Disorders.* Stoneham, MA: Butterworth; 192, 1989.

81. Mayberry JC, Moneta GL, Taylor LM Jr, et al: Nonoperative treatment of venous stasis ulcer. In: Bergan JJ, Yao JST (eds). *Venous Disorders.* Philadelphia: WB Saunders Company; 381, 1991.

82. Ferris EB, Kisner RL: Femoral vein reconstruction and the management of chronic venous insufficiency. *Arch Surg* 117:1571–1579, 1982.

83. Baker SR, Stacey MC, Singh G, et al: Aetiology of chronic leg ulcers. *Eur J Vasc Surg* 6:245–251, 1992.

84. Cornwall JV, Dore CJ, Lewis JD: Leg ulcers: epidemiology and aetiology. *Br J Surg* 73:693–696, 1986.

85. Callam M: Prevalence of chronic leg ulceration and severe chronic venous disease in western countries. *Phlebology* (suppl) 1:6–12, 1992.

86. The Alexander House Group: Consensus paper on venous leg ulcer. *J Dermatol Surg Oncol* 18:592–602, 1992.

87. Cordts PR, Hartono C, LaMorte WW, et al: Physiologic similarities between extremities with varicose veins and chronic venous insufficiency utilizing air-plethysmography. *Am J Surg* 164:260–264, 1992.

88. Ryan TJ, Burnand K: Diseases of the veins and arteries: leg ulcers. In: Champion RH, Burton JL, Ebling FJG (eds). *Textbook of Dermatology.* Oxford, UK: Blackwell Scientific Publication; 1992.

89. Lever W: *Histopathology of the Skin.* Philadelphia: JB Lippincott Company; 1990.

90. Kirsner RS, Pardes P, Eaglstein W, et al: The clinical spectrum of lipodermatosclerosis. *J Am Acad Dermatol* 28:623–627, 1993.

91. Jorizzo JL, White WL, Zanolli MD, et al: Sclerosing panniculitis. *Arch Dermatol* 115:449–452, 1991.

92. Phillips TJ, Bhawan J: unpublished data.

93. Adair HM: Epidermal repair in chronic venous ulcers. *Br J Surg* 64:800–804, 1977.

94. Phillips TJ, Samonte B, Leigh IM, et al: Expression of keratins, involucrin, integrins, and kallinin in acute and chronic wounds. *J Invest Dermatol* 25:547A, 1993.

95. Leu HJ: Morphology of chronic venous insufficiency: light and electron microscopic examinations. *VASA* 20:330–342, 1991.

96. Laaf H, Vanscheidt W, Weiss JM, et al: Immunohisto-chemical investigation of pericytes in chronic venous disease. *VASA* 20:323–328, 1991.

97. Herrick SE, Sloan P, McGurk M, et al: Sequential changes in histologic pattern and extracellular matrix deposition during the healing of chronic venous ulcers. *Am J Pathol* 141:1085–1095, 1992.

98. Frain-Bell W: Atrophie blanche. *Trans St Johns Hosp Dermatol Soc* 42:59–65, 1959.

99. Milstone M, Braverman IM, Lucky A, et al: Classification and therapy of atrophie blanche. *Arch Dermatol* 119:963–969, 1983.

100. Nodl F: Zur Histopathogense der Atrophie Blanche. *Milian Dermatol Wochenschir* 121:193–200, 1950.

101. Browse NL, Burnand KG: The cause of venous ulceration. *Lancet* 11:243–245, 1982.

102. Falanga V, Moosa HH, Nemeth AJ, et al: Dermal peri-capillary fibrin in venous disease and venous ulceration. *Arch Dermatol* 123:620–623, 1987.

103. Vanscheidt W, Laaf H, Wokalek H, et al: Pericapillary fibrin cuff: a histologic sign of venous leg ulceration. *J Cutan Pathol* 17:266–268, 1990.

104. Falanga V, Kirsner R, Katz MH, et al: Pericapillary fibrin cuffs in venous ulceration: persistence with treatment and during ulcer healing. *J Dermatol Surg Oncol* 8:409–414, 1992.

105. Gay J: On varicose disease of the lower extremities. *The Lettsomian Lectures of 1867*. London: Churchill; 1868.

106. Homans J: The operative treatment of varicose veins and ulcers based upon a classification of these lesions. *Surg Gynecol Obstet* 22:143–158, 1916.

107. Bauer J: The aetiology of leg ulcers and their treatment by resection of the popliteal vein. *J Int Chir* 8:937–960, 1948.

108. Krupski WC, Bass A, Dilley RB, et al: Propagation of deep venous thrombosis identified by duplex ultraso-nography. *J Vasc Surg* 12:468–475, 1990.

109. Markel A, Manzo RA, Bergelin RO, et al: Valvular re-flux after deep vein thrombosis: incidence and time of occurrence. *J Vasc Surg* 15:377–384, 1992.

110. Killewich LA, Bedford GR, Beach KW, et al: Sponta-neous lysis of deep venous thrombi: rate and outcome. *J Vasc Surg* 9:89–97, 1989.

111. Raju S, Fredericks R: Valve reconstruction procedures for non-obstructive venous insufficiency: rationale, techniques, and results in 107 procedures with 2- to 8-year follow-up. *J Vasc Surg* 7:301–310, 1988.

112. Train JS, Schanzer H, Peirce EC, et al: Radiological evaluation of the chronic venous stasis syndrome. *JAMA* 258:941–944, 1987.

113. Hanrahan LM, Araki CT, Rodrigues AA, et al: Distri-bution of valvular incompetence in patients with venous stasis ulceration. *J Vasc Surg* 13:805–812, 1991.

114. Shull KC, Nicolaides AN, Fernandes e Fernandes J, et al: Significance of popliteal reflux in relation to ambula-tory venous pressure and ulceration. *Arch Surg* 114:1304–1306, 1979.

115. Hoare MC, Nicolaides AN, Miles CR, et al: The role of primary varicose veins in venous obstruction. *Surgery* 92:450–453, 1982.

116. Sethia KK, Darke SG: Long saphenous incompetence as a cause of venous ulceration. *Br J Surg* 71:754–755, 1984.

117. McEnroe CS, O'Donnell TF Jr, Mackey WC: Correla-tion of clinical findings with venous hemodynamics in 386 patients with chronic venous insufficiency. *AJS* 156:148–152, 1988.

118. Nicolaides AN, Hussein MK, Szendro G, et al: The relation of venous ulceration with ambulatory venous pressure measurements. *J Vasc Surg* 17:414–419, 1993.

119. Raju S, Fredericks R: Hemodynamic basis of stasis ul-ceration: a hypothesis. *J Vasc Surg* 13:491–495, 1991.

120. Van Bemmelen PS, Mattos MA, Hodgson KJ, et al: Does air-plethysmography correlate with duplex scan-ning in patients with chronic venous insufficiency? *J Vasc Surg* 18:796–807, 1993.

121. LaMorte WW, Cordts PR, Hanrahan LM, et al: Leuko-cytes, lipids, and chronic venous insufficiency: a new perspective on an old disease. *Vasc Surg* 1:95–107, 1993.

CHAPTER 15

Cellular Mechanisms in Venous Disease

John J. Bergan, MD

Ultimately, tissue changes of venous insufficiency are expressed on the skin and in subcutaneous tissue. There, cellular events take place which lead to clinical findings. These, in the past, have been termed the "postphlebitic state." Although this term is time-honored, a better term is chronic venous insufficiency (CVI). This may be the end product of obstructive and valvular destructive effects of venous thrombosis. More importantly, all of the chronic changes may be caused by superficial venous incompetence, perforator vein reflux, or primary deep venous incompetence.

A unified theory of the cause of CVI is now conceivable. However, the exact triggering mechanism which differentiates limbs with long-standing varicose veins, but without skin changes, from limbs with identical venous pathophysiology which have severe, late ravages of CVI, has not been identified.[1] It is acknowledged that some extremities wth CVI, and some with only varicose veins, may differ substantially hemodynamically from one another. Air-plethysmography (APG) has proven this; however, APG has shown considerable hemodynamic overlap among limbs with early varicosities, normal limbs, and those with CVI. The Boston group summarized their impressions on this subject saying, " . . . for the most part, one is struck more by the remarkable degree of similarity between extremities with varicose veins and those with chronic venous insufficiency than by their differences."[2]

Progression of venous insufficiency is characteristic in limbs with venous problems. An examination of limbs on the waiting list for surgery revealed what clinicians have long known. Further sources of reflux are identified, lipodermatosclerosis newly develops, and had surgery been undertaken immediately, many patients would have required further interventions.[3] Thus, it is acknowledged that venous insufficiency is progressive, that fundamental pathologic hemodynamic mechanisms are the same across the various ranges of venous insufficiency, and that the triggering mechanism which initiates complications has not been found.

Hemodynamic Forces

Cellular and/or molecular events are inseparable from hemodynamic forces acting in the diseased venous system. Common anatomic patterns of varicose veins suggest two influences. These are easily studied hemodynamically.[4] One is the gravitational influence transmitted through incompetent saphenofemoral and saphenopopliteal junctions and to the unsupported subdermal reticular, flat, blue-green network of veins on the anterior and lateral aspects of the thigh. Gravitational forces are expressed as mm of water pressure. They are equivalent to the weight of a column of blood from the right atrium transmitted through incompetent valves to the point of measurement.

It is gravitational reflux that has been greatly emphasized in prescribing therapy for venous insufficiency. For example, Trendelenburg advocated ligation of the saphenous vein based on the theory that this would decrease distal venous pressure. Gravitational reflux is detected easily by Doppler and duplex ultrasound techniques. These are an important part of the examination of patients with venous insufficiency.[5,6] Gravitational reflux does influence deep venous function (Figure 1). Either primary or secondary failure of

From *The Basic Science of Vascular Disease*. Edited by Sidawy AN, Sumpio BE, and DePalma RG. Armonk, NY: Futura Publishing Company, Inc.; © 1997.

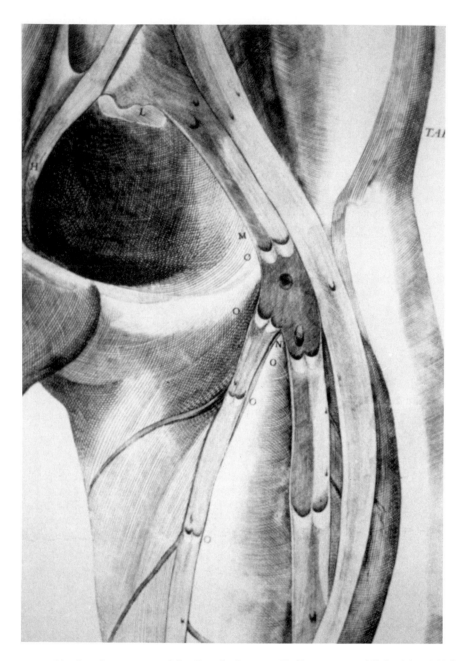

Figure 1. This drawing, executed by Jan Stefan van Kalkan, was published in 1963 in a monograph by Hieronymus Fabricius. The anatomy shown elegantly displays the difference between arteries and veins, and shows the paired valves in the common femoral vein, the saphenous vein, and the superficial femoral vein with the relationship of tributaries to those valves. Notice the important medial posterior tributary to the saphenous vein and the multiple tributaries in the mid-thigh. It is these tributaries that allow persistence of saphenous patency in the refluxing saphenous vein which is surgically interrupted at its saphenofemoral origin. Placement of these valves and the intervals between them were emphasized by Fabricius who said that these were placed to delay the blood from " . . . flooding into the feet . . . and collecting there." (Reproduced with permission from Bergan JJ, Yao JST (eds). *Venous Disorders*. Philadelphia: WB Saunders, Co.; 1989.)

deep valve function permits distribution of the weight of the column of blood more distally. This may play a part in dilation of vein walls to increase further incompetence of distal venous valves. Gravitational reflux appears to be detected better by duplex scanning than by descending phlebography.[7,8]

As important as gravitational reflux is, it is not the only force acting to cause venous insufficiency.[5] The other hemodynamic influence acting on cutaneous and subcutaneous tissues is a powerful hydrodynamic force transmitted from muscular compartments through failed perforator vein check valves.[1] The actual importance of perforating veins and their incompetent valves is a controversial subject. Most observers consider them important. Some even feel that they are of prime importance.[9] Cockett's influence on this subject led to ankle perforating veins being named for him.[10] However, recurrent venous ulcerations occurring after surgical interruption of incompetent perforating veins have cast some doubt on their influence.[11] Nevertheless, it is certain that large perforating veins which permit outward flow are commonly associated with the severe changes of CVI.[12] Clinical observations confirm elegant physiologic studies by Arnoldi which described very high systolic (muscular contraction) pressure in all veins of the lower leg and especially those at the ankle.[13] These studies complement previous work by Bjordal[14] which showed bidirectional flow through perforating veins during ambulation with inward flow during a "foot-lifting" phase (diastole), and an outward flow in the "foot-on-the-ground" phase (systole). Main flow was detected to be inward, but very high systolic pressures were generated in the skin through incompetent superficial veins (Figure 2).

Physiologic studies have focused on calf perforating veins. These transmit pressure externally.[15] In addition, similar dynamic pressure changes are transmitted through failed perforating veins in the thigh[16] and characteristic locations about the knee.[17,18]

Cellular Pathology in the Vein Wall

Histologic studies have shown that the vein walls of the saphenous and jugular systems have a similar arrangement of endothelium, muscle, and fibrous tissue. All layers are much thinner in veins subjected to less pressure.[19–21] In varicose veins, weakness of the venous wall is often localized, occurring in scattered areas and in regions of different magnitude along the various veins of the lower extremities. Histologically, the weaknesses appear to be caused by thinning of the muscular layer of the venous wall which allows dilations clinically apparent as varicosities.[22] Grossly, these changes have been noted at the site of the upper valve of the saphenous vein proximal to the valve and,

importantly, in different areas along the vein even between two normal valves. Such clinical observations, backed up by histology, suggest a hereditary cause for the localized thinning of the muscular layer of the venous wall.[23] This occurs independent of valvular incompetence, but clearly can be influenced by it when present. Valvular incompetence, in such situations, can occur if the valve ring is allowed to dilate because of vein wall weakness. These influences of wall weakness and valve dysfunction can act in axial veins, saphenous systems, tributary veins, and in perforating veins. The upper anteromedial calf perforating veins, distal thigh perforating veins, and Hunterian perforating veins are typical.[24]

Hormonal Influences

The gross and microscopic changes indicated suggest a hereditary influence on the development of varicose veins and venous insufficiency. This has been confirmed in many studies, most recently by Sadick who found 84% of 420 patients had a genetic predisposition.[25] He suggested that the inheritance was a sex-linked autosomal-dominant influence with incomplete penetrance and variable expressivity.

Hormonal influences have been linked to the development of varicose telangiectatic complexes. Pregnancy is the most powerful hormonal event and is dominated by progesterone influences. In pregnancy, at least 30% of patients will detect telangiectasias and varicosities in the first trimester and another 24% during the second. Thus, more than half of varicosities develop before maximal uterine size and blood flow are reached in the final trimester. Sadick said," . . . varicose and telangiectatic veins may occur during the early first trimester of pregnancy, before significant uterine enlargement, suggesting that increased hydrostatic pressure is not the sole mechanism of development of telangiectatic and varicose veins." Since estrogen and progesterone receptors are absent in the vein walls of telangiectasias and varicosities, it has been concluded that estrogen and progestational agents act indirectly on the endothelial vascular complex to induce vasodilation and perhaps even angioproliferative activity.

It is a common misconception that varicose veins are caused by uterine compression on iliac vessels, or inferior vena cava, or by an increase in blood flow through the uterine wall.[26] As indicated, most varicosities appear before the size of the uterus is sufficient to compress pelvic vessels. Sumner has said that "the theory of the influence of sexual hormones actually holds and is confirmed by the observation of a spectacular regression of varicose veins in the immediate postpartum period."[27]

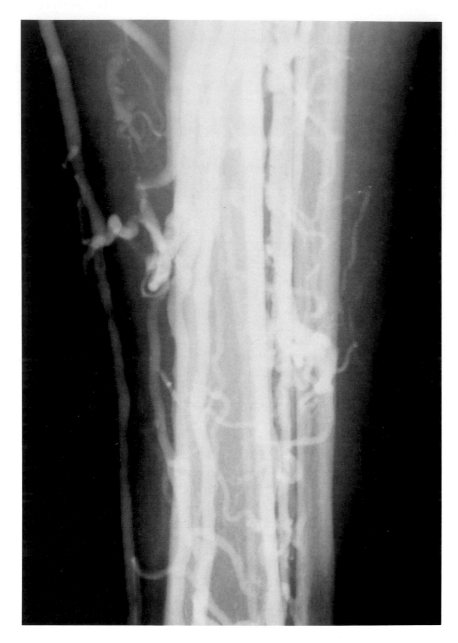

Figure 2A. Medial calf perforating veins are those which allow bidirectional flow, and flow outward during calf muscular contraction, transmitting high muscular intracompartmental pressures to unsupported veins in the subcutaneous tissue and skin. Note the pronounced elongation of the medial calf perforating vein and the absence of changes which would indicate previous deep venous thrombosis in the crural veins.

In an analysis of symptoms of venous insufficiency in correlation with therapeutic doses of estro-progestogen, Vin showed that heaviness, pain, and paresthesias were significantly more common in patients with normal dose pills than patients receiving minimum dose treatment.[28] Medications containing 10 μg estrogen and 500 mg progesterone were particularly culpable. This suggests that estrogens cause an increase in capillary permeability with edema formation, and progesterones produce a loss of muscular tone, particularly in the media. This affects venous compliance. Functional symptomatology of venous insufficiency often precedes actual dilation and clinical evidence of varicosities. Thus, it is interesting to speculate that oral contraceptive agents over time may contribute to the development of varicose veins. This may occur particularly in those patients who have a hereditary predisposition.

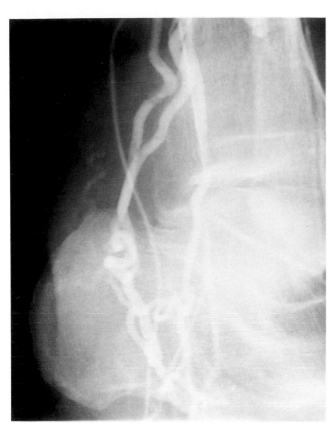

Figure 2B. Perforating veins in the retromalleolar and infra-malleolar position are extremely important as they transmit both gravitational forces and hydrodynamic forces to the unsupported cutaneous and subcutaneous venules.

Estrogen and/or progesterone interactions have been shown by physiologic studies.[29] For example, the venotropic activity of RUSCUS extract appears to be enhanced following exposure to progesterone, but that effect is reversed by the addition of estrogen. The adrenergic component of muscular contraction is enhanced by progesterone and decreased by estrogen. The nonadrenergic component itself is more prominent when serum levels of female steroid hormones are low.

Chronic Venous Insufficiency

The association of deep venous thrombosis with subsequent venous ulceration was recognized in the nineteenth century; hence, the persistence of the term *postphlebitic leg* as used to describe the chronic stigmata of venous insufficiency (Table 1). Homans' 1917 paper on venous ulcerations has been often quoted.[30] He is credited with the concept of tissue anoxia which arises from stagnant, deoxygenated blood causing ulceration. Although de Takats[31] found decreased levels of oxygen in venous blood of limbs with venous ulceration, that report was refuted by Alfred Blalock.[32] Sub-

sequently, many investigators have found a higher venous oxygen content in blood taken from limbs with CVI.[33,34]

Elevated PO_2 in venous blood from limbs with venous insufficiency is probably explained by the opening of thermoregulatory shunts.[35] This is the most likely explanation for the rapid venous filling seen in arteriography of limbs with CVI.[36,37] This is also the most likely explanation for the identified abnormal arteriovenous communications (AVC) detected by Gius[38] and more recent investigators such as Haeger[39] and Schalin.[40] The presence of such abnormal AVC has been refuted by Partsch,[41] but that one report, however influential, does not answer all the questions raised by those who have detected evidence of arterio-

---

Table 1
Proposed Theory of Origin of Skin and Subcutaneous Changes of Chronic Venous Insufficiency

I. Valvular Reflux

  1. Hereditary/hormonal origin
  2. Thrombotic destruction

II. Gravitational Reflux

  1. Superficial venous system
  2. Deep venous system

III. Hydrodynamic Reflux

  1. Perforator valve incompetence
  2. Muscular compartment pressure transmitted to superficial veins

IV. Dilation, Elongation, Tortuosity of Dermal, Subdermal, Subcutaneous Venules

  1. Breakdown of arteriovenous thermoregulatory barrier
  2. Creation of arteriovenous microfistulae
  3. Increased capillary permeability, leakage of fibrinogen

V. Leukocyte Trapping

  1. Leukocyte trapping
  2. Leukocyte activation
  3. Proteolysis
  4. Toxic oxygen destruction of tissue
  5. Defective fibrinolysis

This table proposes to link the various observations that have been made regarding leg ulcers of venous etiology. A description of each of these separate elements is found in the text.

venous shunting in CVI. The question remains open and even unanswered since recent review of the subject by Scott.[42]

Laser Doppler studies[43] have demonstrated increased values of arterial blood flow which do not increase further after local heating. Other methods of blood flow quantitation, including scintigraphy and xenon clearance, confirm an increased blood flow in the region of venous ulcerations. That the hyperdynamic circulation may be dependent upon AVC remains open, as Partsch's study used 30 μm diameter beads, and the shunts themselves may have been even smaller.[44,45]

It may be that sympathetic neuropathy plays a part in the causation of hyperdynamic circulation in venous insufficiency.[46] Certainly, the sympathetically controlled venoarteriolar reflux is impaired in CVI.[47,48] Whatever its effect, or its origin, the presence of excessive circulation in CVI is undoubted. Further investigations of this should prove fruitful.[49]

Fibrin Cuff Theory

After rejecting theories of venous stasis as proposed by Homans, and arteriovenous shunts as mentioned, Browse and Burnand proposed a fibrin cuff theory of tissue hypo-oxygenation.[50] They recognized that high venous pressure was associated with increased permeability of large molecules into the skin of limbs affected by CVI.[51] Fibrinogen was shown to leak significantly faster into the calf skin in limbs in which a high venous pressure had been produced. A close relationship was found between fibrin deposition, capillary proliferation, and venous pump malfunction.[52] Patients with lipodermatosclerosis were found to have defective fibrinolysis, and their plasma fibrinogen proved to be raised even as tissue fibrinolysis was decreased. These findings led to the theory that fibrin cuffs surrounding arterioles constituted a barrier to diffusion of oxygen and other nutrients from the capillaries to the skin. This hypothesis has remained dominant and much quoted throughout the late 1980s and early 1990s. The finding of reduced transcutaneous oxygen tension in lipodermatosclerotic skin supported the ideas proposed by Browse and Burnand.[53–56] The conventional method of measuring tissue oxygen, however, involves heating a Clarke's electrode to 43° or 44°C. At this temperature, the $TcPO_2$ corresponds well to the arterial PO_2 in the thin skin of neonates. It was in this situation that the method was devised. When the probe is heated to 37°C, skin affected by liposclerosis has a higher $TcPO_2$ than the skin of the contralateral leg. Others have found variable tissue oxygen tensions in various situations of venous insufficiency, and many studies show a wide overlap between limbs

with actual disease and normals. Therefore, the Middlesex group has said that "these reservations about the degree to which skin oxygenation is actually impaired in CVI disease have led to the development of alternative hypotheses for skin damage."[57]

White Cell Trapping in Venous Disease

As the search for the triggering event which incites the cutaneous and subcutaneous changes of CVI continues, data accumulate which suggest a new theory of tissue damage (Figure 3). The theory originates in the observations that raised venous pressure is associated with extremity white blood cell trapping.[58] Dormandy's group showed that limbs with venous disease, characterized by lipodermatosclerosis and ulceration, trapped some 30% of circulating white blood cells after 1 hour of dependency. In contrast, only 7% of leukocytes were trapped in the normal limbs.[59] Consequences of such white blood cell trapping can be related immediately to other conditions. It is known that white blood cells are much larger than red cells, deform very slowly on entering the capillary bed, and are responsible for a great deal of the peripheral vascular resistance.[60] According to Schmid-Schonbein, "because the vascular obstruction by granulocytes is a capillary phenomenon, virtually every organ may be afflicted. This phenomenon may be the pathophysiological mechanism in myocardial ischemia, stroke, shock, and many other diseases."[61]

In the theory proposed by Coleridge Smith and Scurr,[62] activation of white cells is inseparable from tissue destruction. Activation results in the release of proteolytic enzymes, superoxide radicals, and chemotactic substances.

White cells, in general, and neutrophils, in particular, are potential mediators of microvascular injury. Neutrophils produce an assortment of agents, including proteases, elastase, collagenase, and cathepsin G. They also produce a variety of toxic oxygen products intended for the destruction of bacteria. These can produce injury to normal microcirculation. Neutrophil adherence to capillary endothelium and neutrophil-to-neutrophil aggregation are thought to play an important part in the occlusion of postcapillary venules (Figure 4). This contributes to ischemia. In sepsis and septic shock, neutrophils act as mediators of organ injury.[63] It may be that they act in the same way in venous insufficiency.

Biopsies have been taken from the skin of patients with varicose veins, lipodermatosclerosis, and a history of ulceration.[64] In uncomplicated varicose veins, a median of six white blood cells per mm^2 was found. In patients with lipodermatosclerosis, there were 45 white blood cells per mm^2, and where there was a his-

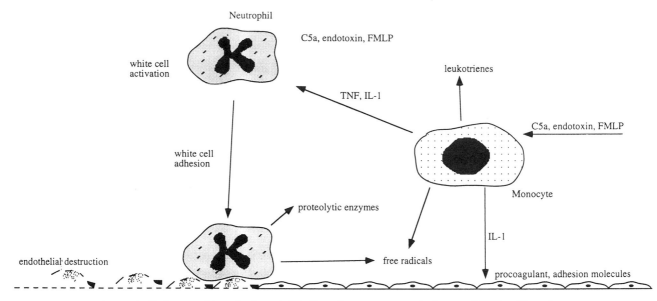

Figure 3. Release of interleuken 1 (IL-1) and tumor necrosis factor (TNF) will activate endothelial cells to release VCAM-1. This interacts with leukocytes, and the adherence of neutrophils to the microvascular endothelium is the initial step in diapedesis. The accumulation of neutrophils is the sine qua non of inflammation which results in phagocytosis and intracellular killing. Importantly, neutrophils release hydrogen peroxide, reactive oxygen intermediates, proteolytic enzymes, and cationic proteins that cause tissue damage. (Reproduced with permission from Philip Coleridge Smith of the Middlesex Hospital Vascular Laboratory.)

tory of ulceration, 217 white blood cells per mm². Further analysis of the cells indicated that the predominant infiltrating cell types were T-lymphocytes and macrophages. B-cells and neutrophils were rarely seen.[65] The number of capillaries were greatly increased in the papillary dermis as has been reported by others.[66] However, the expression of adhesion molecules, in general, and vascular cell adhesion molecules, in particular, was not elevated. "The absence of an increase in ELAM-1 is consistent with the absence of neutrophils from the lesion," said Coleridge Smith. In more severely diseased skin, intercellular adhesion molecule-1 (ICAM-1) expression did increase. This may be related to macrophage and lymphocyte adherence. Curiously, there was no evidence of microvascular occlusion, so it may be that capillary occlusion by white cells does not compromise skin nutrition in venous ulcer disease.

It is uncertain whether the accumulation of macrophages and T-cells in areas of CVI is the cause or effect of CVI. An inflammatory response to tissue damage from any cause could lead to similar findings. Angel's unifying hypothesis deserves further investigation.[66] He points out that normal wound healing is characterized by an inflammatory phase and a healing phase. During the inflammatory phase, there is activation of complement and clotting mechanisms with increased capillary permeability and cellular infiltration. This is much like what is seen in CVI. However, the second

phase of wound healing with its collagen deposition, wound contraction, and epithelialization does not occur in the limb with venous hypertension. It appears that the processes of edema, fibrin deposition, microvascular dysfunction, and perhaps ischemia and free radical production are related in a way that becomes self-perpetuating. Possibly, inflammation generated by activated white blood cells, which accumulate under the influence of venous hypertension, is the key event which is being sought. Bacteria-activated macrophages may cooperate with lymphocytes to initiate a cell-mediated hypersensitivity response in this situation. While this is speculative at present, such a theory would explain findings published by the Middlesex group.[65]

Clearly, answers to the problem of what triggers lipodermatosclerosis and ulceration, the processes which differentiate the limb with CVI from the limb with uncomplicated varicose veins, have yet to be elucidated (Figure 5). Further investigation and development of ideas are necessary to "incorporate the rapidly increasing volume of data on the cellular and microcirculatory abnormalities present in this common, but still mysterious disease."[57]

Clinical Application of Basic Science Investigations

As indicated, there are two main theories of activation processes which lead to CVI and separate this

The White Cell Trapping Hypothesis

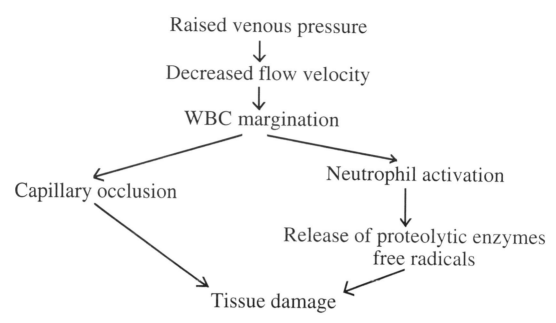

Figure 4. The white cell trapping hypothesis suggests that elevated venous pressure allows white blood cell (**WBC**) margination because of decreased flow velocity. As leukocytes adhere to endothelium and to one another, capillary occlusion may occur. Alternatively, cellular activation will cause the release of proteolytic enzymes and free radicals. The net result of this activity is tissue damage. (Reproduced with permission from Philip Coleridge Smith of the Middlesex Hospital Vascular Laboratory.)

condition from simple venous stasis. These theories depend on the observations of two phenonena: the presence of pericapillary fibrin cuffs, and the observation of white cell trapping and activation in limbs bearing the stigmata of CVI.

At present, there are four classes of drugs which have been advocated to treat such CVI.[67] Because pericapillary fibrin was thought to block oxygen, the anabolic steroid, Stanozolol, was used to promote fibrinolysis. Subjective and objective improvement of lipodermatosclerosis was observed in a pilot study which led to a double-blind crossover trial. The summary findings of this are: leg volumes increased in patients receiving the anabolic steroid; no change was observed in ambulatory venous pressure; and tissue biopsies suggested a reduction in tissue fibrin. Most patients reported subjective improvement even though they were unable to differentiate between treatment with Stanozolol or a placebo.

A separate study looked at ulcer healing comparing Stanozolol to placebo in limbs receiving conventional compression therapy. There was no statistically significant difference in healing between treatment groups. Thus, this agent may be of benefit in symptomatic relief of CVI and possibly in the treatment of lipodermatosclerosis, but it does not improve venous ulcer healing.

On the Continent, hydroxyrutosides have been used for many years. These agents are thought to restore the barrier properties of the fiber matrix between capillary endothelial cells. Prospective, double-blind, placebo-controlled studies have been conducted. A number of parameters have been measured, but the chief findings have been a decrease in leg edema and a subjective reduction in symptoms of tired legs. Thus, these agents appear to be beneficial in relieving symptoms in patients with CVI, but they have no proven role in the management of venous ulcers.

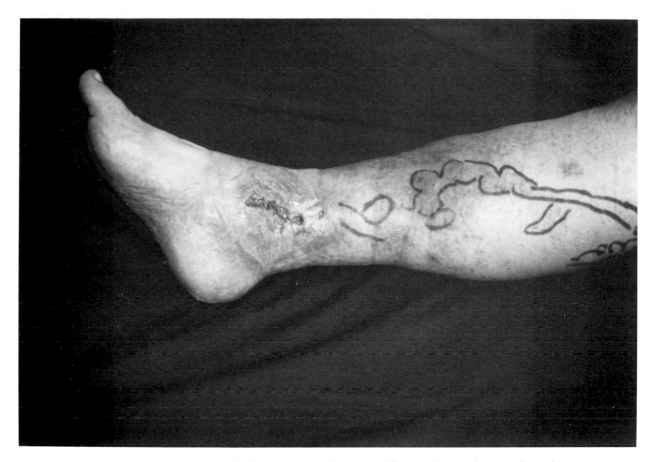

Figure 5. This limb, with its hyperpigmentation, atrophic scarring, and open ulceration refractory to healing, demonstrates all of the elements of chronic venous insufficiency, termed the post-thrombotic state (postphlebitic limb). In fact, all of the changes were produced by superficial venous incompetence without deep venous involvement. These findings were detected on duplex scanning of the superficial and deep venous system. This experience emphasizes the importance of recognition of the superficial venous system in the advanced changes demonstrable on the skin of patients with severe venous insufficiency. It further emphasizes the importance of identification of the triggering mechanism which differentiates a limb such as this one from a limb with varicose veins and no stigmata of chronic venous insufficiency.

Although stable oral analogs of prostaglandin E_1 are not available, this agent has also been tried in treating CVI. The favorable properties of this agent include vasodilation, inhibition of platelet aggregation, and inhibition of neutrophil activation. In treatment of venous ulcerations with intravenous prostaglandin E_1 daily compared to placebo, 8 of 20 patients treated with prostaglandin had complete healing of their ulcers compared with 2 of 22 patients receiving a placebo. Observations were only continued for 6 weeks or until the ulcers healed. Improvement was seen in all parameters of measurement, including ulcer depth, area, and diameter. Edema was significantly improved in patients receiving the active agent. These results are promising and require confirmation by other studies.

Because methylxanthines are said to improve red cell deformability with improvement in oxygen delivery to tissues, these agents have been examined in the treatment of CVI. Methylxanthines reduce white cell aggregation and activation. They also have mild fibrinolytic activity. Pentoxifylline inhibits alterations in the microvasculature induced by interleuken 2 (IL-2). Weitgasser, from the Dermatologic Outpatient Clinic in Graz, Germany, was the first to report a placebo-controlled, double-blind study using pentoxifylline. He included 59 patients with venous ulceration. Twenty-six of the 30 patients on active treatment showed improvement over the study period. This contrasted with only 13 of the 29 patients receiving a placebo. Assessment was objective, comparing photographic data before and after treatment, but no firm data were provided in his study.[68]

Barbarino also performed a double-blind, placebo-controlled study.[69] This was done in only 12 patients with CVI and persistent leg ulcers. Active agent was compared to placebo, and all patients received compression bandaging. Pentoxifylline was administered both intravenously and orally for the first 7 days and then orally for another 60 days. The control group received a matching placebo in an identical regimen. Four of six patients receiving the active agent experienced complete ulcer healing; mean ulcer surface area was reduced. In the controls, only one patient of six experienced complete ulcer healing. Only a moderately reduced ulcer area was observed in the other patients. Other assessments, including continuous-wave Doppler ultrasound, venous pressure at the ankle, valvular competence, and venous reflux intervals, were unchanged.

Subsequently, four outpatient clinics treating leg ulcers in England and Ireland combined their efforts in a double-blind, randomized, prospective, placebo-controlled, parallel group study.[70] In this study, all patients received oxypentifylline, 400 mg three times a day orally, or a matching placebo. The study lasted 6 months or until the reference ulcer healed. Compression bandaging was used in all patients. Primary end points of complete ulcer healing and secondary end points of change in area of the ulcer over the 6-month period were utilized. Complete healing of the reference ulcer occurred in 23 of 38 limbs which were treated by oxypentifylline. Complete ulcer healing only occurred in 12 of the 42 patients treated with placebo. Sixty-four percent (64%) of the treated ulcers healed in 6 months, compared to 34% in the group treated with placebo ($P < 0.01$).

Another approach was undertaken by Salim in Baghdad, Iraq.[71] This investigation was targeted at oxygen-derived free radicals, the hypothesis being that these interfered with the healing of venous ulceration. In this study, free radical scavengers, allopurinol (in 45 patients), or dimethyl sulfoxide (in 44 patients), were used in addition to compression bandaging. Applications were in powder form and applied daily for 7 days and then once weekly until the end of the study period of 3 months. At end points of 4, 8, and 12 weeks, statistically significantly-improved ulcer healing was seen in the treated groups. At 3 months, 93% of allopurinol-treated ulcers were healed, and 95% of dimethyl sulfoxide-treated ulcers were healed.

Salim based his study entirely on the observations of those workers who had linked venous hypertension occurring during muscle contraction to the events of liposclerosis and ulceration. He cited the work of Coleridge Smith and others which showed that raised pressure during standing and walking depressed capillary perfusion pressure which, in turn, led to trapping of white blood cells. His treatment was to block the effects of toxic oxygen metabolites and proteolytic enzymes. He believes that the action of the radical scavengers was achieved by removing the agents that mediate tissue damage and cited that allopurinol is a potent scavenger of hydroxoradicals in addition to its inhibition of the formation of the enzyme xanthine oxidase. He explained that dimethyl sulfoxide scavenges hydroxyl groups and pointed out that the only action the two agents have in common is the scavenging of oxygen-derived free radicals. This was emphasized in his study by the virtually identical healing rates achieved with allopurinol and dimethyl sulfoxide. This study is provocative and singular, but may lead to further investigations which would clarify the etiology and persistence of chronic venous ulcerations.

Conclusions

Cellular mechanisms in CVI act within the vein wall, the venous valve, and in the perivenous tissues. Events that trigger CVI are not precisely defined, although developing observations may prove fruitful. The problem is an important one and increasing numbers of investigators are turning their attention to it.

References

1. Bergan JJ: New developments in surgery of the venous system. *J Cardiovasc Surg* 1:624–631, 1993.
2. Cordts PR, Hartono C, LaMorte WW, et al: Physiologic similarities between extremities with varicose veins and chronic venous insufficiency utilizing air plethysmography. *Am J Surg* 164:260–264, 1992.
3. Sarin S, Shields DA, Farrah J, et al: Does venous function deteriorate in patients waiting for varicose vein surgery? *J Royal Soc Med* 86:21–23, 1993.
4. Bergan JJ: Common anatomic patterns of varicose veins. In: Bergan JJ, Goldman MP (eds). *Varicose Veins and Telangiectasias: Diagnosis and Management*. St. Louis: Quality Medical Publishing, Inc.; 1993.
5. Moulton S, Bergan JJ, Beeman S, et al: Gravitational reflux does not correlate with clinical status of venous stasis. *Phlebology* 8:2–6, 1993.
6. Bergan JJ: Clinical application of duplex testing in treatment of primary venous stasis, varicose veins. In: van Bemmelen PS (ed). *Quantitative Measurement of Venous Incompetence*. Austin, TX: R. Landes Co.; 78–103, 1992.
7. Baker SR, Burnand KG, Sommerfille KM, et al: Comparison of venous refluxes assessed by duplex scanning and descending phlebography in chronic venous disease. *Lancet* 341:400–403, 1993.
8. Ruckley CV: Does venous reflux matter? *Lancet* Editorial 341:411–412, 1993.
9. Negus D: Prevention and treatment of venous ulceration. *Ann Roy Coll Surg Engl* 67:144–148, 1985.
10. Cockett FB, Elgan-Jones DE: The ankle blow-out syndrome. *Lancet* 1:17–23, 1953.
11. Stacey MC, Burnand KG, Layer GT, et al: Calf pump function in patients with healed venous ulcers is not im-

proved by surgery to the communicating veins or by elastic stockings. *Br J Surg* 75:436–439, 1988.

12. Sarin S, Scurr JH, Coleridge Smith PD: Medial calf perforators in venous disease: the significance of outward flow. *J Vasc Surg* 16:40–46, 1992.

13. Arnoldi CC: In: Eklof B, Gjores JE, Thulesius O, Bergqvist D (eds). *Controversies in the Management of Venous Disorders.* London: Butterworth Publishers; 14, 1989.

14. Bjordal RI: Simultaneous pressure flow recordings in varicose veins of the lower extremity. *Acta Chir Scand* 136:309–317, 1970.

15. Sarin S, Scurr JH, Coleridge Smith PD: Medial calf perforators in venous disease: the significance of outward flow. *J Vasc Surg* 16:40–46, 1992.

16. Lea Thomas M: Techniques of phlebography: a review. *Eur J Radiol* 11:125–130, 1990.

17. Lea Thomas M, Bowles JN: Incompetent perforating veins: comparison of varicography and ascending phlebography. *Radiology* 154:619–623, 1985.

18. Weiss RA, Weiss MA: Painful telangiectasias: diagnosis and treatment. In: Bergan JJ, Goldman MP (eds). *Varicose Veins and Telangiectasias: Diagnosis and Management.* St. Louis: Quality Medical Publishing, Inc.; 389–407, 1993.

19. Ham AW: Valves of veins. In: Ham AW (ed). *Histology.* 7th ed. Philadelphia: JB Lippincott; 579, 1974.

20. Crawford T: Arteries, veins, and lymphatics. In: Payling Wright G, St. Clair Symmers W (eds). *Systemic Pathology.* 2nd ed, vol 1. Edinburgh: Churchill Livingstone, Inc.; 152–153, 1976.

21. Gottlob R, May R: Anatomy of venous valves. In: Gottlob R, May R (eds). *Venous Valves.* Berlin: Springer-Verlag; 25–52, 1986.

22. Franklin KJ: Valves and veins: an historical study. *Proc Soc Med* 21:1–17, 1927.

23. Mashiah A, Rose SS, Hod I: The scanning electron microscope in the pathology of varicose veins. *Isr J Med Sci* 27:202–206, 1991.

24. Zukowski AJ, Nicolaides AN, Szendro G, et al: Haemodynamic significance of incompetent calf perforating veins. *Br J Surg* 78:625–629, 1991.

25. Sadick NS: Predisposing factors of varicose and telangiectatic leg veins. *J Dermatol Surg Oncol* 18:883–886, 1992.

26. Tournay R, Wallois P: Les varices de la grossesse et leur traitement principalement par les injections sclerosantes. In: *Expansion Scientifique Francaise.* Paris. 1948.

27. Sumner DS: Venous dynamic varicosities. *Clin Obstet Gynecol* 24:743–760, 1981.

28. Vin F, Aalaert FA, Levardon M: Influence of estrogen and progesterone on the venous system of the lower limbs in women. *J Dermatol Surg Oncol* 18:888–892, 1992.

29. Miller VM, Marcelon G, Vanhoutte PM: Progesterone augments the venoconstrictor effect of RUSCUS without altering adrenergic reactivity. *Phlebology* 6:261–268, 1991.

30. Homans J: The etiology and treatment of varicose ulcer of the leg. *Surg Gynecol Obstet* 24:300–311, 1917.

31. De Takats G, et al: The impairment of the circulation in the varicose extremity. *Arch Surg* 18:671–676, 1929.

32. Blalock A: Oxygen content of blood in patients with varicose veins. *Arch Surg* 19:898–905, 1929.

33. Piulachs P, Vidal-Barraquer F: Pathogenic study of varicose veins. *Angiology* 4:59–100, 1953.

34. Holling HE, Beecher HK, Linton RR: Study of the ten-

dency to oedema formations associated with incompetence of the valves of the communicating veins of the leg: oxygen content of the blood contained in varicose veins. *J Clin Invest* 17:555–561, 1938.

35. Ryan TJ: Microvascular system and the skin. *Br J Hosp Med* 5:741–745, 1970.

36. Piulachs P, Vidal-Barraquer E: Pathogenic study of varicose veins. *Angiology* 4:59–100, 1953.

37. Haimovici H: Abnormal arteriovenous shunts associated with chronic venous insufficiency. *J Cardiovasc Surg* 17:473–482, 1976.

38. Gius JA: Arteriovenous anastomoses and varicose veins. *Arch Surg* 81:299–308, 1960.

39. Haeger KHM: Arteriovenous connections in the calf as a cause of pain and walking difficulties. *J Cardiovasc Surg* 4:124–128, 1963.

40. Schalin L: Arteriovenous communications in varicose veins localised by thermography and identified by operative microscopy. *Acta Chir Scand* 147:409–420, 1981.

41. Lindemayr W, Loefferer O, Mostbeck A, Partsch H: Arteriovenous shunts in primary varicosis: a critical essay. *Vasc Surg* 6:9–13, 1972.

42. Scott HJ: Varicose veins and arteriovenous shunts: a review. *Phlebology* 5:77–83, 1990.

43. Partsch H: Hyperaemic hypoxia in venous ulceration. *Br J Derm* 110:249–251, 1984.

44. Partsch H: Investigations on the pathogenesis of venous leg ulcers. *Acta Chir Scand* 544:25–29, 1988.

45. Loefferer O, Mostbeck A, Partsch H: Arterioveose kurzschlosse der extremitaten. Nuklearmedizinische untersuchungen mit besonderer Berucksichtigung des postthrombotischen unterschenkelgeschwuers. *Zentralbl Phlebol* 8:2–22, 1969.

46. Shami SK, Chittenden SJ, Scurr JH, et al: Skin blood flow in chronic venous insufficiency. *Phlebology* 8:72–76, 1993.

47. Belcaro G, Rulo A, Vasdekis S, et al: Combined evaluation of postphlebitic limbs by laser Doppler flowmetry and transcutaneous PO$_2$/PCO$_2$ measurements. *VASA* 17:257–261, 1988.

48. Allen AJ, Wright DII, McCollum CN, et al: Impaired postural vasoconstriction: a contributory cause for oedema in patients with chronic venous insufficiency. *Phlebology* 3:163–168, 1988.

49. Partsch H: Investigations on the pathogenesis of venous leg ulcers. *Acta Chir Scand* (suppl 1)544:25–29, 1988.

50. Browse NL, Burnand KG: The cause of venous ulceration. *Lancet* ii:243–245, 1982.

51. Burnand KG, Whimster IW, Clemenson G, et al: The relationship between the number of capillaries in the skin of the venous ulcer-bearing area of the leg and the fall in foot vein pressure during exercise. *Br J Surg* 68:297–300, 1981.

52. Burnand KG: The aetiology of venous ulceration. *Acta Chir Scand* 544:21–24, 1988.

53. Clyne CAC, Ramsden WH, Chant ADB, et al: Oxygen tension on the skin of the gaiter area of limbs with venous disease. *Br J Surg* 72:644–647, 1985.

54. Mannarino E, Pasqualini L, Maragoni G, et al: Chronic venous incompetence and transcutaneous oxygen pressure: a controlled study. *VASA* Band 17, Heft 3:159–161, 1988.

55. Kolari PJ, Pekanmaki K, Pohjola RT: Transcutaneous oxygen tension in patients with post-thrombotic leg ulcers: treatment with intermittent pneumatic compression. *Cardiovasc Res* 22:138–141, 1988.

56. Quigley FG, Faris IB: Transcutaneous oxygen potentials in venous disease. *Aust NZ J Surg* 59:165–168, 1989.
57. Cheatle TR, Sarin S, Coleridge Smith PD, et al: The pathogenesis of skin damage in venous disease: a review. *Eur J Vasc Surg* 5:115–123, 1991.
58. Moyses C, Cederholm-Williams SA, Michel CC: Haemoconcentration and the accumulation of white cells in the feet during venous stasis. *Int J Microcirc: Clin Exp* 5:311–320, 1987.
59. Thomas PRS, Nash GB, Dormandy JA: White cell accumulation in the dependent legs of patients with venous hypertension: a possible mechanism for trophic changes in the skin. *Br Med J* 296:1693–1695, 1988.
60. Braide M, Amundson B, Chien S, et al: Quantitative studies of leukocytes on the vascular resistance in a skeletal muscle preparation. *Microvasc Res* 27:331–352, 1984.
61. Schmid-Schonbein GW: Granulocyte: friend and foe. *Nips* 3:6–9, 1988.
62. Scurr JH, Coleridge Smith PD: Pathogenesis of venous ulceration. *Phlebology* (suppl 1)9:13–16, 1992.
63. Mileski WJ: Sepsis: what it is and how to recognize it. *Surg Clin N Am* 71:749–764, 1991.
64. Scott HJ, Coleridge Smith PD, Scurr JH: Histological study of white blood cells and their association with lipodermatosclerosis and venous ulceration. *Br J Surg* 78:210–211, 1991.
65. Wilkinson LS, Bunker C, Edwards JCW, et al: Leukocytes: their role in the etiopathogenesis of skin damage in venous disease. *J Vasc Surg* 17:669–675, 1993.
66. Angel MF, Ramasastry SS, Swartz WM, et al: The causes of skin ulcerations associated with venous insufficiency: a unifying hypothesis. *Plas Reconstruc Surg* 79:289–297, 1987.
67. Colgan MP, Moore DJ, Shanik DG: Drug therapy for venous ulcers: new methods of treatment. *Phlebology* (suppl)9:41–43, 1992.
68. Weitgasser H: The use of pentoxifylline ("Trental 400") in the treatment of leg ulcers: results of a double-blind trial. *Pharmatherapeutica* 3:143–151, 1983.
69. Barbarino C: Pentoxifylline in the treatment of venous leg ulcers. *Curr Med Res Opin* 12:547–551, 1992.
70. Colgan MP, Dormandy JA, Jones PW, et al: Oxypentifylline treatment of venous ulcers of the leg. *Br Med* 300:972–975, 1990.
71. Salim AS: The role of oxygen-derived free radicals in the management of venous (varicose) ulceration: a new approach. *World J Surg* 15:264–269, 1991.

CHAPTER 16

Structure and Function of the Lymphatic System:
Scientific and Clinical Perspectives

Ralph G. DePalma, MD; Mitchel Kanter, MD

The lymphatic system is an intriguing part of the vascular system; many of its functions are incompletely understood, and in contrast to arteries and veins, surgical procedures on the lymphatics are uncommon. In 1784, William Hunter[1] estimated the importance of the lymphatic system, stating, "I think I have proved that the lymphatic vessels are the absorbing vessels all over the body; that they are the same as the lacteals; and that these all together with the thoracic duct constitute one great and general system dispersed through the whole body for absorption; that this system only does absorb and not the veins; that it serves to take up and convey whatever is to make or to be mixed with the blood from the skin, from the intestinal canal, and all the internal cavities whatever."

Hewson, one of Hunter's assistants at his famous anatomic school in London, published in 1774 an important anatomic treatise entitled *The Lymphatic System in the Human Subject and Other Animals*.[2] The book was dedicated to Benjamin Franklin of Philadelphia who just prior to the American Revolution mediated a bitter dispute between Hewson and Hunter. The young anatomist had sought permission from Hunter to retain his personal lymphatic dissection specimens and had been refused. William Hunter believed that the delineation of the lymphatics was a pivotal anatomic and physiologic discovery which

had occurred in his laboratory. He said, "If we mistake not, in proper time, it (the lymphatics) will allow to be the greatest discovery both in physiology and pathology that anatomy has suggested, since the discovery of the circulation."[1] In contrast, William Harvey, whose earlier classic description of circulation, *De Motu Cordis*, was the turning point for modern understanding of cardiovascular physiology, recognized lymphatics but never considered these vessels important. He stated that "lymphatics arose occasionally and by accident, and proceeded from too ample a supply of nourishment,"[3] probably a reference to the prominent intestinal lymphatics filled with chyle after feeding and illustrated by Aselli in 1627[4] (Figures 1 and 2).

Mayerson's teleologic view of the lymphatics[5] is illuminating: "In the mammal it became necessary to evolve a closed high-pressure system with conduits of diminishing thickness carrying blood and oxygen to thin-walled capillaries, but here, nature ran into a snag. The high pressures made the capillaries leaky, and fluid and various substances left the blood stream. It now became necessary to evolve a drainage system to clear the tissue spaces of substances which had leaked out of the blood capillaries and which could not be reabsorbed directly into the blood stream." The transport capacity of the lymphatics is physiologically crucial in homeostasis. Lymphatics play a key role in regulating

From *The Basic Science of Vascular Disease*. Edited by Sidawy AN, Sumpio BE, and DePalma RG. Armonk, NY: Futura Publishing Company, Inc.; © 1997.

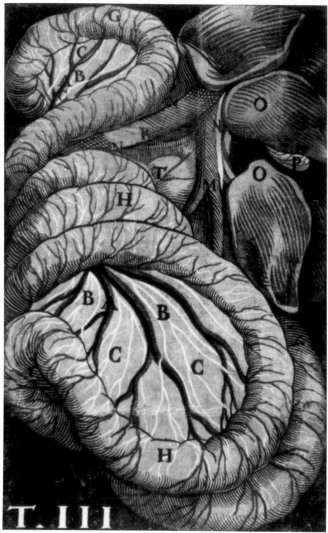

Figure 1. The first known illustration of the lymphatic system showing engorged lacteals in a dog after feeding.[4]

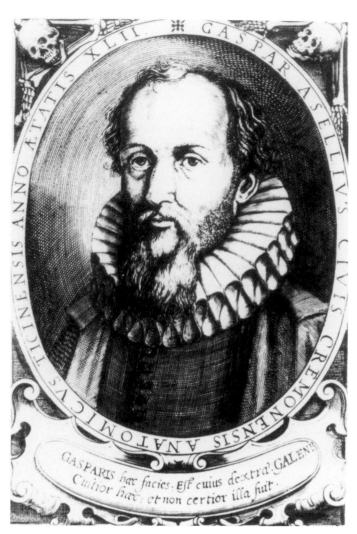

Figure 2. Portrait of Aselli from frontispiece of his monograph published in 1627.

interstitial fluid pressure and maintaining plasma volume. Every 24 hours, the lymphatics return to the veins about 40% of the total plasma protein through the thoracic duct[6]; the total volume of lymph returned to the circulation via the thoracic duct in 24 hours approximates plasma volume.[7]

While recognition of the lymphatic drainage role simplifies comprehension of peripheral obstructive lymphatic disorders, the lymphatic system has many other functions: it removes macromolecules and foreign substances from tissues, and participates in the clearing of debris after tissue injury; as an example, lymph flow increases in scald injuries.[8] The system regulates tissue fluid volume and pressure, and also protects the circulating blood volume by plasma volume repletion. Through its channels, lymphocytes and other important cells reenter the central circulation along with proteins and other large molecules such as chylomicrons and lipoprotein complexes.

Regional lymph nodes are the first mechanical and immunologic sites encountered by viruses, bacteria, neoplastic cells, and foreign proteins. Although the lymphatic network is a secondary circulatory system, certain lymphatics exhibit selective absorptive functions: the blind-ended villous lymphatics of the intestine selectively absorb cholesterol, long chain fatty acids, and triglycerides, accounting for the milky appearance of the intestinal lymph or chyle. Continuous lymphatic absorption of transudative fluid from serous cavities occurs. Regional lymph flow from different organs varies in composition considerably depending on organ activity, motion, fluid balance, and other factors. This chapter reviews basic aspects of lymphatic structure and function. Great potential exists for further advances in understanding the lymphatic system as well as practical information related to the pathophysiology of vascular disease, shock, and crucial immune functions of the lymphatic system.

Embryology

Sabin[9] indicated that lymphatics develop in close relationship to venous structures; this view correlates well with congenital abnormalities later observed in lymphatic vessels. Huntington[10] believed that the systemic lymphatics develop from fusion of perivenous mesenchymal clefts. Lymphatic vessels, in general, course parallel with major veins, and, when obstructed in the adult state, develop variable direct lymphatic venous connections. The existence of these channels reinforces the probable venous origin of the lymphatic system. Figure 3 illustrates the developing lymphatics of human embryos during the fifth through ninth weeks of gestation. By the sixth week, paired jugular lymph sacs appear in the neck and iliac sacs in the lumbar region. By the seventh to ninth weeks, retroperitoneal lymph sacs develop at the root of the mesentery along with the cisterna chylae initially which forms dorsal to the abdominal aorta. The jugular lymph sacs join with the cisterna chylae to produce paired thoracic ducts with numerous anastomoses across the midline. However, in most individuals, the inferior portion of the right lymphatic duct emerges via a cross connection at the level of the fourth to sixth dorsal vertebra to form a dominant left thoracic duct draining into the left subclavian or jugular vein in the root of the neck. The right lymphatic duct or, more commonly, several lymphatic ducts persist on the right side.

Primary lymphatic disorders are developmental abnormalities mainly due to hypoplasia or absence of lymph nodes or ducts. In certain cases, when lymphedema occurs at birth or in early life, the lymph nodes are fibrotic and conducting lymph vessels of the lower extremities are absent or hypoplastic. Less commonly, ductal hyperplasias with valvular incompetence occur. Abnormal growth of the primitive lymph sacs in the area of the jugular buds causes multilocular lymph cysts called cystic hygromas, and, as might be expected, these lesions involve the neck, axillae, and mediastinum of children. Hyperplasia of lymphatic capillaries combines with a variety of congenital vascular tumors such as simple and capillary lymphangiomas and cavernous lymphangiomas. Certain individuals with megalymphatics exhibit both capillary angiomas of the skin and overgrowth of bones in the involved

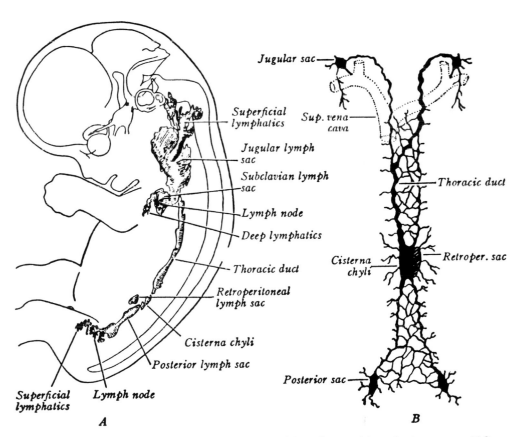

Figure 3. Development of lymphatics and disposition of central lymphatic system. (After Sabin[9] with permission.) **A.** Profile reconstruction of the primitive lymphatic system in an embryo at 9 weeks. **B.** Diagram, in ventral view, of the definitive thoracic duct emerging from a lymphatic plexus. (Reproduced with permission from Arey LB: *Developmental Anatomy*. Philadelphia: W.B. Saunders Company; 371, 1975.)

limb. These disorders are described in Kinmonth's[11] now classic volume on the lymphatic system. Servelle[12] has recently described congenital malformations of intestinal lymphatics, relating these to protein-losing enteropathy, chylous accumulations in body cavities, hypoproteinemia, and actual reflux of visceral chyle into leg lymphatics.

Structure and Function of the Lymphatic System

The lymphatics provide a secondary drainage function accommodating overflow of protein, water, and electrolytes from the blood capillaries. Lymphatic development relates to the high-pressure mammalian arterial circulation which accommodates widely divergent blood flows to different organs and tissues. Consistent with this function, lymphatic capillaries transport lymph to valved collecting vessels; the anatomic arrangements of lymphatics and the composition of lymph vary considerably from organ to organ. Interposed lymph nodes not only act as mechanical filters, but are also sites of immunologic responses. Other lymphoid organs include the spleen, thymus, and mucosal associated lymphatic tissue (MALT), e.g., the adenoidal tonsillar complex and pulmonary lymphatics; also called gut associated lymphatic tissue (GALT)[13] including Peyer's patches and the appendix.

The Peripheral Lymphatic System

Vascular surgeons most commonly encounter primary and secondary lymphedemas involving the peripheral vascular system. Primary lymphedemas are defined as those occurring in the absence of any acquired disease which would damage the lymphatics, and secondary lymphedemas are due to trauma and wounds involving lymph pathways, malignant disease, filariasis, infections, and inflammations, as well as radiation.

The gross anatomy of the peripheral lymphatic system is illustrated in Figures 4 and 5. The microscopic anatomy of peripheral lymphatic capillaries is unique: these are composed of single layers of flat endothelial cells which are slightly larger and thinner than those of blood capillaries. In lymphatic capillaries, the basement membrane is absent or vestigial, facilitating permeability of lymphatic capillaries to large molecules and cells. Caseley-Smith[14] demonstrated in lymph capillaries openings between the endothelial cells of up to 10 microns, a diameter two to five times larger than those of venous capillaries, and an endothelium thicker than that of blood vessels. This endothelium contains vesicles suggesting active endothelial transport; absence of fenestri, and adhesion of plates between inter-

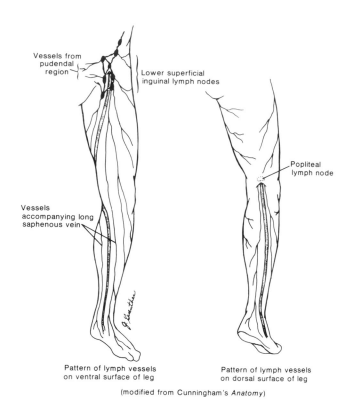

Figure 4. Diagram of superficial lymph vessels and nodes of the lower extremity. (Reproduced with permission from Reference 129.)

cellular junctions, further characterize the lymphatic capillaries. Lymphatic vessels can be distinguished from capillaries by light microscopy in appropriate preparations.[15]

The intercellular junctions and the characteristics of lymph capillaries differ in distinct parts of the body. The lymph capillaries of the extremities end blindly in rounded edges consistent with the closed drainage function of the system. Lymph vessels are absent from the cornea, the central nervous system deep to the meninges, cartilage and tendon, inner ear, placenta, and teeth. While lymphatics exist in intramuscular fascia, they are absent in skeletal muscle bundles; there are no lymphatics in the epidermis of the skin. Fixed epidermal macrophages called Langerhans cells do enter the lymphatic circulation comprising an immune arc the afferent limb of which ends in the regional nodes.[16] These cells are capable of conveying viruses from superficial injury into nodes.

A rich lymphatic network exists just beneath the superficial dermis. It contains abundant lymphatic capillaries without valves. These valveless lymphatics drain into the valved channels of the deep dermis and subcutaneous tissue, illustrated in Figures 4 and 5. The lymphatics of the extremities consist of the dermal plexi, collecting channels, and superficial lymphatic trunks which course with the major veins superficial

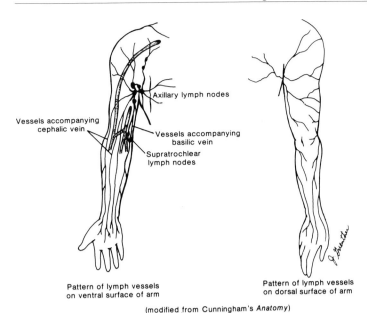

Figure 5. Diagram of superficial lymph vessels and nodes of the upper extremity. (Reproduced with permission from Reference 129.)

to the fascia of the muscles. A few lymphatics pass through scanty popliteal and epitrochlear nodes distally. Most of them pass to the more proximal inguinal and axillary nodes. From this region large efferent trunks arise to course retroperitoneally or in the upper thorax in close relationship with the major vessels. The sparse deep lymphatic system of the intramuscular fascia in humans is believed to communicate only under abnormal conditions[17] with the superficial lymphatic network. The valves of the collecting lymphatics maintain prograde lymphatic drainage, and collecting ducts exhibit an endothelial layer covered by connective tissue, exhibiting both muscular and elastic elements and an adventitia. The larger lymphatic ducts are supplied by their own vasa vasorum. Lymphatic collecting duct walls exhibit well-developed basement membranes, emphasizing conduit rather than exchange functions. Muscular and respiratory activity, as well as pulsatile

forces from neighboring blood vessels, tend to accelerate proximal lymph flow.

Figure 6 illustrates schematically the physiologic relationships between the peripheral lymphatics and capillaries in a subcutaneous location. A long train of physiologic investigation was needed to comprehend the elegant simplicity of these relationships. The role of the lymphatics was emphasized by C. Bernard's[18] ninetheenth-century global concept of mammalian requirements for maintenance of a constant internal milieu bathing all cells. Later in the nineteenth century, Starling[19] clarified the relationship between the hydrostatic pressure of the blood in the capillaries and the colloid osmotic pressure of the plasma protein. Starling's hypothesis[19] and Ludwig's previous insights[20] about capillary circulation led to development of a theory of capillary exchange with the oncotic pressure of plasma proteins functioning as a driving osmotic force

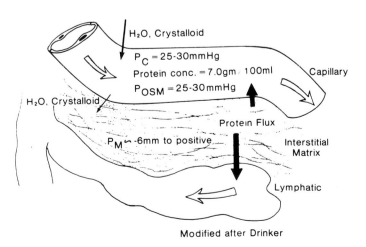

Figure 6. Diagram of relationships between a blood capillary, the interstitium, and a lymph capillary. **Heavy arrows** indicate protein flux. PC = capillary pressure, POSM = osmotic pressure, PM = matrix pressure. (Reproduced with permission from Reference 129.)

in capillaries then thought to be relatively impermeable to protein.

From 1930 to 1941, Drinker and his colleagues[21] measured protein flux from the capillaries into tissues showing that blood capillaries were much leakier than hitherto believed. This finding solidified a physiologic concept of lymphatic capillaries as vessels which serve to return blood protein molecules from the periphery into the central circulation. The diagram shown in Figure 8 illustrates Guyton's current concept[22] based on direct measurement of negative interstitial pressure in the extremities. This idea had not been universally accepted. Some[23] previously stated that interstitial tissue pressure exceeds lymphatic pressure by 0.5 to 1.5 cm water, thus providing a hydrostatic gradient promoting flow into lymphatic capillaries. The negative interstitial pressure concept is now more accepted.

The Formation of Lymph

As shown in Figure 6, the balance of hydrostatic and colloidal osmotic pressures in the arterial side of blood capillaries favors the loss of water and electrolytes into the interstitium; some plasma proteins such as albumin also escape.[14] Then, at the venous side of blood capillaries, the balance of these pressures favor resorption, and this promotes an exchange into the plasma from the extracellular tissue fluid. However, fluid formation and protein leakage on the arteriolar side usually exceed the absorptive rate on the venous side. These excesses are drained by the lymphatic capillaries which coalesce into larger vessels as they travel centrally toward the thoracic duct on the left or the right lymphatic duct on the right. The physiologic necessity to return protein and fluid to the central circulation is a special feature of evolution of the mammalian vascular system. This need is particularly critical for albumin; almost one half of the circulating albumin is recovered daily in this manner.[24] The thoracic duct returns much of the lymph collected in the body to the venous circulation as it enters the left subclavian vein near its junction with the left jugular vein. In addition, lymphatic vessels readily absorb particulate matter from their surrounding interstitial milieu, such as chylomicrons,[25] red blood corpuscles,[26] bacteria, and snake venom.[27]

Interstitial pressure varies in different organs and tissues, increasing with enhanced organ function in response to fluid loading, venous pressure increase, and certain disease states. In the extremities, motion stimulates lymph flow from the periphery. With proximal lymphatic obstruction, continuing protein leak from capillaries causes protein trapping in interstitial spaces. A protein-laden interstitium, in turn, attracts water, attaining a characteristic protein concentration

of subcutaneous lymphedema fluid in the extremities. Lymphatic edema can be distinguished from other causes of swelling as the fluid aspirated in lymphedema exhibits protein concentrations greater than 1.0 to 1.5 grams/100 mL.[28] Protein concentration is lower in edema fluid due to heart failure or early venous obstruction. Clinically, lymphedema is recognized by its characteristic doughy consistency and the slow pitting produced by finger pressure.

Lymph Nodes

It is estimated that 500 to 1000 lymph nodes exist in individual humans.[29] These consist of lymphatic tissue accumulations which vary in size from 1 mm to more than 2 cm. Lymph nodes are always located along the course of lymphatic vessels whose contents pass from the periphery through the regional nodes to the main drainage systems of the thoracic and right lymphatic ducts. In health, lymph nodes are not usually palpable, but can enlarge transiently with heavy exercise in young adult athletes, presumably secondary to increased fluid flux. A prototypical lymph node is illustrated in Figure 7. The hilus of the lymph node contains the efferent lymphatics along with blood vessels, while the afferent lymphatics enter the node at multiple sites over its convex surface. With excision of lymph nodes or their accompanying vessels, there is rapid regeneration by vascular budding or sprouting to produce continuation of lymph flow except when the excision is quite wide or the lymphatics are further damaged by radiation or scar tissue.[30]

While lymph nodes are primary filters for trapping foreign proteins and viral and bacterial particles, they are also important sites of first encounter with the immune system. Malnutrition[31] causes lymphatic atrophy related to immunologic deficiencies of malnutrition and severe injury. Certain foreign proteins selectively enter the peripheral lymphatics to gain access to the central circulation. For example, an ordinarily lethal snake venom experimentally injected into the limb of rabbits with completely divided lymphatics does not result in death.[32] In heavy exercise, red cells enter the peripheral lymphatic capillaries and appear in the thoracic duct in high volume.[26] Once macromolecules enter the collecting lymphatics, there is little exchange with the blood until the lymph enters the venous system. Within lymph nodes of experimental animals, there is no exchange with the blood of molecules greater than a molecular weight of 2300. In a variety of circumstances, labeled soluble antigens or homologous cells can be recovered intact from efferent lymph node ducts.[33]

Migrating cells from the lymphatic ducts pass through "traffic areas" in lymph nodes away from the central germinal centers. Cells destined to remain in

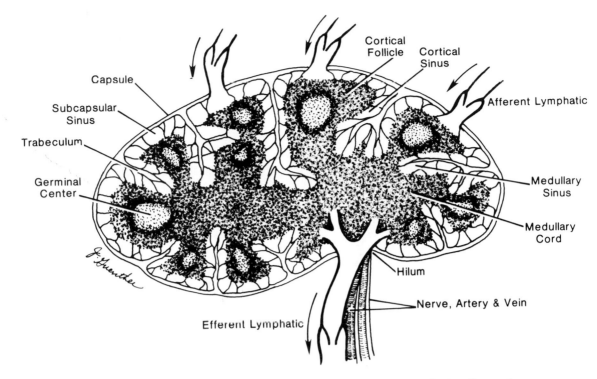

Figure 7. Prototypical lymph node. Note multiple afferent ducts and single efferent duct; "traffic area" for migrating cells in the periphery of the node. (Reproduced with permission from Reference 129.)

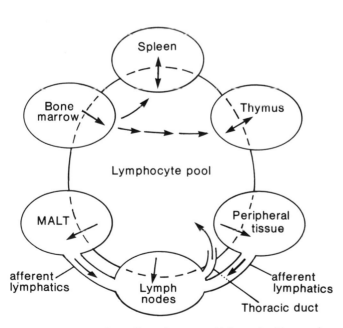

Figure 8. Circulation of lymphocytes. (Adapted with permission from Reference 34.)

the node become distributed throughout the superficial and deep cortex. The proportion of blood-borne versus lymph-borne lymphocytes entering and leaving lymph nodes depends on whether the node is a peripheral or a central one. Less than 10% of the cells leaving peripheral nodes reach the node in the lymph; 90% arrive via the blood stream. The cortex of the node contains mainly aggregates of B cells forming primary and often secondary follicles[34]; a deeper paracortex contains T cells in close apposition to interdigitating antigen presenting cells derived from the blood. The importance of the integrity of the follicular dendritic cell network in maintaining this structure and trapping viruses has been recently appreciated.[35] Lymphocytes enter the node from the blood through specialized high endothelial vessels (HEV) in this zone. The medulla contains both T and B cells as well as plasma cells arranged in cords. Lymphocytes can only exit the node via the efferent lymphatics. The circulation of lymphocytes through the central organs and peripheral lymphatics is illustrated in Figure 8.

Central Lymphatic System

All blood cells arise from a common stem cell precursor in the embryonic yolk sac which migrates to the embryonic liver and then to the bone marrow. Unlike

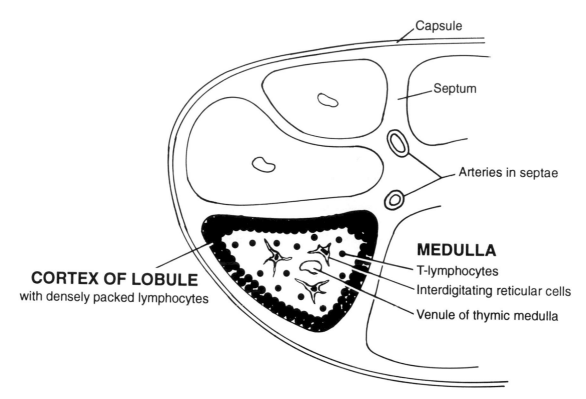

Figure 9. Thymus: a diagrammatic representation. **Cortex** contains immature densely packed T lymphocytes. **Arteries** derived from internal mammary and inferior thyroid arteries give arteriolar branches penetrating lobules. **Medulla** containing smaller, mature, and less densely packed T lymphocytes; interdigitating reticular cells and venule of thymic medulla which drain mature T cells and accompany arteries in septae and drain into innominate and thyroid veins.

other blood cells, however, the "basic" lymphocyte requires further maturation in lymphoid tissue to become an immunocompetent cell. There are two ways in which this immunocompetence may be expressed: 1) the cellular immune response, or 2) the humoral immune response.[36]

The thymus, illustrated in Figure 9, provides a microenvironment for maturation of cells destined to participate in cellular immunity. These lymphocytes, designated as T cells, enter via the blood stream and develop into immunocompetent T lymphocytes. From the thymus, these cells reenter the blood stream and seek lymphatic tissues throughout the body. From these locations they continuously recirculate via both the blood stream and the lymphatic channels until they encounter a specific antigen which they may be preprogrammed to recognize. Then they return to local lymphatic tissue and multiply in an activated form ("lymphoblasts"), which then migrate to the site of the antigenic intruder. At this point, they challenge the antigen with enhanced phagocytic activity ("macrophage"), lymphokines, and direct cytotoxic destruction ("killer T lymphocytes"). A future challenge by the same antigen will evoke an even greater response by "memory cell" T lymphocytes in lymphoid tissues.

The thymus is the first lymphatic organ appearing during fetal life and is most prominent during childhood.[37] Involution begins during adolescence and in adulthood the thymus is largely obliterated. Its only known function is to process lymphocytes into immunocompetent T cells, but the process by which this occurs is not known. The thymus may also influence the development of other lymphoid organs during fetal development. Lymphocytes from the circulation infiltrate its outer cortical layer via blood vessels which travel in the capsule and fibrous septae of the gland. Large and densely packed at the cortex, these immature lymphocytes divide and migrate inward toward the thymic medulla while they acquire immunocompetence. The thymus does not contain lymphatic channels except in the connective tissue septa, and the mature T lymphocytes leave the thymus via the venous capillaries in the medulla.

The second way in which lymphocytes express immunocompetence is the production of antibodies or humoral immune response. Cells destined for this purpose also require a maturation process and a considerable effort has been directed toward determining the site of this differentiation. In 1956, Glick et al[38] observed that operative excision of the bursa of

Fabricius, a lymphoepithelial organ found only in avian species and connected to the gastrointestinal tract, significantly reduced antibody production. Further studies showed that the bursa of Fabricius provides a microenvironment for immature lymphocytes to develop into immunocompetent antibody-producing cells called B cells.

Since the bursa of Fabricius does not exist in mammals, it has been hypothesized that gut associated lymphoid tissue (GALT), including Peyer's patches, appendix, and tonsils, or possibly the spleen play a similar role in man. This hypothesis has not been confirmed; some believe that the bursa equivalent in man might be the bone marrow itself.[39]

Like the T cell, each B cell recognizes a specific antigen and mature cells seed other lymphatic tissues such as the lymph nodes and spleen. Unlike the T cells, however, B cells generally do not circulate. Their contact between antigens occurs via the circulating macrophage, the B cell then becomes activated, and it trans-

forms into the active plasma cell which produces antibodies characterizing the humoral immune response. The antibody, in turn, is circulated by both the blood and lymphatic vascular systems.

Isolated lymphocytes may be found in any tissue, but are usually found in the primary lymphoid organs (lymph nodes, spleen, thymus) or in aggregations such as Peyer's patches. Despite the functional dichotomy of T cell and B cell responses, it should be recognized that a single antigen may evoke both responses.

The spleen, illustrated in Figure 10, is the largest lymphoid organ. Although rich in lymphoid aggregations, the spleen has no afferent lymphatic channels and few efferent lymphatic channels. The organ also sequesters defective red blood cells and particulate matter including bacteria. Just as lymph nodes provide immunologic contact between immunocompetent lymphocytes and afferent lymph, the spleen provides contact between these cells and the blood. T and B cells proliferate in response to the appropriate antigenic stimulus.

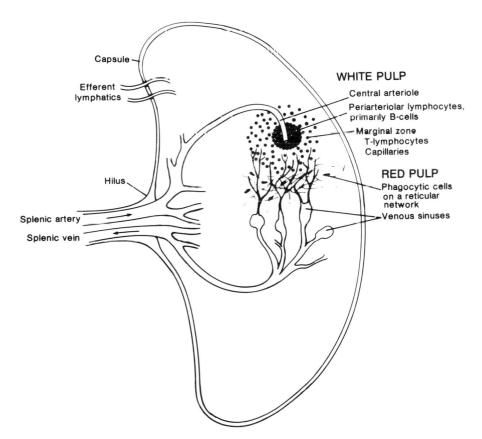

Figure 10. Spleen: a diagrammatic representation. Scant efferent lymphatics exist in capsule and follow trabeculae. **White pulp** named according to the gross appearance on fresh-cut section. Note periarteriolar lymphocytes, primarily B cells, which form germinal centers upon antigenic stimulation. **Marginal zone** contains T lymphocytes and capillaries, and drains into red pulp. **Red pulp** named according to gross appearance on fresh-cut section. Note venous sinuses, phagocytic cells on a reticular network consisting of monocytes and macrophages. Complex circulatory connections occur between the red and white pulp, and red pulp drains into S.V. Destruction of abnormal RBCs occurs in red pulp.

The spleen is an encapsulated organ. From its hilus, the splenic artery divides into smaller arteries and arterioles. Populations of both T and B cell lymphocytes surround the arterioles; these zones correspond macroscopically to the white pulp. Prominent lymphocytic aggregations around the splenic arterioles are sometimes referred to as malpighian corpuscles. In the white pulp, the lymphoid tissue forms sheaths around the arterioles. In addition to these T and B cells, these also contain macrophages, and specialized antigen presenting cells. In contrast to the thymus, germinal centers may be seen in the spleen during B lymphocyte stimulation; such areas may resemble lymph nodes except for the presence of central splenic arterioles. As the arterioles further branch into capillaries, they reconstitute into venules of the red pulp. While the ultrastructural detail of the capillary and venous connections is still controversial, endothelial pores are present. Filtration and sequestration of defective red blood cells as well as phagocytic activities occur via these pores. Venous channels reconstitute into larger veins and drain via the splenic vein into the portal circulation.

Other tissues in the body also store immunocompetent lymphocytes. These range from identifiable organs such as the tonsils and appendix to aggregations of lymphoid tissue in the ileum known as Peyer's patches and other unnamed aggregations of lymphoid tissue. The tonsils surround the oropharynx at its entrance to the hypopharynx. The palatine tonsils are most prominent and are paired structures that lie between the glossopalatine and pharyngopalatine arches. Mitosis in tonsillar lymphoid follicles can be seen, particularly during an activated humoral response. The surface of the tonsil is covered by the stratified squamous epithelium of the oropharynx, and its base is separated from underlying muscle by connective tissue. The tonsils do not have a discrete hilus; multiple blood vessels enter the tonsil along its attached surfaces. Unlike true lymph nodes, efferent lymphatic vessels begin near the tonsillar surfaces. The tonsils contain no afferent lymphatics. Thus, in contradistinction to lymph nodes, the tonsils lie at the beginning of lymphatic vessels and do not filter lymph.

Similar nests of lymphatic tissue lie along the back of the tongue, the lingual tonsils, and the posterior nasopharynx. When the latter become hypertrophied due to chronic inflammation, they are referred to as adenoids. Peyer's patches also represent aggregations of lymphoid tissue in the gastrointestinal tract, particularly in the terminal ileum along the antimesenteric border. They are separated from the gut lumen by one layer of columnar epithelium and extend into the submucosa of the bowel wall.

Cellular Components of the Lymphatic System

Lymphocytes with distinct immunologic functions originate in the central lymphatic organs.[36] Animal experiments and clinical studies on congenitally athymic patients proved that lymphocytes derived from the thymus or T cells mediate cellular immunity. A second class of lymphocytes, the B cells, are generated independently of the thymus. As described previously, these cells produce antibodies mediating humoral immunity. A third division of heterogeneous lymphocytes, known as null or non-B, non-T types, are sources of extramedullary hematopoiesis or can evolve to form specialized cytotoxic cells which kill target cells either in the presence or absence of specific antibodies. The lymphocytes constitute an immunologic memory bank with recall capabilities on antigenic reexposure. The different types of cells associated with the lymphatic system are identified largely by surface markers and, overall, probably more than 38 types of lymphatic cells have been discovered, which can also be classified on the basis of nuclear deoxyribonucleic acids.[40] Current thinking supports the concept of derivation of the lymphocytes from an architecturally arranged system specifically involved with immune competence. These interrelationships are shown schematically in Figure 11.

One of the most important clinical correlates of disordered lymphatic function is depressed immune function. These disorders are characterized by changes in the helper and suppressor lymphocyte numbers and ratios. Profound changes in total number and ratios occur postoperatively after major surgery, in severe trauma, and in burns.[41] Infection of the helper cells with human immunodeficiency virus (HIV) produces acute immune deficiency disease or AIDS. Early in AIDS, lymph nodes are strikingly enlarged.

Exciting information is accumulating regarding the dominant roles of the lymphatic system particularly in HIV infection. HIV infection disrupts the microenvironment of the lymphatic system[35] and its associated immune functions involving complex interactions between peripheral blood and mononuclear cells, increased cytokine production, and the ultimate destruction of the follicular dendritic cells late in the disease. This process is accompanied by viral spillover into the circulation with loss of HIV specific immune responses along with the ability to respond to other pathogens. These events determine the eventual lethal outcome of AIDS. The dominant role of the lymphatic system in HIV disease gives special and poignant relevance to Hunter's 1784 prediction and estimate of the importance of the lymphatic system. As noted by Fauci[35] recently, "the loss of thymic cellular elements . . . in HIV infection provides a compelling argument . . . to

LYMPHATIC SYSTEM INTERFACE WITH THE IMMUNE RESPONSE

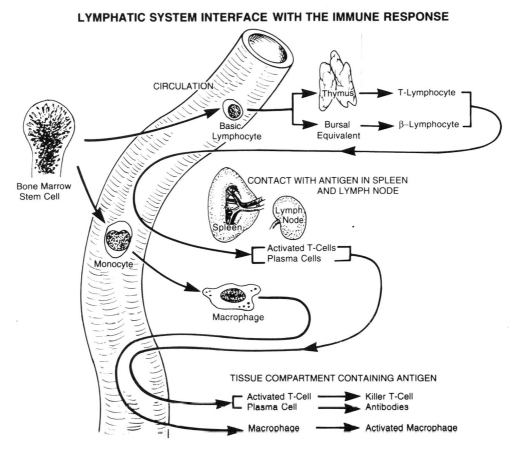

Figure 11. Simplified schema of derivation of T and B cell lymphocytes and their interactions.

pursue (thymic transplantation) . . . as a component of attempts directed at immunologic reconstitution . . . ." This lymphatic affliction might offer surgeons yet another frontier.

Of surgical importance also is the fact that uncontrolled lymphatic leaks from thoracic or other major ducts cause severe hypoproteinemia, malnutrition, and loss of immune competence within days or weeks. In a trial assessing thoracic duct drainage for renal transplant immune suppression, Starzl and associates[42] produced controlled duct drainage in 40 patients. Although this technique is no longer used for this purpose, they drained a daily average of 1.88 ± .9 SE x 10[9] cells and 4.7 liters of lymph for about 2 months. Such lymphatic diversion produced cellular humoral immune suppression in most patients. The fluid components of the lymph loss could be adequately replaced by electrolyte solutions. Most of the cells lost were classified as small lymphocytes, but some of the cell collections were variable, exhibiting as much as 25% monocytes.

Pathophysiology of Lymph Flow

The physiologic role of the lymphatic system in returning extracellular fluid and cells to the central circulation is altered in certain conditions. Stern has provided an important review of many of these states.[43] Obstruction of lymphatics yields variable results depending on the site and extent of blockage. Following lymphatic obstruction, lymphovenous communications open and collaterals also develop.[44] Generally speaking, collaterals are believed to be of sufficient magnitude to correct transient pressure increases after most lymphatic obstructions. When the thoracic duct is ligated on the left, there is collateral development on the right and usually no apparent ill effects.

Whether or not extremity lymphedema develops depends on the extent of lymphatic ablation. As will be discussed, it is quite difficult to produce lymphedema experimentally. When swelling occurs following proximal lymphatics damage, there has been extensive lymphatic interruption. With acute venous obstruction, compensatory lymph flow increases to approximately twice that of normal, returning to baseline levels by about 12 weeks after venous occlusion. According to Chavez,[45] complete venous obstruction is compensated by both increased lymph flow and the opening of venolymphatic shunts.

The lymphatics play a crucial role in restoring protein content and fluid volume during shock. Early in hypovolemic shock there may be a transient increase in lymph flow; however, lymph flow within the thoracic duct promptly decreases to subnormal levels and remains low until plasma and interstitial volume are repleted. Experimentally, in hypovolemic shock with reinfusion of shed blood, lymph flow increases to about 54%[46] above control levels. In hypovolemic animals, the plasma protein concentration increases parallel with the protein contribution of the lymph, showing that plasma albumin repletion occurs via the lymphatic tracts.[47] In the early stages of hypovolemic shock, albumin is retained by the plasma to be liberated as volume repletion occurs. Either blood transfusion or infusion with Ringer's lactate achieves these results.

In experimental endotoxic shock, thoracic duct lymph flow initially increases[48] and red cells often enter thoracic duct lymph. One route of red cell entry is probably via the hepatic lymphatics originating in the space of Disse.[49] Some of the high molecular particles transported by lymph include lysosomal enzymes which increase during shock and probably arise from the liver and the intestine. Thoracic duct external drainage[50–52] in endotoxic shock is said to prolong animal survival by reducing blood levels of myocardial depressant factor and beta glucuronidase.[53,54]

Thus far, changes in thoracic duct lymph flow have been discussed. Lymph egress from various organs varies as to particular functions and anatomic peculiarities. For example, lymphatic intestinal drainage is closely related to arterial flow. Experimentally, superior mesenteric artery ligation causes a marked reduction of lymph flow in the thoracic duct,[50,52] while ligation of the mesenteric vein increases lymph flow to eight times normal. Obstruction of the mesenteric lymphatics produces a number of peculiar sequelae including collateral drainage by submucosal and subserosal regions. In spite of these collaterals, there may be marked edema of the intestine. Clinically, the lacteals supplying intestinal villi can dilate strikingly to cause steatorrhea and lowered serum albumin level, as described over two decades ago by Fish, et al[55] and recently reemphasized by Servelle.[12] Thus, protein-losing gastroenteropathy is primarily a lymphatic abnormality.[56] Intestinal lymphatic obstruction[47] also lowers serum cholesterol levels as these lymphatics specifically transport lipids.

Hepatic lymph is formed by diffusion directly from the hepatic sinusoids into Disse's space. The hepatic lymph approximates 30% of the volume transported by the thoracic duct[58] and the intrahepatic drainage system provides the largest volume of visceral lymph generated. Hepatic lymph exits in the region around the protal vein to join the cisterna chylae and subsequently the thoracic duct. Hepatic lymph is less fatty in composition than that of intestinal lymph; its composition is similar to that of plasma. Hepatic lymph flow is greatly stimulated by intravenous infusion of glucose, food ingestion, and particularly in cirrhosis.

Supradiaphragmatic vena caval obstruction also causes a large increase of hepatic lymph flow with elevated protein content and secondarily increases flow and pressure in the thoracic duct. These changes probably relate to elevated hepatic sinusoidal pressure. In association with cirrhosis and variceal bleeding, it has been found that the thoracic duct is dilated and the lymph might also be hemorrhagic under these conditions.[58] A side-to-side portacaval shunt reduces lymph flow from the cirrhotic liver, while an end-to-side portacaval shunt causes a lesser reduction.[59] It has also been shown[60] that portacaval shunting decreased flow in the thoracic duct and increased its protein content. Biliary tract obstruction caused increased bilirubin content of the hepatic lymph which preceded bilirubin increases in the blood.[61]

A volume by A.J. Miller[62] provides valuable sources of historic, physiologic, and pathologic summaries of the lymphatic system in general and about the heart in particular. The lymphatics in the heart begin in the endocardium. These exist as blind sacs in the interstitial tissues and are quite similar to lymphatics elsewhere. The larger cardiac lymph vessels contain valves and accompany the coronary vessels.[63] The collecting vessels of the heart terminate in a cardiac lymph node which drains mainly into the right lymphatic duct.

Experimentally, the protein content of cardiac lymph has been found to be higher than that of the thoracic duct lymph, while sodium and potassium levels are similar to those of plasma.[64] Obstruction of cardiac lymphatics can produce subendocardial hemorrhage and fibroelastic-like cardiac lesions.[65] Right heart failure causes increased lymph formation; in congestive heart failure generally the thoracic duct is dilated, probably a secondary effect of extracellular fluid excess.[66,67] As in the periphery, when venous return from myocardium is obstructed, cardiac lymph flow and pericardial fluid formation increase.

The pulmonary lymphatics facilitate alveolar clearance of fluid and possibly toxic substances as well. Lauweryns and Baert[68] have provided a comprehensive review of this subject. Lymphatics do not exist in either alveolar walls or interalveolar septa. Terminal pulmonary lymphatic channels begin at the region of terminal bronchioles and are present in pleural, peribronchial, perivascular, and intralobar connective tissue. The terminal lymphatics in relation to terminal bronchioles are called juxta-areolar lymphatics. Extensive pleural lymphatics outline the respiratory lobules and form polyhedral and wide meshed networks. Pleural lymphatics run over the surface of the lung and toward the hilus where they anastomose with central lymphatic ducts and deep plexi which parallel ramifications of the airways to the level of the respiratory bronchioles and small branches of the pulmonary vessels.

Lung lymphatic drainage occurs mainly via the right lymphatic ducts; only the upper lobe of the left lung or some part of it is drained by the thoracic duct.[69,70] Pulmonary lymph resembles cardiac lymph in composition; its protein content is about 3.5 gm.[71,72] It is estimated that in humans a protein leak into the lungs of 5 to 10 grams occurs daily.[71] The pulmonary lymphatics are involved in the removal of fluid and particles from the alveolar lumina. It has been hypothesized that[73] cytotoxic substances are to a larger extent cleared by the lymphatics and are particularly lymphotropic. The removal of nontoxic particles is postulated to occur via the airways and ciliary activity, though this generalization has been extensively qualified.[68]

Pulmonary lymphatic function is clinically relevant in many conditions. For example, radiographic clearance of interstitial pulmonary edema occurs slowly because the pulmonary lymphatics are at some distance before entering the lymphatic capillaries. One important clinical correlate is that positive pressure ventilation decreases lymph flow to some degree,[74] while increasing the resorption of edema fluid by the alveolar capillaries, possibly also an important route for reabsorbing lung fluid. Meyer and coworkers[75] estimated that the efficiency of lymphatic absorption was about 37 times that of blood. Thus, the rate of recovery from pulmonary edema relates to adequate lymphatic drainage.

Lymphatic Visualization

The large collecting ducts of the thorax and abdomen are visualized after feeding with milk or cream rendering readily visible the intestinal lacteals and major duct systems. This simple method can be used clinically to locate major lymph fistulae involving these ducts. Early anatomists used a variety of substances to delineate the lymphatic system. The fatty meal provided the first visualization when Aselli[4] in 1627 discovered the lacteal vessels while dissecting the canine mesentery in search of nerves. Since then, many materials have been used to visualize the lymphatic system such as air, gelatin, turpentine, olive oil, asphalt, benzol, a variety of inks and dyes, and even microorganisms.[76,77] A particularly effective early method was used by Gerota[78] who, in 1896, used a mixture of Prussian blue and turpentine in ether and contributed anatomic knowledge of the collecting vessels.

By the twentieth century, it was clear that the lymphatics were a unique and important network handling fluid and protein transport; little in vivo physiology existed because study methods used examinations in cadavers or anesthetized animals. An important advance was made by Hudak and McMaster[79] at the Rockefeller Institute for Medical Research in 1933. Having observed that vital dyes such as patent blue violet injected intracutaneously stained lymph channels in animals, they used themselves as experimental subjects to demonstrate superficial lymphatic plexuses along the forearm and inner thigh. These investigators described in detail their methods to identify lymphatics; similar methods are still useful today. The technique involves slow injection of patent blue violet with little pressure on the plunger of the syringe in order to minimize interstitial diffusion of dye which might obscure the dermal lymphatic channels. In normal circumstances, the dye was noted to extend along lymphatics up to 8 cm from the site of injection. In clinical practice today, 1% isosulfan blue (Lymphazurin, Hirsch Industries, Cherry Hill, New Jersey) is used in a similar manner.

Hudack and McMasters' observations[79] showed that the lymphatics could be examined under physiologic conditions. By demonstrating the "streamer" effect, they also dispelled the notion that lymph was static in a limb at rest and also showed that lymph flow was greatly augmented by muscular contraction. In addition, increased lymphatic capillary permeability was documented in response to various stimuli, including mild trauma, heat, ultraviolet light, bacterial toxins, and histamine. It was concluded that "participation of the lymphatics in skin lesions must obviously be great." In another interesting experiment performed by Drinker[80] in the preantibiotic era of this century, pneumococci were injected into the blood stream of rabbits. Organisms could be cultured in the thoracic duct in less than 1 hour following bacteremia and were more concentrated in chyle than in blood. Specific antisera capable of sterilizing the blood did not sterilize lymph.

Even in our current era of high technology, one of the primary challenges in studying lymphatics is simply to find them. Probably the best method remains injection of dye into the region drained by the lymphatics to be investigated. Much experience is required to isolate the vessel from its surrounding connective tissue and to gauge how much tension and shearing it can withstand without contracting or tearing. Lymphatics are particularly difficult to identify and isolate in fatty or fibrous tissue. Injection of 1% isosulfan blue is an important aid in identifying lymph channels.

Improved methods of visualization appeared in the wake of the development of improvements in radiologic techniques and the advent of plastic catheters to replace thinly drawn-out glass previously used to cannulate lymph vessels. In 1948, Glenn[81] found a lymphatic vessel in the paw of a dog with the aid of dyes, cannulated the vessel, and injected intravenous pyelography contrast material. He thereby produced a lymphangiogram in the canine leg and groin. Servelle[82] visualized lymphatics in humans suffering from elephantiasis by using a retrograde injection of thorium dioxide (Thorotrast) contrast media in 1951. Visualization of the dilated lymph channels in the diseased leg depended on partial or complete valvular incompetence. Thorotrast, once popular, is no longer used because of its irritant and carcinogenic effects in humans.[83]

Credit for clinical lymphangiography, performed

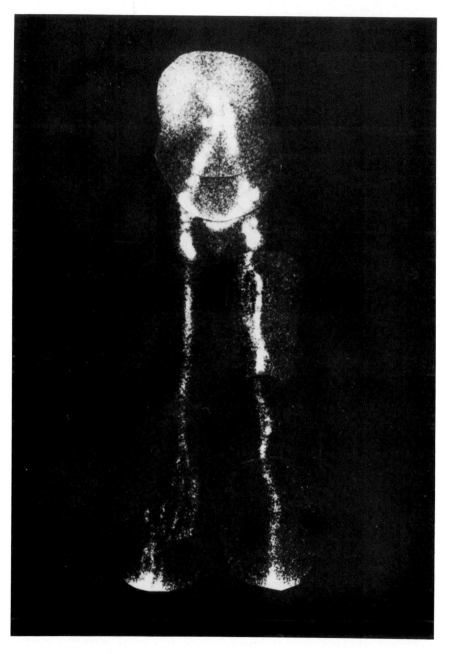

Figure 12A. A radionuclide lymphoscintiscan obtained 3 hours following the intradermal injection of 1 mCi (per injection site) of technetium 99m (Tc 99m) antimony trisulfide colloid at sites overlying the first and fifth metatarsals. This is a 38–year-old female who had a history of right calf edema since childhood and multiple bouts of cellulitis involving the right lower extremity. At 3 hours, we see marked collateralization of the lymph channels over the right anterior tibial region. However, more proximal to this point there is normal drainage bilaterally to the inguinal, internal iliac, common iliac, and para-aortic nodes to the level of the kidneys.

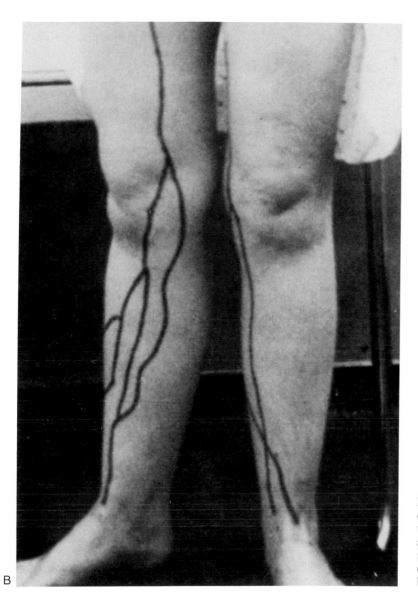

Figure 12B. The location of these channels was defined by external radioactive markers and their position and pathway delineated on the skin as marked. Both of these photos were sent to the microsurgeon for his use in the operating room. (Courtesy of William D. Kaplan, MD, Dana Farber Cancer Institute, Boston, Massachusetts.)

in 1952, also belongs to Kinmonth.[84] Again with the aid of dyes, peripheral lymphatics were isolated in the extremity, cannulated, and injected with a diodone, a water soluble radio-opaque contrast medium. Thus, a clinically applicable and reliable method was established to study the anatomy of the lymphatic system. This led to a clearer understanding of primary and secondary lymphedema.

Kinmonth's procedure,[84] with a few improvements, is the basis of modern lymphangiography. One of these improvements is the use of Ethiodol which is an iodinated, lipid soluble substance derived from poppy seed oil. It disappears less quickly from the lymphatics than its water soluble precursor. Although Ethiodol is safer than older agents, both pulmonary[85] and cerebral[86] embolism may occur. Great care must

be taken to avoid inadvertent intravenous administration.[87,88]

Lymphangiography undoubtedly gives the most detailed anatomic study of the lymphatic system clinically available. Yet it requires isolation and cannulation of a suitable lymphatic vessel for injection, and remains cumbersome. Also, in the presence of obstruction, lymphangiography can produce intense irritation and possibly make this condition worse. These limitations have led to an interest in radionucleotide imaging using interstitial or subcutaneous injections. Lymphatic tissue uptake of radioactive gold was noted as early as 1953,[89] yet only in recent years have clinically useful refinements been developed.[90]

The behavior of a substance injected into the interstitial space depends primarily on particle size. Particles several microns in size are absorbed rapidly by the blood vessel capillaries while larger particles over 100 microns are trapped in the interstitial space. Radio-pharmaceuticals of intermediate size are absorbed by the lymphatics and can be scanned on a standard gamma camera. Gold and colloidal albumin have been used in the past, but presently the preferred compound for lymphoscintigraphy is technetium 99 antimony sulfide colloid. This compound has a particle size of 4 to 11 microns and yields images within 3 hours of subcutaneous injection. While less anatomic detail is shown in a lymphoscintigram in comparison to a lymphangiogram, it is often sufficient to demonstrate lymphatic channels or sites of obstruction. Figure 12 is a lymphoscintoscan of a lymphatic channel obtained in a case of primary lymphedema; such studies can be used to locate lymphatic trunks prior to possible operative interventions. Unfortunately, lymphatico-venous anastomoses have not proved effective clinically; experimentally these have been shown to be marginally feasible, exhibiting shunt patency in only two of six dogs at 8 months.[91] Another microsurgical approach used microsurgical lymphatic lymphatic-anastomoses as reported by Baumeister[92] et al. The long-term results of these procedures require scrutiny.

Animal Models and Experimental Perspectives

While lymphedema due to malignancy, operation, radiation, chronic infection, parasitic infestation, or congenital disorders is familiar to most clinicians, effective treatment of this disorder continues to be a problem. In order to devise definitive treatment, there have been many attempts to reproduce lymphedema in experimental animals. Yet for nearly 100 years, this seemingly simple task has been difficult to accomplish.

In 1888, Meyer,[93] experimenting with dogs, ligated and divided the lymphatic trunks near the saphenous vein in the leg; lymphatic stasis did not occur. Investigating the cause of soft tissue edema, Eloesser[30] reasoned that scar tissue blocked regeneration of lymphatic vessels. This was based on his observations of small lymph vessels stained with India ink in experimental incisions in the rabbit ear, which showed that some degree of lymph blockage persisted for several months. Acting upon a suggestion by William Halsted, Reichert[94] in 1926 attempted to produce experimental lymphedema in dogs by extensive surgical ablation of the lymphatics. His procedure included a circumferential incision around the middle third of the leg and division of the skin, subcutaneous tissue, and muscle tissue. The femoral artery and vein were skeletonized, and a circular cut was made through the periosteum of the femur. Finally, soft tissues were reapproximated.

In this way, it was felt that all lymphatic tissue had been severed. Nevertheless, chronic edema did not develop. As a result, the process of lymphatic regeneration accompanying healing wounds was exquisitely delineated.

Since Reichert's observations,[94] the regenerative capacity of the lymphatic system has been repeatedly documented. This phenomenon accounts for the difficulty in creating a consistent model of experimental lymphedema. Lymphatic regeneration has been demonstrated following skin incisions and sectioning of lymphatic vessels,[95–99] skin grafting,[100–107] tube pedicle flaps,[100] secondary wound healing,[108] sectioning lymphatic vessels and reimplantation onto lymph nodes,[98,109] lymphadenectomy,[106] and organ transplantation.[111–113] In addition, two independent investigators removed the canine small intestine with its mesentery, stored it at a low temperature for several hours, and then replanted it into the animal with vascular and bowel reanastomoses. Lymphatics regenerated across the resected mesentery, despite the fact that no lymphatic anastomosis was attempted.[114,115]

Credit for the first successful attempt to produce experimental chronic lymphedema belongs to Cecil Drinker in 1934.[116] This was accomplished by repeated surgical disruption of the lymphatics in the groin of the dog in staged procedures, combined with intralymphatic injections of a sclerosing solution of silica and quinine. This model for lymphedema is limited by the requirement for systematic destruction of all distal lymphatics. However, this report is notable not only for the reproducibility of edema, but also for quantification of limb swelling over time. While most physicians recognize clinically a swollen extremity, quantification of edema is more difficult and often neglected. Such measurements are essential in experimental models, as well as in the follow-up of patients after treatment. Drinker measured limb circumference in inches: " . . . first at the base of the toes, the second half way to the ankle joint, the third at the ankle joint, and the fourth one inch below the knee."[116]

Three years later, in 1937, Blalock[117] attempted complete surgical interruption of all lymphatic channels in the abdomen and thorax in dogs and cats. Complete interruption was achieved with difficulty, requiring up to seven operations per animal. When complete lymphatic interruption was finally achieved, this state was incompatible with life unless secondary lymphatico-venous anastomoses developed, which occurred in 11 of 20 experiments.

Since the popliteal node is quite prominent in the rat, in 1964 Engeset[118] irradiated the popliteal fossae of rats with 3000 rads. Chronic lymphedema did not occur in any of the several hundred rodents so injured. Burn[119] in 1966 ligated the deep inguinal lymphatics of greyhound dogs; while many developed mild swelling, all extremities returned to normal within 2 weeks. In 1967 Olszewski,[120] also using dogs, performed a circumferential thigh incision similar to that used by Reichert[94] 40 years earlier and added to the procedure a segmental resection of the skin and soft tissues. The resection included at least a 4 cm segment of femoral lymphatic channels and the popliteal lymph node. In addition, he left the wound open. At 1 year, edema persisted in one third of the animals. A year later, Danese[121] performed similar experiments on dogs in one- and two-staged procedures, and again, chronic lymphedema occurred in less than one half of the animals and experimental mortality was high.

A chemical lymphatic ablation, similar to Drinker's[116] earlier experiment with silica and quinine, was reproduced by Pflug and Calnan[122] in 1971 with the use of Neoprene latex. While nearly all dogs developed chronic edema, this model diffusely obliterated all lymphatics. In 1973, Clodius[123] created experimental chronic lymphedema in dogs, using a polyurethane foam sponge to inhibit lymphatic regeneration after circumferential surgical lymphatic ablation and excision in the mid-thigh. Skin bridges across the wound were found to be necessary if the animal were to survive. Otherwise, a "malignant" form of fulminant edema occurred; all animals died or required sacrifice within 3 weeks. In addition, Clodius[123] demonstrated lymphangiographically the greater distensibility of the superficial lymphatic system compared to the deep system. On this basis, he questioned the validity of purportedly "physiologic operations" for lymphedema which were thought to produce drainage of superficial into deep lymphatics. While highly successful in producing lymphedema, this model required several surgical procedures, surgical drains, a dependent apposition of the extremity for several days, and the use of a head basket on the dog. Five months of observation were required before the presence of chronic lymphedema could be securely ascertained.

Canine models of lymphedema can be expensive and, as described, cumbersome. For these reasons, interest in an experimental murine model developed. Kramer[124] reported surgically-induced lymphedema in the limb of the rat, but swelling was not quantitated and all edema resolved by the tenth postoperative day. In another interesting study, Vickery[125] was able to induce chronic lymphedema in immunodeficient mice infested with the parasite *Brugia malayi*. Furthermore, this type of lymphedema could be reversed by removing the worms. Since filariasis is still a major worldwide affliction, this result is of therapeutic interest.

Kanter et al[126] developed a murine chronic lymphedema model using a combination of radiation of the inguinal region, operative excision of superficial lymphatics, and microsurgical division of deep lymphatic channels with the aid of isosulfan blue dye. Edema appears within a relatively short period of time and has been quantified. The reliable production of stable chronic lymphedema for at least 9 months makes this a useful model. This model has the advantages of consistent results in a readily available and inexpensive animal.

Surgical disorders of the lymphatic system are uncommon and surgery of the lymphatics is underdeveloped. Nevertheless, there are subsets of patients with particularly challenging problems possibly amenable to operative treatment. Many operations have been devised to treat chronic lymphedema. However, no operation as yet yields consistent long-term results. Current procedures suffer from a lack of consistent published follow-up data. Recent work by Glovitsky[127] suggests that lympholymphatic anastomoses are more favorable since lymph is less coagulable than blood. Lymphoscintigrams, several months after suprapubic lymphatic grafting, showed patency in two patients. For treatment of lymphedema, modern devices that use sequential compression are particularly useful and are currently the preferred method of therapy.[128]

Reproducible experimental models could be used to evaluate surgical procedures such as direct reconstructions and illuminate conditions favoring successful outcomes. At a basic scientific level, capillary leak syndromes such as acute respiratory distress syndrome have focused mainly on blood capillaries. Little attention has been directed toward lymphatic pathology and the absorptive potential of lymphatic endothelium. The lymphatic endothelial cells are not simply passive barriers between the plasma and the interstitium. Lymphatic endothelial cells actively regulate transport of macromolecules, small solutes, and fluid.[129] More information about these cells and interstitial and plasma fluid fluxes would lead to better understanding and control of a variety of disorders.

References

1. Hunter W: *Two Introductory Lectures in His Last Course of Anatomic Lectures at His Theatre in Windmill Street.* London: J. Johnson; 1784.
2. Hewson W: *The Lymphatic System in the Human Subject and Other Animals.* London: J. Johnson; 1774.
3. Harvey W, quoted in Foster M: *Lectures on the History of Physiology.* Cambridge, England: Cambridge University Press; 1901.
4. Aselli G: *De Factibus sive Lacteis Verris, Quarto Vasorum Mesarai Corum Genere Novo Invento.* Milano: JB Bieldellium, Mediolani; 1627.
5. Mayerson HS: The lymphatic system with particular reference to the kidney. *Surg Gynecol Obstet* 116:259, 1963.
6. Dumont AD, Witte MH: Clinical usefulness of thoracic duct cannulation. *Adv Int Med* 15:51, 1969.
7. Mayerson HS: The physiologic importance of lymph, etc. In: Hamilton WF (ed). *Handbook of Physiology.* Vol II. Washington, DC: American Physiology Society; 1035–1073, 1963.

8. Arturson G, Soeda S: Changes in transcapillary leakage during healing of experimental burns. *Acta Chir Scand* 133:609, 1967.

9. Sabin FR: A critical study of the evidence presented in several recent articles on the development of the lymphatic system. *Anat Rec* 5:417, 1911.

10. Huntington GS: *The Anatomy and Development of the Systemic Lymphatics in the Domestic Cat.* Philadelphia: Wistar Institute Press; 1911.

11. Kinmonth JB: *The Lymphatics: Surgery, Lymphography, and Disease of the Chyle and Lymph System.* 2nd ed. London: Edward Arnold; 1982.

12. Servelle M: Congenital malformation of the lymphatics of the small intestine. *Cardiovasc Surg* 32:159, 1991.

13. Brandtzaeg P, Baklein K: Immunoglobulin producing cells in the intestine in health and disease. *Clin Gastroent* 5:251, 1976.

14. Caseley-Smith JR: The fine structure, properties, and permeabilities of the lymphatic endothelium. In: Collett JM, Jantet G, Schoffeniels E (eds). *New Trends in Basic Lymphology.* Basel: Birkhauser; 19–39, 1967.

15. Wheater PR, Burkitt HG, Daniels VG: *Functional Histology.* New York: Churchill Livingstone, Inc.; 86, 1984.

16. Breathnoch SM: Centenary review: the Langerhans cell. *Brit Dermatol* 119:463, 1988.

17. Malek P, Belan A, Kocandrle UL: The superficial and deep lymphatic system of the lower extremities and their mutual relationship under physiological and pathological conditions. *J Cardiovasc Surg* 5:686, 1964.

18. Bernard C: *Lecons sur les Phenomenes de la vie Communs aux Animaux et aux Vegetaux.* Vol 1. Paris: JB Bailliere et Fils; 1878.

19. Starling EH: On the absorption of fluid from the connective tissue spaces. *J Physiol* (London) 19:312, 1896.

20. Ludwig CFW: *Lehrbuch der Physiologie des Menschen.* 2nd Aufl., Leipzig: 1858.

21. Drinker CK, Field ME: The protein content of mammalian lymph and the relation of lymph to tissue fluid. *Am J Physiol* 97:32, 1931.

22. Guyton AC: A concept of negative interstitial pressure based on pressures in implanted perforated capsules. *Circ Res* 12:399, 1963.

23. McMaster PD: Conditions in the skin influencing interstitial fluid movement, lymph formation, and lymph flow. *Ann NY Acad Sci* 46:743, 1946.

24. Patterson RM, Ballard CJ, Wasserman K, Mayerson HS: Lymphatic permeability to albumin. *Am J Physiol* 194:120, 1958.

25. Morris B, Courtice FC: The origin of chylomicrons in the cervical and hepatic lymph. *Q Jl Exp Physiol* 41:341–348, 1956.

26. Pritchard JA, Weisman R: The absorption of labelled erythrocytes from the peritoneal cavity of humans. *J Lab Clin Med* 49:756, 1957.

27. Burns JM, Trueta J: Absorption of bacteria, toxins, and snake venoms from the tissues. *Lancet* 1:623–626, 1941.

28. Crockett DJ: The protein levels of edema fluid. *Lancet* 1:1179, 1956.

29. Ehrich WE: The role of the lymphocyte in the circulation of lymph. *Ann NY Acad Sci* 46:823, 1946.

30. Eloesser L: Obstruction of lymph channels by scar. *JAMA* 81:1867, 1923.

31. Andreasen E: Studies on the thymolymphatic system. *Acta Path Microbiol Scand* 49, 1943.

32. Barnes JM, Trueta J: Absorption of bacteria, toxins, and snake venoms from the tissues. *Lancet* 1:623, 1941.

33. Sabiston DC, Archer GW, Blalock A: Fate of cells in passage through lymphatics and lymph nodes. *Ann Surg* 158:570, 1963.

34. Roitt I, Brostoff J, Male D: *Immunology.* St. Louis: CV Mosby and Company; 1985.

35. Fauci AS: Multifactorial nature of human immunodeficiency virus disease: implications for therapy. *Science* 262:1011, 1993.

36. Vogler LB, Grossi CE, Cooper MD: Human lymphocyte subpopulations. In: Brown EB (ed). *Progress in Hematology.* Vol XI. New York: Grune and Stratton; 1–46, 1979.

37. Pansky B: *Review of Medical Embryology.* New York: Macmillan; 132, 1982.

38. Glick B, Chang TS, Jaap RG: The bursa of Fabricius and antibody production. *Poultr Sci* 35:224–225, 1956.

39. Wheater PR, Burkitt HG, Daniels VG: *Functional Histology.* New York: Churchill Livingstone; 147, 1984.

40. Cohen RJ, Jaffe ES: Current methods used in the diagnosis and classification of malignant lymphomas. *Updates Oncol* 1:1, 1987.

41. Salo M: Immune response to shock. In: Barrett J, Nyhus LM (eds). *Treatment of Shock: Principles and Practice.* Philadelphia: Lea and Febiger; 179–194, 1986.

42. Starzl TE, Weil R, Koep JL, et al: Thoracic duct fistula and renal transplantation. *Ann Surg* 190:474, 1979.

43. Stern EE: Current concepts of lymphatic transport. *Surg Gynecol Obstet* 138:773, 1974.

44. Neyazaki T, Kupic EA, Marshall WH, Abrams ML: Collateral lymphatico-venous communications after experimental obstruction of the thoracic duct. *Radiology* 85:423, 1965.

45. Chavez CM: The clinical significance of lymphaticovenous anastomoses; its implications in lymphangiography. *Vasc Dis* 5:35, 1968.

46. Clermont HG, Adams JT, Williams JS: Source of lysosomal enzymes acid phosphates in hemorrhagic shock. *Ann Surg* 175:19, 1972.

47. Mayerson HS: The lymphatic system with particular reference to the kidney. *Surg Gynecol Obstet* 116:259, 1963.

48. Rhoda DA, Beisel WR: Lymph production during staphylococcic B. enterotoxemia-induced shock. *Am J Vet Res* 31:1845, 1970.

49. DePalma RG, Coil J, Davis JH, Holden WD: Cellular and ultrastructural changes in endotoxemia: a light and electron microscopic study. *Surgery* 62:505, 1967.

50. Ackay F, Ackerman NB: Effects of operative manipulation on the flow of intestinal lymphatics. *Am J Surg* 122:662, 1971.

51. Berman IR, Moseley RV, Lamborn PB, Sleeman MK: Thoracic duct lymph in shock: gas exchange, acid base balance, and lysosomal enzymes in hemorrhagic and endotoxin shock. *Ann Surg* 169:202, 1969.

52. Dumont AE, Weissman G: Lymphatic transport of betaglucuronidase during hemorrhagic shock. *Nature* 201:1231, 1964.

53. Glenn TM, Lefer AM: Protective effect of thoracic lymph diversion in hemorrhagic shock. *Am J Physiol* 219:1305, 1970.

54. Tice DA, Dumont AE: Lethal factor in thoracic duct lymph following superior mesenteric artery ligation. *Surg Forum* 15:86, 1964.

55. Fish JC, McNeil L, Holaday WJ: Lymphatic obstruc-

tion in the pathogenesis of intestinal mucosal atrophy. *Ann Surg* 169:316, 1969.

56. Danese C, Howard JM, Bower R: Regeneration of lymphatic vessels: a radiographic study. *Ann Surg* 156:61, 1962.

57. Servelle M, Rouffilange F, Andrieux J, et al: Physiopathology of intestinal lymphatic vessels. *J Cardiovasc Surg* 9:310, 1968.

58. Dumont AE, Witte CL, Witte MH, Cole WR: Origin of red blood cells in thoracic duct lymph in hepatic cirrhosis. *Ann Surg* 171:1, 1970.

59. Orloff MJ, Wright PW, DeBendetti MJ, et al: Experimental ascites—VIII: the effects of external drainage of the thoracic duct on ascites and hepatic hemodynamics. *Arch Surg* 93:119, 1966.

60. Witte MH, Dumont AE, Cole WR, et al: Lymph circulation in hepatic cirrhosis; effect of porta caval shunt. *Ann Int Med* 70:303, 1969.

61. Gonzalez-Oddone M: Bilirubin, bromsulfalein, bile acids, alkaline phosphates, and cholesterol of thoracic duct lymph in experimental regurgitation jaundice. *Proc Soc Exp Biol Med* 63:144, 1946.

62. Miller AJ: *Lymphatics of the Heart.* New York: Raven Press; 1982.

63. Kline IK: Lymphatic pathways in the heart. *Arch Pathol* 88:638, 1969.

64. Miller AJ, Ellis A, Katz LH: Cardiac lymph: flow rates and composition in dogs. *Am J Physiol* 206:63, 1964.

65. Miller AJ, Pick R, Katz LN: Ventricular endomyocardial pathology produced by chronic cardiac lymphatic obstruction in the dog. *Circ Res* 6:941, 1960.

66. Dumont AE, Witte MH: Clinical usefulness of thoracic duct cannulation. *Adv Int Med* 15:51, 1969.

67. Dumont AE, Clauss RH, Reed GE, Tice DA: Lymph drainage in patients with congestive heart failure. *N Engl J Med* 269:949, 1963.

68. Lauweryns JM, Baert JH: Alveolar clearance and the role of the pulmonary lymphatics: state of the art. *Am Rev Resp Dis* 115:625, 1977.

69. Rouviere H: *Anatomie des Lymphatiques de l'Homme.* Paris: Masson et Cie; 218, 1932.

70. Warren MD, Drinker CK: The flow of lymph from the lungs of the dog. *Am J Physiol* 136:207, 1942.

71. Courtice FC: Lymph formation in the lungs. *Jap Heart J* 8:729, 1967.

72. Nisimaru Y: Blood and lymph vessels and body fluid flow in the lungs. *Hiroshima J Med Sci* 18:31, 1969.

73. Klosterkotter W: L'elimination des poussieres difficilements soluble hors de la zone respiratoire des poumons (epuration alveolaire). *Poumon Coeur* 23:1229, 1967.

74. Drinker CK: *Pulmonary Edema and Inflammation.* Cambridge, Mass: Harvard University Press; 1950.

75. Meyer EC, Dominguez EA, Bensch KG: Pulmonary lymphatic and blood absorption of albumin from alveoli: a quantitative comparison. *Lab Invest* 20:1, 1969.

76. Fischer E: Lymphgefabuntersuchungen an Serosen Hauten mit Luftfullongmethoden. *Verh Deutsch Pathol Ges* 28:223, 1935.

77. Bartels P: *Das Lymphgefasssystem.* Jena: Verlag um Gustav Fischser; 22–24, 1909.

78. Gerota D: Zur Technik der Lymphgeffasinjektion. *Atat Anzeiger* 12:216, 1896.

79. Hudack SS, McMaster PD: The lymphatic participation in human cutaneous phenomenon. *J Exp Med* 57:751, 1933.

80. Drinker CK, Enders JF, Shaffer MF, Leigh OC: The emigration of pneumococci Type III from the blood into the thoracic duct of rabbits and the survival of these organisms in the lymph following intravenous injection of specific antiserum. *J Exp Med* 62:849–860, 1935.

81. Glenn WLW: The lymphatic system. *Arch Surg* 116:989, 1981.

82. Servelle M, Deyson M: Reflux of intestinal chyle in the lymphatics of the leg. *Ann Surg* 133:234, 1951.

83. Haagensen CD: *Lymphatics in Cancer.* Philadelphia: Saunders and Co.; 26–27, 1972.

84. Kinmonth JB: Lymphangiography in clinical surgery and particularly in the treatment of lymphoedema. *Ann R Coll Surg* 15:300–315, 1954.

85. Bron KM, Baum S, Abrams HL: Oil embolism in lymphangiography: incidence, manifestations, and mechanisms. *Radiology* 80:194–202, 1963.

86. Jay JC, Ludington LG: Neurologic complications following lymphangiography. *Arch Surg* 106:863–864, 1973.

87. Smazal SF, Brown RC: Accidental intravenous injection of ethiodol. *J Can Assoc Radiol* 30:170, 1979.

88. Kinmonth JF: *The Lymphatics: Diseases, Lymphography, and Surgery.* Baltimore: Williams and Wilkins Co; v, 1972.

89. Sherman AI, Ter-Pogossian M: Lymph node concentration of radioactive colloidal gold following interstitial injection. *Cancer* 6:1238–1240, 1953.

90. Ege GN (ed): Lymphoscintigraphy. *Sem Nuc Med 1983* 13(1), 1983.

91. Glovitzki P, Hollier LH, Nora FE, Kaye MP: The natural history of microsurgical lymphovenous anastomoses: an experimental study. *J Vasc Surg* 4:148, 1986.

92. Baumeister R, Siuda S, Bohmert H, Moser E: A microsurgical method for reconstruction of interrupted lymphatic pathways. *Scand J Plast Reconst Surg* 20:141, 1986.

93. Delius: Uber die regeneration der lymphdrusen, dissertation, Bonn, 1888, quoted by Meyer AW: An experimental study on the recurrence of lymphatic glands and the regeneration of lymphatic vessels in the dog. *Bull Johns Hopkins Hosp* 17:185, 1906.

94. Reichert FL: The regeneration of the lymphatics. *Arch Surg* 13:871–881, 1926.

95. Clark ER, Clark EL: Observations of the new growth of lymphatic vessels as seen in transparent chambers introduced into the rabbit ear. *Am JH Anat* 51:49–87, 1932.

96. McMaster PD, Hudack SS: The participation of skin lymphatics in repair of the lesions due to incisions and burns. *J Exp Med* 60:479–501, 1934.

97. Bellman S, Oden B: Regeneration of surgically divided lymph vessels: an experimental study on the rabbit ear. *Acta Chir Scand* 116:99–117, 1959.

98. Manson EM: A study of the powers of reanastomosis of the limb lymphatic vessels and nodes in the dog. *Can J Surg* 5:329–333, 1962.

99. Sigel ME, Fisch UP: The effect of surgery on the cervical lymphatic system. *Laryngoscope* 75:458–474, 1965.

100. Gray JH: Studies of the regeneration of the lymphatic vessels. *J Anat* 74:309–335, 1930–1940.

101. McGregor IA, Conway H: Development of lymph flow from autografts and homografts of skin. *Transplant Bull* 3:46–47, 1956.

102. Scothorne RJ: Lymphatic repair and the genesis of homograft immunity. *Ann NY Acad Sci* 73:673–675, 1958.

103. Oden B: Microlymphangiographic studies of experi-

mental skin autografts. *Acta Chir Scand* 121:129–132, 1961.

104. Oden B: Microlymphangiographic studies of experimental skin homografts. *Acta Chir Scand* 121:233–241, 1961.
105. Vrubel J: Indirect color lymphography in skin grafts. *Folio Biol Praha* 7:131–184, 1961.
106. Weatherley-White RCA, Stark RB, DeForest M: Physiologic evidence of lymphatic repair after skin homotransplantation. *Surgery* 50:784–788, 1961.
107. Psillakis JM: Lymphatic vascularization of skin grafts. *Plast Reconstr Surg* 43:287–291, 1969.
108. Oden B: A microlymphangiographic study of experimental wounds healing by second intention. *Acta Chir Scand* 120:100–114, 1960.
109. Danese CA, Bower R, Howard JM: Experimental anastomoses of lymphatics. *Arch Surg* 84:6–9, 1962.
110. Chiappa SA, Galli G, Luciani L, Severini A: Considerations on the restoration of lymphatic circulation after pelvis lymphadenectomy. *Surg Gynecol Obstet* 120:323–334, 1964.
111. Eraslan S, Turner MD, Hardy JD: Lymphatic regeneration following lung reimplantation in dogs. *Surgery* 56:970–973, 1964.
112. Mobley JE, O'Dell RM: The role of lymphatics in renal transplantation: renal lymphatic regeneration. *J Surg Res* 7:231–233, 1967.
113. Malek P, Vrubel J: Lymphatic system and organ transplantation. *Lymphology* 1:4–22, 1968.
114. Goot B, Lillehei RC, Miller FA: Mesenteric lymphatic regeneration after autografts of small bowel in dogs. *Surgery* 48:571–575, 1960.
115. Kocandrle V, Houttuin E, Prohaska JV: Regeneration of the lymphatics after autotransplantation and homotransplantation of the entire small intestine. *Surg Gynecol Obstet* 122:587–592, 1966.
116. Drinker CK, Field ME, Homans J: The experimental production of edema and elephantiasis as a result of lymphatic obstruction. *Am J Physiol* 108:509, 1934.
117. Blalock A, Robinson SC, Cunningham RS, Gray ME: Experimental studies of lymphatic blockage. *AMA Arch Surg* 34:1049–1071, 1937.
118. Engeset A: Irradiation of lymph nodes and vessels. *Acta Radiol* (Stockholm) (suppl)229, 1964.
119. Burn II, Rivero OR, Pentecost BL, Calnan JS: Lymphographic appearances following lymphatic obstruction in the dog. *Brit J Surg* 53:634, 1966.
120. Olszewski W: The provocation of experimental lymphedema. *Pol Przegl Chir* 9:926, 1967.
121. Danese CA, Georgalas-Bertalsis M, Morales LE: A model for chronic postsurgical lymphedema in dogs' limbs. *Surgery* 64:814–820, 1968.
122. Pflug JJ, Calnan JB: The experimental production of chronic lymphedema. *Brit J Plast Surg* 24:1, 1971.
123. Clodius L, Wirth W: A new experimental model for chronic lymphedema of the extremities. *Chir Plastica* 2:115–132, 1974.
124. Kramer EL, McClaws R, Langer JJ, Shaw W: Lymphedema in the replanted limb of the rat. *Microsurgery* 6:40–45, 1985.
125. Vickery AC, Nayar JK, Albertine KH: Differential pathogenicity of *Brugia Malayi, B. pahangi* in immunodeficient nude mice. *Acta Tropica* 42:353, 1985.
126. Kanter MA, Slavin SA, Kaplan W: A model for experimental chronic lymphedema. *Plastic and Reconstr Surg* 85:573, 1990.
127. Glovitsky P: *Microsurgical Treatment for Chronic Lymphedema: An Unfulfilled Promise in Venous Disorders?* In: Bergan JJ, Yao JST (eds). *Venous Disorders* Philadelphia: WB Saunders; 344–359, 1992.
128. DePalma RG: Disorders of the lymphatic system. In: Sabiston (ed). *Textbook of Surgery: The Biologic Basis of Modern Surgical Practice*. Philadelphia: WB Saunders Co,; 1479–1489, 1991.
129. Symposium presented by the American Physiological Society at the 68th Annual Meeting of the Federation of American Societies for Experimental Biology, St. Louis, Missouri. *Fed Proc* 44:2602–2626, 1984.

II

The Science of Ancillary Disciplines:

The Essential Tools for the Treatment of Vascular Disease

CHAPTER 17

Diabetic Vascular Disease

Bruce A. Jones, MD; Anton N. Sidawy, MD
Frank W. LoGerfo, MD

Introduction and Epidemiology

Diabetes mellitus (DM) affects between 1% and 5% of the general population of the United States.[1,2] The incidence is increasing as the population ages, and is especially high among some subpopulations such as Native Americans and Mexican Americans. Diabetes is associated with a marked increase in cardiovascular disease.[3] In the Framingham study, the incidence of coronary artery disease was 40% in diabetic patients, representing a four- to fivefold increase compared to the nondiabetic population.[4] The incidence of peripheral vascular disease may be as high as 58%.[5] Kreines et al demonstrated an incidence of claudication of 37.7% in men and 24.3% in women 13 years following the diagnosis of non-insulin-dependent diabetes mellitus (NIDDM).[6] The significance of this is emphasized by the observation that nearly 75% of the deaths in the diabetic population occur secondary to cardiovascular disease-associated morbidity.[7]

The diabetic foot with its potential for gangrene and amputation causes patients much anxiety and uncertainty regarding future employability, financial security, and social well-being. Over 50% of nontraumatic amputations in this country are directly related to diabetic vascular disease-associated morbidity, representing a ten- to fifteenfold increased risk.[8,9]

The higher incidence of peripheral vascular disease in NIDDM patients is likely related to many factors, including age of onset of NIDDM (typically later in life) and gender. A higher incidence of vascular disease is seen in diabetic females.[10] The hyperinsulinemia seen in NIDDM patients has been implicated as a major factor in accelerated arterial disease.[11]

The most consistently implicated pathophysiologic findings in patients with diabetic vascular disease are the presence of basement membrane thickening and an accumulation of proteins in the extracellular matrix.[12–17] The resultant microangiopathy is systemic and affects the capillaries of the retina, renal glomerulus, nervous system, and integument. Retinopathy, diabetic nephropathy, and diabetic neuropathy lead to substantial morbidity and mortality. Nephropathy is the leading cause of morbidity in patients with diabetes.[15,18] Our understanding of microangiopathy has increased recently as refined techniques have been developed in the fields of endocrinology and molecular biochemistry.

The most distinguishing feature of atherosclerosis in diabetes is the pattern in which it occurs in the lower extremity arteries. The occlusive process tends to involve the infrageniculate arteries (anterior and posterior tibial arteries, and peroneal artery). One series showed a 63.6% incidence of peripheral vascular disease in the infrageniculate distribution of diabetics compared to a 6.4% incidence of vascular occlusive disease in the more proximal anatomy.[19] There is also a predominance of bilateral peripheral vascular disease when comparing diabetic to nondiabetic patients.

In prospective studies by Strandness[20] and by Menzoian[21] it was noted that the foot arteries were relatively spared of occlusive disease in diabetic amputation specimens even though the tibial arteries in the leg were occluded. In an angiographic study of the pattern of vascular disease, we also demonstrated that

From *The Basic Science of Vascular Disease*. Edited by Sidawy AN, Sumpio BE, and DePalma RG. Armonk, NY: Futura Publishing Company, Inc.; © 1997.

foot vessels, especially the dorsalis pedis, were spared in the diabetic even though the leg arteries were occluded.[21] Recognition of this pattern of vascular occlusion is important because it opens up the possibility of arterial reconstruction with bypass grafts to the inframalleolar vessels, especially the dorsalis pedis artery.[22,23] With this pattern of occlusion, the runoff to the foot should be determined angiographically even when the infrageniculate arteries are occluded. It is a common mistake to terminate the angiogram upon noting that the three infrageniculate arteries are occluded, on the assumption that distal vessels must also be occluded.

The basis for the increased macrovascular disease associated with diabetes may include lipid abnormalities. Lipid abnormalities are common, usually characterized by elevated triglycerides and low HDL cholesterol. LDL cholesterol is not typically elevated although the VLDL component might be high. Elevated triglyceride levels are associated with obesity and hyperinsulinemia. This pattern holds true for nearly all diabetic populations in the United States, i.e., Caucasians, Hispanics, African Americans, Native Americans, Asians, and Indians.

Hypertension is significantly associated with peripheral vascular disease in diabetic patients.[4] Higher mean blood pressures are seen in bilateral above-knee amputees compared to single above-knee amputees.[19,24] Hypertension associated with hyperlipidemia and hyperinsulinemia has been identified and labeled as a diabetic-related syndrome—syndrome X.[11,25,26]

Recent investigation of race and the incidence of peripheral vascular disease in diabetic patients has shown interesting results. Yet we have evaluated 135 patients with peripheral vascular disease, suggesting that DM and hypertension affect the severity of peripheral vascular disease in white patients and show no such influence in the African-American population.[27] As shown in Table 1, when infrageniculate vessels were graded arteriographically using the SVS/ISCVS scoring system, a marked improvement in severity was seen in the white population when hypertension was excluded. An even greater improvement was seen when both hypertension and DM were excluded as factors. No such improvement was seen in the African-American population, suggesting that other factors may be involved in severity of infrageniculate peripheral vascular disease in African-American patients.

Insulin and Glucose Regulation

Insulin is a large polypeptide molecule, synthesized in the β islet cell of the pancreas and responsible for the regulation of carbohydrate metabolism. The structure of insulin is demonstrated in Figure 1. The gene for insulin is found on chromosome 11p.[28] Proinsulin is a polypeptide macromolecule and a product of preproinsulin. Upon cleavage of two basic residues at each end of the molecule, proinsulin yields insulin and C-peptide. Figure 2 illustrates the conversion of proinsulin that occurs within immature secretory granules of β cells in the pancreas. Circulating C-peptide can be measured as an index of insulin secretion.

A relative state of "hyperinsulinemia" is seen in both obese adult patients and patients with NIDDM. Normal-weight patients with impaired glucose tolerance and NIDDM also manifest a hyperinsulinemic response to glucose.[29] The hyperinsulin state seen in NIDDM patients may be a product of both insulin as well as circulating proinsulin and split products of proinsulin. Evidence shows that there is a defect in the pancreatic β cell that impairs the conversion of proinsulin to insulin in the NIDDM patient.[30] Many current radioimmunoassays do not distinguish between proinsulin and insulin and this likely accounts for the findings of hyperinsulinemia.

Standl et al showed that fasting C-peptide levels are elevated in NIDDM patients that demonstrate macrovascular disease.[31] Patients that had the highest fasting C-peptide levels were also more likely to have macrovascular disease including coronary artery disease, peripheral vascular disease, and carotid arterial disease.

As described in 1990, patients with NIDDM also demonstrate resistance to insulin action due to 1) an

Table 1
Hypertension, Diabetes Mellitus, and Race: Relation to the Severity of Peripheral Vascular Disease

	SVS/ISCVS Disease Severity Score: Infragenicular Vessels		
	Total Population	Non-HTN	Non-HTN, Non-DM
African Americans	2.08 ± 0.05	2.10 ± 0.06	2.21 ± 0.09
Caucasians	1.57 ± 0.06	1.42 ± 0.06	1.22 ± 0.19

(Reproduced with permission from Reference 27.)

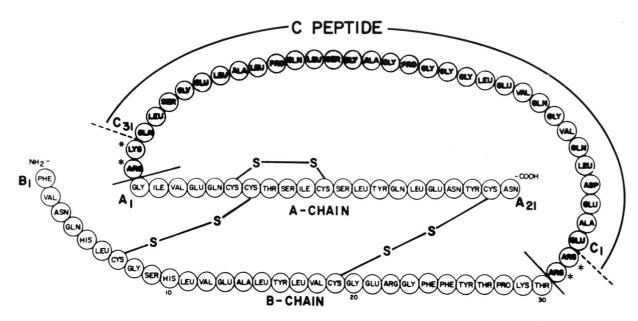

Figure 1. Structure of human insulin. **Shaded circles** indicate the connecting segment. The loss of four basic amino acids during conversion of proinsulin to insulin (**asterisks**) results in formation of equimolar concentrations of C-peptide and insulin. The numbering of the proinsulin molecule for each component of the molecule is designated by **A** for the A chain, **B** for the B chain, and **C** for the C-peptide. The basic amino acids at the two ends of C-peptide are designated by **CA** or **BC** to indicate the residue attached to the A or B chain, respectively. (Reproduced with permission from Reference 32.)

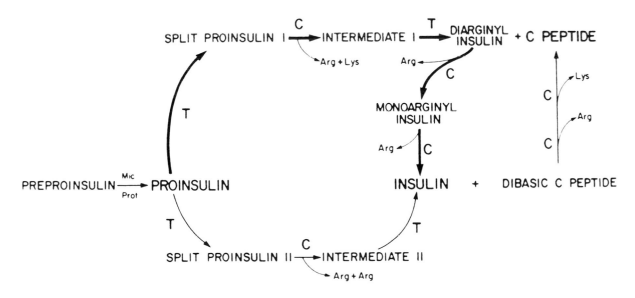

THE THICKER ARROWS DEPICT THE MOST PROBABLE PATHWAY OF INSULIN SYNTHESIS IN MAN.
T = TRYPSIN-LIKE ENZYME.   C = CARBOXYPEPTIDASE-LIKE ENZYME.   Mic Prot = MICROSOMAL PROTEASE.

Figure 2. Schematic presentation of proinsulin conversion sequence. **Heavy arrows** indicate the probable pathway of insulin synthesis in humans. (Reproduced with permission from Reference 32.)

abnormal β cell secretory product; 2) circulating insulin antagonists; or 3) a target tissue defect in insulin action.[32]

Insulin has been demonstrated to play a role in atherosclerosis and is a potent mitogen and growth factor for the proliferation of vascular smooth muscle cells.[33,34] The state of hyperinsulinemia is therefore generally considered to be a key factor in the development of diabetic vascular disease.[11]

Glucose Control and Peripheral Vascular Disease

The tight metabolic control of blood glucose levels in an effort to avoid the development of diabetic peripheral vascular disease remains controversial. Evidence supports the concept that good control of glucose levels can prevent and in fact stabilize diabetic nephropathy. Bilious et al[35] showed that diabetic nephropathy in a recipient allograft is significantly improved and showed less mesangial proliferation following renal-pancreas transplantation as opposed to renal transplantation alone. The stabilization of blood glucose with the pancreatic transplantation is surmised to be the important factor that limits subsequent renal damage.

However, the importance of tight control of blood glucose levels in the prevention and amelioration of diabetic peripheral vascular disease is still controversial. In fact, multiple investigators have shown that the incidence of peripheral vascular calcifications, intermittent claudication, arteriosclerosis obliterans, and the rate of arteriosclerosis does not appear to be different between patients with good diabetic control and those patients with poorly controlled blood glucose levels.[36–38] However, the Diabetes Control and Complications Trial (DCCT) research group has provided evidence that tight blood glucose regulation possibly limits macrovascular disease.[39] This multicenter, randomized clinical trial included 1441 patients with insulin-dependent diabetes mellitus (IDDM), and compared conventional with intensive diabetes therapy with regard to the development and progression of vascular morbidity. Conventional therapy included one or two daily insulin injections, and intensive care consisted of an insulin pump or three or more insulin injections daily. Intensive therapy was designed to maintain preprandial glucose levels between 70 to 120 mg/dL, postprandial levels less than 180 mg/dL, a weekly 3-A.M. glucose level >65 mg/dL, and a monthly hemoglobin A_{1C} within normal range. By measuring the degree of retinopathy, microalbuminuria and albuminuria, and evaluating the degree of clinical neuropathy, significant results were obtained. The evidence shows that intensive therapy does delay the onset and slows the progression of diabetic retinopathy, neuropathy, and nephropathy in patients with IDDM.[39] When peripheral vascular and cardiovascular morbidity were combined, the DCCT group found that intensive therapy reduced the risk of macrovascular disease. A reduction from 0.8 event/100 patient-years to 0.5 event/100 patient-years (a 41% decrease) was seen. Although this was not statistically significant, it does suggest that tight glycemic control limits peripheral vascular and cardiovascular morbidity.[39]

Atherosclerosis

In addition to smooth muscle cell proliferation and migration that is induced by insulin, it has been suggested that insulin plays a role in atherosclerosis.[40–43] Insulin resistance has also been shown to have a direct influence on the atherosclerotic process.[44] Insulin not only stimulates smooth muscle cell and connective tissue synthesis, but also stimulates lipid metabolism in both smooth muscle cells and monocyte macrophages.

Hyperinsulinemia is associated with low HDL cholesterol levels and elevated triglyceride levels.[12,15,46] In fact, a commonly described trio exists in the patient with cardiovascular disease: hyperinsulinemia, high VLDL and triglyceride levels, and a decreased HDL cholesterol level. The importance of this has been proven with coronary heart disease showing a reverse correlation between HDL level and coronary artery disease.[47] However, less evidence exists when determining the significance of a lowered HDL and peripheral vascular disease.

The pig aorta model has demonstrated a high triglyceride level and elevated lipogenic enzyme activity after the injection of insulin.[48,49] It is speculated that insulin may inhibit the breakdown of triglycerides by altering the effect of a triacylglycerol lipase.[50]

Stamler and associates used studies in the chick model to demonstrate the relation of insulin to atherosclerosis.[43] After high cholesterol diets were changed to low cholesterol diets, arterial lesions that normally regressed after diet change were prevented from regressing with the addition of insulin. This study provided later investigators a basis for the pathophysiology behind these findings.

Sato and associates studied an in vivo model of the Wistar rat in which their experimental group was subjected to daily injections of insulin-zinc suspension for a 1-year duration.[40] Light microscopic evaluation after 1 year revealed intimas that were significantly thickened compared to control animals. Similarly, triglyceride content of the aortic intimal lesions in the experimental group was significantly elevated compared to the control group. Electron microscopy of the "atheroma" lesions showed findings consistent with smooth muscle as the cell of origin.

An immune mechanism of atherosclerosis in diabetic patients has also been suggested. Modified lipoproteins are increased in diabetic patients and are thought to stimulate the development of foam cells from macrophages. They induce an immune response with the subsequent formation of antibodies and later immune complexes. These lipoprotein-containing immune complexes are then taken up by the macrophages causing activation and release of humoral mediators (IL-1β and TNF-α) that can contribute to the initiation of atheromatous lesions.[51]

Ruderman and Schneider have suggested that regular exercise can diminish the risk for atherosclerotic vascular disease in NIDDM and obese patients.[52] Although not yet proven, the authors believe that the beneficial effect of exercise comes from its ability to prevent or decrease hyperinsulinemia.

Cultured smooth muscle cells show an increased lipid metabolism when subjected to insulin treatment. A resultant increase in the binding of LDLs to cell membranes and an increased sterol synthesis is seen.[53,54] Smooth muscle cell migration from the media to the intima is essential in the development of the atheroma. When smooth muscle cell migration is induced by 12-L-hydroxy-5,8,10,14-eicosatetraenoic acid (12-HETE), the addition of insulin appears to enhance the cellular migration.[42,55]

The importance of the macrophage-foam cell in the pathogenesis of atherosclerosis is well-known. Krone et al have shown that insulin stimulates LDL binding to the cell membrane of monocytes, likely by increasing the activity of the enzyme 3-hydroxy-3–methylglutaryl-CoA reductase.[56,57] This is the key enzyme responsible for cholesterol metabolism.

Macrophage accumulation of triglyceride-rich lipoproteins are modulated by receptor and nonreceptor mechanisms.[58] Lipoprotein lipase (LpL) enhances the uptake of lipoproteins by the macrophage by utilizing both mechanisms. The macrophage also secretes products that influence lipoprotein uptake and receptor affinity. ApoE is one such product that becomes incorporated into triglyceride-rich lipoproteins and augments their uptake.[59]

There remains much speculation on how diabetes mellitus alters the uptake of lipoproteins by macrophages. Several possibilities are currently under investigation. Although yet to be proven, macrophage LpL and ApoE secretion in the diabetic is thought to be altered and likely diminished.[58] This would lead to a diminished lipoprotein uptake by the LDL receptor, but would allow a prolonged time for the uptake by scavenger receptors.[58]

The hypertriglyceridemia induced by the hyperinsulinemic state provides for an environment conducive to the avid uptake of triglyceride-rich lipoproteins by the macrophage.

Another possibility lies with the HDL cholesterol. Nonenzymatic glycosylation of HDL$_3$ (as occurs in diabetes mellitus) diminishes cholesterol esterification and net efflux of cholesterol from the cell. This was shown in the human monocyte-derived macrophage and human skin fibroblasts[60,61] and may contribute to accelerated atherosclerosis. Similarly, Fievet et al[62] isolated the HDL ApoA-1, which is known to protect against atherosclerosis, from two poorly controlled IDDM patients. Lipoprotein A-1 particles from both patients were separated into glycosylated and nonglycosylated fractions. The results indicate that glycosylated lipoprotein A-1 particles are less effective in cholesterol efflux compared to nonglycosylated fractions.[62]

Lipoprotein (LP) oxidation products exist in atherosclerotic lesions and are hypothesized to contribute to the atherosclerotic process. Oxidized LDL interferes with the relaxation of vascular tissue by the endothelial cell,[63,64] is chemoattractant to monocytes,[65] and augments the production of monocyte chemotactic factors.[66] Hyperglycemia and LP oxidation may be related and have been the topics of intense study.[67,68] Human LDL incubated with high glucose has been shown in vitro to increase lipid perioxidation.[69,70] The combination of glycation and oxidation byproduct accumulation is accelerated in diabetic patients.[71] If, in fact, hyperglycemia does influence LP oxidation in vivo and subsequent acceleration of atherosclerosis, this would provide invaluable assistance to the treatment of diabetic vascular disease with the use of antioxidants, etc. Hypertriglyceridemia, as seen in diabetes mellitus, has been demonstrated to increase superoxide production in mononuclear cells of diabetic patients as compared to controls.[72]

Watanabe et al isolated the LDL cholesterol fraction from 10 patients with IDDM. After incubation with platelets, the degree of aggregation was observed. A positive correlation was seen between the degree of LDL glycosylation and the degree of platelet aggregation, suggesting that this may be a contributory factor. They also found that thromboxane B$_2$ production was increased during aggregation when LDL was isolated from IDDM patients compared to controls.[73]

Mechanism of Action of Insulin

The regulation of insulin release from the pancreatic β cell is mediated by levels of D-glucose in the blood. Insulin action is then dependent upon specific receptor binding on the cell surface with subsequent receptor activation and intracellular signaling.[32]

Cell-surface receptor anatomy has been characterized. The receptor resides within the cell's plasma membrane. The receptor is a polypeptide dimer linked by a disulfide bond and glycosylated before being available for binding.[74] Two subunits, α and β, are linked and provide the sites for glycosylation. The α subunits are entirely outside of the cell membrane while the β subunits provide a transmembrane structure and are the site of the tyrosine kinase domain.[32] The gene for the insulin receptor contains 4.1 kilobases (kb) of coding sequence over 22 exons.[75] It is a member of the src family of tyrosine-specific protein kinases and resides on chromosome 19.[76,77]

Once insulin binds to the receptor, phosphorylation of the tyrosine kinase sites occurs, resulting in increased tyrosine kinase activity and increased insulin action.[78] Kinase activity leads to activation of phosphodiesterase with a diminution of cAMP levels in adipose and hepatic tissue.[79,80] However, sufficient evidence exists that insulin does not alter cAMP levels in many other tissues. This evidence suggests that there is another mechanism of action of insulin besides the alteration in cAMP levels.

Other intracellular mediators include phosphatidylinositol 4,5–biphosphate (PIP$_2$). The PIP$_2$ is degraded and releases 1,4,5–triphosphate (IP$_3$) and 1,2-diacylglycerol (DAG). IP$_3$ raises cytosolic Ca^{2+} which subsequently mediates the action of insulin. DAG when present with Ca^{2+} and phosphatidylserine activate protein kinase C which subsequently mediates the protein phosphorylation necessary.[81]

Recently, other intracellular signaling pathways have been described. Evidence using interferon-α (IFN-α) shows that when IFN-α binds to its cell surface receptor, the associated tyrosine kinase activates a transcription factor inside the cell which then enters the nucleus to activate its own particular set of genes.[82,83] Many speculate that other regulatory molecules such as insulin use similar signaling pathways.

The ultimate action of insulin is the dephosphorylation of key regulatory enzymes in intermediary metabolic pathways. This leads to the increased synthesis of glycogen, protein, and fat by the enzymes glycogen synthase, pyruvate dehydrogenase, and hormone-sensitive lipase.[79,80]

Insulin as a Growth Factor

There is a hyperinsulinemic state present in obese patients and those with NIDDM. An understanding of how insulin acts as a growth factor is essential. Insulin stimulates both proliferation and migration of aortic smooth muscle cells in vitro.[34,41,84,85,156]

Early in vitro studies of the effect of insulin showed that the proliferative effects on the vascular smooth muscle cell were seen with small increases in the concentration of insulin, and increasing concentrations only stimulated the proliferation of fibroblasts in cultured rat aortic smooth muscle cells and monkey aortic smooth muscle cells.[84,86,156] Since these early studies, much has been learned with the use of newer assays and advanced techniques in cell culture.

Insulin acts upon both insulin-like growth factor-1 (IGF-1) receptors and insulin receptors. However, insulin has a one hundredfold less affinity for the IGF-I receptor than does IGF-1.[87,88] The metabolic and proliferative effects of insulin occur at different receptors. Using a polyclonal antibody to the insulin receptor and a monoclonal antibody to the IGF-1 receptor, the proliferative effects of both insulin and IGF-1 have been studied by measuring DNA synthesis with [^{3}H] thymidine labeling.[87] By utilizing a selective blockade of receptors, it has been demonstrated that the proliferative effects of insulin occur through the IGF-1 receptor.

Using cell culture techniques, King et al,[13] isolated endothelial cells and pericytes from bovine retinal capillaries as well as endothelial and smooth muscle cells from bovine vascular smooth muscle. They characterized the receptors and growth-promoting effects of IGF-1 and multiplication-stimulating activity (MSA, an IGF-II). In addition, the growth-promoting effects of insulin were measured and compared using [^{3}H] thymidine labeling techniques as a means to measure DNA synthesis. Retinal vessel cells were used as an example of diabetic microvascular disease and the aortic vessel cells as representative of diabetic macrovascular disease. Their results suggested that insulin and the IGFs play a role in the development of diabetic vascular disease. IGF-I and other growth factors are further delineated and discussed in Chapter 6. In King's study, insulin stimulated [^{3}H] thymidine incorporation in retinal capillary endothelial cells with a maximal effect occurring at a concentration of 10^{-7}M, with a growth-promoting effect over a wide range of concentrations (3 × 10^{-9} to 2 × 10^{-7}M).[13] The vascular supporting cells (retinal capillary pericytes) also showed an enhanced [^{3}H] thymidine incorporation with the addition of insulin (again over a broad range of concentrations with a maximal effect at a concentration of 10^{-7}M).

Aortic endothelial cells reveal a much more modest growth enhancement with the addition of insulin than do the retinal endothelial cells; however, smooth muscle cells from the aorta show remarkable growth with the addition of insulin. With concentrations of 10^{-7}M and 10^{-6}M, insulin has stimulated cell growth by 35% and 51% above basal level.[13] Interestingly, King's studies were also among the first to show that insulin and IGF-I likely use the same cell membrane receptor.[13,89]

Cultured human smooth muscle cells from renal,

popliteal, and tibial sources have been used to characterize receptors and to note growth regulation by insulin and IGF-I.[87] By their origin, these cells may provide better evidence of the in vivo responses of diabetic patients.

Banskota et al estimated cellular proliferation by measuring the proto-oncogene c-myc mRNA levels after induction.[87] The induction of proto-oncogenes is seen in cellular regeneration and as a result of certain growth factors.[90,91] Preliminary evidence has shown that both insulin and IGF-I stimulate the early gene c-myc in vascular smooth muscle cells.[87] Measuring mRNA of c-myc may provide an estimate of cellular proliferation. However, by selective receptor blockade it was noted that the antibody to IGF-I receptor can also stimulate c-myc induction.[87] Therefore, further study is necessary to determine the role of c-myc amplification and its association with DNA synthesis and mitosis.

Recent evidence suggests that insulin and its precursor proinsulin may impair fibrinolysis leading to subsequent diabetic vascular morbidity.[92,93] The endothelial exposure to clot-associated mitogens activates macrophages and causes proliferation of vascular smooth muscle cells. In vitro studies using human hepatoma cells and porcine aortic endothelial cells show an enhanced plasminogen activator inhibitor type-1 (PAI-1, the primary inhibitor of t-PA) expression as well as an enhanced PAI-1 activity when exposed to insulin concentrations seen in NIDDM patients.[93–96] The increase in PAI-1 mRNA expression seen when exposed to insulin is due to its decreased degradation rather than to an increased rate of transcription.[93]

Insulin's Relation to Other Growth Factors

Other peptide growth factors are commonly expressed and prominent when intimal hyperplasia exists. Platelet-derived growth factor, endothelin-1, IGF-I, epidermal growth factor, and growth hormone are all important. Although these factors are discussed in Chapter 6, it is important here to realize that insulin has a joint role with many of these growth factors. The synergy between insulin and the above-mentioned growth factors will be discussed and the complementary roles of each will be presented.

Endothelin-1

Endothelin-1 (ET-1) is the most powerful vasoconstrictor known and has potent mitogenic effects for the vascular smooth muscle cell.[25,97,98] Our understanding of the role that ET-1 plays in atherosclerosis and the development of intimal hyperplasia is evolving, but recent studies indicate that the synthesis and receptor upregulation of ET-1 is influenced by insulin.[25,99–101]

Aortic and kidney afferent artery smooth muscle cells from the Sprague-Dawley rat have been studied in vitro to note the effect of insulin upon ET-1 synthesis.[25] ET-1 receptor binding assays were used to measure receptor number, and [^{3}H] thymidine labeling was used to measure DNA content and ascertain mRNA regulation of the ET-1 receptor gene.[25]

Frank et al found that when cultured vascular smooth muscle cells were incubated with insulin, a time-dependent increase in the expression of ET-1 receptor mRNA was seen (a 2.3 ± 0.3-fold increase versus control, maximal at 4 hours). Binding assays also showed a receptor protein expression increase in those cells incubated with insulin. In a concurrent in vivo study, it was determined that after 11 days of hyperinsulinemia both ET-1 secretion and ET-1 receptor numbers were significantly increased when compared to the control animals.[25]

Under the influence of insulin, bovine endothelial cells manifest similar findings of increased ET-1 secretion and upregulation of gene expression.[99,101] ET-1 secretion was increased to nearly four times normal with the addition of insulin and increased twofold when insulin was at physiologic levels.[99]

By inhibiting tyrosine kinase with genistein, a reduction in ET-1 secretion and gene expression is noted.[99] This supports the hypothesis that it is the insulin receptor, and not the IGF-I receptor, that is used by insulin to augment ET-1 activity.

Growth Hormone

Growth hormone (GH) is known to have mitogenic effects.[102] These mitogenic effects are indirect and have been shown to be mediated by IGF-I.[103]

In vitro studies using human T-lymphoblast cell lines have elicited the relationship between GH and insulin. The mitogenic effects of insulin are attenuated when these cells are preincubated with GH.[104] Subsequently, it was determined that the resistance to the mitogenic effects of insulin by GH are through the action of local IGF-I in a paracrine manner.[105]

Platelet-Derived Growth Factor

As with GH, platelet-derived growth factor (PDGF) stimulates smooth muscle cell migration, contraction, and matrix synthesis.[106] Synergistic effects with insulin have been studied to a limited degree and with a limited number of cell types.

Fayed et al studied the synergistic effects of insulin and PDGF in uterine myometrial cells, leiomyoma cells, and vascular smooth muscle cells.[107] Although no data were presented, when these growth factors were incubated together with the vascular smooth muscle cells obtained from umbilical veins, an increase in DNA synthesis was seen.[107]

Insulin-Like Growth Factor-I

The regulation of IGF-I secretion is closely associated with both insulin and growth hormone levels.[108] This in combination with the fact that IGF-I is also a strong smooth muscle cell mitogen adds to the importance of insulin in the development of diabetic vascular disease.

By studying diabetic animals, it has been shown that the IGF-I levels are markedly elevated when insulin is given to these animals.[109,110] In vitro analysis of smooth muscle cells from humans shows an incremental increase in the IGF-I peptide with varying concentrations of insulin added. Insulin at concentrations between 1 to 10 ng/mL produced the largest response.[108]

The synergy of these two factors continues to be characterized. As mentioned earlier, the mitogenic effect of insulin appears to occur through the IGF-I receptor.[87]

The Microcirculation

Diabetes mellitus is considered as a macro- and microvascular disease to the clinician when treating diabetic vascular morbidity. A close look at the microcirculation in the diabetic patient reveals its overall importance and how the tissue level remains the basis for all diabetic-related diseases.

The Tissue Level

The abnormalities in the microcirculation associated with diabetes are multifold. Vascular occlusion, however, is not always present in the diabetic microcirculation. The most commonly described lesion is a thickening of the capillary basement membrane.[2] Surprisingly, this is not associated with a narrowing of the capillary. In fact, the lumenal capillary diameter in diabetic patients is actually greater than that in nondiabetics.[111,112] In a study of sural nerve biopsies, it was noted that the largest capillary diameters actually occurred in diabetic patients with the greatest degree of neuropathy.[113]

While not an occlusive process, the capillary basement membrane thickening may alter the exchange of nutrients, proteins, and inorganic molecules between the capillary and the interstitium. It has been demonstrated that there is an increased flux of highly charged molecules, most notably albumin, from the capillary.[114] This capillary leak has been attributed to a decreased charge on the basement membrane, due to glycosylation and replacement of sulfur groups, allowing easier movement of highly charged molecules through the membrane.[14] Indeed, Deckert et al have suggested that the increased permeability is due to an altered electrostatic charge of the supporting matrix.[115] However, an in vitro study indicated that the enhanced capillary leak is more a result of glycosylation of albumin rather than the basement membrane.[116] The permeability changes may well have physiologic consequences leading to tissue that is less biologically resistant to the effects of ischemia, pressure, and infection.

It is of note that there does not appear to be any impairment of oxygen diffusion across the capillary basement membrane. In a study of diabetics and nondiabetics presenting with foot ulceration, the transcutaneous PO_2 in the diabetics was actually greater than that in the nondiabetics.[117]

There is probably a complex interplay between microvascular perfusion, neuropathy, and inflammation. Normally the distribution of skin blood flow is regulated by sympathetic tone and by local axon reflexes. Autonomic neuropathy is common in diabetics, usually detectable by absent sinus reflexes in response to the Valsalva maneuver. This may result in increased physiologic ateriovenous (AV) shunting of skin blood flow and a decrease in nutrient flow. When skin is injured, the axon reflexes come into play in what is broadly referred to as the nociceptive response. Stimulation of a sensory axon transmits the impulse to the nerve body at the sensory ganglion (prodromic transmission). Simultaneously, there is a rapid antidromic transmission to other axon branches. Neuro kinins are released, including substance P, which cause release of histamine and initiation of the inflammatory response. Both substance P and calcitonin gene-related peptide (CGRP), which is also released, cause vasodilatation.[118] Normally, CGRP acts to increase capillary permeability, but this response is blunted in streptozotocin-induced diabetes, suggesting a decreased responsiveness in the effector tissue.[118] Similarly, there is a decreased hyperemic response seen in diabetics as compared with nondiabetics which correlates with duration of disease.[119]

The normal vasodilatory response that is attenuated in diabetic patients limits maximal microvascular blood flow. In Tooke's model of arterial occlusion, a diminished capillary flow and pressure is seen following release of arterial occlusion.[120,121] This appears to correlate to the degree of hyalinosis and basement membrane thickening.[119,122]

The acute phase of inflammation is followed by migration of PMN leukocytes, lymphocytes, and monocytes into the injured tissue. A blunted neurogenic inflammatory response is appreciated in diabetic patients. Blunting of this response leaves the skin more susceptible to unrecognized injury and perhaps more susceptible to bacterial invasion. This may explain why deep infections in the diabetic foot are typically accompanied by surprisingly little inflammation and are often overlooked.

Another contribution to microvascular disease may be derived from hyperglycemia. Chronically elevated glucose leads to formation of nonenzymatic advanced glycosylation end-products (AGE) such as HBA1c in the tissues. AGE alters the extracellular matrix which decreases endothelial cell adhesion, increases vascular permeability, inactivates nitric oxide activity, and induces the release of growth-promoting cytokines.[123] This mechanism may also lead to excessive production of extracellular matrix including the basement membrane.[14] Many early glycosylation end-products undergo several rearrangements to form irreversible complexes which accumulate, bound to protein, on blood vessel walls.

AGE also acts as an interface between the basement membrane insoluble matrix proteins and extravasated plasma lipoproteins through covalent cross-linking as shown in Figure 3. As the amount of advanced glycosylation end-products increases, the amount of LDL-collagen cross-linking also increases.[14,124] It has also been shown that other plasma proteins, such as albumin, bind covalently to collagen through these AGEs,[123] and that collagen cross-linking within the matrix is greatly increased in the presence of AGEs.[126,127,157]

The consequences of the accumulation of AGE are shown in Table 2. An increase in vascular permeability and a thickened, inelastic vessel wall occur with many of the permeability changes being irreversible.

Hyperglycemia is also a contributor to the increased elaboration of other extracellular matrix components in vitro in the mesangial cell. When hyperglycemia was introduced to mesangial cell cultures, there was a 50% increase in the amount of type IV collagen, fibronectin, and laminin when measured by enzyme-linked immunosorbent assay (ELISA).[128,129] Fibronectin and type IV collagen are similarly elevated in endothelial cell culture. These findings were shown by Cagliero et al to occur at a concentration of 30 mM glucose for at least 4 days. Interestingly, when media was changed to normal levels of glucose, the mRNA transcripts for both fibronectin and type IV collagen remained high, indicating a type of "memory."[130,131]

Protein kinase C (PKC) activation appears to be a factor that stimulates the elevated levels of these proteins.[132] The hyperglycemia has been shown in vitro to elevate diacylglycerol(DAG) levels either from de novo synthesis or from the breakdown of phosphoino-

sitides.[133] DAG activates the Ca^{2+}-dependent PKC.[4] In addition to stimulating matrix protein production, PKC has also been shown to directly alter membrane permeability in the presence of high glucose.[134,135] By inhibiting PKC with staurosporin, these investigators demonstrated that membrane permeability decreased and, therefore, it was determined that the PKC directly alters membrane permeability.

The normal vasodilatory response to serotonin and acetylcholine is inhibited in diabetes due to an increase in endothelium-derived contracting factor.[136] There also appears to be a diminished release of EDRF in experimental diabetes and in patients with diabetes. This is attributed to a hyperglycemia-induced increase in DAG. This increase in DAG leads to an associated activation of PKC which phosphorylates nitric oxide (NO) synthase.[137] The result is an increase in NO and in endothelin.[138,139]

Diabetes also affects the expression of cellular adhesion receptors on monocytes.[140] An increased level of a circulating form of ICAM-1 has been detected in IDDM patients and relatives.[141] These events are consistent with an ongoing autoimmune process. Pertinent to foot problems, the circulatory adhesion molecules may interfere with normal leukocyte-endothelial interactions or the homing of leukocytes at a point of inflammation.

Hyperglycemia may be a source of vascular dysfunction initiated by increased metabolism via the polyol pathway. Glucose is converted to sorbitol by the enzyme aldose reductase. Sorbitol can be converted to fructose by sorbitol dehydrogenase with production of NADH. This is a relatively slow reaction so sorbitol may accumulate in cells as a consequence of hyperglycemia.[142] Elevated levels of glucose and sorbitol compete for the uptake of myo-inositol. This in turn decreases the levels of myo-inositol and may change the levels of phospholipids involved in normal mechanisms of signal transduction.

With this active polyol pathway seen in hyperglycemia, there is a subsequent diminution in myo-inositol necessary for phosphoinositol synthesis. A defect in the Na^+/K^+ ATPase has been noted in peripheral nerve studies presumably due to a decreased PKC activity.[15,143–145] This likely contributes significantly to the peripheral neuropathy due to the associated decreased nerve conduction velocity.

Similarly, endothelial cells cultured in high glucose also manifest diminished Na^+/K^+ ATPase activity. The consequences of this have not been determined as there is no effect on phosphoinositide metabolism despite elevated sorbitol levels indicating an active polyol pathway in the face of hyperglycemia.[146]

Thus, hyperglycemia may alter arterial wall metabolism by mechanisms other than glycosylation of

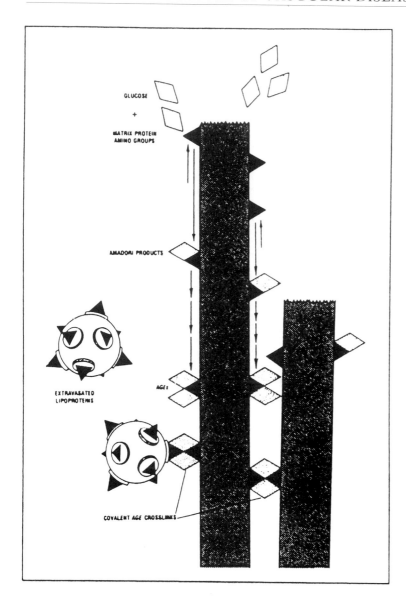

GLUCOSE

+

MATRIX PROTEIN
AMINO GROUPS

AMADORI PRODUCTS

EXTRAVASATED
LIPOPROTEINS

AGEs

COVALENT AGE CROSSLINKS

Figure 3. Formation of cross-links in matrix protein due to advanced glycosylation end-products. The **upper portion** of the figure shows the formation of irreversible advanced glycosylation end-products (AGE). In the **lower part** of the figure, chemically reactive advanced glycosylation end-products accumulate on long-lived matrix proteins as a function of time and glucose concentration. These accumulated end-products form covalent cross-links with other matrix proteins and with extravasated plasma proteins by bonding with amino groups. (Reproduced with permission from Reference 14.)

proteins. The extent to which the polyol pathway for glucose metabolism actually contributes to clinical events is not established. Thus far, it is not clear how the diminished endothelium-dependent relaxation noted in diabetes can be explained by this hypothesis. Experimentally, aldose reductase inhibitors have not been shown to be effective in clinical studies of neuropathy or retinopathy.[147,148]

The Diabetic Foot

The etiology of ulceration in the diabetic foot is multifactorial, involving ischemia, neuropathy, and infection. In the past, there has been some speculation that ischemia in the diabetic foot is a result of an occlusion in the microcirculation. This derives from an observational study of amputation specimens where it was thought that there was a high incidence of arterio-losclerosis in the amputation specimens from diabetic patients.[149] Strandness examined this in a prospective study using blinded histology and was unable to confirm the observation.[20] In a subsequent preoperative anatomic study, Conrad used an arterial casting technique in amputation specimens.[3] Once again, there was no evidence of a small artery or arteriolar occlusive process that was more common in the diabetic amputation specimens than in the nondiabetic.

If diabetics had arteriolosclerosis, they would be expected to have a fixed and high peripheral resistance. Barner tested this hypothesis by injecting papaverine at the conclusion of femoral-popliteal bypass grafting and found no difference in vasodilatation between diabetics and nondiabetics where there was similar tibial runoff.[150] Based on this study, he concluded that arterial reconstruction should not be withheld in diabetics on the mistaken idea that they had an occlusive lesion in the microcirculation.

Table 2
Consequences of the Accumulation of Advanced Glycosylation End-Products in Tissue

Consequences	Mechanism	Tissue Component Involved
Increase in vascular permeability	Response to secreted monokines induced by AGEs (tumor necrosis factor, interleukin-1)	Endothelium
	Decrease in binding of anionic proteoglycans to proteins with AGEs	Extracellular matrix
	Degradation of anionic proteoglycans in response to secreted monokines induced by AGEs	Extracellular matrix
	Abnormal self-assembly of basement-membrane components with AGEs	Extracellular matrix
Thickened, inelastic vessel wall	Resistance of AGE-cross-linked proteins to enzymatic degradation	Extracellular matrix
	Accumulation of plasma protein deposits through AGE cross-linking	Extracellular matrix
	Proliferation of matrix and cells in response to AGE-induced secretion of growth-promoting monokines (from macrophages and endothelial cells)	Vessel wall
	Possibly, proliferation of matrix and cells in response to secretion of PDGF induced by matrix with AGE-cross-linked plasma proteins	Vessel wall

* AGE: advanced glycosylation end-products; PDGF: platelet-derived growth factor.
(Reproduced with permission from Reference 14.)

Using noninvasive techniques, Irwin was also unable to demonstrate physiologic evidence of microvascular occlusive disease associated with diabetes in patients presenting with foot ulceration.[151] Thus, a great deal of evidence argues against the existence of small vessel or arteriolar occlusive disease as being more common in diabetics as compared with nondiabetic patients.[152] If, in fact, there was an occlusive lesion in the microcirculation, treatment of ischemia in the diabetic would be hopeless. In that sense, the term "small vessel disease" can be harmful and inhibits the appropriate care of diabetic foot ulcers.

Diminished sensation, loss of vasomotor control, a blunted inflammatory response, and altered capillary dynamics add up to a highly compromised biology for the diabetic foot. In this setting, relatively moderate ischemia is poorly tolerated. The foot is more susceptible to ulceration and infection as perfusion pressure drops. This is an important concept in understanding the role of vascular reconstruction and the technical approach that optimizes salvage of the foot.

When ischemia occurs in the diabetic foot, it is due to atherosclerotic occlusive disease as discussed previously. Most studies have supported the view that progression of atherosclerosis is more rapid.[116] Calcification of the media is common in diabetes, but it is not associated with arterial occlusive disease either in the periphery or in the heart.[153,154] Calcification can, however, interfere with noninvasive testing and can add to the technical difficulties of arterial reconstruction.

Neuropathy is almost always a contributing factor to ulceration in the diabetic foot. It leads to sensory loss, atrophy of the intrinsic muscles with the development of foot deformities, and increased pressure points, as well as autonomic dysfunction and loss of the nociceptive reflex.[155] When severe, this can lead to ulceration even in the presence of normal arterial circulation. In general, neuropathy makes the foot more susceptible to ulceration even at lesser degrees of ischemia which would not cause ulceration in nondiabetics. In addition, the many effects of hyperglycemia and hyperinsulinemia on tissues and cells lead to a compromised biology. When a diabetic presents with a foot ulceration, an evaluation for ischemia should always be performed even when neuropathy is also a contributing factor. Once the diagnosis of arterial occlusion is made, arteriography should be performed except in those patients with the most superficial ulcerations under circumstances where they can be closely observed with conservative management. It should be emphasized that optimum care of the diabetic foot is a true multidisciplinary effort involving vascular surgeons, podiatrists, orthopedic surgeons, cardiologists, infectious disease specialists, etc. However, in recent years, increased proficiency with extreme distal arterial reconstruction has been the critical advance leading to improved outcome. Surprisingly, the results of arterial reconstruction in diabetics are as good as or better than in nondiabetics.[111] Again this supports the view that there is no occlusive lesion in the microcirculation limiting runoff or impairing graft patency.

Patients with diabetic foot lesions often present complex management problems that extend beyond those of the ischemic foot in nondiabetics. However, an understanding of the pathobiology and in particular the etiology and management of ischemia will be rewarded by a greatly decreased rate of major amputation.

References

1. Giordano JM, Trout HH, DePalma RG: *The Basic Science of Vascular Surgery*. Armonk, NY: Futura Publishing Company, Inc.; 1988.
2. Braunwald E, Isselbacher KJ, Petersdorf RG, Wilson JD, Martin JB, Fauci AS: *Harrison's Principles of Internal Medicine*. New York: McGraw-Hill Book Co.; 1987.
3. Conrad MC: Large and small artery occlusion in diabetics and nondiabetics with severe vascular disease. *Circulation* 36:83–91, 1967.
4. Brand FN, Abbott RD, Kannell WB: Diabetes, intermittent claudication, and risk of cardiovascular events: the Framingham study. *Diabetes* 38:504–509, 1989.
5. Report of the National Commission on Diabetes. Washington, DC: Government Printing Office; 60, 1976. DHEW publication (NIH) 76–1022, Vol 3, Part 2.
6. Kreines K, Johnson E, Albrink M, et al: The course of peripheral vascular disease in non-insulin-dependent diabetes. *Diabetes Care* 8:235–243, 1985.
7. West K: Report of work group on macrovascular disease. In: Report of the National Commission on Diabetes, *DHEW* publication Vol 3, Part 2, 1976.
8. Ganda OP: Pathogenesis of accelerated atherosclerosis in diabetes. In: Kozak GP, Hoar CS, Rowbotham JL, et al (eds). *Management of Diabetic Foot Problems*. Philadelphia: WB Saunders Company; 1984.
9. US Department of Health and Human Services: The treatment and control of diabetes: a national plan to reduce mortality and morbidity. A report of the National Diabetes Advisory Board. Washington, DC: US Government Printing Office; 25, November 1980. NIH Publication 81–2284.
10. Dawber TR: *The Epidemiology of Atherosclerotic Disease: The Framingham Study*. Cambridge, MA: Harvard University Press; 1980.
11. Krolewski AS, Warram JH, Valsania P, et al: Evolving natural history of coronary artery disease in diabetes mellitus. *Am J Med* 20:2A-56–61S, 1991.
12. Siperstein MD, Unger RH, Madison LL: Studies of muscle capillary basement membranes in normal subjects, diabetic, and prediabetic patients. *J Clin Invest* 47:1973–1999, 1968.
13. King GL, Goodman AD, Buzney S, Moses A, Kahn CR: Receptors and growth-promoting effects of insulin and insulin-like growth factors on cells from bovine reti-

nal capillaries and aorta. *J Clin Invest* 75:1028–1036, 1985.
14. Brownlee M, Cerami A, Vlassara H: Advanced glycosylation end products in tissue and the biochemical basis of diabetic complications. *N Engl J Med* 318:1315–1321, 1988.
15. Kreisberg JI: Biology of disease: hyperglycemia and microangiopathy. Direct regulation by glucose of microvascular cells. *Lab Inves* 67:416–426, 1992.
16. Porta M, Townsend C, Clover GM, et al: Evidence for functional endothelial cell damage in early diabetic retinopathy. *Diabetologia* 20:597–601, 1981.
17. Shimomura H, Spiro RG: Studies on macromolecular components of human glomerular basement membrane and alterations in diabetes: decreased levels of heparin sulfate proteoglycan and laminin. *Diabetes* 36:374–381, 1987.
18. United States Renal Data System. 1991 Annual Data Report. U.S. Department of Health & Human Services, PNS, NIH:16.
19. Janka HU, Standl E, Mahnert H: Peripheral vascular disease in diabetes mellitus and its relation to cardiovascular risk factors: screening with the Doppler ultrasonic technique. *Diabetes Care* 3:207, 1980.
20. Strandness Jr DE, Priest RE, Gibbons GE: Combined clinical and pathologic study of diabetic and nondiabetic peripheral arterial disease. *Diabetes* 13:366–372, 1964.
21. Menzoian JO, LaMorte WW, Paniszyn CC, et al: Symptomatology and anatomic patterns of peripheral vascular disease: differing impact of smoking and diabetes. *Ann Vasc Surg* 3:224–228, 1989.
22. Pomposelli FB Jr, Jepsen SJ, Gibbons GW, et al: Efficacy of the dorsalis pedis bypass for limb salvage in diabetic patients: short-term observations. *J Vasc Surg* 11:745–751, 1990.
23. Pomposelli FB Jr, Jepsen SJ, Gibbons GW, et al: A flexible approach to infra-popliteal vein grafts in patients with diabetes mellitus. *Arch Surg* 126:724–727, 1991.
24. Ogbuawa O, Williams JT, Henry WL Jr: Diabetic gangrene in black patients. *South Med J* 75:285–288, 1982.
25. Frank HJL, Levin ER, Hu R-M, Pedram A: Insulin stimulates endothelin binding and action on cultured vascular smooth muscle cells. *Endocrinology* 133:1092–1097, 1993.
26. Kaplan NM: The deadly quartet: upper-body obesity, glucose intolerance, hypertriglyceridemia, and hypertension. *Arch Intern Med* 49:1514–1520, 1989.
27. Sidawy AN, Schweitzer EJ, Nevilte RF, et al: Race as a risk factor in the severity of infragenicular occlusive disease: study of an urban hospital population. *J Vasc Surg* 11:536–543, 1990.
28. Spielman RS, McGinnis RE, Ewens WJ: Transmission test for linkage disequilibrium: the insulin gene region and insulin-dependent diabetes mellitus (IDDM). *Am J Hum Genet* 52:506–516, 1993.
29. Reaven GM, Hollenbeck CB, Chen Y-DI: Relationship between glucose tolerance, insulin secretion, and insulin action in nonobese individuals with varying degrees of glucose tolerance. *Diabetologia* 32:52–55, 1989.
30. Porte D: β-cells in type II diabetes mellitus. *Diabetes* 40:166–180, 1991.
31. Standl E, Janka HU: High serum insulin concentrations in relation to other cardiovascular risk factors in macrovascular disease of type II diabetes. *Horm Metab Res* (suppl)15:46–51, 1985.
32. Katabchi AE, Duckworth WC, Stentz FB: Insulin syn-

thesis, proinsulin, and C-peptides. In: Rifkin H, Porte D Jr (eds). *Diabetes Mellitus: Theory and Practice.* 4th ed. New York: Elsevier; 71–88, 1990.

33. Stout RW: The role of insulin in atherosclerosis in diabetics and nondiabetics: a review. *Diabetes* 30:54–57, 1981.

34. Capron L, Jarnet J, Kazandjian S, Housset E: Growth promoting effects of diabetes and insulin on arteries. *Diabetes* 35:973–978, 1986.

35. Bilious RW, Mauer SM, Sutherland DER, Najarian JS, Goetz FC, Steffes MW: The effects of pancreas transplantation on the glomerular structure of renal allografts in patients with insulin-dependent diabetes. *N Engl J Med* 321:80–85, 1989.

36. Pirart J: Why don't we teach and treat diabetic patients better? *Diabetes Care* 1:139–140, 1978.

37. Beach KW, Standness DE Jr: Arteriosclerosis obliterans and associated risk factors in insulin-dependent and non-insulin-dependent diabetes. *Diabetes* 29:882–888, 1980.

38. University Group Diabetes Program: *Diabetes* 19:789–815, 1970.

39. DCCT Research Group: The effect of intensive treatment of diabetes on the development and progression of long-term complications in insulin-dependent diabetes mellitus. *N Engl J Med* 329:977–986, 1993.

40. Sato Y, Shiraishi S, Oshida Y, Ishiguro T, Sakamoto N: Experimental atherosclerosis-like lesions induced by hyperinsulinism in Wistar rats. *Diabetes* 38:91–96, 1989.

41. Stout RW: Insulin as a mitogenic factor: role in the pathogenesis of cardiovascular disease. *Am J Med* 90: 2A-62S-65S, 1991.

42. Stout RW: Insulin and atheroma: 20-year perspective. *Diabetes Care* 13:631–654, 1990.

43. Stamler J, Pick R, Katz LN: Effect of insulin in the induction and regression of atherosclerosis in the chick. *Circ Res* 8:572–576, 1960.

44. Laakso M, Sarlund H, Salonen R, et al: Asymptomatic atherosclerosis and insulin resistance. *Arterioscler Thromb* 11:1068–1070, 1991.

45. Kuo PT, Feng LY: Studies of serum insulin in atherosclerotic patients with endogenous hypertriglyceridemia (Types III and IV hyperlipoproteinemia). *Metabolism* 19:372–380, 1970.

46. Brown WV: Lipoprotein disorders in diabetes mellitus. *Med Clin North Am* 78:143–161, 1994.

47. Miller NE: Plasma-high-density-lipoprotein concentration and development of ischaemic heart disease. *Lancet* 1:16–19, 1975.

48. Falholt K, Alberti KGMM, Heding LG: Aorta and muscle metabolism in pigs with peripheral hyperinsulinaemia. *Diabetologia* 28:32–37, 1985.

49. Falholt K, Cutfield R, Alejandro R, Heding L, Mintz D: The effects of hyperinsulinemia on arterial wall and peripheral muscle metabolism in dogs. *Metabolism* 34: 1146–1149, 1985.

50. Mahler R: The effect of diabetes and insulin on biochemical reactions of the arterial wall. *Acta Diabet Latinoam* 8:68–83, 1971.

51. Lopes-Virella MF, Virella G: Immune mechanisms of atherosclerosis in diabetes mellitus. *Diabetes* (suppl 2)41:86–91, 1992.

52. Ruderman NB, Schneider SH: Diabetes, exercise, and atherosclerosis. *Diabetes Care* 15:1787–1793, 1992.

53. Young IR, Stout RW: Effects of insulin and glucose on the cells of the arterial wall: interaction of insulin with

dibutyryl cyclic AMP and low density lipoprotein in arterial cells. *Diabete Metab* 13:301–306, 1987.

54. Stout RW: The effect of insulin and glucose on sterol synthesis in cultured rat arterial smooth muscle cells. *Atherosclerosis* 27:271–278, 1977.

55. Nakao J, Ito H, Kanayasu T, Murola S-I: Stimulatory effect of insulin on aortic smooth muscle cell migration induced by 12-L-hydroxy-5,8,10,14-eicosatetraenoic acid and its modulation by elevated extracellular glucose levels. *Diabetes* 34:185–191, 1985.

56. Krone W, Greten H: Evidence for post-transcriptional regulation by insulin of 3-hydroxy-3-methylglutaryl coenzyme. A reductase and sterol synthesis in human mononuclear leucocytes. *Diabetologia* 26:366–369, 1984.

57. Krone W, Nagele H, Behnke B, Greten H: Opposite effects of insulin and catecholamines on LDL-receptor activity in human mononuclear leukocytes. *Diabetes* 37:1386–1391, 1988.

58. Kraemer FB: Role of lipoprotein lipase and apolipoprotein E secretion by macrophages in modulating lipoprotein uptake; possible role in acceleration of atherosclerosis in diabetes. *Diabetes* (suppl)41:77–80, 1992.

59. Ishibashi S, Yamada N, Shimano H, et al: Apolipoprotein-E and lipoprotein lipase secreted from human monocyte-derived macrophages modulate very low density lipoprotein uptake. *J Biol Chem* 265:3040–3047, 1990.

60. Duell PB, Bierman EL: Diabetic HDL has reduced capacity to promote HDL receptor-mediated cholesterol efflux (abstr). *Arteriosclerosis* 10.7689, 1990.

61. Duell PB, Oram JF, Bierman EL: Nonenzymatic glycosylation of HDL and impaired HDL-receptor-mediated cholesterol efflux. *Diabetes* 40:377–384, 1991.

62. Fievet C, Theret N, Shojaee N, et al: Apolipoprotein A-1–containing particles and reverse cholesterol transport in IDDM. *Diabetes* (suppl 2)41:81–85, 1992.

63. Simon BC, Cunningham LD, Cohen RA: Oxidized low density lipoproteins cause contraction and inhibit endothelium-dependent relaxation in the pig coronary artery. *J Clin Invest* 86:75–79, 1990.

64. Jacobs M, Plane F, Bruckdorfer KR: Native and oxidized low-density lipoproteins have different inhibitory effects on endothelium-derived relaxing factor in the rabbit aorta. *Br J Pharmacol* 100:21–26, 1990.

65. Quinn MT, Parthasarathy S, Fonz LG, Steinberg D: Oxidatively modified low density lipoproteins: a potential role in recruitment and retention of monocyte/macrophages during atherogenesis. *Proc Natl Acad Sci USA* 84:2995–2998, 1987.

66. Cushing SD, Berliner JA, Valente AJ, et al: Minimally modified (MCP-1) in human endothelial smooth muscle cells. *Proc Natl Acad Sci USA* 87:5134–5138, 1990.

67. Lyons TJ: Oxidized low-density lipoproteins: a role in the pathogenesis of atherosclerosis in diabetes? *Diabetic Med* 8:411–419, 1991.

68. Baynes JW: Role of oxidative stress in development of complications in diabetes. *Diabetes* 40:405–412, 1991.

69. Hunt JV, Smith CCT, Wolff SP: Autooxidative glycosylation and possible involvement of peroxides and free radicals in LDL modification by glucose. *Diabetes* 39:1420–1424, 1990.

70. Sakurai T, Kimura S, Nakano M, Kimura H: Oxidative modification of glycated low density lipoprotein in the presence of iron. *Biochem Biophys Res Commun* 177:433–439, 1991.

71. Lyons TJ: Glycation and oxidation: a role in the patho-

genesis of atherosclerosis. *Am J Cardiol* 71:26B-31B, 1993.

72. Hiramatsu K, Arimori S: Increased superoxide production by mononuclear cells of patients with hypertriglyceridemia and diabetes. *Diabetes* 37:832–837, 1988.

73. Watanabe J, Wohltmann HJ, Klein RL, Colwell JA, Lopes-Virella MF: Enhancement of platelet aggregation by low-density lipoproteins from IDDM patients. *Diabetes* 37:1652–1657, 1988.

74. Ronnett GV, Knutson VP, Kohanski RA, Simpson TL, Lane MD: Role of glycosylation in the processing of newly translated insulin prorereceptor in 3T3-L1 adipocytes. *J Biol Chem* 259:4566–4575, 1984.

75. O'Rahilly S, Choi WH, Patel P, Turner RC, Flier JS, Moller DE: Detections of mutations in insulin-receptor gene in NIDDM patients by analysis of single-stranded conformation polymorphisms. *Diabetes* 40:777–782, 1991.

76. Ebina Y, Ellis L, Jarnagin K, et al: The human insulin receptor cDNA: the structural basis for hormone-activated transmembrane signalling. *Cell* 40:747–758, 1985.

77. Ullrich A, Bell JR, Chen EY, et al: Human insulin receptor and its relationship to the tyrosine kinase family of oncogenes. *Nature* 313:756–762, 1985.

78. Yu K-T, Czech MP: Tyrosine phosphorylation of the insulin receptor β subunit activates the receptor-associated tyrosine kinase activity. *J Biol Chem* 259: 5277–5286, 1984.

79. Nichols WK, Goldberg ND: The relationship between insulin and apparent glucocorticoid-promoted activation of hepatic glycogen synthetase. *Biochem Biophys Acta* 279:245–259, 1972.

80. Jefferson LS, Exton JH, Butcher RW, et al: Role of adenosine 3'5'-monophosphate in the effects of insulin and anti-insulin serum on liver metabolism. *J Biol Chem* 243:1031–1038, 1968.

81. Olefsky JM, Molina JM: Insulin resistance in man. In: Rifkin H, Porte D Jr (eds). *Diabetes Mellitus: Theory and Practice.* 4th ed. New York: Elsevier; 121–153, 1990.

82. Marx J: Taking a direct path to the genes. *Science* 257: 744–745, 1992.

83. Schindler C, Shuai K, Prezioso VR, Darnell JE: Interferon-dependent tyrosine phosphorylation of a latent cytoplasmic transcription factor. *Science* 257:809–813, 1992.

84. Pfeifle B, Ditschuneit HH, Ditschuneit H: Insulin as a cellular growth regulator of rat arterial smooth muscle cells in vitro. *Horm Metab Res* 12:381–385, 1980.

85. Weinstein R, Stemerman MR, Macias T: Hormonal requirements for growth of arterial smooth muscle cells in vitro: an endocrine approach to atherosclerosis. *Science* 212:818–820, 1981.

86. Turner JL, Bierman EL: Effects of glucose and sorbitol on proliferation of cultured human skin fibroblasts and arterial smooth muscle cells. *Diabetes* 27:583–588, 1978.

87. Banskota NK, Taub R, Zellner K, Olsen P, King GL: Characterization of induction of proto-oncogene c-myc and cellular growth in human vascular smooth muscle cells by insulin and IGF-I. *Diabetes* 38:123–129, 1989.

88. King GL, Kahn CR, Rechler MM, Nissley SP: Direct demonstration of separate receptors for growth and metabolic activities of insulin and multiplication-stimulating activity (an insulin-like growth factor) using antibodies to the insulin receptor. *J Clin Invest* 66:130–140, 1980.

89. Jialal I, Creetaz M, Hachiya HL, et al: Characterization of the receptors for insulin and the insulin-like growth factors on micro- and macrovascular tissues. *Endocrinology* 117:1222–1229, 1985.

90. Armelin HA, Armelin MC, Kelly K, et al: Functional role for c-myc in mitogenic response to platelet-derived growth factor. *Nature* 310:655–660, 1984.

91. Muller R, Bravo R, Buckhardt J, Curran T: Immediate dramatic induction of *c-fos* by growth factors precedes activation of c-myc. *Nature* 312:316–320, 1984.

92. Juhan-Vague I, Alessi MC, Vague P: Increased plasma plasminogen activator inhibitor 1 levels: a possible link between insulin resistance and atherothrombosis. *Diabetologia* 34:457–462, 1991.

93. Schneider DJ, Nordt TK, Sobel BE: Attenuated fibrinolysis and accelerated atherogenesis in type II diabetic patients. *Diabetes* 42:1–7, 1993.

94. Schneider DJ, Nordt TK, Sobel BE: Stimulation by proinsulin of expression of plasminogen activator inhibitor type 1 in endothelial cells. *Diabetes* 41:890–895, 1992.

95. Alessi MC, Juhan-Vague I, Kooistra T, DeClerck PJ, Collen D: Insulin stimulates the synthesis of plasminogen activator inhibitor 1 by the human hepatocellular cell line Hep G2. *Thromb Haemostas* 60:491–494, 1988.

96. Kooistra T, Bosma PJ, Tons HAM, Van Den Berg AP, Meyer P, Princen HMG: Plasminogen activator inhibitor 1: biosynthesis and mRNA level are increased by insulin in cultured human hepatocytes. *Thromb Haemostas* 62:723–728, 1989.

97. Yanagisawa M, Masaki T: Molecular biology and biochemistry of the endothelins. *Trends Pharmacol Sci* 10: 374–378, 1989.

98. Dubin D, Pratt RE, Cooke JP, Dzan VJ: Endothelin, a potent vasoconstrictor, is a vascular smooth muscle mitogen. *J Vasc Med Biol* 1:150–154, 1989.

99. Hu R-M, Levin ER, Pedram A, Frank HJL: Insulin stimulates the production and secretion of endothelin from bovine endothelial cells. *Diabetes* 42:351–358, 1993.

100. Hattori Y, Kasai K, Nakamura T, Emoto T, Shimoda S-I: Effect of glucose and insulin on immunoreactive endothelin-1 release from cultured porcine aortic endothelial cells. *Metabolism* 40:165–169, 1991.

101. Oliver FJ, de laRubia G, Feener EP, et al: Stimulation of endothelin-1 gene expression by insulin in endothelial cells. *J Biol Chem* 266:23251–23256, 1991.

102. Isaksson OGP, Lindahl A, Nilsson A, Isgaard J: Actions of growth hormone: current views. *Acta Paediatric Scand* 343:12–18, 1988.

103. Van Wyk JJ, Lund PK: Autocrine and paracrine effects of the somatomedin/insulin-like growth factors. In: LeRoith D, Raizada MK (eds). *Molecular and Cellular Biology of Insulin-Like Growth Factors and Their Receptors.* New York: Plenum Press; 5–23, 1989.

104. Geffner ME, Bersch N, Golde DW: Growth hormone induces insulin resistance in Laron dwarf cells via lactogenic receptors. *J Clin Endocrinol Metab* 76: 1039–1047, 1993.

105. Geffner ME, Bersch N, Bailey RC, Golde DW: Growth hormone induces resistance to the mitogenic action of insulin through local IGF-I: studies in normal and pygmy T cell lines. *Diabetes* 43:68–72, 1994.

106. Raines EW, Bowen-Pope DF, Ross R: Platelet-derived growth factor. In: Sporn MB, Roberts AB (eds). *Handbook of Experimental Pharmacology: Peptide Growth Factors and their Receptors.* New York: Springer-Verlag; 1989.

107. Fayed YM, Tsibris JCM, Langenberg PW, Robertson Jr. AL: Human uterine leiomyoma cells: binding and growth responses to epidermal growth factor, platelet-derived growth factor, and insulin. *Lab Invest* 60: 30–37, 1989.

108. Pfeifle B, Hamann H, Fubganger R, Ditschuneit H: Insulin as a growth regulator of arterial smooth muscle cells: effect of insulin on IGF-I. *Diabete Metab* 13: 326–330, 1987.

109. Seigenmann JE, Becker M, Kammermann B, et al: Decrease of nonsuppressible insulin-like activity after pancreatectomy and normalization by insulin therapy. *Acta Endo Copenh* 85:818–822, 1977.

110. Scheiwiller E, Guler HP, Merryweather J, et al: Growth restoration of insulin-deficient diabetic rats by recombinant human insulin-like growth factor I. *Nature* 323: 169–171, 1986.

111. Hurley JJ, Auer AI, Hershey FB, et al: Distal arterial reconstruction: patency and limb salvage in diabetics. *J Vasc Surg* 5:796–802, 1987.

112. Katz MA, McCusky P, Beggs JL, Johnson PC, Gaines JA: Relationships between microvascular function and capillary structure in diabetic and nondiabetic human skin. *Diabetes* 38:1245–1250, 1989.

113. Britland ST, Young RJ, Sharma AK, Clarke BF: Relationship of endoneurial capillary abnormalities to type and severity of diabetic polyneuropathy. *Diabetes* 39: 909–913, 1990.

114. Parving HH, Rasmussen SM: Transcapillary escape rate of albumin and plasma volume in short- and long-term juvenile diabetes. *Scand J Clin Lab Invest* 32:81, 1973.

115. Deckert T, Feldt-Rasmussen B, Borch-Johnson K: Albuminuria reflects widespread vascular damage: the Steno hypothesis. *Diabetologia* 32:219–226, 1989.

116. Beach KW, Bedford GR, Bergelin RO, et al: Progression of lower-extremity arterial occlusive disease in type II diabetes mellitus. *Diabetes* 11:464–478, 1988.

117. Wyss CR, Matsen FA, Simmons CW, Burgess EM: Transcutaneous oxygen tension measurements on limbs of diabetic and nondiabetic peripheral vascular disease. *Diabetes* 13:366, 1964.

118. Mathison R, Davison JS: Attenuated plasma extravasation to sensory neuropeptides in diabetic rats. *Agents Actions* 38:55–59, 1993.

119. Rayman G, Malik RA, Day JL, et al: The relationship between transcutaneous oxygen tension and capillary morphology and microvascular blood flow in diabetic skin. *Diabetes* 40:210A, 1991.

120. Tooke JE: A capillary pressure disturbance in young diabetics. *Diabetes* 29:815–819, 1980.

121. Tooke JE, Lins P-E, Ostergren J, Fagrell B: Skin microvascular autoregulatory responses in type I diabetes: the influence of duration and control. *Int J Microcirc* 40:249–256, 1985.

122. Kastrup J, Norgaard T, Parving HH, et al: Impaired autoregulation of blood flow in subcutaneous tissue of long-term type I (insulin-dependent) diabetic patients with microangiopathy: an index of arteriolar dysfunction. *Diabetologia* 28:711–717, 1985.

123. Nakamura Y, Horii Y, Toshihiko N, et al: Immunohistochemical localization of advanced glycosylation end products in coronary atheroma and cardiac tissue in diabetes mellitus. *Am J Pathol* 143:1649–1656, 1993.

124. Brownlee M, Vlassara H, Cerami A: Nonenzymatic glycosylation end products on collagen covalently trap low-density lipoprotein. *Diabetes* 34:938–941, 1985.

125. Brownlee M, Pongor S, Cerami A: Covalent attachment of soluble proteins by nonenzymatically glycosylated collagen: role in the in situ formation of immune complexes. *J Exp Med* 158:1739–1744, 1983.

126. Miller EJ, Gay S: Collagen: an overview. In: Colowick S, Cunningham LW (eds). *Methods in Enzymology*. Vol. 82. Cunningham LW, Fredrikson DW, eds. Structural and contractile proteins. Part A. Extracellular matrix. New York: Academic Press; 3–32, 1982.

127. Miller EJ, Rhodes RK: Preparation and characterization of the different types of collagen. In: Colowick S, Cunningham LW, (eds). *Methods in Enzymology*. Vol 82. Cunningham LW, Frederiksen DW, eds. Structural and contractile proteins. Part A. Extracellular matrix. New York: Academic Press; 3–32, 1982.

128. Ayo SH, Radnik RA, Garoni J, Glass NF, Kreisberg JI: High glucose causes an increase in extracellular matrix proteins in cultured mesangial cells. *Am J Pathol* 136: 1339–1348, 1990.

129. Ayo SH, Radnik RA, Glass WF, et al: Increased extracellular matrix synthesis and mRNA in mesangial cells grown in high glucose medium. *Am J Physiol* 260:F185-F191, 1991.

130. Cagliero E, Maiello M, Boeri D, Roy S, Lorenzi M: Increased expression of basement membrane components in human endothelial cells cultured in high glucose. *J Clin Invest* 82:735–738, 1988.

131. Cagliero E, Roth T, Roy S, Lorenzi M: Characteristics and mechanisms of high-glucose-induced overexpression of basement membrane components in cultured human endothelial cells. *Diabetes* 40:102–110, 1991.

132. Ayo SH, Radnik R, Garoni J, Troyer DA, Kreisbery JI: High glucose increases diacylglycerol mass and activates protein kinase C in mesangial cell cultures. *Am J Physiol* 261:F571-F577, 1991.

133. Lee TS, Saltsman KA, Ohashi H, King GL: Activation of protein kinase C by elevation of glucose concentration: proposal for a mechanism in the development of diabetic vascular complications. *Proc Natl Acad Sci USA* 86:5141–5145, 1989.

134. Wolf BA, Williamson JR, Easom RA, Chang K, Sherman WR, Turk J: Diacylglycerol accumulation and microvascular abnormalities induced by elevated glucose levels. *J Clin Invest* 87:31–38, 1991.

135. Lynch JJ, Ferro TJ, Blumenstock FA, Brockenauer AM, Malik AB: Increased endothelial albumin permeability mediated by protein kinase C activation. *J Clin Invest* 85:1991–1998, 1990.

136. Ware JA, Heistad DD: Platelet-endothelial interactions. *N Engl J Med* 328:628–635, 1993.

137. Tesfamariam B, Brown ML, Cohen KA: Elevated glucose impairs endothelium-dependent relaxation by activating protein kinase C. *J Clin Invest* 87:1643–1648, 1991.

138. Tilton RG, Chang K, Hason KS, Smith SR, et al: Prevention of diabetic vascular dysfunction by guanidines: inhibition of nitric oxide synthase versus advanced glycation end-product formation. *Diabetes* 42:221–232, 1993.

139. Takahashi K, Ghatei MA, Lam HC, O'Halloran DJ, Bloom SR: Elevated plasma endothelin in patients with diabetes mellitus. *Diabetologia* 33:306–310, 1990.

140. Radoff S, Vlassara H, Cerami A: Isolation of a macrophage receptor for proteins modified by advanced glycosylation end products (AGE) (abstr). *Fed Proc* 46: 2116, 1987.

141. Lampeter ER, Kishimoto TK, Rothlein R, Mainolfi EA,

et al: Elevated levels of circulating adhesion molecules in NIDDM patients and in subjects at risk for NIDDM. *Diabetes* 41:1668–1671, 1992.

142. Hawthorne GC, Barblett K, Hetherington CS, Alberti KG: The effect of high glucose on polyol pathway activity and myoinositol mechanism in cultured human endothelial cells. *Diabetologia* 32:163–166, 1989.

143. Lattimer SA, Sima AAF, Greene DA: In vitro correction of impaired Na$^+$-K$^+$-ATPase in diabetic nerve by protein kinase C agonists. *Am J Physiol* 256:E264-E269, 1989.

144. Greene DA, Lattimer SA, Sima AAF: Pathogenesis and prevention of diabetic neuropathy. *Diabetes Metab Rev* 4:201–221, 1988.

145. Simpson DMF, Hawthorne JN: Reduced Na$^+$-K$^+$-ATPase activity in peripheral nerve of streptozotocin-diabetic rats: a role for protein kinase C? *Diabetologia* 31:297–303, 1988.

146. Lee TS, Mac Gregor LC, Fluharty JJ, King GL: Differential regulation of protein kinase C and (Na$^+$,K$^+$)-adenosine triphosphatase activities by elevated glucose levels in retinal capillary endothelial cells. *J Clin Invest* 83:90–94, 1989.

147. Frank RN: Aldose reductase inhibition: the chemical key to the control of diabetic retinopathy? *Arch Ophthalmol* 108:1229–1231, 1990.

148. Judzewitsch RG, Jaspan JB, Polonsky KS, et al: Aldose reductase inhibition improves nerve conduction velocity in diabetic patients. *N Engl J Med* 308:110–125, 1983.

149. Goldenberg SG, Alex M, Joshi RA, Blumenthal HT: Nonatheromatous peripheral vascular disease of the lower extremity in diabetes mellitus. *Diabetes* 8: 261–273, 1959.

150. Barner HB, Kaiser GC, Willman VL: Blood flow in the diabetic leg. *Circulation* 43:391–394, 1971.

151. Irwin ST, Gilmore J, McGrann S, Hood J, Allen JA: Blood flow in diabetics with foot lesions due to "small vessel disease." *Br J Surg* 75:1201–1206, 1988.

152. LoGerfo FW, Coffman JD: Vascular and microvascular disease of the diabetic foot in diabetes: implications for foot care. *N Engl J Med* 311:1615–1619, 1984.

153. Maser RE, Wolfson SK Jr, Ellis D, et al: Cardiovascular disease and arterial calcification in insulin-dependent diabetes mellitus: interrelations and risk factor profiles. *Arterioscler Thromb* 11:958–965, 1991.

154. Chantelau E, Ma XY, Herrnberger S, Dohmen C, Trappe P, Baba T: Effect of medial arterial calcification on O$_2$ supply to exercising diabetic feet. *Diabetes* 39: 938–941, 1990.

155. LoGerfo FW, Gibbons GW, Pomposelli FB Jr, et al: Trends in the care of the diabetic foot: expanded role of arterial reconstruction. *Arch Surg* 127:617–621, 1992.

156. Stout RW, Bierman EL, Ross R: The effect of insulin on the proliferation of cultured primate arterial smooth muscle cells. *Circ Res* 36:319–327, 1975.

157. Brownlee M, Vlassara H, Kooney A, Ulrich P, Cerami A: Aminoguanidine prevents diabetes-induced arterial wall protein cross-linking. *Science* 232:1629–1632, 1986.

CHAPTER 18

Plasma Lipoproteins and Vascular Disease

John C. LaRosa, MD

The pivotal role of lipoprotein metabolism in atherosclerosis is well-known. This chapter reviews current knowledge about normal and abnormal lipoprotein metabolism and the evidence linking dyslipoproteinemic states to the development and treatment of atherosclerotic vascular disease.

Lipoproteins

Lipoproteins are large, complex macromolecules that facilitate transport of large amounts of neutral (nonpolar) fats in plasma water, a charged (polar) solvent. Lipoproteins are thought to be spheres with an inner core of neutral fat (triglyceride and esterified cholesterol) covered with polar substances—proteins, phospholipids, and unesterified cholesterol—that solubilize the particles in plasma. All lipoproteins contain the same four basic ingredients: cholesterol (either free or esterified), triglyceride, phospholipid, and protein. They differ in the relative amount of each of these constituents and in the nature of the protein on the lipoprotein surface. The surface proteins are called apolipoproteins (apoproteins).[1,2]

Lipoproteins can be classified according to their electrophoretic mobility, charge, or density. There are five major categories (Table 1). Chylomicrons are large, triglyceride-carrying particles formed in the intestine after a fatty meal. They have very little surface charge and migrate poorly on electrophoresis strips. They have the lowest density of any of the lipoproteins.

Very low density lipoproteins (VLDL) are not as large as chylomicrons and are somewhat more dense. They carry triglyceride and other fats synthesized in the liver. On electrophoresis, they migrate just forward of the beta-globulin region and are known as prebeta lipoproteins.

Intermediate density lipoproteins (IDL) are formed when some of the triglyceride is removed from VLDL. These lipoproteins are smaller in diameter than VLDL and more dense. Under ordinary circumstances, they are so rapidly removed from plasma that their concentration is quite low, and they are not detectable on electrophoresis. In certain disease states, these IDL particles may accumulate. On electrophoresis, they migrate in a broad band through the beta and prebeta globulin region and are referred to as beta (β)-VLDL, or broad-beta lipoproteins.

Low density lipoproteins (LDL) normally are formed from the catabolism of VLDL. In some disease states, they may be formed de novo by the liver. These are the major carriers of cholesterol in the plasma. On electrophoresis, they migrate in the beta-globulin region and are known as beta (β)-lipoproteins.

Lipoprotein(a) [Lp(a)] is a form of LDL to which a peptide similar to plasminogen, apoprotein(a) or apo(a), is attached by a single desulfide bond. Like VLDL, Lp(a) migrates in the prebeta region. Its origin and function is unclear.[3]

Finally, high density lipoproteins (HDL) are the smallest and most dense of the lipoproteins. Derived from a variety of sources, including de novo synthesis as well as chylomicron and VLDL catabolism, they have a higher protein and phospholipid content than any other lipoprotein. On electrophoresis, they migrate in the alpha-globulin region and are known as alpha (α)-lipoproteins.

For clinical purposes, lipoprotein concentrations

From *The Basic Science of Vascular Disease*. Edited by Sidawy AN, Sumpio BE, and DePalma RG. Armonk, NY: Futura Publishing Company, Inc.; © 1997.

Table 1
Characteristics of Plasma Lipoproteins

Lipoproteins	Electrophoretic Mobility	Hydrated Density (g/mL)	Diameter (Å)	Composition (%)				Associated Apoproteins
				CH	TG	PL	PT	
Chylomicrons	origin	<1.006	750–12,000	5	90	3	2	A, B, C, E
VLDL	pre-β (α₂)-globulin region	<1.006	500–700	20	60	14	6	A, B, C, E
IDL	β to pre-β	1.006–1.019	300–500	40	20	22	18	B, E
LDL	β	1.019–1.063	225	50	7	22	21	B
HDL	α	1.063–1.21	100–150	25	5	26	44	A, C

CH: cholesterol; TG: triglyceride; PL: phospholipid; PT: protein; VLDL: very low density lipoprotein; IDL: intermediate density lipoprotein; LDL: low density lipoprotein; HDL: high density lipoprotein.

are measured in terms of their cholesterol content. Thus, unless otherwise specified, LDL, HDL, and VLDL levels refer to the portion of the total plasma cholesterol carried in each of these lipoprotein fractions.

Apolipoproteins

Apolipoproteins or apoproteins,[1,4] the surface protein of lipoprotein particles, have the unique ability to be both soluble in plasma and able to bind lipids. In circulating plasma, small fractions of some of these apoproteins may exist unbound, but most are bound to lipoproteins. Apoproteins freely exchange between lipoprotein fractions at various stages of their metabolism. The most widely accepted nomenclature for apoproteins is alphabetical. For example, "A" apoproteins are associated predominantely with HDL fractions. [An exception to this is apo(a), which is linked to LDL in lipoprotein(a).] "B" apoproteins are associated with LDL, VLDL, IDL, and chylomicrons. Table 2 provides a summary of some of the known characteristics of apoproteins.

In addition to packaging the neutral lipids for transport in plasma, apoproteins have specific metabolic roles. Some act as activators or inhibitors of enzymes that act on lipoproteins. Others form sites on the lipoprotein surface that are recognized by specific receptors on the surface of cells. Some may facilitate intravascular transport of lipids from one lipoprotein fraction to another. Abnormalities in these apoproteins are the basis for many of the genetic abnormalities of lipoprotein metabolism that are currently described.

Normal Lipoprotein Metabolism[1-5]

Chylomicrons

Under ordinary circumstances, ingested fat (predominantly triglyceride by weight) is taken up by intes-

tinal mucosal cells and formed into chylomicrons (Figure 1). Chylomicrons are transported by intestinal lymphatics via the thoracic duct to the peripheral circulation. At peripheral sites, such as adipose tissue and muscle, chylomicrons are acted on by the enzyme lipoprotein lipase, which is bound to capillary endothelium by a mucopolysaccharide and does not normally circulate. A portion of the core of triglyceride is removed, transported as free fatty acid and glycerol into the adipose tissue cells, reformed into triglyceride, and stored.

After removal of much, but not all, of the core triglyceride, a smaller sphere, termed a chylomicron remnant, remains. In the process of remnant formation, some of the surface material, consisting of free cholesterol, apoprotein C (particularly apoCII), and phospholipid, becomes redundant and breaks away, joining the HDL fraction. The remaining remnant is enriched in apoprotein E and apoprotein B-48. These remnants are recognized by specific apoE (remnant) receptors in the liver, rapidly removed from the plasma, and catabolized in hepatic cells. If these receptors are saturated, chylomicron remnants may be taken up by receptors on the surface of macrophages.

VLDL, IDL, and LDL

VLDL is formed in the liver (Figure 2). Like chylomicrons, VLDL carries a core of neutral triglyceride. This triglyceride, however, has been formed from plasma carbohydrate and free fatty acids delivered to the liver to be transformed into fatty acids, which can be stored in adipose tissue.

VLDL secreted by the liver circulates to peripheral cells where it is acted on by lipoprotein lipase. When redundant surface material from VLDL breaks away (again consisting of apoC, free cholesterol, and phospholipid), a particle enriched in apoprotein E and B-100 remains. These particles of IDL are analogous

Table 2
Characteristics of Major Apolipoproteins

Apoprotein	Molecular Weight	Associated Lipoproteins	Functions	Associated Clinical Disorders
A-I	28,300	chylomicrons, HDL	-structural protein -activates LCAT	-Tangier disease -ApoA-I/C-III deficiency -Other apoA-I variants
A-II	17,400	chylomicrons, HDL	-structural protein -activates hepatic TGL	?
A-IV	46,000	chylomicrons	?	?
B-100	250,000	VLDL, IDL, LDL	-structural protein -binding to apoE/B-100 receptors	-abetalipoproteinemias -hypobetalipoproteinemia
B-48	120,000	chylomicrons	-structural protein	?
C-I	6,300	chylomicrons, VLDL, HDL	-LCAT cofactor	?
C-II	8,800	chylomicrons, VLDL, HDL	-lipoprotein lipase cofactor	-familial apoC-II deficiency (chylomicronemia)
C-III	8,800	chylomicrons, VLDL, HDL	-inhibits lipoprotein lipase	-apoA-I/C-III deficiency
D	22,000	HDL	-assists reverse cholesterol transport	?
E_2-E_4	37,000	chylomicrons, VLDL, IDL, HDL$_c$	-binding to apoE/B-100 and apoE/B-48 receptors	-type III dyslipoproteinemia

VLDL: very low density lipoproteins; IDL: intermediate density lipoproteins; LDL: low density lipoproteins; HDL: high density lipoproteins; HDL$_c$: apoE containing HDL; LCAT: lecithin-cholesterol-acyl-transferase; TGL: triglyceride lipase.

to chylomicron remnants. Like chylomicron remnants, they are transported to the liver, but are taken up by apoE/B-100 (or LDL) receptors. While chylomicron remnants are thought to be completely catabolized in the liver, some of these IDL particles are only partially catabolized and are released back into plasma as LDL. In the process, apoCII and apoE are transferred to HDL. This reaction may be catalyzed by another non-circulating tissue-bound lipase, called hepatic triglyceride lipase (H-TGL). It is possible that this conversion of IDL to LDL may also occur entirely in the plasma, without a hepatic phase. Under circumstances in which hepatic receptors are saturated, some IDL may be taken up by receptors on the surface of macrophages.

Under normal circumstances, all plasma LDL can be accounted for by VLDL catabolism. LDL is the major means by which cholesterol is transported to peripheral cells for cell membrane synthesis and for the formation of adrenal and gonadal hormones. These cells remove LDL from the plasma by binding to cell surface receptors. About 70% of these receptors occur in the liver. The rest are found on peripheral cells.

Once LDL is bound to cell surface receptors, it is internalized by endocytosis, combined with lyzosomes, and broken down to cholesterol, amino acids, and other components.

Saturation of receptors with LDL leads to intracellular inhibition of the enzyme 3-hydroxy-3-methylglutaryl coenzyme A reductase or HMG-CoA-reductase. This enzyme catalyzes the rate-limiting step in cholesterol synthesis. Thus, a cell that obtains cholesterol from LDL is inhibited from manufacturing its own. When LDL cholesterol is not available, however, HMG-CoA-reductase activity is high and intracellular synthesis proceeds. If LDL cell surface receptors are saturated, either because they are low in number or LDL levels are overwhelmingly high, excess LDL may be taken up by the scavenger cells, including macrophages and, perhaps, by smooth muscle cells in the arterial intima.[5,6] In vitro evidence demonstrates that scavenger cell uptake occurs most readily when LDL has been oxidized or otherwise chemically altered. It has been suggested that when LDL is not efficiently removed from plasma, it undergoes chemical changes, particularly oxidation, that allow it to bind more easily to scavenger cells.[1]

CHYLOMICRON METABOLISM

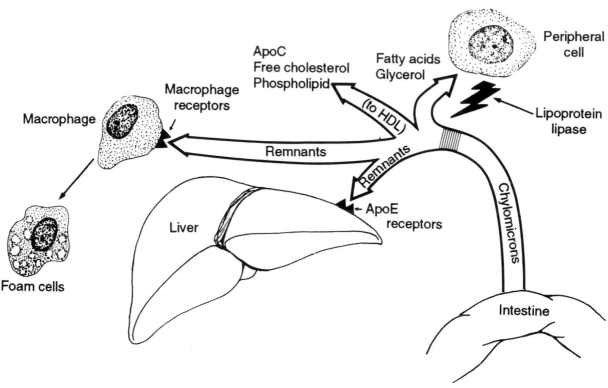

Figure 1. Chylomicron metabolism (see text for discussion). In this and other figures and in the text, hepatic and peripheral receptors are identified by the apoproteins that they recognize. ApoE receptors are also known as remnant receptors. HDL = high density lipoproteins.

HDL

HDL is the lipoprotein responsible for transporting cholesterol from cells to other lipoprotein or catabolic sites (Figure 3). HDL may be formed de novo in the liver and intestines, intravascularly from the redundant surface material of chylomicrons and VLDL (see above) and, perhaps, by peripheral cells as well. Newly formed or nascent HDL is a disc consisting of free cholesterol, phospholipid, and apoproteins. Free cholesterol from cells and perhaps from other lipoproteins reacts in plasma with a complex containing the enzyme lecithin-cholesterol-acetyl-transferase (LCAT), apoprotein A-I (apoA-I), and a cholesterol exchange protein currently thought to be an HDL-associated apoprotein (apoD). This complex attaches to the surface of the disc, and the cholesterol is esterified under the influence of LCAT. As nonpolar esterified cholesterol migrates to the interior of the disc, a sphere, consisting of an outer coating of free cholesterol, phospholipid, and protein and an inner core of esterified cholesterol and small amounts of triglyceride is formed.[7] This is a mature HDL particle. Recent work indicates that the

fraction of HDL containing only apoA-I, termed lipoprotein A-I or LpA-I, is most active in cholesterol binding.[8]

HDL can be divided into two fractions, HDL_3 and HDL_2. HDL_3 is the early disc form. When converted to spherical particles with a neutral fat core, it becomes HDL_2. HDL_2 may transfer some of its cholesterol ester to other lipoproteins in exchange for triglyceride via a protein called cholesterol ester transfer protein (CETP) or may carry it to the liver where HDL is recognized by specific receptors and removed from the plasma.

HDL_2 may be converted to another HDL fraction, called HDL_c or HDL_1 or apoE-containing HDL. This occurs under conditions in which dietary cholesterol is high and macrophages become laden with excess chylomicron remnants that cannot be readily taken up by hepatic apoE (remnant) receptors. It is hypothesized that macrophages that have become laden with cholesterol then transfer free cholesterol (converted to esterified cholesterol by LCAT) and apoprotein E (apoE) to HDL_2, forming HDL_c. HDL_c, unlike other forms of HDL, can be removed from the plasma by receptors that recognize apoE.[1,5,6] The precise steps

VLDL METABOLISM

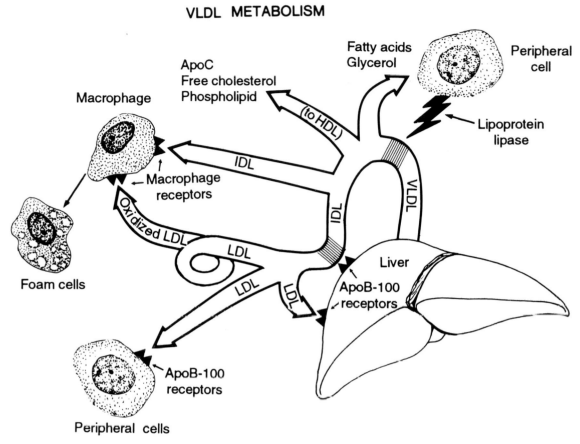

Figure 2. VLDL metabolism (see text for discussion). Hepatic and peripheral receptors are identified by the apoproteins that they recognize. ApoB-100 receptors are also known as LDL receptors. VLDL = very low density lipoproteins; IDL = intermediate density lipoproteins; HDL = high density lipoproteins; LDL = low density lipoproteins.

by which HDL is catabolized in the liver are not completely understood.

Abnormal Lipoprotein Metabolism [1,2,4,9,10]

Lipoprotein metabolism may be altered at many points. These alterations may be of genetic or acquired origin. Although these abnormalities will be reviewed with reference to the normal pathways just discussed, it should be remembered that lipoprotein classes do not exist as isolated entities. Rather, they form a continuous spectrum of particles that are highly interactive in exchanging lipid and protein components.

Abnormal Chylomicron Metabolism

Chylomicrons, as well as other apoB-containing lipoproteins, may fail to form altogether, due to an apparent defect in intracellular lipoprotein assembly (although apoB appears to be normally synthesized). A

recessive genetic abnormality, abetalipoproteinemia, results in fat malabsorption and in very low levels of cholesterol and triglycerides. The profound deficiency of circulating cholesterol affects cell membranes, resulting in acanthocytosis (abnormal crenated red blood cells), retinitis pigmentosa, and a variety of severe neurologic developmental abnormalities. An autosomal dominant disorder, homozygous hypobetalipoproteinemia, may also result in an absence of apoB-containing lipoproteins, resulting from a defect in apoB synthesis. A number of other genetic defects of apoB-48 or apoB-100 have also been described, resulting in deficiency of chylomicron formation and fat malabsorption or low plasma LDL levels, respectively.

When lipoprotein lipase is deficient, chylomicrons may be formed in the intestine and reach peripheral tissue normally, but not be efficiently catabolized. Under such circumstances, chylomicrons accumulate in the plasma (type I hyperlipoproteinemia). This abnormality is inherited as a recessive trait. In another familial recessive disorder, apoprotein C-II (apoC-II), a necessary cofactor for lipoprotein lipase activity, is

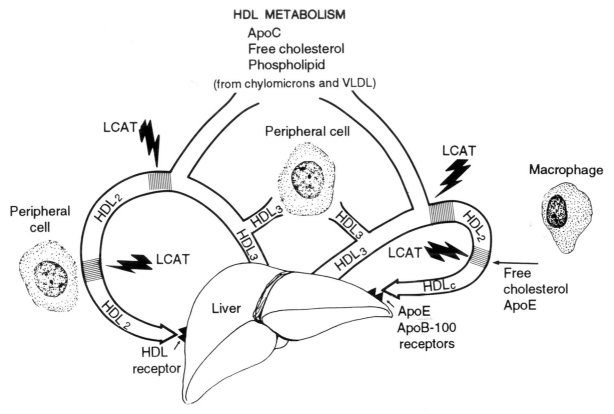

Figure 3. HDL metabolism (see text for discussion). Hepatic and peripheral receptors are identified by the apoproteins that they recognize. ApoE receptors are also known as remnant receptors. ApoB-100 receotors are also known as LDL receptors. VLDL = very low density lipoproteins; HDL = high density lipoproteins; HDL$_2$ and HDL$_3$ = apoE-containing HDL; HDL$_c$ = apoE-containing HDL; LCAT = lecithin-cholesterol-acetyl-transferase.

missing, and plasma chylomicrons and VLDL accumulate (type V hyperlipoproteinemia). In both disorders, the signs and symptoms of excess chylomicrons in the plasma may develop. These include pancreatitis, hepatosplenomegaly (due to uptake of chylomicron particles by scavenger cells in the liver and spleen), cutaneous eruptive xanthomas, and lipemia retinalis (pink-white coloring of the retinal vessels).

Lipoprotein lipase activity may be inhibited by a variety of acquired conditions. For example, an antibody against lipoprotein lipase may be formed in systemic lupus erythematosis and other dysgammaglobulinemias. Since lipoprotein lipase synthesis is insulin-dependent, insulinopenic diabetes may result in lipoprotein lipase deficiency and chylomicronemia. Finally, in chronic renal failure, circulating inhibitors of lipoprotein lipase may be present.

If chylomicrons are successfully converted to chylomicron remnants, the catabolism of the remnants themselves may be blocked if apoprotein E-III (apoE-III), which is necessary for recognition of the remnant by hepatic receptors, is deficient. This may occur in two major genetic abnormalities, one in which apoE-III is not synthesized but other apoproteins in the E series (apoE-II and apoE-IV) are substituted,[11] and another in which no apoprotein E is made.[12] A number of other genetic variants of apoE that result in deficient chylomicron remnant catabolism have also been described.[10] These abnormalities only result in hyperlipoproteinemia (type III) if another genetic abnormality, which results in overproduction of VLDL, also exists (see below). Then, when the normal catabolism of IDL and chylomicron remnants is blocked (Figures 2 and 3), hyperlipoproteinemia occurs. Both IDL and chylomicron remnants are atherogenic (see below), and patients with remnant removal disorders (type III hyperlipoproteinemia) develop atherosclerosis. For reasons that are not well understood, such patients are particularly susceptible to the development of large extremities, as well as coronary and arterial disease. Genetic deficiency of apoE-III is relatively common, but the combination of apoE-III deficiency with genetic VLDL overproduction is not, so that type III hyperlipoproteinemia is relatively uncommon.

The type III abnormality may be aggravated by acquired diseases, such as thyroxine and estrogen deficiency, but acquired forms of apoE-III deficiency have not been described.

Abnormal VLDL Metabolism[1,2,4,10,11]

As noted above, failure to produce apoB may result in a deficiency of VLDL and profound hypolipidemia. Conditions in which apoB and VLDL are overproduced, however, are more commonly seen. The genetic mechanisms involved are poorly understood. One such abnormality is familial combined hyperlipidemia (FCHL). In this condition, apoB-containing lipoproteins are apparently overproduced by the liver. Affected individuals may exhibit elevated levels of VLDL (type IV hyperlipoproteinemia), LDL (type IIa), or both (type IIb).[13] The mechanisms by which one or another of these phenotypes is expressed are unknown. The genetics of this abnormality are not clear, although a working hypothesis is that it represents a single gene disorder inherited as a dominant trait. There is probably a close relationship between FCHL, genetic syndromes in which a small, dense form of LDL predominates,[14] familial disorders characterized by elevated apoB[15] with or without abnormally high LDL cholesterol, and genetic disorders in which combined hyperlipidemia occurs in conjunction with hypertension.[16] Susceptibility to atherosclerosis in individuals with these syndromes appears to be most closely related to elevated apoB levels and occurs even when cholesterol and triglyceride levels fall within normal limits.

Another genetic disorder that results in accumulation of VLDL is familial hypertriglyceridemia (familial type IV hyperlipoproteinemia).[13] This disorder is even less well understood. It is not clear whether it is a single or multiple gene disorder. As in familial combined hyperlipidemia, VLDL production is high. ApoB levels, however, are not disproportionately elevated.

Susceptibility to atherosclerosis in familial hypertriglyceridemia is uncertain. Some have suggested that patients with this disorder are not likely to develop atherosclerosis and that it is the elevation of apoB that identifies patients, with or without hypertriglyceridemia, who do have such susceptibility.[17] If true, this dichotomy may explain the confusion that has surrounded the role of elevated plasma triglyceride as a risk factor for atherosclerotic vascular disease. Accumulation of VLDL may occur in a variety of circumstances secondary to other diseases. In insulinopenic diabetes, lipoprotein lipase, dependent on insulin for synthesis, may be deficient. VLDL overproduction in the liver, however, may occur in response to excessive circulating insulin under circumstances in which peripheral insulin resistance is high. Examples include noninsulinopenic diabetes, obesity, and chronic renal failure. Alcohol can stimulate hepatic VLDL synthesis and inhibit catabolism by a variety of mechanisms. Abnormal globulins, by combining with VLDL or chylomicron particles, may render them inaccessible to catabolic sites.[9]

Abnormal LDL Metabolism

LDL represents the final product of VLDL catabolism. Thus, in abetalipoproteinemia, LDL, like other apoB-containing proteins, is absent. LDL levels also may be deficient in other inherited abnormalities, such as familial hypobetalipoproteinemia. These are presumed to be the result of defects in apoB synthesis, although their mechanisms are not well understood.

Some of the mechanisms by which LDL accumulates in plasma, however, have been clearly elucidated. If LDL receptors are deficient or defective, then LDL cannot be efficiently removed from the plasma.[18] Intracellular cholesterol synthesis, moreover, is not as effectively inhibited when receptors are deficient, and some of the excess cholesterol produced eventually finds its way to LDL. The various genetic defects of apoE/B-100 (LDL) receptors are collectively referred to as familial hypercholesterolemia (FH). They represent single gene disorders with an autosomal dominant inheritance.[19]

Because LDL carries most of the total plasma cholesterol, heterozygotes, which have about one half the normal complements of receptors, are likely to have total cholesterol levels between 300 and 500 mg/dL (7.7—13 mmol/L). Males exhibit coronary and other vascular disease by the fourth decade, females about a decade later. FH may exhibit tendon and cutaneous xanthomas, xanthelasma, and corneal arcus.

Homozygotes for FH have cholesterol levels above 500 mg/dL (13 mmol/L) and xanthomas and atherosclerosis manifest as early as the first or second decade of life. Some cases of valvular heart disease related to valvular cholesterol deposition have also been described.

Unfortunately, the gene for FH is rather common. The heterozygous state occurs in one out of every 500 live births. The homozygous state is much less common, occurring in one in every one million live births.

Patients with FH may exhibit either phenotype IIa hyperlipoproteinema (accumulation of LDL alone) or, less commonly, IIb (accumulation of LDL and VLDL). The presence of xanthomas, although not detected in all cases, helps to separate these individuals from those with FCHL, who may have the same lipoprotein phenotype. Exceptionally high cholesterol levels and a strong family history of coronary disease also help to distinguish patients with FH from those with FCHL.

LDL may also accumulate because of a variant from defective apoB-100 structure, which consists of the substitution of one glutamine molecule by arginine at position 3500. The molecule apoB-100 loses most of its ability to bind to LDL receptors. The result is an increase in total cholesterol of about 80 mg/dL (2.1 mmol/L), all in the LDL fraction.[20]

Accumulation of LDL may also result from several acquired abnormalities. High fat diets may saturate hepatic cells with cholesterol and reduce the number of apoE/B-100 (LDL) receptors that the cell produces. Age may also reduce the number of these receptors.

A number of diseases may diminish LDL receptor activity.[9] In hypothyroidism, LDL accumulates because of decreased LDL metabolism and perhaps because of a separate unexplained effect of elevated thyroid-stimulating hormone (TSH).

LDL elevations may also occur in a nephrosis. Overproduction of apoB-containing lipoproteins in the liver is a by-product of a general increase in hepatic protein synthesis stimulated by the loss of smaller proteins through the diseased glomerulus. LDL may also accumulate in dysgammaglobulinemia due to a combination of LDL with abnormal gammaglobulins that interfere with LDL clearance. Similarly, in diabetes, LDL apoB may be glycosylated and rendered inaccessible to normal cell-surface receptors.[21]

Abnormal HDL Metabolism

HDL levels are inversely related to vascular disease. Elevations of HDL, then, are generally not thought of as pathologic states. HDL elevations may result from a genetic condition, familial hyperalphalipoproteinemia, that is not yet well understood. Families with this genetic trait are characterized by their longevity.[22]

Deficiencies of HDL may result from a variety of familial disorders.[10] The most completely described of these are rare disorders of apoprotein A-I (apoA-I) synthesis such as Tangier disease, in which abnormal apoA-I is produced that cannot combine with lipids to form HDL and is rapidly catabolized. Others include disorders of cholesterol esterification, such as familial LCAT deficiency and fish eye disease, in which mature cholesterol-ester-enriched HDL is not formed. Apoprotein A-I/C-III deficiency is another genetic abnormality in which both of these apoproteins are genetically deficient, resulting in reduced HDL synthesis. Individuals with apoA-I/C-III deficiency are very susceptible to premature atherosclerosis. Those with Tangier disease, however, are not susceptible, perhaps because their LDL levels are also relatively low. Other rare mutations of apoA-I have been described.[23]

HDL may be present but in diminished quantities (familial hypoalphalipoproteinemia).[24] It is unlikely that this syndrome represents a single genetic disorder. Nevertheless, it is increasingly clear that there are many individuals whose only lipoprotein abnormality is a deficiency of HDL. Because such individuals will not be detected on routine cholesterol screening, it is recommended that HDL, as well as total cholesterol, be measured in adults.[25]

HDL deficiency may also be a result of the influence of several other environmental, genetic, and acquired factors. Male sex, poorly controlled diabetes, cigarette smoking, obesity, and lack of exercise all are associated with low HDL levels.[26]

Drugs may also affect HDL levels. Use of beta-blocking agents, widely used to treat hypertension, is associated with low HDL levels. Estrogen, alcohol, and phenytoin use is associated with elevated levels.[27]

It should be remembered that most of the data relating HDL levels to other factors are cross-sectional. Less is known about prospective changes in HDL. While it is tempting to promote changes in lifestyle because of their association with HDL levels, it is not certain whether changes in these factors will alter HDL levels or how such changes will affect atherosclerotic risk.

Therapeutic Interventions in Abnormal Lipoprotein Metabolism

It is beyond the scope of this chapter to review therapy for dyslipoproteinemia in detail; however, a brief review of available therapeutic modalities and, where known, their mechanism of action is presented. Lipoprotein levels may be altered by three kinds of therapeutic manipulation: diet, drugs, and surgical procedures.

Diet[28]

Several dietary factors, including total caloric intake, dietary cholesterol content, and the relative amounts of saturated, monounsaturated, and polyunsaturated dietary fat, affect lipoprotein levels. In addition, other dietary factors, including total carbohydrate intake, alcohol intake, and the source of dietary protein, may be of importance.

Up to an intake of 400 mg (10.3 mmol/L) per day, dietary cholesterol raises blood cholesterol levels in linear fashion. Conversely, reduction of dietary cholesterol below this intake is reflected in lower plasma levels. These effects are mediated, in part, through hepatic receptors. High cholesterol diets, which saturate hepatic cells with cholesterol, reduce the number of receptors and allow LDL to accumulate in the plasma.

If dietary cholesterol intake is low, however, receptors will be activated and LDL cleared from the plasma.

The mechanisms by which saturated fats raise cholesterol levels and polyunsaturated fats lower them are still incompletely understood. Both dietary cholesterol and saturated fat apparently decrease LDL receptor activity, although not necessarily by the same mechanism.[29] Several lines of evidence indicate that polyunsaturated fats interfere with cholesterol absorption and accelerate catabolism of cholesterol-containing lipoproteins. It is interesting to note that when polyunsaturates are substituted for saturated fat, lower levels of both LDL and HDL in the plasma result. This may simply be the result of a concomitant decline in saturated fat intake. In some studies, however, substitution of saturated fat by monounsaturated fat results in less HDL decline.[30] Not all monounsaturates have identical effects. When monounsaturates are formed by commercial hydrogenation of polyunsaturated fats, a form known as "trans" fatty acids are produced. These "trans" forms do not lower LDL and appear to raise levels of Lp(a), both of which may increase coronary artery disease risk.[31]

Reduction of total calories, carbohydrates, and alcohol intake all lower cholesterol and triglyceride levels primarily by decreasing the production of VLDL. LDL levels may also fall in some individuals.

In the last several years, much interest has been focused on the omega-3 fatty acids (named for the distance from the methyl carbon of the first double bond). These fats are derived primarily from fish oils. They have been demonstrated to lower plasma triglyceride levels and raise HDL levels. Their effects on LDL and cholesterol are more variable, in some cases resulting in higher LDL levels.[32]

Because of their effects on prostaglandins, omega-3 fatty acids have been associated with a decrease in platelet adhesiveness. In one study, a population that had historically consumed high levels of fish oil was shown to have a lower rate of coronary disease.[33] This, however, may simply be the result of lower saturated fat intake.

Drug Therapy

Several lipid-lowering drugs are currently available. Some of their properties are summarized in Table 3. LDL cholesterol-lowering drugs include those (like the bile acid sequestrants, cholestyramine and colestipol) that bind bile salts, interrupt the enterohepatic circulation of bile, and stimulate the hepatic production of apo-B (LDL) receptors in order that hepatocytes may obtain cholesterol for the formation of bile. This effect is demonstrable even in individuals heterozygous for familial hypercholesterolemia, who, under basal circumstances, lack the normal complement of receptors.

Lovastatin, pravastatin, and simvastatin are all newer drugs that competitively inhibit HMG-CoA-reductase. By limiting the availability of intracellular cholesterol, they also stimulate the cell to produce more receptors.

Drugs such as nicotinic acid interfere with the synthesis of VLDL in the liver and in this way lower VLDL and LDL levels.

Probucol has a unique effect on LDL. It appears to combine with the LDL particle in the plasma and make it more susceptible to removal. Unfortunately, probucol also appears to inhibit hepatic synthesis of apoA-I and HDL. Whether the fall in LDL is worthwhile if accompanied by a fall in HDL remains unclear, although there is evidence that treatment with probucol can mobilize cholesterol deposits in cutaneous and tendinous xanthomas.

Probucol has another, potentially important, effect in inhibiting the oxidation of LDL. Prevention of oxidation may be important in inhibiting LDL uptake into atheromas (see below). Other antioxidants, such as beta-carotene and vitamin E, have also been associated with decreased risk of clinical atherosclerosis.[34,35]

Drugs used to lower triglyceride apparently act primarily by enhancing activity of lipoprotein lipase and accelerating clearance of triglyceride-carrying lipoproteins, particularly VLDL, from the plasma. Usually, as triglycerides fall, HDL levels rise, so that these drugs often promote both effects. Both nicotinic acid and the fibric acid derivatives, of which clofibrate and gemfibrozil are available in the United States, promote this action.[36]

Surgical Therapy

Surgical procedures in the treatment of dyslipoproteinemia have all been directed to patients with FH. Partial ileal bypass surgery has been advocated as a means of interrupting biliary enterohepatic circulation, similar to the accomplishment of bile acid sequestrants.[37] The advantage of such surgery is that drug compliance is not a problem, and greater and more sustained cholesterol reductions can be achieved. In a trial involving 838 survivors of a first myocardial infarction, deaths due to CAD and recurrent myocardial infarction were decreased by 35% in the surgical group. This was associated with a 37.7% fall in LDL levels and arrest of progression of atherosclerosis in a subsample studied with repeat coronary angiography.[38] The availability of HMG-CoA-reductase inhibitors, which can produce such drops in LDL without surgery, make the indications for this procedure problematic.

In patients with homozygous FH, who have a

Table 3
Lipid Lowering Drugs

	Nicotinic Acid	Bile Acid Sequestrants	Probucol	HMG-CoA-Reductase Inhibitors*	Clofibrate	Gemfibrozil
Lipoprotein effects						
Chylomicrons	?↓	?	→	→	→	?↓
VLDL	↓	→ or ↑	→	→	↓	↓
IDL	↓	→ or ↑	→	?	↓	↓
LDL	↓	↓	↓	↓	→ or ↑	→ or ↑
HDL	↑	→ or ↑	↓	→	→ or ↑	→ or ↑
Side effects	Flushing; rash; acanthosis nigricians; GI cramping; nausea; abdominal pain; abnormal liver function tests; ↓ glucose tolerance; ↑ uric acid; ↑ atrial arrhythmias	Bloating; constipation; binding of vitamins and medications; hyperchloremic acidosis (in children)	Loose stools; flatulence; diarrhea; abdominal pain	Abnormal liver function tests; myositis (rare)	Myositis; cholelithiasis; coumadin potentiation;	Similar to clofibrate
Daily dosage	1.0–3.0 (1.0–2.0 g TID)	12–24 g/d (cholestyramine); 15–30 g/d (colestipol); (in BID or TID dosage ½ hr before meals)	1,200 mg (600 mg BID)	20 mg (lovastatin) 20–40 mg (pravastatin) 10–20 mg (simvastatin)	1,000 mg (500 mg BID)	1,200 mg (600 mg BID)

VLDL: very low density lipoproteins; IDL: intermediate density lipoproteins; LDL: low density lipoproteins; HDL: high density lipoproteins.
* (lovastatin, pravastatin, simvastatin)

complete absence of functional apoB (LDL) receptors, portacaval shunting has sometimes been effective in lowering LDL cholesterol levels.[39] The mechanism by which this procedure lowers cholesterol is not clear. The cholesterol-lowering achieved has not been sufficient to normalize levels in these severely afflicted patients.

Finally, mention should be made of one case in which a young girl with homozygous FH and severe vascular and valvular heart disease was treated with combined heart and liver transplantation.[40] This procedure provided her with a liver capable of synthesizing receptors. In terms of LDL metabolism, the surgery was a complete success. Her total and LDL cholesterol levels were lowered, although not to normal levels. Eventually, the long-term benefits of such a procedure must be weighed against the substantial risks of chronic immunosuppression. In perhaps the not-too-distant future, well-defined LDL-receptor deficiency diseases may be candidates for gene therapy, although to date no such experiments have been performed.

The Relationship of Lipoproteins to Atherogenesis[6,18]

A broad discussion of the process of atherogenesis is beyond the scope of this chapter. The role of lipopro-

tein metabolism in that process is of special interest here.

Atherogenesis appears to proceed under one of three lipoprotein states:[41,42] 1) when low density lipoproteins are elevated, as in FH and other forms of type II hyperlipoproteinemia; 2) when VLDL and chylomicron remnants are elevated, as in the combination of apoE-III deficiency and VLDL overproduction states, collectively known as type III hyperlipoproteinemia; and 3) when HDL is deficient. In addition, elevation of Lp(a) (see above) may play a role, although that role has not yet been clearly defined.

LDL

When LDL levels are elevated and receptors are either saturated or deficient, it can be demonstrated that scavenger cells in arterial intima and other tissues take up the excess (Figure 2). Recent experiments have indicated, however, that LDL uptake is most likely to occur when LDL has been oxidized.[43,44] LDL oxidation, moreover, is more likely if LDL is small and dense, such as that which accumulates in the presence of hypertriglyceridemia,[14] or if it is glycosylated, such as occurs in diabetes with hyperglycemia. It has been shown in vitro that these cells have a receptor on this surface that does not recognize normal LDL, but can recognize and bind LDL that has been oxidized. As they accumulate cholesterol, these scavenger cells become the foam cells of the atherosclerotic plaque.

The nature of these scavenger cells is unclear. It was once thought that they were the smooth muscle cells of the arterial intima. Smooth muscle cells, however, appear to contain normal LDL receptors, but not receptors that bind oxidized LDL. A more likely candidate now appears to be the macrophage or a stem cell that has the potential to develop into either a smooth muscle cell or a macrophage that can bind such abnormal lipoproteins. Thus, when LDL is not efficiently removed from the plasma because of a genetic abnormality, it may infiltrate into the arterial intima and undergo changes that render it accessible for binding to scavenger cells. These cells may then form the nidus of an atherosclerotic plaque.

Whether Lp(a) plays a role in this process, perhaps by binding LDL to subendothelial tissues, or whether Lp(a) itself is oxidized and taken up by macrophages is unclear.

VLDL and Chylomicron Remnants

Ingestion of high levels of cholesterol in both animals and humans has been shown to increase concentrations of VLDL and chylomicron remnants. This is thought to occur when the hepatic removal system for remnants becomes saturated. Accumulation of these remnants is not necessarily associated with detectable elevations of total plasma cholesterol levels, so that it is possible that high cholesterol diets may produce atherogenic particles without substantially increasing levels of total cholesterol.

It is clear from animal experiments that these potentially atherogenic particles bind not only to the apoprotein E receptors of the liver, but also to the receptors on the surface of macrophages. Like altered LDL, they convert macrophages into foam cells and, perhaps, form the nidus of an atherosclerotic plaque.

HDL

Plasma HDL levels are inversely associated with atherosclerosis and its complications. HDL can be subdivided into HDL particles containing apoprotein E (HDL$_c$) and those not containing apoprotein E (HDL$_3$ and HDL$_2$, see above and Figure 3). The fraction of HDL containing only apoA-I (Lp A-I, see above) is broadly similar to HDL$_2$ and appears to be most active in binding to cells and initiating reverse cholesterol transport.[45]

When animals or humans are fed high cholesterol diets, the plasma level of apoE-containing HDL increases. A plausible, but unproven, hypothesis is that this occurs as HDL takes up excess cholesterol from the scavenger cells that have become laden with cholesterol. Macrophages that bind oxidized LDL and remnants can synthesize and secrete large quantities of apoE. They are thought to be the source of both apoE and cholesterol, which is added to HDL$_2$ in its conversion to HDL$_c$. Thus HDL$_2$, by taking up apoE and cholesterol, can prevent the permanent conversion of the macrophage to a foam cell. The HDL$_c$ formed can be recognized by hepatic apoE receptors (Figure 3) and removed from the plasma. Alternatively, the cholesterol can be transferred to other lipoproteins by binding first to CETP.

Conditions in which plasma HDL levels are low inhibit this process. Scavenger cells are left without a means of ridding themselves of excess cholesterol and become the foam cells of the atherosclerotic plaque.

One or more of these mechanisms may be operative in individuals who develop atherosclerosis. It is important to remember that at least two of these conditions, formation of remnants and low levels of HDL, may *not* be reflected in elevated levels of total cholesterol.

The Relationship of Lipoproteins to Clinical Vascular Disease

Over the years, a wealth of evidence has linked atherosclerosis, particularly in the coronary arteries, to elevated levels of both dietary and blood cholesterol levels.[46] Since LDL is the major carrier of cholesterol in the plasma, it is not surprising that in populations in which it has been investigated, there is a strong relationship between elevated LDL levels and coronary vascular disease. In fact, a case can be made that in populations in which LDL is low (below 100 mg/dL—2.6 mmol/L), atherosclerosis does not occur, even in the presence of other risk factors.[47]

More recently, it has become apparent that low levels of HDL are also predictive of coronary vascular disease.[45] Low HDL levels, moreover, are also strongly associated with atherosclerosis in the cerebral and peripheral beds where total and LDL cholesterol levels are not as strongly predictive.[48]

Of the three lipoprotein abnormalities experimentally associated with atherogenesis, elevation of LDL, depressed levels of HDL, and accumulation of lipoprotein remnants in the plasma, only the first two have been correlated in population studies with vascular disease. Elevated Lp(a), as noted, has also demonstrated such associations. The role of chylomicron and VLDL remnants in the overall population burden of atherosclerosis, however, is difficult to assess because of the technical difficulty of measuring these remnants. In patients with type III hyperlipoproteinemia, who accumulate such remnants because of the genetic defects, there is no doubt that vascular disease is a prominent complication.

Whether more subtle forms of remnant accumulations, such as may occur after ingestion of high cholesterol diets, also contribute to vascular disease in humans is not known. Given the wealth of animal evidence that links postprandial accumulations of these remnants to experimental atherosclerosis, that conclusion would not be surprising. Accumulation of such remnants without elevation of plasma cholesterol in individuals on high cholesterol diets, a phenomenon known to occur, may be a partial explanation for the difficulty in linking dietary cholesterol to plasma cholesterol levels and to atherosclerosis.

The most important question is what effect the treatment of dyslipoproteinemia has on vascular disease. Regression of atherosclerotic lesions has been demonstrated clearly in a variety of experimental animal models, including subhuman primates, dogs, and swine.[49] More recently, a number of human regression studies have also been reported and demonstrate the same findings. These studies show as well that regression is associated with a lower risk of coronary events.[50] In general, the levels of total plasma cholesterol associated with significant regression (150 to 180 mg/dL—3.9 to 4.7 mmol/L) are the same as those that have been shown in populations to be associated with a low risk of atherosclerotic cardiovascular disease.

In recent years, several large-scale clinical trials have demonstrated the value of lowering cholesterol by either dietary or pharmacologic means.[51] While these trials have sometimes been hampered by deficiencies in design, the results have all pointed in the same direction. Cholesterol lowering is associated with decline in morbid and mortal complications of atherosclerosis, including fatal and nonfatal myocardial infarction. Beneficial effects on *total* mortality, while present in some studies, have been difficult to demonstrate consistently, due largely to limits of sample size and study duration.[52] The effects of cholesterol lowering on peripheral vascular disease have been less well documented, but available trials indicate that the progress of femoral atherosclerosis can be retarded.[53,54]

As a result of this accumulated evidence, guidelines for the detection, evaluation, and treatment of high blood cholesterol (and associated disorders) have been issued by the National Cholesterol Education Program (NCEP). They identify LDL cholesterol lowering as the chief therapeutic intervention to be attempted. HDL and triglyceride levels are seen not so much as therapeutic targets, but as additional risk factors to be taken into account in planning therapy. In defining a total cholesterol of 240 mg/dL (6.2 meq/L)

as "high," they define 25% of the US adult population as in need of additional evaluation and, in some cases, intervention. They particularly target aggressive cholesterol lowering (to levels less than 180 mg/dL—4.6 meq/L) to those with clinically apparent atherosclerotic disease.[25]

These recommendations have been, and will continue to be, subject to debate. Nevertheless, there is little question that for those individuals with elevated LDL, the benefits of treatment are substantial. It is less clear, however, whether attempts should be made to raise HDL levels by other than hygienic means. Clearly, some of those factors associated with low HDL levels such as obesity, lack of exercise, and cigarette smoking can and should be changed whenever possible. The value of pharmacologically-induced elevations in HDL, however, is still unclear.

Summary

In this chapter, the relationship of normal and abnormal lipoprotein metabolism to atherogenesis, the principles of treatment of dyslipoproteinemia, and the relationship between dyslipoproteinemia and clinical vascular diseases have been presented. Our understanding of these issues is not complete. Nevertheless, there is substantial evidence that links abnormal lipoprotein metabolism to the atherosclerotic process. In particular, accumulations of low density lipoprotein, remnants of very low density lipoprotein and chylomicron catabolism, and deficiencies of high density lipoprotein are associated experimentally with atherogenesis and clinically with atherosclerotic vascular disease in humans.

Evidence that correction of these abnormalities leads to arrest or reversal of atherosclerosis is incomplete. Lowering of LDL cholesterol has been the most extensively studied. There seems to be little doubt that it is beneficial in reducing both coronary and peripheral vascular disease manifestations. Evidence that treatment of remnant accumulation is of benefit has been hampered by an inability to easily detect these particles. Experimental animal models, however, clearly indicate the value of reducing accumulations of such lipoprotein remnants.

While there are strong correlations between HDL cholesterol levels and vascular disease, prospective evidence of the value of raising HDL levels is scanty and only suggestive. Nevertheless, many of the recommendations that would be made to an individual with a risk of vascular disease, such as weight reduction, cessation of smoking, and the institution of regular exercise, will probably be effective in raising HDL cholesterol levels.

No attempt has been made in this chapter to systematically review treatment regimens for dyslipopro-teinemia. It is evident, however, that such treatment has the potential to substantially reduce the cata-strophic risks of atherosclerosis even in middle-aged individuals who may have been exposed to those risks for many years.

References

1. Ginsberg HN: Lipoprotein physiology and its relation-ship to atherogenesis. *Endocrinol Metab Clin North Am* 19:211, 1990.
2. Brewer HB Jr, Gregg RE, Hoeg JM, et al: Apolipopro-teins and lipoproteins in human plasma: an overview. *Clin Chem* 34/8:B4, 1988.
3. Scanu AM (ed): *Lipoprotein(a)*. New York, NY, Aca-demic Press, Inc., Harcourt Brace Jovanovich; 1990.
4. Gotto AM Jr: Apolipoproteins and metabolism in athero-sclerosis. *Trans Am Clin Climatol Assoc* 101:46, 1989.
5. Mahley RW: Apolipoprotein E: cholesterol transport protein with expanding role in cell biology. *Science* 240:622, 1988.
6. Brown MS, Goldstein JL: Lipoprotein metabolism in the macrophage: implications for cholesterol deposition in atherosclerosis. *Am Review Biochem* 52:223, 1983.
7. Schonfeld G: Disorders of lipid transport. *Prog Cardio-vasc Dis* XXVI:89, 1983.
8. Brewer HB Jr, Rader DJ, Hoeg JM, et al: Recent ad-vances in lipoprotein metabolism and the genetic dysli-poproteinemias. In: Malmendier CL, Alaupovic P, Brewer HB Jr (eds). *Adv Exp Med Biol* New York: Plenum Press; 237, 1990.
9. LaRosa JC: Dyslipoproteinemia secondary to common clinical disorders: mechanisms and treatment. *Cardio-vasc Risk Factors* 1:52, 1990.
10. Schonfeld G: Inherited disorders of lipid transport. *En-docrinol Metab Clin North Am* 19:229, 1990.
11. Havel RJ: Familial dysbetalipoproteinemia: new aspects of pathogenesis and diagnosis. *Med Clin North Am* 66:441, 1982.
12. Ghisselli G, Schaefer EJ, Gascon P, et al: Type III hyper-lipo-proteinemia associated with apolipoprotein E defi-ciency. *Science* 214:1239, 1981.
13. Brunzell JD, Albers JJ, Chait A, et al: Plasma lipopro-teins in familial combined hyperlipidemia and monogenic familial hypertriglyceridemia. *J Lipid Res* 24:147, 1983.
14. Krauss RM: The tangled web of coronary risk factors. *Am J Med* (suppl 2A)90:36S, 1991.
15. Kwiterovich PO: Biochemical, clinical, genetic, and metabolic studies of hyperapo-β-lipoproteinemia. *J Inher Metab Dis I* (suppl II)57, 1988.
16. Williams RR, Hunt SC, Hopkins PN, et al: Familial dys-lipidemic hypertension: evidence from 58 Utah families for a syndrome present in approximately 12% of patients with essential hyper-tension. *JAMA* 259:3579, 1988.
17. Sniderman AD, Silberg J: Is it time to measure apolipo-protein B? *Arterioscler Thromb* 10:665, 1990.
18. Goldstein JL, Rita R, Brown MS: Defect in lipoprotein receptors and atherosclerosis: lessons from an animal counterpart of familial hypercholesterolemia. *N Engl J Med* 309:288, 1983.
19. Russell DW, Esser V, Hobbs HH: Molecular basis of familial hypercholesterolemia. *Arteriosclerosis* (suppl I)9:8, 1989.
20. Tybjaerg-Hansen A, Humphries SE: Familial defective apolipoprotein B-100: a single mutation that causes hy-percholesterolemia and premature coronary artery dis-ease. *Atherosclerosis* 96:91, 1992.
21. Curtiss LK, Witztum JL: Plasma apolipoproteins A-I, A-II, B, C-II and E are glycosylated in hyperglycemic diabetic subjects. *Diabetes* 34:452, 1985.
22. Glueck CJ, Fallat RW, Millet F, et al: Familial hyperal-phalipoproteinemia: studies in eighteen kindreds. *Me-tabolism* 24:1243, 1975.
23. Schaefer EJ: Clinical, biochemical, and genetic features in familial disorders of high density lipoprotein defi-ciency. *Arteriosclerosis* 4:303, 1984.
24. Vergani C, Bettale G: Familial hypoalphalipoproteine-mia. *Clin Chim Acta* 114:45, 1984.
25. Summary of the second report of the National Choles-terol Education Program (NCEP) Expert Panel on detec-tion, evaluation, and treatment of high blood cholesterol in adults (Adult Treatment Panel II). *JAMA* 269:3015, 1993.
26. Levy RI, Rifkind BM: The structure, function and me-tabolism of high-density lipoproteins: a status report. *Circulation* 62(suppl IV)62:14, 1980.
27. Wallace RB, Hunninghake DB, Reiland S, et al: Altera-tions in plasma high density lipoprotein levels associated with consumption of selected medications. *Circulation* (suppl IV)62: IV, 1980.
28. Stone NJ: Diet, lipids, and coronary heart disease. *Endo-crinol Metab Clin North Am* 19:321, 1990.
29. Kris-Etherton PM, Krummel D, Dreon D, et al: The ef-fect of diet on plasma lipids, lipoproteins, and coronary heart disease. *J Am Diet Assoc* 88:1373, 1988.
30. Grundy SM, Nix D, Whelan MF, et al: Comparison of three cholesterol-lowering diets in normolipidemic men. *JAMA* 256: 2351, 1986.
31. Mensink RP, Katan MB: Effect of dietary trans fatty acids on high-density and low-density lipoprotein choles-terol levels in healthy subjects. *N Engl J Med* 323:439, 1990.
32. Harris WS: Fish oils and plasma lipid and lipoprotein metabolism in humans: a critical review. *J Lipid Res* 30:785, 1989.
33. Kromhout D, Bosscheiter EB, Coulander C: The inverse relation between fish consumption and 20-year mortality from coronary heart disease. *N Engl J Med* 312:1205, 1985.
34. Gwynne JT: Probucol. In: LaRosa JC (ed). *Practical Management of Lipid Disorders*. Fort Lee, NJ: Health Care Communications, Inc.; 91, 1992.
35. Jackson RL, Ku G, Thomas CE: Antioxidants: a biologi-cal defense mechanism for the prevention of atheroscle-rosis. *Med Res Rev* 13:161, 1992.
36. Hunninghake DB: Drug treatment of dyslipoproteine-mia. *Endocrinol Metab Clin North Am* 19:345, 1990.
37. Buchwald H, Moorehead RB, Vareo R: Ten years clini-cal experience with partial ileal bypass in management of the hyperlipidemias. *Ann Surg* 180:384, 1974.
38. Buchwald H, Long JM, Pearce MB, et al: Effect of par-tial ileal bypass surgery on mortality and morbidity from coronary heart disease in patients with hypercholesterol-emia: report of the Program on the Surgical Control of the Hyperlipidemias (POSCH). *N Engl J Med* 323:946, 1990.
39. Starzl TE, Chase P, Ahrens EH, et al: Portocaval shunt in patients with familial hypercholesterolemia. *Ann Surg* 198:273, 1983.
40. Bilheimer DW, Goldstein JL, Grundy SM, et al: Liver transplantation to provide low-density-lipoprotein recep-

tors and lower plasma cholesterol in a child with homozygous familial hypercholesterolemia. *N Engl J Med* 311: 1658, 1984.

41. Steinberg D, Fielding C, Sniderman AD: Lipoproteins and the pathogenesis of atherosclerosis. *Circulation* 80: 719, 1989.
42. Breslow JL: The genetic basis of lipoprotein disorders. *J Internal Med* 231:627, 1992.
43. Davies MJ, Woolf N: Atherosclerosis: what is it and why does it occur? *Br Heart J* (suppl)69:S-3, 1993.
44. Witztum JL: Role of oxidised low density lipoprotein in atherogenesis. *Br Heart J* (suppl)69:S-12, 1993.
45. Tribble DL, Krauss RM: HDL and coronary artery disease. *Adv Intern Med* 38:1, 1993.
46. LaRosa JC: Cholesterol and cardiovascular disease: how strong is the evidence? *Clin Cardiol* (suppl II)15:III-2, 1992.
47. Roberts WC: Factors linking cholesterol to atherosclerotic plaques. *Am J Cardiol* 62:495, 1988.
48. Vigna GB, Bolzan M, Romagnoni R, et al: Lipids and other risk factors selected by discriminant analysis in symptomatic patients with supra-aortic and peripheral atherosclerosis. *Circulation* 85:2205, 1992.
49. St. Clair RSW: Atherosclerosis regression in animal models: current concepts of cellular and biochemical mechanisms. *Prog Cardiovasc Dis* XXVI:109, 1983.
50. Brown BG, Zhao X-Q, Sacco DE, et al: Arteriographic view of treatment to achieve regression of coronary atherosclerosis and to prevent plaque disruption and clinical cardiovascular events. *Br Heart J* (suppl)69:S-48, 1993.
51. Holme I: Relation of coronary heart disease incidence and total mortality to plasma cholesterol reduction in randomised trials: use of meta-analysis. *Br Heart J* (suppl)69:S-42, 1993.
52. LaRosa JC: Cholesterol lowering, low cholesterol, and mortality. *Am J Cardiol* 72:776–786, 1993.
53. Blankenhorn DH, Azen SP, Crawford DW, et al: Effects of colestipol-niacin therapy on human femoral atherosclerosis. *Circulation* 83:438, 1991.
54. Duffield RGM, Miller NE, Brunt JNH, et al: Treatment of hyperlipidaemia retards progression of symptomatic femoral atherosclerosis. *Lancet* 8351:639, 1983.

CHAPTER 19

Cigarette Smoking
and
Vascular Disease

Joseph M. Giordano, MD

Introduction and Epidemiology

Cigarette smoking is the single most preventable cause of morbidity and mortality in the United States. An association between early death and cigarette smoking was first reported in 1938.[1] The Surgeon General, in a report released in 1964, documented the adverse effects of smoking.[2] Since then, clinical, epidemiologic, pathologic, and laboratory findings have consistently verified a relationship between smoking and cancer, chronic obstructive pulmonary disease, and cardiovascular disease.[3,4]

Despite impressive efforts to inform the public about the hazards of cigarette smoking, in 1987,[5] 31.7% of adult men and 26.8% of adult women continued to smoke. However, this represents a significant downward trend; in 1965, 52% of men and 34% of women smoked cigarettes.[5] Data from national health interview surveys project smoking prevalence in the year 2000 to be 20% of men and 23% of women.[6] Socioeconomic subgroups are important determinants of smokers, with 30% of adults having a high school diploma, but less than 10% of college graduates smoking in the year 2000. Annual per capita sales of manufactured cigarettes decreased from 4325 cigarettes in 1963 to 3196 in 1987, a 26% reduction.[5] Total cigarette sales fell from 640 billion cigarettes in 1981 to 574 billion in 1987.

Cigarette smoking has a profound effect on morbidity and mortality.[7–10] In Western societies, people who smoke have twice the overall death rate as non-smokers. It is estimated that more than 350000 people die each year in the United States from smoking cigarettes.[11] Approximately 30% to 40% of the 565000 deaths from coronary artery disease can be attributed to smoking.[12] Men who smoke more than one pack of cigarettes a day, at the time of initial examination, have a risk for a first major coronary event that is two to three times as great as that of a nonsmoker.[13,14] Of all the clinical manifestations of coronary heart disease, sudden death is most strongly related to cigarette smoking.[14] Patients with angiographic-proven coronary artery disease who continue to smoke have a 5-year mortality of 22% compared to 15% for those who stop smoking.[15] Most of the increased mortality is due to myocardial infarction or sudden cardiac death.

The relationship between smoking and cerebrovascular disease is controversial. The Framingham Study reported that for stroke in general and cerebral infarction in particular, cigarette smoking was a weak risk factor confined to men and women under the age of 65.[14] Abbott, however, reported that male smokers had two to three times the risk of thromboembolic or hemorrhagic stroke after control for age, diastolic blood pressure, coronary heart disease, and other risk factors.[16] Smoking has also been identified as a strong independent risk factor for atherosclerosis of the extracranial and intracranial carotid arteries.[17,18]

Cigarette smoking is a highly significant risk factor for the development of peripheral arterial occlusive disease.[14] Heavy smokers have three times the risk of developing intermittent claudication compared to non-

From *The Basic Science of Vascular Disease*. Edited by Sidawy AN, Sumpio BE, and DePalma RG. Armonk, NY: Futura Publishing Company, Inc.; © 1997.

smokers.[19] Nonsmokers present with symptomatic vascular disease much later than smokers, more than 11 years later in one study.[20] Ninety percent of patients with aortoiliac disease and 91% with femoropopliteal disease have a history of heavy cigarette smoking.[21] Patients with a diagnosis of intermittent claudication treated conservatively have a high amputation rate in the follow-up period if they continue to smoke cigarettes.[22] Patients with severe ischemic vascular disease of the lower extremity who undergo bypass procedures have a lower patency rate in the postoperative period if they continue to smoke.[23] Smokers undergo amputation eight years sooner than nonsmokers.[24] Even if the patient was a former smoker, amputation occurs one year sooner than in patients who never smoked.

The risk for the development of vascular disease in smokers may be different for women than men. Kannel, on the basis of the Framingham Study, states that the incidence of vascular problems is more pronounced in men than women with a difference most apparent in coronary artery disease and less obvious in peripheral arterial occlusive disease.[3] Reports from the Office of the Surgeon General in 1980 and 1983, however, disputed these data, noting that women with similar smoking patterns as men have the same risk of death from coronary artery disease.[12,25] For women who take oral contraceptives or estrogen-containing medications, smoking cigarettes markedly increases their risk of cardiovascular disease.[26–28] There is a tenfold increase in coronary artery disease and a higher incidence of stroke in women who smoke and use oral contraceptives as compared to female smokers not using oral contraceptives.

The increased risk of vascular disease from smoking, with the possible exception of cerebral infarction, is dose-dependent.[29] The more cigarettes a person smokes, and the more frequently and deeply he or she inhales, directly increase the risks of vascular disease. People who smoke cigars or pipes do not inhale as much as those who smoke cigarettes and therefore have a reduced incidence of coronary heart disease compared to cigarette smokers.[25] However, the incidence of vascular disease in pipe and cigar smokers increases when compared to nonsmokers. People exposed to passive smoke, i.e., tobacco smoke in a closed room, show an increase in their blood carbon monoxide and nicotine levels equal to levels found in people who smoke five cigarettes a day.[30] Studies have not shown an increase in vascular disease for patients exposed to passive smoke, but exercise tolerance is decreased in patients with angina or intermittent claudication exposed to a smoky environment.[31,32]

Low tar nicotine cigarettes or cigarettes with filters have reduced the incidence of cancer, but have not reduced the incidence of vascular disease.[33] The Framingham Study did not show reduced coronary

heart disease in patients who switched to filter cigarettes.[34] Nonperforated filter cigarettes may actually deliver more carbon monoxide than nonfilter cigarettes.[35] Finally, recent studies have suggested that cigarette smokers who use low nicotine or filtered cigarettes alter their smoking habits to increase the inhaled amounts of tar and nicotine to compensate for the lower amounts of these substances in the low-yield cigarettes.[36,37]

Smoking and the Development of Atherosclerosis

Development of atherosclerosis is an extremely complex process that has been extensively studied, but incompletely understood. As discussed, cigarette smoking influences and enhances development of atherosclerosis. The finding of the mechanism is complicated by the 4000 chemical compounds found in smoke from cigarettes, the majority of which have not been studied. Nevertheless, there is considerable information on the effect of smoking on important components in the pathogenesis of atherosclerotic disease: endothelial cells, hyperlipidemia, platelets, and white blood cells.

Endothelial Cells

The effect of cigarette smoking on endothelial cells has been studied in human umbilical cord arteries.[38,39] Comparing umbilical arteries in smoking and nonsmoking women, endothelial wall changes including cell swelling with bleb formation, subendothelial edema with opening of the intracellular junctions, and basement membrane thickening have been documented in the smoking group. Experimentally, cigarette smoke alters endothelium in both rabbits and rats.[40,41] The endothelium appears swollen and irregular with blebs and microvilli-like projections on the luminal membrane of the cell. Platelets are adherent to the endothelium, perhaps indicating early mural thrombus formed over an injured endothelial surface. Both nicotine and carbon monoxide have been studied individually and have been shown to cause endothelial changes similar to those just described.[42,43] In addition to these morphologic studies, other studies have shown that cigarette smoke reduces prostaglandin synthesis by endothelial cells, upsetting the balance between prostaglandin and thromboxane A_2, and thereby reducing the antithrombotic potential of the endothelial surface.[41] Long-term smokers have reduced reproductive capacity of freshly harvested endothelial cells.[44] Smoking has been shown to actively impair vascular dilatation in both the saphenous vein and the brachial artery.[45,46] These studies all suggest that cigarette smoke not only damages the endothelium creating the injury that is the initial event in the development of atherosclerosis, but also functionally impairs the endothelial cells.

Plasma Lipoproteins

Smoking can affect the incidence of vascular disease by altering the levels of plasma lipoproteins.[47] It has been well documented that smokers have different concentrations of plasma lipoproteins compared to nonsmokers. Specifically, low density lipoproteins (LDL), intermediate density lipoproteins (IDL), and very low density lipoproteins (VLDL) are increased. High density lipoproteins (HDL), also, are found to be lower in the smoking population compared to nonsmokers. Also, cessation of smoking is associated with a relatively rapid increase in the serum concentration of HDL, less than 30 days after an individual stopped smoking, according to one report.[48] This adds support to the concept that smoking has an effect on plasma lipoproteins, although the mechanism of this relationship is unknown. However, it does not appear to be related to the diet or physical activity of smokers as compared to nonsmokers.

Platelet Function and Acute Myocardial Infarction

A relationship between acute myocardial infarction and smoking has been established.[49] Since myocardial infarction usually occurs from a coronary artery thrombotic event, smoking has been implicated as a cause of the coronary artery thrombosis.[50] Marked reduction in the incidence of acute myocardial infarction following cessation of smoking supports its role in acute myocardial events. The benefit of aspirin in reducing myocardial infarction supports a role for platelets as a mediator of coronary thrombosis.[51] These facts have stimulated an enormous research effort to delineate the effects of smoking on platelet function. However, these studies have produced conflicting results due to the complexity of platelet function, the myriad of tests used to evaluate platelet function, and the difficulty in establishing in vivo models of platelet vascular wall interaction. The timing of smoke inhalation and its effects on platelet function also is not clear. How long after smoking a cigarette is platelet function compromised, or whether chronic smokers sustain a change in platelet function remain unanswered. Nevertheless, despite these problems, a consensus is emerging that smoking induces a marked, but perhaps short increase in platelet aggregability.[52-54] Simply stated, smoking then is implicated as a major cause of acute

myocardial infarction by increasing platelet aggregability causing coronary artery thrombosis.

White Blood Cells

Elevated white blood cell counts (WBC) have been associated with vascular and coronary artery disease.[55-57] Although the exact mechanism is unclear, elevated WBC may act as mediator in the development of atherosclerosis. Since smoking increases WBC, the atherogenic effects of cigarettes may occur at least partially through their effects on WBC either by direct vascular damage or through microcirculatory occlusion by the increased WBC aggregation.

Pharmacology of Nicotine

Nicotine has been studied extensively for its relationship to vascular disease.[58] Nicotine enters the blood stream through the lungs and within 30 seconds of inhalation is distributed to the brain. Nicotine blood levels reach a similar magnitude from tobacco that is absorbed through the mouth. The levels of nicotine progressively rise and accumulate in the body with each cigarette smoked. A heavy smoker absorbs enough nicotine during the day so that high levels persist throughout the night, giving a heavy smoker nicotine effects for a full 24 hours. It is important to note that both low- and high-yield cigarettes contain the same amount of nicotine. Nicotine acts throughout the body with effects on the skeletal muscles, endocrine organs, and cardiovascular system. It interacts with specific receptors throughout the nervous system, altering brain metabolism. It increases catecholamines, serotonin, corticosteroids, and pituitary hormones.

Nicotine acutely increases cardiac output, heart rate, systolic arterial pressures, and causes continuous vasoconstriction, all of which increase the work of the heart.[59-61] Nicotine also reduces cerebral blood flow and increases platelet aggregation, and possibly stimulates spontaneous thrombosis.[62-64] Carbon monoxide, as compared to oxygen, has a markedly increased affinity for hemoglobin. The resulting carboxyhemoglobin compound thus reduces the oxygen-carrying capacity of hemoglobin. Nicotine and carbon monoxide together then could trigger a cardiac arrest in a patient with preexisting coronary disease by increasing the myocardial oxygen demand and reducing oxygen delivery. These factors probably account for the strong association between sudden cardiac death and cigarette smoking.

Cigarette smoking because of nicotine is addictive, and has all the characteristics and qualities of drug dependence.[58] Nicotine alters mood, causing pleasurable effects. Like most addictive drugs, tolerance develops so that diminished response occurs with repeated use of the drug. For similar effects from cigarettes, increased doses of nicotine must be absorbed. Since nicotine causes physical dependence, cessation of cigarette smoking is accompanied by a withdrawal syndrome. Restlessness, irritability, difficulty concentrating, increased appetite, increased food intake, and weight gain are withdrawal symptoms reported by exsmokers. The pharmacologic and behavioral characteristics of tobacco addiction are similar to addictions produced by heroin and cocaine. However, tobacco dependence can be treated successfully either with behavioral approaches alone, or behavioral approaches with adjunctive pharmacologic treatment.

Cessation of Smoking

A decrease in the percentage of men and women who smoke, as well as the more recent decrease in the annual per capita consumption of cigarettes, have been reported. It is suggested that a decrease in smoking reduces the incidence of cardiovascular disease.[10,65] The degree of this reduction depends on the amount smoked, the duration of smoking, and the age of cessation. In a massive study of the smoking habits of 34000 British physicians followed for over 20 years, a reduction of ischemic heart disease was noted in men 30 to 40 years old at the time they stopped smoking.[66] The reduction in heart disease in men who stopped smoking at the age of 55 was less impressive; no reduction was reported in men over 65 who stopped smoking. In the same study, physicians who stopped smoking before the age of 30, with an average smoking history of seven years, had the same mortality as physicians who never smoked.

Smoking clearly is pivotal in the development of vascular disease. For the vascular surgeon, the smoking habit has other implications. It interferes with the conservative treatment of claudication and reduces patency of lower extremity bypass grafts. As the primary physician treating vascular disease, the vascular surgeon must appreciate the addictive properties of cigarette smoke. Effective approaches toward this dependency should be part of his or her armamentarium.

References

1. Pearl R: Tobacco smoking and longevity. *Science* 87: 216, 1938.
2. US Public Health Service: *Smoking and health: report of the advisory committee to the surgeon general of the public health service* (PHS publication, No. 1103). Department of Health, Education and Welfare, Public Health Service, Center for Disease Control, Atlanta, GA 1964.
3. Kannel WB: Update on the role of cigarette smoking in coronary artery disease. *Am Heart J* 101:319, 1981.
4. Fielding JE: Smoking health effects and control. *N Engl J Med* 313:491, 1985.
5. US Public Health Service: *The Surgeon General's 1989 report on reducing the health consequence of smoking: 25 years of progress.* Department of Health and Human Services, Center for Disease Control, Atlanta, GA MMWR 1989:38 (suppl No. S-2).
6. Pierce JP, Fiore MC, Novotny TE, et al: Trends in cigarette smoking in the United States: projection to the year 2000. *JAMA* 261:61, 1989.
7. Friedman GD, Dales LG, Ury HK: Mortality in middle-aged smokers and nonsmokers. *N Engl J Med* 300:213, 1979.
8. Doll R, Hill AB: Mortality in relation to smoking: ten years observations of British doctors. *Br Med J* 1:1339, 1964.
9. Hammond EC: Smoking in relation to the death rate of one million men and women. *Natl Cancer Inst Managr* 19:127, 1966.
10. Kahn HA: The Dorn study of smoking and mortality among US veterans: report of eight and one-half years of observations. *Natl Cancer Inst Managr* 19:1, 1966.
11. Warner KE: The economics of smoking: dollars and sense. *NY State J Med* 83:1273, 1983.
12. *The health consequences of smoking: cardiovascular disease. A report of the Surgeon General.* Department of Health and Human Services, Rockville, MD, 1983.
13. The Pooling Project Research Group: Relationship of blood pressure, serum cholesterol, smoking habit, relative weight, and ECG abnormalities to incidence of major coronary events: final report of the pooling project. *J Chronic Dis* 31:201, 1978.
14. Dawber TR: *The Epidemiology of Atherosclerotic Disease: The Framingham Study.* Cambridge, MA: Harvard University Press, 1980.
15. Vliestra RE, Kronmal RA, Oberman A, et al: Effect of cigarette smoking on survival of patients with angiographically documented coronary artery disease. *JAMA* 255:1023, 1986.
16. Abbott RD, Yin Yin MA, Reed DM, et al: Risk of stroke in male cigarette smokers. *N Engl J Med* 315:717, 1986.
17. Ingall TJ, Homer D, Baker HL Jr, et al: Prediction of intracranial carotid artery atherosclerosis. *Arch Neurol* 48:687, 1991.
18. Tell GS, Howard G, McKinney WM, et al: Cigarette smoking cessation and extracranial carotid atherosclerosis. *JAMA* 261:1178, 1989.
19. Kannel WB, Shurtleff D: Cigarettes and the development of intermittent claudication: the Framingham Study. *Geriatrics* 28:61, 1973.
20. Menzoian JO, La Morte WW, Paniszyn CS, et al: Symptomatology and anatomic patterns of peripheral vascular disease: differing impact of smoking and diabetes. *Ann Vasc Surg* 3:224, 1989.
21. Tomatis LA, Fierens EE, Verbrugge GP: Evaluation of surgical risk in peripheral vascular disease by coronary artriography, a series of 100 cases. *Surgery* 71:429, 1972.
22. Juergens JL, Barker NW, Hines EA Jr: Arteriosclerosis obliterans: review of 520 cases with special reference to pathogenic and prognostic factors. *Circulation* 21:188, 1960.
23. Meyers KA, King RB, Scott DF, et al: The effect of smoking on the late patency of arterial reconstructions in the legs. *Br J Surg* 65:267, 1978.
24. Eneroth M, Persson BM: Risk factors for failed healing in amputation for vascular disease. *Acta Orthop Scan* 64(3):369, 1993.

25. A Report of the Surgeon General: *The health consequences of smoking for women.* Department of Health and Human Services, Rockville, Maryland, 1980.

26. Shapiro S, Rosenberg L, Slone D, et al: Oral contraceptive use in relation to myocardial infarction. *Lancet* 1: 743, 1979.

27. Mann JI, Doll R, Thorogood DM, et al: Risk factors for myocardial infarction in young women. *Br J Prevent Soc Med* 30:94, 1976.

28. Petitti DB, Wingerd J: Use of oral contraceptives, cigarette smoking, and risk of subarachnoid hemorrhage. *Lancet* 2:234, 1978.

29. Kleinman JC, Feldman JJ, Monk MA: Trends in smoking and ischemic heart disease mortality: recent trends of major coronary risk factors and CHD mortality in the USA and other industrialized countries. In: Kleiman JC, Feldman JJ, Monk MA (eds). *Proceedings of a NHLBl Conference on the Decline in CHD Mortality.* US Department of Health, Education, and Welfare, NIH Public No. 79–1610, 1979.

30. Seppanen A: Smoking in a closed space and its effect on carboxy-haemoglobin saturation of smoking and non-smoking subjects. *Ann Clin Res* 9:281, 1977.

31. Frishman WH: Involuntary smoking: cardiovascular effects of smoke on non-smokers. *Cardiovasc Med* 4:289, 1979.

32. Aronow WS: Effect of passive smoking on angina pectoris. *N Engl J Med* 299:21, 1978.

33. Lee PN, Garfinkel L: Mortality and type of cigarette smoked. *J Epidemiol Comm Health* 35:16, 1981.

34. Castelli WP, Dawber TR, Feileib M, et al: The filter cigarette and coronary heart disease: the Framingham Study. *Lancet* 2:109, 1981.

35. Wald N, Idle M, Smith PG, et al: Carboxyhemoglobin levels in smokers of filter and plain cigarettes. *Lancet* 1: 110, 1977.

36. Hoffmann D, Adams J, Haley NJ: Reported cigarette smoke values: a closer look. *Am J Pub Health* 73:1050, 1983.

37. Rickert WS, Robin JC, Young JC, et al: A comparison of the yields of nicotine and carbon monoxide of thirty-six brands of Canadian cigarettes tested under three conditions. *Prev Med* 12:682, 1983.

38. Asmussen I, Kjeldsen K: Intimal ultrastructure from newborn children of smoking and non-smoking mothers. *Circ Res* 36:577, 1975.

39. Bylork A, Bondjers G, Jansson I, et al: Surface ultrastructure of human arteries with special reference to the effects of smoking. *Acta Path Microbiol Scand* Sect A. 87:201, 1979.

40. Wolf N, Wilson-Holt N: Cigarette smoking and atherosclerosis. In: Greenhalgh RM (ed). *Smoking and Arterial Disease.* Barth, England: Pitman Medical

41. Pitillo RM, Mackie IJ, Rowles PM, et al: Effects of cigarette smoking on the ultrastructure of rat: thoracic aorta and its ability to produce prostacyclin. *Thromb Haemostas* 48:173, 1982.

42. Boayse FM, Osikowicz G, Quarfoot AJ: Effects of chronic oral consumption of nicotine on the rabbit aortic endothelium. *Am J Pathol* 102:229, 1981.

43. Kjeldsen K, Astrup P, Wanstrup J: Ultrastructural intimal changes in the rabbit aorta after a moderate carbon monoxide exposure. *Atherosclerosis* 16:67, 1972.

44. Zilla P, Sudler S, Fasal R, et al: Reduced reproductive capacity of freshly harvested endothelial cells in smok-

ers: a possible shortcoming in the success of seeding? *J Vasc Surg* 10:143, 1989.

45. Celermajer DS, Sorensen DE, Georgakopoulos D, et al: Cigarette smoking is associated with closely related and potentially reversible impairment of endothelium-dependent dilatation in healthy young adults. *Circulation* 88: 2149, 1993.

46. Higman DJ, Greenhalgh RM, Powell JT: Smoking impairs endothelium-dependent relaxation of saphenous vein. *Br J Surg* 80:1242, 1993.

47. Olsson AG, Molgaard J: Relations between smoking, food intake, and plasma lipoproteins. In: Diana JN (ed). *Tobacco Smoking and Atherosclerosis.* New York: Plenum Press; 1990.

48. Moffatt RJ: Normalization of high density lipoprotein cholesterol following cessation from cigarette smoking. tobacco smoking and atherosclerosis. In: Diana JN (ed). *Tobacco Smoking and Atherosclerosis.* New York: Plenum Press; 1990.

49. Kannel WB: Cigarettes, coronary occlusion, and myocardial infarction. *JAMA* 246:871, 1981.

50. DeWood MA, Spores J, Notske R: Prevalence of total coronary occlusion during the early hours of transmural myocardial infarction. *N Engl J Med* 303:897, 1980.

51. Fuster V, Cohen M, Halpern J: Aspirin in the prevention of coronary disease. *N Engl J Med* 321:183, 1989.

52. Levine P: An acute effect of cigarette smoking on platelet function. *Circulation* 48:619, 1973.

53. Gugnani G, Gamba G, Ascair E: Cigarette smoking effect on platelet function. *Thromb Haemostas* 37:442, 1977.

54. Rinaud S, Blacke D, Dumont E, et al: Platelet function after cigarette smoking in relation to nicotine and carbon monoxide. *Clin Pharmacol Ther* 36:389, 1984.

55. Ernst E, Hammerschmidt DE, Bagge U, et al: Leukocytes and the risk of ischaemic disease. *JAMA* 257:2318, 1987.

56. Friedman GD, Klotsky AL, Siegilab AB: The leukocyte count as a predictor of myocardial infarction. *N Engl J Med* 290:1275, 1970.

57. Zalokar JB, Richard JL, Claude JR: Leukocyte count, smoking, and myocardial infarction. *N Engl J Med* 304: 465, 1981.

58. US Public Health Service: *The Health Consequence of Smoking and Nicotine Addiction: A Report of the Surgeon General.* US Department of Health and Human Services. Rockville, MD; 1988.

59. Tachmes L, Fernandez RJ, Sadmer MA: Hemodynamic effects of smoking cigarettes of high and low nicotine content. *Chest* 74:243, 1978.

60. Aronowy WS, Dendinger J, Rokaw SN: Heart rate and carbon monoxide level after smoking high, low, and non-nicotine cigarettes. *Ann Int Med* 74:697, 1971.

61. Ball K, Turner R: Smoking and the heart: the basis for action. *Lancet* ii:822, 1974.

62. Rogers RL, Meyer JS, Shaw TG, et al: Cigarette smoking decreases cerebral blood suggesting increased risk for stroke. *JAMA* 250:2796, 1983.

63. Rogers RL, Meyer JS, Judd BW, et al: Abstention from cigarette smoking improves cerebral blood flow among elderly chronic smokers. *JAMA* 253:2970, 1985.

64. Hawkins RI: Smoking, platelets, and thrombosis. *Nature* 236:450, 1972.

65. Gordon T, Kannel WB, McGee D, et al: Death and coronary attack in men after giving up cigarette smoking: a report from the Framingham Study. *Lancet* 2:1345, 1974.

66. Doll R, Peto R: Mortality in relation to smoking: 20 years of observations on male British doctors. *Br Med J* 2: 1525, 1976.

CHAPTER 20

Coagulation and Disorders of Hemostasis

Thomas W. Wakefield, MD

Basic Mechanisms of Coagulation

The initiating events in hemostasis involve collagen and tissue factor (Figure 1). Tissue factor is released from injured cells activating the extrinsic pathway of coagulation, while disruption of the endothelium of blood vessels exposes the underlying collagen to platelets, activating these elements. In the blood, tissue factor complexes with activated factor VII (VIIa), activating factors IX and X to factors IXa and Xa (activated factors IX and X). The tissue factor-factor VII complex may also have low coagulant activity on its own.[1] The enzyme responsible for the initial activation of factor VII is unknown. However, factors Xa and VIIa both catalyze activation of factor VII, so there is a possible potential amplification for the formation of factor VIIa.[2] At the same time, activated platelets change shape, with their procoagulant phospholipid (termed platelet factor 3 [PF-3]) buried on the inner side of the surface membrane, spreading to allow for the externalization of PF-3 activity. This allows for the coagulation cascade proteins to assemble on the surface of platelets, accelerating the coagulation reactions (Figure 2).[3] Platelet membranes contribute to critical surfaces for coagulation assembly. Activated, but not resting, platelets express binding sites for coagulation factors and during platelet activation in vitro, microparticles are released from the platelet rich in receptors for factors Va and VIIIa.[4,5] von Willebrand factor (vWF) plays an important role in platelet adhesion through binding to glycoprotein (Gp) Ib,[6] while fibrinogen forms a bridge between activated platelets by binding to GpIIb/IIIa on adjacent stimulated platelets[7]; unstimulated platelets attach to immobilized fibrinogen by the same receptor.[8]

Once the platelet plug has formed, the stage is set for the coagulation proteins to assemble. Activated factor X (Xa), activated factor V (Va), ionized calcium, and factor II (prothrombin) assemble on the platelet phospholipid surface to form the prothrombinase complex, which catalyzes the formation of thrombin faster than can be achieved with activated factor X alone (Figure 3).[3] When the amount of tissue factor is limited, activation of factor IX, rather than factor X, is favored.[9,10] This allows for tissue factor activation in situations of low tissue factor concentration. The pathway so described up to this point corresponds to the extrinsic pathway. The formation of thrombin is central to all of coagulation. Among the many functions of thrombin, two small peptides from fibrinogen are removed, fibrinopeptide A (FPA) from the alpha-chain and fibrinopeptide B (FPB) from the beta-chain.[11] This cleavage leads to the release of four fibrinopeptides and new fibrin monomers. These monomers then cross-link with each other, leading to fibrin polymerization. Thrombin also activates factor XIII to factor XIIIa which then catalyzes the cross-linking of fibrin to make the clot firm,[12] activates platelets increasing platelet aggregation, and activates factors V and factors VIII, two nonenzymatic cofactors, to Va and VIIIa.[3] Factor XIIIa also cross-links other plasma proteins such as fibronectin and α_2-antitrypsin to the

From *The Basic Science of Vascular Disease*. Edited by Sidawy AN, Sumpio BE, and DePalma RG. Armonk, NY: Futura Publishing Company, Inc.; © 1997.

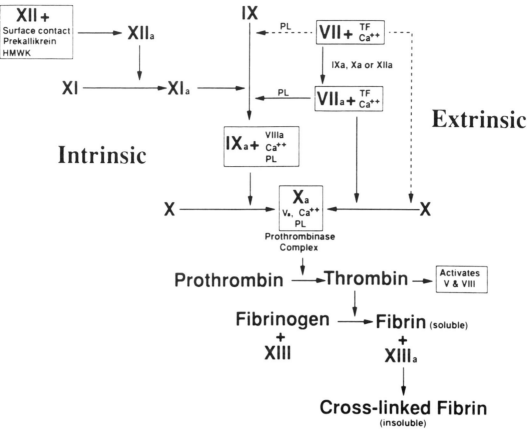

Figure 1. Extrinsic/intrinsic pathways of coagulation. (Reproduced with permission from Hoch JR, Silver D: Hemostasis and thrombosis. In: Moore WS (ed). *Vascular Surgery: A Comprehensive Review*. Philadelphia: WB Saunders, Co.; 66, 1991.)

alpha-chains of fibrin, resulting in their incorporation into clot.[13]

The intrinsic pathway of blood coagulation requires activation of factor XI to factor XIa. This activation may occur by both the contact activation system through activation of factor XII, plasma prekallikrein, and high-molecular weight kininogen, and through the presence of thrombin with negatively-charged surfaces.[14] Factor XIa will activate factor XI in an autocatalytic nature,[14] and also catalyze the conversion of factor IX to factor IXa.[15] Factor IXa, X, ionized calcium, and thrombin activated factor VIII (VIIIa) then assemble on the platelet surface (the Xase complex) to catalyze the activation of factor X to activated factor X (Xa, Figure 3).[3] Factor Xa then enters into the prothrombinase complex for further amplification of thrombin formation. Activated factor VIII (VIIIa), and not nonenzymatic cofactor VIII, plays a major role in this amplification process as does activated factor V (Va) and not nonenzymatic cofactor V in the prothrombinase complex. Since thrombin generation activates both nonenzymatic cofactors V and VIII to activated V (Va) and VIII (VIIIa) through minor proteolysis, thrombin mediates its own generation.[3] The impor-

tance of a mechanism of factor XI activation, independent of the contact activation system, is significant as patients deficient in factor XI bleed, while patients deficient in factor XII, prekallikren, and high-molecular weight kininogen (contact activation system) do not usually bleed.[13]

Natural Anticoagulant Mechanisms

At the same time that thrombin formation proceeds, the body has natural mechanisms which oppose further thrombin formation. Since thrombin generation is the key element in coagulation, antithrombin III is the most central of the natural anticoagulant proteins. This is a glycoprotein of approximately MW 70000 which binds to thrombin, preventing the removal of FPA and FPB from fibrinogen,[16] preventing the activation of factors V and VIII to Va and VIIIa, and inhibiting its activation and aggregation of platelets. In addition, antithrombin III inhibits factors IXa,[17] Xa, and XIa.[18] Another natural anticoagulant is activated protein C (APC [protein Ca]) which inactivates factors Va[19,20] and VIIIa.[21] This inactivation reduces the abil-

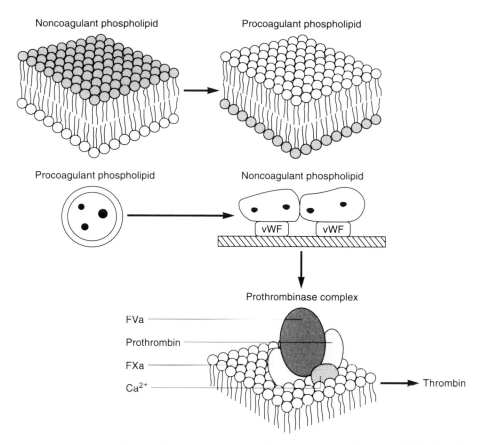

Figure 2. Formation of coagulation cascade assembly on the platelet phospholipid surface. (Reproduced with permission from Wakefield TW: Hemostasis. In: Greenfield LJ, Mulholland MW, Oldham KT, Zelenock GB (eds). *Surgery: Scientific Principles and Practice.* Philadelphia: JB Lippincott; 103, 1993; and modified with permission from Hassouna HI: Laboratory evaluation of hemostatic disorders. In: Penner JA, Hassouna HI, (eds). *Coagulation Disorders II.* Hematology/Oncology Clinics of North America; 1188, 1993.)

ity of the Xase complex and prothrombinase complex to accelerate the rate of thrombin formation. A central role of thrombin for protein C activation is also evident. In the circulation, protein C is activated to protein Ca on endothelial cell surfaces by thrombin complexed with one of its receptors, thrombomodulin,[22–24] (Figure 4) in a one-to-one complex.[25] The formation of this thrombin-thrombomodulin complex greatly speeds the activation of protein C as compared to thrombin alone. Thrombin at the same time, by its binding to thrombomodulin, loses its platelet-activating activity,[26] as well as its enzymatic activity for fibrinogen and factor V.[27] Protein S is a cofactor for protein Ca.[28] A third natural anticoagulant is heparin cofactor II.[29] Its concentration in plasma is estimated to be significantly lower than antithrombin III, and its action is implicated primarily in the regulation of thrombin formation in extravascular tissues. Finally, as appropriate for thrombin in its central role in coagulation, thrombin is inactivated by becoming incorporated into the clot itself.

The extrinsic pathway is short-lived, due to the presence of an inhibitor known as lipoprotein-associated coagulation inhibitor (LACI),[30] or extrinsic pathway inhibitor (EPI).[31] This protein inactivates the tissue factor-factor VIIa complex activation of factor X to factor Xa, but not of factor IX to factor IXa,[13] thus shifting much of the coagulation cascade from the extrinsic to the intrinsic system. This inhibitor has also been termed *tissue factor pathway inhibitor.*

During the process of thrombus formation, there is a constant process of clot lysis which prevents thrombus formation from leading to massive intravascular thrombosis. Plasminogen, tissue plasminogen activator (tPA), and alpha-2-antiplasmin (α_2-AP) are incorporated into the fibrin clot as it forms (Figure 5).[3] In fact, thrombin (both alpha and gamma) promotes the release of tPA from endothelial cells, as well as induces the production of plasminogen activator inhibitor (PAI-1) from endothelial cells.[32,33] tPA catalyzes the conversion of plasminogen to plasmin, the main fibrinolytic enzyme in the body. This is a serine protease whose main substrates include not only fibrin and fibrinogen, but other factors of the coagulation path-

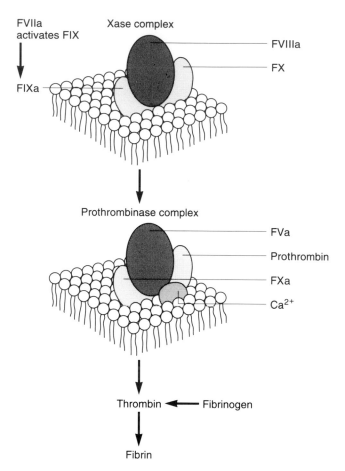

Figure 3. Formation of the Xase complex and prothrombinase complex with amplification of thrombin and fibrin formation. (Reproduced with permission from Wakefield TW: Hemostasis. In: Greenfield LJ, Mulholland MW, Oldham KT, Zelenock GB (eds). *Surgery: Scientific Principles and Practice*. Philadelphia: JB Lippincott; 104, 1993; and modified with permission from Hassouna HI: Laboratory evaluation of hemostatic disorders. In: Penner JA, Hassouna HI (eds). *Coagulation Disorders II*. Hematology/Oncology Clinics of North America; 1177, 1993.)

way. Plasmin also interferes with the adhesion function of vWF by proteolysis of Gp Ib.[34] Fibrin, when digested by plasmin, yields one molecule of fragment E and two molecules of fragment D. In physiologic clot formation, fragment D is released in dimeric form (D-dimer).[3] The D-dimer fragment is a marker for ongoing thrombosis and fibrinolysis of formed thrombus. The natural inhibitor of excess plasmin is α_2-AP, also secreted by endothelial cells. In physiologic fibrinolysis, these substances are bound to fibrin, and plasmin is readily inactivated. However, in fibrinolytic states and during treatment with fibrinolytic agents (termed *fibrinogenolysis*), circulating fibrinogen in addition to clot-bound fibrin is digested by circulating plasmin which is not readily inactivated by α_2-AP. Circulating fibrinogen is digested by removal of FPB and the carboxyl terminal portion of the alpha-chain yielding frag-

ment X which clots slowly.[35] This fragment is further degraded to one molecule of fragment D and a fragment Y, neither of which clot thrombin; further degradation results in two molecules of fragment D and one molecule of fragment E (Figure 6).[3] In these nonphysiologic fibrinolytic states, the fragments D are not cross-linked and little D-dimer is formed. The large fragments Y and D are potent inhibitors of fibrin formation.

The endothelial cell itself appears to have three

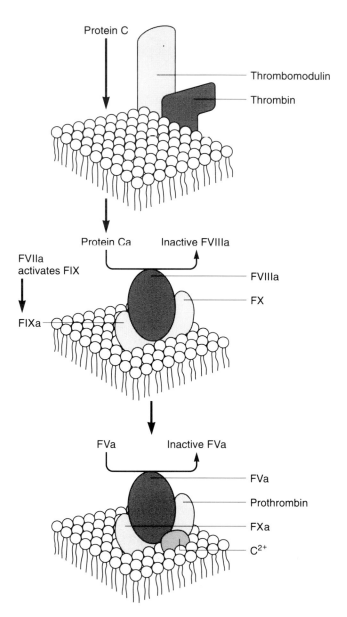

Figure 4. Activation of protein C by thrombin-thrombomodulin interaction. (Reproduced with permission from Wakefield TW: Hemostasis. In: Greenfield LJ, Mulholland MW, Oldham KT, Zelenock GB (eds). *Surgery: Scientific Principles and Practice*. Philadelphia: JB Lippincott; 104, 1993; and modified with permission from Hassouna HI: Laboratory evaluation of hemostatic disorders. In: Penner JA, Hassouna HI (eds). *Coagulation Disorders II*. Hematology/Oncology Clinics of North America; 1175, 1993.

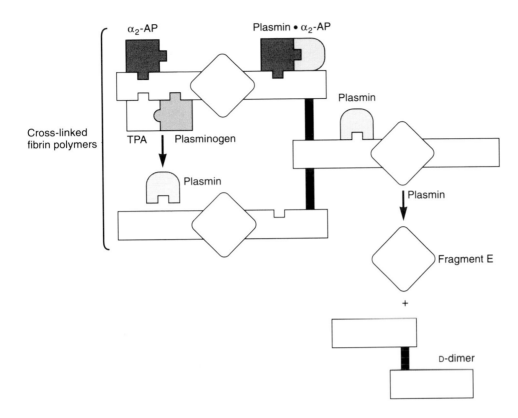

Figure 5. Incorporation of plasminogen, tissue plasminogen activator (tPA), and alpha-2-antiplasmin (α_2-AP) into the fibrin clot as it forms with production of D-dimer fragments. (Reproduced with permission from Wakefield TW: Hemostasis. In: Greenfield LJ, Mulholland MW, Oldham KT, Zelenock GB (eds). *Surgery: Scientific Principles and Practice*. Philadelphia: JB Lippincott; 105, 1993; and modified with permission from Hassouna HI: Laboratory evaluation of hemostatic disorders. In: Penner JA, Hassouna HI (eds). *Coagulation Disorders II*. Hematology/Oncology Clinics of North America; 1186, 1993.)

systems for the promotion of a nonthrombotic surface including thrombin-thrombomodulin interaction, heparin-antithrombin III binding, and a recently described membrane-bound fibrinolytic system. Circulating plasminogen exits in an N-terminal glutamic acid form (Glu-Plg). On the endothelial cell surface, Glu-Plg is converted to its N-terminal lysine form (Lys-Plg) by plasmin, which is generated locally through the natural tPA elaborated by endothelial cells.[36] Local cell concentrations of tPA may be great enough to saturate high-affinity receptors, elaborate small amounts of plasmin, and promote conversion of Glu-Plg to Lys-Plg. Lys-Plg is then converted to plasmin with improved catalytic efficiency, resulting in a local fibrinolytic response.

The major categories of plasminogen activators include exogenous such as streptokinase, endogenous such as tPA and urokinase, and intrinsic factors.[3] These intrinsic factors include factor XII, prekallikrein, and high-molecular weight kininogen which appear more important in their function of clot lysis than thrombus formation. Activated forms of factor XII, kallikrein, and factor XI independently can convert plasminogen to plasmin.[37] These enzymes also have the ability to liberate bradykinin from high-molecular weight kininogen; this liberation causes increased vascular permeability, prostacyclin liberation, and tPA secretion. Finally, APC (factor Ca) has been found to proteolytically inactivate tPA inhibitor, thus promoting tPA activity and fibrinolysis.[25]

In summary, coagulation is an ongoing process of thrombus formation and thrombus dissolution, with activation complexes speeding the process. The central mediator of coagulation is thrombin.[3] Abnormalities in coagulation occur when one process, either thrombus formation, thrombus inhibition, or fibrinolysis, overcomes the others and becomes dominant in the normal delicate balance that is hemostasis.

Thrombosis and Inflammation

Thrombosis and inflammation are closely linked. Tumor necrosis factor (TNF), a polypeptide cytokine of stimulated macrophages released in response to inflammation and sepsis, down-regulates thrombomodulin expression. This is likely through endocytosis and degradation of thrombomodulin, leading to a hypercoagulable state.[38] TNF increases the level of C4b-binding protein, thus decreasing the amount of free protein S available to function as a cofactor for protein C. Additionally, TNF induces the expression of tissue factor on the surface of vascular endothelium. In a recent study from the Netherlands of six normal human volunteers given TNF, factor X was activated to factor Xa early after administration, followed by the activation of prothrombin in a more gradual and prolonged pattern of increase noted hours after maximal concentrations of factor Xa had been reached.[39] TNF also inhibits the fibrinolytic system by suppressing the re-

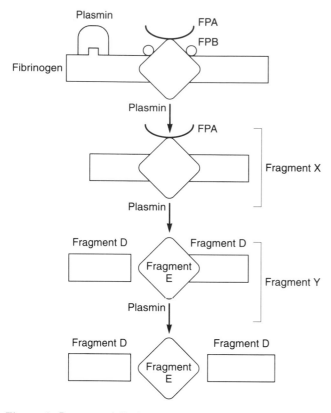

Figure 6. Process of fibrinogenolysis and formation of non-cross-linked fragments D. (Reproduced with permission from Wakefield TW. Hemostasis. In: Greenfield LJ, Mulholland MW, Oldham KT, Zelenock GB (eds). *Surgery: Scientific Principles and Practice*. Philadelphia: JB Lippincott; 106, 1993; and modified with permission from Hassouna HI: Laboratory evaluation of hemostatic disorders. In: Penner JA, Hassouna HI (eds). *Coagulation Disorders II*. Hematology/Oncology Clinics of North America; 1193, 1993.)

lease of tPA and inducing the expression of PAI-1.[40–45] In vivo, TNF initially causes an increase in overall plasma plasminogen activator activity followed by an even greater rise in PAI-1 antigen, leading to an inhibition of the fibrinolytic system.[46] Additionally, by down-regulating thrombomodulin, TNF decreases the production of protein C which normally inhibits PAI, also decreasing the fibrinolytic potential of the blood. Along with its effects on coagulation, TNF is in a unique position to facilitate the production of an inflammatory response. TNF and other cytokines stimulate adherence proteins on endothelial cells[47–50] for leukocytes, and induce endothelial and vascular wall smooth muscle cell (SMC) production of interleukin-8 (IL-8) gene expression and monocyte chemotactic protein-1 (MCP-1) mRNA expression[51] among others. These latter cytokines activate neutrophils in vitro and induce neutrophil movement in vivo (IL-8) along with monocyte movement (MCP-1). They are also involved in the process of cytokine networking, in which one cytokine activates other cytokines to produce a physio-

logic response. Clearly, the association between TNF and activation of the coagulation and inflammatory pathways has been firmly established.

A model for the possible interactions between the thrombotic episode and the inflammatory response has been proposed (Figure 7).[52] In this model, vascular injury causes circulating platelets to marginate along the vessel wall, probably mediated by vWF. The platelets then activate and aggregate in an interaction mediated by fibrinogen, leading to platelet plug formation. Blood clotting is stimulated by the expression of tissue factor, and the clotting complexes are propagated on the phospholipid surfaces of activated platelets as described earlier. These coagulation complexes result in the formation of a fibrin clot. Circulating neutrophils and monocytes then interact with the platelets through P-selectin and with the endothelial cells through P-selectin and E-selectin, events that lead to the stable interaction of white blood cells and platelets at the thrombus-wall interface. Neutrophils and monocytes, thus, participate in the local inflammatory response, and monocytes may contribute to clot formation by further tissue factor expression on their surface. This has been suggested in a recent study of fibrin formation under the influence of a monoclonal antibody to P-selectin.[53]

In the venous circulation, a series of steps linking thrombosis and inflammation has been suggested.[54] In step 1, thrombus formation with platelets and neutrophils is initiated at venous confluences, saccules, and valve pockets. In step 2, adherent neutrophils and platelets are activated, releasing substances such as ADP (platelets) and neutrophil-activating peptide-2 (NAP-2, platelets and neutrophils) that activate and attract more platelets and neutrophils. Catepsin G, secreted from activated neutrophils, is capable of converting B-thromboglobulin (BTG, secreted from platelets) into NAP-2 by proteolytic cleavage.[55] This NAP-2 can stimulate more catepsin G secretion which, in turn, can stimulate more platelet secretion,[56,57] providing more substrate for NAP-2 and causing a feedback activation for the recruitment of more platelets and neutrophils. In step 3, coagulation is initiated and promoted on the phospholipid surface the platelets provide. Finally, in step 4, new layers of neutrophils and platelets form on the surface of fibrin, activate, and begin another new round of the clotting process. In a baboon model of deep vein thrombosis (DVT) induced by stasis, the presence of a venous catheter for a short period of time, and the administration of the thrombogenic reagents TNF and antibody to protein C (HPC$_4$), it has been noted by direct protein ELISA measurements and immunohistochemical tissue staining the presence of inflammatory cytokines in the vein wall directly beneath the luminal thrombus, especially when the thrombus was practically occlusive, including IL-8, IL-6, MCP-1, ENA, and MIP-1a.[58] In a simi-

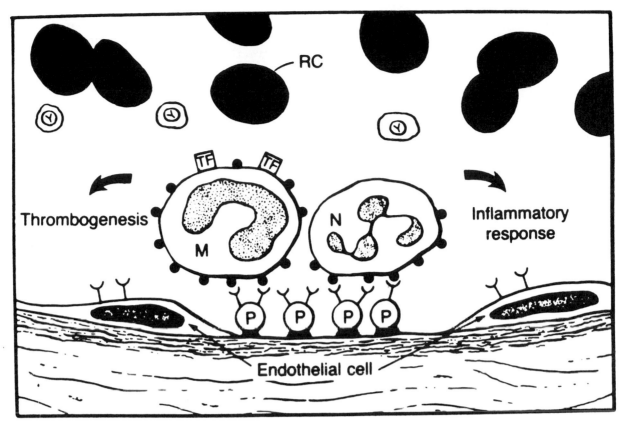

Figure 7. Cellular basis for blood coagulation: platelets (**P**), neutrophils (**N**), monocytes (**M**), P-selectin (**Y**), red blood cells (**RC**). (Reproduced with permission from Reference 52.)

lar fashion in a model of stasis-induced thrombosis in the rat, an initial infiltration of neutrophils into the vein wall early after thrombosis, followed by monocytes/macrophages and lymphocytes in a typical pattern of acute to chronic inflammation, has also been found.[59] This suggests that the proposed sequence may lead to a full-blown inflammatory response in the vein wall. An exciting area for further research will involve the determination of the ability to interfere with the inflammatory response and the subsequent effect this interference may have on the detrimental interactions between the thrombus and the vein wall and valves, the organization and maturation of the thrombus, and the propagation of the thrombotic process once the clot has formed. Approaches to interfere with the inflammatory response include blocking initial white blood cell adhesion, subsequent activation, or a combination of both initial adhesion and subsequent activation.

Hypercoagulable States

There are a number of conditions that can lead to a hypercoagulable state including heparin-associated thrombocytopenia, antithrombin III deficiency, protein C and S deficiency, resistance to APC, dysfibrino-

genemia, lupus anticoagulant and the presence of antiphospholipid antibodies, abnormalities of fibrinolysis, hyperhomocyteinemia, elevated lipoprotein a, malignancy, pregnancy, myeloproliferative syndromes, and paroxysmal nocturnal hemoglobinuria. The most important of these conditions will be discussed.

Heparin-associated thrombocytopenia occurs in 0.6% to 30% of patients who receive heparin, although severe thrombocytopenia (platelet counts less than 100000 mm³) is seen in fewer than 10% of patients treated with heparin.[60] It is caused by a plasma factor, most likely a heparin-dependent platelet antibody that causes platelet aggregation when exposed to heparin. Activation of platelets in this setting results in thrombocytopenia, thrombosis, and embolic episodes which can lead to death. Morbidity and mortality rates as high as 61% and 23% have been noted.[61] Both bovine and porcine heparin have been associated with this syndrome, although bovine heparin seems to be more frequently associated. The syndrome usually begins 5 to 15 days after heparin therapy begins, although it may begin earlier if the patient has been exposed to heparin in the past. Arterial and venous thromboses have all been noted in this syndrome and are more likely to occur in diseased or traumatized vessels. Even minimal exposure, as with heparin coating on pulmonary artery catheters, has been reported to lead to this condition.

Heparin-associated thrombocytopenia should be suspected in a patient when thrombosis occurs while receiving heparin. Suspicion of this diagnosis includes a fall in platelet count to less than 100000/mm^3, or evidence of recurrent or unexplained thrombosis while receiving heparin. The laboratory diagnosis is made by demonstrating 20% or greater platelet aggregation within 15 minutes or 6% ^{14}C serotonin release within 45 minutes when heparin is added to a mixture of donor platelets and the patient's own platelet-poor plasma. If the patient's platelet count is >100000/mm^3, the patient's own platelet-rich plasma may be used. If the platelet count is <100000/mm^3, alternative platelet-rich plasma from another patient not treated with antiplatelet agents must be used. Other coagulation parameters are usually normal in these patients. Treatment consists of cautious administration of protamine for heparin reversal if active thrombosis has occurred, or stoppage of heparin, allowing its effects to wear off followed by use of another anticoagulant such as dextran sulfate while beginning coumadin therapy. Aspirin has been used with limited success, while iloprost, a prostacyclin analog, has been found useful in management of these patients[62] (although it is not available at this time for compassionate use due to its potential for causing extreme vasodilatation and hypotension). Other possible anticoagulants that have been suggested include ancrod, hirudin, and low-molecular weight heparins.

Antithrombin III deficiency accounts for approximately 2% of venous thrombotic events, although this deficiency has been described in pulmonary embolism, mesenteric venous thrombosis, lower extremity venous thrombosis, arterial thrombosis, and dialysis fistula failure. Antithrombin III deficiency was first noted to be associated with arterial thrombosis in 1981 with four cases of thrombosis after arterial reconstruction and two cases of spontaneous arterial thrombosis,[63] although DVT is much more common in this disorder. Antithrombin III is a serine protease inhibitor of thrombin and factors Xa, IXa, and XIa. This protein, present in normal plasma, is an alpha-2-globulin with a half-life of 2.8 days. As one of the main actions of heparin is to potentiate the anticoagulant effects of antithrombin III by changing its shape, a patient with this deficiency usually presents with thrombosis while on heparin, or shows an inability to become adequately anticoagulated with heparin. This deficiency may be either congenital or acquired. Most cases become apparent between 10 and 35 years of age, and by age 50, 85% of patients will have suffered at least one thrombotic event, usually in the venous circulation. Homozygous individuals usually die in infancy, while heterozygous individuals show a decreased plasma level,

usually less than approximately 70% to 85%. Acquired deficits occur with inadequate production as in liver disease, malignancy, nephrotic syndrome, disseminated intravascular coagulation, malnutrition, or increased protein catabolism.[64] There appears to be a clear temporal relationship between antithrombin III levels and protein metabolism. Additionally, a second less frequent condition exists in which patients make an abnormal defective antithrombin III with normal levels quantitatively, and a third less frequent condition in which there is an abnormal interaction between antithrombin III and heparin. Thrombotic episodes are often related to predisposing factors such as operations, childbirth, and infections, and recurrent episodes are common. The diagnosis is made by measuring antithrombin III levels, preferably with the patient off anticoagulants. Heparin has been shown to decrease antithrombin III levels, while coumadin will increase these levels. In addition, measuring the level during acute thrombotic events may be misleading, as the level of antithrombin III may be low due to thrombotic consumption. Once the diagnosis is established, fresh frozen plasma should be administered beginning with two units every 8 hours and decreasing over 72 hours to one unit every 12 hours, followed by long-term coumadin. Antithrombin III concentrates are now available and may be useful during situations when heparin use is necessary for a short period of time in patients with antithrombin III deficiency.

Protein C and S deficiencies are frequently described as causes of the hypercoagulable state. As mentioned above, protein Ca inactivates factors Va and VIIIa. Protein C is activated to protein Ca 20000 times faster than by thrombin alone through the interaction of thrombomodulin and thrombin on the endothelial cell surface.[65] In addition, protein C proteolytically inactivates the inhibitor to tissue plasminogen activator, thus increasing the natural fibrinolytic activity of plasma; protein S is a cofactor for protein C. Although the majority of reports describe venous thrombosis with deficiencies of protein C and S, noted in as many as 4% and 5% of young patients with venous thrombotic disorders, arterial thrombosis has recently been reported in these deficiency states; in young patients under 51 years of age requiring arterial revascularization, protein S deficiency was found in 20%, and protein C deficiency was noted in 15% of cases.[66] The half-life of protein C is approximately 6 hours, and deficiency can be either on a congenital or acquired basis. Likewise, deficiency of protein S (which also has a short half-life) may be either on a congenital or acquired basis. In the congenital conditions, those homozygous for protein C deficiency usually die in infancy from unrestricted clotting of the microvasculature (purpura fulminans), while those heterozygous have protein C levels less than 55% of normal. Levels between 55% and 65% are consistent with either heterozygous deficiency or the lower end of the distribution of normal values.[3] Both protein C antigen levels and protein C activity should be measured, while only protein S antigen levels are measured. The range for protein S levels is 70% to 100% of normal. Acquired deficiencies usually follow along with conditions that interfere with hepatic synthetic functions, as these factors are produced in the liver along with the other vitamin-K dependent factors. The onset of episodes of thrombosis, especially venous thrombotic events, is typically between 15 and 30 years of age. The treatment for patients with thrombotic events is lifelong coumadin therapy. Not all patients with these deficiencies will experience episodes of thrombosis, and low levels of either factor by itself in an asymptomatic patient are not an indication for anticoagulation. In a large population of blood donors, 0.3% have been found to have low protein C levels without any overt clinical thrombotic episodes, while many heterozygous family members of homozygous protein C-deficient infants are clinically unaffected.[67] It has been reported that protein C deficiency may also be associated with an abnormality in the protein C molecule itself, resulting in the generation of minimal enzymatic activity. Thus, qualitative abnormalities in the protein C system may also result in a hypercoagulable state in addition to the more typical quantitative abnormalities.

A dangerous paradox may occur with the administration of oral anticoagulants in patients with protein C and S deficiency. When oral anticoagulants are used, protein C levels often decline more rapidly than most of the other vitamin K-dependent liver factors which have half-lives of 5 to 7 days (II, IX, and X), thus rendering the patient receiving the coumadin hypercoagulable for a short period of time. This can result in coumadin-induced skin necrosis from clotting in the microcirculation from this hypercoagulable state.[68] The best way to avoid this devastating complication, which leads to full-thickness necrosis of the skin and subcutaneous tissues on fatty areas of the body (but has been seen over all parts of the body including the extremities), involves full anticoagulation with heparin, while beginning coumadin therapy until the vitamin-K-dependent liver factors have all reached low levels, or using very low doses of coumadin to initiate oral anticoagulation, thus protecting the patient from thrombosis.

Resistance to activated protein C involves a recently described syndrome that may explain up to 40% of patients who present with idiopathic DVT in which no other causes can be found.[69-71] The activated partial thromboplastin time (aPTT) is measured with the addition of APC and calcium chloride to the patient's serum and the result then compared to the same test without the presence of the APC. This defect has been found to be related to an abnormality of factor V and its expression has been found to be consistent with incomplete penetrance.[72] Treatment issues are not resolved at this time, although the general recommendation has been to use anticoagulants only after a thrombotic event.[73]

The lupus anticoagulant/antiphospholipid syndrome involves one of a number of antiphospholipid antibodies which may cause a hypercoagulable state, or be associated with liberated cellular phospholipid antigen from thrombosis (such as cardiolipin) and act as a marker for ongoing coagulation.[74] The antiphospholipid syndrome (APS) is defined by the presence of antiphospholipid antibody or the lupus anticoagulant, along with any or all of the following clinical events: recurrent thromboses, recurrent fetal losses, thrombocytopenia, and livedo reticularis. A prolonged activated partial thromboplastin time, not corrected by normal plasma in the face of other standard coagulation tests being normal, is considered to be indicative of this problem, in addition to a direct measurement of the antiphospholipid or anticardiolipin antibody. In fact, the abnormality in the aPTT is a laboratory artifact as phospholipid is added to the test system, and the antiphospholipid antibody and lupus anticoagulant IgG or IgM immunoglobulins are specifically directed against anionic phospholipid. Thrombosis-promoting antibodies are most often of the IgG isotype. In addition, the antiphospholipid antibody may cross-react with cardiolipin, the antigen used in blood screening for syphilis, producing a false-positive syphilis serology.

There is imperfect concordance among those tests used to identify the abnormality responsible for APS. Approximately 80% of patients with the lupus anticoagulant have a positive ELISA antiphospholipid antibody, but only 10% to 50% of patients with a positive ELISA antiphospholipid antibody have a lupus anticoagulant.[75] The antiphospholipid antibody measured by ELISA, and the lupus anticoagulant identified by coagulation tests, can be physically separated, and patients have been identified who have one without the other. Patients with both appear to have a similar prognosis as those with either alone. Possible mechanisms for the hypercoagulable state associated with the APS which have been proposed include inhibition of prostacyclin synthesis or release from endothelial cells, inhibition of protein C activation by the thrombin-thrombomodulin complex on the surface of endothelial cells, inhibition of plasminogen activator synthesis, or plasminogen activator release from endothelial or other cells, and direct activation of platelets. Although the lupus anticoagulant has been reported to exist in approximately 5% to 40% of patients with systemic lupus erythematosus (SLE), the condition can exist in patients without SLE, can be induced by medications, and can be seen in patients with cancer and certain infectious disorders. Current evidence suggests that the lupus anticoagulant is a better predictor of thrombotic events, while a high titer antiphospholipid antibody measured by ELISA (>40 units) is more sensitive for identifying pregnancies at risk for fetal loss. A low titer ELISA test (5 to 40 units) is a common, nonspecific finding of no clinical significance.[75]

Thrombosis may involve both the venous and the arterial circulation, especially the peripheral vessels of the extremities, although aortic occlusion has been reported in association with the lupus anticoagulant. Antibodies to phospholipids and cardiolipin have also been documented in the cerebral circulation of young stroke victims. Less common manifestations include livedo reticularis, pulmonary hypertension, vascular heart disease, labile hypertension, migraine headaches, chorea, the Guillain-Barre syndrome, positive Coombs test, lesions of the multiple sclerosis type, digital gangrene, coronary thrombosis, epilepsy, repeated strokes, and subacute lupus erythematosus. At least one third of patients with the lupus anticoagulant have a history of one or more thrombotic events, with 70% of these events in the venous circulation.[69] Arterial thrombosis can also occur with this abnormality and, in a recent study, 50% of 18 vascular procedures were associated with thrombosis in patients positive for antiphospholipid antibodies versus only 2 of 33 nonvascular procedures in this same group of patients.[76] In another series of 158 patients with peripheral vascular disease, including 27 with abdominal aortic aneurysms, 1 with renovascular hypertension, 28 with cerebrovascular insufficiency, 31 with aortoiliac occlusive disease, and 71 with infrainguinal occlusive disease, 137 patients underwent peripheral vascular surgical procedures.[77] Fifteen patients were identified with hypercoagulable states, including 5 with protein C and protein S deficiency, and 5 with a lupus-like anticoagulant. Of the patients undergoing 137 vascular procedures, 5 suffered from thrombosis within 30 days including 3/14 (21%) with either a lupus anticoagulant or heparin-associated thrombocytopenia, as opposed to only 2/123 (1.6%) with no hypercoagulable state identified (p<0.01). A particular problem reported with this syndrome has been the occurrence of recurrent spontaneous abortions associated with both the lupus anticoagulant and other antiphospholipid and anticardiolipin antibodies due to thrombosis of placental vessels. Approximately 10% of women with two or more unexplained fetal losses are found to have a positive antiphospholipid antibody. Treatment for thrombosis associated with APS includes heparin for the acute thrombotic event and long-term coumadin therapy. It is unfortunate that this entity has been misnamed as an anticoagulant, and it is important to realize that it is one of the entities associated with the hypercoagulable state.

Defective fibrinolytic activity is another cause of the hypercoagulable state. Plasminogen is a normal plasma protein consisting of a single polypeptide chain, molecular weight approximately 90000. It exists in 10 different forms. An abnormal plasminogen functional activity has been demonstrated in over 30 cases of spontaneous arterial or venous thromboses, and may affect 10% of the normal population, but only becomes clinically evident once a thrombotic-prone event occurs.[78] Once this diagnosis is made, treatment is long-term coumadin therapy. Fibrinogen itself, as a marker of disease states, has been found more useful as an indicator for the development of atherosclerosis in a number of studies than as a marker for a hypercoagulable state.[79]

Fibrinolytic activity of blood is derived from plasminogen activators which are produced in the endothelium of small blood vessels and are continuously presented to the bloodstream, including tPA in response to thrombin, histamine, and bradykinin, and the binding of thrombin to thrombomodulin on the surface of endothelial cells enhancing fibrinolysis by APC which inactivates PAI.[67,80] In addition, factors of the contact system of coagulation are intrinsic activators of plasminogen as indicated above. Defective fibrinolytic activity may be due to either a decreased content of plasminogen activators, their decreased release, or an increase in the level of their inhibitors. In a study of 100 patients with recurrent DVT or pulmonary embolism and no other known underlying disease, 67 were found to have normal tPA levels after a venous occlusion test, while 22 patients were found to have increased PAI in their serum and 11 had low activator levels.[81] It has been commonly observed that fibrinolytic activity is reduced postoperatively for a 7- to 10-day period, which may result from an altered relationship between tPA and its inhibitor. Recent studies have demonstrated that pneumatic-compression devices may exhibit their antithrombotic effects systemically through prevention of this fibrinolytic shut-down. Arterial graft thrombosis has also been associated with plasminogen deficiency. Major inhibitors of the fibrinolytic system include α_2-AP and PAI. As secretion of endothelial cell-derived tPA inhibitor is stimulated by thrombin, endotoxin, and IL-1, elevated levels of PAI have been found circulating during certain infections.[82] Also, TNF down-regulates the activity of protein C. Down-regulated protein C is less able to inactivate PAI, shifting the balance in the direction of thrombosis and linking the coagulation system with sepsis.

Abnormal platelet aggregation has been seen in two definite clinical situations separate from heparin-associated abnormal platelet aggregation. The first is advanced malignancy, especially of the lung and uterus, and the second is in the occasional patient who undergoes carotid endarterectomy and then experiences thrombosis of the endarterectomy site due to platelet activation and aggregation. Additionally, hyperreactive platelets have been associated with arterial graft thrombosis in patients undergoing peripheral vascular reconstructions.[66] However, platelet function may be more dependent on external factors, such as the circulating level of fibrinogen or the production of thrombin, rather than an intrinsic feature of the platelets themselves, suggesting that antiplatelet agents alone will be unlikely to totally eliminate a thrombogenic potential.[83]

Disseminated intravascular coagulation (DIC) is the primary form of acute thrombosis. Causes of this syndrome include abruptio placentae, gram-positive and gram-negative sepsis, endotoxemia, malignant tumors, pelvic operations, certain snake bites, hematologic malignancies, and hepatic failure.[3] Coagulation is activated by the release into the circulation of tissue factor which activates factor VII to VIIa, leading to massive thrombin production and fibrin generation. Fibrinolysis then becomes activated in turn, leading to bleeding in the later stages of the syndrome due to the consumption of clotting factors, depletion of fibrinogen, and unchecked plasmin activity. Laboratory values in DIC usually show a decline in the platelet count and fibrinogen level and a concomitant elevation in fibrin split products. A more chronic form of DIC has been noted with the release of small amounts of tissue factor into the circulation in such conditions as tumors of the prostate, diabetes mellitus, the use of factor IX concentrates, total hip replacement, and abdominal aortic aneurysm.[3] In a prospective study of 76 patients with extensive aortic aneurysms, 4% (especially those with thoracoabdominal involvement) exhibited clinically overt DIC preoperatively.[84] In this more chronic form of DIC, fibrinogen levels tend to remain within the normal range (since fibrinogen is an acute phase reactant), and the laboratory diagnosis depends more on the inhibitory capacity of the plasma.

In summary, there are a number of conditions that potentially can lead to a hypercoagulable state. A hypercoagulable screen should include routine coagulation tests such as the activated partial thromboplastin time and platelet count, antithrombin III activity assay, protein C antigen and activity levels, protein S antigen level, APC resistance test, mixing studies to identify a lupus anticoagulant (if indicated), and an antiphospholipid antibody screen including anticardiolipin antibody, fibrinogen level, functional plasminogen assay, and platelet aggregation testing, if possible. It is important to remember that although conditions exist that potentially lead to these hypercoagulable states, only 10% to 15% of patients with DVT will be found to have one of the above conditions, the most frequent condition involving abnormalities in protein C and protein

S. The newly described syndrome of APC resistance will likely increase the percentage of patients in which an abnormality of the blood will be able to be demonstrated. Thus, not every patient with a thrombotic event should be screened. However, patients with a strong positive family history, young patients with arterial and venous thromboses without obvious cause, and patients with multiple episodes of thrombosis without underlying anatomic abnormality should be screened.

Bleeding Disorders

Although the surgeon deals more often with hypercoagulable states than bleeding disorders, it is important to recognize these disorders when they occur.

Coagulation factor deficiency states exist as important causes of abnormal bleeding. Factor VIII and IX deficiency states are involved in hemophilia A and B and type I von Willebrand disease. Hemophilia A is inherited as a sex-linked recessive deficiency of factor VIII, with a minority of cases secondary to spontaneous mutation. The incidence of this abnormality is approximately 1/10000 births. Clinical findings range from bleeding into joints and muscles, epistaxis, hematuria, and bleeding after minor trauma to prolonged postoperative bleeding, retroperitoneal bleeding, and intramural bowel hemorrhage. Laboratory screening tests will usually reveal a prolongation of aPTT, with other tests being normal. The minimum level of factor VIII required for hemostasis is 30%, while spontaneous bleeding is uncommon with factor VIII levels greater than 5% to 10% of normal.[85] In severe genetic deficiency states, levels as low as 1% have been noted. Although the half-life of factor VIII is 2.9 days in normal individuals, the half-life of factor VIII concentrates is only 9 to 18 hours.[3] Levels between 80% to 100% of normal should be attained for surgical bleeding or life-threatening hemorrhage. Acquired deficiency has been reported to occur with the development of antibodies to factor VIII following therapy. Approximately 10% to 15% of patients with hemophilia A will develop inhibitor antibodies, although the incidence of antibody formation may be much higher in previously untreated patients. A new recombinant factor VIII preparation has been developed and tested in children and infants, and despite the development of low levels of inhibitors in 20% of children at a mean of 9 days after first administration, these inhibitors either disappeared or remained at low levels.[86] Because of the fact that this recombinant preparation is virus-free, the benefits outweigh the risks of low levels of inhibitor development for the treatment of hemophilia A. Factor IX deficiency (Christmas factor) is also known as hemophilia B. This disease is transmitted as an X-linked recessive trait. It may also be acquired due to enhanced factor

IX clearance in states such as the nephrotic syndrome, abnormal protein synthesis in vitamin K deficiency, and due to acquired specific inhibitors to factor IX in various autoimmune diseases such as SLE. It is clinically indistinguishable from hemophilia A, and laboratory screening tests again reveal a prolonged aPTT, with other tests normal. Severe deficiency (approximately 30% of cases) is defined as a level of activity less than 4% of normal, while moderate deficiency is noted with activity levels between 20% and 40%.[3] Treatment consists of plasma or factor IX concentrates and vitamin K. It has been recommended to achieve levels greater than 30% for hemostasis.[85]

vWF mediates platelet adhesion to collagen. It also forms a complex with factor VIII in the blood. Produced in endothelial cells and megakaryocytes (versus the liver for factor VIII), it has a circulating half-life of 6 to 20 hours.[3] A number of different subtypes have been identified for its deficiency state, and the syndrome is transmitted as both autosomal dominant (heterozygous) and autosomal recessive (homozygous). It is most likely as common as hemophilia A, although the true incidence may be greater than generally appreciated since many mild cases may remain undiagnosed. The classic syndrome is caused by a reduction of factor VIII activity (although not as great as in hemophilia A) and vWF (vWF-factor VIII complex). Clinical manifestations include epistaxis, gingival bleeding, menorrhagia, rare joint or muscle bleeding, and subcutaneous bleeding.[3] Spontaneous bleeding is not as common as in hemophilia A. Screening laboratory tests include a prolonged aPTT, with other coagulation tests normal. In addition, due to the importance of this factor in platelet adhesion, patients will display a prolonged bleeding time, there will be a decreased level of factor VIII activity, decreased immunoreactive levels of the vWF, and an abnormal platelet aggregation response to ristocetin.[3] The most reliable source of vWF is cryoprecipitate. Levels of 25% to 50% are needed for hemostasis.[85]

Other specific factor deficiencies are much less common and will receive only a brief overview. Factor XI (plasma thromboplastin antecedent) is complexed to high-molecular weight kininogen in the plasma and has a half-life of 40 to 80 hours.[3] Deficiency of this factor carries an autosomal recessive inheritance. Homozygous individuals will demonstrate levels as low as 20% of normal, while heterozygous patients will normally show levels between 30% and 60% of normal.[3] The incidence of this syndrome is particularly great in certain ethnic groups such as Ashkenazi Jews. Screening tests include a prolonged aPTT and whole blood clotting time, with other coagulation tests normal. A factor XI assay is the definitive test for the diagnosis of this syndrome. Treatment includes administration of fresh frozen plasma, and hemostasis requires at least 25% of normal factor XI activity.[85] Fac-

tor V (proaccelerin) deficiency is rare. This liver-produced factor has a half-life of 12 to 36 hours and its deficiency is inherited as autosomal recessive.[3] Severe deficiency (called parahemophilia) occurs with 1% plasma activity, while moderate deficiency is characterized by 25% plasma activity.[3] Dysfunctional factor V syndrome has also been described, and an acquired deficiency syndrome has been seen in patients with acute and chronic liver disease.[3] Screening tests include prolonged aPTT, partial time (PT), and whole blood clotting times; levels of factor V may be measured. Treatment consists of fresh frozen plasma and levels at least 15% of normal are needed for hemostasis.[85]

Factor VII (proconvertin) deficiency is inherited as autosomal recessive with intermediate penetrance. Homozygous deficiency is found with levels of 10% of normal, while heterozygous individuals have levels of 40% to 60% normal.[3] A dysfunctional syndrome has also been described with normal levels of factor VII and decreased enzymatic activity. Again, this deficiency state can also be acquired in the presence of liver disease and vitamin K deficiency. Heterozygous individuals are usually asymptomatic, while homozygous patients often display bleeding signs. Screening tests include a prolonged PT with other coagulation tests normal. A factor VII assay will confirm the diagnosis and treatment involves the administration of fresh frozen plasma. Levels as low as 10% of normal will allow for hemostasis.[85] Factor X (Stuart-Prower Factor) deficiency is transmitted as an autosomal recessive-heterogeneous, incomplete recessive trait.[3] Homozygous individuals with severe deficiency have less than 1% normal plasma activity, while those with moderate deficiency have levels of 10% to 20% of normal plasma activity.[3] Acquired deficiency states have been described. Screening tests include a prolonged aPTT, PT, and whole blood clotting time with a normal thrombin clotting time (TCT) while a specific factor X assay exists.[3] Clinical findings again include minor or more major bleeding episodes. Treatment involves the use of fresh frozen plasma. Plasma levels should be maintained above 10% of normal to prevent bleeding.[85] The most rare of the inherited disorders of bleeding is factor II deficiency. This deficiency, transmitted as an autosomal recessive trait, can also be related to liver disease, oral anticoagulation, and the newborn period. Screening tests include a prolonged aPTT and PT with normal TCT and platelet function.[3] Factor II has a half-life of 2 to 5 days and treatment of this deficiency syndrome involves fresh frozen plasma and prothrombin concentrates; levels of 40% are needed for hemostasis.[85]

Deficiencies of fibrinogen can also lead to bleeding disorders. This is the only factor deficiency state in which the TCT will be prolonged. It is generally believed that a fibrinogen level of 100 mg/mL should be achieved to stop bleeding associated with low levels of fibrinogen. Fibrinogen deficiency may also occur from consumption during DIC and primary fibrinolytic states.

Platelet disorders are another important cause of bleeding. Platelets have three major roles in coagulation, including initial adhesion to areas of endothelial denudation, externalization of the phospholipid surface allowing for coagulation complexes to assemble, accelerating the speed of coagulation, and platelet aggregation. Platelet function can be related to three distinct zones in these anucleate cells. The outer zone contains the glycoprotein (Gp) receptors responsible for platelet adhesion (GpIb), platelet aggregation (GpIIb/IIIa), receptor activity for fibrinogen, vWF and fibronectin (GpIIb/IIIa), and the receptor for thrombospondin (GpIIIb).[3] The second zone, the sol-gel zone, contains those elements that allow platelet contraction, while the third zone, the organelle zone, contains electron dense bodies that store Ca^{2+}, serotonin, ADP, and ATP, and the nondense alpha granules that store markers for platelet activation.[3] Bleeding disorders associated with platelets usually include mucosal bleeding (epistaxis), easy bruisability, petechiae, purpura, and menorrhagia.

Extracorporeal bypass circuits such as cardiopulmonary bypass and ECMO activate platelets (regardless of the type of oxygenator employed) and can produce abnormal bleeding. During cardiopulmonary bypass, after fibrinogen and IgG become absorbed onto the bypass circuit, platelets are immediately activated. These activated platelets change their shape, aggregate, and adhere to the fibrinogen surface through multiple interactions between the GpIIb/IIIa and the exposed binding sites on the C-terminus of the gamma chain of fibrinogen and the Fc regions of IgG antibodies. Furthermore, fibrinogen can induce in nonactivated platelets both platelet activation and aggregation. Platelets release granule contents such as PF-4, beta-thromboglobulin, serotonin, adenine nucleotides, and thromboxane. Sensitivity to various platelet agonists decreases. Some adherent platelets break away and leave membrane fragments on the surface of the extracorporeal circuit. Platelet aggregates form, new larger platelets arrive from the bone marrow, and a diluted heterogeneous mixture of fragments, degranulated platelets, resealed platelets with damaged membranes, reversibly activated, and new platelets occurs.[87] Thus, bleeding time increases are frequently noted. In addition, cardiopulmonary bypass activates factor XII and complement leading to neutrophil activation, release of lysosomal enzymes, generation of oxygen free radicals, and the harmful "inflammatory" response noted with extracorporeal circuits. Prosthetic vascular grafts likewise are known to activate platelets, and platelet uptake on both Dacron and polytetrafluoroethylene (ePTFE) grafts has been noted in a number of animal models, but importantly also in patients for up to 6 months to 10 years after graft implantation.[88] This appears to be mostly a phenomenon of platelet recruitment with three different pathways for recruitment available, including the release of ADP from activated platelets, the production of thromboxane from activated platelets, and the generation of thrombin.

Inherited defects of platelet receptors include GpIIb/IIIa called Glanzmann's thrombasthenia characterized by an inability of platelet binding to vWF, fibrinogen and fibronectin, and GpIb called Bernard-Soulier syndrome in which the absolute number of platelets is decreased, the platelets are larger, and aggregation and adhesion are abnormal.[3] Acquired deficits can be seen in uremia when both GpIb and GpIIb/IIIa are defective, resulting in impaired adhesion and aggregation and in those who have received platelet transfusions in the past and who develop immune-mediated platelet antibodies. Patients with Glanzmann's thrombasthenia also show an abnormality in the sol-gel zone, and their platelets lack the ability to contract and retract. A number of platelet disorders associated with abnormalities of the organelle zone have been described.

Abnormalities in fibrinolysis may play a role in abnormal bleeding disorders. Genetic or acquired deficiencies in α_2-AP may be associated with bleeding, while deficiency in factor XIII (fibrin stabilizing factor) may lead to clot which is susceptible to rapid lysis by plasmin. Treatment of α_2-AP deficiency is best with epsilon aminocaproic acid (EACA) or transexamic acid. Homozygous individuals for factor XIII deficiency with less than 1% of normal plasma activity will often display bleeding from the umbilical cord at birth, bleeding following trauma or surgery, and delayed bleeding 24 to 36 hours later.[3] A high incidence of intracranial bleeding has been noted. Screening tests include a shortened euglobulin lysis time, while the presence of clot solubility in 5 M urea, 2% acetic acid, or 1% monochloroacetic acid will help confirm this diagnosis.[3] A specific assay for factor XIII activity does exist. Treatment consists of fresh frozen plasma, cryoprecipitate, and factor XIII concentrates. Finally, a deficiency of PAI has been described which may lead to abnormal bleeding.

Pharmacologic/Nonpharmacologic Interventions

Heparin, first discovered by Jay McLean in 1916 while working in the laboratory of William Henry Howell, is a heterogeneous mixture of sulfated polysaccharide molecules of varying molecular weights. Heparin catalytically accelerates the reaction between thrombin and antithrombin III, accelerating the inhibition of thrombin and other serine proteases by antithrombin III. Additionally, heparin directly binds to and inhibits coagulation proteases and is important for another selective inhibitor of thrombin (heparin cofactor II). After an intravenous bolus, heparin has a half-life of approximately 90 to 120 minutes, although the half-life tends to be dependent on the amount injected. Activated factor X and activated factor II are the clotting factors most sensitive to the heparin-antithrombin III complex. Heparin is not excreted through the kidney or liver, but is cleared through the reticuloendothelial system. Heparin does not cross the placental barrier. Commercial heparin is obtained from pork or beef lung or intestine. Clinical use of heparin in DVT, pulmonary embolism, and as a prophylactic agent has been established.[89] A lower frequency of bleeding complications has been found with continuous infusion rather than bolus injections. In addition, a lesser degree of thrombin accumulation has been found with continuous rather than intermittent heparin administration. In monitoring the heparin effect, an aPTT of 1.5 times control or a TCT of 2 times control reflect adequate anticoagulation, while whole blood activated clotting times in a range of 150 to 200 seconds also suggest adequate anticoagulation. It has been demonstrated that in many situations, direct measurement of heparin levels does not correlate with the actual level of anticoagulation as measured by the aPTT. Although heparin may decrease platelet aggregability at the same time that it enhances the generation of thromboxane from platelets,[90] noncoagulant high-molecular weight heparin fragments may also potentiate platelet aggregation and, as mentioned above, heparin-associated thrombocytopenia from an immune mechanism is a potential complication of heparin usage. Any patient undergoing heparin therapy should have a platelet count measured every other day after the fourth day of therapy, or earlier if known to have been exposed to heparin in the past. The most common complication of heparin therapy is bleeding. The risk of hemorrhage is increased in the elderly, postmenopausal women, and patients with preexisting abnormalities of the coagulation system, thrombocytopenia, or uremia. Long-term therapy may be associated with alopecia and osteoporosis; osteoporosis has been noted in patients receiving large doses of heparin for greater than 6 months.

Heparin as used in venous thrombosis prophylaxis has received considerable attention. Low-dose heparin is thought to protect against DVT through three different mechanisms. First, antithrombin III activity with its inhibition of factor Xa is enhanced by trace amounts of heparin; second, there may be a decrease in thrombin availability which prevents its activation and, thus, its fibrin stabilizing effect; and third, small doses of heparin may inhibit the second wave of platelet aggre-

gation and the subsequent platelet release reaction. In a review of 27 clinical trials concerning the use of low-dose heparin for venous thromboembolism prophylaxis, the incidence of DVT in the control group averaged 25% versus only 7% in those receiving low-dose heparin.[91] Additionally, thrombi likely to produce major pulmonary embolism were decreased from 6% in the control group to 0.6% in the group treated with low-dose heparin. Also low-dose heparin was found to decrease the incidence of massive pulmonary embolism noted at autopsy. However, low-dose heparin does carry an increased risk of wound hematoma and, therefore, only high-risk patients should be treated. The sodium and calcium salts of heparin seem to be equally effective for prophylaxis, and the incidence of wound hematoma does not appear to be related to the type of salt in the heparin preparation. In addition, there is only a slight advantage to giving 5000 units three times a day, rather than twice a day.

The use of low-dose heparin therapy has been endorsed for a number of applications by the National Institutes of Health Consensus Conference on venous thrombosis prophylaxis,[92] and in a recent meta-analysis of 70 randomized trials in 16000 patients comparing low-dose heparin prophylaxis with standard therapy, the odds of developing DVT with low-dose heparin prophylaxis decreased 67 + 4%, while for pulmonary embolism (both fatal and nonfatal), the odds decreased 47 + 10%.[93] For fatal pulmonary embolism, the odds reduction was even greater (64 + 15%). No increase in mortality from other causes was found in those patients treated with low-dose heparin. Importantly, these reductions were noted not only in patients undergoing general surgical procedures, but were also seen in urologic, elective orthopedic, and traumatic orthopedic procedures. This is somewhat at variance with accepted clinical doctrine concerning urologic and orthopedic procedures, but may reflect previous errors in interpretation of studies with small numbers of patients, (type II error). Bleeding complications were more frequent in the heparin-treated patients, with no difference between 5000 units two times a day and 5000 units three times a day, as was the effectiveness of the prophylaxis not influenced by either two times a day administration or three times a day dosage. Low-dose heparin prophylaxis appears to be a good means of preventing venous thromboembolic events during many surgical procedures, but should be confined to those patients known to be at high risk due to the potential for increased bleeding complications associated with its use. Other methods of pharmacologic prophylaxis will not be reviewed here, but suffice it to say that heparin, plus other agents such as dihydroergotamine, coumadin, dextran, and aspirin, along with mechanical measures, have been evaluated and are nicely categorized in the National Institute of Health Consensus Conference report.[92]

Due to the bleeding complications related to low-dose heparin, a number of investigations evaluating the role of low-molecular weight heparin for venous thrombosis prophylaxis have commenced. Standard heparin is a mixture of polysaccharide molecules that vary in MW from 2000 to 40000 d. The anticoagulant effect is primarily centered over the lower end of the molecular weight spectrum. Maximal heparin effect requires a three-way complex between heparin, antithrombin III, and thrombin. However, a two-way complex between antithrombin III and thrombin with heparin binding to antithrombin III, but not thrombin (due to its small size in low-molecular form) will allow for anti-Xa activity with less inhibition of thrombin, and, theoretically, a decrease in systemic bleeding complications. In addition, with MW below 5000 to 8000 d, heparin cannot bind to both antithrombin III and platelets at the same time, thus decreasing the antiplatelet effect of the drug and the potential bleeding complications associated with platelet abnormalities. Although there are many types of low-molecular weight heparin available, in general they are eliminated from the bloodstream more slowly than standard heparin, have a half-life approximately twice as long as standard heparin, have a rate of disappearance from the bloodstream which is not dose-dependent, and their reversal by protamine sulfate is not complete as measured by anti-Xa activity.[94] In addition, low-molecular weight heparins are readily absorbed from the subcutaneous injection sites and do not cross the placental barrier. Although promising studies on the use of low-molecular weight heparins in thromboembolism prophylaxis have been reported, bleeding complications still have been reported and in the aggregate are not appreciably different than with standard heparin prophylaxis.[94] Clearly, more work with low-molecular weight heparin is necessary, not only for venous thrombosis prophylaxis, but also for its routine use in other cardiovascular applications such as during extracorporeal bypass. Low-molecular weight heparins will undoubtedly become very important in various applications in this country, as they have in Europe and Canada.

Reversal of heparin anticoagulation with protamine sulfate is often associated with adverse hemodynamic and hematologic side effects including hypotension, bradycardia, pulmonary artery hypertension or hypotension, declines in oxygen consumption, leukopenia, and thrombocytopenia.[95,96] Although the pulmonary changes have been observed in up to 3% to 4% of cases, hypotension is a more frequent problem and deaths have been reported following the use of this drug, with noncardiogenic pulmonary edema and right heart failure accompanying the most severe reactions. In a recent survey sent to members of the Society for Vascular Surgery (SVS) and European Society for Vascular Surgery (ESVS), the incidence of significant protamine-related side effects was significant at 4% to 5% as reported by approximately 650 surgeons. The most likely cause of the hypotension appears to involve the elaboration of a vasodilator factor, such as nitric oxide (NO), as well as a direct depression of myocardial function, including the development of bradycardia.[97,98] Pulmonary artery hypertension, on the other hand, is thought to result from thromboxane release from nonplatelet sources in the pulmonary circulation.[99] Lastly, thrombocytopenia and leukopenia are most likely the result of a direct effect of protamine on phospholipid membranes of these blood elements.[100] In addition to these side effects, immunologic reactions may also occur in patients with prior exposure to protamine, especially important in diabetics taking NPH insulin which contains protamine to allow for more prolonged absorption, or those exposed to protamine in the past. Unfortunately, at this time no other effective and safe agent for heparin neutralization exists, and in those situations when heparin must be neutralized such as at the completion of major aortic reconstructions and cardiopulmonary bypass, protamine must be given. Although some have suggested that the rate of administration is the most crucial factor in protamine-related reactions, clearly declines in hemodynamic parameters and oxygen consumption still occur with slow administration.[96] We have recently demonstrated that total cationic charge appears to be an important determinant for both anticoagulation reversal and hemodynamic toxicity.[101] Effective and less toxic alternatives to protamine for both standard unfractionated heparin and low-molecular weight heparin anticoagulation reversal should be possible in the future.

Oral anticoagulant therapy is recommended for chronic treatment of venous thromboembolism. Warfarin interferes with the vitamin K-dependent factors II, VII, IX, and X, protein C, and protein S. In the liver, these factors are transported to the hepatocyte endoplasmic reticulum where they are gamma-carboxylated in a reaction catalyzed by reduced vitamin K. During this reaction, 10 to 12 glutamic acid residues are converted to gamma carboxy-glutamic acid residues. When these factors are released from the liver, they are secreted as active proteins.[3] The carboxy-glutamic acid residues allow for these proteins to bind to phospholipid membranes, especially important for the formation of the Xase and prothrombinase complexes on the surface of activated platelets. Warfarin blocks the reduction of vitamin K once it has functioned as a cofactor for the gamma-carboxylation. Two classes of compounds possess anticoagulant effects, 4-hydroxycoumarins (of which crystalline warfarin sodium, [Coumadin[R]], is the most common) and the 2-substituted 1,3-indandiones.[3] Using the one-stage prothrombin time measurement, the prothrombin time should be kept at 1.3 to 1.4 times control for effective anticoagulation. At higher levels, there is nearly a fivefold increase in the frequency of bleeding complications, as the rate of bleeding complications with the lower prothrombin time has been found to be 4% versus 22%, with the prothrombin time 1.5 to 2.0 times control.[102]

Due to variations in the thromboplastins used for the prothrombin time determinations in various countries, a new system has been developed called the international normalized ratio (INR) in which the sensitivity of thromboplastins can be standardized and prothrombin times thus compared accurately.[103] Using this system, the proper INR ratio for treatment of DVT by warfarin is 2 to 3. Major complications of sodium warfarin therapy include recurrent thrombosis and bleeding. It is recommended that warfarin be continued 4 to 6 months after an initial episode of DVT. Between 10 weeks and 4 months after DVT, there is a recurrent thrombosis rate of 8.3 episodes per 1000 patient months. Between 4 months and 3 years, this incidence falls to 4 episodes per 1000 patient months. At 4 months, the risk of bleeding matches and exceeds the benefit from anticoagulant therapy and, thus, is the basis for discontinuing warfarin administration at this time. However, with recurrent DVT, the thrombotic risk is greater and sustained anticoagulation is appropriate; recurrent DVT has been found in up to 20% of patients with recurrent DVT who are treated with only a short 6-month course of warfarin.[104] Patients at highest risk for bleeding during warfarin therapy include the elderly, those with gynecologic or urologic disorders, women after childbirth, and patients given large loading doses of warfarin. A final important complication of warfarin is skin necrosis in patients with protein C deficiency, as discussed above. This usually involves full thickness skin sloughing over fatty areas such as the breasts and buttocks, but can also be seen in other anatomic distributions.

Antiplatelet agents are commonly used in an attempt to prevent cardiovascular events such as coronary thrombosis and neointimal hyperplasia. Platelet aggregation is mediated by a number of receptors on the platelet surface. Many of these receptors are part of the mammalian integrin family including the beta$_1$ family (very late lymphocyte-activation antigen— VLA) mediating interactions between platelets and other cells and collagen, fibronectin, and laminin; beta$_2$ family (LeuCAM) present on leukocytes mediating interactions important in inflammation and immune reactions; and beta$_3$ family (cytoadhesions) including the megakaryocyte specific GpIIb/IIIa complex and the vitronectin receptor present on platelets and other cells.[105] Receptors involved in adhesion (except GpIIb/ IIIa) appear to be functional on resting platelets, whereas aggregation is mediated by GpIIb/IIIa which binds fibrinogen, vWF, fibronectin, vitronectin, and thrombospondin to activated platelets. These high-density receptors are hidden on unactivated platelets while they become present on the surface of activated platelets, although more recent evidence suggests that fibrinogen on the surface of biomaterials can also bind to these receptors and activate platelets. Fibrinogen's dimeric structure allows for platelet-platelet interactions and platelet aggregation, while at high shear rates, vWF may mediate platelet aggregation. The GpIIb/IIIa receptor contains a binding site for the tripeptide sequence arginine-glycine-aspartic acid which is common to many of the above receptor proteins. Platelet agonists expose this receptor and allow for aggregation in addition to initiating the release of arachadonic acid, leading to thromboxane A$_2$ (TxA$_2$) release and further platelet aggregation. Arachadonic acid release is not mandatory for the occurrence of aggregation as most all agonists can directly expose GpIIb/IIIa. In addition, platelet adhesion is a stimulus for platelet aggregation and receptor exposure.

Platelet aggregation can, thus, theoretically be inhibited by 1) blocking cyclooxygenase (which is the first step converting arachadonic acid to thromboxane and prostacyclin); 2) blocking thromboxane synthase (the enzyme specifically leading to the production of TxA$_2$; 3) blocking the receptor for TxA$_2$, 4) increasing intraplatelet levels of adenosine 3′,5′-cycle monophosphate (cAMP) or cyclic quanosine 3′,5′-monophosphate (cGMP) (which inhibits the exposure of GpIIb/ IIIa); and 5) directly blocking GpIIb/IIIa. Aspirin inhibits cyclooxygenase as does indomethacin. Although aspirin inhibits the generation of thromboxane, it also inhibits prostacyclin. In clinical situations, the use of low-dose aspirin in the hopes of inhibiting thromboxane, but preserving prostacyclin generation has not been sustained. Methylxanthines, such as dipyridamole, inhibit phosphodiesterase (which normally degrades cAMP leading to a higher level of cAMP), endothelium-derived relaxing factor (EDRF, nitric acid), nitroglycerin, and nitroprusside-mediated platelet aggregation through modulation of cGMP, and monoclonal antibodies to the GpIIb/IIIa receptor itself or synthetic peptide blockers of this receptor containing the arginine-glycine-aspartic amino acid residue sequence or the fibrinogen gamma-chain carboxy-terminal sequence which directly interfer with the function of this receptor. Receptor blockage is the most specific way to inhibit aggregation, and when this receptor is blocked, even high concentrations of agonists are not able to stimulate platelets. In models of prosthetic vascular graft-platelet interactions, thromboxane synthase inhibitors appear less effective than aspirin, suggesting that endoperoxide intermediates PgG$_2$ and PgH$_2$ are proaggregatory and can interact at the platelet thromboxane receptor, thus subverting the potential anti-aggregatory effect of thromboxane reduction. Thromboxane receptor antagonists should rectify this situation and even have a synergistic effect with thromboxane synthase inhibitors. Thromboxane synthase inhibitors and not thromboxane receptor antagonists are associated with a decreased urinary excretion of thromboxane metabolites and a marked increase in prostacyclin generation. Combined compounds with both thromboxane synthase inhibition and receptor antagonism have been developed with the intent of enhancing prostacyclin production from endoperoxide intermediates (anti-aggregatory) while preventing these intermediates from combining with the thromboxane receptor augmenting platelet aggregation. Ticlopidine, a new antiplatelet agent, appears to inhibit the exposure of the GpIIb/IIIa receptor. However, this agent takes several days of therapy to become effective. Other agents with the possibility of inhibiting the generation of platelet thrombi include monoclonal antibodies to vWF, inhibitors of thrombin production such as APC, and direct thrombin inhibitors such as hirudin. APC has appeal as it may not increase the bleeding time as many of the other agents do.

Hirudin (obtained from the saliva of leeches) is a single-chain, polypeptide composed of 65 amino acids, with 3 disulfide bonds and a MW of 8000 to 9000. It is fast and highly specific for thrombin inhibition. It has a short half-life and is excreted unchanged in the urine. It has no natural inhibitors (versus heparin with the natural inhibitors PF-4 and fibrin II-monomer). As an inhibitor of thrombin, hirudin prevents fibrinogen conversion to fibrin, thrombin catalyzed activation of factors V, VIII, and XIII, and importantly, thrombin-induced platelet aggregation. In addition to its small size and high potency for thrombin, hirudin has a dominant antiplatelet effect, even on platelet-rich thrombi. Compared to heparin, hirudin has been found to be more effective in reducing platelet deposition and mural thrombosis at similar aPTT levels.[106] Levels of aPTT of two to three times control (0.7 to 1.0 mg/kg hirudin) appear effective in limiting arterial thrombosis and platelet deposition. Hirudin prevents thrombus growth at high and low shear rates of blood flow, and has been found to stop thrombus growth even in severe stenoses. However, the high incidence of bleeding complications from this drug may limit its clinical usefulness. The gene for hirudin was cloned in 1986 and a recombinant hirudin has now been produced called Hirulog. Hirulog, a 20-amino acid polypeptide, has two domains, one that inhibits the active site of thrombin and a second that prevents the binding of thrombin to fibrinogen.

One area of great potential benefit for all prosthetic surfaces ranging from cardiopulmonary bypass and ECMO circuits to prosthetic vascular grafts is the ability to "passivate" the surface, lessening platelet-surface interactions in addition to leukocyte activation. Inhibition of platelet function during cardiopulmonary bypass has been accomplished using iloprost, but due to its vasodilatory properties, vasoconstrictors are often needed to maintain systemic arterial blood pressure.[107] "Passivation" of the circuit lasts far beyond the time when the drug is present in the circulation. Other compounds that have been suggested for this purpose include a new class of reversible platelet-fibrinogen receptor inhibitors, the RGD-containing peptides called disintegrins obtained from viper venon that inhibit receptors associated with platelet GpIIb/IIIa receptor complexes.[108,109] In sheep, disintegrins protect platelet numbers, preserve platelet responsiveness to ADP, attenuate release of PF-4, and decrease the Gp-IIIa antigen associated with a 24-hour ECMO circuit surface.[109] Inhibitors of the contact activation portion of extracorporeal systems are less well described. Factor XII is activated by cardiopulmonary bypass. Corn trypsin inhibitor is a weak inhibitor of factor XII activation,[87] while aprotinin inhibits prekallikrein, kallikrein, fibrinolysis, and preserves platelet function (perhaps by inhibiting the high deleterious levels of plasmin).[110] The inhibition of prekallikrein and kallikrein produces an anticoagulant state, while the inhibition of plasmin prevents fibrinolysis. However, aprotinin has a greater affinity for plasmin than kallikrein and only at very high doses will an anticoagulant effect be noted.[111] This agent has successfully reduced transfusion requirements and blood loss in open-heart surgery.[112] Another agent which has been suggested to preserve platelet function is desmopressin acetate (DDAVP). DDAVP, a synthetic analog of vasopressin, has been found to trigger the release of preformed vWF from storage sites (Weibel-Palade bodies) in endothelial cells.[113] vWF then stimulates the production of factor VIII coagulant protein, stabilizes its structure, and forms a circulating noncovalent complex with factor VIII. This vWF:factor VIII complex supports platelet adhesion and improves platelet-platelet interactions. The activated partial thromboplastin time shortens, and prothrombin consumption increases due to the increase in factor VIII coagulant protein. Additionally, DDAVP alters the distribution of vWF multimers of various sizes, elevating the plasma levels of the larger multimers which are more effective. Finally, tPA secretion is stimulated by DDAVP. DDAVP corrects the hemorrhage tendency in mild hemophilia A, von Willebrand's disease, and has been found to reduce blood loss and the need for transfusion by 30% to 40% in complex cardiac operations, excluding simple coronary artery bypass procedures. Additionally, the qualitative platelet defects in uremia and cirrhosis of the liver may be corrected transiently.[114] The platelet lesion caused by small doses of aspirin may also be corrected by DDAVP. DDAVP has not been shown to increase the risk of thrombosis.

Another anticoagulant which has been used in place of heparin for anticoagulation in infrainguinal bypass procedures is ancrod, a thrombin-like enzyme derived from the Malayan pit viper.[115] This substance produces a controlled decrease in fibrinogen levels by depleting FPA from fibrinogen but not FPB, and the fibrin monomers that result are felt to stimulate the local production of tPA. Both of these actions lead to anticoagulation. However, the amount of fibrinogen depletion must be carefully titrated to prevent bleeding.

Fibrinolytic agents act directly or indirectly as activators of plasminogen, the inactive proteolytic enzyme of plasma which binds to fibrin during the formation of thrombus. Fibrin-bound plasminogen is more susceptible to activation than is plasminogen free in plasma. Streptokinase, a nonenzymatic protein isolated from group C beta-hemolytic streptococci, and acylated plasminogen-streptokinase (APSAC) act through a streptokinase-plasmin complex; urokinase, single-chain urokinase-type plasminogen activator (scuPA), and recombinant tissue plasminogen activator (rtPA) act directly on plasmin without an intermediate drug-plasmin complex.[116] tPA (originally isolated from a melanoma cell line and now manufactured with recombinant DNA technology), APSAC and scuPA are termed "fibrin-selective" agents because of their high ratio of activity for fibrin-bound plasminogen to circulating plasma plasminogen. Acylation of the streptokinase-plasminogen complex on the active serine moiety on the light chain stabilizes the catalytic serine site making this complex inert to circulating plasminogen. Binding occurs by virtue of the heavy chain lysine-plasminogen portions to fibrin and, over time, the acetyl group leaves the complex resulting in a fibrin-specific thrombolytic effect. Urokinase, a two-chain polypeptide, is formed by the cleavage of scuPA by plasmin, produced by the epithelial cells of urinary origin. scuPA (a pro-enzyme-like substance) is fibrin-specific through a mechanism whereby scuPA activates plasminogen at the fibrin surface (tenfold more active than in circulating blood) converting it to plasmin. Thus, only the fibrin-bound plasminogen is converted to plasmin for selective thrombolysis at the fibrin clot surface. tPA occurs in two forms, a single and double polypeptide chain form. tPA has a fibrin binding site and a catalytic site, widely separated from each other. This separation allows tPA to be activated to its fibrin target, thus establishing its fibrin-specific nature. The level of the lytic state is greatest with streptokinase and APSAC, intermediate with urokinase, less with scuPA and least with single-chain tPA.[110] Half-lives also vary among different agents from 5 minutes for single-chain

rtPA to 90 minutes for APSAC.[110] Streptokinase, as a bacterial protein produced by group C beta-hemolytic streptococci, is antigenic along with APSAC, while urokinase and scuPA, produced from human fetal kidney cells in tissue culture, are nonantigenic. Allergic reactions to streptokinase have been reported in from 2% to 20% of cases. In addition, an unusual serum sickness also has been reported with streptokinase.

Bleeding complications associated with fibrinolytic agents (reported in up to 50% of patients receiving systemic fibrinolytic agents for DVT) appear related to the invasive diagnostic or therapeutic procedures associated with drug therapy. Therapy induces a hemostatic defect through a combination of factors. Hypofibrinogenemia and fibrin degradation products inhibit fibrin polymerization and, in combination with a decrease in the clotting factors V and VIII (from excess plasmin not neutralized by α_2-AP), inhibit the ability of the blood to clot. Although coagulation tests in general do not correlate with bleeding complications, a fibrinogen level less than 100 mg/dL is associated with an increased risk and severity of bleeding. In addition, newly-formed thrombi are easily lysed as they are formed. Platelets are both inhibited and stimulated by fibrinolytic agents. As fibrinogen is a necessary cofactor for ADP-induced platelet aggregation, low fibrinogen levels will aggravate a platelet defect. At the same time, activation of plasminogen bound to platelets leads to impaired adhesion and a decrease in their ability to aggregate. Plasmin-induced cleavage of adhesive proteins such as thrombospondin, fibronectin, and fibrin also disrupt platelet aggregates, leading to platelet disaggregation. In addition, plasmin formed on the endothelial cell surface impairs platelet adhesion, resulting in poor platelet adhesion to areas of vascular injury. Despite the above mechanisms, most suggesting a decrease in the ability of the blood to clot during fibrinolytic therapy, it has been shown that these agents promote reocclusion in up to 30% of cases early after thrombolysis through platelet activation, such that platelet activation occurs early after lysis and platelet inhibition occurs later.[38] Additionally, increased synthesis of endothelial cell PAI-1 has been demonstrated experimentally after treatment with tPA, another mechanism that would contribute to early thrombotic reocclusion.[117]

Indications for thrombolytic therapy remain controversial. Clearly, in DVT, fibrinolytic agents allow for complete clot lysis more frequently than heparin therapy and help preserve valve function to a greater degree, but at the risk of a higher degree of bleeding complications.[118] Thirteen studies of thrombolytic therapy for acute DVT have been compiled from the literature.[119] In these studies, patients were assessed with venography. Of those treated with anticoagulants, only 4% had complete lysis and 14% revealed partial lysis, while 45% of those patients treated with thrombolytic agents showed significant or complete clot lysis and an additional 18% revealed partial clearing. Two studies have evaluated the long-term success of thrombolytic therapy compared to anticoagulation for DVT. In 39 patients with follow-up of 1.6 to 5 years, 21% of those treated with heparin had no evidence of postthrombotic symptoms, while 64% of those treated with streptokinase were asymptomatic.[120,121] In a similar fashion, significant functional benefits 5 to 10 years after therapy in patients with significant clot lysis as measured by PPG and foot volumetry were noted, although the PPG did not normalize in the lysis group. On the contrary, in a large prospective study in patients followed for 2 years after DVT after either heparin or streptokinase, no major improvement in deep venous valvular competence was found with lytic agents, and venous functional preservation appeared the same whether clot lysis was complete or incomplete.[122] In addition, although it has been documented that approximately 50% of patients with their first episode of DVT who begin lytic therapy within 72 hours of the onset of symptoms may achieve complete dissolution of their thrombus, only approximately 15% of patients who acutely present with lower extremity DVT would fit into this category. Thus, the practicality of using this therapy must be questioned.[123] Controversy remains about the use of thrombolytic therapy in the setting of DVT.

If one decides to use lytic therapy for DVT, then which agent, what dose, and for how long? In a comparison of streptokinase and urokinase in DVT, little cost difference was found after considering the longer infusion time and greater bleeding complications associated with streptokinase compared to urokinase.[124] Turpie has reported on the use of tPA 0.5 mg/kg over 4 hours or over 8 hours times 2 with heparin versus placebo plus heparin for proximal DVT. He has demonstrated greater than 50% total clot lysis in 58% of a group of patients treated over 4 hours, 23% in a group treated for 8 hours, and only 7% complete clot lysis in the placebo-treated group.[125] Follow-up in those patients with greater than 50% clot lysis revealed evidence of chronic venous insufficiency (CVI) in only 25% versus 56% of those with less than 50% clot lysis, a difference that was close to but not statistically different (p = 0.07). This study suggests that further investigation into the use of the new fibrin-specific agents for proximal DVT may be enlightening. Fibrinolytic therapy has been suggested for use in upper extremity effort DVT, catheter-induced DVT, Paget-Schroetter syndrome, and superior vena caval thrombosis. An interesting approach combining thrombolytic therapy and thoracic outlet decompression has been suggested.[126] Thrombolytic therapy is initiated locally

with urokinase (250000 IU bolus, then 1000 to 4000 IU/min) by a small catheter positioned from a basilic vein. After lysis, anticoagulation is continued for 3 months with heparin/coumadin to allow for thrombophlebitis (the inflammatory response in the vein which occurs due to the thrombus) to resolve, and then thoracic outlet decompression is performed. Percutaneous transluminal angioplasty is not successful in the presence of an anatomic defect. Long-term results have been reported to be excellent and correlated well with the initial ability to clear the thrombus.

Thrombolytic therapy in pulmonary embolism has been extensively studied. Two carefully designed studies have evaluated the use of either urokinase or streptokinase. Although both agents were capable of rapidly lysing clots and improving pulmonary hemodynamics, there was no difference in patient mortality or recurrence rate of pulmonary embolism when compared to heparin therapy alone.[127,128] Urokinase dissolved pulmonary arterial clots within 24 hours of treatment, and in certain instances, reversed clinical shock. By 7 days, both the thrombolytic and heparin-treated patients revealed equal improvement in pulmonary hemodynamics, and there was no difference in lung scan improvement. No difference between urokinase and streptokinase was noted. In addition, bleeding complications were more frequent in the thrombolytic group. Patients receiving urokinase responded better if they were younger, the embolus was less than 48 hours old, or the embolus was large. Thrombolytic therapy for pulmonary embolism should be considered when there is angiographically documented lobar or greater pulmonary embolism, which is responsible for the production of acute pulmonary hypertension and shock; lesser degrees of pulmonary embolism should be treated with standard heparin anticoagulation.

Turpie has also reported on the use of tPA, 0.6 mg/kg over 2 minutes, plus heparin, versus placebo plus heparin for patients with pulmonary embolism, using lung scans at 24 hours and 7 days to document treatment efficacy.[125] No increase in bleeding complications was noted, and lysis was significantly improved at 24 hours in the tPA group (34.4%) versus the placebo group (12%), p = 0.026. However, the advantage for tPA had disappeared by 7 days (59% lysis as compared to 56% lysis). The benefit for tPA, thus, would be expected only early in the 11% of patients who die as a result of massive pulmonary embolism in the first hour after the embolus occurs.

Thrombolytic therapy for peripheral arterial applications is becoming more frequently used, especially when the agent(s) are given intra-arterially rather than intravenously in a systemic fashion. The method of McNamara has gained the most recognition.[129] This method involves passing a guidewire through the thrombus and then infusing a high dose of urokinase at 4000 U/min for 1 to 2 hours directly into the clot. If progress is made, further fibrinolytic therapy is given at 1000 to 2000 U/min for a 6- to 12-hour period or until complete clot lysis has occurred. Using this technique, the mean infusion time was found to be 18 hours, and the incidence of bleeding complications was significantly lessened. McNamara and Fischer compared these results to those of streptokinase from the literature and found a 13% incidence of severe bleeding complications with streptokinase and only a 4% incidence with high-dose intra-arterial urokinase therapy. McNamara and Bomberger reported on their first 100 cases of selective intra-arterial infusion of urokinase and noted complete clot lysis in 77%, with native arterial occlusions responding better than arterial graft occlusions (71% versus 41% success) at 6-month follow-up.[130] However, as has been reported in a number of series, after thrombolytic therapy has reopened an occluded vessel or graft, radiologic or surgical correction of the lesion responsible for the thrombosis initially forming must be addressed for any hope of long-term success. A 1-year graft patency rate of 89% in those grafts in which an underlying lesion was successfully repaired, compared to 23% in grafts without a correctable lesion, has been reported.[131] At 2 years, this difference was even greater, 79% compared to 10%.

Complications associated with thrombolytic therapy for arterial thrombosis include bleeding, rethrombosis, embolization (treated with further thrombolytic therapy), and sepsis from prolonged catheter placement. The most recent innovation in intra-arterial thrombolytic therapy involves the technique of lacing the entire length of the thrombus with high-dose urokinase prior to continuous infusion and then using initial pulse-spray techniques. The use of tPA in peripheral vascular cases has been reported with promising results, yet 17% of patients still responded with a decrease in systemic fibrinogen levels to less than 100 mg/dL; three developed groin hematomas, and one developed a stroke soon after therapy had been completed. Although fibrin-specific, tPA can still cause a systemic thrombolytic effect.

Recently, the use of intraoperative thrombolytic therapy for those situations where complete clot evacuation cannot be accomplished, as may be seen in up to 40% of patients undergoing balloon embolectomy with an embolectomy catheter for acute arterial occlusion, or when the distal vasculature is occluded and precludes appropriate inflow patency, has been advocated.[118] One method involves giving urokinase distal to an occluding clamp, infused at 250000 units combined with 1000 units of heparin in 250 cc saline, and allowed to remain for a 30-minute period. If necessary, another 125000 units is infused for 30 minutes. Using this regimen, 70% of limbs with critical ischemia at the completion of successful balloon embolectomy were spared amputation with only one bleeding complication.[132] For patients who have multivessel occlusions or for whom any degree of systemic fibrinolysis would be too risky, a new high-dose isolated limb perfusion technique has been described. This technique involves anticoagulation, limb exsanguination with an Esmarch bandage, application of a proximal tourniquet, and direct arterial infusion of 1000000 units or more of urokinase for 45 to 60 minutes, with direct drainage of the venous effluent out in front of the tourniquet.

Although much work has been carried out on the use of thrombolytic agents in acute myocardial infarction, this area is also evolving. In general, the use of streptokinase will reduce in-hospital mortality by 30%, although prospective comparisons between various thrombolytic agents has not as yet been reported.[133] The clinical benefits associated with coronary thrombolysis most likely are determined by the rapidity of coronary artery reperfusion. Platelet-mediated thrombotic events may be responsible for those unsuccessful cases (25% to 30%) with the currently used agents and protocols. Recent studies have suggested that heparin therapy added to tPA improves the efficacy of this thrombolytic agent during coronary thrombolysis and helps to prevent reocclusion after thrombolysis is completed.

Contraindications to thrombolytic therapy, whether regional or systemic, consist of active internal bleeding, recent surgery or trauma (generally within 10 days of infusion), a recent cerebrovascular accident (within 2 months), or documented left-heart thrombus. Relative contraindications include recent surgery, gastrointestinal bleeding or trauma, severe hypertension, mitral valve disease, endocarditis, a history of a defect in hemostasis, or pregnancy.

Dextran is a high-molecular weight polysaccharide produced from sucrose by the action of *Leuconostoc mesenteroides*. Fractionation and hydrolysis produce a product with a molecular weight of either 40000 (dextran 40; Rheomacrodex) or 70000 (dextran 70). Dextran 40 has been studied in detail for its ability to augment patency of lower extremity bypass grafts in the early postoperative period. Dextran 40 acts as a volume-expanding agent and causes hemodilution-decreasing blood viscosity, decreases platelet adhesiveness, reduces factor VIII activity, and increases the lysability of clot.[134] In addition, dextran has been found to coat endothelial cell surfaces, decreasing their electronegativity. Two 500 mL bottles on the day of bypass surgery, followed by one on each of the succeeding 3 postoperative days at 75 mL/hour (except for 100 mL/hour during surgery), were found to increase bypass patency 1 day, 1 week, and 1 month postoperatively for femorotibial bypass and all infrainguinal bypasses in which autologous vein was not used. A number of other applications for dextran 40 have been suggested based on experimental observations including vascular trauma, endarterectomy, arterial and venous thrombectomy, venous reconstruction, and as a prophylactic agent for DVT. However, none of these other indications has been substantiated by a clinical study such as in the case of difficult lower extremity bypass procedures.

Mechanical measures are utilized primarily for the prevention of DVT during operative procedures or in those patients who cannot be given pharmacologic prophylaxis. These measures have included early ambulation, elastic stockings, electrical calf muscle stimulation, and external pneumatic compression, either with uniform-pressure leggings or graded-pressure leggings. In many well-controlled studies of venous prophylaxis, intermittent pneumatic compression has been found to be as effective as low-dose heparin therapy. In addition to augmentation of venous return with these devices, local and systemic fibrinolysis appears to be stimulated. The length of time that intermittent pneumatic compression should be used has not been adequately determined, but most available data would suggest that at least 5 days application, or longer in the face of prolonged immobilization, may be optimal.

Vena caval interruption for venous thromboembolism is appropriate if traditional methods of anticoagulation fail, or the use of anticoagulant agents is contraindicated. Early results with vena cava ligation resulted in a high incidence of lower extremity venous complications and an unacceptably high rate of recurrent embolization and, thus, intraoperative caval compartmentalization and clip devices, followed by intravascular venous clot-trapping devices, were developed. These devices have resulted in a lower incidence of venous stasis complications. The most effective device currently available is the Greenfield vena cava filter, a cone-shaped device initially constructed of stainless steel. The cone shape allows for 85% of the device to contain clot and still maintain flow, allowing for natural fibrinolysis to take place. Indications for vena caval filters include DVT or pulmonary embolism in a patient with a contraindication to anticoagulation, a complication during anticoagulation, recurrent pulmonary embolism in the presence of adequate anticoagulation, chronic pulmonary embolism with associated pulmonary hypertension and cor pulmonale, and immediately following pulmonary embolectomy. Free-floating iliofemoral DVT may be associated with a 60% incidence of pulmonary embolism despite adequate anticoagulation,[135] while free-floating inferior vena caval thrombi show a 27% incidence of pulmonary embolism despite anticoagulation,[136] and bilateral free-floating femoral thrombi have a 43% incidence of pulmonary embolism despite adequate anticoagulation,[137] all additional indications for filter placement. In 469 patients

reported in the largest experience in the literature to date with the Greenfield filter, a contraindication to anticoagulation was the most frequent reason for filter insertion (38% of cases), followed by failure of anticoagulation (27% of cases).[138] Recurrent pulmonary embolism was noted in only 4% of patients over a 12-year follow-up, the long-term inferior vena caval patency rate was 98% independent of anticoagulation, and venous ulceration was noted in only 3% of patients. No patient with suprarenal filter placement (32 cases) was found to have occluded their inferior vena cava or renal veins over the follow-up period.

Percutaneous insertion, rather than insertion by open surgical technique, offers a number of advantages including decreased patient discomfort, decreased time of insertion, and decreased cost. Using a percutaneous approach, the incidence of DVT at the insertion site has been reported to be as high as 41%.[139] In response to this problem, a titanium Greenfield filter with modified hooks was developed which reduces to a size of 12 F in a 14 F sheath. Testing of this filter in 186 patients revealed 97% successful placement and a recurrent pulmonary embolism rate of only 3%.[140] The thrombosis rate at the insertion site was only 8.7%.

Surgical approaches for pulmonary thromboembolism are indicated in patients who have massive embolism with hypotension and who require large doses of vasopressors. Open pulmonary embolectomy as practiced in the past is associated with high morbidity and mortality. Today, open pulmonary embolectomy or the placement on ECMO is limited to those patients who require cardiac massage manually for hypotension or those who fail catheter pulmonary embolectomy. A catheter device for the removal of pulmonary emboli has also been developed. Catheter pulmonary embolectomy is performed by operative insertion under local anesthesia from either the jugular or common femoral vein. The cup catheter is inserted through a transverse venotomy, and the radiopaque catheter is then visualized under fluoroscopy as it is guided into the right side of the heart, aided by medial angulation and anterior deflection which then allows the cup to enter the pulmonary artery. The left main pulmonary artery is entered most easily. The cup is juxtaposed to the embolus and syringe suction is then used to aspirate the clot into the cup and the entire catheter and clot are withdrawn. Entry into the right main pulmonary artery is performed by deflecting the cup in that direction as it reaches the superior edge of the cardiac shadow. Multiple retrievals may be necessary to remove enough thrombus to improve the pulmonary hemodynamics. In a series of 46 patients treated with this device, emboli were extracted in 76% of cases and the 30-day survival was 70%.[141] Embolectomy was most successful for major pulmonary embolism and massive pulmonary embolism and least helpful for chronic pulmonary embolism. Successful embolectomy predicted long-term survival.

References

1. Zur M, Radcliffe RD, Oberdick J, et al: The dual role of factor VII in blood coagulation: initiation and inhibition of a proteolytic system by a zymogen. *J Biol Chem* 257:5623, 1982.

2. Radcliffe R, Nemerson Y: Mechanism of activation of bovine factor VII: products of cleavage by factor Xa. *J Biol Chem* 251:4749, 1976.

3. Hassouna HI: The laboratory evaluation of hemostatic disorders. In: Penner JA, Hassouna HI (eds). *Coagulation Disorders II*: Philadelphia: Hematology/Oncology Clinics of North America. 7:1161, 1993.

4. Sims PJ, Faioni EM, Wiedmer T, et al: Complement proteins C5b-9 cause release of membrane vesicles from the platelet surface that are enriched in the membrane receptor for coagulation factor Va and express prothrombinase activity. *J Biol Chem* 263:18205, 1988.

5. Gilbert GE, Sims PJ, Wiedmer T, et al: Platelet-derived microparticles express high affinity receptors for factor VIII. *J Biol Chem* 266:17261, 1991.

6. Hickey MJ, Williams SA, Roth GA: Human platelet glycoprotein IX: an adhesive prototype of leucine-rich glycoproteins with flank-center-flank structures. *Proc Natl Acad Sci USA* 86:6773, 1989.

7. Bennett JS, Vilaire G, Cines DB: Identification of the fibrinogen receptor on human platelets by photoaffinity labeling. *J Biol Chem* 257:8049, 1982.

8. Savage B, Ruggeri ZM: Selective recognition of adhesive sites in surface-bound fibrinogen by glycoprotein IIb/IIIa on nonactivated platelets. *J Biol Chem* 266: 11277, 1991.

9. Osterud B, Rapaport SI: Activation of factor IX by the reaction product of tissue factor and factor VIII: additional pathway for initiating blood coagulation. *Proc Natl Acad Sci USA* 74:5260, 1977.

10. Bauer KA, Kass BL, ten Care H, et al: Factor IX is activated in vivo by the tissue factor mechanism. *Blood* 76:731, 1990.

11. Blomback, B, Blomback M: The molecular structure of fibrinogen. *Ann NY Acad Sci* 202:77, 1972.

12. Folk JE, Finlayson JS: The epsilon-(gamma-glutamyl) lysine cross-link and the catalytic role of transglutamines. *Adv Protein Chem* 31:1, 1977.

13. Davie EW, Fujikawa K, Kisiel W: The coagulation cascade: initiation, maintenance, and regulation. *Biochemistry* 30:10363, 1991.

14. Naito K, Fujikawa K: Activation of human blood coagulation factor XI independent of factor XII: factor XI is activated by thrombin and factor XIa in the presence of negatively charged surfaces. *J Biol Chem* 266:7353, 1991.

15. DiScipio RG, Kurachi K, Davie EW: Activation of human factor IX (Christmas factor). *J Clin Invest* 61: 1528, 1978.

16. Rosenberg RD, Damus PS: The purfication and mechanism of action of human antithrombin-heparin cofactor. *J Biol Chem* 248:6490, 1973.

17. Kurachi K, Fujikawa K, Schmer G, et al: Inhibition of bovine factor IXa and factor Xab by antithrombin III. *Biochemistry* 15:373, 1976.

18. Kurachi K, Davie EW: Activation of human factor XI (plasma thrombo-plastin antecedent) by factor XIIa (activated Hageman factor). *Biochemistry* 16:5831, 1977.

19. Kisiel W, Canfield WM, Ericsson LH, et al: Anticoagulant properties of bovine plasma protein C following activation by thrombin. *Biochemistry* 16:5824, 1977.

20. Marlar RA, Kleiss AJ, Griffin JH: Mechanism of action of human activated protein C, a thrombin-dependent anticoagulant enzyme. *Blood* 59:1067, 1982.

21. Vehar GA, Davie EW: Preparation and properties of bovine factor VIII (antihemophilic factor). *Biochemistry* 19:401, 1980.

22. Esmon CT, Owen WG: Identification of an endothelial cell cofactor for thrombin-catalyzed activation of protein C. *Proc Natl Acad Sci USA* 78:2249, 1981.

23. Owen WG, Esmon CT: Functional properties of an endothelial cell cofactor for thrombin-catalyzed activation of protein C. *J Biol Chem* 256:5532, 1981.

24. Esmon NL, Owen WG, Esmon CT: Isolation of a membrane-bound cofactor for thrombin-catalyzed activation of protein C. *J Biol Chem* 257:859, 1982.

25. Esmon CT: The regulation of natural anticoagulant pathways. *Science* 235:1348, 1987.

26. Esmon NL, Carroll RC, Esmon CT: Thrombomodulin blocks the ability of thrombin to activate platelets. *J Biol Chem* 258:12238, 1983.

27. Esmon CT, Esmon NL, Harris KW: Complex formation between thrombin and thrombomodulin inhibits both thrombin-catalyzed fibrin formation and factor V activation. *J Biol Chem* 257:7944, 1982.

28. Walker FJ: Regulation of activated protein C by a new protein: a possible function for bovine protein S. *J Biol Chem* 255:5521, 1980.

29. Tollefsen DM, Majerus PW, Blank MK: Heparin cofactor II: purification and properties of a heparin-dependent inhibitor of thrombin in human plasma. *J Biol Chem* 257:2162, 1982.

30. Broze GJ, Girard TJ, Novotny WF: Regulation of coagulation by a multivalent Kunitz-type inhibitor. *Biochemistry* 29:7539, 1990.

31. Rapaport SI: Inhibition of factor VIIa/tissue factor-induced blood coagulation, with particular emphasis upon a factor Xa-dependent inhibitory mechanism. *Blood* 73: 359, 1989.

32. Gelehrter TD, Sznycer-Laszuk R: Thrombin induction of plasminogen activator inhibitor in cultured human endothelial cells. *J Clin Invest* 77:165, 1986.

33. Dichek D, Quertermous T: Thrombin regulation of mRNA levels of tissue plasminogen activator and plasminogen activator inhibitor-1 in cultured human umbilical vein endothelial cells. *Blood* 74:222, 1989.

34. Adelman B, Michelson AD, Loscalzo J, et al: Plasmin effect on platelet glycoprotein Ib-von Willebrand factor interactions. *Blood* 65:32, 1985.

35. Schmaier AH: Disseminated intravascular coagulation: pathogenesis and management. *J Intensive Care Med* 6:209, 1991.

36. Hajjar KA, Nachman RL: Endothelial cell-mediated conversion of Glu-plasminogen to Lys-plasminogen: further evidence for assembly of the fibrinolytic system on the endothelial cell surface. *J Clin Invest* 82:1769, 1988.

37. Coleman RW: Activation of plasminogen by human plasma kallikrein. *Biochem Biophys Res Commun* 35: 273, 1969.

38. Esmon NL, Esmon CT: Protein C and the endothelium. *Sem Thromb Haemost* 14:210, 1988.

39. Van der Poll T, Buller HR, ten Cate H, et al: Activation of coagulation after administration of tumor necrosis factor to normal subjects. *N Engl J Med* 322:1622, 1990.

40. Nawroth PP, Stern DM: Modulation of endothelial cell hemostatic properties by tumor necrosis factor. *J Exp Med* 163:740, 1986.

41. Bevilacqua MP, Pober JS, Majeau GR, et al: Recombinant tumor necrosis factor induces procoagulant activity in cultured human vascular endothelium: characterization and comparison with the actions of interleukin-1. *Proc Natl Acad Sci USA* 83:4533, 1986.

42. Conway EM, Bach R, Rosenberg RD, et al: Tumor necrosis factor enhances expression of tissue factor mRNA in endothelial cells. *Thromb Res* 53:231, 1989.

43. Schleef RR, Bevilacqua MP, Sawdey M, et al: Cytokine activation of vascular endothelium: effects on tissue-type plasminogen activator and type I plasminogen inhibitor. *J Biol Chem* 263:5797, 1988.

44. Van Hinsbergh VW, Kooistra T, van den Berg EA, et al: Tumor necrosis factor increases production of plasminogen activator inhibitor in human endothelial cells in vitro and rats in vivo. *Blood* 72:1467, 1988.

45. Medina R, Schocher SH, Han JH: Interleukin-1, endotoxin, or tumor necrosis factor/cachectin enhance the level of plasminogen activator messenger RNA in bovine aortic endothelial cells. *Thromb Res* 54:41, 1989.

46. Van der Poll T, Levi M, Buller HR, et al: Fibrinolytic response to tumor necrosis factor in healthy subjects. *J Exp Med* 174:729, 1991.

47. Pohlman TH, Stanness KA, Beatty PG, et al: An endothelial cell surface factor(s) induced in vitro by lipopolysaccharide, interleukin-1, and tumor necrosis factor-alpha increases neutrophil adherence by CD18-dependent mechanism. *J Immunol* 136:4548, 1986.

48. Schleimer RP, Rutledge BK: Cultured human endothelial cells acquire adhesiveness for neutrophils after stimulation with interleukin-1, endotoxin, and tumor-promoting phorbol diesters. *J Immunol* 136:649, 1986.

49. Rothlein R, Dustin ML, Marlin SD, et al: A human intercellular adhesion molecule (ICAM-1) distinct from LFA-1. *J Immunol* 137:1270, 1986.

50. Bevilacqua MP, Stengelin S, Gimbrone MA, et al: Endothelial leukocyte adhesion molecule 1: an inducible receptor for neutrophils related to complement regulatory proteins and lectins. *Science* 243:1160, 1989.

51. Kunkel SL, Standiford T, Metinko AP, et al: Endothelial cell-derived novel chemotactic cytokines. In: Johson A, Ferro TJ (eds). *Lung Vascular Injury: Molecular and Cellular Response*. New York: Marcel Dekker, Inc.; 213, 1992.

52. Furie B, Furie BC: Molecular and cell biology of blood coagulation. *N Engl J Med* 326:800, 1992.

53. Palabrica T, Lobb R, Furie BC: Leukocyte accumulation promoting fibrin deposition is mediated in vivo by P-selectin on adherent platelets. *Nature* 359:848, 1992.

54. Stewart GJ: Neutrophils and deep venous thrombosis. *Haemostasis* 23:127, 1993.

55. Holt JC, Yan Z, Lu W, et al: Isolation, characterization, and immunological detection of neutrophil-activating peptide 2: a proteolytic degradation product of platelet basic protein. *Proc Soc Exp Biol Med* 199:171, 1992.

56. Ferrer-Lopez P, Renesto P, Schattner M, et al: Activation of human platelets by C5a-stimulated neutrophils: a role for catepsin G. *Am J Physiol* 258:C1100, 1990.

57. Evangelista V, Rajtar G, de Gaetano G, et al: Platelet activation by FMLP-stimulated polymorphonuclear leukocytes: the activity of catepsin G is not prevented by antiproteases. *Blood* 77:2379, 1991.

58. Wakefield TW, Greenfield LJ, Rolfe MW, et al: Inflammatory and procoagulant mediator interactions in an experimental baboon model of venous thrombosis. *Thromb Haemost* 69:164, 1993.

59. Wakefield TW, Streiter RM, Wilke CA, et al: Venous thrombosis-associated inflammation and attenuation with neutralizing antibodies to cytokines and adhesion molecules. *Arterioscler Thromb Vasc Biol* 15:258, 1995.

60. Ansell JE, Price JM, Shah S, et al: Heparin-induced thrombocytopenia: what is its real frequency? *Chest* 88:878, 1985.

61. Silver D, Kapsch DN, Tsoi EK: Heparin-induced thrombocytopenia, thrombosis, and hemorrhage. *Am Surg* 198:301, 1983.

62. Kappa JR, Fisher CA, Berkowitz HD, et al: Heparin-induced platelet activation in sixteen surgical patients: diagnosis and management. *J Vasc Surg* 5:101, 1987.

63. Towne JB, Bernhard VM, Hussey C, et al: Antithrombin deficiency: a cause of unexplained thrombosis in vascular surgery. *Surgery* 89:735, 1981.

64. Flinn WR, McDaniel MD, Yao JST, et al: Antithrombin III deficiency as a reflection of dynamic protein metabolism in patients undergoing vascular reconstruction. *J Vasc Surg* 1:888, 1984.

65. Clouse LH, Comp PC: The regulation of hemostasis: the protein C system. *N Engl J Med* 314:1298, 1986.

66. Eldrup-Jorgensen J, Flanigan DP, Brace L, et al: Hypercoagulable states and lower limb ischemia in young adults. *J Vasc Surg* 9:334, 1989.

67. Esmon CY: The regulation of natural anticoagulant pathways. *Science* 235:1348, 1987.

68. Cole MS, Minifee PK, Wolma FJ: Coumadin necrosis: a review of the literature. *Surgery* 103:271, 1988.

69. Svensson PJ, Dahlback B: Resistance to activated protein C as a basis for venous thrombosis. *New Engl J Med* 330:517, 1994.

70. Koster T, Rosendaal FR, deRonde H, et al: Venous thrombosis due to poor anticoagulant response to activated protein C: leiden thrombophilia study. *Lancet* 342:1503, 1993.

71. Griffin JH, Evatt B, Wideman C, et al: Anticoagulant protein C pathway defective in majority of thrombophilic patients. *Blood* 82:1989, 1993.

72. Greengard JS, Eichinger S, Griffin JH, Bauer KA: Variability of thrombosis among homozygous siblings with resistance to activated protein C due to an arg-gln mutation in the gene for factor V. *New Engl J Med* 331:1559, 1994.

73. Bauer KA: Hypercoagulability: a new cofactor in the protein C anticoagulant pathway (editorial). *New Engl J Med* 330:566, 1994.

74. Greenfield LJ: Lupus-like anticoagulants and thrombosis. *J Vasc Surg* 7:818, 1988.

75. Lockshin MD: Antiphospholipid antibody syndrome. *JAMA* 268:1451, 1992.

76. Ahn SS, Kalunian K, Rosove M, et al: Postoperative thrombotic complications in patients with the lupus anticoagulant: increased risk after vascular procedures. *J Vasc Surg* 7:749, 1988.

77. Donaldson MC, Weinberg DS, Belkin M, et al: Screening for hypercoagulable states in vascular surgical practice: a preliminary study. *J Vasc Surg* 11:825, 1990.

78. Towne JB, Bandyk DF, Hussey CV, et al: Abnormal

plasminogen: a genetically determined cause of hyper-coagulability. *J Vasc Surg* 1:896, 1984.

79. Wu KW: Hypercoagulability in arterial thrombosis: new perspectives from epidemiologic studies. *J Vasc Surg* 12:208, 1990.

80. Rodgers GM: Hemostatic properties of normal and perturbed vascular cells. *FASEB J* 2:116, 1988.

81. Nilsson IM, Ljungner H, Tengborn L: Two different mechanisms in patients with venous thrombosis and defective fibrinolysis: low concentrations of plasminogen activator or increased concentration of plasminogen activator inhibitor. *Br Med J* 290:1453, 1985.

82. Madden RM, Levin EG, Marlar RA: Thrombin and the thrombin-thrombomodulin complex interaction with plasminogen activator inhibitor Type-I. *Blood Coagul Fibrinolysis* 2:471, 1991.

83. Meade TW, Vickers MV, Thompson SG, et al: Epidemiological characteristics of platelet aggregability. *Br Med J* 290:428, 1985.

84. Fisher DF Jr, Yawn DH, Crawford ES: Preoperative disseminated intravascular coagulation associated with aortic aneurysms: a prospective study of 76 cases. *Arch Surg* 118:1252, 1983.

85. Collins JA: Blood transfusion and disorders of surgical bleeding. In: Sabiston DC (ed). *Textbook of Surgery.* 14th ed. Philadelphia: WB Saunders, Co.; 85, 1991.

86. Lusher JM, Arkin S, Abildgaard CF, et al: Recombinant factor VIII for the treatment of previously untreated patients with hemophilia A: safety, efficacy, and development of inhibitors. *N Engl J Med* 328:453, 1993.

87. Edmunds LH: Blood contact activation during cardiopulmonary bypass. *J Vasc Surg* 12:213, 1990.

88. Wakefield TW, Shulkin BL, Fellows EP, et al: Platelet reactivity in human aortic grafts: a prospective randomized midterm study of platelet adherence and release products in Dacron and ePTFE grafts. *J Vasc Surg* 9:234, 1989.

89. Hirsh J: Heparin. *N Engl J Med* 324:1565, 1991.

90. Saba HI, Saba SR, Morelli GA: Effect of heparin on platelet aggregation. *Am J Hematol* 17:295, 1984.

91. Kakkar VV: The current status of low-dose heparin in the prophylaxis of thrombophlebitis and pulmonary embolism. *World J Surg* 2:3, 1978.

92. Consensus Conference: Prevention of venous thrombosis and pulmonary embolism. *JAMA* 256:744, 1986.

93. Collins R, Scrigmeour A, Yusuf S, et al: Reduction in fatal pulmonary embolism and venous thrombosis by perioperative administration of subcutaneous heparin: overview of results of randomized trials in general, orthopedic, and urologic surgery. *N Engl J Med* 318:1162, 1988.

94. Salzman EW: Low-molecular weight heparin: is small beautiful? *N Engl J Med* (editorial) 315:957, 1986.

95. Horrow JC: Protamine: a review of its toxicity. *Anesth Analg* 64:348, 1985.

96. Wakefield TW, Ucros I, Kresowik TF, et al: Decreased oxygen consumption as a toxic manifestation of protamine sulfate reversal of heparin anticoagulation. *J Vasc Surg* 9:772, 1989.

97. Pearson PJ, Evora RR, Ayrancioglu K, et al: Protamine releases endothelium-derived relaxing factor from systemic arteries: a possible mechanism of hypotension during heparin neutralization. *Circulation* 86:289, 1992.

98. Wakefield TW, Bies LE, Wrobleski SK, et al: Impaired myocardial function and oxygen utilization due to protamine sulfate in an isolated rabbit heart preparation. *Ann Surg* 212:387, 1990.

99. Morel DR, Zapol WM, Thomas SJ, et al: C5a and thromboxane generation associated with pulmonary vaso- and broncho-constriction during protamine reversal of heparin. *Anesthesiology* 66:597, 1987.

100. Eika C: On the mechanism of platelet aggregation induced by heparin, protamine, and polybrene. *Scand J Haemat* 9:248, 1972.

101. DeLucia A, Wakefield TW, Andrews PC, et al: Efficacy and toxicity of differently charged polycationic protamine-like peptides for heparin anticoagulation reversal. *J Vasc Surg* 18:49–60, 1993.

102. Coon WW: Anticoagulant therapy. *Am J Surg* 150:45, 1985.

103. Hirsh J: Oral anticoagulant drugs. *N Engl J Med* 324:1865, 1991.

104. Hull R, Carter C, Jay R, et al: The diagnosis of acute, recurrent, deep-vein thrombosis: a diagnostic challenge. *Circulation* 67:901, 1983.

105. Coller BS: Platelets and thrombolytic therapy. *N Engl J Med* 322:33, 1990.

106. Jang IK, Gold HK, Ziskind AA, et al: Prevention of platelet-rich arterial thrombosis by selective thrombin inhibition. *Circulation* 81:219, 1990.

107. Addonzio VP Jr, Fisher CA, Jenkin BK, et al: Iloprost (ZK 36 374), a stable analogue of prostacyclin, preserves platelets during simulated extracorporeal circulation. *J Thorac Cardiovasc Surg* 89:926, 1985.

108. Musial J, Niewiarowski S, Rucinski B, et al: Inhibition of platelet adhesion to surfaces of extracorporeal circuits by disintegrins: RGD-containing peptides from viper venoms. *Circulation* 82:261, 1990.

109. Shigeta O, Gluszko P, Downing SW, et al: Protection of platelets during long-term extracorporeal membrane oxygenation in sheep with a single dose of a disintegrin. *Circulation* (suppl II)86:II 398, 1992.

110. Mohr R, Goor DA, Lusky A, et al: Aprotinin prevents cardiopulmonary bypass-induced platelet dysfunction: a scanning electron microscope study. *Circulation* (suppl II)86:II 405, 1992.

111. Quereshi A, Lamont J, Burke P, et al: Aprotinin: the ideal anti-coagulant? *Eur J Vasc Surg* 6:317, 1992.

112. Royston D, Bidstrup BP, Taylor KM, et al: Effect of aprotinin on need for blood transfusion after repeat open-heart surgery. *Lancet* 2:1289, 1987.

113. Salzman EW, Weinstein MJ, Reilly D, et al: Adventures in hemostasis: desmopressin in cardiac surgery. *Arch Surg* 128:212, 1993.

114. Mannucci PM: Desmopressin: a nontransfusional form of treatment for congenital and acquired bleeding disorders. *Blood* 72:1449, 1988.

115. Cole CW, Bormanis J, Luna GK, et al: Ancrod versus heparin for anticoagulation during vascular surgical procedures. *J Vasc Surg* 17:288, 1993.

116. Marder VJ, Sherry S: Thrombolytic therapy: current status (first of two parts). *N Engl J Med* 318:1512, 1988.

117. Fuji S, Sawa H, Saffitz JE, et al: Induction of endothelial cell expression of the plasminogen activator inhibitor type I gene by thrombosis in vivo. *Circulation* 86:2000, 1992.

118. Quinones-Baldrich WJ, Gomes AS: Thrombolytic therapy. In: Rutherford RB (ed). *Vascular Surgery.* 3rd ed. Philadelphia: WB Saunders, Co.; 313, 1989.

119. Comerota AJ, Aldridge SC: Thrombolytic therapy for acute deep vein thrombosis. *Sem Vasc Surg* 5:76:1992.

120. Elliot MS, Immelman EJ, Jeffrey P, et al: A comparative randomized trial of heparin versus streptokinase in the treatment of acute proximal venous thrombosis: an

interim report of a prospective trial. *Br J Surg* 66:838, 1979.

121. Arnsen H, Hoiseth A, Ly B: Streptokinase or heparin in the treatment of deep vein thrombosis: follow-up results of a prospective study. *Acta Med Scand* 211:65, 1982.

122. Kakkar VV, Lawrence D: Hemodynamic and clinical assessment after therapy for acute deep vein thrombosis: a prospective study. *Am J Surg* 150:54, 1985.

123. Porter JM, Taylor LM: Current status of thrombolytic therapy. *J Vasc Surg* 2:239, 1985.

124. Graor RA, Young JR, Risius B: Comparison of cost effectiveness of streptokinase and urokinase in the treatment of deep vein thrombosis. *Ann Vasc Surg* 1:524, 1987.

125. Turpie AGG: Thrombolytic agents in venous thrombosis. *J Vasc Surg* 12:196, 1990.

126. Machleder HI: Evaluation of a new treatment strategy for Paget-Schroetter syndrome: spontaneous thrombosis of the axillary-subclavian vein. *J Vasc Surg* 17:305, 1993.

127. National Heart and Lung Institute Cooperative Study Group: Urokinase pulmonary embolism trial: phase 1 results. *JAMA* 214:2163, 1970.

128. National Heart and Lung Institute Cooperative Study Group: Urokinase-streptokinase embolism trial: phase 2 results. *JAMA* 229:1606, 1974.

129. McNamara TO, Fischer JR: Thrombolysis of peripheral arterial and graft occlusions: improved results using high-dose urokinase. *Am J Roentgenol* 144:769, 1985.

130. McNamara TO, Bomberger RA: Factors affecting initial and 6-month patency rates after intra-arterial thrombolysis with high-dose urokinase. *Am J Surg* 152:709, 1986.

131. Gardiner GA, Sullivan KL: Catheter-directed thrombolysis for the failed lower extremity bypass graft. *Sem in Vasc Surg* 5:99, 1992.

132. Comerota AJ, White JV: Intraoperative, intra-arterial thrombolytic therapy as an adjunct to revascularization in patients with residual and distal arterial thrombus. *Sem in Vasc Surg* 5:110, 1992.

133. Doorey AJ, Michelson EL, Topol EJ: Thrombolytic therapy for acute myocardial infarction: keeping the unfulfilled promises. *JAMA* 268:3108, 1992.

134. Rutherford RB, Jones DN: The role of Dextran-40 in preventing early graft thrombosis. In: Bergqvist D, Lindblad B (eds). *Pharmacological Intervention to Increase Patency after Arterial Reconstructions*. Malmo: ICM AB; 44, 1989.

135. Norris CS, Greenfield LJ, Herrmann JB: Free-floating iliofemoral thrombus: a risk for pulmonary embolism. *Arch Surg* 120:806, 1985.

136. Radomski JA, Jarrell BE, Carabasi RA, Yang SL, Koolpe H: Risk of pulmonary embolus with inferior vena cava thrombosis. *Ann Surg* 53:97, 1987.

137. Berry RE, George JE, Shaver WA: Free-floating deep venous thrombosis: a retrospective analysis. *Ann Surg* 211:719, 1990.

138. Greenfield LJ, Michna BA: Twelve-year clinical experience with the Greenfield vena caval filter. *Surgery* 104:706, 1988.

139. Kantor A, Glanz S, Gordon DH, et al: Percutaneous insertion of the Kimray-Greenfield filter: incidence of femoral vein thrombosis. *AJR* 149:1065, 1987.

140. Greenfield LJ, Cho KJ, Proctor M, et al: Results of a multicenter study of the the modified hook-titanium Greenfield filter. *J Vasc Surg* 14:253, 1991.

141. Greenfield LJ, Proctor MC, Williams DM, et al: Long-term experience with transvenous catheter pulmonary embolectomy. *J Vasc Surg* 18:450, 1993.

CHAPTER 21

Blood Rheology and the Microcirculation

Joseph Kurantsin-Mills, PhD

Blood Rheology

Since William Harvey described the functional principles of the cardiovascular system, there has been a steady progress towards a quantitative analysis of its dynamics and kinetics under physiologic and pathologic conditions. The blood, which subserves the body by supplying nutrients to all cells and removing metabolic wastes for disposal during flow through the microcirculation, has unique physical properties. The study of these physical properties in relation to its flow characteristics is the concern of the science of rheology. The term ''rheology'' was coined by E. C. Bingham[1] to describe the study of the deformation and flow of a material; in other words, the interrelationships of the forces acting on the material, the deformation, strain or flow produced in the material, and the time element involved. All real fluids have internal friction. It is this internal friction that can be quantified as viscosity that distinguishes the flow behavior of different fluids subject to the same pressure (e.g., water and motor oil). Blood is a complex fluid composed of a suspension of cells in plasma. Its flow properties and transport function in the cardiovascular system and particularly in the microcirculation, therefore, depend upon the physical properties of its constituents. The rheological properties of plasma, erythrocytes, leukocytes, and whole blood, and the functional characteristics of the microcirculation under physiologic conditions are discussed in this chapter.

Rheologic Parameters: Definitions

1) Shear stress (τ) is the force (F) acting per unit area (A) in a tangential direction to a surface. Its units are dynes per cm^2 (dyn/cm^2), or Newtons per m^2 (N/m^2), or Pascal (Pa).

2) Shear rate (also referred to as shear strain rate or velocity gradient (γ) is the rate of change of velocity in a moving fluid in a direction of the shear stress with respect to the distance perpendicular to the plane of the shear (Figure 1). Its unit is cm/sec/cm = sec^{-1}.

(3) Viscosity (η) is a measure of the internal resistance of a fluid to flow and is expressed in Newton's law for viscous substances as the ratio:

$$\frac{\text{shear stress} (\tau) \text{dynes cm}^{-2}}{\text{shear rate} (\gamma) \text{sec}^{-1}} \quad \text{or} \quad \frac{\text{dynes.sec}}{\text{cm}^2} \quad \text{or} \quad \text{Poise} \tag{1}$$

One centipoise (cP) = 1/100 poise or 1 mPa.sec.

(4) Newtonian fluids have a constant viscosity at a constant temperature. Therefore, a change in the shear stress applied to the flowing fluid will produce an exactly proportional change in the shear rate. Thus, the viscosity of real Newtonian fluids is independent of flow (shear) rate or tube size. Such fluids include water, physiologic buffers, mercury, and normal plasma.

(5) Non-Newtonian fluids are characterized by the fact that as the shear stress decreases, the resulting shear rate decreases out of proportion. Therefore, the viscosity increases as the shear rate decreases. Blood is a non-Newtonian fluid because, like other suspensions of colloidal particles, its viscosity increases when the flow decreases to very low levels (Figure 2).

(6) Yield Stress. The flow of a fluid such as blood

From *The Basic Science of Vascular Disease.* Edited by Sidawy AN, Sumpio BE, and DePalma RG. Armonk, NY: Futura Publishing Company, Inc.; © 1997.

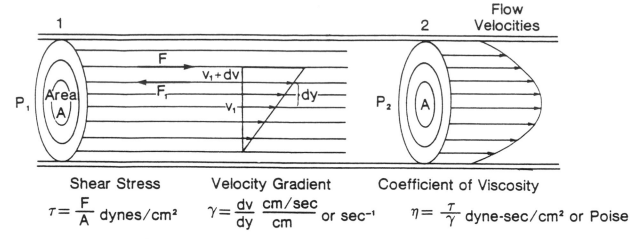

Shear Stress $\quad$ Velocity Gradient $\quad$ Coefficient of Viscosity

$$\tau = \frac{F}{A} \text{ dynes/cm}^2 \qquad \gamma = \frac{dv}{dy} \frac{\text{cm/sec}}{\text{cm}} \text{ or sec}^{-1} \qquad \eta = \frac{\tau}{\gamma} \text{ dyne-sec/cm}^2 \text{ or Poise}$$

Figure 1. Diagram showing the laminar flow of a viscous fluid through a cylindrical tube and a parabolic distribution of velocities. Velocity and flow are maximal along the central axis of the tube and zero at the wall. [The maximum velocity, $V_m = (P_1 - P_2)(R^2)/4\eta$.] The **arrows** indicate that flow is laminar, and that the fluid comprises an infinite number of layers (laminae) that slide past each other without mixing. The velocity gradient in the fluid and the tangential force (**F**) between laminae of fluid are also shown.

is shear- and time-dependent as evidenced by the non-linearity of the shear stress-shear rate curve. Therefore, blood does not flow until a critical shear stress, the yield stress, is exceeded. Such fluids are said to have a yield value or a gel strength and are sometimes described as pseudoplastic. The deformation and flow of materials can be reversible (in which case it is described as elastic) or irreversible (whereby, the material exhibits flow or viscous behavior), or a combination of both properties which is viscoelastic.

(7) Hagen-Poiseuille Law. The relationship between the volumetric flow rate of a homogeneous fluid (viscosity η) in a small cylindrical tube (length, L, radius, r) due to a pressure gradient (P_1-P_2) across the tube (Figure 1) is expressed by the Hagen-Poiseuille law or equation:

$$Q = \frac{(P_1-P_2)\ \pi\ r^4}{8L\eta} \qquad (2)$$

Equation (2) states that the pressure gradient (P_1-P_2) is directly proportional to the volumetric flow rate (Q) when L, r, η are constant. Usually, the equation is simplified as $P_1-P_2 = RQ$, where R is the resistance to flow and is given by:

$$R = \frac{8L\eta}{\pi r4} \qquad (3)$$

Since resistance is the product of blood viscosity and vessel geometry, in the circulation, the contribution of vascular geometry is termed vascular hindrance (Z):

$$Z = R/\eta \qquad (4)$$

or

$$Z \ \alpha \ 1/r^4 \qquad (5)$$

Resistance to blood flow is, therefore, higher in the capillaries where erythrocytes and leukocytes need to deform during entry and transit, and where Z is greater.

(8) Reynold's Number, R_n. The flow of a fluid from point 1 to point 2 (Figure 1) also depends on (a) viscous forces (or laminar viscous energy); (b) inertial forces; (c) the change in kinetic energy; and (d) the difference in potential energy. The flow in the tube may be laminar (or streamlined), or irregular motion of the fluid elements may develop, in which case the flow is described as turbulent. Laminar or turbulent flow in a tube under a given condition may be predicted by Reynold's number, R_n, defined as:

$$R_n = \frac{\rho dv}{\eta}, \qquad (6)$$

where ρ is the density of the fluid, d is the diameter of the tube, v is the mean velocity, and η is the viscosity. Laminar flow is common for $R_n < 2000$; turbulent flow is common for $R_n > 3000$. Therefore, when the viscous term (η) predominates, R_n is low and the fluid flow is laminar. Similarly, when the inertial term (ρdv) is high, R_n is higher and turbulence develops. In the microcirculation, d and v are considerably smaller; R_n is usually less than 1, and flow is laminar.

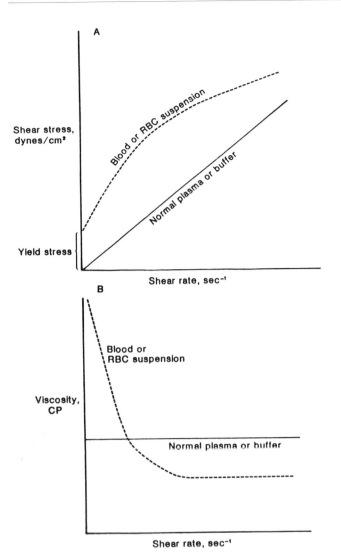

Figure 2. Graphical illustration of the relationship between (**A**) shear stress and shear rate, and (**B**) coefficient of viscosity and shear rate for a Newtonian fluid (plasma or buffered saline) and a non-Newtonian fluid (blood or red blood cell suspension).

Measurement of Viscosity

The viscosity of a fluid can be measured using a variety of viscometers.[2,3] Rotational instruments use one of two basic methods to obtain data. In one method, a sample is placed between two surfaces; one surface is rotated at a fixed speed and the torsional force generated on the other surface is measured. This controlled-rate system utilizes rotational speed as the independent variable, while the measured torque is the dependent variable. In the second method, a torque is applied to one surface, and the rotational speed of the surface is measured. In this case, the torque is the independent variable while the measured motion is the dependent variable. By ramping either the applied torque or rotational speed, the viscosity of a fluid can be mea-

sured. In the definition of viscosity (equation 1), the shear stress is proportional to the torque and the shear rate is proportional to the rotational speed.

The viscometers currently available for such measurements are (a) the rotating cylindrical viscometers, and (b) the cone on plate viscometers. An example of the first group is the Weissenberg Rheogoniometer, a research tool of considerable complexity and cost. It requires large sample volumes and expertise to operate. The Contraves LS-3O (Couette geometry) is a rotational viscometer that is considered precise by many investigators.[4,5] The Carri-Med Controlled Stress Rheometer (of double concentric cylinder geometry) is an instrument that is clinically attractive.[6] However, for several years, the Wells-Brookfield microviscometer (cone and plate geometry) has been the most common device used in research and clinical laboratories (Figure 3).[7] It will be used to illustrate the principles of operation of the viscometer. One study compared the precision and responsiveness of all three viscometers under a variety of flow conditions.[5]

The Wells-Brookfield cone on plate microviscometer consists of a flat stainless steel plate and a stainless steel cone with a very obtuse angle (Figure 3). The apex of the cone is separated from the plate surface by a gap of a few microns and the fluid under study fills

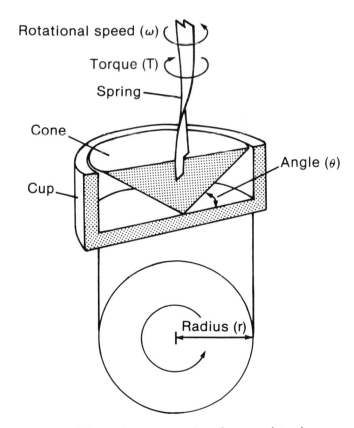

Figure 3. Schematic representation of a cone-plate viscometer (Wells-Brookfield).

this gap. The gap width increases linearly with radial distance as does the linear velocity on the rotating cone. When the cone is rotated at a constant speed (ω), and the flow is tangential, the shear rate and shear stress in a Newtonian fluid are uniform at all points in the gap. If the angle (θ) of the gap is less than 4°, the shear rate is related to the cone rotational speed (ω), and the gap width (c) at any radial distance (r) from the center of the rotating cone. Since the ratio r/c is constant for any value of r and c is maximum at the cone radius (r), the shear rate is given by:

$$\text{Shear rate } (\gamma) = \frac{\omega}{\text{sine } \theta} \text{ sec}^{-1}. \tag{7}$$

The shear stress is equal to the summation of the torque (T) over the conical surface.

$$\text{Shear stress } (\tau) = \frac{3\ T}{2\pi r^3} \text{ dynes/cm}^2 \tag{8}$$

The viscosity (η) is τ/π dynes.sec/cm² or Poise.

Viscosity of Plasma

The major determinants of the rheologic behavior of blood are the plasma, the erythrocytes, and the leukocytes. Plasma is a complex fluid that contains proteins, lipids, and carbohydrates in an aqueous medium of salts, organic chemicals, and various other metabolic products. Serum is the liquid extruded when plasma clots, as thrombin cleaves two pairs of α- and β-chains of soluble fibrinogen to convert it into insoluble and contracting fibrin threads that entrap red cells, platelets, and plasma. Therefore, plasma and serum are distinctly different. Table 1 summarizes the normal concentration and some molecular characteristics of plasma proteins, and the effect of the major proteins on blood viscosity. The viscosity of plasma can be calculated from the measurements of shear stress and

shear rate. It is shear-independent. The plasma viscosity of healthy adult subjects is fairly constant in the basal state.[8,9] This constancy implies a strict dynamic equilibrium between the synthesis and release of new plasma proteins and the continual catabolism of these proteins. The viscosity of a protein solution depends more on the molecular shape of the protein than on its size. The less symmetrical the molecule, the greater effect it exerts on the viscosity of its solution. As shown in Table 1, the concentration of albumin is about 15 times greater than that of fibrinogen. Yet fibrinogen with an axial ratio of 18.75 has a substantial effect on the viscosity of plasma, compared to albumin with an axial ratio of 3.95.[10] Since the plasma viscosity is primarily a function of plasma protein concentration, the mechanisms by which plasma protein cause the change in the plasma viscosity can be attributed to the hydrodynamic influence of the protein molecules.

This influence is the function of the volume concentration of the proteins and the hydrodynamic variation of the effective molecular volume. Among the plasma proteins, fibrinogen is a molecule with a large axial asymmetry, and it is a major determinant of plasma viscosity. However, there are clinical states such as hyperglobulinemia in which the globulins contribute significantly to the plasma viscosity. The protein molecules may be regarded essentially as rigid particles, with effective hydrodynamic volumes that do not change significantly with shearing. Therefore, the plasma viscosity is shear-independent and does not show significant elastic properties.[10] In terms of blood viscosity, the interaction of plasma protein with red blood cells, rather than the proteins themselves, is more significant.

Viscoelastic Properties of Erythrocytes and Leukocytes

The viscosity of blood is defined in terms of the macrorheologic relations between shear stress and

Table 1
Protein Fractions in Human Plasma: Normal Concentrations, Molecular Characteristics and Effect on Viscosity

Protein	Average Conc g/dL	Molecular Weight daltons × 1000	Axial Ratio L/D%	Percent of Total	% Effect on Viscosity
Total	7.5	—	—	100	99
Albumin	4.6	69	3.95	58	30–41
Globulin	2.5	—	—	41	40–42
α_1-globulin	0.2	44–200	4.60	3.0	—
α_2-globulin	0.6	85–820	4.60	10.0	—
β-globulin	0.9	90–20,000	2.33	14.0	—
γ-globulin	0.5	150–960	4.00	12.0	—
Fibrinogen	0.3	340	18.75	3.8	22–24

shear rate. However, these parameters have a microrheologic basis. The microrheologic behavior of erythrocytes and leukocytes plays an important role in governing the flow dynamics of the blood in the microcirculation. Knowledge of the microrheologic properties of these blood cells is, therefore, essential for the understanding of their functional behavior. This includes their deformation during their release from the bone marrow; motion and deformation in blood vessels; the aggregation and disaggregation of red cells; the rolling of leukocytes, for example, on the vascular endothelium; their migration through the venular wall into the interstitium; and their deformation during phagocytosis. The analysis of the microrheologic behavior of erythrocytes and leukocytes requires quantitative knowledge of the morphologic characteristics including volume, surface area, membrane area of the cells and the nucleus. Knowledge of the flow behavior of erythrocytes and leukocytes has been obtained by (a) a technique that involves filtration of the cells through polycarbonate sieves[11-13]; (b) flow through narrow glass capillary tubes[14]; (c) a flow channel where the red blood cells attached to a coverslip are elongated by fluid shear stress[15]; (d) micropipette aspirations[16,17]; and (e) intravital microscopy of the living microcirculation.[18,19] However, quantitative understanding of the cellular mechanics during flow has been obtained mainly by means of micropipette aspiration techniques.

The mechanical properties of blood cells have been studied by measuring their deformation in response to micropipette aspiration under a constant negative pressure. Details of the micropipette technique have been described elsewhere.[16,17] Briefly, the experimental apparatus consists of an inverted microscope whose stage supports a small thermostated chamber filled with about 1 mL of dilute erythrocyte or leukocyte suspension. The microscope is interfaced with a videocamera connected to the eyepiece, a videotimer, and a videomonitor. Micropipettes with internal diameter of about 2 to 4 μm are filled with phosphate buffered saline, pH 7.4, and mounted on a hydraulic micromanipulator. The opposite wide end of the micropipette is connected to an assembly of a pressure tank, a transducer, and a manometer. Using small aspiration pressures (50 to 300 dynes/cm^2), a hemispherical portion of a membrane, or whole cells (in the case of erythrocytes) is aspirated and recorded for analysis. In the case of leukocytes, a theoretical model is applied which treats the cells as a standard solid consisting of an elastic element, K_1, in parallel with a Maxwell element (an elastic element, K_2, in series with a viscous element, μ).[20] The data are analyzed by theoretical modeling, and the rheologic coefficients of the respective cells can be calculated. Table 2 summarizes the geometric characteristics and the viscoelastic coefficients of erythrocytes and leukocytes under small deformation in the micropipette experiments. These mechanical measurements of the physical properties of leukocytes and erythrocytes have confirmed the in situ observations that leukocytes are relatively stiffer than erythrocytes and deform more slowly during capillary flow.[18] These mechanical properties of leukocytes contribute to their flow (rolling) behavior in microvessels.[21]

The filtration technique has also been useful in the determination of microrheologic characteristics of blood cells, as they are filtered through polycarbonate sieves (nuclepore membranes). An attractive presumption of this technique is that it simulates the flow of the cells through capillaries.[11,12] A variety of approaches have been used to determine the rheologic index for these cells in this model flow system. In some techniques, the pressure generated to filter the given volume of cells of known concentration is measured at a constant flow. In others, the volume filtered per unit time under constant pressure is determined. Some in-

Table 2
Geometric and Viscoelastic Characteristics of Erythrocytes and Leukocytes

Cell	Vol. μm^3	Surface Area μm^2	Surface Area Excess	D_{min}[a]	Cellular Viscosity η (Poise) or mPa-sec
Erythrocytes	90	140	44	2.7	0.06
Neutrophils	190	300	84	2.6	130
Eosinophils	206	324	92	2.6	—
Lymphocyte	120	270	130	1.8	
B	—	—	—	—	145
T	—	—	—	—	206
Monocytes	230	430	137	2.2	—

[a] This is the minimum diameter of the cell, with a cylindrical shape and hemispherical caps at a constant area and volume. In the case of leukocytes, the effect of the nucleus is excluded in the calculations. (Summarized with permission from Chien et al.[14])

vestigators measured the time required for the filtration of a known volume of cell suspension.[3] The reliance on a single index for the deformability of these cells has obscured the complexity of the filtration technique. This transient process has various phases which are influenced by several factors including entrance effect at the pores, contaminating leukocytes if red cells are being filtered, clogging of the pores by the leukocytes that are less deformable, and air bubbles that are a constant problem in all such flow systems. A theoretical model for analyzing the pressure-time curve under constant flow rate during filtration of red cells or leukocytes has been developed by Skalak and colleagues.[21] This model allows an accurate estimation of the rheologic index that probably reflects the microrheologic behavior of a homogeneous cell suspension during flow through the pores.

The filterability or flow resistance of erythrocytes or leukocytes through polycarbonate sieves (nuclepore membranes) is measured under constant flow or variable flow. Fresh cell suspension of various proportions in buffered physiologic medium (e.g., phosphate buffered saline or tris-buffered Ringer's solutions pH 7.4, 295 to 300 mosm/kg, containing 0.5 g/dL serum albumin) is pumped through the sieves and the filtration pressure (P_i) recorded as a function of time by means of a transducer and a physiograph recorder. The filtration pressure (P_o) of the buffer solution alone is also recorded. The ratio P_i/P_o is proportional to the cell concentration in the suspension. The mechanical deformation of cells can be visually examined by fixing the nuclepore membrane and processing it for electron microscopy.

Thus, it has been shown that suspensions of leukocytes exhibit much greater flow resistance than equivalent proportions of erythrocytes. As illustrated in Figure 4, the pressure-time curve for a dilute suspension of normal human erythrocytes assessed in the filtration device at a constant flow rate is greater than the suspending buffer. The pore diameter of the filters used for the filtration of the red cells averaged 4.75 ± 0.55 μm and the pore density was $(4.0 \pm 0.1) \times 10^5$ per cm^2 in an effective filtration area of 0.78 cm^2. At the flow rate of 29.5 μL/sec, the cell flux through the pores was 6.43×10^5 cell/sec.

Therefore, during the initial second of the filtration process, the cells-to-pores ratio was about 2.0. The pressure generated by 0.2% erythrocytes suspension, or the buffer alone in PBS flowing through the polycarbonate filters at a constant flow rate of 29.5 μL/sec, is displayed as a function of time. The pressure-time curves for the buffer and the normal erythrocytes are biphasic, and the steady-state pressure values, P_o and P_i, were obtained in about 1 to 2 seconds. Since the buffer and the cell suspension have been pumped through the nuclepore membranes at the same flow rate, the initial pressure values (P_o and P_i) can be nor-

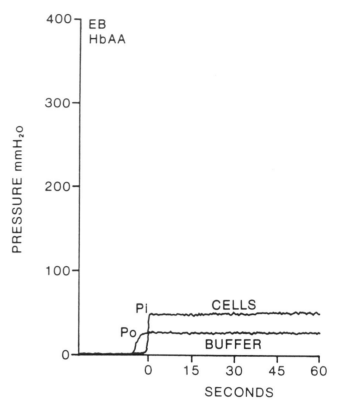

Figure 4. Pressure-time recordings of 0.2% normal human red blood cell suspension in PBS flowing through nuclepore filters, with mean pore diameter of 4.7 ± 0.5 μm at a flow rate 29.5 μL/sec. The pressure-time curves of the buffer are also shown. Po indicates the initial steady-state pressure attained by the buffer, and Pi is that of the suspension. The concentration of leukocytes in all cell suspensions was about 5/mm^3.

malized as the ratio P_i/P_o to reflect the flow resistance of the red cells.[11,13,21] The P_o values at a flow rate of 29.5 μL/sec averaged 26.5 ± 3.5 mm H$_2$O for all filters used in these experiments. Alternatively, the relative resistance of an individual red cell in a pore of the nuclepore membrane is defined by a dimensionless parameter, β, which is the ratio of resistance in a pore bearing a cell to that in a pore filled with suspending buffer only. The reciprocal of β is an index of erythrocyte deformability. From the various dimensionless quantities defined by Skalak et al,[12,13,21] relating pore radius, pore length, red cell volume, (white cell volume), equivalent pore length, and RBC/pore volume ratio (WBC/pore volume ratio), the following equation can be derived in the absence of leukocytes in the buffer medium:

$$\beta = 1 + [(P_i/P_o) - 1]V/h \qquad (9)$$

where V is RBC/pore volume ratio, and h is the fractional volume of cells in the suspension. Because equation 9 was developed for homogeneous cell suspension, modifications may be necessary for mixed blood suspensions in which there are abnormal cells (e.g., sickle cell disease with rigid, irreversibly sickled red cells or leukemia with rigid blast leukemic cells). Figure 5 illustrates the morphology of normal erythrocytes during

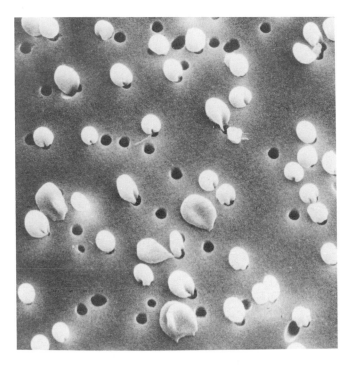

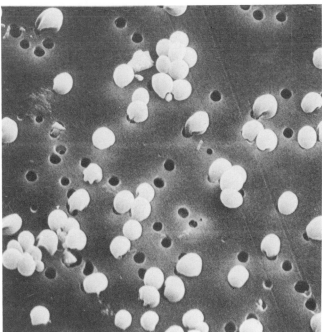

Figure 5. Scanning electron micrographs showing the dynamic deformation of erythrocytes though 5 μm pores of nuclepore membranes. (**Top**) At the entrance side of the filter, and (**bottom**) at the exit side of the same filter where the cells present a bouquet formation from a single pore.

deformation through nuclepore filter pores in a positive pressure filtration device.

In most studies, the red cell deformability is measured in buffer solutions. However, in vivo red blood cells in plasma interact with plasma proteins. The interaction of these proteins with the red cell membrane can change its mechanical properties. Some studies[22] have compared red cell deformability in plasma and phosphate-buffered saline with 1 g/L bovine serum albumin. Red cell deformability was measured using the micropipette and the flow channel techniques. When the micropipette technique is employed, the shear modulus of the membrane is determined by measuring the aspirated length of a red blood cell in a 1 μm pipette at various pressures. The shear modulus of the cells showed 70 $\pm$ 10% increase in plasma as compared with buffer, indicating that the membrane is stiffer in plasma. Red blood cells attached to a glass coverslip elongate due to a shear force induced by a transversal flow of fluid. Red blood cell elongation due to plasma or buffer was measured by means of microscopic video analysis or light transmission through the cells (monolayer technique). The relaxation time was decreased in plasma, and higher stresses were needed to induce the same elongation as in buffer, suggesting that both the dynamic and the static deformabilities were decreased in the presence of plasma. The results of the experiments suggest that red blood cells are less deformable in plasma as compared with buffer.[22]

The average deformability of circulating leukocyte populations has also been assessed by means of the filtration technique. The deformability was estimated in terms of the yield pressure required to dislodge leukocytes trapped in polycarbonate filter (nuclepore) membranes with median pore diameter of 5 μm, and related to the effective mean yield pressure anticipated across an equivalent in vivo capillary network. The computed in vivo yield pressure was significantly lower than the in vitro estimates, due to the larger mean diameter of the capillaries compared to the filter pores, and also their comparatively broader statistical distribution.[22a]

Viscosity of Blood

Because blood is not a homogeneous fluid, its flow behavior depends on the rheologic properties of the plasma and the cells, and the interactions of plasma proteins with red cells. Leukocytes and platelets normally exist in such low fractional volumes that they do not contribute significantly to whole blood viscosity. Under normal physiologic conditions, the apparent viscosity of blood is a function of plasma protein concentration, and the red cell concentration, which is determined by the true cell concentration or the fractional volume of cells due to the variations in cell shape, cell deformability, and cell aggregation.[9,23]

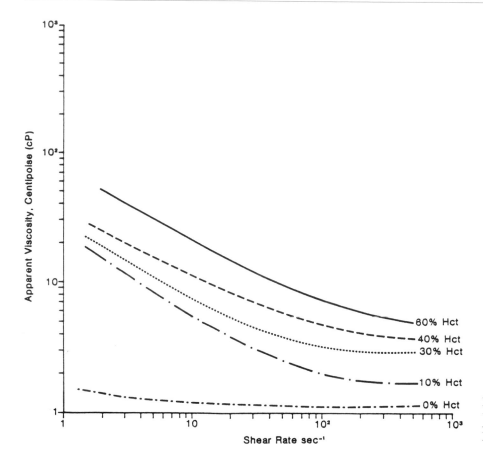

Figure 6. The relation between apparent viscosity and shear rate (Log-log plot) for normal human blood of varying fractional volume of erythrocytes.

As shown in Figure 6, the viscosity of blood within the normal range of arterial or venous hematocrit (e.g., 40% to 45%) increases curvilinearly as the shear rate decreases from 500 sec^{-1} to near zero. This rheologic behavior of the red cells in the flow field is attributed to the shear-dependent changes in their deformation and aggregation.[14,23,24] At very low shear rates (less than 10 sec^{-1}), the red cells form rouleaux due to the bridging of adjacent cells by fibrinogen, globulins, and other large molecules.[23] Accordingly, the energy of aggregation (E_a) represents an algebraic balance of energies between macromolecular bridging energy (E_m) and the electrostatic repulsive energy (E_r) at the cell surface (due to exposed sialic acids of membrane glycoproteins), the mechanical shear energy (E_s), and the energy of cell membrane bending (E_{mb}).[24] Therefore:

$$E_a = E_m - E_r - E_s - E_{mb} \qquad (10)$$

The blood viscosity is also dependent on the concentration of red cells (Figure 7). The relationship between apparent viscosity and hematocrit is curvilinear and convex to the hematocrit axis, with a sharp rise in viscosity as the hematocrit exceeds 40%. A rise in hematocrit from 40% to 60 or 70% that occurs in poly-

cythemia results in more than a tenfold increase in apparent viscosity, with a proportionate effect on the flow resistance of blood. Under low flow states (e.g., 5 to 50 sec^{-1}), the viscosity of blood with a 60% hematocrit will increase more than tenfold, due partly to aggregation of the cells and the shear-dependent reduced deformability. The major factors that influence whole blood viscosity are plasma protein concentration, the red cell concentration, the red cell deformation or deformability, and red cell aggregation (Table 3).[9,23,24]

Variations in the red cell deformability and red cell aggregation contribute quite strongly to the dependence of blood viscosity on shear rate. The time constants for these two processes, namely red cell deformation and red cell aggregation, can be characterized from more or less direct observations.

Micropipette experiments on individual red cells and observations of microcirculatory blood flow indicate that the characteristic red cell deformation time is relatively short, approximately 60 msec or less. The processes of aggregation and disaggregation of red blood cells are probably not symmetrical. The factors that influence the rate of red cell aggregation include cell and aggregate collision frequency, which is itself

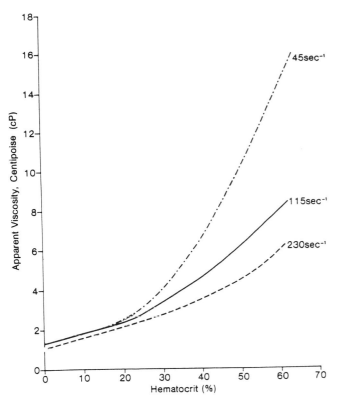

Figure 7. The relation between apparent viscosity of blood and increasing hematocrit illustrated for shear rates of 46 sec^{-1}, 1.15 sec^{-1}, and 230 sec^{-1}. Temperature, 37°C.

a function of hematocrit, shear rate and concentration of fibrinogen, globulins, or other factors, such as red cell shape, deformability, and surface charge. Disaggregation depends on the rate of development of local forces on the aggregate during changes in flow conditions and the shear rate. It is known that stresses greater than 0.1 dyn/cm^2 cause rouleaux disaggregation.[14] These observations suggest that the relatively high shear rates existing in the normal circulation keep the blood viscosity rather low by preventing red cell aggregation and inducing deformation. The ability of the normal red blood cell to deform in response to the fluid shear stresses stems from the fluid nature of the internal hemoglobin solution, the flexibility of the red cell membrane, and the existence of an excess membrane area relative to the cell volume. Such properties make it possible for the normal discoid erythrocytes with a major diameter of about 8 μm to traverse small channels, such as capillaries in the heart and skeletal muscle, with an average diameter of about 5 μm

Effects of Vessel Diameter

The viscosity of blood is also related to the diameter of the blood vessel. Studies of laminar blood flow through cylindrical tubes of various sizes have shown a decrease in blood viscosity in tubes with internal di-

Table 3
The Major Factors that Influence Blood Viscosity

Factor	Effect on Blood Viscosity
Plasma proteins	Concentration-dependent: an increase causes a rise in blood viscosity due to hydrodynamic variations of the effective molecular volume, e.g., fibrinogen with a large axial asymmetry increases plasma viscosity more than albumin (globular shape) at the same plasma concentration.
Cell concentration	A rise in the true fractional volume of red cells increases blood viscosity. The viscosity increases exponentially as the fractional volume of cells (hematocrit) approaches 60%. The blood viscosity also rises steeply as the true fraction of leukocytes approaches 20%.
Cell deformation	The deformability of red cells reduces blood viscosity in large vessels. Cell deformability is itself determined by cell concentration, cell geometry, membrane viscoelasticity, internal fluid viscosity, and mean shear rate.
Cell aggregation	Red cell aggregation is the result of bridging of adjacent (rouleaux) cells by fibrinogen and globulins absorbed to the surfaces. Under low shear rate, rouleaux formation is favored and blood viscosity increases. When the shear rate is increased, the rouleaux are broken down to shorter rouleaux resulting in a decrease in blood viscosity.

ameters less 300 μm.[25] This decrease in the blood viscosity in these tubes is explained by a decrease in the tube hematocrit, as compared with the feed hematocrit. This reduction in the tube hematocrit results from the screening of cells at the tube entrance and/or faster transit of red blood cells than plasma. This occurs because the cells travel preferentially in the center of the tube, a phenomenon called axial streaming or the Fahraeus-Lindqvist effect.[26] The concentration of red cells at the center of the tube or vessel during laminar flow results from the rapid rate of change in velocity profiles near the wall. This velocity gradient pulls the long axis of the erythrocyte parallel to the direction of the flow, and forces the cell toward the center of the tube where the flow is more stable. The process leaves a relatively cell-free layer of plasma near the wall and leads to a phenomenon Krogh[27] termed "plasma skimming." The phenomenon is further illustrated by experiments conducted by Barbee and Cokelet.[26] The relative hematocrit of blood flowing from a feed reservoir through narrow capillary tubes (inner diameter 25 to 800 μm) was determined. The relative hematocrit is the ratio of the hematocrit in the capillary tube to that of the feed tube. A graph of relative hematocrit, as a function of capillary tube diameter, showed that for tubes of 500 μm or greater, the relative hematocrit was about 1.0. As the diameter of the capillary tubes decreased, there was a progressive decline in the relative hematocrit. For 30 μm capillary tubes, the relative hematocrit was about 0.6. Axial streaming does not occur in vessels or tubes with inner diameters equal to or greater than 1000 μm because the velocity changes rather slowly. As a result, forces associated with the velocity gradient are insufficient to realign the cells from random radial collisions. When the tube diameter is further reduced below 8 μ, which approximates the diameter of human red blood cells, the blood viscosity increases. This inverse Fahraeus-Lindqvist effect can be explained by the necessity of the red blood cells to deform during passage through these narrow channels. Therefore, the Fahraeus-Lindqvist effect plays a significant role in decreasing blood viscosity in arterioles and venules, but the phenomenon is not significant in capillaries where the deformability of red blood cells becomes predominant.

Physiologic Variations in Plasma and Blood Viscosity

Longitudinal studies have shown that healthy individuals maintain their own plasma viscosity value remarkably constant for several years. However, the blood viscosity shows individual variations under different physiologic conditions. The viscosity of plasma in a healthy adult population falls within a restricted range of about 1.16 to 1.35 cP at 37°C. A small change of 0.03 to 0.05 cP may occur in response to certain physiologic stimuli. The normal physiologic variations in blood viscosity can be attributed to changes in plasma protein concentration and/or hematocrit. Table 4 summarizes the effects of various factors on normal plasma and blood viscosities.

The Microcirculation

Topographic Features

So far, our discussion has been restricted to aspects of the systemic circulation where there is an interplay of inertial forces, pressure forces, and viscous forces during flow. Some of the fluid dynamic phenomena associated with the microcirculation will now be described.

The microcirculation is a collective term used to describe the smallest components of the cardiovascular system, namely the arterioles, the capillaries, and the venules. Each component of the microcirculation has its own characteristic structure and function. In most microvascular beds, the network architecture is designed such that there is a succession of branching arterioles and a sequential division of arterioles into smaller diameter branches that are characterized as bifurcations or branch points. This branching pattern has also been described as dichotomous because from each parent arteriole emerge two offspring, and each offspring gives rise to two additional offspring, and so on. There is also a decrease in the diameter of the microvessels with each successive division. This dichotomously branching system of arterioles and precapillaries is, therefore, divergent and culminates at the capillaries. The venous collecting microvessels then emerge from the capillaries as confluent systems which would be the mirror image of the arterial distribution system (Figure 8).

The lymphatic capillaries constitute extravascular closed-end networks intermeshed with the blood capillaries. Although the lymphatics are not ordinarily considered a structural part of the microcirculation, they are conceptually a functional component of the microcirculation. The blood capillaries, the lymphatic capillaries, and the interstitial spaces of tissue that constitute the functional microcirculation are often referred to as the microvascular bed. Each organ of the body exhibits its own characteristic architectural organization of the microcirculatory bed.[35,36] Therefore, it is not correct to assume that the information obtained on one organ system would necessarily apply to another

Table 4
Physiologic Factors that Affect Plasma and Blood Viscosities

Factor	Effect on Viscosity	Reference
Neonate:	At birth, lower plasma protein concentration results in lower plasma viscosity; however, highter Hct of 50–54% and low RBC deformability results in higher viscosity than adult blood. Viscosity falls in the neonate until 5 months of age due the decline in Hct. The Hct rises gradually from 5 months to 18 years, with parallel changes in viscosity.	28
13–18 yrs	Gender differences in viscosity appear due to Hct.	
18–80 yrs	There are differences in viscosity within the sexes. Females 56–80 yrs. have slightly higher blood viscosity vs 15–35-year-olds due to higher plasma fibrinogen concentration.	8 29
Sex	Males have higher Hct (45–47%) than females (40–42%) and, therefore, higher blood viscosity.	
Menstruation	The current literature suggests that both plasma and blood viscosities in healthy young women show temporal variations in the menstrual cycle. Plasma and blood viscosities show a significant premenstrual rise. Plasma viscosity rises, with fibrinogen levels during the luteal phase, and then declines throughout the cycle. Blood viscosity also falls during menstruation. These variations correspond to changes in Hct, red cell deformability, and aggregation.	30 31
Oral Contraception	Plasma viscosity rises slightly from strongly progestagenic combined pills due to elevated fibrinogen levels. However, whole blood viscosity is not significantly altered by the pill.	31 32
Pregnancy	Plasma fibrinogen and viscosity both rise during the first trimester. However, plasma viscosity decreases to the non-pregnant level by term, while fibrinogen concentration peaks at 36 weeks. Whole blood viscosity declines significantly during pregnancy, corresponding to the decrease in the Hct (physiologic anemia).	30 32 34
Diurnal	Blood viscosity exhibits rhythmic, temporal variations during the 24-hr cycle. It peaks at 8:00 a.m., decreases to a minimum between 12:00 a.m. and 3:40 a.m. There are corresponding variations in plasma protein concentration and Hct.	23 33
Exercise	Severe exercise is accompanied by dehydration, a decrease in plasma volume, and an increase in plasma viscosity. The resulting hemoconcentration may also increase blood viscosity. The average plasma viscosity of a group of joggers was lower than the value for a matched group of non-joggers measured at rest.	23 34
Food	The consumption of ordinary amounts of food and drink does not affect plasma and blood viscosities. Ingestion of a high-fat diet does not alter blood or plasma viscosity. However, in the light of the interaction between blood lipids and red cells, and the circulatory flow dynamics, this subject requires further study. Ingestion of large volumes of water (e.g., 1 liter saline) causes hemodilution and a decrease of 0.05–0.08 cP in plasma viscosity.	23 34

Hct = Hematocrit

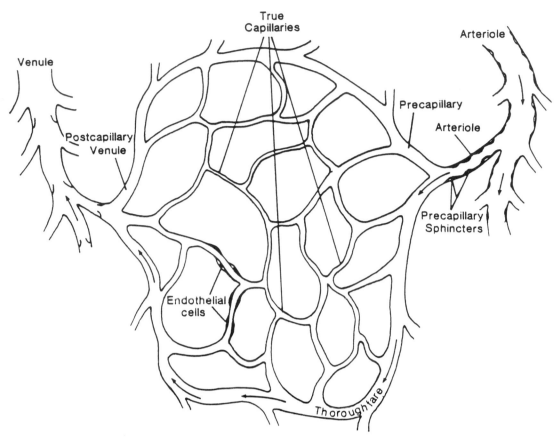

Figure 8. Schematic diagram of a microvascular bed showing the complex, dichotomous branching system and topography of arterioles, capillaries, and venules. The assumed complete symmetry does not require that all pressure-flow statistics and rheologic parameters at corresponding branch points be equal. This representation is idealized and differs significantly from any microvascular bed found in vivo.

organ system. In spite of the organizational and architectural heterogeneity that is seen among the different microvascular beds, the knowledge we have gained during the past several decades has forced upon us certain basic concepts of the independent nature of microcirculatory behavior.[35–37]

The conceptual framework ascribes certain basic attributes to the microcirculation. These attributes are: a) the network between the feeding arteriole and the collecting venule has an overall modular design; b) the blood flow is determined by the balance of viscous stresses and pressure gradient; c) the individuality of the blood cells can be recognized as seen in intravital microscopy; d) the capillary endothelium provides a unique barrier for blood-tissue exchange of materials along simple diffusion and osmotic gradients; e) within a given tissue, exchange of fluid and dissolved solutes between the blood and the interstitium is adjusted to meet local demand; and f) the smooth muscle of the microvasculature orchestrates the regulation of blood flow locally.[36,37] The determinants of microcirculatory

blood flow are, therefore, the vascular factors and the blood rheologic factors and the complex interreaction between them. The blood rheologic factors include the blood velocity (i.e., shear rates), the pressure gradient, the hematocrit, viscosity, and leukocyte count as they apply to the single unbranched microvessels and the network branch points. The determinants of this relationship have been shown to include red cell deformability and aggregation, leukocyte deformability, and leukocyte endothelial interaction, all of which contribute to the specification of blood viscosity in vivo. The vascular factors are the topographic features of the network organization from the arterioles to the venules. Direct topographic effects on the resistance to flow within an individual microvessel are the summation of the alterations in the microvascular luminal diameter brought about by regulatory mechanisms within the module. Furthermore, the branching of the network plays an important part in dictating the resistance to flow within the network and the local apportionment of the overall distribution of pressure and flow.[36,37]

Early Studies

Earlier, in vitro studies that have formed the conceptual framework for the rheology of blood, namely the role of viscosity and shear rate in the flow of blood, were discussed. The following paragraphs relate these in vitro rheologic measurements to the in vivo microvascular behavior. Whittaker and Winton attempted one of the earliest studies in the early 1930s to determine in vivo viscosity of blood.[38] These investigators perfused the isolated hindlimb of dogs with physiologic fluids and red cell suspensions, and calculated the in vivo pressure flow data, the relative resistance, and the relative viscosity of the suspensions. The in vivo viscosity was always less than that measured in a tube viscometer. Whittaker and Winton attributed this discrepancy to the Fahraeus-Lindqvist effect. However, later studies by Benis et al[39] corrected for the inertial effect of the initial experiment and observed a good agreement between the relative viscosity determined in vivo and that measured in vitro using the cylindrical viscometer. Perfusion studies of this type have provided significant information on the pressure-flow relationships in an organ or tissue between the supplying artery and the draining vein. Such studies have also provided insight into the sites of resistance in a microvascular network in a particular organ, and the contribution of these sites to the modulation of the overall arteriovenous resistance to blood flow by vasomotor adjustments or rheologic parameters of the blood. With the development of new technology for in vivo measurements of rheologic parameters, it is now possible to study pressure-flow relationships and the effects of hematocrit, hemoglobin oxygen saturation, microvessel diameter, and other variables in single vessels, and relate the data to the network topography, the microcirculation, and the macrocirculation. Such studies have been pursued by several investigators.[37]

Measurement of Microvascular Hemodynamics

Microvessel Pressures

Pressures in microvessels have been measured by two methods. The first is direct cannulation of these vessels (5 to 100 μm) with glass micropipettes. The second method is indirect mechanical obstruction of the vessels and release until flow reappears under known pressures.[40-44] Accurate estimates of microvessel pressures were first obtained by E. M. Landis[40,41] using micropipettes filled with a dyed salt solution inserted into the mesenteric vessels of frogs, rats, and guinea pigs, as well as human nailfold capillaries. The micropipette was linked to a hydraulic micropressure sensor system. By observing the dye-plasma interface in micropipettes until the interface did not move, Landis measured average microvascular pressures. Modern methods for microvascular pressures are based on this same principle. Microvessels are cannulated with glass micropipettes (2 to 4 μm i.d.) filled with 1.2 M NaCl which has an electrical resistivity much less than that of blood. The micropipette is connected to a micromanipulator interfaced with a low compliance pressure transducer and an electronic servo-controlled micropressure measuring system.[42-44]

Microvessel Blood Flow

Microvessel blood velocity has been measured by: a) direct or supplemented visual methods; b) photographic methods; c) cinematographic methods; d) electro-optical methods; and e) laser-Doppler techniques. The first two methods are antiquated and only of historical interest. Cinematographic methods are sometimes used under certain experimental conditions, but will not be considered further. Current techniques that have given us some insight into microvascular blood flow are the electro-optical and the laser-Doppler techniques.[44-50]

Electro-optical Techniques: The electro-optical technique has been available for about three decades. It is based on the principle that differences in the light transmitted by red cells and plasma during flow vary in intensity. Therefore, if the temporal variation in light intensity is converted into electrical signals, the amplitude of the signal will be proportional to the instantaneous light detected by a phototransistor sensor, after appropriate amplification. In 1967, Wayland and Johnson[47] reported a method in which two photosensors were positioned in the center of a blood vessel image separated by a distance, d. In arterioles, capillaries, and venules, approximately the same temporal signs was recorded by the sensors. In an ideal situation, the upstream $f_u(t)$ and the downstream $f_d(t)$ signals should be identical in amplitude, frequency, and waveform, except for displacement in time which is equal to the transit time (T) between the photosensors. Therefore, the velocity of red cells should be d mm/T sec.

In reality, the photosensor responses are not identical due to radial distribution of red cells in the vessel, blood velocity, vessel diameter, the distance between $f_u(t)$ and $f_d(t)$, signal-to-noise ratio, and other factors. These limitations were corrected by cross-correlation involving mathematical and electronic processes used to evaluate the degree of similarity between the two signals.[48] The computation of red cell transit time (T) involves storage and delay of the

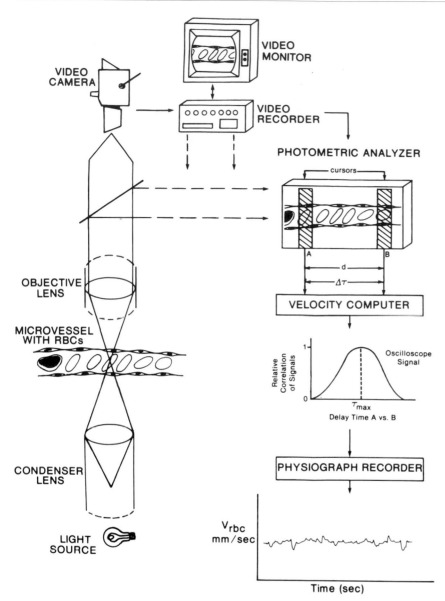

Figure 9. Schematic representation of the principles of operation of the dual-slit velocity measuring device used in intravital video-microscopy observatory for studying microvascular flow dynamics in an experimental animal. (Reproduced with permission from Reference 50.)

$f_u(t)$ relative to $f_d(t)$. When the two signals are multiplied by each other, the product will be maximum when a specific delay causes the greatest coincidence and similarities between the two signals. The cross-correlation function $\phi_{ud}(\tau)$ for the maximum similarity of $f_u(t)$ and $f_d(t)$ has been expressed by Silva and Intaglietta[49] as:

$$\phi_{ud}(\tau) = \frac{\lim}{T} \frac{1}{T} f_u(t)f_d(t + \tau)dt. \qquad (11)$$

where T is the duration for matching the signals, and is far greater than τ, the delay time required to maximize the value of $\phi_{ud}(\tau)$ relative to some initial time, t. A velocity correlation computer calculates the correlation function for various time delays less than T, and displays the results on an oscilloscope for visual check for τ max. The velocity, d/τ_{max} is then computed, and registered on a meter and a recorder (Figure 9). The technique has been called two-slit or dual-slit temporal correlation method. A variation of the technique is the videometric dual-window method.[49] In spite of the complex electronic instrumentation and engineering involved in the technique, the instrument that is commercially available (Instrumentation for Physiology and Medicine Inc., San Diego, CA) is relatively easy to use. Figure 9 illustrates an experimental setup of intravital video-microscope observatory for studying microvascular flow dynamics in tissues such as the mesentery and muscle of experimental animals.

Laser-Doppler Flowmeter

In laser-Doppler flowmetry (LDF), two coherent laser rays are superimposed by crossing them within the microvessel under study and, thereby, causing interference fringes, resulting in scattered light from the beams. The laser light scattered by the flowing red cells is shifted in frequency, and this Doppler frequency shift is proportional to the velocity of the red cells.[46] Mishina and associates[51] proposed a laser-Doppler microscope that used 1 mW He-Ne laser to produce two parallel beams. With appropriate optics, the two beams crossed at a focal plane that determined the sample volume. Blood cells flowing through this focal plane scattered the light from both beams. Alternatively, a simple incident He-Ne laser beam may be used to illuminate the blood vessel and then compared to a reference beam in order to measure the Doppler frequency shift. In the laser microscope, the scattered light is collected by the objective and focused onto a phototransistor sensor as a pulse signal with a history of a few milliseconds required for the transit of the red cells through the interference fringes. The wave period, ω, of the pulse signal is related to mean flow velocity, V, of the red cells as follows:

$$1/\omega = f = 2V.\sin(\theta/2\lambda) \qquad (12)$$

where f is the frequency of a pulse signal, θ is the intersecting angle of the beams, and λ is the wavelength of the incident laser beams. The laser beams can be made as small as 5 μm in diameter to permit measurement in very small capillaries. Stern[52] introduced a specific laser-Doppler technique for measuring skin microcirculation which was based on the same principles discussed above. Holloway and Watkins[53] and later Nilsson et al[54] and Bonner et al[55] refined the method to make it practical and clinically useful. A low power He-Ne laser generates a single frequency of 632.8 nm light via an optical fiber onto a 1 mm^2 area of the skin surface and to a depth of about 1.0 to 1.5 mm. The change in frequency (the Doppler shift) is received by a second optical fiber and transmitted to a photosensor for amplification and signal processing. The method has been applied extensively to several different types of biomedical and clinical research.[46,56,57] Although the output of the laser-Doppler velocimeter is in millivolts, it provides relative correlation with plethysmography, microspheres, and ^{133}xenon washout techniques in which skin blood flow is expressed as mL/min^{-1} or mL/min^{-1} 100 g^{-1} tissue.[58] However, fundamental differences exist in the parameters measured by these methods. Commercial models of the LDF for measuring blood flow of the skin and also internal organs are currently available from Transonic Systems Inc., Ith-aca, NY 14850 (as ALF 21 Laser-Doppler Microvascular Perfusion Monitor); PERIMED, Stockholm, Sweden PERIMED Laser-Doppler flowmeter [as PeriFlux PF3 & PF4]; and TSI Inc. St. Paul, MN 55164 (as LASERFLO Blood Perfusion Monitor BPM 403).

Pressure-Flow Relations in the Microcirculation

Systematic insight into the characteristics of intravascular pressures and red cell velocities in small vessels resulted from the work of Zweifach, Lipowsky, Johnson and associates, among others.[59] These studies have elucidated the functional distribution of pressure, velocity, volumetric flow, and hematocrit within successive segments of the network hierarchy in various tissues such as the mesentery, the omentum, and muscle. Figure 10 illustrates the arteriovenous distribution of intravascular pressures as measured by the servo-null micropressure method and red cell velocity as measured by the "two-slit" photometric technique as a function of microvascular luminal diameter. The red cell flow (Q) can be calculated from the mean flow velocity (V_{mean}) using the corrected ratio ($V_{ibc} = 1.6$ V_{mean}) and multiplied by the cross-sectional area ($Q = V_{mean} \pi D^2/4$) of the vessel. The diameters of the vessel indicated in the horizontal axis refer to the position of the vessel within the successive hierarchy of the network. Figure 10 also illustrates the functional apportionment of pressure and flow in dissimilar microvasculatures of two splanchnic beds (the mesentery and omentum) and two skeletal muscles (tenuissimus and spino-trapezius). The data, obtained from animals whose arterial pressure were in the normal range, emphasize the variations in the distribution of these hemodynamic parameters in the different tissues, which is dependent upon the characteristic network topography, the overall arteriovenous pressure drop and the rheologic properties of blood. The microvascular hemodynamics of the mesentery (modular network) show a rapid decline in the pressure within the 15 to 35 μm arterioles, and a minimum blood flow in the 10 to 15 μm postcapillary vessels. In the omentum (dichotomizing network), the pressure and flow exhibit maximum decline in the capillaries. The tenuissimus and the spino-trapezius muscles both exhibit maximum pressure and flow decline at the true capillary level. Thus, the pressure drops in the arterioles of the skeletal muscle are larger than those of the splanchnic beds. The pressure gradient, dP/dL, measured by inserting two pressure micropipettes, separated by a distance, L, into side branches of a given vessel, increased curvilinearly as the vessel size decreased.[59,60]

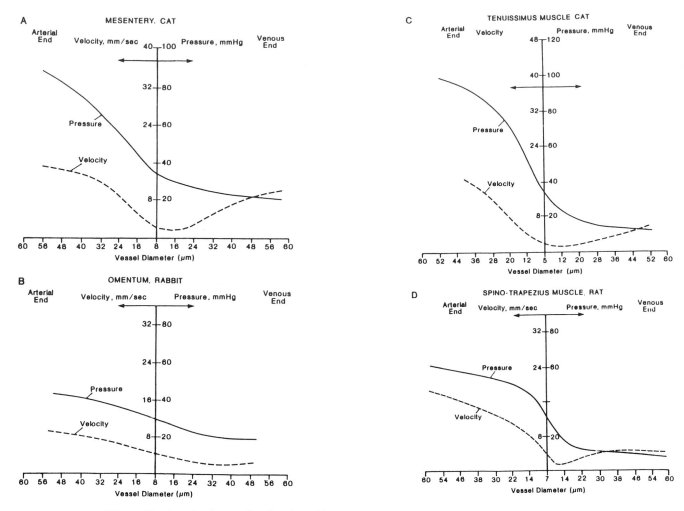

Figure 10. Arteriovenous distribution of intravascular pressure (by servo-null method) and red cell velocities (two-slit photometric technique) as a function of microvessel luminal diameter. (Adapted with permission from References 59 and 60.)

The pressures recorded in these microvessels also show temporal oscillations with normal amplitudes of 1 to 2 mm Hg. Other oscillations with high amplitudes and higher periodicity are also detectable. These pressure variations indicate that the cardiac pulses propagate ripples to the capillary level that are dissipated by the dominance of viscous stresses.[59]

Furthermore, the resistance of the blood during flow in these vessels rises sharply as the blood courses the precapillary network and achieves a maximum value at the true capillary level. The flow of the blood is also minimal in the true capillaries. Further calculation of the resistance per unit length of vessel shows that the fourth power function of the relationship, as predicted by the Poiseuille's equation, is dominant as the blood flows through various segments of the network with varying ranges of vessel diameters. Therefore, it appears that in the normal flow state, the fourth power radius relationship is the dominant factor in specifying intravascular resistance both at the network

level and at the global level within the microvasculature. Variations from this rule may be attributed to local variations in the mechanisms regulating of flow within the microvascular bed.[59]

Microvessel Hematocrit and Apparent Viscosity

Hematocrit is an important factor in the flow of blood in microvessels, in the delivery of oxygen to tissues, and as a determinant of the apparent viscosity of blood in various segments of microcirculation. In recognition of this fact, several studies have evaluated the systemic and microvascular distribution of hematocrit. As a consequence of these numerous studies, two basic concepts relating to microvascular hematocrit are now accepted.[61,62] The first is the actual microvessel or dynamic hematocrit which refers to the value that can be determined by instantaneously stopping the

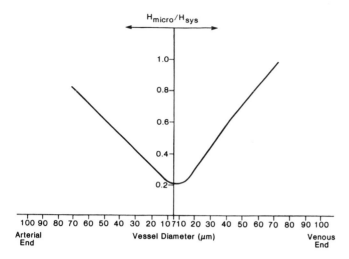

Figure 11. Arteriovenous distribution of microvessel hematocrit (Hmicro) in cat mesentery normalized with respect to systemic values (Hsys) and plotted as a function of vessel diameter. (Adapted with permission from Reference 62.)

flow of blood in a vessel and measuring the packed fractional volume of cells as done in centrifugation. The second is the discharge hematocrit or outflow hematocrit which is defined as that value obtained by collecting the effluent of blood flowing in a vessel into the hypothetical mixing cup and determining its packed fractional volume of cells.

In spite of these conceptual differences, actual measurements of the hematocrit in microvessels have shown that the intravascular hematocrit value decreases progressively from the large arteries through the arterioles to capillaries, and shows the lowest values in the true capillaries. The value of the hematocrit then increases from the venules progressively to the values measured in the large veins. Figure 11 shows the diagram of the arteriole-venous distribution of microvessel hematocrit in the normal flow state of the mesenteric microvasculature of the cat. For microvessels larger than 20 μm in diameter, the microvessel hematocrit was determined by the optical density method. In smaller microvessels, the hematocrit was determined by micro-occlusion technique, that is, rapid occlusion of the vessels and cell counting. The solid curve is a piece-wise cubic spline smoothing (a statistical procedure) of the 150 individual measurements completed in several animals. Arteriolar hematocrits averaged 15.9%, venular hematocrits averaged 17.3%, and capillary hematocrit averaged 8% to 10%. Such experimental data have been obtained using the cheek pouch of the hamster, the rat and cat mesentery, and the rat cremaster muscle.[59,60–62] One reason for the unsteadiness and the wide scatter of hematocrit in these microvessels is the unsteadiness of velocity in these vessels. Because many factors influence the relationship between velocity and hematocrit in vivo, only

simple model studies have been used to obtain definitive mathematical relationships between the two.[63–66]

The apparent viscosity of blood in individual microvessels has been determined by simultaneous measurements of the pressure difference and flow within individual microvessels of the mesentery by Lipowsky et al.[60,62] Together with the geometric parameters of length and radius, the apparent blood viscosity of blood in these vessels was then estimated using Poiseuille's equation (equation 2). The apparent viscosity declined slowly from 3 to 4 cP in the 60 μm arterioles to approximately 2 cP in the precapillaries, and showed a slight rise to about 3 cP in the postcapillary vessels. The slight elevation of viscosity in the small venules may be due to higher hematocrits, red cell aggregation, adhesion of the leukocytes to the endothelium, and lower shear rates. A graph of in vivo viscosity as a function of microvessels luminal diameter showed that the lowest apparent viscosity observed in the precapillaries and capillaries was about 60% of the value in the large vessels. However, it appears that the integrated apparent viscosity in the microvascular bed would be higher than the lowest values in single vessels.[62] It should be noted that the apparent viscosity deduced by these microvascular techniques most probably underestimates the true values, due to the inability to estimate vessels with no cells flowing through them or those with too low a hematocrit and, hence, viscosity to be accessible for accurate measurements.

Other studies[62] were undertaken to investigate the variability of the apparent viscosity with hematocrit in arterioles, with luminal diameters ranging from 24 μm to 47 μm. The measurements were conducted in the mesentery of the cat at high shear rates averaging 2430 sec⁻¹, and no leukocyte adhesion to the endothelium. Within a 95% confidence limit, the values of apparent viscosity calculated from the Poiseuille equation were 1.5 to 2.5 cP for hematocrits ranging from 2% to 36%. These results were reasonably similar to data obtained in vitro using the cone-plate Weissenberg rheogoniometer at a shear rate of 2000 sec⁻¹. Therefore, at comparable hematocrits and shear rates, the apparent viscosity of blood will be essentially the same in most vessels regardless of their size.[26,62]

Blood Flow Through Bifurcations or Branch Points

A characteristic feature of the microvascular hemodynamics is the continuous nonhomogeneity of the blood flow. It has been observed many times that the velocity, direction of movement of blood cells, and the number of capillaries with active red cell flow in any microvascular network exhibit significant temporal and spatial fluctuations, and heterogeneity. The dichotomous configuration of most networks, involving segmental and successive branching of arterioles into smaller diameter offspring vessels, influences the distribution of pressure, flow, and hematocrit at the bifurcations. A number of studies,[63–66] have demonstrated that red cell distribution at arteriolar and capillary bifurcations is determined by the following parameters: diameter ratio of the cells and vessels, shape and deformability of the cells, the hematocrit in the parent vessel, pressure and shear stress distribution at the branch point, and the ratio of flow velocities in the offspring vessels downstream. Thus, for example, measurement of intravascular pressures in an arteriolar network, with diameters ranging from 50 to 20 μm, showed that the magnitude of the pressure drop from an arteriole to the branching vessels increased remarkably with a decrease in the ratio of their respective diameters.[59,60]

Theoretical and experimental studies using both model systems,[63,64] as well as the living microcirculation,[65,66] have shown that the distribution of red cells at bifurcations depends on the pressure distribution and the shear stress acting on the cell at the time when it is located at the branch point of the vessel. The cell is always pulled into the branch vessel with the faster stream. These studies confirmed a nonlinear relationship between hematocrit ratio and velocity ratio, as well as a critical flow ratio beyond which red cells enter the branch vessel with faster stream. Furthermore, the entrance of a red cell or leukocyte into a branch vessel at a bifurcation causes an increase in local resistance and decreases the flow in that vessel, such that the next red cell enters the other branch vessel. Therefore, red cells flowing to a bifurcation alternate the entrance into the two branch vessels and, thereby, adjust their distribution. In the case of a leukocyte entering a branch vessel, its high coefficient of viscosity, lower deformability, and larger effective volume causes a more substantial increase in the local resistance than the red cell. As a result, subsequent red cells arriving at such a bifurcation are diverted into the other branch vessel due to the difference in viscosity between the leukocyte and the red cells. This process continues until there is a balance in the resistance in the branch vessels. According to Schmid-Schonbein et al,[66] every leukocyte entering a branch vessel where the ratio of cell diameter/vessel diameter is 0.85 may be equivalent to 20 to 30 red cells in terms of resistance change. Therefore, the entry and distribution of leukocytes into the capillary network can exert a considerably large effect on the distribution of red cells.

Leukocyte-Endothelial Cell Adhesion

Under normal physiologic conditions, erythrocytes and platelets in the bloodstream do not adhere to the vascular endothelium. On the other hand, intravital microscopy has revealed neutrophils rolling along the endothelial lining of postcapillary venules.[67] Several studies have reported that there are hemodynamic and network topographic features that affect leukocyte distribution throughout the microvasculature.[59,67] It is, therefore, widely recognized that leukocyte margination, or their outward radial migration within the microvascular lumen, is an essential initial step for the initial contact between the leukocyte and endothelium, described as leukocyte rolling, and the firm stationary leukocyte adhesion to the endothelium. Adherence of circulating neutrophils to the microvascular endothelium is, therefore, the initial step in diapedesis, the process by which leukocytes emigrate through microvessels and accumulate at sites of tissue injury. Microvascular studies in vivo have demonstrated that hydrodynamic forces due to blood flow velocity and shear rates exert substantial influence on leukocyte-endothelial cell interaction in arterioles and venules.[67] An interesting and consistent observation is that leukocyte margination or leukocyte-endothelial interactions in vivo are mainly confined to the postcapillary venules of the microcirculation and are rarely observed in the arterioles.[59,67,68] Studies by several investigators have provided some explanations for the preferential margination of leukocytes along the venular endothelium: a) the existence of lower shear rates in the venules compared to the arterioles, b) radial shear forces that act in concert with the topographic convergence of capillaries into venules to augment the rolling of leukocytes along the venular walls[59,67,68]; the heterogeneous distribution of receptors or adhesion molecules between arterioles and venules.[69]

Several studies have documented that leukocyte rolling in vivo depends on the function of the selectin family of adhesion receptors, which comprises three molecules sharing common structural features including a functionally important NH_2-terminal lectin domain. Adhesion molecules are cell surface substances that primarily determine the migration of cells, but also affect other cell functions, such as cytotoxicity and antigen presentation.[70,71] Adhesion molecules are divided into a number of distinct families (Table 5). The selectins include lectins that bind to sialylated fucosylated tetrasaccharides, such as sialylated Lewis x. Current experimental data suggest that they act in the initial phases of leukocyte adhesion to attract them from the circulation onto the vascular endothelium. This interaction is momentary, unless additional adhesive molecules are activated.

The immunoglobulin superfamily (IGSF) adhesive molecules (adhesins: ICAM-1, VCAM1) are the ligands primarily for β_1 and β_2 integrins. These adhesive pairs of molecules are involved in establishing the firm adhesion of leukocytes to the vascular endothelium,

Table 5
Principal Families of Adhesion Molecules, Examples of Family Members
and Ligands

Adhesion Molecule Family	Members	Ligand
Selectin Family	E-Selectin	Sialylated
	P-Selectin	Fucosylated
	L-Selectin	Tetrasaccharides
Immunoglobulin Superfamily	ICAM-1	LFA-1, Mac-1
	ICAM-2	LFA-1
	ICAM-3	LFA-1
	VCAM-1	VLA-4
	MadCAM-1	β_7,α_4,L-Selectin
	PECAM-1	PECAM-1
Integrins β_1 Family	VLA-4 β_1,α_4,	VCAM-1, Fibronectin
β_2 Family	LFA-1 β_2,α_L	ICAM-1,ICAM-2,ICAM-3
	Mac-1, β_2,α_M	ICAM-1,Fibrinogen,C3bi C3bi
	p150 95,β_2,α_x	

ICAM: intracellular adhesion molecule; VCAM: vascular cell adhesion molecule; LFA: lymphocyte function associated antigen; VLA: very late antigen; PECAM: platelet endothelial cell adhesion.

following the initial selectin-mediated interaction and the subsequent emigration of leukocytes into tissues (diapedesis). The activation and cytolytic function of lymphocytes is also dependent on the efficient cell contact mediated by ICAM/integrin pairs. L-selectin which is constitutively expressed on all granulocytes, monocytes, and most lymphocytes. P-selectin is stored in the α-granules of platelets and Weibel-Palade bodies of endothelial cells from where it can be rapidly expressed on the plasma membrane when induced by mediators such as histamine or thrombin.[70,71] Induction of leukocyte rolling in vivo also occurs much faster than expression of E-selectin on endothelial cells both in vitro or in vivo. In an indirect histologic study, leukocyte accumulation has been observed to start as early as 3 minutes after exteriorization of the mesentery.

In other experimental designs using the cat mesentery, there was a linear decline in leukocyte rolling (V_{wbc}) as red blood cell velocity (V_{rbc}) was reduced. Moreover, a reduction in shear stress was associated with increased leukocyte adhesion to the endothelium, particularly when V_{rbc} was reduced below 50 μm/s. A decrease in the wall shear rate below 500 s^{-1} in arterioles resulted in 1 to 3 leukocytes adhering per 100 μm length of the vessel, whereas exposure of venules to similar shear conditions resulted in 5 to 16 adherent leukocytes.[69] Furthermore, pretreatment of the vessels with monoclonal antibodies against leukocyte endothelial cell adhesion glycoprotein CD11/CD18 increased

leukocyte rolling velocity in venules by approximately 20 μm/s. These studies support the notion that there are molecular factors that contribute to the greater propensity of leukocyte rolling and adhesion in venules than arterioles, not just differences in shear rates between the two types of vessels.[69]

Recent studies[72] have also reported that histamine can induce leukocyte rolling in vivo via H$_2$ receptors, most likely by inducing endothelial expression of P-selectin. Additionally, mediators other than histamine released from mast cells and/or other cells are likely to promote sustained leukocyte rolling.

This phenomenon of leukocyte rolling along venular endothelium and adhesion is particularly evident during the early stages of an acute inflammatory process where rolling neutrophils usually change their shape and undergo diapedesis. The adhesion molecules are important components of this physiologic process. The pathophysiologic significance of the selectins and integrins in mediating adhesive interactions between neutrophils and endothelial cells is currently being investigated.

Neutrophils have also been implicated in ischemia-reperfusion injury in a variety of different vascular beds after both local and hemorrhage-induced ischemia. Evidence supporting the involvement of neutrophils in reperfusion injury has been obtained from several quantitative studies in which there was a decrease in leukocyte rolling velocity, and there was an increased leukocyte adhesion and emigration in the venules. Furthermore, monoclonal antibodies against either leukocyte or endothelial cell adhesion glycoprotein CD11/CD18 significantly attenuated ischemia-reperfusion-induced leukocyte adhesion regardless of whether the antibody was administered before or after the ischemic insult.[68] Leukocyte-endothelial cell adhesion and an altered metabolism of endothelial cell-derived nitric oxide (NO) have been implicated in the microvascular dysfunction associated with ischemia/reperfusion.

Capillary Blood Flow in Humans

Thus far, we have discussed invasive experimental approaches to an understanding of the functions of the microcirculation. In situ measurements of blood flow in human microcirculation have been made in only a few tissues such as the skin, the conjunctiva, and the retina. Using a standard slit-lamp microscope with a magnification of 62x, Lee and Holze[73] identified the arterioles, collecting venules, true capillaries, and arteriovenous anastomoses in the human conjunctiva. The blood velocity was estimated to be 0.12 mm/sec in 10 to 14 μm arterioles. Spontaneous vasomotion was also recorded at the precapillary region. The vasomotion was characterized by a total constriction of the arterioles lasting 2 to 3 minutes, followed by a 1- to 5-minute period of relaxation prior to the next contractile phase. Recent reports of erythrocyte flow velocity in the conjunctival capillaries of healthy subjects record values of 0.59 to 0.24 mm/sec in 8 μm capillaries.[74] Induction of local hypoxia in these subjects increased the red cell flow velocity by 30%. Using intravital biomicroscopy interfaced with video recording techniques, we obtained similar results for the time-averaged flow velocity of erythrocytes in the conjunctival microvessels of normal, healthy subjects. However, patients with sickle cell disease (hemoglobin SS and hemoglobin SC diseases) showed a decrease in flow velocity.[75]

It is important to recognize that effective automated morphometric analysis of microvessels in video or photographic images obtained by transillumination requires extensive knowledge about the relationship between image intensity values and the object being imaged. Recently, Wick, Lowe, and Kurantsin-Mills have developed a comprehensive model that was undertaken to determine the component intensity-value relationships present in an image of the microvessels of translucent tissues such as the mesentery, cremaster muscle, or bulbar conjunctiva. Experiments were conducted during the modeling process to account for all the illumination effects for evaluation of the microvessels. There was an excellent agreement between the model and the experiment that provides a foundation for the detection and precise measurement of mi-

crovessel dimensions within a diffuse medium such as the sclera of the conjunctiva. The ability to compute relative depth of a microvessel, from a single view, also permits discrimination between neighboring microvessels in complex images.[76]

Plethysmographic determinations of limb blood flow have provided the basis for the elucidation of reflex and local control of skin blood flow in humans. However, Bagge and Branemark[77] introduced the titanium arm chamber technique, combined with intravital video microscopy for studies of blood flow in human skin microcirculation. Although the technique is invasive, it has provided significant insight into the microvascular rheologic behavior of erythrocytes, leukocytes, platelets, and their interactions. Skin blood flow is currently measured by a variety of noninvasive techniques such as vital capillaroscopy, dynamic capillaroscopy, fluorescein microangiography, and laser-Doppler technique. Among these techniques, the laser-Doppler is the easiest to use under experimental and clinical conditions. Figure 12 shows representative results of finger blood flow measured with the LDF under a variety of conditions and maneuvers in a normal healthy subject. These data illustrate some of the physiologic mechanisms that may influence finger blood flow in normal individuals under ambient conditions.

Effect of Red Cell Concentration on Oxygen Transport

A fundamental function of the microcirculation is to facilitate the transport of oxygen and nutrients to subserve the metabolic needs of the tissues. This ability of the microcirculation to deliver oxygen to the tissues depends on the volumetric flux of red blood cells (Q_{rbc}) throughout the hierarchy of microvascular divisions. The volumetric flux of red blood cells is itself determined by the network of values of bulk volumetric flow (Q) of the cells and plasma. At the microcirculatory level, the volumetric flow of oxygen (QO_2) is a function of the product of blood flow (Q_b) and arterial oxygen content (Art O_2). Furthermore, an important parameter governing blood flow through various tissues (e.g., myocardium and brain) is the hematocrit.[78] Within the physiologic range of hematocrit, there is ample evidence[9,14,39,62] that blood viscosity varies linearly with hematocrit in the range 0% < Hct < 30% and thereafter rises exponentially with increasing hematocrit (Figure 6). Because of this nonlinear relationship between blood viscosity and hematocrit, the concept of an optimum hematocrit has evolved to express the value that maximizes Q_{rbc} and, hence, QO_2.

Under normal physiologic conditions, the red blood cell mass is maintained precisely, by production and elimination processes, at approximately 30 mL/kg body weight. Therefore, the physiologic responses to acute or long-term alterations in terms of systemic, re-

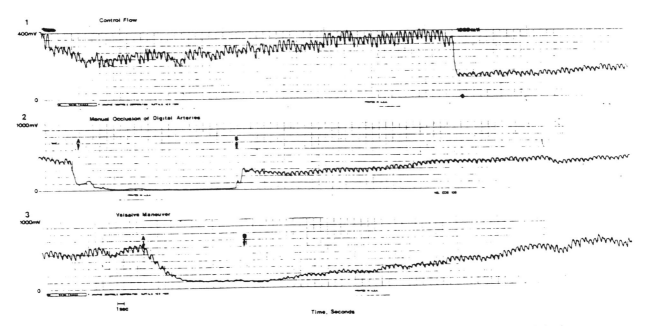

Figure 12. Recordings of the waveforms of finger blood flow under varied physiologic conditions using a laser-Doppler velocimeter. Note the oscillations that reflect pulsations of microvascular flow within a microvascular area of 1 mm² and a depth of approximately 1 mm. The large oscillations reflect respiration.

gional, or microvascular hemodynamics, blood viscosity, and oxygen transport have attracted much attention.[23,62,79–81] The singular effect of hematocrit (Hct) on blood flow and, hence, volumetric oxygen flux can be deduced from the following relationships proposed by Chien.[23]

$$QO_2 = Q_b \times (Art\ O_2) \tag{13}$$

Under normal physiologic conditions (i.e., normal RBC mass, MCHC, and hemoglobin O_2 saturation) the arterial oxygen content depends on hemoglobin (Hb) concentration and its percent O_2 saturation (Sat); therefore:

$$(Art\ O_2) = K\ (Sat\ HbO_2)(Hct) \tag{14}$$

where K is the oxygen capacity of hemoglobin and a proportionality constant (i.e., 1.34 mL O_2/g hemoglobin; for MCHC of 33 g/dL, K = 44.22 mL O_2/100 mLRBC). The blood flow can be derived from the Hagen-Poiseuille equation (Equation 2):

$$Q_b = \Delta P/R \tag{15}$$

where ∇P is the pressure difference $(P_1 - P_2)$ and R is the resistance term that is the product of the blood viscosity (η) and vascular hindrance (Z):

$$Q_b = \Delta P/R \tag{16}$$

Therefore, for a given arterial pressure and flow resistance, the volumetric flux of oxygen is related to hematocrit as follows:

$$QO_2 = K(Sat\ HbO_2)(Hct)\frac{\Delta P}{Z}\frac{Hct}{\eta} \tag{17}$$

As described by Chien (See Figure 53 of Reference 23), the rate of oxygen transport varies directly with the hematocrit and inversely with the blood viscosity. Furthermore, as discussed therein, the curve relating oxygen transport (a function of C_{rbc}/η to hematocrit (C_{rbc}) is bell-shaped, with a peak corresponding to the optimum hematocrit of about 40%, at a shear stress of 10 dynes/cm² or higher (i.e., normal arterial pressure). Admittedly, the above discussion simplifies complex physiologic responses. Nonetheless, assuming normal respiratory function, normal hemoglobin oxygenation and O_2 saturation, normal red cell number, and a constant vascular hindrance, subsequent experimental investigations in the dog have supported these theoretical considerations.[80]

These subsequent studies were done by systematic isovolumetric stepwise hemodilution using homologous plasma or hemoconcentration with red cells in plasma and measuring systemic and regional hemodynamics, oxygen transport, and blood viscosity. The results demonstrated that a change in hematocrit resulted in corresponding alterations in blood viscosity that caused an inverse variation in blood flow (Figure 13). The rate of oxygen transport showed a bell-shaped

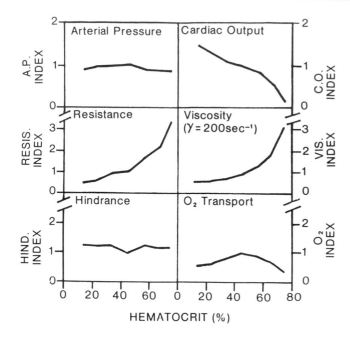

Figure 13. Response of systemic arterial pressure, cardiac output, total peripheral resistance, blood viscosity, peripheral vascular hindrance, and overall systemic oxygen transport to hemodilution or hemoconcentration. Indices were normalized by dividing various values by those obtained at a hematocrit of 45%. (Adapted with permission from Reference 78.)

The rate of oxygen transport showed a bell-shaped curve with a plateau within the 30% to 60% hematocrit range. Figure 14 shows an example of this study in which the effect of hematocrit alterations on the oxygen transport rate and blood flow to the myocardium, brain, intestines, liver with its hepatic artery, kidney, and spleen were measured. Oxygen transport rate index as obtained in these studies was measured as the product of blood flow rate and arterial oxygen content. The results reveal that all organs are supplied with the most adequate oxygen at hematocrits ranging from 25% to 45%. This observation is in agreement with the value predicted from the theoretical calculations. During experimental hemorrhagic hypotension, the microvessel hematocrit decreases in parallel with the systemic hematocrit. There is a strong vasoconstriction causing the vascular hindrance to increase and the microvascular flow to decrease. The resultant reduction in microvascular flow also leads to a sharp decline in red cell flux. This reduction in flux is also observed in the overall systemic circulation. The systemic effects observed in this study were an integrated response to regional compensatory vasomotor adjustments to the blood rheologic changes and the rate of oxygen transport.

Furthermore, these regional hemodynamic responses are due to the summated effects of the trends in red cell delivery for individual microvessels within the successive network topography of the respective

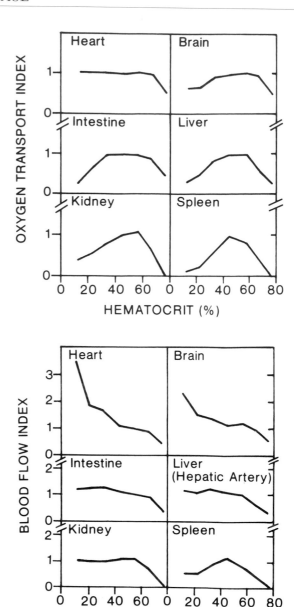

Figure 14. Effect of hemodilution and hemoconcentration on regional blood flow and oxygen transport through the myocardium, the brain, the intestine, the liver, the kidney, and the spleen. Blood flow index was normalized by dividing flow values by those measured at a hematocrit of 45%. (Adapted with permission from Reference 78.)

tissues, during the hemodilution or hemoconcentration maneuvers.[79] Microvascular hemodynamics following systemic hemodilution and hemoconcentration have been investigated by measurements of intravascular pressure, red blood cell velocity, leukocyte velocity, adherent leukocytes on the endothelium, and microvessel hematocrit in arterioles and venules of the cat mesentery.[79] The results of the study demonstrated a heterogeneous behavior of red cell flux within individual microvessels that affected the distribution of red cells throughout the more distal regions of the network.

The summation of these numerous heterogeneous responses resulted in the effective optimization of red cell flux within the range of systemic hematocrit. This range of systemic hematocrit, $28\% < Hct_{sys} < 46\%$, for the maximization of red cell volumetric flux for the mesentery is consistent with the studies of regional circulation.[78]

It is now widely recognized that within the microcirculation, oxygen exchange occurs not only across the capillaries, but also across the walls of the arteriolar network.[82,83] Using video microspectrophotometric technique, Duling, Pittman, and coworkers determined oxygen saturation in red blood cells in the capillaries of several tissues.[82,83] These studies have demonstrated that there is transmural oxygen flux in most microvessels, and that it is erroneous to assume that oxygen saturation in precapillary vessels is equal to that in systemic arterial blood, or that oxygen saturation in postcapillary vessels is comparable to that of systemic mixed venous blood.

Regulation of Blood Flow in the Microcirculation

A remarkable property of the microcirculation is that most tissues regulate their own rates of perfusion by means of mechanisms intrinsic to the particular tissue. The microcirculation of organs such as the skin is related largely to their specialized functions. In other organs (e.g., kidneys, brain), however, there is autoregulation of blood flow, which refers to the tendency of certain microvascular beds to maintain a relatively constant flow, despite changes in perfusion pressure. In addition, other microvascular beds have the intrinsic ability to change their flow despite the relatively constant perfusion pressure. The basic mechanisms for the regulation of tissue microcirculation may be divided into three types: local regulation, nervous regulation, and humoral and biochemical regulation.

Local Regulation

Local regulation of the microcirculation is confined within a single organ or tissue, and may be due to acute responses to the metabolic needs of the tissue, or long-term adaptation of the tissue to increased metabolic demands. Induction of local mechanisms for increased tissue blood flow is usually a compensatory response to increased demand for oxygen and other nutrients such as glucose, amino acids, and fatty acids. This mechanism has been described as the nutrient demand theory (or the oxygen demand theory, because oxygen is a strong stimulus for increased local blood flow). However, increased tissue metabolism results in the formation of by-products such as carbon dioxide, lactic acid, adenosine, adenosine phosphates, hydrogen ions, potassium ions, some prostaglandins, and

histamine. These by-products have intense vasodilator effects on vascular smooth muscle. As a result, when their tissue levels increase beyond a critical threshold concentration, vasodilation of the resistance vessels increases blood flow. This compensatory response also increases the volumetric flux of oxygen, washes the vasoactive metabolites out of the local or regional microvasculature, and restores their concentration to the basal level and blood flow back toward normal. These processes form the physiologic basis of reactive hyperemia and the metabolic theory of local blood flow regulation.[74]

Another explanation for local regulation of blood flow is considered in the myogenic theory. The theory postulates that the smooth muscle of the terminal arterioles and precapillary sphincters have unstable resting membrane potentials, and undergo spontaneous oscillatory spike depolarizations that may spread to adjacent cells to induce mass contraction. The theory postulates that the pacemaker (or spike depolarization) properties of the smooth muscle cells can be related to the perfusion pressure (P) in the microcirculation and the tension (T) in the vessel wall according to the law of Laplace. Laplace's law describes the forces present in the wall of a cylindrical tube or blood vessel at equilibrium and can be stated as follows: the distending pressure (P) (or transmural pressure) in a hollow elastic system at equilibrium equals the wall tension (T) divided by the two principal radii of curvature of that system. $P = T/(r_1 - r_2)$, where r_1 and r_2 are the two principal radii of the vessel. In a cylinder or a blood vessel, one radius is infinite, hence the relationship becomes $P = T/r$. Thus, increases in P lead to decreases in r and vice versa, so that T is restored, resulting in regular sequence of opening and closing of the sphincter (vasomotion).[75] The advocates of the theory suggest that when the pressure in the microvessels increases, for example, as a result of high arterial pressure, vascular constriction stretches the vessel and reduces blood flow toward the normal range. However, low pressure reduces the stretch of the smooth muscle, relaxes it, and allows increased blood flow to distal sites. The myogenic theory is supported by the experimental observation that passive stretch increases the rate of depolarization of the vascular smooth muscle unit and its contractility. This ability of many blood vessels to maintain nearly normal levels of blood flow, despite significant fluctuations in arterial pressure, is called myogenic autoregulation. The phenomenon is well developed in renal vessels, but is also present in the brain, heart, liver, intestines, and skeletal muscles. Autoregulatory responses have not been observed in the cutaneous circulation.[75,76]

Long-term regulation of tissue blood flow is a physiologic compensatory adaptation to meet a change in the metabolic demands of a tissue. This long-term response occurs over a period of hours, days, and weeks, in addition to the acute mechanism. If the metabolism of a tissue (e.g., skeletal muscle) increases for several days or weeks, the number and sizes of vessels in the tissue increases and vice versa. Therefore, there is a continual reconstruction of the microvasculature to subserve the needs of tissues. These processes occur rapidly in young animals and new tissue (e.g., cancerous tissue or a scar). The reconstruction is relatively slow, however, in well-established tissues and in tissues of older people. The physiologic stimulus for increased or decreased tissue vascularity may be oxygen. This fact is supported by observations such as the increased tissue vascularity in animals exposed to high altitudes or those who live at heights where the partial pressure of oxygen is lower. The theory that oxygen is the stimulus is also supported by clinical conditions such as retrolental fibroplasia.[84]

An angiogenesis factor has been isolated from several tissues including tumors. This factor induces the growth and proliferation of new hemovascular networks in several tissues that exhibit excessive metabolic activity. The factor has been isolated from the retina of the eye and from solid tumors. Lack of oxygen or excessive metabolic activity are primary stimuli for the synthesis of the angiogenesis factor.[85] The factor may be significant in the neovasculization found in proliferative retinopathy of hemoglobinopathies and diabetes mellitus.

The development of collateral vessels to facilitate continual tissue perfusion when the parent vessel is blocked is another example of long-term local regulation. The opening of collateral vessels may be initiated by vascular occlusion at proximal sites, resulting in reduced volumetric flux of oxygen. The enlargement of the collateral vessels usually satisfies the long-term flow requirements of the tissue in question. These microvascular adaptations to pressure-flow perturbations, metabolic changes, or oxygen flux suggest that the vascularity of most tissues is directly related to the local metabolism.[86]

Nervous Regulation

Superimposed onto the basal vasomotor tone of arterioles are neural inputs that originate from the anterolateral reticular substance of the medulla and lower third of the pons (C-1 area) in the central nervous system. Sympathetic vasoconstrictor fibers from this vasomotor (or vasoconstrictor) center innervate arterioles and precapillaries of most of the microcirculation. The microvessels of the skeletal muscle, kidneys, spleen, skin, and the splanchnic area have a much richer distribution of these nerve fibers than do the coronary and cerebral microvasculature. A second central locus is the vasodilator (or A-1 area) which is located bilaterally in the anterolateral portions of the lower medulla. The neurons emerging from the A-1

area project to the C-1 area and modulate the rate of vasoconstrictor impulses from the latter, thereby inducing vasodilation in the resistance vessels. A group of neurons located bilaterally in the tractus solitarius of the posterolateral area of the medulla and lower pons also receive sensory impulses from the vagus and glossopharyngeal nerves. The efferent impulses from this sensory area modulate the arterioles of the vasomotor center.[75,76,78,79]

In general, there is a continuous flow of impulses from the vasoconstrictor nerves at a rate of 1 to 2/sec, in response to signals from the vasomotor center, that maintains precapillary arterioles in a contracted state. This is called sympathetic vasoconstrictor tone or vasomotor tone. Norepinephrine is the neurotransmitter released at the neuroeffector junction of the fibers and vascular smooth muscle. This neurotransmitter interacts with receptors on the smooth muscle membrane, which leads to increased transmembrane conduction of ions (e.g., $Na+$, $K+$, $Cl-$), increased frequency of action potentials, and an increase in vascular tone.[76,79] The vasomotor center is also controlled by higher nervous system centers including: a) the mesencephalon, diencephalon, and the reticular substance of the pons; b) the hypothalamus; and c) several areas of the cerebral cortex, all of which can either excite or inhibit the vasomotor center. There are also cholinergic vasodilatory fibers that travel with the cranial nerves to the precapillary arterioles of the tongue and salivary glands. Others innervate the bladder and genital microvasculature. In the salivary glands, the vasodilatory transmitter appears to be bradykinin; in other tissues, acetylcholine may activate cholinergic receptor sites. These receptors may induce hyperpolarization of the smooth muscle cell membrane, probably by selective increase in membrane permeability to potassium. The net result is inhibition of the frequency of action potentials and tone of the vascular muscle cells.[76]

Humoral and Biochemical Regulation

In addition to the local and nervous regulation of the microcirculation, there are several biochemical compounds that modulate specific regional microcirculation when infused into experimental animals or human subjects. All of these compounds are found in body fluids. Some are synthesized in endocrine cells and then transported by the blood to distant sites where they exert their physiologic effects. Others are synthesized and released at specific, local areas within the microvascular bed. Regulation of blood flow in the microcirculation by such substances is described as humoral (or biochemical) regulation.[78,79] Table 6 summarizes some important humoral and biochemical factors that have significant regulatory effect on the microcirculation.

Table 6
Humoral and Biochemical Factors that Affect Blood Flow in the Microcirculation

Factor	Effect on Blood Flow
Histamine	Released in tissue damage by mast cells and basophils; relaxes arterioles; increases capillary permeability, inhibits norepinephrine release; decreases sympathetic tone; induces vasodilation.
Serotonin	Present in chromaffin tissue; regulatory role in blood flow is unknown. Vasoconstrictor effect in some tissues, vasodilator effect in skeletal muscle, mesentery, and brain.
Bradykinin	A product of the kallikrein-kinin system, it induces a very strong arteriolar dilatation and increases capillary permeability. Role in the control of local blood flow is unknown.
Angiotensin	A product of the renin-angiotensin system, it is one of the most potent biologic vasoconstrictors known. It has vasoconstrictor effect on most blood vessels, especially skin, splanchnic, and renal vessels. The effect is less in the heart, brain, and skeletal muscle where blood flow may increase.
Vasopressin	Shows vasoconstrictor effect in high concentration; rat mesenteric arterioles show more sensitivity to it than angiotensin; may potentiate action of catecholamines.
Oxytocin	Direct vasoconstrictor effect on microvessels of male rats; more sensitive than female rats.
Catecholamines	Effect on vascular smooth muscle via α-receptors (vaso-constriction) and β-receptors (vasodilation). Type of response depends on tissue and concentration; in skin, epinephrine causes only vasoconstriction. Precapillary sphincters show greatest sensitivity to the vasoconstrictor action.
Prostaglandins	Present in every tissue, some cause vasoconstriction; most induce vasodilation. Their specific role is unclear; however, their ubiquitous distribution makes them physiologically ideal candidates for the fine regulation of the microcirculation.
Thromboxane and Leukotrienes	These compounds have a vasoconstrictor effect on blood vessels
Others	Biochemicals such as intermediates of the TCA cycle, glucagon, cholecystokinin, and secretin are known to induce vasodilation that may be physiologically significant in local control of blood flow for tissue metabolism.

Capillary-Lymphatic Dynamics, Transport, and Exchange

The capillaries of the microcirculatory bed form an anastomosing network of variable length, topography, and density that may branch off a 50 μm arteriole or a 15 μm precapillary arteriole, and eventually coalesce into the postcapillary venules. Capillaries consists of endothelial cylinders with luminal diameters of about 5 μm to 9 μm. The wall thickness and its ultrastructure vary considerably in different tissues, and suggest the existence of several potential transport pathways. The lymphatic vessels also constitute a special extravascular closed-end network of endothelial tubes. The design allows them to collect extra interstitial fluid and protein, and transport them to the vascular system via the thoracic duct.[87–89] Therefore, the capillary-lymphatic dynamics provide a mechanism for the maintenance of tissue homeostasis, and entail the essential aspects of

the functioning microvascular bed. These include the following: a) the physical transport of the blood by the microcirculation; b) the exchange of nutrients and waste materials across the capillary endothelium by the process of diffusion, osmosis, and bulk transport; c) the transport of excess capillary filtrate by the lymphatic system into the vascular compartment; and d) the maintenance of the pressure-flow equilibrium within the interstitial space.

The movement of water and other molecules across the capillary endothelium proceeds by diffusion, bulk flow (or filtration), and osmosis. The most important of these transport processes is diffusion. Lipid-soluble molecules, such as oxygen and carbon dioxide, diffuse directly through the cell membranes of the endothelial cell. Water molecules, water-soluble substances, and plasma proteins are transported at intracellular junctions by combined convection and restricted diffusion, and also rapidly through the intercellular clefts. However, lipid-insoluble molecules such as sodium, chloride ions, glucose, and others require specialized membrane-integral protein which binds the solute and facilitates its transport across the capillary membrane. The permeability of the capillary pores for different substances varies with their molecular size.[90] The rate of diffusion of a single molecular species is described by Fick's law, which states:

$$Q_s = -DA \frac{(dc)}{(dx)} \tag{18}$$

where Q_s is the rate of flow of the molecule at right angle to the endothelial cell membrane, dc/dx is the concentration gradient across the blood-endothelium-tissue interface, A is the cross-sectional area of the diffusion path, and D is the diffusion coefficient whose value depends on the temperature, properties of the molecular species, and the endothelial membrane. The negative sign indicates that molecules migrate from areas of high concentration to areas of low concentration.

The free movement of water and solutes across the capillary membrane is also strongly influenced by the capillary hydrostatic pressure difference across the endothelial barrier. In the presence of such a pressure difference, water and solute flow as a unit through the capillary pores, a phenomenon called bulk flow or filtration. The capillary hydrostatic pressure is variable and dependent on a) the arterial pressure; b) the venous pressure; and c) the precapillary (arteriolar plus precapillary sphincter) and postcapillary venular resistances. The algebraic effect of these forces on capillary hydrostatic pressure and hence filtration may be summarized by the following relationship:

$$P_c = \frac{(R_v/R_a)P_a + P_v}{1 + (R_v/R_a)} \tag{19}$$

where P_c is capillary hydrostatic pressure, P_a is the arterial pressure, P_v is the venous pressure, R_a and R_v are the precapillary and postcapillary resistances respectively.[87-89] The interstitial fluid exerts a negative pressure (P_i) of about -6 mm Hg that opposes the capillary hydrostatic pressure. Therefore, it is the differential pressure P_c-P_i that constitutes the filtration pressure at the arterial end of the capillaries. It should be clear from equation 19 that changes in any one of the variables will change the value of P_c.

In order to maintain a semivacuum in the interstitial space and avoid accumulation of the plasma ultrafiltrate, 90% of the filtered fluid is reabsorbed at the venous end of the capillary back to the vascular system. The force that restrains the accumulation of interstitial fluid is the osmotic pressure of plasma proteins, also called colloid osmotic pressure or oncotic pressure. The colloid osmotic pressure of plasma is partly explained by van't Hoff's law as a function of the number of particles (molecular species) in the solution. Albumin, being the smallest, mW 69,000 d, and the most concentrated protein in plasma (4.6 g/dL), provides about 68% of the total oncotic pressure. Globulins and fibrinogen provide about 6% and 1%, respectively, of the oncotic pressure. The remaining solutes provide about 25% of the pressure.

The plasma ultrafiltrate that is not reabsorbed at the venous end of the capillaries contains about 2 gm/dL protein that exerts an osmotic pressure of approximately 6 mm Hg. Therefore, the effective plasma oncotic pressure is the difference between plasma protein oncotic pressure and the interstitial fluid oncotic pressure. Although the magnitude of the effective plasma oncotic pressure varies in different microvascular beds, because of the variation of interstitial fluid protein concentration, it averages about 20 to 26 mm Hg. The balance of the hydrostatic and oncotic forces regulates the transport and exchange of fluid in the microcirculation. This fact was first recognized by Ernest Starling in 1896 and, hence, called the Starling hypothesis or the Starling equilibrium of capillary exchange. This equilibrium may be expressed mathematically as:

$$V = k[P_c + II_i - P_i - II_p] \tag{20}$$

where V is fluid filtered or reabsorbed per minute (it is positive for filtration and negative for reabsorption), P_c is capillary hydrostatic pressure, P_i is the interstitial fluid pressure, II_p is the plasma osmotic pressure, II_i is the interstitial fluid osmotic pressure, and k is a filtration constant for the capillary endothelial barrier, with the units milliliter fluid per mm Hg pressure in 100 gm tissue per minute at 37°C.

The filtration-reabsorption equilibrium expressed in the Starling hypothesis simplifies rather complicated physiologic mechanisms that maintain capillary dynamics. The equilibrium may not exist at all times in any one microvascular bed. The equilibrium depends on the forces mentioned, the status of precapillary and postcapillary resistance vessels, the network topography of the capillaries, the surface area of the capillaries available for filtration and for reabsorption, the distance across the capillary wall, the viscosity of the filtrate, and the functional state of the lymphatic system.

The regulation of water and solute exchange in microvessel endothelium has been extensively studied in single perfused capillaries.[91,92] The technology applied to these studies include single capillary techniques, transport theory, electron microscopy, tracer techniques, fluorescence techniques, and confocal microscopy. These studies have demonstrated that the rate that substances cross the capillary wall depend on the permeability properties of the capillary barrier and the net driving forces for solute exchange. Thus, the transcapillary solute flux of a solute (J_s/S), in terms of the driving force (which are $\Delta C = C_1 - C_2$, the concentration gradient for the test solute, and the frictional drag due to water flow on diffusing solute or solvent drag), for transcapillary solute flux through a porous membrane, can be expressed as follows:[92]

$$J_s/S = P_s(C_1 - C_2).Z + (J_v/S)/(1 - \sigma_s)C_1 \quad (21)$$

where

$$Z = P_e(\exp P_e - 1) \text{ and } P_e = (J_v/S)/(1 - \sigma_s)/P_s \quad (22)$$

Furthermore,

$$J_s/S = L_p(\Delta P - \sigma_p\Pi - \sigma_s RT\Delta C). \quad (23)$$

Therefore, the flux of a tracer through single porous membrane is determined by at least two mechanisms: diffusion and solvent drag (equation 21). The relative magnitude of the diffusion and the solvent drag terms is not constant, but is dependent on the solute diffusion velocity in the pore relative to water velocity, as measured by the dimensionless term, P_e. Experimental measurements of the transcapillary flux of α-lactalbumin and the hydrostatic pressure in the microvessel lumen in individually perfused frog mesentery show that solvent drag dominates exchange when $P_e > 3$.[92]

The interstitium constitutes the spaces between cells and comprises approximately 16% of the body. It is composed of collagen fiber bundles and proteoglycan filaments. The collagen fiber bundles provide the tensional strength that binds cells together, whereas the coiled proteoglycan filaments, composed of 98% hyaluronic acid and 2% protein, connect into an extremely fine reticular filament that fills the minute interstices of the tissues.[88,89] The fluid in these spaces is the interstitial fluid and it is an ultrafiltrate of plasma derived from the balance of the filtration and reabsorption at the capillaries. This fluid containing protein and other substances (blood cells, bacteria, and other solutes and particles) diffuses through the gaps in between the valves of the terminal lymphatic capillaries. The fluid then flows into larger lymphatic vessels facilitated by the transmitted pulsations from adjacent small arteries and skeletal muscle, contractions of the lymphatic vessels, and the extensive one-way lymphatic valves. The lymphatic vessels eventually drain their contents into the right and left subclavian veins at the junctions of the internal jugular vein, respectively. The rate of lymph flow in the thoracic duct in a resting man is about 1.3 mL per kilogram body weight per hour. Despite this low lymph flow, it is the only means of removal of the 10% excess ultrafiltrate of plasma (proteins and fluids) and its transport to the circulatory system. Therefore, the recycling of interstitial fluid and protein back to the vascular compartment is essential for the maintenance of normal negative interstitial fluid pressure and volume, and hence tissue homeostasis. The significance of these delicate lymphatic dynamics is evident from conditions in which the volume of interstitial fluid exceeds the capacity of the lymphatics and the lymphatic vessels become blocked, resulting in clinical edema.

Summary

The rheologic properties of plasma, erythrocytes, leukocytes, and whole blood have been described. The rheologic characteristics of whole blood, under normal physiologic conditions, is a complex function of plasma viscosity, (which depends on plasma protein concentration), erythrocyte concentration, erythrocyte aggregation, and erythrocyte deformation. The deformation of erythrocytes is determined by: a) intracellular viscosity (which is a function of mean corpuscular hemoglobin concentration); b) membrane material properties (including elasticity and viscosity); c) cellular geometry (surface area to volume ratio, and morphology); and d) the shear stresses acting on the cell surface. Erythrocyte aggregation represents an algebraic balance of energies. These energies are the bridging energy due to fibrinogen and the globulins, the electrostatic repulsive energy at the cell surface, and the mechanical shear energy due to cell deformability and cell membrane bending. The plasma viscosity of a healthy population is stable for a long time, although it may fluctuate in response to a variety physiologic stimuli and challenges.

A number of in vitro and in vivo studies have established that the flow properties of erythrocytes and leukocytes are dependent upon their viscoelastic characteristics. These viscoelastic characteristics, which can be quantitated by micropipette aspiration techniques, also determine the cell transit through the microcirculation. The microcirculation is the smallest terminal segment of the cardiovascular system consisting of arterioles, capillaries, and postcapillary venules. The architectural and topographic organization of the microcirculation is characteristic for the respective tissues and organs, although certain common anatomic and physiologic features can be identified in some microvascular beds. The gains in our fund of information and knowledge, and the technologic developments in microcirculatory investigation during the past several decades, have fostered the concept of the independent nature of microcirculatory behavior. Within the microcirculation, the architectural organization of the feeding arterioles, the network of capillaries, and the collecting venules have an overall modular design. Therefore, vascular and topographic features, and blood rheologic factors influence the distribution of

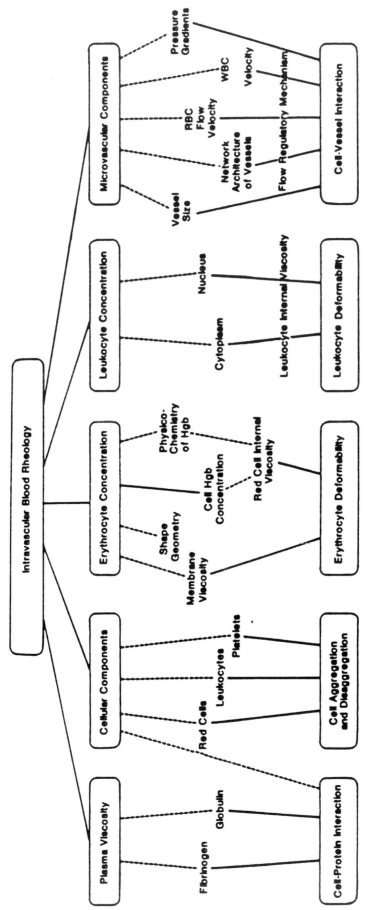

Figure 15. Schematic representation of the components of blood rheology and microvascular hemodynamics.

pressure-flow values within the module. These, in turn, determine the local apportionment of erythrocytes and, hence, their volumetric flux through various tissues (Figure 15).

Current microcirculatory technology has permitted in situ determination of pressure-flow relationships, apparent viscosity, and hematocrit in individual microvessels. These in situ measurements have provided microcirculatory interpretation to macrocirculatory observations in organs such as the myocardium, skeletal muscle, splanchnic microcirculation, and the kidney. The combined efforts of researchers from different disciplines, including anatomy, physiology, engineering, biochemistry, immunology, surgery, and pathology are providing significant insights into the mechanisms that regulate microvascular functions. For example, the recent discovery of the role of adhesion molecules in leukocyte-endothelial interactions has yielded a fresh understanding about the molecular distribution of adhesion molecules in arterioles and venules, and their significance in both local and hemorrhage-induced ischemia, as well as ischemia-reperfusion. Most microvascular beds can regulate their local blood flow through mechanisms that dilate or constrict local arterioles. Nervous and humoral mechanisms superimposed on these local controls provide the fine and increased compensatory responses that are needed during cardiovascular challenges such as exercise or hemorrhage.

The arteriovenous distribution of pressures and the ratio of precapillary to postcapillary resistances determine capillary hydrostatic pressure. The sum of capillary pressure and interstitial colloid osmotic pressure determine the filtration of fluid at the arterial end of the capillary. These forces are counterbalanced by the interstitial fluid hydrostatic pressure and plasma colloid osmotic pressure, as expounded in Starling's hypothesis. The rate of transport of fluid across the capillary endothelium is also dependent on the area of the endothelial wall, the distance across the capillary wall, the viscosity of the filtrate, and a filtration constant characteristic of the endothelial membrane. The significance of these capillary and lymphatic dynamics in relation to the fluid movements is twofold: a) to satisfy the exchange of nutrients and waste materials between the blood and the tissues, and b) to regulate interstitial fluid volume, the pressure within the interstitium, and tissue homeostasis.

Acknowledgments

This work was supported in part by NIH-NHLBI Grant No R29-HL38521. The author is grateful to Dr. Marie M. Cassidy and the editors for helpful suggestions and discussions on the manuscript. The author also appreciates the assistance of Judy Gunther of the Biomedical Communications Department of the George Washington University Medical Center for the preparation of the figures.

References

1. Bayliss LE: The rheology of blood. In: Hamilton WF (ed). *Handbook of Physiology, Circulation* Vol 1. Sec 2. Washington, DC: American Physiological Society; 137–150, 1962.
2. Barnes HA, Hutton JF, Walters K: *An Introduction to Rheology*. New York: Elsevier Science Publishing; 1989.
3. Stolz JF, Puchelle E (eds). New methods in biorheology. *Biorheology* (suppl 1):1, 1984.
4. Davenport, Roath S: A variable shear stress viscometer. *Clin Hemorheol* 2:280, 1982.
5. Monshausen CEE, Matrai A: Blood viscosity: a comparative study on three rotational instruments. *Biorheology* 22:471, 1985.
6. Dormandy JA: Measurement of whole blood viscosity. In: Lowe ADO, Barbenel JC, Forbes CD (eds). *Clinical Viscosity and Cell Deformability*. New York: Springer-Verlag; 67–78, 1981.
7. Wells RE, Denton R, Merrill EW: Measurement of viscosity of biological fluids by cone and plate viscometer. *J Lab Clin Med* 57:646, 1961.
8. Ditzel J, Kampmann J: Whole blood viscosity, hematocrit, and plasma protein in normal subjects at different ages. *Acta Physiol Scand* 81:264, 1971.
9. Chien S: Present state of blood rheology. In: Messmer K, Schmid-Schonbein H (eds). *Hemodilution: Theoretical Basis and Clinical Application*. Basel: Rottach-Egern, Karger; 1–40, 1972.
10. Usami S: Physiological significance of blood rheology. *Biorheology* 19:29, 1982.
11. Lessin LS, Kurantsin-Mills J, Weems HB: Deformability of normal and sickle erythrocytes in a pressure flow filtration system. *Blood Cells* 3:241, 1977.
12. Chien S, Schmalzer EA, Lee MML, et al: Role of white blood cells in filtration of blood cell suspension. *Biorheology* 20:29, 1983.
13. Schmalzer EA, Skalak R, Usami S, et al: Influence of red cell concentration on filtration of blood cell suspensions. *Biorheology* 20:29, 1983.
14. Chien S, Usami S, Skalak R: Blood flow in small tubes. In: Renkin EM, Michel C (eds). *Handbook of Physiology. Sec 2. The Cardiovascular System. Vol IV. Microcirculation. Part 1*. Bethesda, MD: American Physiological Society; 217–249, 1984.
15. Bronkhorst PJH, Berends HG, Nijhof EJ: A flow channel for measuring erythrocyte deformability under fluid shear stress. *Biorheology* 29:476–478, 1992.
16. Evans E, Mohandas N, Leung A: Static and dynamic rigidities of normal and sickle cells. *J Clin Invest* 73:4777, 1984.
17. Evans EA, Hochmuth RM: Mechanochemical properties of membranes. *Curr Top Memb Trans* 10:1, 1978.
18. Branemark PI: *Intravascular Anatomy of Blood Cells in Man*. Basel: Karger, 1971.
19. Wiedeman MP, Tuma RF, Mayrovitz HN: *An Introduction to Microcirculation*, New York: Academic Press, Inc.; 1981.
20. Schmid-Schonbein GW, Sung KLP, Tozeren H, et al:

Passive mechanical properties of human leukocytes. *Biophys J* 236–243, 1981.

21. Skalak R, Impelluso T, Schmalzer EA, et al: Theoretical modeling of filtration of blood cell suspensions. *Biorheology* 20:41, 1983.

22. Bronkhorst PJH, Berends HG, Nijhof EJ, Sixma JJ: Red cell deformability (RCD) in plasma as compared with phosphate-buffered saline. *Int J Microcirc Clin Exp* 14: 235–236, 1994.

22a. Eppihimer MJ, Lipowsky HH: Experimental and analytical characterization of in vitro and in vivo filtrability of leukocyte population. *FASEB* 8:A1039, 1994.

23. Chien S: Biophysical behavior of red cells in suspensions. In: MacNamara D, Surgenor D (eds). *The Red Blood Cell*. Vol II. Orlando, FL: Academic Press Inc.; 1031–1133, 1975.

24. Chien S: Aggregation of red blood cells: an electrochemical and colloid chemical problem. In: Blank M (ed). *Bioelectrochemistry: Ions, Surfaces, Membranes*. Washington, DC: American Chemical Society; 3–38, 1980.

25. Fahraeus R, Lindqvist T: The viscosity of blood in narrow capillary tubes. *Am J Physiol* 96:562, 1931.

26. Barbee J, Cokelet GR: The Fahraeus effect. *Microvasc Res* 3:6, 1971.

27. Krogh A: *The Anatomy and Physiology of Capillaries*. New Haven, CT: Yale University Press, 1929.

28. Walker CHM, Mackintosh TF: The treatment of hyperviscosity syndromes in the newborn with hemodilution. In: Messmer K, Schmid-Schonbein H (eds). *Hemodilution: Theoretical Basis and Clinical Application*. Basel: Rottach-Egern Karger; 271–288, 1972.

29. Rosenblatt G, Stokes J, Bassett DR: Whole blood viscosity, hematocrit, and serum lipid levels in normal subjects and patients with coronary heart disease. *J Lab Clin Med* 65:202, 1965.

30. Buchan PC, Macdonald HN: Rheological studies in obstetrics and gynecology. In: Lowe GDO, Forbes (eds). *Clinical Aspects of Blood Viscosity and Cell Deformability*. Berlin: Springer-Verlag; 175–192, 1981.

31. Poller L: Oral contraceptives, blood clotting, and thrombosis. *Br Med Bull* 34:151, 1978.

32. Aronson HB, Magora F, Schenker JG: Effect of oral contraceptives on blood viscosity, *Am J Obstet Gynecol* 110:997, 1971.

33. Seaman GVF, Engel R, Swan RL, et al: Circadian periodicity in some physiochemical parameters of circulating blood. *Nature* 207:833, 1965.

34. Charm SE, Paz H, Kurland GS: Reduced plasma viscosity among joggers compared to non-joggers. *Biorheology* 6:185, 1979.

35. Wiedeman MP: Patterns of the arteriovenous pathways: In: Hamilton WF, Dow P (eds). *Handbook of Physiology. Circulation II*. Sec 2. Vol II. Washington, DC: American Physiological Society; 891–933, 1963.

36. Wiedeman MP: *Architecture*. In: Renkin E, Michel C. (eds). *Handbook of Physiology*. Sec. 2. *The Cardiovascular System*. Vol IV. *Microcirculation*. Part I. Bethesda, MD: American Physiological Society; 11–40, 1984.

37. Baker C, Nasfuk WL (eds). *Microcirculatory Technology*. Orlando, FL: Academic Press, Inc; 1–534, 1986.

38. Whittaker SRF, Winton FR: The apparent viscosity of blood flowing in the isolated hindlimb of the dog and its variation with corpuscular concentration. *J Physiol* 78: 339, 1933.

39. Benis AM, Usami S, Chien S: A reappraisal of Whittaker

and Winton's results on the basis of inertial losses. *Biorheology* 11:153, 1974.

40. Landis EM: The capillary pressure in frog mesentery as determined by microinjection methods. *Am J Physiol* 75:548, 1926.

41. Landis EM: Microinjection studies of capillary blood pressure in human skin. *Heart* 15:207, 1930.

42. Wiederhielm CA, Woodbury JW, Kirk S, et al: Pulsatile pressures in the microcirculation of frog's mesentery. *Am J Physiol* 225:992, 1973.

43. Intaglietta M, Tompkins WR: Pressure measurements in the mammalian microvasculature. *Microvasc Res* 2:212, 1970.

44. Intaglietta M: Pressure measurements in the microvasculature with active and passive transducers. *Microvasc Res* 5:317, 1973.

45. Slaaf DW, Arts T, Jeurens JM, et al: Electronic measurement of red blood cell velocity and volume flow in microvessels. In: Chayen J, Bitensky L (eds). *Investigative Microtechniques in Medicine and Biology*. New York: Marcel Dekker; 327–384, 1984.

46. Bonner R, Nossal R: Model for laser-Doppler measurements of blood flow in tissue. *Appl Optics* 20:2097, 1981.

47. Wayland H, Johnson PC: Erythrocyte velocity measurement in microvessels by a two-slit photometric method. *J Appl Physiol* 22:333, 1967.

48. Wayland H: Photosensor methods of flow measurements in the microcirculation. *Microvasc Res* 5:336, 1973.

49. Silva J, Intaglietta M: The correlation of photometric signals derived from in vivo red blood cell flow in microvessels. *Microvasc Res* 1:156, 1974.

50. Kurantsin-Mills J, Lessin LS: Cellular and rheological factors contributing to sickle cell microvascular occlusion. *Blood Cells* 12:249, 1986.

51. Mishina H, Koyama T, Asakura T: Velocity measurements of blood flow in the capillary and vein using a laser-Doppler microscope. *Appl Optics* 14:2326, 1975.

52. Stern MD: In vivo evaluation of microcirculation by coherent light scattering. *Nature* 254:56, 1975.

53. Holloway GA, Watkins DW: Laser-Doppler measurement of cutaneous blood flow. *J Investig Dermatol* 69: 306, 1977.

54. Nilsson GE, Tenland T, Obert PA: A new instrument for continuous measurement of tissue blood flow by light beating spectroscopy. *IEEE Transactions Biomedical Engineering (BME)* 27:12, 1980.

55. Bonner RF, Clem TR, Bowen PD, et al: Laser-Doppler continuous real-time monitor of pulsatile and mean blood flow in tissue microcirculation. In: Chen SH, Che Baird Nossal R (eds). *Scattering Techniques Applied to Supramolecular and Nonequilibrium Systems*. New York: Plenum Press; 685–701, 1981.

56. Johnson JM, Taylor WF, Shepher AP, et al: Laser-Doppler measurement of skin blood flow: comparison with plethysmography. *J Appl Physiol* 56:798, 1984.

57. Sherpherd AP, Oberg PA (eds). *Laser-Doppler Blood Flowmetry*. Hingham, MA: Kluwer Academic Publishers; 1–416, 1990.

58. Englehart M, Kristensen JK: Evaluation of cutaneous blood flow responses by [133]Xenon washout and laser-Doppler flowmeter. *J Investig Derm* 80:2, 1983.

59. Zweifach BW, Lipowsky HH: Pressure-flow relations in blood and lymph microcirculation. In: Renkin EM, Michel C (eds). *Handbook of Physiology*. Sec 2. *The Cardiovascular System* Vol IV. *Microcirculation*. Part 1. Bethesda, MD: American Physiological Society; 251–307, 1984.

60. Lipowsky HH, Kovalcheck S, Zweifach BW: The distribution of blood rheological parameters in the microvasculature of cat mesentery. *Circ Res* 43:738, 1978.

61. House SD, Lipowsky HH: Microvascular hematocrit and red cell flux in rat cremaster muscle. *Am J Physiol* 252:H2111, 1987.

62. Lipowsky HH, Usami S, Chien S: In vivo measurements of hematocrit and apparent viscosity in the microvasculature of cat mesentery. *Microvasc Res* 19:297, 1980.

63. Yen RT, Fung YC: Effect of velocity distribution on red cell distribution in capillary blood vessels. *Am J Physiol* 235:H251, 1978.

64. Chien S, Twetenstrand CD, Epstein AF, et al: Model studies on distribution of blood cells at microvascular bifurcations. *Am J Physiol* 248:H568, 1985.

65. Klitzman B, Johnson PC: Capillary network geometry and red cell distribution in the master cremaster muscle. *Am J Physiol* 242:H211, 1982.

66. Schmid-Schoenbein GW, Usami S, Skalak R, et al: Cell distribution in capillary networks. *Microvasc Res* 19:18, 1980.

67. House SD, Lipowsky HH: Leukocyte-endothelium adhesion: microhemodynamics in mesentery of the cat. *Microvasc Res* 34:363–379, 1987.

68. Perry MA, Granger DN: Leukocyte adhesion in local versus hemorrhage-induced ischemia. *Am J Physiol* 263 (*Heart Circ Physiol* 32):H810–H815, 1992.

69. Perry MA, Granger DN: The role of CD11/CD18 in shear rate-dependent leukocyte-endothelial cell interactions in cat mesenteric venules. *J Clin Investig* 87:1798–1804, 1991.

70. Harlan JM, Liu DY: Adhesion: its role in inflammatory disease. New York: WH Freeman and Co; 1992.

71. Pigott C, Power C: *Adhesion Molecule Fact Book*. Orlando, FL: Academic Press, Inc; 1993.

72. Ley, Klaus: Histamine can induce leukocyte rolling in rat mesenteric venules. *Am J Physiol* 267: (*Heart Circ Physiol* 36): H1017–H1023, 1994.

73. Korber N, Jung F, Kiesewetter H, et al: Microcirculation in the conjunctival capillary of healthy and hypertensive patients. *Klin Wochenschr* 64:953, 1986.

74. Grunwald JE, Riva CE, Brucker AJ, et al: Effect of panretinal photocoagulation on retinal blood flow in proliferative diabetic retinopathy. *Ophthalmology* 93:590, 1986.

75. Kurantsin-Mills J, Cohen SB, Van Hoten P, et al: Morphometry and flow dynamics of conjunctival microcirculation in sickle cell disease. *Ann NY Acad Sci* 565: 418–421, 1989.

76. Wick CE, Loew MH, Kurantsin-Mills J: Understanding microvessels in two and three dimensions. In: Chen CH, Pan LF, Wong PSP (eds). *Handbook in Pattern Recognition and Computer Vision*. New York: World Scientific Publishing Co., 667–693, 1993.

77. Bagge U, Branemark PI: White cell rheology: an intravital study in man. *Adv Microcirc* 7:1, 1977.

78. Fan FC, Chen RYZ, Schuessler GB, et al: Effects of hematocrit variations on regional hemodynamics and oxygen transport in the dog. *Am J Physiol* 238:H545, 1980.

79. Lipowsky, Firrell JC: Microvascular hemodynamics during systemic hemodilution and hemoconcentration. *Am J Physiol* 250:H908, 1986.

80. Duling BR, Klitzman B: Local control of microvascular function: role in tissue oxygen supply. *Ann Rev Physiol* 42373, 1980.

81. Guyton AC, Coleman TG, Granger J: Circulation: overall regulation. *Ann Rev Physiol* 3413, 1972.

82. Pittman RN: Microvessel blood oxygen measurement techniques. In: Baker C, Nasfuk WL (eds). *Microcirculatory Technology*. Orlando, FL: Academic Press, Inc: 367–389, 1986.

83. Stein JC, Ellis CG, Ellsworth M: Relationship between capillary and systemic venous P_{O_2} during nonhypoxic and hypoxic ventilation. *Am J Physiol* 265 (*Heart Circ Physiol* 34):H537–H542, 1993.

84. Guyton AC: Local control of blood flow by the tissue, and nervous and humoral regulation. In: Guyton AC (ed). *Textbook of Medical Physiology*. 7th ed. Philadelphia: WB Saunders, Co; 230–243, 1986.

85. Valleel BL, Riordan JF, Lobb RR, et al: Tumor-derived angiogenesis factors from rat. Walker 256 carcinoma: an experimental investigation and review. *Experimentia* 41: 1, 1985.

86. Altura BM: Humoral hormonal myogenic mechanisms in microciculatory regulation. In: Kaley G, Altura BM (eds). *Microcirculation*. Vol II. Baltimore, MD: University Park Press; 431–502, 1978.

87. Renkin EM: Control of microcirculation and blood tissue exchange. In: Renkin EM, Michel CC (eds): *Handbook of Physiology*. Sec. 2. Vol II. Bethesda, MD: American Physiological Society; 627–687, 1984.

88. Bert JL, Pearce RH: The interstitium and microvascular exchange. In: Renkin EM, Michel CC (eds). *Handbook of Physiology*. Sec 2. Vol IV. Bethesda, MD: American Physiological Society; 521–547, 1984.

89. Aukland, Nicoloysen G: Interstitial fluid volume: local regulatory mechanism. *Physiolog Rev* 61:556, 1981.

90. Pappenheimer JR: Passes of molecules through capillary walls. *Physiol Rev* 33:387, 1953.

91. Curry FE, Joyner WL: Modulation of capillary permeability methods and measurements in individually-perused mammalian and frog microvessels. In: Ryan U (ed). *Endothelial Cells*. Vol 1. Boca Raton, FL: CRC Press; 3–17, 1988.

92. Curry FE: Regulation of water and solute exchange in microvessel endothelium: studies in single perfused capillaries. *Microcirc* 1:11–26, 1994.

CHAPTER 22

Drugs in Vascular Disease

James M. Edwards, MD; Lloyd M. Taylor Jr., MD
John M. Porter, MD

Practicing vascular surgeons need to be knowledgeable about an increasing number of drugs. This chapter reviews the basic pharmacology and mechanism of action of a number of drugs of current interest to vascular surgeons, as well as selected new and promising drugs presently in clinical trials. A large number of drugs such as antibiotics, analgesics, and cardiac active drugs that are essential, but not specific to vascular surgery will not be considered in this chapter.

The drugs reviewed in this chapter are grouped into four sections: anticoagulants, thrombolytic agents, antiplatelet agents, and drugs of potential usefulness in the treatment of claudication, including vasodilators (Table 1). Drugs with multiple effects will be discussed with the group in which they have their primary action. Obviously, the present discussion of clinical usefulness, mechanisms of action, and complications of drug use are meant as a review for the practicing vascular surgeon, and are limited to what we feel are the most important and interesting features of these drugs. The reader may consult more comprehensive pharmacologic reviews of each drug as needed.

Anticoagulants

Heparin

Heparin was discovered by MacLean in 1916 and has been used extensively in clinical practice for over 40 years.[1] During this time, many of the complex chemical and pharmacologic properties of heparin have become well recognized, although incompletely understood. Heparin is the most widely used anticoagulant, and it has been estimated that more than 6 metric tons of heparin were used in approximately 10 million patients in clinical practice in a recent year.[2]

Heparin occurs naturally in varying amounts in many tissues where it is concentrated in the mast cells. It is obtained commercially from bovine lung or porcine intestine. Heparin is actually a group of substances rather than a single compound. Chemically, heparin consists of mixtures of polymers of sulfonated mucopolysaccharide chains containing multiple acidic groups. The length of the polymers and their molecular weights vary, an observation that explains the variable biologic activity of each heparin batch. Because of this variability, the activity of heparin is measured in international units rather than by weight. As strong organic acids, the heparins increase the negative charge of the cell surfaces to which they attach, especially the endothelium, where injected heparin is selectively concentrated more than 100 times greater than in the circulating plasma.[2]

Using an isoelectric focusing technique, beef lung heparin can be separated into at least 21 components with the same charge, but with molecular weights that range from 3000 to 37500 d (2 to 22 hexasaccharides). Pork intestine heparin has the same 21 components, as well as dimers of each of the 21 components. The individual components exhibit distinct chemical and biologic activity. They can be separated using affinity chromatography with such substrates as antithrombin III, platelet factor 4, protamine, fibronectin, and on

From *The Basic Science of Vascular Disease*. Edited by Sidawy AN, Sumpio BE, and DePalma RG. Armonk, NY: Futura Publishing Company, Inc.; © 1997.

Table 1
Drugs Discussed in This Chapter

Anticoagulants
    Heparin
    Low molecular weight heparin
    Warfarin

Thrombolytic Drugs
    Streptokinase
    Anistreplase
    Urokinase
    Single-chain urokinase plasminogen activator
    Tissue plasminogen activator

Antiplatelet Drugs
    Aspirin
    Sulfinpyrazone
    Dipyridamole
    Ticlopidine
    Thromboxane synthetase inhibitors
        Picotamide

Claudication Drugs
    Pentoxifylline
    Dextran
    L-carnitine
    L-propionylcarnitine
    Cilostazol

Serotonergic agents
    Ketanserin
    Sumatriptan

Vasodilators
    Papaverine
    Isoxuprine
    Guanethidine
    Phenoxybenzamine
    Prazosin
    Tolazoline
    Phentolamine
    Cyclandelate
    Calcium channel blockers
    Nitrates
    Prostaglandins
        Iloprost

the basis of size and charge density. Approximately 10% of the fragments in available heparin possess 90% of the anticoagulant activity.[2,3] The specific anticoagulant activity of heparin fragments appears generally dependent upon molecular weight.[4,5]

Many heparin fractions have no detectable anticoagulant activity. Interestingly, both the anticoagulant and nonanticoagulant fractions of heparin have been shown to inhibit smooth muscle proliferation within the vascular wall.[6] Inhibition of myointimal growth appears dependent on the quantity of heparin administered, and not on the anticoagulant activity of the heparin. This effect appears specific for heparin and apparently is not secondary to the interaction of heparin with other substances such as platelet-derived growth factor (PDGF).

Heparin is not absorbed from the gastrointestinal tract or sublingually because of its polarity and large molecular size. It is well absorbed as a deep subcutaneous, intrafat, or intramuscular injection. It may also be administered intravenously or intra-arterially.

The dose of heparin is dependent on the condition being treated. For thrombosis prophylaxis, heparin may be given subcutaneously or as an "ultra low-dose" intravenous infusion.[7] For the treatment of an established thrombosis, heparin usually is given as a continuous intravenous infusion, but it may also be given intermittently either intravenously or subcutaneously. Evidence, however, indicates the superiority of the intravenous route.[8]

The anticoagulant activity of heparin follows apparent first-order kinetics, yet the half-life is dependent on the dose; increasing doses of heparin have an increased half-life that ranges from 1 to 5 hours.[9] It may take longer than 48 hours to reach steady state levels because of the dose-dependent kinetics. Heparin is metabolized in the liver by heparinase. It may be excreted unchanged in the urine after large doses. Patients with hepatic or renal failure display a prolonged heparin half-life.

Low-Molecular Weight Heparin

As noted, the anticoagulant activity of heparin fragments is generally dependent on their molecular weight. The interest in low-molecular weight heparins was stimulated by the observation that they are less likely to cause hemorrhage in animal models, but still maintain the ability to inhibit factor Xa. Low-molecular weight heparins specifically inhibit activated factor X, while larger molecular weight heparins appear to have a primary effect on other components of the coagulation system.[10,11] This difference is apparently due to the fact that for full anticoagulant action, a three-way complex of heparin, antithrombin III, and thrombin is required. Low-molecular weight heparins are too small to form this three-part complex and instead only bind to antithrombin III. The resulting low-molecular weight heparin-antithrombin III complex retains the ability to inhibit factor Xa, but has a limited effect on inhibition of thrombin.

Mechanism of Action

The conversion of factor X to factor Xa (activated Stuart-Prower factor) is the essential step in clot forma-

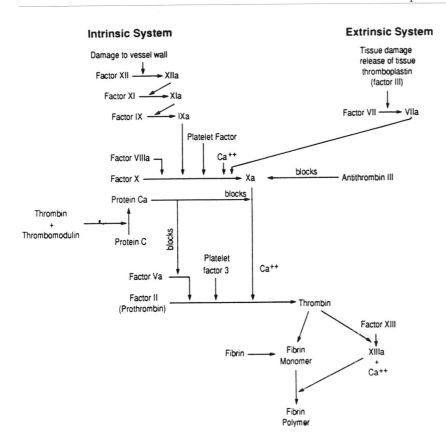

Figure 1. Diagrammatic representation of the human coagulation system showing the intrinsic and extrinsic coagulation pathway.

tion. Factor Xa begins the second stage of clotting, the conversion of prothrombin to thrombin that converts fibrinogen to fibrin, the polymerization of which results in a clot (Figure 1). Heparin affects this clotting cascade at two points. Certain of the heparin modalities combine with a circulating globulin known as antithrombin III, or heparin cofactor. The primary biologic action of antithrombin III is the inactivation of activated factor X. Heparin greatly accentuates the enzyme-inhibiting activity of antithrombin III, which results in the inactivation of factor Xa. This action apparently results from a conformational molecular change of the antithrombin III.

Only a tiny amount of antithrombin III is required to neutralize a much larger amount of Xa, markedly reducing the formation of thrombin. This cascade effect forms the basis for the effectiveness of low-dose heparin therapy. In addition, by interfering with factor XI, heparin inhibits the conversion of factor IX (Christmas factor) to factor IXa, which normally converts X to Xa. The second stage of clotting, the conversion of prothrombin to thrombin, is also inhibited by heparin blockade of the effect of factor V (proaccelerin). Heparin appears to have no significant effect on platelet function.[12]

Heparin may exert a protective effect on injured endothelium. Under normal conditions, the endothelium possesses a negative charge of approximately -90 mV. Injury to the endothelium reduces the negativity or may convert the charge to positive. This renders the endothelium far more thrombogenic as it begins to attract the negatively charged, formed elements of the blood. Heparin restores endothelial electronegativity, thus reinforcing endothelial antithrombotic activity.[2]

The use of heparin in the prophylaxis of venous thrombosis is dependent upon its ability to enhance the action of antithrombin III.[13] As no excess of factor Xa exists in the prethrombotic state, low-dose heparin is sufficient to neutralize small amounts of Xa that may be formed. In the treatment of existing thrombosis, a large excess of Xa is always present and the use of low-dose heparin is totally inappropriate.

Clinical Uses

Heparin is used for the prophylaxis and treatment of deep venous thrombosis, the treatment of pulmonary emboli and some forms of disseminated intravascular coagulation, and as an adjunct to prevent thrombosis on indwelling artificial surfaces such as central venous catheters. Low-molecular weight heparins appear to be at least as effective as conventional heparin in the prevention of deep venous thrombosis.[14] They have also been studied for the treatment of deep venous thrombosis and appear to be efficacious, although they are not yet approved in this country for that use.[15] In comparison to standard heparin therapy for deep venous thrombosis, treatment with low-molecular weight heparin involves subcutaneous injections and minimal laboratory monitoring which means that patients may be treated as outpatients. Heparin also is used in vascular surgery before cross-clamping arteries for prolonged periods of time and has been suggested as the first line of treatment for arterial thrombosis, a position which is controversial.[16]

Complications of Heparin

The most common complication of heparin therapy is bleeding, which occurs frequently enough to require transfusion in about 5% of patients receiving therapeutic heparin anticoagulation. The incidence of heparin-related bleeding increases in patients with liver disease and blood dyscrasia, and in the elderly, and in patients receiving heparin in the postoperative period or after trauma.[17] The incidence of serious bleeding with low-molecular weight heparin appears to be dose-dependent, and there are conflicting reports demonstrating both higher and lower bleeding complication rates when compared to standard heparin therapy.

Cutaneous necrosis frequently occurs at the site of subcutaneous heparin injection; cutaneous necrosis rarely occurs at remote sites.[18] This unusual but striking complication may be due to idiosyncratic stimulation of platelet aggregation by heparin with resulting intravascular thrombosis. It has been suggested that the tissue of origin of heparin may play a role in this complication, but this is not certain as conflicting evidence has been presented.

Osteoporosis as a complication of heparin therapy, first described by Griffith in 1965, appears to be related to the total dosage and duration of therapy.[19,20] As yet, there is no satisfactory explanation of the mechanism of this effect. Heparin-induced osteoporosis usually affects the vertebral column, although the ribs also may be involved. Fractures of these bones may occur in a period as short as 4 months and in patients receiving less than 10000 units/day. Bone pain invariably precedes x-ray evidence of osteoporosis. The occurrence of bone pain in patients on long-term heparin constitutes a clear indication to discontinue the drug regardless of x-ray findings.

Significant thrombocytopenia during heparin administration (heparin-associated thrombocytopenia [HAT]) has been reported in a variable percentage of patients, ranging in reported series from 1% to 30%.[21-23] In rare cases, such thrombocytopenia may appear after a single dose, but in most susceptible patients it occurs days after the initiation of heparin administration. HAT is caused by an antiheparin anti-

body. It has been suggested that this complication may be significantly related to the animal source of the administered heparin, but the supporting evidence is unconvincing. In most patients, HAT is mild and asymptomatic. In a few patients, the syndrome is associated with life-threatening symptoms.

Symptomatic HAT usually begins with increasing heparin resistance that paradoxically is frequently associated with bleeding. Many patients who experience severe HAT develop arterial occlusions that seem to be composed primarily of platelets. This has been termed "white clot syndrome." It is a serious occurrence which frequently leads to loss of a limb or death.[24-27] It has been widely recommended that all patients receiving heparin anticoagulation for more than 5 days have daily platelet counts and that the drug be discontinued at the first sign of a decreasing count.[22] Low-molecular weight heparin therapy has been reported to be an effective treatment for HAT as it does not induce platelet aggregation.[28]

Heparin in Pregnancy

By far, the most common disease for which heparin is given in pregnancy is deep venous thrombosis. Heparin does not cross the placenta, while warfarin does. Warfarin has been widely reported to cause possible teratogenic effects during the first trimester of pregnancy. This effect is not specific to warfarin, however, and the use of either drug carries obvious risks during this formative time.[18,29-31] Significant controversy surrounds the optimal method to achieve safe anticoagulation beyond the first trimester. While some feel that warfarin is safe in such a setting, others prefer to continue heparin.[33-35]

Warfarin

Although several hydroxycoumarin and indanedione derivatives are available for clinical use as anticoagulants, the coumarin, sodium warfarin, is the most commonly used. The coumarins were discovered in 1939 by Link, who identified these agents as causing a hemorrhagic cattle disease associated with improperly cured sweet clover fodder.[36] Warfarin initially was used as a rodenticide as it was felt to be too toxic for humans. Only after a man survived repeated doses in a suicide attempt were clinical trials of warfarin undertaken.[37]

Warfarin is rapidly and completely absorbed, with peak plasma concentrations reached within 1 hour of ingestion. Circulating warfarin is almost completely bound to albumin and its half-life is approximately 37 hours. Warfarin is metabolized in the liver into inactive metabolites that are excreted in the stool and urine.

Warfarin metabolism may be accelerated with induction of hepatic microsomal enzymes by drugs such as the barbiturates. Other drugs, such as disulfiram and cimetidine, may inhibit warfarin metabolism. Drugs such as phenylbutazone and chloral hydrate may displace warfarin from albumin and increase free plasma warfarin levels.

The mode of action of warfarin is through interference with vitamin K metabolism. Specifically, warfarin causes the sequential depression of the four fat-soluble coagulation factors II, VII, IX, and X. Factor VII, with a plasma half-life of approximately 6 hours, is the first to become depressed, although a lowered level of this factor is not associated with a significant antithrombotic effect. Factors II, IX, and X have plasma half-lives of between 1 and 5 days. Thus, therapeutic anticoagulation with the vitamin K antagonists requires 3 to 5 days. In hepatic microsomes, vitamin K must be reduced before the prothrombin precursor, desoxyprothrombin, can be activated by carboxylation to prothrombin. Warfarin blocks vitamin K reduction, thus blocking prothrombin production.[38]

The effect of warfarin on clotting, although usually constant in an individual, varies between patients. Therefore, the dosage must be adjusted accordingly. In addition to the effects of liver disease and drugs, other factors, including age, nutrition, diet, and general health of the patient, may affect the dosage of warfarin. At the conclusion of treatment, the dose should be tapered over a period of days because of reports of rebound hypercoagulability.[39,40]

Clinical Uses

Warfarin is most commonly used for the treatment and prophylaxis of deep vein thrombosis. It also is used in patients with artificial heart valves to decrease the incidence of embolization. Warfarin has been used in the treatment of claudication and transient ischemic attacks, although its efficacy has never been established. There is increasing interest in the use of warfarin as an adjunct to peripheral arterial bypass to prevent graft thrombosis. This is the subject of an ongoing Veterans Affairs multicenter trial.

Complications of Warfarin

The most frequent complication associated with warfarin therapy is significant bleeding, which occurs in 10% of patients. This can be reduced by careful monitoring of the prothrombin time. Elderly patients have a higher incidence of bleeding complications, in part due to changes in drug metabolism; therefore, the use of warfarin in this patient group must be carefully considered.[41]

Cutaneous necrosis is a rare, but well-described complication of warfarin therapy.[42,43] Generally, wide areas of skin necrosis usually localized to the lower half of the body occur on the third to fifth day of warfarin therapy. The mechanism underlying cutaneous necrosis accompanying warfarin administration has been described. Protein C is a vitamin K-dependent protein that is activated during clotting by the binding of thrombin to an endothelial protein termed thrombomodulin. Activated protein C acts as a potent inhibitor of coagulation by inactivating factors V and VIII and enhancing the fibrinolytic capacity of circulating blood. Thus, the physiologic role of this substance appears to be the limitation and modulation of intravascular clotting. The half-life of protein C is only 30 minutes.

Homozygous protein C deficiency is associated with massive venous thrombosis or purpura fulminans neonatalis and usually results in death in infancy.[44] Patients with heterozygous protein C deficiency have levels of protein C about 50% of normal. It has been postulated that, in these patients, the administration of warfarin causes a rapid drop in protein C levels to near homozygous deficient levels before the anticoagulant effect of diminished factors II, VII, IX, and X is established.[45] If these patients are not treated with other anticoagulants when their protein C levels drop, a pronounced hypercoagulable state develops. The cutaneous necrosis appears to result from thrombosis of the nutrient skin vessels.

Thrombolytic Drugs

Streptokinase, urokinase, and tissue plasminogen activator (tPA) are the thrombolytic drugs currently available in the United States. These three drugs act on the same portion of the fibrinolytic reaction (Figure 2). Two other agents, anistreplase and single-chain urokinase plasminogen activator (scuPA), will also be discussed.

Streptokinase

Streptokinase is a protein with a molecular weight of 47000 d produced by group C beta-hemolytic streptococci. The half-life of streptokinase is biphasic, with an initial fast half-life of about 12 to 16 minutes due to antibodies, and a slow half-life of 83 minutes in the absence of antibodies. Streptokinase has no intrinsic enzymatic activity. After administration, however, streptokinase binds to plasminogen. The resulting complex has protease activity and converts additional plasminogen to plasmin. The affinity of streptokinase for plasminogen is higher than that of the streptokinase-plasminogen complex. This leads to the curious

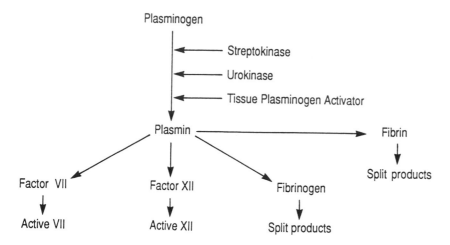

Figure 2. Schematic diagram of the in vivo thrombolysis. Streptokinase, urokinase, and tissue plasminogen activator all act to convert plasminogen to plasmin.

observation that one theoretically possible treatment for bleeding complications due to streptokinase is the administration of additional streptokinase that will result in the binding of all available plasminogen, leaving none available for conversion to plasmin, the active proteolytic enzyme. This, however, is not the standard treatment of bleeding caused by excess streptokinase.

Because streptokinase is derived from streptococci, most patients have some antistreptokinase antibodies in their serum. Ten percent of patients receiving streptokinase have an allergic reaction of hives, swelling, and itching, and an estimated 2% to 3% of patients have an anaphylactic reaction requiring emergency treatment. Antibody production after streptokinase administration begins within 1 week and titers peak at 2 to 3 weeks. Because of persistence of antibodies, redosing of streptokinase is not recommended within 1 year.[46]

Anistreplase

Anistreplase is an acylated plasminogen streptokinase complex (APSAC) in which the active enzymatic site is temporarily inactivated by the acylation. This inactivation leads to both decreased degradation by the normal plasma inhibitors alpha-2-antiplasmin and alpha-2-macroglobulin, as well as minimal plasma thrombolytic activity.[47] APSAC has a high affinity for fibrin, and in its presence becomes active. The theoretic benefit of decreased systemic activity has not been established in human studies, as a systemic fibrinolytic state is seen with standard dosing.

The half-life of APSAC is in the range of 105 to 120 minutes.[48] APSAC, like streptokinase, is antigenic, with a similar incidence of allergic reaction and antibody response.

Urokinase

Urokinase is a proteolytic enzyme found in human urine which is synthesized and secreted by the renal tubular cells.[49,50] The initial urokinase for clinical use was extracted from human urine. Presently, urokinase is produced from human embryonic renal cells in tissue culture. One of the advantages of urokinase is that it is totally nonallergenic in humans.

Two molecular forms exist: Sl, which has a molecular weight of 34500 ± 2000 d and is the most active form; and S2, which has a molecular weight of 54000 d. The Sl form is probably a breakdown product of urokinase formed during purification. Urokinase has a short half-life of approximately 30 minutes. It is cleared predominantly by the kidneys, although there is some hepatic metabolism.

Urokinase, unlike streptokinase, is a direct plasminogen activator. Its only known substrate is plasminogen, which it converts directly by cleavage into plasmin. Urokinase appears to have a higher affinity for fibrin-bound plasminogen than for free plasminogen. This gives it a theoretical advantage over streptokinase in that it should preferentially stimulate fibrinolysis in areas of ongoing thrombosis. This advantage has not been apparent in clinical use, and a systemic lytic state is invariably produced when using systemic urokinase.

Single-Chain Urokinase Plasminogen Activator

scuPA, or prourokinase, is a single-chain glycoprotein consisting of 411 amino acid residues which occurs naturally and is produced commercially from tissue culture or more recently by using recombinant DNA technology.[51] The thrombolytic activity of scuPA is almost completely fibrin-specific.[52] When exposed to fibrin, scuPA slowly converts plasminogen to plasmin, which in turn converts scuPA to plasminogen activator, which leads to a rapid increase in the amount of plasminogen activator. There is a circulating scuPA inhibitor that prevents this reaction in the absence of fibrin.

The half-life of scuPA is quite short, with 90% cleared in 3 to 6 minutes, and the remaining 10% cleared with a half-life of 20 minutes.[53] Heparin appears to increase the fibrinolytic activity of scuPA.[54] As with urokinase, scuPA is nonallergenic.

Tissue Plasminogen Activator

tPA is produced by human endothelial cells and has an extremely high affinity for fibrin-bound plasminogen. Initially, tPA was produced from human melanoma cells in tissue culture. Recent advances in genetic engineering have allowed the cloning and large-scale production of tPA by *Escherichia coli*.

The theoretical advantage of tPA is that in vitro it appears to only activate fibrin-bound plasminogen. Thus, it theoretically should activate thrombolysis only in areas of active thrombosis and should not degrade plasma fibrinogen or cause bleeding. This theoretical advantage has not been apparent in clinical use, and clinical reports of this agent have described a prominent systemic lytic effect.[55] It is quite potent, and clinical lysis with local infusion has been noted within 30 to 60 minutes.

Experimental Agents

Autologous plasmin solution has been tested in a limited fashion in animals and has been shown to produce thrombolysis at least as effectively as urokinase.[56] A combination of tPA and scuPA produced by recombinant DNA engineering called K1K2PU has also undergone limited testing in animals and appears to be effective.[57] Another strategy for improving thrombolysis is to insure an adequate supply of plasminogen by concurrent infusion of plasminogen. Experimentally, infusion of lys-plasminogen with urokinase has demonstrated greater thrombolysis.[58]

Clinical Uses of Thrombolytic Agents

There are four areas in which thrombolytic therapy has been used. The first is in the treatment of acute coronary artery thrombosis. Other uses include the treatment of deep vein thrombosis, pulmonary emboli, and arterial occlusions.

All thrombolytic drugs require parenteral administration, and all have extremely short half-lives. These agents have been given intravenously and intra-arterially in low and high doses. In the treatment of arterial occlusions, it has become common to impact a catheter into the arterial clot and administer "low-dose" thrombolytic therapy in this manner. Despite theoretical considerations to the contrary, it must be noted that this almost invariably results in a systemic lytic state.

In a number of studies, thrombolytic therapy has been shown to preserve venous valve architecture and function as determined by venography.[59,60] It would follow that thrombolytic therapy may be indicated in selected patients who present shortly after the onset of their first episode of thrombosis and have no contraindication to drug use. A study by Kakkar revealed that even those patients who were treated with streptokinase and had normal phlebograms after treatment had the same vascular laboratory abnormalities as patients treated with heparin.[61] These data suggest there may be little or no role for thrombolytic therapy in the treatment of lower extremity deep vein thromboses, although we and others have found it useful in the treatment of upper extremity deep vein thrombosis.[62–64]

The role of thrombolytic therapy in the treatment of pulmonary emboli is not totally clear, but currently we recommend it only for patients with massive pulmonary emboli who are sufficiently hemodynamically unstable to require pressor agents.

Thrombolytic therapy initially was used with great enthusiasm by vascular surgeons in the treatment of arterial thrombosis. It has become clear, however, that thrombolytic therapy is not the panacea many hoped it would be. The modest success rate, coupled with a significant incidence of complications, have led most authorities to recommend routine thrombolytic therapy only for arterial occlusions for which there are no good surgical alternatives, such as a thrombosed popliteal aneurysm with obliteration of the outflow tract.[65,66] There remains no consensus on the best agent, optimal dose, method of delivery, or clinical situation for thrombolysis of the peripheral arteries.[67]

Complications of Thrombolytic Therapy

The major complication of thrombolytic therapy is bleeding, which requires transfusion in about 10% of patients. Bleeding frequently accompanies low-dose intra-arterial drug administration, despite theoretical considerations to the contrary. The usual treatment of such bleeding is cessation of drug administration and the use of fresh frozen plasma. Streptokinase has the additional complication of allergic reaction.

Antiplatelet Medications

The platelet may play a central role in the development of arteriosclerosis, as well as in the induction of arterial thrombosis. The role of antiplatelet drugs in the primary prevention and treatment of arteriosclerosis, as well as an adjunct to improve the result of vascular surgery, is under intense evaluation.

The four drugs in widespread clinical use in the United States as antiplatelet agents include aspirin, sulfinpyrazone, dipyridamole, and ticlopidine. Other drugs or families of drugs that appear to have significant antiplatelet action include thromboxane synthetase inhibitors, prostaglandins, and serotonergic agents. The latter two will be discussed in later sections.

Aspirin

Aspirin (acetylsalicylic acid) is rapidly absorbed from the proximal intestine and secondarily from the stomach. Rectal absorption occurs, but is slower, incomplete, and unreliable. Aspirin is rapidly converted to salicylate. Salicylate levels peak about 2 hours after ingestion. The half-life of aspirin in plasma is about 15 minutes, and that of salicylate is 2 to 3 hours in low doses, and 2 to 15 hours at the high doses used for an anti-inflammatory effect.

Aspirin blocks the platelet production of thromboxane A_2 by irreversibly acetylating and, thereby, inactivating the enzyme cyclooxygenase (Figure 3). This eliminates an important stimulus for platelet aggregation and release.[68] Aspirin does not affect platelet adhesion. As platelets have no nucleus, they cannot synthesize new cyclooxygenase, so the effect of aspirin persists for the entire 7-to-10-day life span of platelets following a single dose.

Aspirin also blocks endothelial cell cyclooxygenase, thus inhibiting the endothelial cell production of prostacyclin PGI_2, a potent vasodilator and platelet antiaggregator. However, these cells have nuclei and rapidly synthesize new supplies of the enzyme, leading to an apparent reversibility of aspirin's effect. Numerous investigators have attempted to precisely adjust the dose of aspirin to produce selective blockage of thromboxane TxA_2 synthesis while sparing PGI_2. This has not been achieved to date.[69] There is some evidence that 80 mg of aspirin daily may produce levels high enough in the portal circulation to block TxA_2 synthesis, but has negligible spillover into the systemic circulation, thus sparing PGI_2 production. Further studies in this area are needed.

Sulfinpyrazone

Sulfinpyrazone, marketed as a uricosuric agent, also inhibits platelet cyclooxygenase, but its effect is weaker than that of aspirin and, more importantly, is

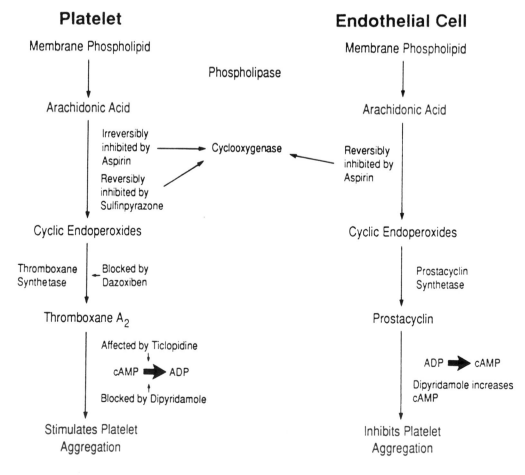

Figure 3. Diagram of the important biochemical reactions leading to the production of thromboxane A_2 and prostacyclin PGI_2.

reversible. Sulfinpyrazone is well absorbed after oral administration and is strongly bound to plasma albumin. It may displace other drugs from albumin. The half-life after intravenous administration is 2 to 3 hours, although its effects may be present for 10 hours after a single oral dose. It is primarily excreted unchanged in the urine.

Dipyridamole

Dipyridamole inhibits platelet phosphodiesterase, which causes an increase in the intraplatelet level of cyclic adenosine monophosphate phosphodiesterase (cAMP) (Figure 3). This in turn retards the platelet membrane-cytoplasm calcium shift, resulting in inhibition of platelet adhesion, release, and aggregation.[70]

Dipyridamole is variably absorbed after oral ingestion, with one third to two thirds of the dose eventually being absorbed. It is tightly bound to serum proteins. Excretion is mainly biliary, with about 20% of the drug undergoing enterohepatic recirculation.

Ticlopidine

Ticlopidine is a new antiplatelet drug which is now available in Europe and North America. The mechanism of action is through a decrease in platelet aggregation caused by inhibition of platelet ADP receptors.[71] The early clinical trials have shown prominent platelet inhibition in humans.[72] The onset of action of ticlopidine is within 24 to 48 hours of initiation of therapy and maximal action is not seen until 3 to 5 days. Platelet inhibition is still present 3 days after a final dose. Ticlopidine is rapidly absorbed orally and its metabolites are also active.[73] The most common side effects are gastrointestinal distress which affects 10% to 15% of patients. Agranulocytosis has been reported and white blood cell counts should be monitored after initiating therapy.

Thromboxane Synthetase Inhibitors

TxA_2 is formed by the action of the enzyme TxA_2 synthetase upon the cyclic endoperoxide intermediates PGE_2 and PGH_2 (Figure 3). TxA_2 is a powerful stimulator of platelet aggregation and release, and a powerful vasoconstrictor. TxA_2 has a half-life of only 30 seconds and is converted to the more stable, but less active thromboxane B_2. The putative benefit of TxA_2 synthetase inhibition is the shift of the PGE^2 synthetic pathway toward the production of PGI^2, which should be protective. Several low-molecular weight imidazole compounds selectively block the action of ^{TxA2} synthetase. Interestingly, while these compounds do indeed block TxA_2 synthetase, an increase in the amount of PGI_2 and its metabolites has not been consistently noted.[74] Pyridine compounds termed OKYs also block TxA_2 synthesis and are under intensive study. It has been postulated that the optimal antiplatelet medication in the future may prove to be a combination of a TxA^2 synthetase inhibitor plus low-dose aspirin.[75]

Picotamide, which acts as both a TxA_2 synthetase inhibitor and receptor antagonist, has undergone limited clinical trials.[76,77] Picotamide is an effective antithrombotic agent and has also been shown to decrease exercise-induced microalbuminuria in diabetic patients.[78] Its ultimate clinical utility remains to be determined.

Clinical Use of Antiplatelet Drugs

The antiplatelet agents have been shown to be effective in the treatment of transient ischemic attacks and unstable angina. Aspirin is effective in increasing graft patency rates in patients undergoing coronary artery bypass, and the same benefits probably apply to patients undergoing peripheral vascular surgery. The addition of sulfinpyrazone or dipyridamole in this setting has not been demonstrated to confer additional protection. Ticlopidine is slightly more effective than aspirin in preventing stroke and death in patients with recent neurologic events.[79,80] However, because the toxicity of ticlopidine is greater than that of aspirin, the current recommendation is to treat patients with ticlopidine if they either cannot tolerate aspirin or if there has been a neurologic event while on aspirin. Many other potential clinical uses, including the treatment of claudication and the prevention of stroke and myocardial infarction in atherosclerotic patients, are being investigated.[81]

Complications of Antiplatelet Drugs

In animal models, aspirin in combination with dipyridamole retards endothelial healing and causes increased platelet accumulation on injured arterial surfaces.[82] In addition, at least one study has suggested that aspirin may be important in the production of carotid artery intraplaque hemorrhage, with subsequent production of neurologic symptoms. These potentially harmful side effects must be considered when prescribing aspirin.[83] Ticlopidine administration is associated with diarrhea in 10%, rash in 5%, gastritis or ulcer in 2% to 3%, and severe but reversible neutropenia in approximately 1% of patients.

Claudication Drugs

Historically, the treatment of claudication has centered around vasodilators. The fields of hemorheology, the microcirculation, and metabolic enhancement are now the main targets in the search for new treatments for claudication.

It is important to keep in mind the natural history of claudicants when discussing pharmacologic treatment. The belief of some clinicians that patients presenting with claudication will have an inexorable progression of their disease culminating in amputation is incorrect. Only 10% to 15% of patients with claudication as their presenting symptom ever require amputation as a result of progression of their disease. A majority of claudicants experience stabilization of their disease or spontaneous improvement without any specific therapy. Thus, the natural perturbations of the disease must be considered when evaluating any treatment program, including pharmacologic therapy.

The drugs whose effects have been intensively studied in the areas of hemorheology and metabolic enhancement are pentoxifylline, the dextrans, and L-carnitine.

Pentoxifylline

Theobromine, a methylxanthine, was first investigated as a vasodilator over 50 years ago. The usefulness of the product was never established and it was withdrawn. A German pharmaceutical firm, Hoechst AG, initiated a synthetic theobromine investigative program in the 1960s, including studies of the drug pentifylline. The first studies showed that pentifylline was rapidly metabolized to pentoxifylline. This, then, became the focus of the study.

In 1976, Reid et al and Ehrly independently observed that erythrocytes (RBC) from patients with peripheral vascular disease appeared more rigid, or less flexible, than those from matched control individuals without vascular disease. This obviously is important, as RBCs with an 8 μm diameter must pass regularly through capillaries that are 4 to 5 μm in diameter.[84,85]

At about the same time that Ehrly showed that RBCs from patients with vascular disease were less flexible than normal, he found that pentoxifylline added to blood obtained from claudicants resulted in an increase in blood filterability as measured by the timed volume flow of blood under constant pressure through microporous material. This led Ehrly to conclude that the pentoxifylline caused an increase in RBC flexibility.[86]

The impairment of RBC flexibility in patients with vascular disease was felt to be caused by regional hyperosmolality and acidosis. These conditions occur in ischemic regions as a result of the local accumulation of metabolic products of anaerobic glycolysis. Under these conditions, there is a decrease in RBC content of cAMP and ATP. It has been suggested that this decrease occurs in association with an increase in calcium-dependent cross-linkage of RBC membrane proteins, leading to greater membrane rigidity. The resulting increased RBC rigidity may then compound preexisting ischemia by preventing or impeding RBC passage through regional capillaries in ischemic areas.

A number of investigators have noted that a single oral dose of pentoxifylline results in a measurable reduction in whole blood viscosity. The relative contribution of increased RBC flexibility to the observed decrease in blood viscosity is difficult to determine, however, since the drug also reduces plasma fibrinogen and retards platelet aggregation, both of which may affect blood viscosity. Further studies have shown that pentoxifylline increases normal RBC filterability to supranormal levels. The drug also appears to markedly affect leukocyte function.

Pentoxifylline is well absorbed after oral ingestion. The drug binds to the RBC membrane, with a half-life of approximately 30 minutes, and that of its major metabolites of approximately 90 minutes. While the half-life of pentoxifylline is measured in minutes, the time to onset of maximal clinical benefit is 6 to 8 weeks. Pentoxifylline is metabolized by the RBC and the liver, and the metabolites are excreted by the kidney.

Clinical Uses of Pentoxifylline

Pentoxifylline is the first and remains the only drug approved by the US Food and Drug Administration for the treatment of intermittent claudication. Several randomized studies have demonstrated the efficacy of pentoxifylline in the healing of venous ulceration.[87,88] It has also been suggested that pentoxifylline may be useful in the treatment of Raynaud's syndrome and transient ischemic attacks.[89] Studies in these areas are continuing.

Complications of Pentoxifylline

The most frequent complication noted with pentoxifylline is nausea. This has never been a major problem, and has been recently reduced by a change in the formula by the manufacturer.

Dextran

The dextrans are a group of long-chain carbohydrates of varying molecular weight formed by polymerization of glucose subunits. The two dextrans available in the United States are dextran 40 and dextran 70. Dextran 40 has a mean molecular weight of 40000 d, and 90% of its molecules have a molecular weight between 10000 and 90000 d. Dextran 70 has a mean molecular weight of 70000 d and a similar range of molecular weights. The clinical utility of the dextrans resides in the three properties of plasma volume expansion, microcirculatory blood flow enhancement, and antithrombotic effect.

The dextrans can be used only intravenously. The polymers of less than 50000 d are primarily excreted in the urine. The larger polymers are secreted into the digestive tract where they are hydrolyzed into simple sugars. About 50% of dextran 40 and 30% of dextran 70 is excreted in 4 hours, while 80% of dextran 40 but only 40% of dextran 70 is excreted in 24 hours.

The dextrans are potent intravascular hydrophilic agents that cause rapid plasma volume expansion. This appears to be the major cause of microvascular flow enhancement because of a lowering of blood viscosity associated with plasma volume expansion. In the mid ranges of red cell volume, an 8% drop in hematocrit will decrease blood viscosity by one half.[90]

The effects of dextrans on clotting mechanisms have been studied extensively. Dextran coats the endothelial lining of the blood vessel and the formed elements of the blood. The coating enhances the normal electronegative charge of these structures, producing mutual repulsion and discouraging thrombus formation. Dextran also forms complexes with some of the plasma proteins necessary for clotting, thereby interfering with their actions.[91] The dextrans decrease the level of factor VIII activity, which produces a coagulopathy similar to von Willebrand's disease. During active clotting, dextran will polymerize with fibrin monomers resulting in an alteration of the composition and structure of the subsequent clot, thus rendering it more susceptible to thrombolysis.

Clinical Uses of Dextran

Dextran has been used as a volume expander in trauma, a use that will not be discussed here. There is some evidence that dextran can improve the patency rates of low flow peripheral bypasses, an effect that appears to be mediated through a combination of dextran's effects on the coagulation mechanism and through its improvement of flow characteristics.[89]

Complications of Dextran Therapy

Increased bleeding occurs after treatment with dextran. Dextran also coats RBCs, potentially making subsequent transfusion cross-matching difficult. Allergies to dextran are not uncommon, and anaphylactic reactions have been reported.

L-Carnitine, L-Propionylcarnitine

L-Carnitine is a naturally occurring substance that plays an essential role in fatty acid metabolism and the Krebs cycle. Patients with peripheral vascular disease have a deficiency of carnitine in their leg muscles and may also have abnormal carnitine metabolism.[92,93] Numerous trials in Europe have demonstrated that oral supplementation of L-carnitine results in increased circulatory reserve and walking distance.[94,95] L-propionylcarnitine appears to be more effective on a molar basis than L-carnitine.[96] A phase III clinical trial with L-propionylcarnitine is currently underway in the United States.

Complications of L-carnitine and L-propionylcarnitine Therapy

L-carnitine and L-propionylcarnitine side effects appear to be limited to mild gastrointestinal upset at high doses in a few patients.

Cilostazol

Cilostazol is a selective inhibitor of cAMP which produces relaxation of vascular smooth muscle and also functions as an antiplatelet agent.[97,98] In preliminary testing, cilostazol has been shown to increase the walking distance in claudicants although the mechanism by which the drug is effective is not clear. It is currently undergoing a phase III trial in the United States.

Serotonergic Agents

In 1948, Page and associates showed that during coagulation the powerful vasoconstrictor serotonin is released into serum from intraplatelet stores. In addition to its marked vasoconstrictive properties, serotonin is a potent platelet aggregator.

Two cellular serotonergic binding sites have been defined, termed S1 and S2. Serotonin interacts with blood vessels, bronchi, and platelets through the S2 binding site. A selective S2 blocking agent, ketanserin, is currently undergoing clinical trials. Sumatriptan is a selective agonist at the S1 site.

Ketanserin is a quinazoline derivative, of which about 50% is absorbed after oral ingestion. Peak levels are seen 1 to 2 hours after ingestion and the half-life is about 18 hours. Ketanserin is metabolized by reduction, as well as oxidation with the metabolites excreted mainly in the urine. Ketanserin consistently improves the hemorheologic properties of blood in patients with essential hypertension, myocardial infarction, or peripheral vascular disease by increasing red blood cell deformability and decreasing white blood cell sludging.

Sumatriptan is an S1 agonist which has recently been approved in an injectable form for the treatment of migraine headaches.[99] Oral and intranasal formulations are also being studied.[100,101] The mechanism of action of sumatriptan appears to be vasoconstriction of intracerebral vessels, thus validating the vasodilation as the cause of migraine pain theory.

Clinical Uses of Serotonergic Agents

Ketanserin is an effective antihypertensive agent. While early studies revealed ketanserin to be effective in the treatment of claudication, subsequent studies have not been able to duplicate these results.[102,103] A statistician, while reviewing the results of all the trials conducted with ketanserin, noted that patients receiving a placebo had the expected number of cardiovascular morbid events, but the patients receiving ketanserin had one third the number of expected events. An international placebo-controlled trial of ketanserin in the reduction of stroke, myocardial infarction, and the prevention of progression of peripheral vascular disease did not confirm this finding. As noted above, sumatriptan is an effective form of migraine therapy.

Complications of Serotonergic Agents

Ketanserin, in addition to causing dizziness from a decrease in blood pressure, has been noted to produce nausea in some patients. It may also cause prolongation of the QT interval. The clinical significance of this is unclear, although sudden death has been associated with this finding. Sumatriptan causes coronary vasoconstriction and an increase in pulmonary and systemic arterial pressures.[104] Myocardial infarction has been reported after sumatriptan administration, and its use is contraindicated in patients with known heart disease or previous complicated migraine.[105]

Vasodilators

Many drugs have vasodilation as a primary or secondary effect. Rather than consider all drugs that cause vasodilation, the present discussion focuses upon the most commonly used vasodilators. The vasodilators can be divided into direct-acting drugs (cyclandelate, nicotinic acid, papaverine); beta-receptor stimulating drugs (nylidrin and possibly isoxuprine); drugs that interfere with adrenergic neuromuscular synaptic transmission (ethyl alcohol, guanethidine, methyldopa, phenoxybenzamine, reserpine, and tolazoline); calcium

Table 2
Vasodilator Drugs

Direct Acting Drugs
  Papaverine
  Isoxuprine
  Cyclandelate

α-Adrenergic Blockers
  Guanethidine
  Phenoxybenzamine
  Prazosin
  Tolazoline
  Phentolamine

Prostaglandins
  PGE, PGI

β Stimulating Drugs
  Nylidrin

Calcium Channel Blockers
  Nifedipine
  Verapamil
  Diltiazem
  Amlodipine
  Felodipine
  Isradipine
  Nicardipine
  Nimodipine

Nitrates
  Nitroprusside

channel blockers; nitrates; and prostaglandins (Table 2).

While the exact mechanism of vasodilation of each drug is not known with certainty, an understanding of the cellular mechanisms of vasodilation is rapidly increasing. In vascular smooth muscle, the major mediator of contraction appears to be calcium (Figure 4). Intracellular calcium levels are controlled by regulation of calcium entry into the cell and sequestration of calcium in intracellular membranes. Inositol, cAMP, and calmodulin are important mediators of calcium-controlled vasoconstriction, and their relative role probably varies from tissue to tissue.[106,107]

Papaverine

Papaverine is an alkaloid present in crude opium, yet it is chemically and pharmacologically unrelated to the opioid alkaloids. It is a nonspecific smooth muscle relaxant whose mechanism of action appears to be the inhibition of cyclic nucleotide phosphodiesterase, with

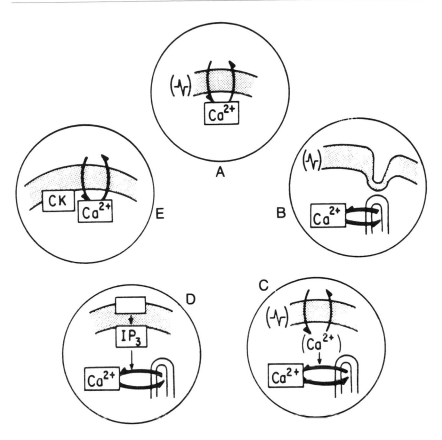

Figure 4. Alternative models of Ca^{++} messenger function. **A.** Depolarization of membrane leads to Ca^{2+} movement across the membrane. **B.** Depolarization of membrane leads to Ca^{2+} movement across intracellular membranes. **C.** Depolarization leads to movement of Ca^{2+} across both the membrane and intracellular membranes. **D.** Binding of cell surface receptor activates inositol triphosphate (IP_3) which regulates intracellular membrane Ca^{2+} movement. **E.** Ca^{2+} movement across membranes regulates activity of protein kinase C (CK). (Modified with permission from Reference 107.)

a subsequent increase of cAMP and decrease of calcium flux.

Isoxuprine

Isoxuprine is chemically similar to the sympathomimetic amines and is usually classified as a beta-adrenergic agonist, although its vasodilating effects are not blocked by propanolol. The drug probably has direct vasodilating properties similar to papaverine.

Guanethidine

Guanethidine is poorly absorbed after oral ingestion and, while it is cleared rapidly from plasma by the kidney, small amounts remain in the body for weeks. Guanethidine is taken up and stored in adrenergic nerves. It accumulates in and displaces norepinephrine from intraneuronal storage granules, thereby inhibiting responses to stimulation of sympathetic nerves by decreasing release of the neurotransmitter norepinephrine.

Phenoxybenzamine

Phenoxybenzamine is an alpha-adrenergic blocking agent that is moderately selective for alpha-1 recep-

tors. It is incompletely and inconsistently absorbed after oral ingestion. It is highly lipid-soluble at physiologic pH, and while the half-life is around 12 hours, small amounts remain for days.

Phenoxybenzamine blocks the alpha-1 receptor on smooth muscle, thus preventing stimulation (and vasoconstriction) by epinephrine and, to a lesser extent, norepinephrine.

Prazosin

Prazosin is moderately well absorbed and has a half-life of 2.5 hours. It is extensively metabolized in the liver with many of the metabolites having longer half-lives. It is a selective alpha-1 receptor blocker and selectively blocks the action of epinephrine on smooth muscle.

Tolazoline and Phentolamine

Tolazoline and phentolamine are substituted imidazolines that have many actions, including alpha-1 adrenergic blocking properties. Tolazoline is well absorbed after intravenous and oral administration. Absorption from the gastrointestinal tract is slower than renal excretion, so high serum concentrations are not usually obtainable with oral use; it is excreted unchanged by the kidney. Phentolamine is not well absorbed after oral administration; it is excreted primarily as metabolites.

Cyclandelate

Cyclandelate is a direct-acting vasodilator. It may cause gastrointestinal upset, as well as flushing and tingling.

Clinical Uses of Vasodilators

Certain of the vasodilators listed above, including guanethidine and prazosin, have a clinical role in the treatment of hypertension, and this action will not be further considered here.

The vasodilators represent important mileposts in our quest for effective claudication drugs. Early clinicians, seeing the blanched feet of claudicants, intuitively assumed that vasoconstriction must play a role in limb ischemia. This belief initiated a 50-year quest for a clinically effective vasodilator to treat claudication. We now know that the blanching in claudicants results from the selective redistribution of the limited blood entering the ischemic limb to the dilated proximal muscle circulatory bed, and that, in fact, the local accumulation of the products of anaerobic metabolism are among the most powerful vasodilators known. The fallacy of the use of vasodilators in the treatment of claudication has been widely recognized and eloquently described.[108]

Available evidence, however, suggests caution in dismissing all vasodilators. Certainly some of these drugs have conveyed anecdotal benefits for almost a half century. The absence of requisite randomized placebo-controlled data resulted in part from the time period in which these drugs were studied. Our penchant for carefully controlled clinical studies was not in place in those early years. Additionally, multicenter clinical trials with isoxuprine and cyclandelate have shown benefits very similar to pentoxifylline. Most, if not all, of these drugs have multiple actions including hemorheologic effects. It is unfortunate that until recently only the vasodilator effects had been recognized. It is interesting to recall that pentoxifylline was produced as a vasodilator, and until the recent recognition of its hemorheologic properties was classified only as a vasodilator.

Complications of Vasodilators

While each vasodilator may have idiosyncratic reactions, the main complication of the vasodilating agents is hypotension caused by too large a dose or increased patient sensitivity.

Calcium Channel-Blocking Agents

Since the first edition of this book, at which time there were only three calcium channel-blocking agents in the United States (nifedipine, verapamil, and diltiazem), many new calcium channel blockers have been approved for use including amlodipine, felodipine, isradipine, nicardipine, and nimodipine.

Nifedipine is well absorbed with sublingual administration, but only about one half of an oral dose is absorbed. Its half-life is 3 to 4 hours. Nifedipine is extensively bound to plasma proteins and excreted as inactive metabolites by the kidneys. Other members of the dihydropyridines include felodipine, isradipine, and nicardipine. This family of calcium channel blockers is more likely to cause at least an initial reflex tachycardia.

Verapamil, diltiazem, and amlodipine usually do not affect the heart rate but may adversely affect atrioventricular node conduction and should be used cautiously in combination with beta-blockers.

Smooth muscle contraction is dependent on an increase in free intracellular cytoplasmic calcium, which either comes through the membrane or is released from intracellular stores. The calcium channel-blocking drugs affect influx of calcium from the extracellular milieu. The site of action and the tissue type specificity varies from drug to drug.[109]

Clinical Uses of Calcium Channel Blockers

The calcium channel blockers are widely used in the treatment of hypertension and ischemic heart disease. They are also used in the prophylaxis and treatment of migraine as well as for the treatment of certain cardiac arrhythmias. These uses will not be further discussed here.

There are two uses of this class of drugs that are of interest to vascular surgeons. The first is in the treatment of claudication. Verapamil anecdotally has been reported to be effective in treating claudicants, and clinical trials of various calcium channel blockers are ongoing. It is not clear if the purported beneficial effects of calcium channel blockers result from vasodilation, improvements in hemorheology, or an as yet undescribed mechanism. The other area in which calcium channel blockers are proven to be effective is in the treatment of upper extremity vasospasm, manifested clinically as Raynaud's syndrome. We have found that nifedipine, either alone or in combination with diltiazem, produces symptomatic relief without intolerable side effects in over half of the patients with Raynaud's syndrome of sufficient severity to require drug treatment.

Complications of Calcium Channel Blockers

In addition to the risk of hypotension, the calcium channel blockers, particularly the dihydropyridines, may cause headache and ankle swelling, the mechanism of which is unknown. Fatigue is a rare but well-recognized complication of the calcium channel blockers which resolves upon discontinuation of the drug.

Nitrates

Many nitrate formulations are available, but the two most commonly prescribed by vascular surgeons are nitroglycerine and nitroprusside. Nitroglycerine is rapidly absorbed after sublingual or cutaneous application. It has a half-life of about 2 minutes and is metabolized to the much less active dinitrates, which have a half-life of 40 minutes.

Sodium nitroprusside is converted rapidly by erythrocytes to cyanide, and then to thiocyanate. Thiocyanate is excreted by the kidneys and has a half-life of 4 to 7 days. Toxic levels may be reached rapidly in patients with renal disease.

The nitrates activate guanylate cyclase, causing an increase in available cyclic monophosphate (cGMP) in smooth muscle. The activation is apparently caused by the reaction of the free radical nitric oxide ($NO\Sigma$) with guanylate cyclase. Increased cGMP levels in smooth muscle cause sequestration of calcium, which prevents contraction.

Clinical Uses of Nitrates

The nitrates are most commonly used in the treatment and prophylaxis of coronary ischemia. The nitrates can be extremely useful to vascular surgeons in two areas. One is the acute treatment of hypertension, particularly in the postoperative patient, and the second is in the acute treatment of ergotism, the incidence of which may be on the rise with the widespread use of ergots such as dihydroergotamine-heparin for the prophylaxis of venous thrombosis.

Complications of Nitrates

The nitrates may cause the rapid onset of profound hypotension, especially in patients with depleted intravascular volume. The accumulation of thiocyanate, a toxic metabolite of nitroprusside, must be considered when treating patients for more than 24 to 48 hours.

Prostaglandins

The prostaglandins are a family of naturally occurring 20 carbon chain fatty acids. The substances that have attracted the most attention in relationship to the cardiovascular system are prostaglandins PGE_1 and PGI_2.

The biologic half-life of prostaglandins in the bloodstream is approximately 20 seconds. Both PGE_1 and PGI_2 bind to membrane receptors. The binding results in elevation of adenylate cyclase and an increase in cAMP. Increased intracellular cAMP levels lead to calcium sequestration and inhibit contraction of vascular smooth muscle and platelets.

Iloprost

Iloprost is a stable analog of PGI_2 which is now available in both oral and intravenous forms, although neither preparation is approved for use in the United States. Iloprost has been extensively tested in Europe in peripheral arterial disease.

Clinical Uses of Prostaglandins

It was initially hoped that the vasodilator and antiplatelet properties of PGE_1 would result in widespread clinical usefulness. Indeed, numerous early anecdotal reports described apparent remarkable benefits in the treatment of ischemic limb ulcers and Raynaud's syndrome. Unfortunately, subsequent controlled studies failed to show benefit.[110,111] Iloprost appears to have clinical utility in peripheral arterial disease and has been demonstrated to improve both treadmill walking distance and ischemic ulcer healing.[112,113] Iloprost has also been used to treat patients with Buerger's disease and Raynaud's syndrome with digital artery obstruction due to scleroderma.[114,115]

References

1. MacLean J: Thromboplastic action of cephalin. *Am J Physiol* 41:250, 1916.
2. Jacques LB: Heparin: an old drug with a new paradigm. *Science* 206:528, 1979.
3. Fareed J: Heparin: its fractions, fragments, and derivatives. *Semin Thromb Hemostasis* 11:1, 1985.
4. Cifonelli JA: The relationship of molecular weight, and sulfate content and distribution to anticoagulant activity of heparin preparations. *Carbohydr Res* 37:145, 1974.
5. Laurent TC, Tengblad A, Thunberg L, et al: The molecular weight dependence of the anticoagulant activity of heparin. *Biochem J* 175:691, 1978.
6. Guyton J, Rosenberg RD, Clowes AW, et al: Inhibition of rat arterial smooth muscle cell proliferation by heparin. Part I: In vivo studies with anticoagulant and non-anticoagulant heparin. *Circ Res* 45:625, 1980.

7. Negus D, Friedgood A, Cox SJ, et al: Ultra-low dose intravenous heparin in the prevention of postoperative deep-vein thrombosis. *Lancet* 1:891, 1980.

8. Salzman EW, Deykin D, Mayer Shapiro R, et al: Management of heparin therapy. *N Engl J Med* 292:1046, 1975.

9. Estes JW: Clinical pharmacokinetics of heparin. *Clin Pharmacokinet* 5:204, 1980.

10. Andersson LC, Barrowcliffe TW, Holmes E, et al: Anticoagulant properties of heparin fractionated by affinity chromatography on matrix-bound anti-thrombin-III and by gel filtration. *Thromb Res* 9:575, 1976.

11. Andersson LC, Barrowcliffe TW, Holmes E, et al: Molecular weight dependency of the heparin potentiated inhibition of thrombin and activated factor X. *Thromb Res* 15:531, 1979.

12. Salzman EW: The limitations of heparin therapy after arterial reconstruction *Surgery* 57:131, 1965.

13. Kakkar W, Corrigan TP, Fossard DP: Prevention of fatal postoperative pulmonary embolism by low doses of heparin: an international multicenter trial. *Lancet* 2: 7924, 1975.

14. Hirsh J: From unfractionated heparins to low molecular weight heparins. *Acta Chir Scan* (suppl)556:42–50, 1990.

15. Prandoni P, Lensing AWA, Büller HR, et al: Comparison of subcutaneous low molecular weight heparin with intravenous standard heparin in proximal deep venous thrombosis. *Lancet* 339:441–445, 1992.

16. Blaisdell FW, Steele M, Allen RE: Management of acute lower extremity arterial ischemia due to embolism and thrombosis. *Surgery* 84:822, 1978.

17. Joist JH: Laboratory control, prevention, and management of complications of anticoagulant therapy. In: Joist JH, Sherman LA (eds). *Venous and Arterial Thrombosis: Pathogenesis, Diagnosis, Prevention, and Therapy*. New York: Grune & Stratton; 173, 1979.

18. Kelly RA, Gelfraud JA, Pincus SH: Cutaneous necrosis caused by systemically administered heparin. *JAMA* 246:1582, 1981.

19. Griffith GC, Nichols G, Asher JD: Heparin osteoporosis. *JAMA* 193:85, 1965.

20. Squires JW, Pinch LW: Heparin-induced spinal fractures. *JAMA* 241:2417, 1979.

21. Powers PJ, Cuthbert D, Hirsch J: Thrombocytopenia found uncommonly during heparin therapy. *JAMA* 241: 2396, 1979.

22. Towne JB, Bernhardt VM, Hussy C, et al: White clot syndrome: peripheral vascular complications of heparin therapy. *Arch Surg* 114:372, 1979.

23. Kapsch DN, Adelstein EH, Rhodes GR, et al: Heparin induced thrombocytopenia, thrombosis, and hemorrhage. *Surgery* 86:148, 1979.

24. Weissman RD, Tobin RW: Arterial embolism occurring during systemic heparin therapy. *Arch Surg* 76:219, 1958.

25. Roberts B, Rosato F, Rosato E: Heparin: a cause of arterial emboli? *Surgery* 55:803, 1964.

26. Rhodes GR, Dixon RH, Silver D: Heparin-induced thrombocytopenia. *Ann Surg* 186:752, 1977.

27. Bell W, Royall RM: Heparin-associated thrombocytopenia: a comparison of three heparin preparations. *N Engl J Med* 303:902, 1980.

28. Vitoux J-F, Mathieu J-F, Roncato M, et al: Heparin associated thrombocytopenia treatment with low molecular weight heparin. *Thromb Haemost* 55:37–39, 1986.

29. Coon WW: Anticoagulant therapy for venous thromboembolism. *Postgrad Med* 63:157, 1978.

30. Hall JG, Pauli RM, Wilson KM: Maternal and fetal sequelae of anticoagulation during pregnancy. *Am J Med* 68:122, 1980.

31. Tawes RL, Kennedy PA, Harris EJ, et al: Management of deep vein thrombosis and pulmonary embolism during pregnancy. *Ann J Surg* 144:141, 1982.

32. Walsh PN: Oral anticoagulation therapy. *Hosp Pract* Jan:101, 1983.

33. Poller L: Oral anticoagulant therapy. In: Bloom AL, Duncan PT (eds). *Hemostasis and Thrombosis*. New York: Churchill Livingstone; 725, 1981.

34. Hirsh J, Cade JF, Gallus AS: Anticoagulation in pregnancy: a review of indications and complications. *Am Heart J* 83:301, 1972.

35. Baskin HF, Munay JM, Harris RE: Low dose heparin for prevention of thromboembolic disease in pregnancy. *Am J Obstet Gynecol* 129:590, 1977.

36. Link KP: The anticoagulant from spoiled sweet clover hay. *Harvey Lect* 39:162, 1943–1944.

37. Link KP: Discovery of dicumarol and its sequels. *Circulation* 19:97, 1959.

38. Whitlon DS, Sadowski JA, Suttie JW: Mechanism of coumarin action: significance of vitamin K epoxide reductase inhibition. *Biochemistry* 17:1371, 1978.

39. Poller L, Thompson J: Reduction of "rebound" hypercoagulability by gradual withdrawal ("trailing off") of oral anti-coagulants. *Br Med J* 1:1475, 1965.

40. Michaels L: Incidence of thromboembolism after stopping anticoagulation therapy. *JAMA* 215:595, 1971.

41. Routledge PA, Chapman PA, Davies DM: Factors affecting warfarin requirement. *Eur J Clin Pharm* 15:319, 1979.

42. Chua FS, Chiscano AD, Wukasch DC, et al: Dermal gangrene. *J Thorac Cardiovas Surg* 65:238, 1973.

43. Bahadir I, James EC, Feede CW: Soft tissue necrosis and gangrene complicating treatment with the coumadin derivatives. *Surg Gynecol Obstet* 145:497, 1977.

44. Seligsohn U, Berger A, Abend M, et al: Homozygous protein C deficiency manifested by massive venous thrombosis in the newborn. *New Engl J Med* 310:559, 1984.

45. Broekmans AW, Bertina RM, Loeliger EA, et al: Protein C and the development of skin necrosis during anticoagulant therapy. *Thromb Haemost* 49:244, 1983.

46. Jalihal S, Morris JK: Antistreptokinase titers after intravenous streptokinase. *Lancet* 335:184–186, 1990.

47. Matsuo O, Collen D, Verstraete M: On the fibrinolytic and thrombolytic properties of active site P-anisolated streptokinase plasminogen complex (BRL 26921).*Thromb Res* 24:347–358, 1981.

48. Nunn B, Esmail E, Fears R, et al: Pharmacokinetic properties of anisolated plasminogen streptokinase activator and other thrombolytic agents in animals and humans. *Drugs* (suppl 3)33:88–92, 1987.

49. MacFarlane RG, Pilling J: Fibrinolytic activity of normal urine. *Nature* 159:779, 1947.

50. Aoki N, Von Kaulla KN: Dissimilarity of human vascular plasminogen activation and human urokinase. *J Lab Clin Med* 78:354, 1971.

51. Gunzler WA, Cramer J, Frankus E, et al: Biological and thrombolytic properties of proenzyme and active forms of human urokinase-1, fibrinolytic and fibrinogenolytic properties in human plasma in vitro of urokinases obtained from human urine or by recombinant DNA technology. *Thromb Haemost* 52:19, 1984.

52. Flohe L: Single-chain urokinase type plasminogen activators: new hopes for specific clot lysis. *Eur Heart J* 6:905–908, 1985.

53. Hillis WS, Gemmill JD, Bhargava B: Thrombolytic therapy in arterial disease. 1: Available agents. *Vasc Med Rev* 3:145–156, 1992.

54. Lijnen HR, Collen D: Stimulation by heparin of the plasmin-mediated conversion of single-chain to two-chain urokinase-type plasminogen activator. *Thromb Res* 43:687, 1986.

55. Graor RA, Risius B, Young JR, et al: Peripheral artery and bypass graft thrombolysis with recombinant human tissue-type plasminogen activator. *J Vasc Surg* 3:115, 1986.

56. Mizutani M, Kobayashi T, Makita M, et al: Potential thrombolysis under selective infusion of autologous plasmin (AP) solution. *JPN Heart J* 30:723–732, 1989.

57. Lu HR, Wu Z, Pauwels P, et al: Comparative thrombolytic properties of tissue type plasminogen activator (t-PA), single-chain urokinase-type plasminogen activator (scu-PA), and K1K2Pu (a t-PA/scu-PA chimera) in a combined arterial and venous model in dogs. *J Am Coll Cardiol* 19:1350–1359, 1992.

58. Badylak SF, Voytik SL, Henkin J, et al: The beneficial effect of lys-plasminogen upon the thrombolytic efficacy of urokinase in a dog model of peripheral arterial thrombosis. *Thromb Haemost* 21:278–285, 1991.

59. Porter JM, Seaman AJ, Common HH, et al: Comparison of heparin and streptokinase in the treatment of venous thrombosis. *Am J Surg* 41:511, 1975.

60. Kakkar W, Flanc C, Howe CT: Treatment of deep vein thrombosis: a trial of heparin, streptokinase, and arvin. *Br Med J* 1:806, 1969.

61. Kakkar W, Lawrence D: Hemodynamic and clinical assessment after therapy for acute vein thrombosis. *Am J Surg* 150(4a):54, 1985.

62. Taylor LM, McAlister WR, Dennis DL, et al: Thrombolytic therapy followed by first rib resection for spontaneous ("effort") subclavian vein thrombosis. *Am J Surg* 149:644, 1985.

63. Druy EM, Trout HH, Giordano JM, et al: Lytic therapy in the treatment of axillary and subclavian vein thrombosis. *J Vasc Surg* 2:721, 1985.

64. Use of thrombolytic drugs in noncoronary disorders. *Drugs* 38:801–821, 1989.

65. Porter JM, Taylor LM: Current status of thrombolytic therapy. *J Vasc Surg* 2:239, 1985.

66. Hallett JW, Greenwood LH, Yrizarry JM, et al: Statistical determinants of success and complications of thrombolytic therapy for arterial occlusion of the lower extremity. *Surg Gynecol Obstet* 161:431, 1985.

67. Andaz S, Shields DA, Scurr JH, Coleridge Smith PD: Thrombolysis in acute lower limb ischemia. *Eur J Vasc Surg* 7:595–603, 1993.

68. Roth GJ, Majerus PW: The mechanism of the effect of aspirin on human platelets. 1. Acetylation of particulate fraction protein. *J Clin Invest* 56:624, 1975.

69. Preston FE, Whipps S, Jackson CA, et al: Inhibition of prostacyclin and platelet thromboxane A2 after low dose aspirin. *N Engl J Med* 304:76, 1981.

70. Mills DCB, Smith JB: The influence on platelet aggregation of drugs that affect the accumulation of adenosine 3'5' cyclic monophosphate in platelets. *Biochem J* 121:185, 1971.

71. Lips JPM, Sixma JJ, Schiphorst ME: The effect of ticlopidine administration to humans on the binding of adenosine diphosphate to blood platelets. *Thromb Res* 17:19, 1980.

72. Berglund U, Von Schenck H, Walletin L: Effects of ticlopidine on platelet function in men with stable angina pectoris. *Thromb Haemost* 54:808, 1985.

73. Saltiel E, Ward A: Ticlopidine: a review of its pharmacodynamic and pharmacokinetic properties, and therapeutic efficacy in platelet-dependent disease states. *Drugs* 34:222–262, 1987.

74. Vermylen J, Carreras LO, Schaeren JV, et al: Thromboxane synthetase inhibition as anti-thrombotic strategy. *Lancet* 1:1073, 1981.

75. Bertele V, Falanga A, Tomasiak, et al: Platelet thromboxane synthetase inhibitors with low doses of aspirin: possible resolution of the "aspirin dilemma." *Science* 220:517, 1983.

76. Coto V, Cocozza M, Oliviero U, et al: Clinical efficacy of picotamide in long-term treatment of intermittent claudication. *Angiology* 40:880–885, 1989.

77. Balsano F, Violo F: Effect of picotamide on the clinical progression of peripheral vascular disease: a double-blind placebo-controlled study: the ADEP Group. *Circulation* 87(5):1563–1569, 1993.

78. Giustina A, Bossoni S, Cimino A, et al: Picotamide, a dual TXB synthetase inhibitor and TXB receptor antagonist, reduces exercise-induced albuminuria in microalbuminuric patients with NIDDM. *Diabetes* 42(1):178–182, 1993.

79. Hass WK, Easton JD, Adams HP Jr, et al: A randomized trail comparing ticlopidine hydrochloride with aspirin for the prevention of stroke in high-risk patients: ticlopidine aspirin stroke study group. *N Engl J Med* 321:501–507, 1989.

80. Gent M, Blakely JA, Easton JD, et al: The Canadian American Ticlopidine Study (CATS) in thromboembolic stroke. *Lancet* 1 (8649)1215–1220, 1989.

81. Jazon L, Bergqvist D, Boberg J, et al: Prevention of myocardial infarction and stroke in patients with intermittent claudication: results from STIMS, the Swedish Ticlopidine Multicenter Study. *J Int Med* 227:301–308, 1990.

82. Bomberger RA, DePalma RG, Ambrose TA, et al: Aspirin and dipyridamole inhibit endothelial healing. *Arch Surg* 117:1459, 1982.

83. Carson SN, Demling RH, Esquivel CO: Aspirin failure in symptomatic atherosclerotic carotid artery disease. *Surgery* 90:1084, 1981.

84. Reid HL, Dormandy JA, Barnes AJ, et al: Impaired red cell deformability in peripheral vascular disease. *Lancet* 1:666, 1976.

85. Ehrly AM: Improvement of the flow properties of blood: a new therapeutical approach in occlusive arterial disease. *Angiology* 188, 1976.

86. Johnson G Jr, Keagy BA, Rodd DW, et al: Viscous factors in peripheral tissue perfusion. *J Vasc Surg* 2:530, 1985.

87. Colgan MP, Dormandy JA, Jones PW, et al: Oxpentifylline treatment of venous ulcers of the leg. *Br Med J* 300(6730):972–975, 1990.

88. Barbarino C: Pentoxifylline in the treatment of venous leg ulcers. *Curr Med Res Opinion* 12:547–551, 1991.

89. Jones NF: Acute and chronic ischemia of the hand: pathophysiology, treatment, and prognosis. *J Hand Surg* 16:1074–1083, 1991.

90. Litwin MS: Blood viscosity changes after trauma. *Crit Care Med* 4:67, 1976.

91. Rutherford RB, Jones DN, Bergentz, et al: The efficacy

of dextran 40 in preventing early postoperative thrombosis following difficult lower extremity bypass. *J Vasc Surg* 1:765, 1984.

92. Brevetti G, Angelini C, Rosa M, et al: Muscle carnitine deficiency in patients with severe peripheral vascular disease. *Circulation* 84(4):1490–1495, 1991.

93. Hiatt WR, Nawaz D, Brass EP: Carnitine metabolism during exercise in patients with peripheral vascular disease. *J Appl Physiol* 62(6):2383–2387, 1987.

94. Brevetti G, Attisano T, Perna S, et al: Effect of L-carnitine on the reactive hyperemia in patients affected by peripheral vascular disease: a double-blind, crossover study. *Angiology* 40(10):857–862, 1989.

95. Brevetti G, Chiariello, M, Ferulano G, et al: Increases in walking distance in patients with peripheral vascular disease treated with L-carnitine: a double-blind, crossover study. *Circulation* 77(4):767–773, 1988.

96. Brevetti G, Perna S, Sabba C, et al: Superiority of L-propionylcarnitine versus L-carnitine in improving walking capacity in patients with peripheral vascular disease: an acute, intravenous, double-blind, crossover study. *Eur Heart J* 13(2):251–255, 1992.

97. Tanaka T, Ishikawa T, Hagiwara M, et al: Effects of cilostazol, a selective cAMP phosphodiesterase inhibitor on the contraction of vascular smooth muscle. *Pharmacology* 36(5):313–320, 1988.

98. Igawa T, Tani T, Chijiwa T, et al: Potentiation of antiplatelet aggregating activity of cilostazol with vascular endothelial cells. *Thromb Res* 15;57(4):617–623, 1990.

99. Tansey MJ, Pilgrim AJ, Lloyd K: Sumatriptan in the acute treatment of migraine. *J Neurol Sci* 114:109–116, 1993.

100. The Finnish Sumatriptan Group and the Cardiovascular Clinical Research Group: A placebo-controlled study of intranasal sumatriptan for the acute treatment of migraine. *Eur Neurol* 131:332–338, 1991.

101. The Multinational Oral Sumatriptan and Cafergot Comparative Study Group: A randomized, double-blind comparison of sumatriptan and cafergot in the acute treatment of migraine. *Eur Neurol* 31:314–322, 1991.

102. DeCree J, Lcempocls J, Geukens H, et al: Placebo-controlled double-blind trial of ketanserin in treatment of intermittent claudication. *Lancet* 2:775, 1984.

103. Bounameaux H, Holditch T, Hellemans H, et al: Placebo-controlled double-blind two-centre trial of ketanserin in intermittent claudication. *Lancet* 2:1268, 1985.

104. Macintyre PD, Bhargava B, Hogg KJ, et al: The effect of i.v. sumatriptan, a selective 5-HT1-receptor agonist on central haemodynamics and the coronary circulation. *Br J Clin Pharmacol* 34:541–546, 1992.

105. Ottervanger JP, Paalman HJ, Boxma GL, Stricker BH: Transmural myocardial infarction with sumatriptan. *Lancet* 341(8849):861–862, 1993.

106. Rasmussen H: The calcium messenger system. Part 1. *N Engl J Med* 314:1094, 1986.

107. Rasmussen H: The calcium messenger system. Part 2. *N Engl J Med* 314:1164, 1986.

108. Coffman JD: Vasodilator drugs in peripheral vascular disease. *N Engl J Med* 300:713, 1979.

109. Snyder SH, Reynolds IJ: Calcium channel antagonist drugs. *New Engl J Med* 313:995, 1985.

110. Schuler JJ, Flanigan DP, Holcroft JW, et al: Efficacy of prostaglandin El in the treatment of lower extremity ischemic ulcers secondary to peripheral vascular occlusive disease. *J Vasc Surg* 1:160, 1984.

111. Mohrland JS, Porter JM, Smith EA, et al: A multiclinic, placebo-controlled, double-blind study of prostaglandin El in Raynaud's syndrome. *Ann Rheum Dis* 44:754, 1985.

112. Brevetti G, Rossini A, Perna S, et al: Beneficial effect of a new prostacyclin derivative on the walking capacity in patients with peripheral arterial insufficiency. *Angiology* 40(10):907–913, 1989.

113. U.K. Severe Limb Ischaemia Study Group: Treatment of limb-threatening ischemia with intravenous iloprost: a randomized, double-blind, placebo-controlled study. *Eur J Vasc Surg* 5:511–516, 1991.

114. Fiessinger JN, Schafer M: Trial of iloprost versus aspirin treatment for critical limb ischaemia of thromboangitis obliterans: The TAO Study. *Lancet* 335(8689):555, 1990.

115. Kyle MV, Belcher G, Hazleman BL: Placebo-controlled study showing therapeutic benefit of iloprost in the treatment of Raynaud's phenomenon. *J Rheumatol* 19(9):1403–1406, 1992.

CHAPTER 23

Scientific Basis for Balloon Embolectomy

Philip B. Dobrin, MD, PhD

Introduction

Before 1963, emboli and thrombi were extracted from arteries by direct surgical intervention.[1] This required general anesthesia, was limited to relatively large accessible vessels, often involved extensive dissection, and in many cases caused narrowing of the arteries following closure of the arteriotomies. A variety of methods were used to remove emboli from small arteries and extract residual thrombus that was adherent to the vessel wall. These methods included retrograde flushing,[2] application of compression bandages,[3] insertion of curved and corkscrew-shaped wires,[4] and the use of intraluminal suction.[5] In 1963, Fogarty et al[6] published their use of an embolectomy catheter with an inflatable balloon. This technique permitted extraction of thrombus by means of a single incision in a large vessel, thereby avoiding excessive dissection and the need to incise a small distal vessel. It also permitted extraction of emboli and thrombi with the patient under local anesthesia, a distinct advantage in the aged or unstable patient.

Currently, lytic therapy has also become a method for clearing thrombus from arteries and vascular grafts.[7-9] However, there are conditions where lytic therapy is contraindicated. These include surgery within 1 week, a recent cerebrovascular event, and a variety of conditions in which patients are predisposed to bleeding. Under these conditions, balloon embolectomy remains the treatment of choice. This chapter examines the mechanical aspects of balloon embolectomy, the injuries produced by embolectomy, and techniques that can be used to prevent them.

Balloon Embolectomy Induced Injuries

The use of balloon embolectomy catheters generally is effective; however, their use also may cause vessel injury. Six types of acute vessel injury have been described[10-40] and are illustrated in Figure 1. These include: a) perforation of the vessel wall with the catheter tip; b) perforation of the vessel by overdistention of the balloon; c) elevation of an intimal flap; d) raising of an atherosclerotic plaque into the flowing stream; e) rupture of the balloon with embolization of balloon fragments; and f) detachment of the balloon or catheter tip with embolization of these materials.

Perforation of the vessel wall may lead to extravascular bleeding. Elevation of an intimal flap or of an atherosclerotic plaque may cause intraoperative or postoperative thrombosis. A dramatic example of arterial perforation by an embolectomy balloon is illustrated in Figure 2.

Table 1 summarizes clinical injuries produced by embolectomy described in the surgical literature.[10-40] The incidence or rate of balloon catheter-induced injuries cannot be computed because the denominator, i.e., the total number of embolectomies performed in patients, is unknown. However, of those complications reported before 1976, Schweitzer et al[37] reported that arterial perforation by the catheter tip accounted for 25.7%, rupture of the artery by an

From *The Basic Science of Vascular Disease*. Edited by Sidawy AN, Sumpio BE, and DePalma RG. Armonk, NY: Futura Publishing Company, Inc.; © 1997.

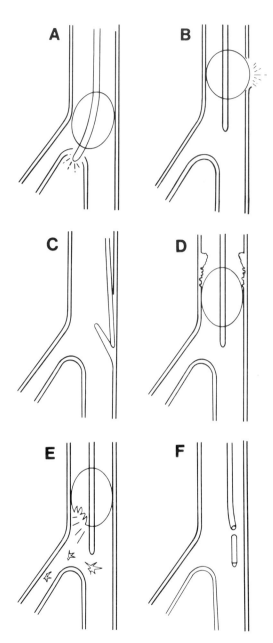

Figure 1. Six mechanisms of injury to blood vessels caused by balloon embolectomy catheters and inflated balloons. (Expanded with permission from Reference 10; reproduced with permission from Reference 11.)

Table 1
Acute Clinical Complications of Balloon Embolectomy Injury to Arteries

Perforation of artery with catheter tip.
Rupture of artery by overinflated balloon.
Arteriovenous fistula.
Intimal dissection.
Dissection of a plaque.
Bursting of balloons, leaving balloon fragments.
Separation of catheter tip and/or balloons.

One way to be certain that an adequate embolectomy has been performed and that the arteries have not been grossly injured is to obtain an arteriogram on the operating table at the completion of embolectomy. A normal arteriogram after embolectomy is also valuable for medical-legal purposes. If an injury is observed, immediate treatment may be necessary. A small injury to a vessel that is not actively bleeding may not require surgical intervention, but a large injury usually does require repair. Major perforations, intimal flaps, and arteriovenous fistulas should be corrected at the time of recognition in order to prevent ischemia to the involved extremity. Rupture of the balloon mandates immediate retrieval of balloon fragments. Patients who manifest a compartment syndrome should undergo fasciotomy in order to prevent neuromuscular injury.

An injury not illustrated in Figure 1 is trauma to the intima which denudes it of endothelium. This alters physiologic control of the vascular muscle, causes loss of nitric oxide-dependent relaxation, increases procoagulant activity, and increases vasoconstrictor responses to norepinephrine.[41-46] All of these reactions dispose to vessel thrombosis. Denudation of the intima also may lead to the development of intimal hyperplasia,[47,48] especially if there is injury to the underlying media.[49,50] In fact, injury to the intima with balloons is a method frequently used in experimental animals to deliberately produce intimal hyperplasia[49-51] and accelerated atherogenesis.[52] In patients, intimal hyperplasia may not become apparent until several months after embolectomy. In fact, it is likely that catheter-induced injuries to the intima often occur during surgical embolectomy but, because of the delay, are not recognized as sequelae of the procedure. Bowles et al[53] described five patients with lower extremity ischemia appearing 2 to 4 months after embolectomy. None of these patients had had clinical evidence of disease prior to embolectomy, and all had normal vessels demonstrated arteriographically at the time of embolectomy. Pathologic specimens available in two of the patients demonstrated marked intimal hyperplasia in regions of

overdistended balloon accounted for 13.5%, elevation of an intimal flap accounted for 2.2%, and rupture of the balloon with loss of the balloon fragments accounted for 4.1%. In addition, two complications that can result from perforation of the vessel, i.e., the development of an arteriovenous fistula and the development of a compartment syndrome, in combination accounted for 13.6% of complications. Injuries that occur after some delay, such as the development of intimal hyperplasia, accelerated atherosclerosis, or the development of a pseudoaneurysm were not included in Schweitzer's review.

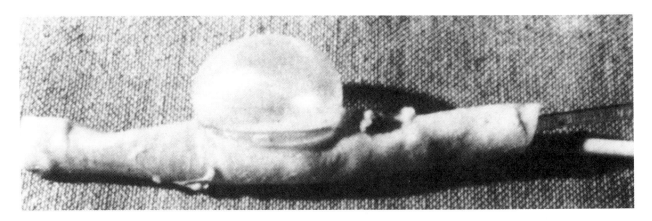

Figure 2. Overinflated embolectomy balloon perforating an artery in a dog. (Reproduced with permission from Reference 12.)

the arterial tree that had been exposed to the distended embolectomy balloon.

Mechanics of Balloon Embolectomy

Experimental studies have demonstrated the importance of two mechanical parameters associated with embolectomy. These are *lateral wall pressure* and balloon-artery *shear force*. The following sections describe these mechanical factors, methods used to measure them, their histologic effects, and the techniques that may be used to control them.

Lateral Wall Pressure

When an embolectomy catheter is inserted into an artery, but the balloon is not inflated, it exerts no force or pressure laterally against the wall of the vessel. When the balloon is inflated to just fill the lumen, it still exerts little or no pressure against the wall. Nevertheless, because of the elastic characteristics of the balloon itself, high pressure is developed within the balloon. Further inflation of the balloon within the lumen causes it to distend the artery and apply force against the vessel wall. If this force is divided by the area over which that force is exerted, i.e., the area of contact between the balloon and the wall, one obtains the force per unit area or lateral wall pressure. When performing an embolectomy in a patient, the balloon must be distended sufficiently to extract thrombus from the lumen and remove that which may be adherent to the wall. Under these conditions, the balloon inevitably distends the artery and exerts lateral pressure against the wall. However, because of the stiffness of the balloon itself, the pressure within the balloon cannot be used as an indicator of the lateral wall pressure exerted against the vessel wall. Although easily understood, lateral wall pressure cannot be measured

directly. No matter how carefully a slender gauge might be inserted between the balloon and the artery, the measurement device will be subjected to artifactually high compressive forces as it is squeezed as a space-occupying object between the balloon and the vessel wall. In order to determine lateral wall pressure, an in vitro method was developed in our laboratory. This is illustrated in Figures 3 through 5. An artery is excised from an anesthetized animal such as a dog. The vessel is catheterized at both ends and is placed in a tissue bath in a horizontal position. One end of the

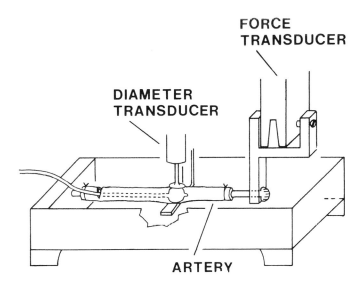

Figure 3. Apparatus used to study lateral wall pressure and shear forces exerted by embolectomy balloons. Arteries are mounted in a tissue bath in vitro, bathed in buffered Krebs-Ringer solution, and held at 37°C and pH 7.4. Balloon catheter is inserted through an arteriotomy. Artery diameter is measured with linear displacement transducer to determine lateral wall presure. Shear force exerted during catheter withdrawal is measured by force gauge. (Reproduced with permission from Reference 54.)

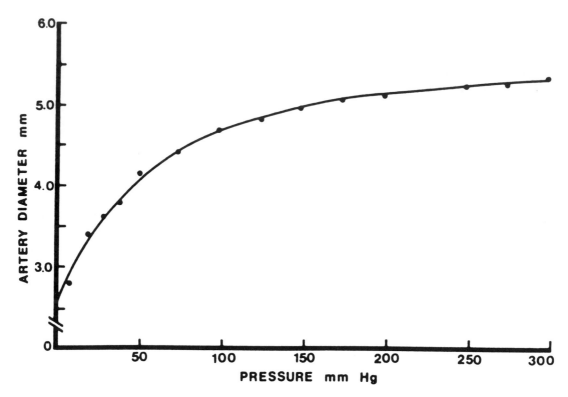

Figure 4. Pressure-diameter curve recorded for intact vessel in tissue bath shown in Figure 3. (Reproduced with permission from Reference 54.)

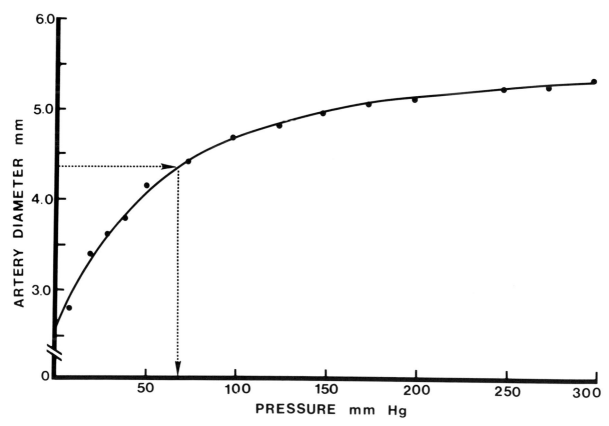

Figure 5. Diameter (**Y axis**) recorded after catheter has been inserted and balloon has been inflated. Projecting this diameter to the pressure-diameter curve (**horizontal broken line**) discloses the lateral wall pressure exerted by the inflated balloon (**vertical broken line**). (Reproduced with permission from Reference 55.)

vessel is sealed and is suspended from a force gauge (Figure 3). The artery is extended to in situ length. The lumen of the vessel is subjected to pressure in steps up to 300 mm Hg while the external diameter is measured with a linear displacement transducer. After several stepwise cycles to relax the vessel, reproducible pressure-diameter curves are obtained (Figure 4). The slope and coordinates of this curve are determined by the elastic characteristics of the artery. An arteriotomy then is made near the end of the vessel that is away from the force gauge. An embolectomy catheter is introduced into the lumen and fluid is injected into the balloon while the diameter of the vessel is measured. The previously obtained pressure-diameter curve (Figure 4) is referenced in order to determine the pressure in the intact vessel that would be associated with each diameter recorded for that same vessel while it is distended by the balloon. This pressure is in fact the lateral wall pressure exerted by the balloon. This rises with each step increase in volume injected into the balloon. In this way, the elastic properties of the artery itself are used to determine the lateral wall pressure. Figure 5 illustrates one such estimate. In the example shown, the balloon produced a diameter which corresponded to 70 mm Hg pressure. This method requires that a pressure-diameter curve be obtained for each individual vessel. It cannot be used to measure lateral wall pressure in vivo, but it does permit laboratory analysis of the mechanics of embolectomy from which insight and principles of the surgical procedure may be obtained.

Balloon Pressure Versus Lateral Wall Pressure

When an embolectomy catheter has been inserted into an artery and the balloon is distended, pressure rises markedly within the balloon even before the balloon has come into contact with the wall. The rise in pressure occurs because of the stiffness of the balloon itself. After the balloon has filled the lumen and the vessel is distended, the pressure in the balloon may increase somewhat further due to the resistance offered by the artery wall. Nevertheless, the pressure in the balloon is very high and is not related to the pressure exerted against the vessel wall (Figure 6). Therefore, the pressure within the balloon *cannot* be used as an indication of lateral wall pressure. For this reason, balloon pressure is not a useful way to judge whether or not the balloon is filling the lumen. The lateral wall pressure produced by the balloon depends on the size of the balloon relative to the size of the surrounding artery.[54] A large balloon will readily fill a small vessel and will exert a great deal of lateral wall pressure against it. A very small balloon in a large artery must be greatly inflated before it encounters the vessel wall and exerts lateral wall pressure. In both cases, there will be a marked rise in balloon

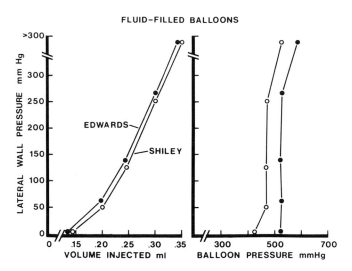

Figure 6. Left: Lateral wall pressure plotted against injected volume. Volume is proportional to balloon diameter. Increasing balloon diameter distends the artery raising lateral wall pressure. **Right**: Many values of lateral wall pressure correspond to few values of balloon pressure, i.e., lateral wall pressure is not determined by balloon pressure. (Reproduced with permission from Reference 54.)

pressure with inflation of the balloon. In the operating room, the adequacy of balloon volume is determined subjectively by the surgeon as he or she injects volume and attempts to withdraw the catheter. Experimental studies have shown that when balloons are filled to give subjectively satisfactory levels of drag, the balloons distend the artery to produce lateral wall pressures of about 60 mm Hg.[47] However, we also have found that if, after inflating the balloon to apparently satisfactory levels, one slightly deflates the balloon, lower lateral wall pressures can be obtained while still retaining satisfactory contact with the wall (Table 2).[55–56] This provides a lower potential for injury.

Balloon-Artery Shear Forces

When an embolectomy catheter is withdrawn with the balloon distended, it produces a shearing force between the balloon and the artery wall. This manifests as

Table 2
Lateral Wall Pressure in Millimeters of Mercury (mm Hg) Exerted by Fluid-Filled and Gas-Filled Balloons After Inflation and After Deflation

Balloon State	1 cc Fluid	1 cc Air
Inflation	54.4 ± 8.0	95.2 ± 13.8
Deflation	28.1 ± 5.7	34.2 ± 7.1*

* 3/14 balloons collapsed spontaneously to 0 mm Hg

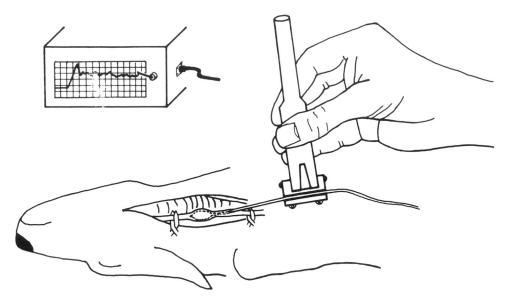

Figure 7. Method of holding force gauge by hand to permit measurement of shear forces in vivo. (Reproduced with permission from Reference 47.)

drag felt subjectively by the surgeon. When this shear *force* is divided by the area of contact between the balloon and the artery, the shear *stress* is obtained. This stress tends to de-endothelialize the intima and, if excessive, also can damage the internal elastic lamella and media.[47] Shear forces can be measured by a force gauge in vitro as illustrated in Figure 3 or by attaching the catheter to a force gauge when performing embolectomy in vivo as shown in Figure 7. Figure 8 illustrates shear force recordings obtained with an Edwards embolectomy catheter in an artery in vitro. The balloon was distended in steps to generate lateral wall pressures of 25, 75, 175, and 200 mm Hg. It is evident from this figure that the shear force exerted by the balloon increases more or less linearly with increasing lateral wall pressure. This means that any comparison of products or techniques that may influence shear force *must* be performed at the same lateral wall pressure.

Figure 8 shows that there are two components to the shear force. As catheter motion is initiated, there is

a high force as the balloon overcomes *initial* or *static* friction. After motion is under way, the force falls to a lower steady value as the balloon overcomes *dynamic* friction. This is analogous to what is experienced subjectively when pulling a child on a sled over snow. At first it is difficult to begin motion; once motion has begun, it is easier to keep the sled moving. The high initial value may be termed "initial shear force," and the subsequent lower shear force may be termed "dynamic shear force." Shear forces could be measured in the operating room by surgeons by attaching the proximal end of balloon catheters to force gauges such as that shown in Figure 7. In addition, shear forces could be controlled automatically by attaching the catheter to a device that would slip whenever excessive shear forces were produced. However, the effectiveness of such devices would be limited because higher shear forces are produced when balloons are pulled through large vessels than when they are pulled through small ones. This results largely from the greater balloon-artery surface area of contact in the larger vessels.

Histologic Effects of Embolectomy

The histologic reactions to embolectomy have been studied and are illustrated in Figures 9A through 9E for arteries subjected to single catheter withdrawals.[47] Control artery without catheter insertion showed no measurable injury (Figure 9A). Two days after catheter passage with the balloon inflated, the intima was found to be denuded of endothelium and was covered with platelets (Figure 9B). Seven and 14 days after catheter passage, the intima was found to be hypercellular, con-

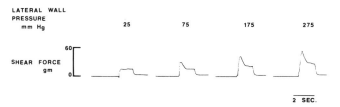

Figure 8. Shear forces recorded with an embolectomy catheter withdrawn through a vessel in vitro. Shear forces rise with increasing lateral wall pressure. Shear forces have a high initial or static component and a lower dynamic component. (Reproduced with permission from Reference 54.)

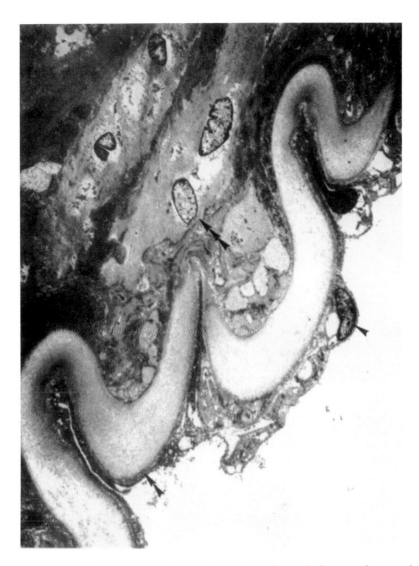

Figure 9A. Transmission electron microscopic section of vessel after arteriotomy, but without catheter insertion. Endothelium is one cell thick (**single arrow**). Internal elastic lamella (**double arrow**) and medial smooth muscle cells (**triple arrow**) are intact. (Reproduced with permission from Reference 47.)

taining up to four myointimal cell layers in thickness (Figure 9C). This histologic response was seen when the artery was exposed to shear forces greater than 60 grams, but less than 200 grams. Exposure to less than 60 grams shear force produced less intimal injury and incomplete endothelial denudation. Although these responses appeared to be localized to the intima, during the recovery period the smooth muscle cells in the media exhibited increased numbers of ribosomes and increased amounts of rough endoplasmic reticulum. These changes reflect increased cellular metabolic activity as part of the reparative process. The internal elastic lamella and the media in these vessels showed no evidence of direct injury unless 200 grams shear force was applied (Figure 9E). Disruption of the elastic lamellae may not appear until quite late after embolectomy,[57] so

there may be a delay between injury and histologic response. Mononuclear cells have been observed adhering to the site of balloon catheter injury.[58] This may be a critical step because monocytes/macrophages are known to release growth factors that may stimulate the development of intimal hyperplasia.[59] A shear force of 50 grams elicits less intimal hyperplasia than does a shear force of 100 to 200 grams,[48] and for all levels of shear force, repeated withdrawals with embolectomy catheters produce greater intimal hyperplasia than do single catheter withdrawals (p <.05).[48]

Summary of Mechanics

The above discussion highlights some important mechanical principles relevant to balloon catheter em-

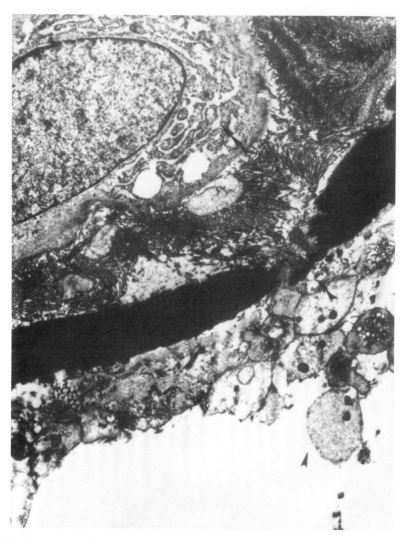

Figure 9B. Dog carotid artery subjected to 60 grams shear force, excised after 2 days. Endothelial cells have been removed and are replaced by platelets (**single arrow**). Intimal elastic lamella is present and contains normal fenestration (**double arrow**). Medial smooth muscle cells exhibit increased ribosomes (**triple arrow**) suggesting increased reparative activity. (Reproduced with permission from Reference 47.)

bolectomy. First, lateral wall pressure is not determined by the pressure within the balloon, but instead is determined by the size of the balloon relative to that of the surrounding artery. In fact, there is little relationship between the pressure in the balloon and the pressure the balloon exerts against the artery. Second, when the catheter is withdrawn through the artery with the balloon distended, a high initial shear force is developed between the balloon and the artery wall; this is followed by a lower dynamic shear force. As the lateral wall pressure is increased by increasing the size of the balloon, the shear force rises in an approximately linear fashion. Shear force is a prime determinant of arterial injury and of the development at intimal hyperplasia. Therefore, it is imperative for the surgeon to precisely

control the shear force exerted by the balloon during embolectomy. In turn, this requires control of lateral wall pressure.

Determinants of Lateral Wall Pressure and Shear Force

Laboratory studies performed in vitro and in vivo have identified several factors that determine lateral wall pressure and balloon-artery shear force. The remainder of this chapter summarizes the results of those experiments and provides guidance for the technique of performing embolectomy in patients.

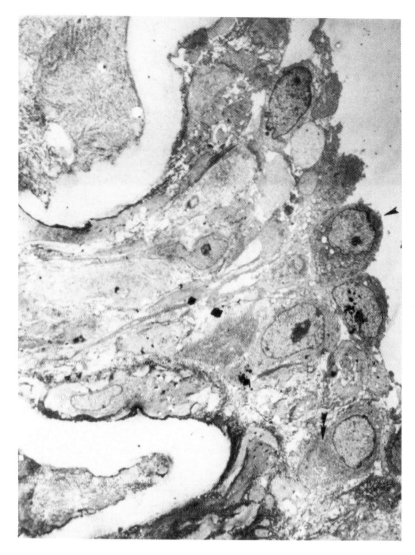

Figure 9C. Dog carotid artery after 90 grams shear force, excised after 14 days. Intima is three to four cells thick (**single arrow**). Some of these exhibit increased ribosomes (**double arrow**). (Reproduced with permission from Reference 47.)

Catheter Size

Canine arteries were mounted in a tissue bath in vitro as illustrated in Figure 3. Different size catheters (3F, 4F, and 5F) were inserted into the vessels, distended with saline to predetermined lateral wall pressures, and then were withdrawn to simulate an embolectomy. Shear forces measured during withdrawal were significantly different with different size catheters, i.e., 3F<4F<5F (p <.05).[54] This was found for lateral wall pressures of both 25 mm Hg and 75 mm Hg, and was found with both Edwards and Shiley catheters. It also was found for small (2.9 mm diameter) and larger (3.7 mm diameter) arteries (Figure 10). It also has been found for different size catheters pulled through plastic tubes.[12] Radiographs obtained of the

balloons within arteries demonstrated that the balloons on the larger catheters had a larger area of balloon-artery contact,[54] explaining why large catheters exert more shear force than do small catheters. These data indicate that when performing embolectomy in patients, one should select the smallest catheter size that will be effective.

Brands of Catheters

A variety of experiments were performed to evaluate and compare different brands of commercially available catheters.[60] In order to study the shear forces developed by these devices, arteries were mounted in a tissue bath in vitro and four brands of catheters were

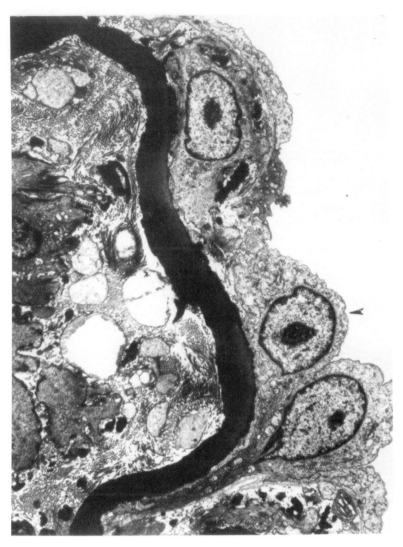

Figure 9D. Dog carotid artery after 90 grams shear force, excised after 28 days. Intima has returned to normal one-cell thickness (**single arrow**). Elastic lamella and media appear normal. (Reproduced with permission from Reference 47.)

studied. They were: Fogarty catheter (American Edwards Laboratories, Santa Ana, CA); Multi-Pro catheter (Shiley, Inc., Irving, CA); Elecath catheter (Electro-Catheter Corp., Rahway, NJ); and Bard-Parker catheter (Becton-Dickinson, East Rutherford, NJ). All of the balloons were latex except for that manufactured by Becton-Dickinson; these balloons were silicone. These studies demonstrated that at lateral wall pressures of 50 mm Hg and 100 mm Hg, initial shear forces were significantly different for the four catheters; Becton-Dickinson>Edwards>Shiley>Elecath-catheter (p <.05). In contrast, during catheter withdrawal dynamic shear forces were not significantly different among the four brands of catheters.

Balloon emptying times also were studied in vitro. Emptying time reflects the rapidity with which a bal-

loon can decrease in diameter. This is a measure of how quickly a balloon can be made to accommodate to a narrowed region in a vessel that might suddenly be encountered during catheter withdrawal. Balloons were filled with fluid, and then opened to air to permit them to empty. Results showed that because of the compliant balloon, the Becton-Dickinson balloon required more than twice the time to empty (5.7 ± 1.2 seconds) as the other three latex balloons (1.6 to 2.4 ± 0.3 sec). These differences were statistically significant (p <.05). Forceful suction-emptying gave similar results.

In vitro studies also were undertaken to examine the ''sharpness'' of catheter tips. Experiments were performed on strips of rabbit aorta to examine the force required to penetrate a vessel wall with the tips of the

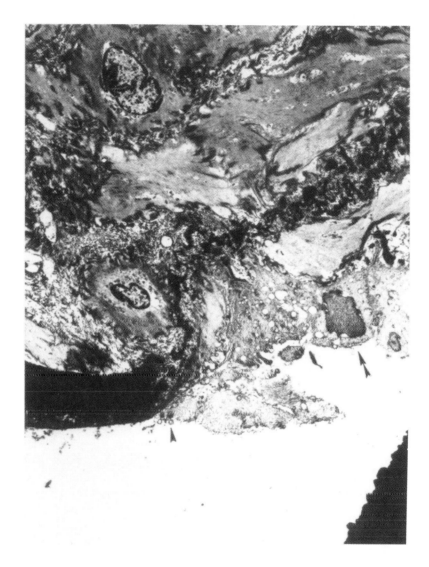

Figure 9E. Dog femoral artery after 200 grams shear force, excised after 6 months. Artery exhibits fractured elastic lamella (**single arrow**). Elastin and collagen fibrils are covered with myointimal cells (**double arrow**). (Reproduced with permission from Reference 47.)

four brands of catheters. Results showed that the puncture force required was greatest for the Shiley catheter (295 ± 22 gm), and lower for Elecath (270 ± 18 gm), Becton-Dickinson (225 ± 13 gm), and Edwards (217 ± 11 gm) catheters. The Shiley catheter was significantly greater ($p < .05$) than the Becton-Dickinson and Edwards catheters. The higher the penetration force required, the less likely the catheter is to penetrate the vessel wall.

The four brands of catheters also were examined with respect to eccentricity of the balloons. Although the silicone Becton-Dickinson was more eccentric (2.2:1) than the other three brands of catheters (1.1:1 to 1.3:1), differences between the four brands of catheters were not statistically significant. As discussed below, balloon eccentricity can be an important factor in producing injury to the artery wall.

Finally, in vivo studies were carried out in dogs to determine the intimal hyperplasia produced by the different brands of catheters. Histologic examination of the vessels 3 months after they had been exposed to 50, 100, and 200 gm shear forces showed that intimal hyperplasia increased with rising shear forces for all four catheters ($p < .05$), but that there were no differences in the intimal hyperplasia elicited by the different brands.

In conclusion, there are some clear differences between the different catheters, but most of these are not critical with respect to their use in patients. Moreover, one catheter is not consistently superior or inferior to all of the others with respect to all of the parameters tested. However, one particularly important feature is the slow emptying time of the silicone balloon on the Becton-Dickinson catheter. This is likely to be a disad-

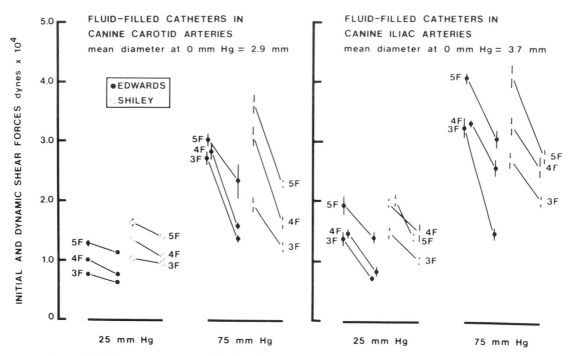

Figure 10. Shear forces recorded for different size catheters at two lateral wall pressures. Data show that smaller catheters produce lower shear forces than do large catheters at each level of lateral wall pressure (3F<4F<5F<, p <.05). (Reproduced with permission from Reference 54.)

vantage during catheter withdrawal through an uneven blood vessel. The silicone balloons on these catheters also are highly prone to rupture and did so frequently during the tests. When they ruptured, they simply broke without leaving balloon fragments. Overall, these results suggest that catheters with latex balloons appear to be preferable to silicone balloons.

Balloon Eccentricity

When balloons are filled they may deform eccentrically, bulging more to one side than to the other (Figure 11). Experimental studies were performed in order to study the importance of this phenomenon.[61] First, balloon eccentricity was measured with catheters in air and after the same catheters were inserted into vessels in vitro and distended to lateral wall pressures of 25, 75, and 100 mm Hg. Eccentricity was expressed as the ratio of the larger radius (R) to the lesser radius (r) (Figure 12). Results demonstrated a high correlation (r=0.88) between balloon eccentricity in air and balloon eccentricity in arteries (Figure 13). This demonstrates that the presence of an artery surrounding an eccentric balloon does not reduce or abolish the eccentricity. Measurements then were performed to evaluate the effect of eccentricity on shear forces. Catheters were inserted into vessels in vitro and the balloons were distended to lateral wall pressures of 25, 75, and

125 mm Hg. Regression analysis demonstrated that there was a 10 percent increase in shear force for every unit increase in eccentricity, i.e., increase in the R:r ratio (Figure 14). In vivo experiments also were performed in dogs using eccentric balloons. Histologic studies of tissues harvested 2 and 14 days after embolectomy showed that when the balloon was extremely eccentric (R:r=8:1), severe damage was observed in the vessel wall from the bulging balloon pushing the catheter through the internal elastic lamella into the media (Figure 15). The catheter gouged a trough over the length of the vessel. Medial edema was observed when the balloon was moderately eccentric, i.e., R:r=3:1.

Fluid-Filled Versus Gas-Filled Balloons

Experiments were performed in vitro to study the effects of using fluid versus using gas to fill embolectomy balloons.[56] One might predict *a priori* that, because a gas-filled balloon is compressible, it is more likely to comply with an irregular lumen, and this may be true for static conditions.[62] However, results of experiments showed that lateral wall pressures were precisely controlled with fluid, but were poorly controlled with gas because gas-filled balloons exhibited spontaneous changes in diameter. This occurs because the mechanical properties of gas or fluid in the balloon in-

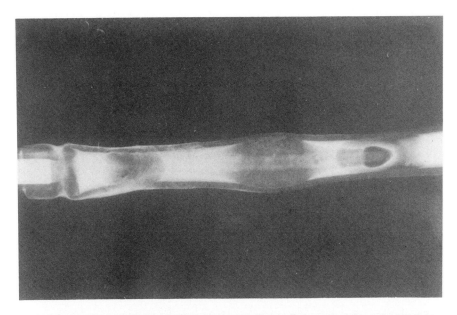

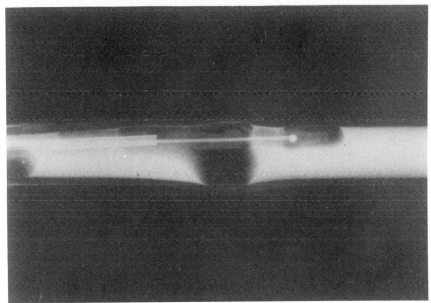

Figure 11. Arteriograms with embolectomy catheters within arteries. **Top** shows catheter with a concentric balloon. **Bottom** shows catheter with an eccentric balloon. (Reproduced with permission from Reference 61.)

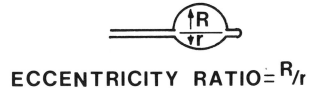

ECCENTRICITY RATIO= $^R/_r$

Figure 12. Eccentricity ratio (R/r) computed as ratio of larger radius (R) to smaller radius (r). (Reproduced with permission from Refernence 61.)

teract with the material properties of the balloon itself. Fluid is virtually incompressible. If a given volume of incompressible saline is injected into an embolectomy balloon, the pressure in the balloon first rises steeply, then falls, and then rises again. The first two phases of this process are shown in Figure 16. These unusual curves reflect the unique elastic properties of the large deformation polymers used to fabricate the balloons. The curves depicted in Figure 16 are for Edwards and Shiley latex balloons filled with fluid, and reflect the elastic characteristics of latex. Highly compliant silicone balloons exhibit similar curves, but with lower absolute pressures in the balloon at each level of injected volume, and of course, lower peak pressures as well. The *slopes* of the curves shown in Figure 16 re-

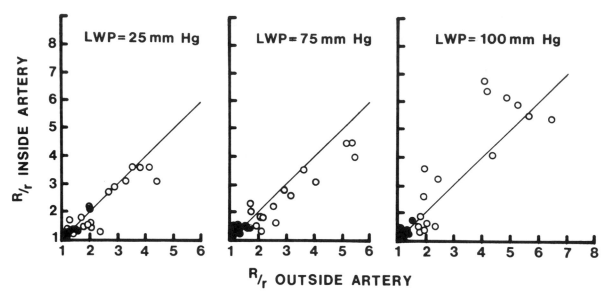

Figure 13. Eccentricity ratio of balloons in air and within arteries. High correlation indicates that artery surrounding the balloon does not reduce eccentricity. (Reproduced with permission from Reference 61.)

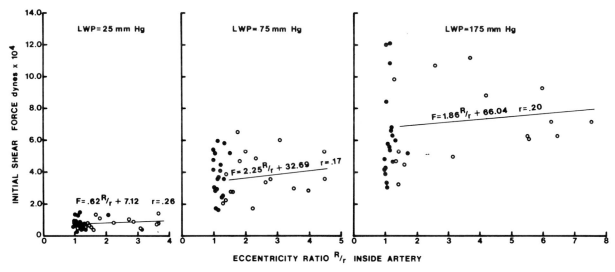

Figure 14. Shear force rises with increasing balloon eccentricity. (Reproduced with permission from Reference 61.).

flect the *stiffness* of the balloon material. As can be seen, the balloon is at first very stiff as indicated by the initial steep rising slope. It then becomes exceedingly compliant as indicated by the subsequent falling slope. Finally, it again becomes very stiff, although this is not shown in Figure 16. This three-phase stiffness characteristic is known intuitively to anyone who has tried to blow into a balloon in order to inflate it. At first it is difficult to inflate the balloon, then it becomes much easier, and finally it becomes more difficult.

When an embolectomy balloon is filled with an incompressible fluid such as water or saline, the pres-

sure developed in the balloon is determined by the volume of fluid injected and the elastic characteristics of the balloon. With the injection of fluid, the volume of the balloon is dictated by the amount of incompressible fluid injected. By comparison, gas is compressible and follows Boyle's Law. When a given volume of gas is injected into a balloon, for example 1 cc, the actual volume present in the balloon is compressed by the rising pressure to less than 1 cc. As more gas is injected, the pressure in the balloon increases, then decreases, and then increases again as mandated by the elastic characteristics of the balloon (Figure 16). Be-

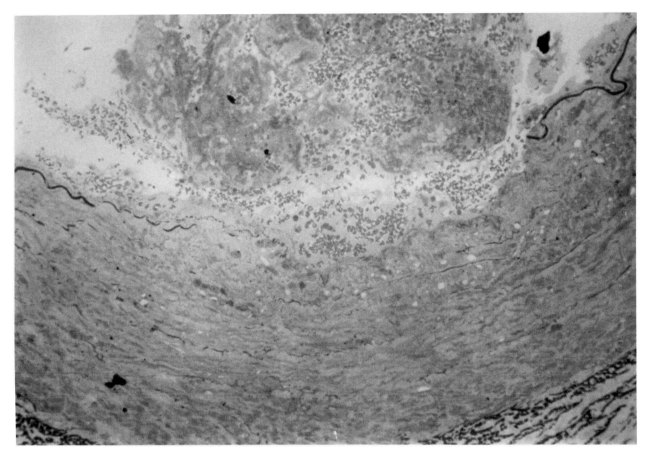

Figure 15. Arterial injury resulting from eccentric balloon pushing catheter into the vessel wall. (Reproduced with permission from Reference 61.)

cause of the interactions between the compressibility of the gas and the discontinuous stiffness characteristics of the balloon, the diameter of the balloon may vary and will not be under precise control by the surgeon. In fact, gas-filled balloons actually change diameter spontaneously as the catheter is withdrawn down the length of the vessel. These erratic volume changes are seen with gas; they are not seen when a balloon is filled with fluid.

Experiments were carried out in arteries to measure the lateral wall pressure exerted by fluid-filled and gas-filled balloons. Dog arteries were mounted in a tissue bath in vitro and catheters were inserted through an arteriotomy. Fluid or gas was injected into the balloons without catheter withdrawal. Results showed that fluid-filled balloons consistently exerted lower lateral wall pressures than did gas-filled balloons. In addition, 20% or more of the balloons filled with gas collapsed and, in vivo, would have left residual thrombus. This thrombus would require repeated passage of the catheter. Repeated passages of the catheter are associated with the development of intimal hyperplasia.[48] Another 20% of the balloons dilated spontaneously to maximum

dimensions, wedging themselves in the vessel. Exerting traction on this catheter would certainly damage the vessel wall. It is evident from these data that fluid-filled balloons are more predictable and controllable than gas-filled balloons.[56]

Experiments then were performed in vessels in vitro to assess the effect of fluid- and gas-filled balloons on shear forces generated during catheter withdrawal. An artery was mounted in the tissue bath and a single suture was placed through the vessel to narrow the lumen 50%. Withdrawing catheters with gas-filled balloons produced 9% less shear force than did fluid-filled balloons (Figure 17), but only at low lateral wall pressures (25 mm Hg and 75 mm Hg) where injury potential is small. At higher lateral wall pressures (125 mm Hg to 175 mm Hg), gas-filled balloons produced no reduction in shear force.

In conclusion, these studies demonstrate only a slight decrease in shear force (9%) with gas-filled balloons, and only at low lateral wall pressures. However, the cost for obtaining this slight reduction in shear force is not inconsequential because gas-filled balloons are so much less controllable than fluid-filled balloons.

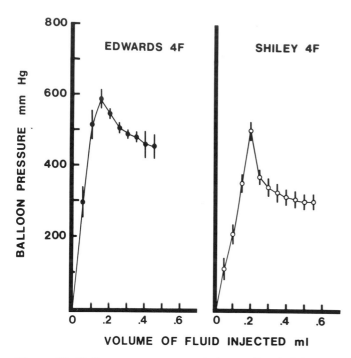

Figure 16. Balloon pressure recorded as saline is injected into Edwards and Shiley balloons. At small injected volumes balloons are extremely stiff (**steep initial slopes**). They then became highly compliant (**falling slopes**). At extremely large injected volumes balloons became stiff with rising slopes (not shown). (Reproduced with permission from Reference 56.)

During catheter motion, gas-filled balloons tend to collapse completely or enlarge to maximum dimensions, wedging themselves in the vessel lumen. These data suggest that fluid-filled balloons, not gas-filled balloons, should be used in patients. Parenthetically, because of the resistance offered by the lumen of small catheters, it may be necessary to use gas in very small catheters, e.g., 2F.

Syringe Size

When performing an embolectomy, it is necessary to select the size of the syringe. Ideally, a syringe that provides precise control of balloon diameter and therefore permits maximum control of lateral wall pressure should be used. This is most readily accomplished using a small-bore, long-stroke syringe, as this will produce the smallest changes in balloon dimension for a given advancement of the syringe plunger. We have found that a tuberculin syringe is ideal with small catheters such as 2F, 3F, and 4F. A larger-bore syringe, for example 2 cc, may be needed to fill larger balloons. However, one must be extremely careful, because a given advancement of the plunger of a larger syringe produces disproportionately larger changes in balloon volume. In fact, for a given advancement of the plunger of any syringe, the volume injected will increase as the *square of the radius* of the syringe plunger. These considerations dictate that, whenever possible, a small-diameter syringe should be used in order to obtain maximum control during embolectomy.

Velocity of Catheter Motion

Because there are static and dynamic components to the balloon-artery shear force (Figure 8), studies were undertaken to examine the effect of velocity of catheter motion on the shear forces that are developed.[54] Experiments were performed by mounting dog arteries in vitro in a tissue bath, inserting embolectomy catheters into their lumens, inflating the balloons, and withdrawing the catheters at 1, 6, or 12 cm/sec. These studies were carried out at lateral wall pressures of 25, 75, 175, and 275 mm Hg. Shear forces were recorded. Rapid motion decreased the shear force, but reduced only the dynamic component, and then only slightly, not the larger initial or static component (Figure 18). Initial shear force is the higher and potentially more injurious component. Therefore, there is little to be gained by moving the catheter rapidly. Moreover, rapid motion gives less time for the surgeon to adjust the balloon volume if he or she suddenly encounters an unsuspected stenosis or atherosclerotic plaque protruding into the lumen. Therefore, during embolectomy the catheter should be withdrawn slowly and, if

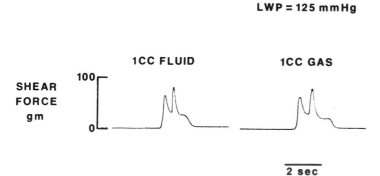

Figure 17. Shear forces recorded as fluid-filled and gas-filled balloons are withdrawn through an artery with a 50% stenosis. Gas-filled balloons decreased peak shear force 9%. (Reproduced with permission from Reference 56.)

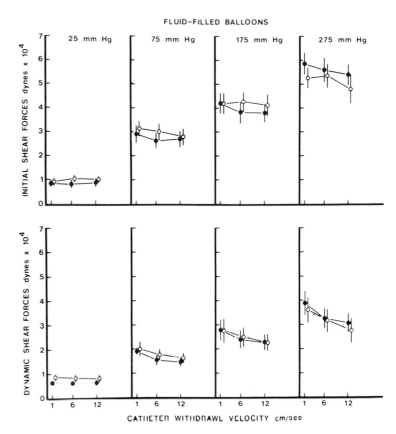

Figure 18. Shear forces recorded with embolectomy catheters withdrawn at different velocities. Rapid motion decreased the shear force, but only the dynamic component, not the more injurious static component. (Reproduced with permission from Reference 54.)

possible, continuously. Keeping the catheter in motion avoids having to reinitate motion and, once again, overcome the initial static friction.

Blood in the Vessel Lumen

It is not uncommon during embolectomy for blood from collateral vessels to enter the vessel lumen and produce minor backbleeding. Blood alters the friction between the balloon and the intima. In order to examine the effects of blood, experiments were performed in dog arteries in vitro at lateral wall pressures of 25, 75, and 125 mm Hg.[63] Results showed that, for all lateral wall pressures, during catheter withdrawal blood in the lumen substantially lowered the recorded shear forces. Decreased balloon-artery friction results from the thickness of the blood lubricating the balloon, as well as the multiphasic composition of cells, protein, and plasma in blood. Experiments performed to systematically vary the hematocrit between 0% and 50% demonstrated clear evidence that shear forces decreased with increasing hematocrit (Figure 19). Therefore, the presence of blood in the vessel lumen is of little concern provided the patient has received adequate anticoagulation.

Inflating Balloons at Rest and During Catheter Motion

Initial shear forces are higher than dynamic shear forces (Figure 8). Because of this, experiments were

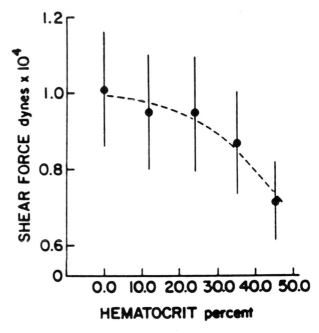

Figure 19. Shear forces recorded with balloons held at constant lateral wall pressure during catheter withdrawal. Lumen was lubricated with blood diluted with saline to various hematocrits. (Reproduced with permission from Reference 62.)

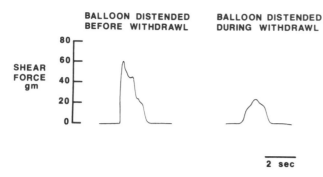

Figure 20. Technique to avoid high initial shear forces. Distending balloon *during* catheter withdrawal avoids high initial shear force and produces only the lower dynamic shear force. (Reproduced with permission from Reference 62.)

undertaken to examine the effects of timing of balloon inflation on the shear forces that are developed.[63] Vessels were mounted in a tissue bath in vitro. A balloon catheter was inserted into the lumen through an arteriotomy and the balloon was inflated *before* or *during* catheter withdrawal. Figure 20 shows shear forces recorded with the balloon filled to a lateral wall pressure of 150 mm Hg. Filling the balloon before motion was initiated produced the usual biphasic pattern of shear forces. This is shown on the left. By contrast, filling the balloon during catheter motion markedly reduced the shear force by avoiding the high initial or static component of shear force. This is shown on the right. This is comparable to a child running with a sled over snow to gain velocity before leaping onto it for sledding. Filling a balloon while the catheter is in motion has its greatest benefits at high lateral wall pressures. This is indeed fortunate, for the potential for injury is greatest with high lateral wall pressures where high shear forces are generated. For example, filling the balloon during catheter motion at 25 mm Hg lateral wall pressure reduced the shear force 23% (p <.05) as compared with filling the balloon before motion had begun. By contrast, filling the balloon during catheter motion at 125 mm Hg lateral wall pressure reduced the shear force 53% (p <.05) as compared with that observed with filling the balloon before catheter motion had begun. Thus, it is evident that the balloon should be filled while the catheter is in motion. Of course, care must be taken not to leave residual thrombus beyond the catheter tip. In most cases, this can be avoided by filling the balloon immediately upon initiating catheter motion so that the balloon is distended within the first few millimeters of passage.

Summary and Clinical Recommendations

This chapter reviews the mechanisms and spectrum of clinical injuries produced by balloon catheter embolectomy. Presented are the concepts of lateral wall pressure and of balloon-artery shear forces, and the histologic consequences of passage of embolectomy catheters. Experimental studies are summarized and, based on the results of these investigations, technical recommendations are made regarding the performance of embolectomy in patients. Attention to these technical aspects of the procedure will provide the operating surgeon with optimal control of the balloon, and will help prevent excessive lateral wall pressures and elevated shear forces. This will reduce the risk of arterial injury. The following are recommendations for performance of balloon embolectomy in patients:

1) Select the smallest size catheter that can be passed and will be effective. Small catheters produce lower shear forces than do large catheters.

2) Use a small-bore, long-stroke syringe. This will provide maximum control over balloon volume, diameter, and lateral wall pressure. Shear force increases with increasing lateral wall pressure.

3) Fill embolectomy balloons with fluid rather than with air. Fluid provides greater control of balloon volume and lateral wall pressure. It may not be possible to use fluid in a very small catheter such as 2F.

4) Before inserting the catheter into a vessel, fill the balloon to check for leaks and for balloon eccentricity. Reject balloons which leak or are more than slightly eccentric.

5) Insert the catheter into the vessel taking care to enter the true lumen. Do not create a false passage. Do not force the catheter against resistance as this may cause perforation or the formation of a false passage.

6) Begin to withdraw the catheter before the balloon is inflated, but fill the balloon within the first few mm of catheter motion. After the balloon has been inflated sufficiently to produce resistance, reduce the volume in the balloon slightly. In most cases, the balloon will continue to be in contact with the wall, but will exert less lateral wall pressures and lower shear forces.

7) Withdraw the catheter slowly and, if possible, continuously.

8) Repeat the embolectomy process until the lumen is clear, but do not pass the catheter an excessive number of times because this will cause the subsequent development of intimal hyperplasia.

9) Obtain an intraoperative completion arteriogram to be sure that thrombus does not remain, and that injury has not been produced.

References

1. Barker WF: Arterial embolism: acute arterial occlusion. In: Barker WF(ed). *Surgical Treatment of Peripheral Vascular Disease.* New York: McGraw-Hill; 235–249, 1961.

2. Lerman J, Miller FR, Lund CC: Arterial embolism and embolectomy retrograde flushing. *JAMA* 94:1128–1130, 1980.

3. Keeley JL, Rooney JA: Retrograde milking: an adjunct in technique of embolectomy. *Ann Surg* 134:1022–1026, 1951.

4. Shaw RS: A method for the removal of the adherent distal thrombus. *Surg Gynecol Obstet* 110:25–56, 1960.

5. Dale WA: Endovascular suction catheters. *J Thorac Cardiovasc Surg* 44:557–558, 1962.

6. Fogarty TJ, Cranley JJ, Krause RJ, et al: A method for extraction of arterial emboli and thrombi. *Surg Gynecol Obstet* 116:241–244, 1963.

7. Belkin M, Belkin BA, Bucknam CA, et al: Intra-arterial fibrinolytic therapy: efficacy of streptokinase versus urokinase. *Arch Surg* 121:769–773, 1986.

8. Towne JB, Bandyk DF: Application of thrombolytic therapy in vascular occlusive disease. *Am J Surg* 154:548–559, 1987.

9. DeMaioribus CA, Mills JL, Fujitani RM, et al: A reevaluation of intra-arterial thrombolytic therapy for acute lower extremity ischemia. *J Vasc Surg* 17:888–895, 1993.

10. Foster JH, Carter HW, Graham CP, et al: Arterial injuries secondary to the use of the Fogarty catheter. *Ann Surg* 171:971–978, 1970.

11. Dobrin PB: Mechanisms and prevention of arterial injuries caused by balloon embolectomy. *Surgery* 106:457–466, 1989.

12. O'Donnell JA, Hobson RW II: Balloon and lateral wall pressures during use of balloon embolectomy catheters. *Surgery* 84:583–587, 1978.

13. Fogarty TJ, Cranley JJ: Catheter technique for arterial embolectomy. *Ann Surg* 161:325–330, 1965.

14. Krause RJ, Cranley JJ, Strasser ES, et al: Further experience with a new embolectomy catheter. *Surgery* 5:81–87, 1966.

15. Hogg GR, MacDougall JT: An accident of embolectomy associated with the use of the Fogarty catheter. *Surgery* 61:716–718, 1967.

16. Stoney RJ, Ehrenfeld WK, Wylie EJ: Arterial rupture during insertion of a Fogarty catheter. *Am J Surg* 115:830–831, 1968.

17. Lord RSA, Ehrenfeld WK, Wylie EJ: Arterial injuries from the Fogarty catheter. *Med J Australia* 2:70–71, 1986.

18. Barker WF, Stern WE, Krayenbuchl H, et al: Carotid endarterectomy complicated by carotid cavernous sinus fistula. *J Cardiovasc Surg* 169:568–572, 1968.

19. Cranley JJ, Krause RJ, Strasser ES, et al: Complication with the use of the Fogarty balloon catheter for arterial embolectomy. *J Cardiovasc Surg* 10:407–409, 1969.

20. Inberg MV, Scheinen TM, Vanttinen EA: Surgical experiences in acute peripheral ischemia. *J Cardiovasc Surg* 11:114–121, 1970.

21. Proven JL, Ransford AO: The role of the Fogarty embolectomy catheter in the treatment of arterial embolism in the limbs. *Br J Surg* 57:59–62, 1970.

22. Colas JL, Castonguay Y, Grondin P: Faux aneurisme arterial tibial anterieur après thrombo-embolectomie avec un cathete de Fogarty. *Union Med Can* 99:1276–1294, 1970.

23. Davie JC, Richardson R: Distal internal carotid thromboendarterectomy using a Fogarty catheter in total occlusion. *J Neurosurg* 27:171–177, 1971.

24. Rob C, Battler S: Arteriovenous fistula following use of Fogarty balloon catheter. *Arch Surg* 102:144–145, 1971.

25. Dainko E: Complications of the Fogarty balloon catheter. *Arch Surg* 105:79–82, 1972.

26. Gaspar DJ, Gaspar MR: Arteriovenous fistula after Fogarty catheter thrombectomy. *Arch Surg* 105:90–92, 1972.

27. Mavor GE, Walker MC, Dahl DP, et al: Damage from the Fogarty balloon catheter. *Br J Surg* 59:389–391, 1972.

28. Ochlert WH: A complication of the Fogarty arterial embolectomy catheter. *Am Heart J* 84:484–486, 1972.

29. Parsa F, Owens ML, Wilson SE: Arteriovenous fistula following use of Fogarty catheter. *Vasc Surg* 105:90–92, 1972.

30. Fogarty TJ: Complications of arterial embolectomy. In: Beebe HG (ed). *Complications in Vascular Surgery*. Philadelphia: JB Lippincott; 95–102, 1973.

31. Love L, Marsan R: Carotid cavernous fistula. *Angiology* 25:231–236, 1974.

32. Holm J, Schersten T: Subintimal dissection secondary to the use of the Fogarty catheter. *J Cardiovasc Surg* 15:684–686, 1974.

33. Tringaud R, Masse C, Boissieras P, et al: Les traumatismes vasculaires consectufs à l'utilization de sonde de fogarty. *Lyon Chir* 58:369–374, 1974.

34. Bradley EL III, Salem AD: Peroneal arteriovenous fistula: an unusual iatrogenic complication of Fogarty catheter thromboendarterectomy. *Vasc Surg* 9:63–66, 1975.

35. Green RM, DeWeese JA, Robb CG: Arterial embolectomy before and after the Fogarty catheter. *Surgery* 77:24–33, 1975.

36. Byrnes G, MacGowan WAL: The injury potential of Fogarty balloon catheters. *J Cardiovasc Surg* 16:590–593, 1975.

37. Schweitzer DL, Aguam AS, Wilde JR: Complications encountered during arterial embolectomy with the Fogarty balloon catheter. *Vasc Surg* 10:144–156, 1976.

38. Dujovny M, Laha RK, Barriouneuvo P: Endothelial changes secondary to use of Fogarty catheter. *Surg Neurol* 7:39–41, 1977.

39. Eggers EG, Anner H, Levy P, et al: Iatrogenic carotid-cavernous fistula following Fogarty catheter thromboendarterectomy. *J Neurosurg* 51:543–545, 1979.

40. Shifrin EG, Anner H, Levy P, et al: Arteriovenous fistula in the lower limb in consequence of Fogarty balloon catheter embolectomy. *J Cardiovasc Surg* 26:310–313, 1985.

41. Makhoul RG, O'Malley MK, Hagen PO, et al: Selective supersensitivity to norepinephrine in intimal thickened rabbit aorta. *Blood Vessels* 22:252–256, 1985.

42. O'Malley MK, Hagan P-O, Mikat EM, et al: Contraction and sensitivity to norepinephrine after endothelial denudation is inhibited by prazosin. *Surgery* 99:36–43, 1986.

43. Liu MW, Roubin GS, King SB: Restenosis after coronary angioplasty: potential biologic determinants and the role of intimal hyperplasia. *Circulation* 79:1374–1387, 1989.

44. Shimokawa H, Flavahan HA, Vanhoutte PM: Natural course of the impairment of endothelium-dependent relaxations after endothelium removal in porcine arteries: possible dysfunction of a pertussis toxin-sensitive G-protein. *Circ Res* 65:740–753, 1989.

45. O'Malley MK, Cotecchia S, Hagen P-O: Increased receptor agonist affinity and responsiveness of phosphatidylinositol turnover: a possible mechanism for catecholamine supersensitivity in rabbit aortic intimal hyperplasia. *J Surg Res* 51:148–153, 1991.

46. Cartier R, Pearson PJ, Lin PJ, Schaff HV: Time course and extent of recovery of endothelium-dependent con-

tractions and relaxation after direct arterial injury. *J Thorac Cardiovasc Surg* 102:371–377, 1991.

47. Jorgensen RA, Dobrin PB: Balloon embolectomy catheters in small arteries IV. *Surgery* 93:798–810, 1983.
48. Schwarcz TH, Dobrin PB, Mrkvicka R, et al: Early myointimal hyperplasia following balloon catheter embolectomy: effect of shear forces and multiple withdrawals. *J Vasc Surg* 74:495–499, 1988.
49. Dobrin PB, Gray JL, Schwarcz TH: In vivo models used to study intimal hyperplasia. In: Dobrin PB (ed). *Intimal Hyperplasia*. Austin, TX: RG Landes; 75–84, 1994.
50. Fischell A, Grant G, Johnson DE: Determinants of smooth muscle injury during balloon angioplasty. *Circulation* 82:2170–2184, 1990.
51. Baumgartner HR, Studer A, Golgen AM: Des Gefass Kaheterismus: Normo und Hypercholesterinaemischen Kaninchen. *Pathol Micro Biol* 29:393–405, 1966.
52. Chidi CC, Depalma RG: Atherogenic potential of the embolectomy catheter. *Surgery* 83:549–557, 1978.
53. Bowles CR, Olcott C, Pakter RL, et al: Diffuse arterial narrowing as a result of intimal proliferation: a delayed complication of embolectomy with the Fogarty balloon catheter. *J Vasc Surg* 7:4:487–494, 1988.
54. Dobrin PB: Balloon embolectomy catheters in small arteries I. Lateral wall pressures and shear forces. *Surgery* 90:177–185, 1981.
55. Dobrin PB, Littooy FN: Arterial injuries caused by balloon catheter embolectomy: causes and prevention. In:

Bunt TJ (ed). *Iatrogenic Vascular Injury: A Discourse on Surgical Techniques*. Armonk, NY: Futura Publishing Company, Inc.; 101–125, 1990.
56. Dobrin PB: Balloon embolectomy catheters in small arteries II. Comparison of fluid-filled and gas-filled balloons. *Surgery* 91:671–679, 1982.
57. Goldberg EM, Goldberg MC, Choudhury LN, et al: The effects of embolectomy-thrombectomy catheters on vascular architecture. *J Cardivasc Surg* 24:74–80, 1983.
58. Lucas JF III, Makhoul RG, Cole CW, et al: Mononuclear cells adhere to sites of vascular balloon catheter injury. *Curr Surg* 43:112–115, 1986.
59. Greisler HP: The role of monocytes/macrophages in the formation of intimal hyperplasia. In: Dobrin PB (ed). *Intimal Hyperplasia*. Austin, TX: RG Landes; 193–210, 1994.
60. Schwarcz TH, Dobrin PB, Mrkvicka R, et al: Balloon embolectomy catheter induced arterial injury: a comparison of four catheters. *J Vasc Surg* 11:382–388, 1990.
61. Dobrin PB, Jorgensen RA: Balloon embolectomy catheters in small arteries III. Surgical significance of eccentric balloons. *Surgery* 93:402–408, 1983.
62. Burdick JF, Williams GM: A study of lateral wall pressure exerted by balloon-tipped catheters. *Surgery* 84:638–644, 1980.
63. Dobrin PB, Jorgensen RA: Balloon embolectomy catheters in small arteries: a technique to prevent excessive shear forces. *J Vasc Surg* 2:692–696, 1985.

CHAPTER 24

Basic Principles Underlying the Function of Endovascular Devices

Richard F. Neville, MD; Anton N. Sidawy, MD

Introduction

Dr. Charles Dotter performed the first endovascular procedure by dilating an iliac artery stenosis with the sequential passage of progressively larger catheters across the lesion. This technique of percutaneous arterial dilation was subsequently used in 11 patients in the first reported series of percutaneous angioplasty.[1] Dr. Andreas Gruntzig increased the applicability of percutaneous catheter-based vascular dilation by introducing the concept of a double-lumen balloon catheter.[2] Balloon catheters allowed vascular dilation through a puncture site remote from the target lesion. Flexible wires were developed to guide catheter-based devices through smaller, tortuous arteries previously considered not approachable.[3] These "over-the-wire" techniques utilized a coaxial catheter design with independent movement of the guidewire and treatment catheter. These developments have led to an explosion in the development and application of intraluminal, catheter-based devices for the diagnosis and treatment of vascular occlusive disease in coronary, peripheral, renal, and mesenteric circulation.

An understanding of the catheter-based devices and how they function is important to those involved in the treatment of vascular disease. This chapter is not intended to discuss the clinical implications of these devices, nor explore the results obtained through their application. The focus is placed on the principles underlying device function, and the mechanism of action of different endovascular instruments including balloon angioplasty, laser angioplasty, atherectomy, intravascular stents, and imaging devices such as intravascular ultrasound and angioscopy.

Transluminal Balloon Angioplasty

Clinical Overview

Although clinical evaluation of endovascular devices is not the focus of this discussion, several of the clinical implications of balloon angioplasty must be considered in order to place into context the development of endovascular devices. Transluminal balloon angioplasty is an increasingly common endovascular procedure performed in the aorta, iliac, femoral, tibial, and coronary arteries with varying degrees of success. Several characteristics of the target lesion impact on the success of balloon dilatation including anatomic site, plaque composition, and lesion configuration. Balloon angioplasty is most successful in larger, proximal arteries such as the aortoiliac system, less so in the femoral and popliteal arteries, and least in the smaller,

From *The Basic Science of Vascular Disease.* Edited by Sidawy AN, Sumpio BE, and DePalma RG. Armonk, NY: Futura Publishing Company, Inc.; © 1997.

distal tibial arteries.[4-7] Variability in atheroma composition affects the mechanical responses to balloon inflation. Favorable lesion configuration includes focal stenoses or short occlusions, as opposed to diffuse disease or chronic, total occlusions. Therefore, patients with claudication have better success rates than do those treated for limb salvage with more extensive disease.[5,6,8-10] However, objective interpretation of results is difficult due to a lack of uniform reporting standards including a variability of indications for treatment, differing patient populations, exclusion of initial failures, and a variety of methods used to evaluate therapeutic success.

The objective of balloon angioplasty is to expand a narrowed arterial segment in a manner that retains the luminal expansion, thereby improving blood flow through that arterial segment. As will be discussed later, angioplasty causes trauma to the arterial wall and intimal surface and, therefore, elicits a healing response. A favorable healing response appears crucial for the long-term patency of successfully dilated arteries. The difference between favorable and unfavorable healing is associated with restenosis, with the relative importance of elastic recoil, vasospasm, myointimal hyperplasia, and collagen formation still poorly understood. Many of the "second generation" devices, such as atherectomy catheters and laser angioplasty, were designed to more effectively debulk atheroma and decrease the adverse healing response which results in restenosis. The remainder of this chapter addresses some of the principles involved in the intraluminal dilatation of arterial lesions, the mechanism by which dilatation exerts its effect, and some of the characteristics of balloon catheter construction and design.

Forces of Transluminal Vascular Dilatation

The Dotter technique using tapered, rigid catheters to dilate an arterial stenosis transmits the pushing force of the operator to the distal end of a stiff catheter. A radial component of the pushing force is created as the catheter is advanced across the lesion. A forward-directed longitudinal shearing force is also exerted on the lesion. Unfortunately, these radial and longitudinal forces act on "normal segments" wherever the advancing tip contacts the arterial wall (e.g., curved segments proximal to the lesion).

Balloon angioplasty functions by exerting a circumferential force on the arterial wall as the balloon expands. Balloon catheters modeled after those pioneered by Andreas Gruntzig generate focal forces in the area of the stenosis, which are not dissipated by the tangential motion of the original "Dottering" technique. However, in resistant lesions there will be a longitudinal component of the force acting on the ste-

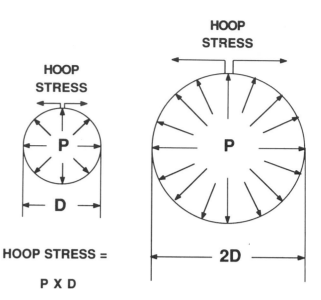

Figure 1. Hoop stress is directly proportional to the distending pressure of the balloon and its cross-sectional diameter. At equal distending pressure, hoop stress is increased by larger diameter balloons. (Reproduced with permission from Reference 12.)

nosis. The circumferential "stretching" force generated during balloon dilatation results from pressure generated by fluid forced into the contained space of the balloon. The pressure within the expanding balloon is transmitted to the adjacent artery, thereby generating circumferential stretching forces on the arterial wall.

The circumferential stretching force acting on the balloon surface is called hoop stress (Figure 1). The average of this force is reflected as a corollary of Laplace's law:

$$\text{Hoop stress} = (\text{hydrostatic pressure}) \times (\text{balloon diameter})$$
$$\text{Hoop stress} = P \times D$$

Hoop stress generates both longitudinal and radial force vectors, with the radial force vector being the dilating force (Figure 2A). The radial force vector is proportional to the diameter of the fully-inflated balloon and the pressure used for balloon inflation measured in atmospheres.[11] Therefore, the radial force vector is greater than the pure hydrostatic force generated by fluid injection into the catheter to inflate the balloon. Angioplasty increases the intraluminal pressure and radius with resultant increase in tangential tension keeping the arterial wall expanded and preventing collapse. If the radius of dilatation is insufficient, or the intraluminal pressure exerted is not sufficient, the appropriate tangential tension will not be produced to prevent arterial recoil and inefficient dilatation.

Balloon expansion will occur as long as the hoop stress generates a radial force vector greater than the intrinsic wall tension of the artery. When arterial wall tension equals hoop stress, balloon expansion is halted. Due to the effect of diameter on hoop stress, larger balloons are able to generate increased forces with dilatation. Therefore, these larger balloons must be made of a material strong enough to withstand the higher hoop stresses which are generated. Although larger balloons have greater dilating power, when the balloon catheter is properly sized inside the artery, less hydrostatic pressure on the balloon is needed to generate a sufficient hoop stress which equals and overcomes the intrinsic wall tension. There are also differences in the force generated by the balloon in the stenotic area, as compared to the fully-dilated areas of the balloon. The radial force vectors are greatest where the stenosis is greatest, decreasing as the fully dilated portions of the balloon are reached (Figure 2B).[11,12] When the balloon is fully inflated, the hoop stress equalizes as the balloon wall becomes taut and the force is transmitted to the point of indentation created by the stenosis.

The generated hoop stress also acts on the artery adjacent to the lesion. The compliant adjacent arterial wall undergoes elastic stretching upon exposure to dilating forces. The inelastic stenotic site may resist deformation at balloon pressures which dilate adjacent compliant segments. In such cases, the hoop stress acting on the nonstenotic artery exceeds that acting on the stenotic site. Angioplasty balloons are made to be noncompliant so that once inflated they maintain a constant diameter and do not elastically stretch. Compliant balloons transmit hoop stress to the adjacent compliant arterial segment more rapidly than in the area of stenosis. This can lead to overdistension and injury or rupture of the nonstenotic adjacent segments at pressures generated to dilate the inelastic stenosis. Noncompliant balloons retain diameter as the pressure is increased, thereby protecting the adjacent segments from uncontrolled overstretching (Figure 3).

If the circumferential hoop stress was the only force acting on narrow stenoses, dilatation might require enormous pressures due to the small diameter of the stenotic area. Large hoop stresses in the adjacent balloon segments could result in balloon rupture. However, the membrane of a pressurized, noncompliant balloon becomes taut, creating a tension equal in all directions within the plane of the membrane, longitudinal as well as circumferential. These longitudinal membrane forces exhibit strong radial components at points where the diameter of the balloon is changing rapidly along the axial direction. This radial force is equal to the "greatest hoop stress" times the radial slope of the balloon indentation. The force is largest where the stenosis is most severe (i.e., the slope of the balloon indentation is the greatest) and becomes the principal dilating force acting on severe, focal stenoses. Conversely, in a longer stenosis with a more gentle radial slope, greater balloon pressures are required to generate the same radial force component.

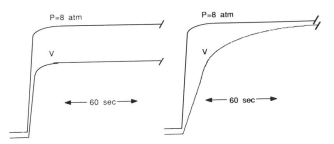

Figure 3. Noncompliant balloon materials (**left**) rapidly maintain a given volume (**V**) and shape with dilating pressures (**P**). Compliant balloon materials (**right**) more slowly reach given volumes (**V**) with dilating pressure (**P**) and may overdistend leading to the possibility of balloon rupture. (Reproduced with permission from Reference 11.)

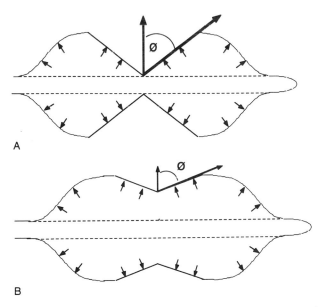

Figure 2 A. Longitudinal and radial force vectors generated by dilating force. The force vectors are greatest in areas of severe stenosis. **B.** Dilating vector forces when the stenosis is partially dilated and balloon deformability is decreased. (Reproduced with permission from Yeatman LA: Angioplasty balloons, guidewires, and other equipment. In: Moore WS, Ahn SS (eds). *Endovascular Surgery*. Philadelphia: WB Saunders, Co.; 20–22, 1989.)

Mechanism of Transluminal Dilatation

Dotter attributed the effect of angioplasty to plaque compression and consequent volume reduction. An avid mountain climber, Dotter likened the process to footprints left in the compacted snow while mountain climbing. Histologic evidence of plaque compression as proposed by Dotter is difficult to find. Fogarty has attributed only 1% to 2% of angioplasty's effect to plaque compression, with 85% to 93% due to arterial wall plaque disruption, and 6% to 12% to fluid extrusion from the plaque.[13] Much work has been done with animal models, autopsy specimens, atherectomy specimens, and intravascular ultrasound, trying to better define the actual effect of transluminal balloon dilatation.[14–18]

Although successfully dilated stenoses generally appear angiographically smooth with uniform flow, significant intimal tears and dissections in the arterial wall and atheroma result from inelastic deformation of the lesion.[14,17] When a balloon catheter is placed across a fibrocalcific plaque and dilated, the radial force vectors separate the inelastic plaque from adjacent compliant arterial tissue which can stretch with dilation. Shearing forces at the interface between the stiff plaque and the compliant arterial wall, usually the media, lead to separation at these boundaries (Figure 4). The separation creates a dissection and the forces generated by the

inflated balloon rapidly extend the tear radially as the balloon expands. The separation begins at the luminal edge of the inelastic atheroma and extends both longitudinally and radially, creating a dissection limited by several factors including balloon size. The plaque remains attached to the arterial wall proximally and distally, with these points of attachment maintaining arterial patency despite plaque dissection. The underlying arterial wall can then be stretched effecting an increase in luminal size. These benign dissections are generally necessary for the irreversible expansion of the arterial lumen, but are not fundamentally unlike the severe or unstable dissections which can lead to abrupt luminal occlusion. Therefore, successful balloon dilatation requires inelastic deformation or focal disruption of the narrowed arterial segment which is not reversible. This initiates a healing process and arterial remodeling so that the dissection planes are often no longer angiographically visible as quickly as 3 to 30 days postdilatation.[14,18–20]

An adaptive arterial response to atherosclerosis may also play a prominent role in the explanation of

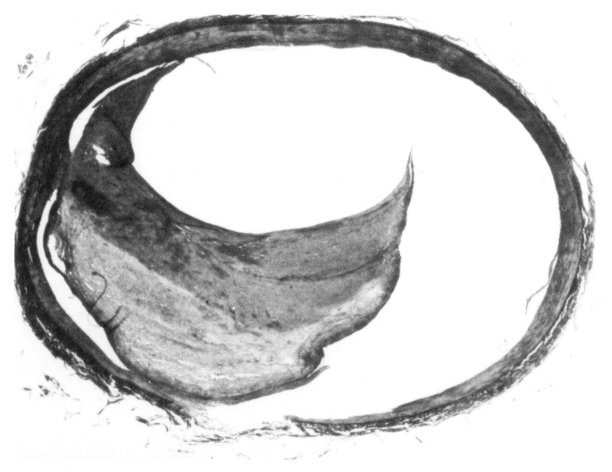

Figure 4. Cross-section of human superficial femoral artery after balloon dilatation. Dissection plane has developed between the plaque and the arterial media. (Reproduced with permission from Reference 19.)

angioplasty's effect on atherosclerotic arteries. The arterial wall dilates in response to early encroachment by atherosclerotic plaque. The effective luminal stenosis of the initial atherosclerotic plaque is negligible due to this arterial enlargement and dilatation. However, the adaptive response is blunted when plaque becomes voluminous (40% of the cross-sectional arterial area), or the arterial wall becomes stiffened by calcium or fibrous plaque so that the arterial lumen can no longer adapt by enlarging.[21,22] When the atherosclerotic plaque becomes circumferential in the arterial wall, the lumen is encased, preventing dilation in response to the development of further atherosclerosis. Angioplasty may crack and separate this atherosclerotic shell from a significant arc of underlying media, thereby allowing the media to resume again its adaptive response to the atherosclerotic process.

Characteristics of Balloon Construction

Several properties are important for optimal balloon catheter function. These properties include catheter pushability, trackability, and crossability, as well as the previously mentioned balloon compliance. Catheter pushability reflects the column strength of the catheter and the coefficient of friction of the catheter's surface material. Optimal pushability results from a strong catheter with a low coefficient of friction, and assures consistent performance at the catheter tip in response to a force exerted on the proximal end of the catheter. Trackability involves the flexibility of the

catheter material, with optimal trackability allowing catheters to be maneuvered through tortuous arteries, often over guidewires. Crossability pertains to catheter diameter and profile. Optimal crossability results from a low, smooth profile and a low coefficient of friction for maneuverability across tight stenoses. Crossability depends on the ratio of the inflated to the deflated balloon diameter or the expansion ratio. A high expansion ratio indicates a smaller cross-sectional area in the deflated state among balloon catheters with a given inflated diameter. Therefore, catheters with a high expansion ratio have good crossability and are easier to advance across an arterial stenosis.

Balloon compliance is a critical property for balloon catheter function. Compliance is the amount of stretch induced by a given force and determines the response of the balloon to the hoop stress exerted by hydrostatic pressure.[11] Early balloons were made with compliant material and exhibited a number of drawbacks that led to the development of newer generations of balloons that are virtually noncompliant even at high pressures. A compliant balloon stretches beyond its nominal diameter and may significantly overstretch when exposed to high inflation pressures. This occurs because hoop stress increases with diameter as well as pressure. A compliant balloon allows overstretch in areas not constrained by the arterial stenosis. The unconstrained balloon may then continue to expand despite a fixed pressure, creating ever greater hoop stress in the unconstrained portion of the balloon with the associated risk of balloon rupture (Figure 5). Compliant balloons also exhibit nonuniform expansion and

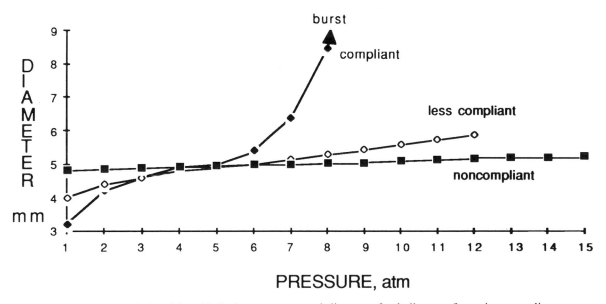

Figure 5. Relationship of inflation pressure and diameter for balloons of varying compliance. (Reproduced with permission from Yeatman LA: Angioplasty balloons, guidewires, and other equipment. In: Moore WS, Ahn SS (eds). *Endovascular Surgery*. Philadelphia: WB Saunders, Co.; 1989.)

nonuniform tension within the balloon membrane, thereby lessening the radial force exerted against the focal stenosis. As an analogy, a child's compliant latex balloon can be partially collapsed by compressing the middle. The collapsed segment exhibits lower wall tension as compared to the adjacent, bulging inflated segments at either end. On the other hand, a noncompliant balloon maintains a constant volume as pressure increases. This limits the likelihood that a correctly-sized balloon will overstretch an artery, and insures that the maximal hoop stress within the balloon wall at a given inflation pressure will be more predictable, thus avoiding rupture. The tension in the wall of the inflated balloon will be uniform, creating a large radial force at the site of the focal indentation caused by a constraining arterial wall stenosis.

Construction material is an important determinant of balloon characteristics. The chosen material must possess adequate tensile strength to allow both expansion and dilatation without rupture. The materials most commonly used are polyvinyl chloride (PVC) and polyethylene (PET). PVC is an elastomeric material with a significant degree of compliance. Therefore, the radial forces generated by dilatation are lessened at the point of maximal arterial stenosis and the balloon stretches beyond its nominal diameter at higher pressures. PVC is also not suitable for high inflation pressures due to limited tensile strength. PET is nonelastomeric, with radial forces which are not dissipated by overstretch around a critical stenosis. This allows the construction of so-called high-pressure balloons. Dilatation of resistant stenoses may be enhanced with the use of high-pressure balloons, as increasing dilation pressure can occur without oversizing of the balloon in adjacent arterial segments. However, oversizing may lead to disruption of adjacent segments, as well as arterial dissections once the resistant lesion yields to the balloon forces. PET has poor memory and does not maintain a low profile, resulting in poor crossability after deflation.

Characteristics of Catheter Design

Catheters for balloon angioplasty have been designed in several different configurations, most commonly coaxial or multilumen configurations. The coaxial catheter design consists of concentric tubes inside the catheter (Figure 6A). The inner tube is for guidewire placement in over-the-wire techniques, and the outer catheter shaft forms a space for the injected liquid which inflates the balloon. The advantages of a coaxial design include less catheter material needed to construct the shaft with resulting increased trackability. However, there is decreased strength and pushability with a coaxial catheter. Multilumen catheters have

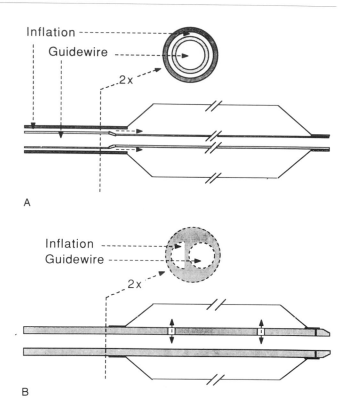

Figure 6. Coaxial (**A**) and dual lumen (**B**) catheter design. (Reproduced with permission from Yeatman LA: Angioplasty balloons, guidewires, and other equipment. In: Moore WS, Ahn SS (eds). *Endovascular Surgery*. Philadelphia: WB Saunders, Co.; 1989.)

two parallel channels (Figure 6B). One channel is a guidewire port, with the second channel used for balloon inflation. This dual lumen configuration results in increased strength and pushability, but decreased trackability and decreased crossability owing to the increased catheter profile, as the balloon must be attached to the outer wall of the catheter.

The extrusion balloon catheter relies on a different catheter design.[23] This catheter consists of a nonelastomeric balloon located inside the tip of a catheter with a separate lumen for guidewire placement. A given amount of fluid is injected proximally, extruding the balloon from the end of the catheter to a predetermined pressure. This allows the balloon to exert a radial expansion force at a known balloon diameter. Theoretically, there are minimal linear shear forces exerted as the balloon emerges from the catheter and dilates.[24] An additional advantage to this catheter is the decreased dependence on fluoroscopic guidance as the balloon seeks the path of least resistance with extrusion and subsequent inflation.

Guidewires have become important, as most balloon catheters are used with over-the-wire guidance for transluminal angioplasty. Guidewire technology has advanced with the advent of steerable wires and smooth "glide" wires, which are hydrophilic and allow the wire to insinuate itself through very tight occlusions. In such cases, the crossability of the low profile balloon catheter advanced over this guidewire is critical to perform reliable angioplasty.

Pathophysiology of the Complications of Transluminal Dilation

Complications associated with transluminal dilation include balloon rupture, arterial rupture or dissection, embolization, acute thrombosis, and restenosis. Balloon rupture occurs when the inflation tension exceeds the balloon's tensile strength. Balloon rupture usually occurs after arterial rupture, thereby releasing the physical restraint on the balloon by the intact arterial wall.[25] The balloon distends beyond its limits with a resultant force exceeding its tensile strength. Currently available noncompliant balloons rarely rupture when properly sized, despite high inflation pressures. However, these noncompliant balloons may develop a tear in the balloon material at its attachment to the catheter shaft at high inflation pressures. These tears result in jagged edges that may injure the artery at the site of dilation, as well as injure the artery upon removal of the catheter through the insertion site. Primary arterial rupture can result from balloon overdistension, especially when large balloons are used in an attempt to increase the radial dilating force for a more effective angioplasty result. Overstretch by 50% may lead to an increased incidence of arterial wall injury and rupture.[26] Current balloons are limited to 25% beyond their designated size in order to minimize the risk of arterial rupture, even with above normal inflation pressures.

Arterial injury also occurs with plaque disruption and the creation of intimal tears and flaps. Intimal flaps are raised with partial plaque separation from the compliant arterial wall. Some degree of intimal flap or dissection is noted in approximately 60% of postangioplasty arteriograms.[19] Embolization of large and small particulate matter from the angioplasty site rarely occurs and is most common after recanalization of total occlusions.[27]

Early angioplasty failures are due to arterial thrombosis or ineffective dilation. Thrombosis can occur after extensive intimal dissection obstructs the lumen. Insufficient stretch of the arterial wall leads to recoil and suboptimal plaque separation resulting in ineffective dilation.

Late failures are due to accelerated atherosclerosis and arterial restenosis in proximity to the angioplasty site. Restenosis is a major problem associated with balloon angioplasty. The problem of restenosis has stimulated the development of other catheter-based devices in order to decrease the impact of this adverse reaction of the arterial wall to dilatation. Although a full discussion of restenosis is beyond the scope of this chapter, restenosis can be characterized as an unfavorable healing response of the arterial wall to the trauma of angioplasty. Early restenosis suggests ineffective initial dilatation or elastic stretching of the arterial media with subsequent recoil.[28] This is especially likely with eccentric lesions in which the arc of "normal" arterial wall not bound by obvious atheromatous plaque is compliant and may be stretched, while the less compliant arc of arterial wall encased in atheroma is left unaffected. Late restenosis is associated with arterial injury involving platelet deposition, vasospasm, myointimal hyperplasia, and accelerated atherosclerosis.[28–31] The histologic process is similar to that which plagues surgical bypass grafts. Myointimal hyperplasia appears to be the histologic process involved and is characterized by the migration and proliferation of smooth muscle cells.[32] However, it has not been clearly demonstrated how such hyperplasia differs from the process allowing dilated arteries to heal favorably. The process of myointimal hyperplasia is fully discussed in another chapter.

Endoluminal Stents

Endoluminal stents are metallic cylinders which were developed in an attempt to increase the effectiveness of balloon dilatation by tacking down intimal flaps and providing support against the elastic recoil which may contribute to early restenosis. Stents provide the endoluminal support necessary to overcome fibroelastic recoil, thereby improving the results of angioplasty, especially the dilatation of hyperplastic lesions. A variety of designs have been developed including balloon expandable stents, self-expanding spirals, and thermal memory alloys. Initial stent designs were bulky and associated with thrombosis.[33] These problems were thought to be related to stent rigidity and the large amount of foreign material exposed to circulating blood elements. Recent technology has produced stents composed of thin wire filaments, reducing total surface area and providing flexibility while maintaining reliable expansible properties.

Balloon Expandable Stents

Balloon expandable stents are mounted on standard balloon angioplasty catheters for deployment across the target lesion as the balloon is inflated. The Palmaz-Schatz stent, Strecker stent, and Roubin-Gianturco coil are examples of balloon expandable stents. The Palmaz stent (Johnson and Johnson) is stainless steel with staggered parallel slots formed by the intersection of thin, filamentous struts.[34] The wall thickness of the individual struts is 0.015 mm. The stent is placed over a balloon and "crimped" in place to maintain a low profile. The balloon catheter is positioned across the target lesion and inflated. The stent is thus deployed against the atherosclerotic lesion with the balloon subsequently deflated and withdrawn.

The Strecker stent (Boston Scientific) is made of a single tantalum wire filament. The wire is configured in a series of connected loops which result in excellent longitudinal and radial flexibility. The Roubin-Gianturco stent is stainless steel with the configuration of an interdigitating coil.[35] The Roubin stent is also mounted on the end of a balloon angioplasty catheter for deployment. The particular advantage of this stent is its extreme flexibility in the longitudinal axis allowing maneuverability around curves and bend points in the arterial tree. Disadvantages include stent recoil after balloon expansion which can be avoided with a small degree of overexpansion. Migration after deployment and a decrease in rapidity of endothelialization has been noted in animal work.[36] However, balloon expandable stents have demonstrated reasonable patency, endothelialization, and an acceptable chronic arterial wall response in clinical trials.[37,38] The Palmaz stent is currently approved by the FDA for use in the iliac arteries, although the role of stent deployment beyond that of angioplasty alone remains to be completely defined.

Self-Expanding Stents

Self-expanding stents do not rely on balloon inflation for deployment, but expand to a predetermined size upon release from the delivery system. These stents are more flexible in the longitudinal axis, allowing easier maneuverability across bend points in the arterial tree, and are deployed through smaller diameter delivery systems. The Sigwart (Medivent) and Wallstent (Schneider) are tubular self-expanding stents. The Wallstent standard configuration has stainless steel wire struts in an unconnected, crisscrossing tubular pattern perpendicular to the longitudinal axis which shortens upon expansion. A Wallstent braid is available that results in less shortening for more predictable positioning during expansion. Several thermal self-expanding stents have also been investigated. These devices are composed of thermal alloys which expand in response to body heat upon deployment. The Cragg stent is composed of nitinol, a nickel-titanium alloy. This alloy can be heated (450° to 500°C) in a desired configuration and then becomes deformable at cooler temperatures. Upon rewarming to the alloy's transition temperature (30° to 60°C), the material returns to the predetermined shape.[39]

Parameters of Proper Stent Deployment

Properties crucial to optimal stent deployment include longitudinal flexibility, ease of fluoroscopic visibility, reliable expansion, and appropriate mechanical deformation. Mechanical deformation is extremely important for proper stent function, involving the properties of stress and strain specific to different materials. Stress is the force applied to a material per unit area (gm/cm^2), while strain is the permanent change or fractional deformation that results in the stressed material. Elastic deformation is the reversible change with stress which occurs in a given material as a linear relationship between stress and strain (Figure 7). The slope of this linear relationship is the modulus of elasticity (Y, Young's modulus) for the material and is a reflection of the material's degree of stiffness; stiffer materials have a greater Y value. Plastic deformation is the irreversible change that occurs when a material is stressed (Figure 8). As a material is stressed, an initial elastic phase occurs with a linear stress-strain relationship. At the material's yield point, the relationship becomes nonlinear. The yield point is that degree of stress at which the deformation becomes permanent for the given material. A higher yield point signifies a greater resistance to plastic deformation.[40]

The combination of a high expansion ratio with a low profile shape allows the stent/catheter system to maneuver through the arterial tree to the target site, and deploy the stent with incremental expansion over a wide range of arterial diameters. Biocompatibility depends on low thrombogenicity, with an acceptable chronic response of the arterial wall to stent deployment. Incorporation into the arterial wall must occur without the formation of excessive myointimal hyperplasia. Stent compliance may also impact on acute deployment and the chronic arterial wall response.

The chronic response of the arterial wall to stent deployment is a major factor of stent efficacy and success. Neointimal coverage of stent struts occurs with the patency of side branches maintained, as much of the space taken up by stents in the expanded state is open area.[34,41] Neointimal coverage of stent struts is under way, but incomplete at 3 weeks; however, by 8 weeks, strut coverage is significant, with complete coverage by 6 months postdeployment. Neointimal coverage seems dependent on metal element thickness and stent porosity. As metal thickness increases or porosity decreases, more fibrin and less neointima develop between the stent struts over time.[42] Arterial wall contact is another important deployment parameter to enhance stent neointimal coverage, as increased neointimal coverage occurs with complete stent-arterial wall contact.[36]

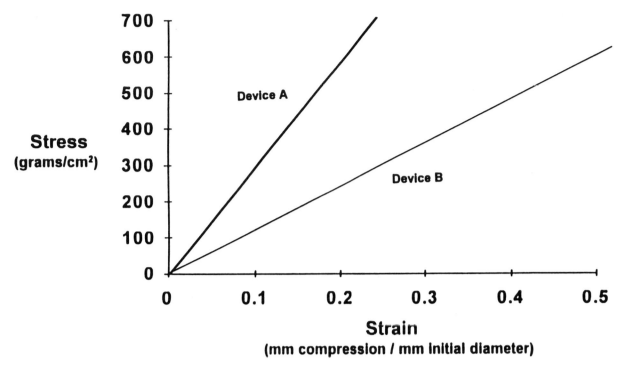

Figure 7. Stress-strain relationship of two elastic materials. The modulus of elasticity (**slope**) for device **A** is greater than device **B**, indicating greater resistance to deformation (stiffness). (Reproduced with permission from Reference 44.)

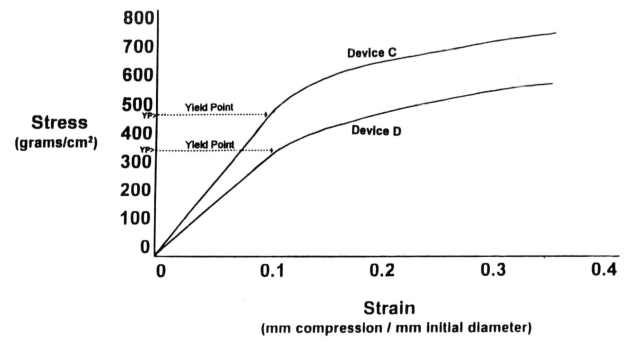

Figure 8. Stress-strain relationship of two materials with both elastic and plastic deformation. The transition to the nonlinear portion of the curve (**yield point**) is higher for device **C** than device **D**, indicating greater resistance to permanent plastic deformation. (Reproduced with permission from Reference 44.)

Complications of Stent Deployment

Complications of stent deployment include thrombosis, migration, and the development of stenosis. Stented arterial segments can thrombose and heparin has been advocated for use during initial deployment.[33] Stent migration distal to the site of deployment can occur with incomplete arterial wall contact at deployment.[36] Stenosis and occlusion of stented arteries can occur with the accumulation of neointimal hyperplasia and subsequent thrombosis. Balloon expandable stents lack radial compliance, and the compliance mismatch at the stent-arterial border may contribute to the hyperplastic response.[34,43] Extrinsic compression may play a role with stents deployed in exposed peripheral locations. The balloon expandable stents may be particularly prone to suffer plastic deformation and collapse, with external compression in unprotected areas of the vascular tree.[44] Stent-arterial wall contact appears to be an important factor in preventing complications. Intravascular ultrasound can demonstrate those stent struts not in contact with the arterial wall (Figure 9). After complete stent expansion, the stent struts can be identified as bright echo reflections seemingly embedded in the arterial wall (Figure 10).[36] This technology may become an important method to assess stent deployment and optimize deployment parameters to minimize complications.

Stented Grafts for Intraluminal Bypass: The Future?

Advances in stent design have led to a recent surge of interest in the combination of an endoluminal stent and a prosthetic graft to create an intraluminal vascular bypass. This concept employs a stent to secure the proximal, and often the distal, end of a prosthetic graft placed inside an artery in order to bypass aneurysmal or occlusive disease. The technology to perform this procedure, percutaneously or by surgical dissection, remains under development. Appropriate clinical indications remain to be defined along with the success rates and durability of this form of revascularization.

Atherectomy

Atherectomy catheters have been developed as a way to debulk atherosclerotic lesions without the use of balloon dilatation. Ideally, this would decrease the rate of restenosis documented with the use of balloon

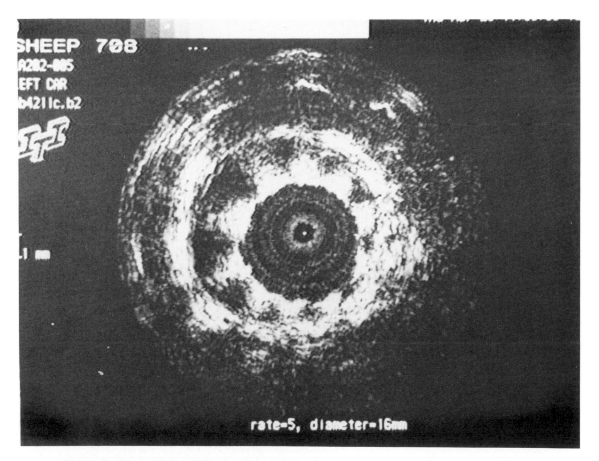

Figure 9. Intravascular ultrasound image of slotted stent after partial expansion in the artery. (Reproduced with permission from Reference 36.)

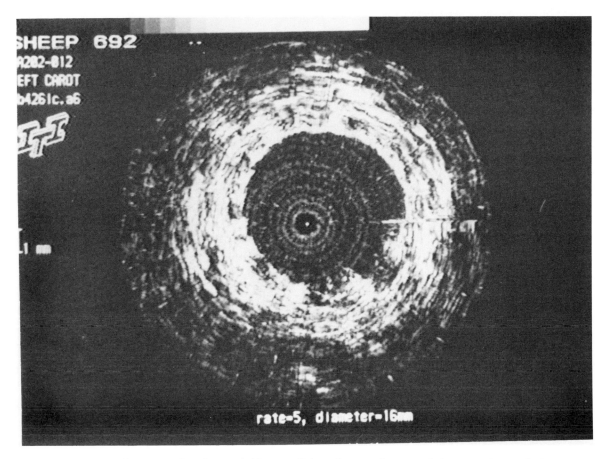

Figure 10. Intravascular ultrasound image of slotted stent after complete expansion so that struts are embedded in the arterial wall. (Reproduced with permission from Reference 36.)

angioplasty. Atherectomy is based on the same principles as surgical endarterectomy. The results of surgical endarterectomy are dependent on the pattern of disease, indication for the procedure, lesion length, and lesion location. The results of atherectomy to date have paralleled these findings. Claudicants fare better than those with rest pain or tissue gangrene; shorter lesions respond better than diffuse disease, and proximal iliofemoral lesions respond better than distal lesions or below-knee lesions. Additionally, certain factors concerning technique are similar between the two modalities. Both modalities attempt to remove atheroma through the development of a plane within the medial portion of the arterial wall, with a smooth transition to normal intima at the distal end point. Additionally, a luminal surface free of thrombotic debris and a widely patent lumen are important factors. Several catheter devices have been developed to, in effect, perform a catheter-based endarterectomy known as atherectomy.

Kensey Catheter

The Kensey device consists of a rotating cam tip at the end of a flexible catheter. Theoretically, as the catheter rotates, it preferentially destroys calcified and fibrotic atheroma, while the normal arterial wall is deflected out of the way of the cam tip. The cam tip rotates at 100,000 rpm, with channels available for the continuous infusion of fluid in the form of lateral jet sprays. The fluid theoretically cools the tip of the catheter and maintains the catheter in a coaxial position inside the arterial lumen. This catheter does not use over-the-wire techniques for guidance and ranges in size from 5 to 9 F. Work with cadaveric arterial segments demonstrates atheroma debulking; however, there is also damage to the intima and hemorrhage into the media and plaque remnants.[45] Clinical use of the catheter has resulted in a significant number of unsuccessful procedures, thromboses, and arterial perforations.[46]

Auth Rotoblator

The Auth rotary atherectomy device, or Rotoblator, also functions with a rotating tip. The tip is composed of a brass burr covered with diamond chips ranging in size from 30 to 120 μm and coating the distal portion of the burr. The brass burr ranges in size from 2.5 to 4.5 mm and is attached to a flexible drive shaft that rotates at 100,000 rpm. This over-the-wire system allows the catheter to track over the guidewire while rotating. Theoretical advantages of this device include the preferential attack of calcified and fibrous atheroma, while the elasticity of the normal arterial wall allows it to deflect out of the path of the rotating burr. The postatherectomy surface is relatively smooth and denuded of intimal and endothelial elements, although the surface is traumatized and a possible source of hyperplasia.[47] The ablated atheroma is ground into small particles so that embolization does not become clinically manifest.[47] However, the aggregate particulate load may be significant, as atherectomized calcific particles have caused ischemia in canine myocardium when injected directly into the coronary arteries.[48]

Simpson Atherectomy Catheter

The Simpson atherectomy catheter, or Atherocath, consists of a rotational blade contained in a cylindrical housing at the end of a catheter. A balloon is positioned on the catheter opposite the opening in the cylindrical housing. The catheter ranges in size from 7 to 11 F. The catheter is deployed across the target lesion and the balloon is gently inflated to stabilize the housing and push the open window in the housing around the atheroma. The rotational blade is then moved back and forth in the housing, shaving the atheroma, and catching the shavings in the distal portion of the cylindrical housing. There is a fixed guidewire at the tip of the housing for an added measure of guidance. Theoretically, this catheter debulks atherosclerotic lesions, leaving a smooth luminal surface with minimal arterial wall effect due to the balloon dilation. The device is designed to debulk atheroma without the need for concomitant balloon dilation and angioplasty. Embolization does not occur, as the shavings are caught in the metallic housing, and the atheromatous material is retrievable for histologic study. Use of the catheter is tedious, less effective with diffuse disease, and cannot treat total occlusions. However, this catheter has been used to make major contributions to the histologic study of atherosclerotic lesions.[16] Initial clinical work demonstrates good initial success rates for focal stenoses; however, restenosis is still in the 30% range with no real advantage over standard balloon angioplasty.[49] The catheter may be best suited for focal calcific or hyperplastic lesions which do not respond to dilatation.

Transluminal Extraction Catheter

The transluminal extraction catheter (TEC) catheter has a motorized cutting head consisting of triangular blades at the tip of a catheter. The catheter rotates at 750 rpm and has a lumen for a guidewire as an over-the-wire system for control inside the artery. There is a suction apparatus to remove the excised atherosclerotic tissue. The embolic material is suctioned out of the body through the catheter. However, the TEC device cannot cross total occlusions, and balloon dilatation has been required in many cases with restenosis noted at follow-up.[50]

Laser Angioplasty

Lasers have been proposed as an energy source for atheroma ablation, because laser light delivers precisely focused, intense energy. The energy can be generated outside the body and transmitted through optical fibers virtually without loss to the target tissue. Ideally, laser energy would vaporize atheroma without damage to surrounding arterial tissue with a favorable healing response.

Laser Physics

In 1960, T.H. Maiman first used a ruby crystal to create a laser beam with a 0.694 μm wavelength. Since then, a variety of lasing media have been used to produce laser light with wavelengths varying in the spectrum from ultraviolet to infrared. Laser is an acronym for *light amplification by the stimulated emission of radiation*. The stimulated emission of radiation upon which laser physics is based takes advantage of the excitation of ground state electrons. Electrons of atoms in the lasing medium are excited by a secondary energy source. The electrons are temporarily raised to an excited singlet state before dropping into a metastable state. Materials chosen to serve as the lasing media must have the metastable state in their electron structure. As metastable electrons return to the ground state, photons of light are emitted. These photons interact with other atoms in the metastable state, generating additional coherent photons in an increasing cascade. Reflective surfaces used to house the lasing medium cause the photons to oscillate back and forth at the speed of light. This accelerates the photon cascade until monochromatic, coherent laser light exits as a laser beam (Figure 11). To adequately amplify the cascade for the spontaneous emission of light, the normal distribution of energy states (ground state > excited state) must become reversed (excited state > ground state) in what is called a population inversion.[51–53]

A unique property of light is its ability to behave as both a particle and a wave. The properties of light as a particle, or photon, are most important to medical laser applications. These properties include coherence, monochromicity, and intensity. Coherent photons

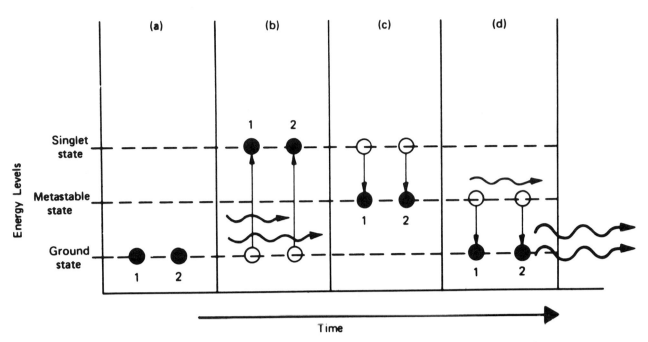

Figure 11. Electron activity in lasing medium: **A.** Ground state electrons; **B.** Excitation to the singlet state by an outside energy source (electrical, chemical, radiofrequency); **C.** Rapid transition to the metastable state; **D.** Random return to the ground state with the emission of coherent photons which impact other electrons in the metastable state until a monochromatic, coherent laser beam is generated. (Reproduced with permission from Reference 67.)

have wavelengths that are in phase and in parallel along the course of the light beam. There is no loss of intensity as coherent light travels over a given distance. Monochromatic light is of a single wavelength, and visually one color. Monochromatic light allows for selective absorption by chromophores in target tissue. The laser energy leads to excited states of the chromophore molecules that rapidly decay in less than a nanosecond. The chromophores decay to their original state, with the energy converted to vibrational energy manifest as heat. Light intensity is described in terms of photons per unit area. Lasers can be adjusted to deliver variable intensity and number of photons per unit target tissue.

The wavelength of laser light is determined by the lasing medium. Wavelengths of 100 to 400 nm fall in the ultraviolet range, 400 to 700 nm in the visible range, and greater than 700 nm in the infrared range. Lasing media include solid state crystals such as ruby or yttrium/aluminum/garnet (YAG); gas media such as helium-neon, argon, and CO_2; liquid media such as the organic dyes; and semiconductors such as gallium arsenide. Additional wavelengths of laser light may be generated by the process of harmonic generation. As coherent, monochromatic photons are passed through asymmetric crystals, frequency and wavelength are altered, increasing the number of possible laser wavelengths.

Dosimetry

Principles of dosimetry determine the target tissue response to laser energy and involve the incident power, beam area, and exposure time. Laser energy is measured in joules (J), while power is measured in watts (W) or joules per unit time (J/s). The intensity of the laser energy is equivalent to the energy per unit area per time, or joules per square millimeter (J/mm^2). Spot size is that radius from the center of the beam to the point at which the power density has dropped to $1/e^2$ that of the beam's center with penetration depth (D) equivalent to the tissue thickness in which 63% of the radiant energy is attenuated. However, if the distance from the laser to the target is increased, divergence increases the spot size and decreases the incident energy density. Absorption of laser energy and penetration depth is dependent on the tissue-specific absorption (a) and scattering (B) coefficients which also vary with laser wavelength[54]:

$$D = 1/a + B$$

Power density is the power applied per unit area of target tissue (W/mm^2). Power density determines the total energy delivered to the target. Fluence is the energy density or concentration delivered, described as joules per square millimeter (J/mm^2). Fluence is determined by the total incident energy, the unit area exposed, and the duration of exposure:

$$Fluence = incident\ power(W) \times \frac{exposure\ time(s)}{beam\ area(mm^2)}$$

$$Fluence = power\ density(W/mm^2) \times time(s)$$

Fluence threshold is the minimum energy required to ablate tissue of a given volume and is dependent on power, exposure time, and spot size, as well as penetration depth of the incident laser beam.[54-56]

Laser energy can be delivered as a continuous or pulsed wave. The continuous-wave mode delivers a steady flow of radiant energy resulting in efficient tissue ablation only when the thermal effect is greater than the thermal losses to the surrounding tissue. Thermal losses through diffusion and convection can be quite large in a liquid field such as blood. Delivery of pulsed laser energy can be more effective. The pulse repetition rate is the number of pulses per second, and the pulse width is equal to the individual pulse duration. The average power of the pulsed wave is determined by the pulse power (W), the repetition rate (s^{-1}), and the pulse width (s). Pulsed laser energy can reduce the extent of surrounding tissue damage and thermal effects by allowing the tissue to cool between individual laser pulses. This interval between pulses is the relaxation time. However, not all wavelengths are amenable to pulsed delivery, and a high repetition rate can decrease the relaxation time so that thermal damage occurs as with continuous-wave energy.[57]

Optical Fibers

A major advance in the development of laser angioplasty is the advent of optical fibers that can carry laser energy without breakage. Optical fibers contain a transparent core, an outer cladding, and a protective outer coating or sheath. The core has a higher refractive index than the surrounding cladding, so that light incident on the core-cladding interface is internally reflected. Snell's law of refraction establishes light propagation at the interface of different media:

$$n_1 \sin(a) = n_2 \sin(a^-)$$

where n is the refractive index of the media, a is the angle of incidence, and a^- is the angle of refraction (Figure 12). The critical angle of incidence (0_c) above which all light is internally reflected can be determined:

$$\sin\{0_c\} = n_{cladding}/n_{core}$$

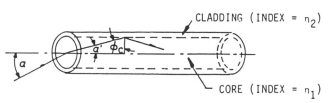

Figure 12. Optical fiber in which the refractive index of the core (n_1) is greater than the refractive index of the cladding (n_2) so that incident light is internally reflected along the fiber; a is the angle of incidence, a^- is the angle of refraction, 0_c is the critical angle of incidence for internal reflection. (Reproduced with permission from Gilbert CE, et al: *Progress in Hemostasis and Thrombosis*, Vol 4. New York: Grune and Stratton, Inc.; 1982.)

where $n_{cladding}$ and n_{core} are the refractive indices of the cladding and core. Thus, an appropriate choice of materials for the core and cladding allows light to travel within the fiber in a coaxial direction without energy loss upon impact with the cladding.[52,53]

In order to maximize the transmission of energy to the distal tip of an optical fiber, laser wavelengths are chosen to generate high quality beams with low divergence that can be focused onto a single optical fiber. At lower and higher wavelengths, light absorption heats the fiber with fiber breakage at high powers. This becomes especially important with newer lasers which utilize short, high power pulses such as the excimer laser.

The numerical aperture determines the cone of light accepted into the fiber's proximal end as well as that emerging from the distal end of the fiber. The proper numeric aperture is especially important for coupling the laser beam with the fiberoptic. Diameter determines the radius of curvature and, thus, the fiber's break point. Fiber diameter (d) also determines the degree of stiffness (d^4) and flexibility ($1/d$). The power transmitting capacity increases with d^2. However, as diameter increases, beam divergence also increases, thereby decreasing beam intensity and ablation efficiency. The fiber damage threshold is the level of pulse energy at which the transmission capability is exceeded and fiber breakdown occurs. The laser operating range is that range of pulse energy densities between the threshold for tissue ablation and that of fiber damage. Ideally, the operating range of the system should be five times the tissue ablation threshold of the chosen laser.[51-53]

Laser Effects on Target Tissue

Laser light incident on target tissue causes a variety of effects dependent on the concentration of energy delivered to the tissue and the interval of energy exposure. Laser energy produces photothermal, photo-

Laser-Tissue Interactions

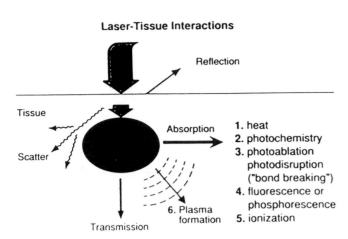

Figure 13. Various types of interactions that occur when laser light impacts biologic tissue. (Reproduced with permission from Reference 67.)

chemical, photoacoustic, and nonlinear effects that result in tissue ablation, fluorescence, ionization, and plasma formation (Figure 13).

Photothermal

The dominant effect between laser energy and biologic tissue is a photothermal reaction. Tissue chromophores preferentially absorb the laser light with conversion to thermal energy. The degree of molecular absorption also depends on the wavelength-specific absorption coefficient (a) and light scattering (B) by the target tissue. A high absorption coefficient favors efficient thermal ablation at lower energy densities with decreased surrounding zones of thermal injury. Ultraviolet and far-infrared laser wavelengths have the highest absorption coefficients for atheromatous tissue.

Several other factors affect the degree to which tissue is heated by laser energy including diffusion, convection, relaxation time, and energy intensity. Diffusion is the transfer of thermal energy to nearby molecules in the target tissue, with thermal conductivity measured in cm²/s. Convection is heat dissipation through a fluid medium such as blood. Therefore, many laser angioplasty systems are designed to maintain contact between the optical fiber and target tissue to minimize convective energy losses. When the optical fiber is in complete contact with the tissue, diffusion is the principle cause of reduced lasing efficiency and is responsible for thermal tissue injury in border zones surrounding sites of laser vaporization.[55,58] Zones of thermal damage around the point of impact are a function of penetration depth and spot size. Carbonization, vacuolization, and edema can be seen histologically in these zones, indicative of coagulation necrosis. Tissue coagulation occurs as structural proteins are denatured

secondary to photothermal heating. Melting occurs when the solid or gelatinous tissue is converted to liquid form, and vaporization occurs when high energy photons cause disruption of chemical bonds as the heat of vaporization is realized (~2J/mm³), generating local temperatures greater than 100°C. Melting and carbonization is more prominent with low intensity photons, especially with a prolonged exposure time and a large spot size. Heat diffuses radially, allowing spatial temperature curves to be constructed for specific laser wavelengths. Thermal relaxation time is the time required for the target tissue to cool to 50% of the maximal temperature after laser exposure. Relaxation time varies directly with the square of the diameter of the cone of tissue impacted and the absorption depth. Surrounding thermal damage can be minimized by using shorter pulse widths to increase the relaxation time.[59]

The intensity threshold, I_0 (J/s/mm², W/mm²) represents the energy required to increase the local tissue temperature sufficiently to cause tissue ablation. Heating must exceed the losses due to diffusion and convection in order to cause tissue ablation. The practical intensity threshold, I, is that energy intensity needed for predictable and reproducible ablation, and is often much greater than the threshold of intensity (I_0). Tissue ablation is proportional to the practical intensity threshold and exposure time. Time threshold (t_0) is the minimum time for ablation to occur at the practical intensity threshold. If the practical intensity threshold is greater than the threshold of intensity ($I > I_0$), then the time threshold for exposure may be decreased, maintaining efficient tissue ablation and minimizing surrounding tissue damage.[54,59]

Early thermal lasers heated the atheroma and arterial wall in order to coagulate or "weld" the artery in an open, dilated position.[60] The destruction of endothelium and vascular smooth muscle was initially deemed beneficial for the inhibition of thrombosis and restenosis. Laser light was transmitted through a fiberoptic with a diffusion tip for circumferential energy distribution within the artery. Laser wavelengths with a high degree of scattering relative to absorption were used so that the laser energy was absorbed diffusely over a large tissue volume. Long exposure times (30 sec) also allowed radial diffusion of heat. Subsequent laser angioplasty systems have emphasized the use of laser energy for the direct ablation of atheroma, with minimal thermal damage to surrounding tissue.

Photochemical

Laser energy can directly disrupt chemical bonds in long chain biomolecules (proteins, DNA), thereby fragmenting cells into a "molecular soup." This photochemical effect occurs as molecular chromophores in target tissue absorb wavelength-specific laser energy with energy transfer to intracellular oxygen. Highly reactive singlet oxygen is generated resulting in intracellular oxidative processes and cytotoxic reactive molecules without the generation of thermal energy. Certain laser wavelengths (excimer) cause tissue ablation through this direct breaking of chemical bonds by high energy photons. The direct transfer of energy can also exceed the molecular bonding energy of the target tissue with the disruption of the molecular bonds and tissue ablation. Photochemical changes make possible photodynamic therapy, which is the process of selective photosensitization through the use of externally administered chromophores and subsequent administration of the appropriate laser light.

Photoacoustic

Several laser wavelengths (excimer, pulsed dye, Ho:YAG) produce high peak powers with short pulse durations (< 200 μsec) causing the rapid formation of vapor bubbles, or an electron cloud (plasma). Both the vapor bubbles and plasma create transient increases in local tissue pressure to hundreds of atmospheres. These high pressure transients induced by steep thermal gradients and rapidly expanding vapor bubbles disrupt or tear the tissue. These pressure transients last less than a msec and can disrupt tissue volumes larger than the tissue directly ablated.

This acoustic trauma or shock wave depends on the power density of the laser system, the total energy applied to the target, the number of laser pulses delivered in one target area, the lasing media (blood, contrast, or crystalloid), and the target tissue composition (normal arterial tissue, fibrocalcific plaque, or thrombus). Intraluminal cavitation bubbles, studied using time-resolved flash photography, expand rapidly within 75 to 250 μsec achieving diameters up to 2.5 mm. The magnitude of these acoustic transients varies inversely with the distance from the bubble center and ranges from 100 to 1200 atm at 0.5 mm to 10 to 100 atm at 5 mm. Pulsed laser systems generate acoustic transients sufficient to cause dissections and perforations, with tissue disruption uniformly distributed along the "lased" arterial segment in contrast to the focal disruption of balloon angioplasty. The pressure transients caused by laser pulses are so short (<1 msec) that the arterial wall does not experience the slow, steady stretching observed with balloon angioplasty. Photoacoustic or shock wave transients result in tissue ablation and disruption contributing to both desired results and complications associated with pulsed laser angioplasty.

Nonlinear

At high power densities, nonlinear absorption of laser energy occurs leading to complex tissue interactions such as ionization, plasma formation, and tissue fluorescence. Nonlinear effects are most often noted after short, high energy laser pulses such as q-switched (nanosecond pulses) and mode-locked (picosecond pulse) delivery which result in extremely high power densities. Ionization is the loss of electrons by atoms of the target tissue. This requires multiphoton absorption, and lasers currently in clinical use do not possess enough energy to create this effect. Plasma formation is the generation of a mass of free electrons. As this gaseous cloud of free electrons is produced, an acoustic shock wave is generated resulting in photoacoustic destruction of the tissue. Tissue fluorescence is energy dissipation through the reemission of light by the target tissue. The energy of the reemitted fluorescent photon is always lower than that of the absorbed photon and, therefore, of a longer wavelength. Laser-stimulated fluorescence can be used to differentiate normal arterial tissue from plaque. The amount and the color of the fluorescent light depend on the reemitted wavelength, which is based on the composition of the target material.[61,62]

Specific Laser Systems

The versatility of laser light has led to a variety of laser angioplasty systems with different theoretical design advantages. Each laser system attempts to effectively and precisely vaporize variable composition atheroma, while minimizing injury to the adjacent arterial wall. A number of laser angioplasty systems have been developed and used in clinical trials. It is important to understand the mechanism of action of each system in order to determine the advantages and disadvantages as compared to other interventional devices, and to improve the methodology for future systems.

Nd:YAG Laser

The Nd:YAG laser uses a yttrium:aluminum:garnet crystal with a neodymium doping element for initial flash lamp excitation. Nd:YAG laser light has a wavelength in the near-infrared spectrum (1.06 μm) and can function in continuous or pulsed modalities. Nd:YAG light is easily coupled to fiberoptic delivery systems with a wide operating range and high maximum power output near 100 W. Tissue ablation with the Nd:YAG laser is primarily through photothermal effects with a deep thermal injury due to the lack of a specific tissue chromophore for Nd:YAG energy. Nd:YAG energy is poorly absorbed by atheromatous plaque, producing deep tissue penetration and considerable thermal damage. Calcified plaque is not ablated by Nd:YAG laser energy, but is shattered at very high energies due to prominent nonlinear photoacoustic effects. Therefore, the ablation efficiency of direct Nd:YAG laser energy is low and unpredictable.[63]

Other near-infrared YAG lasers have been developed including holmium:YAG (2.1 μm) and erbium: YAG (2.94 μm). The holmium:YAG laser has a weak water absorption peak and a relatively high absorption coefficient with atheromatous tissue. This results in improved ablation efficiency, as compared to the Nd: YAG laser with a similar operating range. However, the holmium:YAG laser requires target tissue contact, as the energy is quickly dissipated in a medium with water such as blood. The erbium:YAG laser has a stronger water absorption peak and also requires direct contact for tissue ablation. Both of these YAG lasers can be utilized in the pulse mode and generate less thermal damage to surrounding arterial tissue than the Nd:YAG laser.

Argon Laser

Argon laser energy is generated as a burst of electricity is passed through argon gas inside a laser chamber. The argon laser system operates in the blue/green visible spectrum over a range of wavelengths (457 to 514 nm) with 80% of argon energy generated at the 488 nm and 514 nm peaks. Argon energy has a maximum power between 16 W and 20 W and can function in continuous or pulsed wave modes. Argon laser light is easily coupled to standard optical fibers. There is no need for mechanical contact between the fiberoptic and the target tissue, as the argon laser energy can directly irradiate the tissue through a blood medium. The argon laser has a wide operating range and argon gas is safe to work with.

Tissue ablation occurs through photothermal effects with minimal direct vaporization and a relatively low ablation efficiency, despite the presence of hemoglobin and melanin which are tissue chromophores for argon laser energy. However, absorption is often higher in normal arterial tissue than in the atheroma, leading to considerable thermal damage in surrounding arterial tissue. A relatively high power output is required for tissue ablation, and calcified and fibrotic lesions respond poorly to argon laser energy given the absence of hemoglobin chromophores.[64]

Excimer Laser

Excimer is derived from "excited dimer," referring to the use of a two-molecule complex (dimer) as the lasing medium. Dimers used to generate laser light include XeF, KrF, ArF, and XeCl. Laser light produced by excitation of these dimers is in the ultraviolet spectrum with wavelengths ranging between 157 and 351 nm. Chromophores for excimer energy exist in the form of cellular proteins and nucleic acids, with absorption strong in atherosclerotic plaque. Due to the presence of chromophores, the primary laser-tissue interaction is a photochemical effect causing the disassociation of molecular bonds with the disruption of approximately one molecular bond per photon of laser energy absorbed.[65] Excimer tissue ablation is precise, with well-defined craters and minimal thermal damage to surrounding tissue.[66] However, the increased pulse frequencies utilized in most excimer laser systems generate thermal effects due to the manner in which the energy is delivered. As pulse frequency increases and relaxation time decreases, energy deposited in surrounding tissue results in thermal damage. The excimer wavelength noted to produce the most thermal damage is 351 nm, with the highest absorption coefficient and optimal tissue ablation at 308 nm. Calcified plaque is photoresistant to all wavelengths of excimer laser energy, making ablation of calcific lesions problematic.

Excimer lasers are difficult to couple into currently available optical fibers. Pulse energies required for tissue ablation damage optical fibers. In order to transmit excimer energy, catheters must be large, stiff single fibers, or multiple, small-diameter fibers. Fluence, pulse width, and repetition rate must be limited because of the narrow, safe operating range of the system. Also affecting system safety, toxic gases can be produced and, although contained in the laser system, pose a potential hazard. There have also been reports of ultraviolet energy being mutagenic, especially in the 308 nm range which is most often utilized for excimer laser angioplasty.[67]

CO$_2$ Laser

CO$_2$ laser systems use a mixture of carbon dioxide, nitrogen, and helium as the lasing medium, producing energy in the far infrared spectrum (10.6 μm). Electricity stimulates the nitrogen in the lasing medium and, as the electrons return to their ground state, the energy is transferred to the CO$_2$. CO$_2$ decays, emitting infrared laser energy as it returns to its ground state which impacts the helium atoms. CO$_2$ laser energy has a high water absorption peak, leading to rapid local heat absorption and vaporization. However, this laser energy is not transmitted by conventional fiberoptic catheters and requires a series of reflecting mirrors and lenses. Continuous mode CO$_2$ energy generates significant thermal injury and is unable to ablate calcified lesions. The pulsed mode has higher ablation efficiency and is somewhat more effective against calcified lesions.

However, due to the difficulty of transmission through conventional fiberoptics and the high water absorption peak which makes lasing through a fluid medium such as blood more difficult, the CO_2 laser has not gained wide acceptance in vascular interventions.

Intravascular Ultrasound

Basic Properties of Sound

Sound waves are mechanical disturbances in a gas, liquid, or solid medium. The waves travel outward from the source of the mechanical disturbance at a specific velocity in the form of vibrations that are local changes in pressure. A relative increase in pressure, as compared to atmospheric pressure, is a compression. A decrease is a rarefaction. Sound wavelength (w) is determined by the distance from one peak compression to the next. Sound waves consist of a series of compressions and rarefaction, with one compression and rarefaction considered a cycle measured in hertz (Hz, cycles per second) (Figure 14). Frequency (f) is the number of cycles per unit time with the velocity (v) of sound determined by frequency and wavelength:

$$v = f \times w$$

Velocity of sound through a given medium is also dependent on the density of the medium, as sound travels faster through denser media. Velocity is also dependent on temperature; however, this parameter is fairly constant in dealing with biomedical applications. Therefore, frequency and wavelength are inversely related. Frequencies below 20 Hz are below the range of normal hearing and are classified as infrasound. Frequencies between 20 Hz and 20,000 Hz (20 KHz) are in the audible range of sound. Ultrasound represents those frequencies greater than 20 KHz.[52,68]

Sound intensity is considered the energy related to sound waves passing through 1 square meter of media in 1 second. Sound intensity is measured in bels, which is a comparison of intensities between media:

$$1 \text{ bel} = \log 10 \text{ intensity}^2 / \text{intensity}^1$$

One decibel is equal to 10 bels, with 120 decibels the most intense sound the ear can tolerate without pain.[52] Intensity of sound is related to acoustic impedance (Z) which is determined by the angular frequency (w) and the maximum displacement amplitude (A) of the sound wave:

$$w = 2 \pi \times f$$

Acoustic impedance is determined by the density (p) of the media and the velocity of the sound waves:

$$Z = p \times v$$

Intensity is then equal to $1/2 \ Z(Aw)^2$, with A the maximum displacement amplitude and w the angular frequency.[69]

As mentioned, acoustic impedance (Z) is deter-

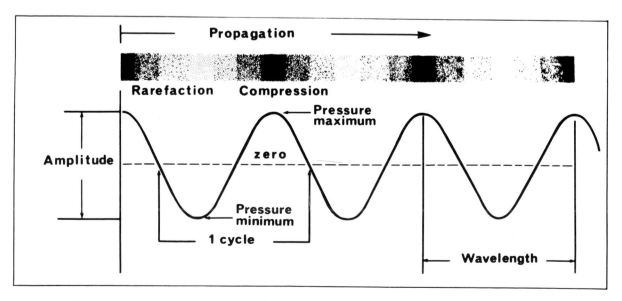

Figure 14. Sound wave represented as a series of compressions and rarefactions. One compression and one rarefaction is considered a cycle, and the distance from corresponding points on consecutive cycles is a wavelength. (Reproduced with permission from Feigenbaum H: *Echocardiography.* Philadelphia: Lea and Febiger; 2, 1994.)

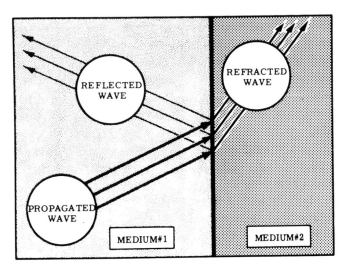

Figure 15. Ultrasound waves are reflected and refracted by the interface of two media with different acoustic impedances. (Reproduced with permission from Feigenbaum H: *Echocardiography.* Philadelphia: Lea and Febiger; 1994.)

mined by the density of the medium and the velocity of the sound through the medium. As the sound strikes an interface between two media with different acoustic impedances, both reflection and refraction of the sound occur (Figure 15). The relative degree of reflection and refraction depend on the difference in acoustic impedances between the two media. A larger mismatch in impedance leads to increased sound wave reflection as opposed to refraction. Therefore, more sound is reflected from a gas-solid interface then from a liquid-solid interface. The incident amplitude (A), the reflected amplitude (R), and the refracted or transmitted amplitude (T) are important considerations in discussing reflection and refraction of sound waves at the interface of materials with different acoustic impedances. The incident amplitude and the reflected amplitude depend on the acoustic impedance of the two different media comprising the reflective interface.[68,70] This is manifest in the equation:

$$R/A = Z_1 - Z_2 / Z_1 + Z_2$$

If the acoustic impedances of the media involved are equal ($Z_1 = Z_2$), then complete transmission occurs without sound reflection. If the two acoustic impedances are different, there is sound wave reflection.[52] The transmitted or refracted amplitude can be determined from the following:

$$T/A = 2(Z_2/Z_1 + Z_2)$$

These equations assume a perpendicular angle of incident impact of the sound at the interface. These equations and theoretic considerations become greatly complicated if the angle of incidence is not 90°. However, the above discussion addresses the basic concepts governing reflected and refracted sound waves from an interface of media with differing acoustic impedances, resulting in the ability to apply the properties of sound waves for biomedical purposes.

The angle of incidence with which sound waves strike an acoustic interface is a major determinant of reflection and refraction from the interface. Similar to the properties of light, the incident angle (O_i) equals the reflected angle between media of differing acoustic impedances. The angle of refraction (O_r) in the target media depends on the incident angle and the velocity difference of the sound waves in the two media[52]:

$$\sin O_i / v_1 = \sin O_r / v_2$$

Impedance matching can be performed to choose materials with similar acoustic impedances for the ready transmission of sound.

Attenuation of sound waves traveling through a given medium is dependent on frictional losses, absorption, and divergence. Energy losses occur due to friction as sound travels through the medium with a resultant decrease in the amplitude of the sound wave. The relationship between the amplitude of the initial sound wave and that of the resultant sound wave after decrease in amplitude is expressed by the equation[70]:

$$A = A_0 E^{-a X}$$

(A is the amplitude of the sound wave at depth X, A_0 is the initial amplitude when X is zero, X is the depth which the sound wave has traversed in the medium, and a is the absorption coefficient for that medium at a given frequency.) Sound wave intensity (I) in a given medium follows a similar pattern[70]:

$$I = I_0 E^{-2 a X}$$

Note that intensity decreases more rapidly with changes in depth than the amplitude of a corresponding sound wave. Sound energy and intensity are also attenuated by absorption. Absorption and scattering of sound waves occur even as sound travels through a homogeneous medium. Sound waves with increased frequencies (ultrasound) have increased absorption and scattering. Sound waves spread radially, or diverge, as distance from the sound source increases. Sound wave intensity is proportional to $1/d^2$ (d = distance from the source).[52] Attenuation of sound in tissue is expressed as half value thickness, which is the tissue thickness required to attenuate the intensity or the amplitude of the sound wave to half its original value.[68] Half value thickness decreases with increasing frequency because of greater tissue absorption at increased frequencies. This limits the maximum frequencies that can be used clinically to insonate deep tissue planes.

Reflection also plays an important role in the clinical utility of sound. Specular reflection occurs from objects which are large, compared to the wavelength of the sound wave. This reflection is dependent on the angle of incidence and the shape and orientation of the interface from which the sound is reflected. Scattered reflection occurs from smaller and irregular interfaces and surfaces. This reflection occurs in multiple directions, with few of the echoes returning to the transducer for interpretation. However, some echoes return to the transducer by chance, as scattered reflection is not dependent on the angle of incidence.[68]

In order for sound waves to reflect from a tissue interface, the total thickness of the object from which the reflection occurs must be at least one-quarter the wavelength of the sound wave.[71] Therefore, increased frequencies allow reflection from small tissue surfaces with greater resolution; however, as mentioned, these higher frequencies are limited in the depth of penetration. A 20 MHz sound wave can distinguish tissue interfaces 1 mm apart. This is the range of frequency commonly employed by catheter-based ultrasound. Acoustic shadowing is also an important consideration. A tissue interface which completely attenuates sound waves due to complete reflection creates an acoustic shadow behind this interface. Objects located in the acoustic shadow are not identified or recorded by the sound waves returning to the transducer.[68]

Interpretation of reflected sound waves is in large measure dependent on the Doppler shift effect. The Doppler shift is based on the increasing pitch of a sound wave if the source is moving toward the listener, and the decreased pitch if the source is moving away from the listener. This occurs due to a change in frequency with motion of the sound wave source or the listener. Sound waves are compressed when the source and listener approach each other with a relative increase in sound wave frequency. This change in frequency is represented by the equation[52]:

$$f \text{ change} = 2F_0 (V/v) \text{ cosine } 0$$

F_0 is the initial frequency of the source of the sound waves, V is the velocity of the moving insonated object, such as RBC, v is the sound wave velocity, and 0 is the angle between the sound wave and the longitudinal axis of the object being insonated, such as an artery. If the frequency of the sound wave at the source and the frequency received by the listener are known, then the object's velocity (RBC in an artery) can be determined.

Instrumentation of Intravascular Ultrasound

The use of ultrasound in medicine is based on the use of piezoelectric crystals. In 1880, Jacques and Pierre Curie discovered the piezoelectric or "pressure electric" effect. Material can change shape under the influence of an electrical field. Certain materials, especially crystals such as quartz, can be cut so that an oscillating electrical voltage will produce similar oscillatory vibrations in the crystal. These oscillatory vibrations generate sound waves of very specific frequencies. These piezoelectric crystals have been applied in biomedical areas as ultrasound transducers, making the biomedical application of ultrasound practical. The piezoelectric crystal must be in contact with the surface to be insonated, as a gaseous interface (air) will result in marked attenuation of the ultrasound. Gels or water are used as an interface between the piezoelectric crystal and the insonated surface to eliminate air interfaces and optimize the acoustic impedance match at the interface.

After the piezoelectric crystal produces an ultrasound wave, echoes are reflected from the tissue interface and returned to the transducer housing the crystal. The crystal vibrates in response to the frequency of the returning sound waves, regenerating an electrical voltage. This voltage signal is amplified and displayed on an oscilloscope. The same piezoelectric crystal functions in the transducer as both the transmitter and the detector. The most intensely detected signals return in a perpendicular direction to the incident beam generated by the transducer. In this capacity, the transducer functions as a receiver of ultrasound approximately 95% of the time with only 5% being used to generate incident ultrasound waves. The transmitter component of the ultrasound system regulates the transducer by controlling the duration and frequency of pulses which are generated. The receiver accepts the electrical impulses generated by the piezoelectric crystal from the returning echoes. The receiver then passes the electrical signal to an amplifier which increases the signal for display on a cathode ray tube or oscilloscope.

Several different display modes are utilized to convert the reflected ultrasound into a signal for interpretation. The A-mode, or amplitude mode, uses the time of receiving the reflected ultrasound as a measure of the proportional depth of structures. Attenuated echoes from deeper tissue structures can be electronically amplified to become more visible for analysis. The ultrasound intensity, as an indication of depth from the transducer to the tissue interface, is reflected as the amplitude of a spike on the oscilloscope. B-mode, or brightness mode, converts the reflected ultrasound signal into two-dimensional images. The signal converts intensity into the brightness of a specific point on the oscilloscope. As the transducer is moved, each reflected wave becomes a dot on the image corresponding to the position of the reflected interface. Storage and analysis of these reflected data allow a composite image in two dimensions. Gray scale images consist of electronically manipulated returning ultrasound to vary the brightness on the oscilloscope, with stronger echoes displayed as brighter than weaker echoes. Color display and digital computer display greatly increase the range of echoes which can be interpreted and reflected on the screen. B-mode images are spatially oriented and can generate cross-sectional or two-dimensional images, as well as real-time images which change with motion of the transducer or motion of the object being insonated. M-mode, or motion mode, utilizes a stationary transducer, much as the A-mode, with the reflected echoes appearing on the screen as brightness dots as in the B-mode. The echo tracing itself moves as a function of time. This is most often utilized in echocardiography.[68]

Several transducer types are utilized for biomedical application. Most ultrasound systems utilize single or phased array transducers. Each single transducer has a natural resonant frequency of vibration and oscillation. Resonant frequency increases as transducer thickness decreases. Smaller transducers produce a ripple wave, whereas larger transducers generate a compact linear wave front composed of multiple smaller waves. Phased array systems use multiple small transducers generating multiple small waves combined to form a linear front. The small transducers can be fired individually or in sequence to optimally manipulate the composite ultrasound beam for focusing and resolution. The sound wave produced by each transducer has a principal longitudinal wave in the direction of propagation. The series of longitudinal composite wave fronts is the ultrasound beam. Shear waves move tangentially outward from the principal wave causing artifactual returning echoes which make interpretation more difficult. These shear waves are produced least with a single large transducer and most with a single small transducer.[72]

An ultrasound beam is composed of a series of longitudinal wave fronts traveling in parallel. At a certain distance, these parallel wave fronts begin to diverge. The area in which they remain parallel is called the near field or Fresenel zone. As the wave fronts begin to diverge, they travel into the far field or Fraunhofer zone.[68] Insonation of objects in the near field is best for ultrasound imaging. Reflection in the near field occurs perpendicular to the composite beam with greater intensity of the returning echoes. The length of the near field is dependent on the ultrasound wavelength (w) and the radius (r) of the transducer:

$$\text{length of the near field} = r^2 / w$$

To increase the near field length, one may increase the ultrasound frequency, thereby decreasing the wavelength, or increase the size of the transducer. In order to focus the ultrasound beam, an acoustic lens is often used, or electronic focusing with phased array systems by electronically-timed firing of the transducers. A three-dimensional image may be generated by a cylindrical single transducer or rectangular phased array composite system. These types of transducers generate both axial and lateral returning echoes with vertical and horizontal axes in the lateral projection. Again, using an acoustic lens or electronic focusing, the lateral dimensions in the vertical and horizontal axis may be manipulated to produce a three-dimensional image.[68,72]

Practical Application of Ultrasound

Intravascular ultrasound (IVUS) is a catheter-based imaging modality that can delineate vessel wall architecture, the location and composition of atherosclerotic disease, and the precise extent of cross-sectional luminal narrowing. IVUS accurately determines arterial wall thickness, lumen diameter, lumen area, and plaque composition.[73–75] As a real-time guidance system, IVUS has the potential to direct endovascular therapeutic devices such as intra-arterial stents, atherectomy catheters, and laser angioplasty, as well as supply important diagnostic information to aid the performance and assessment of complex vascular reconstructions. The evolution of ultrasound technology from rigid, metallic probes to a flexible, catheter-based system has improved the safety and expanded the application of this endovascular imaging modality.

Intravascular ultrasound catheters contain an acoustic subassembly at the end of the catheter that houses the ultrasound transducer in a phased array or single transducer configuration. The transducer crystals serve as both the transmitter and receiver of the ultrasound beam. Single transducer systems employ a flexible torque shaft that couples the transducer to an analog-to-digital converter which is connected to a gray scale video monitor through a computer interface. Positional orientation of the catheter is defined by potentiometers attached to the proximal torque shaft.

The transducers are small piezoelectric crystals (1 mm outside diameter) with a high center frequency (20 to 45 MHz). Specular reflection, producing high resolution images, requires tissue thickness to be one-fourth the wavelength of the ultrasound beam. Therefore, high frequency ultrasound with short wavelengths produces greater image resolution from smaller tissue surfaces. However, this results in decreased tissue penetration as compared to lower frequencies with longer wavelengths. While external beam ultrasound operates

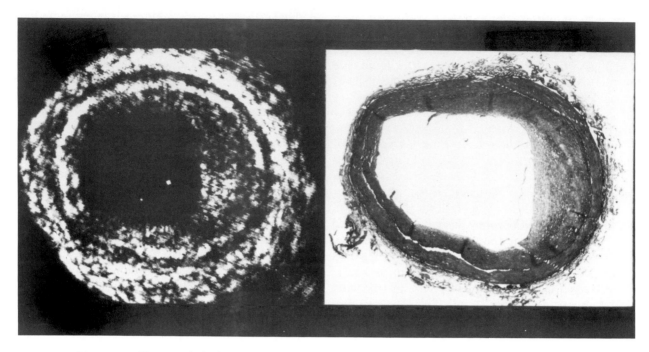

Figure 16. Characteristic intravascular ultrasound image (**left**) with histologic section of corresponding arterial segment (**right**). The cross-sectional ultrasound image demonstrates three distinct, concentric layers around an echo-free lumen: an inner echo-reflective layer (intima), an echo-lucent middle layer (media), and an echo-dense outer layer (adventitia). A fibrotic atherosclerotic plaque is noted along the right side of the arterial wall.

in the 2 to 10 MHz range, catheter-based IVUS operates at 20 to 45 MHz, allowing greater definition of the many small interfaces present in human vascular tissue.

Characteristic IVUS images are two-dimensional, 360°, uniplanar cross-sectional images of the arterial wall demonstrating three distinct concentric layers around a central echo-free lumen, a highly reflective inner layer, an echo-free middle layer, and an echo-dense outer layer (Figure 16). Corresponding to the intima, media, and adventitia of the arterial wall, these layers delineate the acoustic transitions at the lumen-intima, intima-media, and media-adventitia interfaces. The differences in echo-reflectivity from these biologic interfaces are determined by changes in acoustic impedance associated with the composition and structure of the tissue: echo-reflective collagen and elastin, and echo-lucent smooth muscle. The lumen-intima interface results from the bright specular reflection of the internal elastic membrane. The media-adventitia interface is less distinct because the adventitia, while echo dense, is inhomogeneous, resulting in internal scattering of ultrasound with less backscatter received by the transducer.[75]

Standard arteriography is limited in its ability to delineate plaque composition, arterial wall architecture, or thickness. IVUS delivers this information while maintaining blood flow through the artery without requiring blood clearance for quality images. IVUS allows the precise calculation of lumen diameter and area as well as clinically relevant information such as atheroma composition, intimal integrity, and the presence of intimal flaps or residual thrombus.[75,76] IVUS images after stent deployment differentiate between partial and complete stent expansion, allowing the determination of the degree of stent-artery wall contact.[36] While the degree of contact can only be estimated by conventional arteriographic assessment, IVUS images provide precise determination of this important stent deployment parameter. These types of on-line data may prove important for the guidance of therapeutic devices such as intraluminal stents, atherectomy catheters, laser angioplasty, and balloon angioplasty.

Angioscopy

Angioscopy is the process of intraluminal visualization using flexible fiberoptic catheters. Rhea and Walker first used a rigid tube to visualize cardiac structures at operative thoracotomy in 1913. By 1966, the rapid advancement of fiberoptics and the development of flexible fiberoptic bundles allowed the intraluminal visualization of canine peripheral arteries. Since then, angioscopy has rapidly progressed to be used percutaneously and intraoperatively to visualize the lumen of distant portions of the arterial tree. Angioscopes have been used to directly examine the lumen and endothelial surface of bypass grafts at the anastomotic site, and to guide and assess valve lysis and ligation of side branches during in situ bypass. Arterial and venous thromboembolectomy has been evaluated angioscopically as has the endarterectomy site after carotid surgery. The angioscope has also been used to evaluate and guide the repair of arterial intimal injuries.

Principles of Light Transmission

Catheter-based, fiberoptic visualization is based on the physics of light transmission. As previously mentioned, light has the unique ability to behave as both a wave and a particle. Unlike laser angioplasty, angioscopy is primarily dependent on light transmission and properties as a wave. Light waves travel unimpeded at a given speed until they are reflected or refracted upon impact with the surface of a given material. Light waves are bent, or refracted, when the surface is not impacted in a perpendicular direction. The index of refraction is the ratio of the speed of light in vacuum to the speed of light in the given material. Retraction can be utilized to allow precise focusing of light waves. Light is reflected to some degree upon impact with any surface. Two types of reflection occur dependent on the surface of impact. Specular reflection is orderly reflection from smooth surfaces and is dependent on the angle of incidence. Specular reflection is predictable and more useful than diffuse reflection, which occurs upon impact with rough surfaces, scattering light waves in different directions.[52]

Light travels through fiberoptic fibers being constantly reflected from the internal surfaces of the fiber. Light reflection at a critical angle allows loss of light externally through the fiber. Therefore, the angle of reflection must be small enough so that light waves internally reflect and continue to travel down the fiberoptic, much as a stone skims across the surface of a lake. The proper index of refraction allows a larger angle of incidence resulting in the total internal reflection of light waves along the fiberoptic. Cladding is a thin coating applied to the surface of optical fibers and is composed of a material with the desired low index of refraction. This insulates the fiber so that light energy is not dissipated or extracted by another fiber or contaminants such as oil and dust.[52 53]

Certain lens configurations are important to image transmission using optical fibers. A convex input lens captures light from the object to be visualized and focuses the light waves on the fiberoptic bundle composed of coherently arranged optical fibers. The alignment of these fibers is preserved throughout the course of the fiberoptic bundle. The output lens at the opposite end of the fiberoptic contains a magnifying lens with coupling to a video monitor. The image generated by the output lens may be transformed into a digital or electronic signal for recording.

Optical resolution is based on several factors. The number of individual optical fibers in the catheter bundle determines the number of pixels or picture elements. An increased number of pixels improves image resolution. Currently used optical fibers (6 μm in diameter) arranged in a 1 mm in diameter fiberoptic bundle have approximately 160 pixels, whereas the average television screen has 525 pixels. Therefore, currently available fiberoptic catheters have slightly diminished optical resolution as compared to standard television images. Optical resolution may be further reduced as blurring occurs if the optical fibers are in close proximity in the fiberoptic catheter and are impacted by light with varying intensities because of improper spacing between the fibers. Finally, light loss occurs as the light exits from the output lens of the fiberoptic catheter. This light exits tangential to the eyepiece and is lost. Additional light may be lost if two fiberoptic bundles are used in sequence and any bundle mismatching occurs.

The Angioscopic System

Angioscopic systems consist of the angioscope or fiberoptic catheter, an irrigation system, a light source, a video camera, and a video monitor. The angioscope includes a bundle of flexible optical fibers usually composed of glass or silica. Several of the fibers are designated as the viewing fibers and several are designated as the illumination fibers through which the light source operates. There are various bundle arrangements. Often there is the addition of a working channel, which is an open space the length of the angioscope used for irrigation or to place small flexible microinstruments. Many systems incorporate the ability for catheter guidance as an "over-the-wire" system, or for using wires connected to the catheter tip for steerability through wire deflection.

Irrigation systems are crucial to proper use of an angioscope in order to clear the field of blood for proper visualization. Most irrigation systems operate in a coaxial fashion through the working port of the angioscope, or through the introducing catheter with the irrigation solution infused around the angioscope. Parallel systems have also been developed with a separate catheter along the angioscope for irrigation. All irrigation systems operate using high-pressure infusion pumps and the amount of fluid infused should be monitored during clinical use.

Light sources must generate great intensity due to the small diameter of angioscopic catheters. Quartz-halogen and xenon systems are most commonly used to generate 150 and 300 W, respectively. Couplers guarantee precise alignment between the light source and the fiberoptic bundles for proper alignment between the illumination component of the catheter and the light source. Computerized video cameras are utilized at the output viewing lens of the fiberoptic catheter and images are displayed on video monitors.

References

1. Dotter CT, Judkins MP: Transluminal treatment of arteriosclerotic obstruction: description of a new technique and a preliminary report of its application. *Circulation* 30:654–670, 1964.
2. Gruntzig AR, Senning A, Siegenthaler WE: Nonoperative dilatation of coronary artery stenosis: percutaneous transluminal angioplasty. *N Engl J Med* 301:61–68, 1979.
3. Simpson JB, Baim DS, Robert EW, Harrison DC: A new catheter system for coronary angioplasty. *Am J Cardiol* 49:1216–1222, 1982.
4. Bakal CW, Sprayregen S, Scheinbaum K, et al: Percutaneous transluminal angioplasty of the infrapopliteal arteries: results in 53 patients. *AJR* 154:171–174, 1990.
5. Becker G, Katzen B, Dake M: Noncoronary angioplasty. *Radiology* 170:921–940, 1989.
6. Wilson SE, Wolf GL, Cross AP, et al: Percutaneous transluminal angioplasty vs operation for peripheral arteriosclerosis: report of a prospective randomized trial in a selected group of patients. *J Vasc Surg* 9:1–9, 1989.
7. Johnston KW, Rae M, Hogg-Johnston SA, et al: 5-year results of a prospective study of percutaneous transluminal angioplasty. *Ann Surg* 206:403–413, 1987.
8. Murray R, Hewes R, White R, et al: Long-segment femoropopliteal stenoses: is angioplasty a boon or a bust? *Radiology* 162:473–476, 1987.
9. Milford MA, Weaver FA, Lundell CJ, Yellin AE: Femoropopliteal percutaneous transluminal angioplasty for limb salvage. *J Vasc Surg* 8:292–299, 1988.
10. Blair JM, Gewertz BL, Moosa H, et al: Percutaneous transluminal angioplasty vs surgery for limb-threatening ischemia. *J Vasc Surg* 9:698–703, 1989.
11. Castenada-Zuniga WR, Tadavarthy SM: Transluminal angioplasty. In: Castenada-Zuniga WR, Tadavarthy SM (eds). *Interventional Radiology* Baltimore: Williams and Wilkins; 243–275, 1985.
12. Abele JE: Balloon catheters and transluminal dilatation: technical considerations. *AJR* 135:901–906, 1980.
13. Kinney TB, Chin AK, Rurik GW, et al: Transluminal angioplasty: a mechanical pathophysiological correlation of its physical mechanisms. *Radiology* 153:85–89, 1984.
14. Castenada-Zuniga WR, Formanek A, Tadavarthy M, et al: The mechanism of balloon angioplasty. *Radiology* 135:565–571, 1980.
15. Gussenhoven EJ, Zhong Y, Li W, et al: Effect of balloon angioplasty on femoral artery evaluated with intravascular ultrasound imaging. *Circulation* 85:483–493, 1992.
16. Johnson DE, Selmon MR, Simpson JB: Primary stenosis and restenosis excised by peripheral atherectomy: a histologic study. *J Am Coll Card* 11:173A, 1988.
17. Block PC, Myler RK, Stertzer S, et al: Morphology after transluminal angioplasty in human beings. *N Engl J Med* 305:382–385, 1981.
18. Lyon RT, Zarins CK, Lu CT: Vessel, plaque, and lumen morphology after transluminal balloon angioplasty: quantitative study in distended human arteries. *Arteriosclerosis* 7:306–314, 1987.
19. Zarins CK, Lu CT, Gewertz BL, et al: Arterial disruption and remodeling following balloon dilatation. *Surgery* 92:1086–1095, 1982.
20. Steele PM, Cheseboro JH, Stanson AW, et al: Balloon angioplasty: natural history of the pathophysiologic response to injury in a pig model. *Circ Res* 57:105–112, 1985.
21. Zarins CK, Weisenberg E, Kolettis G, et al: Differential enlargement of artery segments in response to enlarging atherosclerotic plaques. *J Vasc Surg* 7:386–394, 1988.
22. Glagov S, Weisenberg E, Zarins CK, et al: Compensatory enlargement of human atherosclerotic coronary arteries. *N Eng J Med* 316:1371–1375, 1987.
23. Fogarty TJ, Chin A, Shoor PS, et al: Adjunctive intraoperative arterial dilation: simplified instrumentation technique. *Arch Surg* 116:1391–1398, 1981.
24. Kinney TB, Fan M, Chin AK, et al: Shear force in angioplasty: its relation to catheter design and function. *AJR* 144:115–122, 1985.
25. Bergovist D, Jonsson K, Weibull H: Complications after percutaneous transluminal angioplasty. *Acta Radiol* 28(1):3–12, 1987.
26. Zollikofer CL, Salomonowitz E, Castaneda-Zuniga WR: The relationship between arterial and balloon rupture in experimental angioplasty. *AJR* 144:777–779, 1985.
27. Ring EJ, Freiman DB, McLean GK, Schwartz W: Percutaneous recanalization of common iliac artery occlusions: an unacceptable complication rate? *AJR* 139:587–589, 1988.
28. Waller BF: "Crackers, breakers, stretchers, drillers, scrapers, shavers, burners, welders and melters-the future treatment of atherosclerotic coronary artery disease? A clinical morphologic assessment. *J Am Coll Card* 13:969–987, 1989.
29. Cheseboro JH, Lam J, Badimon L, Fuster V: Restenosis after arterial angioplasty: a hemorrheologic response. *Am J Card* 60:10–16, 1987.
30. Ip JH, Fuster V, Badimaon L: Syndromes of accelerated atherosclerosis: role of vascular injury and smooth muscle proliferation. *J Am Coll Card* 15:1667–1687, 1990.
31. Fanelli C, Aronoff R: Restenosis following coronary angioplasty. *Am Heart J* 119:357–368, 1990.
32. Neville RF, Sidawy AN, Foegh ML: The molecular biology of vein graft atherosclerosis and myointimal hyperplasia. *Ann Cardiac Surg* 6:95, 103, 1993.
33. Sigwart U, Golf S, Kaufmann U, et al: Analysis of complications associated with coronary stenting. *J Am Coll Card* 11:66A, 1988.
34. Palmaz JC, Sibbett RR, Reuter SR, et al: Expandable intraluminal graft: a preliminary study. *Radiology* 156:73–77, 1985.
35. Roubin GS, Robinson KA, King SB, et al: Acute and late results of intracoronary arterial stenting after coronary angioplasty in dogs. *Circulation* 76:891–897, 1987.
36. Neville RF, Bartorelli AL, Sidawy AN, Leon MB: Vascular stent deployment in vein bypass grafts: observations in an animal model. *Surgery* 116(1):55–61, 1994.
37. Palmaz JC, Richter GM, Noeldge G, et al: Intraluminal stents in atherosclerotic iliac artery stenosis: preliminary report of a multicenter study. *Radiology* 168:727–731, 1988.
38. Bonn J, Gardiner GA, Shapiro MJ, et al: Palmaz vascular stent: initial clinical experience. *Radiology* 174:741–745, 1990.

39. Cragg A, Lund G, Rysavy J: Nonsurgical placement of arterial endoprostheses: a new technique using nitinol wire. *Radiology* 147:261–263, 1983.

40. Van Lack LH: *Elements of Materials Science and Engineering*. 4th ed. Reading, MA: Addison Wesley; 341–349, 1980.

41. Wright KC, Wallace S, Charnsangavi C, et al: Percutaneous endovascular stents: an experimental evaluation. *Radiology* 156:69–72, 1985.

42. Sigwart U: Nonsurgical implantation of a new intravascular stent prosthesis. In: *Interventional Cardiology: Future Directions*. Vogel JH, King SB (eds). St. Louis: CV Mosby; 328–341, 1989.

43. Palmaz JC, Windeler SA, Gariea, et al: Atherosclerotic rabbit aortas: expandable intraluminal grafting. *Radiology* 160:723–726, 1986.

44. Lossef SV, Lutz RJ, Mundorf J, Barth KH: Comparison of mechanical deformation properties of metallic stents with use of stress-strain analysis. *J Vasc and Inter Rad* 5(2):341–349, 1994.

45. Kensey KR, Nash JE, Abrahams C, Zarins CK: Recanalization of obstructed arteries with a flexible, rotating tip catheter. *Radiology* 165:387–389, 1987.

46. Snyder SO, Wheeler JR, Gregory RT, et al: The Kensey catheter: preliminary results with a transluminal tool. *J Vasc Surg* 8:541–543, 1988.

47. Ahn SS, Auth DC, Marcus DR, Moore WS: Removal of focal atheromatous lesions by angioscopically guided high-speed rotary atherectomy: preliminary experimental observations. *J Vasc Surg* 7:292–300, 1988.

48. Prevosti LG, Cook JA, Unger EF, et al: Particulate debris from rotational atherectomy: size, distribution and physiologic effect. *Circulation* 78:II–83, 1988.

49. Simpson JB, Selmon MR, Robertson GC, et al: Transluminal atherectomy for occlusive peripheral vascular disease. *Am J Card* 61:96–101, 1988.

50. Stack RS, Califf RM, Phillips HR, et al: The transluminal extraction catheter. *Am J Card* 62:18–21, 1988.

51. Goldman L, Rockwell RJ: *Lasers in Medicine*. New York: Gordon and Breach; 1971.

52. Cameron JR, Skofronick JG: *Medical Physics*. New York: John Wiley & Sons; 328–332, 1978.

53. O'Shea DC, Callen WR, Rhodes WT: *Introduction to Lasers and Their Applications*. Menlo Park, CA: Addison Welsey; 4–34, 1978.

54. Strikwerda S, Kramer JR, Partovi F, Feld MS: Considerations of dosimetry for laser-tissue ablation. In: *Interventional Cardiology: Future Directions*. Vogel JH, King SB (eds). St. Louis: CV Mosby; 54–56, 1989.

55. Cummins L, Nauenberg M: Effects of laser radiation in biological tissue. *Biophys J* 42:99, 1983.

56. Sliney DH: Laser-tissue interactions. *Clin Chest Med* 6: 203, 1985.

57. Deckelbaum LI, Isner JM, Donaldson RF, et al: Use of pulsed energy delivery to minimize tissue injury resulting from carbon dioxide laser irradiation of cardiovascular tissues. *J Am Coll Card* 7(4):898–908, 1986.

58. Welch AJ, Valvano JW, Pearce JA, et al: Effect of laser radiation on tissue during laser angioplasty. *Lasers Surg Med* 5:251, 1985.

59. Partovi F, Izatt JA, Kittrell CW, et al: Thermal ablation of tissue by laser radiation. In: *Interventional Cardiology: Future Directions*. Vogel JH, King SB (eds). St. Louis: CV Mosby; 67–81, 1989.

60. Sanborn TA, Cumberland DC, Greenfield AJ, et al: Percutaneous laser thermal angioplasty: initial results and 1 year follow-up in 129 femoropopliteal lesions. *Radiology* 168:121–125, 1988.

61. Boulnois JL: Photophysical processes in recent medical laser developments: a review. *Lasers Med Sci* 1:47–66, 1986.

62. Calmettes PP, Berns MW: Laser-induced multiphoton processes in living cells. *Proc Natl Acad Sci* 80: 7197–7199, 1983.

63. Geschwind J, Fabre M, Chaitman BR, et al: Histopathology after Nd: YAG laser percutaneous transluminal angioplasty of peripheral arteries. *J Am Coll Card* 8: 1089–95, 1988.

64. Prince MR, Deutsch TF, Mathews-Roth MM, et al: Preferential light absorption in atheromas in vitro: implications for laser angioplasty. *J Clin Invest* 78:295–302, 1986.

65. Srinivasan R: Ablation of polymers and biological tissue by ultraviolet lasers. *Science* 234:559–565, 1986.

66. Isner JM, Donaldson RF, Deckelbaum LI, et al: The excimer laser: gross, light microscopic, and ultrastructural analysis of potential advantages for use on laser therapy of cardiovascular disease. *J Am Coll Card* 6(5): 1102–1109, 1985.

67. Nelson JS, Wright WH, Eugene J, Berns MW: Introduction to laser physics and laser-tissue interactions. In: *Endovascular Surgery*. Moore WS, Ahn SS (eds). Philadelphia: WB Saunders, Co; 339–357, 1989.

68. Feigenbaum H: *Echocardiography*. 5th ed. Lea and Febeiger: Philadelphia: 1994.

69. Gregg EC, Palogallo GL: Acoustic impedance of tissue. *Invest Radiol* 4:357, 1969.

70. Dunn F, Edmonds P, Fry W: Absorption and dispersion of ultrasound in biological media. *Biological Engineering* In: Schwan HP (ed). New York: McGraw-Hill; 1–10, 1969.

71. Goss SA, Frizzell LA, Dunn F: Ultrasonic absorption and attenuation in mammalian tissues. *Ultra Med Biol* 5:181–186, 1979.

72. Vogel J, Bom N, Ridder J: Transducer design considerations in dynamic focusing. *Ultra Med Biol* 5:187–192, 1979.

73. Bartorelli AL, Potkin BN, Almagor Y, et al: Intravascular ultrasound imaging of atherosclerotic coronary arteries. *J Am Coll Card* 2:54, 1989.

74. Pandian NG, Andreas K, Brockway B, et al: Ultrasound angioscopy: real-time, two-dimensional, intraluminal ultrasound imaging of blood vessels. *Am J Card* 62: 493–494, 1988.

75. Neville RF, Hobson RW, Jamil Z, et al: Intravascular ultrasound: validation studies and preliminary intraoperative observations. *J Vasc Surg* 13(2):274–283, 1991.

76. Neville RF, Yasuhara H, Watanabe B, et al: Endovascular management of arterial intimal defects:, an experimental comparison by arteriography, angioscopy, and intravascular ultrasound. *J Vasc Surg* 13(4):496–502, 1991.

CHAPTER 25

Vascular Grafts

Steven S. Kang, MD; Howard P. Greisler, MD

Forty years of intense research in synthetic and biologic vascular grafts have passed since the initial report by Voorhees[1] of the first successful synthetic prosthesis, made of Vinyon "N" cloth. The early research in vascular graft development was conducted during an era when an artery was considered by most investigators to be a simple conduit through which blood passed. The majority of the research was based philosophically on an attempt to develop an inert replacement for this simple conduit. However, recent knowledge gained in cell and molecular biology has documented that an exceedingly complex set of metabolic activities occurs within and around the artery. We now know that the clinical efficacy of a vascular graft is dependent upon the tissue response that it elicits, particularly in small diameter, low flow arterial segments. This is true not only for synthetic materials, but also for biologic grafts, as well as for other vascular interventions such as endarterectomy, atherectomy, angioplasty, stents, etc. Thus, it is critical that those interested in understanding the currently available vascular prostheses, or in developing new prosthetic devices, fully understand the healing reactions that occur at the blood/material and tissue/material interfaces. With this in mind, we will provide an overview of the basic science of vascular graft healing and then specifically examine the healing, and thus the performance, of certain biologic, hybrid, and synthetic grafts.

Vascular Graft Interfacial Histology

Specific characteristics of prosthetic composition and construction may modulate aspects of the tissue reactions that occur following graft implantation. However, all known prosthetic materials, both synthetic and biologic, elicit a number of common histologic reactions.

Protein Adsorption

Protein adsorption to the prosthetic surface begins instantaneously upon establishment of circulation through the implanted graft. Initial protein adsorption is determined by the relative concentrations of different proteins in blood and their diffusion coefficients. The proteins with the highest concentrations are albumin, immune globulin gamma (IgG), and fibrinogen, and thus these have the greatest initial interaction with the surface.[2] However, the various proteins have different affinities for different surfaces, and an initial low affinity interaction may result in subsequent protein desorption followed by a second round of adsorption of a different protein. This dynamic redistribution of proteins, known as the Vroman Effect,[3] is modulated by surface electrochemical activity and textural characteristics. Roohk,[4] in 1976, showed differential fibrinogen adsorption to a variety of surfaces. Since fibrinogen contains the arg-gly-asp (RGD) sequence to which the platelet membrane glycoprotein GP IIb/IIIa receptor complex binds, the relative concentration of this protein on the surface may modulate the extent of platelet adhesion and subsequent activation and degranulation.

The prosthetic surface also interacts with the plasma proteins involved in the complement pathways. All known biomaterial surfaces are capable of activating both the classic and alternative complement pathways leading to C5a generation. The extent of complement activation varies with biomaterial type. Dacron, for example, activates complement to a greater extent than does expanded polytetrafluoroethylene (ePTFE).[5] This activation of complement has long-term effects. Generated C5a is a potent chemoattractant for monocytes and, thus, may modulate the ensuing cascade of histopathologic events.

From *The Basic Science of Vascular Disease*. Edited by Sidawy AN, Sumpio BE, and DePalma RG. Armonk, NY: Futura Publishing Company, Inc.; © 1997.

Platelet Adhesion

Initiation of platelet adhesion occurs rapidly and is mediated either by receptor recognition of a binding domain on an adsorbed protein, or by surface-induced conformational changes, or by partial denaturation of a platelet membrane glycoprotein. These events themselves are modulated by the initial protein adsorption, as well as by the local hemodynamic characteristics.

The initial platelet adhesion is regulated by interaction between von Willebrand Factor and platelet membrane glycoprotein GPIb. Platelet adhesion and aggregation then proceed rapidly with glycoprotein GPIIb/IIIa receptor complex interactions, with adhesion molecules containing the RGD sequence (Figure 1). Platelet cytoskeletal reorganization, seen as pseudopod formation on scanning electron microscopy, follows adhesion. This "activated" platelet degranulates and releases numerous bioactive substances from both the alpha granules and the dense bodies. This generalized platelet release reaction results in still greater platelet deposition due to an increased local concentration of platelet agonists such as serotonin, epinephrine, and adenosine diphosphate, as well as an increased local concentration of alpha granule adhesive glycoproteins such as fibrinogen, beta-thromboglobulin, thrombospondin, fibronectin, and von Willebrand Factor. Also released are thromboxane A_2, resulting in vasoconstriction and platelet aggregation, as well as neutrophil adhesion, and platelet factor 4, causing increased platelet aggregation and the inhibition of circulating proteases. Platelet-derived growth factor (PDGF) is released from the alpha granules and probably plays a major role in graft healing.

Platelet adhesion to the blood/tissue interface continues chronically at an elevated rate. Ito et al[6] reported an elevated thromboxane B_2 (the stable metabolite of thromboxane A_2) release, as well as depressed systemic platelet counts 1 year after implantation of Dacron grafts into canine models. Using [111]Indium-labeled platelets, investigators have also demonstrated increased platelet adhesion at late times following graft implantation into humans.[7-9] However, it should be understood that the initial differential adhesion of labeled platelets to a surface does not necessarily correlate with long-term patency rates. Attempts to decrease the early deposition of platelets may or may not affect the long-term clinical efficacy of small diameter vascular grafts.

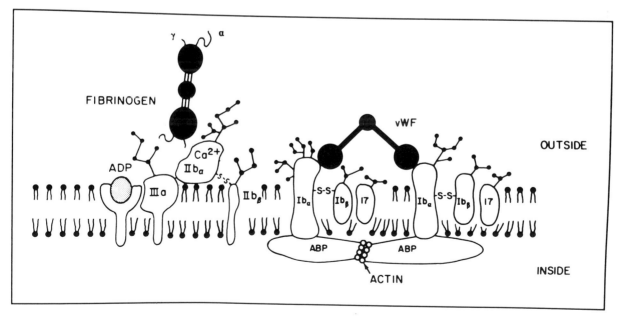

Figure 1. Schematic presentation of the platelet membrane interacting on the outside with vWF and with fibrinogen. vWF, made of two subunits (vWF dimer), is shown to bind through its amino terminal regions to two platelet-membrane GPIb complexes, interfacing on the inside of the platelet with membrane cytoskeleton (actin-binding protein [ABP] and actin). Fibrinogen, shown as a trinodular structure, interacts through the carboxy-terminal segments of the alpha and gamma chains with the platelet membrane GPIIb-IIIa complex, rearranged into a binding mode by the activation of platelets with ADP, shown to occupy its own receptor on the platelet membrane. (Reproduced with permission from Hawiger J: The interaction of platelets and other cellular elements with the vessel wall. In: Loscalzo J, Creager MA, Dzau VJ (eds). *Vascular Medicine*. Boston: Little, Brown and Company; 209, 1992.)

Neutrophil Infiltration

The infiltration of circulating neutrophils into the area of the implanted biomaterial is an invariable hallmark of the acute inflammatory response that biomaterials necessarily elicit. These neutrophils are attracted both to the fibrin coagulum present along the blood-contacting surface and to the endothelial cells present in the peri-anastomotic regions, and potentially throughout the graft, such as when endothelial cell seeding is employed. Compared to other cell types, neutrophils adhere preferentially in vitro to endothelial cells,[10] and this is consistent with the in vivo phenomenon of neutrophil margination within capillaries, primarily in areas of inflammatory processes. Among the most potent neutrophil chemoattractants are C5a, leukotriene B_4 (LTB_4), and platelet-activating factor, all of which enhance endothelial cell-neutrophil adhesion by a direct effect on the neutrophil. Endothelial cells may also increase their affinity for neutrophils, mediated in part by the cytokines interleukin 1 (IL-1) and tumor necrosis factor (TNF).

After their adherence to the endothelial surface, neutrophils, as well as monocytes, penetrate the endothelial layer and enter the subendothelial connective tissues. This process is quite complex. Neutrophil secretion of proteolytic enzymes results in matrix degradation, which allows subsequent neutrophil locomotion through the extracellular matrix. This locomotion occurs along a chemical gradient of neutrophil chemotactic substances.

Neutrophils attach to foreign bodies devoid of overlying endothelium, using a variety of mechanisms. When biomaterials are coated by activated complement factor C3b and IgG, both neutrophils and macrophages may attach through specific adhesion receptors. Following attachment and activation, neutrophils, unable to phagocytize large synthetic biomaterials, release lysosomal enzymes, proteases, and oxygen free radicals, which may inhibit re-endothelialization and tissue incorporation of the implanted biomaterial.

Monocyte Recruitment

Circulating monocytes are attracted to the implanted biomaterial by a variety of chemoattractants and then undergo differentiation progressively into inflammatory monocytes, macrophages, and finally activated macrophages. The presence of a large number of macrophages is a hallmark of chronic inflammation. The degree of macrophage infiltration is dependent in part on such biomaterial characteristics as surface roughness. However, the regulation of monocyte recruitment is highly complex and is affected by products of plasma, of other local cell types, and of the graft material itself.

PDGF is a potent chemotactic agent for monocytes and is produced not only by platelets, but also by endothelial cells, smooth muscle cells, and macrophages themselves. Monocytes preferentially adhere in vitro to areas of injured or regenerating endothelium,[11] and the chronically elevated rate of cell division found in the endothelial cells adjacent to the anastomosis[12] suggests a chronic endothelial cell injury. Macrophages also preferentially adhere to endothelium that has been preactivated by exposure to IL-1, which may be produced by macrophages present in the foreign body reaction. Other potent cell-derived monocyte recruitment factors include LTB_4 and platelet factor 4. Plasma-derived monocyte chemotactic factors include the aforementioned complement-derived peptide C5a, as well as thrombin and the fibrinopeptides. Extracellular matrix products chemotactic for monocytes include fragments of elastin, fibronectin, and collagen, all present within the area of pannus ingrowth.

Macrophages may further modulate healing by releasing neutral proteases, such as collagenase and elastase, and by producing oxygen free radicals. The presence of a nonresorbable biomaterial could result in the chronic release of these proteases by activated macrophages and/or by foreign body giant cells. Macrophage-derived leukotriene B_4 is chemotactic for both neutrophils and monocytes, and increases neutrophil adhesion to endothelial cells, perpetuating the inflammatory response. Macrophage-derived fibronectin may similarly affect cell/matrix interactions as a result of its chemoattractant activity for fibroblasts.

Endothelial Cell and Smooth Muscle Cell Ingrowth

Unlike the case with animal models, humans do not spontaneously endothelialize currently available vascular grafts along their entire lengths. Trans-anastomotic pannus ingrowth results in an endothelialized surface within 1 to 2 centimeters of the anastomoses. This pannus ingrowth is a result of both migration and proliferation of the endothelial cells from the adjacent artery. Smooth muscle cell proliferation occurs predominantly in areas with an apparently confluent endothelial lining, the peri-anastomotic region. This suggests that chronically injured endothelial cells may induce smooth muscle cell proliferation and intimal thickening.

Transinterstitial capillary infiltration resulting in endothelialization of the blood-contacting surface has recently been documented in two animal models with two different experimental vascular prostheses. Clowes[13] demonstrated capillary ingrowth through 60 μ internodal distance ePTFE grafts in baboons yielding complete endothelialization from islands of ingrowing endothelial cells. Such transinterstitial capillary ingrowth did not occur through standard 30 μ internodal distance ePTFE grafts in the same animal model. Unfortunately, no diminution in [111]Indium-labeled platelet deposition was seen following the implantation of such 60 μ internodal distance ePTFE grafts in humans, which is indirect evidence that significant endothelialization did not occur.[14] Studies from our own laboratory have demonstrated capillary ingrowth through the interstices of bioresorbable lactide/glycolide prostheses implanted into both rabbit and canine models, yielding complete endothelialization from islands of ingrowing endothelial cells.[15,16] Our group has also demonstrated a significantly increased rate of endothelialization following the implantation of 60 μ ePTFE grafts pretreated with a fibrin glue suspension containing acidic fibroblast growth factor (FGF-1) into dogs.[17,18] It is thus possible that the combination of appropriate bioactive substances and suitably configured prosthetic material may yield enhanced capillary ingrowth and spontaneous endothelialization in humans.

Mechanisms of Vascular Graft Healing

The histologic reactions that occur following the implantation of vascular grafts reflect the chronic dynamic interfacial phenomena that begin with the initial protein adsorption. All of the various components of these histologic reactions have a role in the healing of vascular grafts.

The Role of Platelets

Following adhesion, activated platelets release the contents of their alpha granules and dense bodies resulting in an increased concentration of bioactive molecules. Locally released growth factors, whether from platelets or from monocytes, endothelial cells, or smooth muscle cells, act predominantly in a paracrine fashion. The mechanisms by which many growth factors exert their myriad effects is only now being elucidated. Some growth factors, for example PDGF, covalently bind to a tyrosine specific protein kinase, triggering a secondary messenger system. In this case, the growth factor does not need to be internalized. However, other growth factors probably do require internalization and have been identified on intracellular organelles including the nucleus.[19] In addition, cell-derived growth factors may theoretically act in an autocrine fashion, either by activating a cytoplasmic or membrane-bound receptor, or via nuclear translocation (often referred to as "intracrine" activity). These distinctions are relevant to the current investigations in several laboratories of affixation of growth factors to biomaterial surfaces.

Growth factors can be divided into competence factors and progression factors. The former stimulate the entrance of the cell into the S phase (DNA synthesis) only in the presence of additional factors generally found in serum. By contrast, progression factors may promote passage into the S phase without the need for additional substances. Insulin-like growth factor and epidermal growth factor are progression factors. PDGF is a competence factor and requires plasma proteins to induce DNA synthesis.

The cationic (pI 9.5–10.4) PDGF has strong mitogenic activity for smooth muscle cells and fibroblasts in culture and binds with high affinity (K_D 10^{-11} M) to these cells, but not to endothelial cells, which lack PDGF receptors. Two PDGF receptors have been identified, alpha and beta. PDGF itself is composed of two polypeptide chains, either A or B, held together by disulfide bonds, and the three isoforms (AA, AB, and BB) are all potent mitogens. Receptor specificity exists with the PDGF alpha receptor recognizing both PDGF A and PDGF B, while the PDGF beta receptor recognizes only PDGF B chain.

PDGF probably exerts its effect only locally due to rapid proteolysis in circulation (half life < 2 minutes).[20] Only brief exposure to PDGF is required to induce cell competence.[21] In addition to its mitogenic and chemoattractant properties, PDGF causes a rapid decline in membrane phosphatidylinositol, resulting in arachidonic acid release and local thromboresistance.[22] Intracellular cyclo-oxygenase also increases following PDGF exposure, resulting in increased prostaglandin production.[23] It is unclear, however, whether PDGF exerts these effects in vivo. Following mechanical de-endothelialization of rat and rabbit arteries, smooth muscle cell proliferation was not inhibited by the use of antiplatelet medications.[24] Similarly, Fingerle[25] found that balloon de-endothelialization of thrombocytopenic rat carotid arteries resulted in less intimal thickening, but no diminution in thymidine labeling. Recent studies[26,27] have demonstrated that balloon de-endothelialization, followed by intravenous PDGF infusion, resulted in an increased smooth muscle cell migration from the media to the intima, but had no effect on smooth muscle cell proliferation. Conversely, antibody blockade of PDGF did not diminish the first wave of smooth muscle cell proliferation (i.e., cell proliferation within the media prior to migration into the intima).

Activated platelets also release epidermal growth factor which is mitogenic for some lines of endothelial cells and vascular smooth muscle cells in culture and is a vasoconstrictor. Platelet-derived transforming growth factor-β (TGF-β) may stimulate fibroblast and smooth muscle cell collagen deposition, as well as modulate the proliferative activity of these cells in an apparent dose-dependent bimodal fashion. However, the role of these growth factors in vascular healing in vivo remains speculative.

The Role of Macrophages

Inflammatory processes likely play a central role in regulating both the early and long-term mesenchymal cell reactions to implanted biomaterials. Monocyte infiltration is stimulated by a host of monocyte recruitment factors as detailed above. The initial differentiation from circulating to inflammatory monocyte may result from the binding of the monocyte to fibronectin by a high affinity magnesium-dependent plasma membrane receptor.[28] Later aspects of the differentiation into the activated macrophage may also involve an interaction with both interferon and bacterial products including lipopolysaccharide.

Macrophages likely play a central role in stimulating vascular healing and remodeling following graft implantation via their production of a variety of bioactive molecules including PDGF, acidic FGF-1 and basic FGF-2, TGF-β, TNF-α, and IL-1 and IL-6. Shimokado[29] first demonstrated macrophage production of PDGF via a neutralizing anti-PDGF antibody technique and a radioreceptor assay. In addition, this group demonstrated PDGF B chain mRNA within macrophages using Northern blot techniques. Baird[30] demonstrated FGF-2 release by activated macrophages using immunoreactivity and biochemical analyses. This basic FGF is a potent mitogen for endothelial cells, as well as smooth muscle cells and fibroblasts.

Studies in our laboratory have demonstrated that experimental bioresorbable vascular prostheses implanted into rabbit and dog models elicit significantly more cellular inner capsules than is seen with similarly implanted Dacron or ePTFE grafts,[31,32] and the rate of tissue ingrowth parallels the rate of macrophage-mediated prosthetic resorption.[33] Autoradiographic analysis of mitotic activity of the myofibroblasts within these inner capsules revealed a high rate of cell division with a rapidly resorbed polymer, polyglactin 910 (PG910), 3 weeks after implantation, and this rate progressively decreased through 12 weeks at which time the prosthetic material and macrophage population were gone. Similarly, in a more slowly resorbed material, polydioxanone, inner capsular myofibroblast mitotic activity remained high for longer periods, until total resorption of the biomaterial and diminution in the macrophage population had occurred.

In order to evaluate the role of macrophage production of growth factors following their activation by biomaterials, New Zealand white rabbit peritoneal macrophages were exposed in vitro to either Dacron or PG910, and the media was analyzed for mitogenic activity using quiescent BALB c/3T3 fibroblasts, rabbit aortic smooth muscle cells, and murine capillary lung LE-II endothelial cells. The macrophages exposed to PG910 released into the media significantly more mitogenic activity for all three cell lines as compared to macrophages exposed either to Dacron or to neither biomaterial.[34] The smooth muscle cell growth assays were then repeated following preincubation of the media with a neutralizing anti-FGF-2 antibody which resulted in significant diminution of this mitogenic activity. Western blotting techniques also demonstrated the media to be immunoreactive to anti-FGF-2 antibody. Similar studies also demonstrated the presence of significantly greater amounts of TGF-β₁ in the media of macrophages exposed to Dacron.[35] One might speculate as to the role of macrophage-derived TGF-β in stimulating peri-anastomotic smooth muscle and fibroblast proliferation, increased collagen deposition, and inhibiting endothelial cell proliferation, all potentially relevant to the pathophysiology of anastomotic pseudointimal hyperplasia.

The Role of Endothelial Cells and Smooth Muscle Cells

Stimuli for endothelial cell migration include soluble attractants (chemotaxis), basement membrane-bound components (haptotaxis), and in the situation of angiogenesis, a three-dimensional extracellular matrix (contact guidance). Mass movement of endothelial cells must involve cell proliferation as well as migration. Quiescent uninjured endothelium has a low rate of cell turnover, 10^{-3} to 10^{-4} replications/day.[36] Following wounding, such as with graft implantation, endarterectomy, or atherectomy, endothelial cell turnover in the adjacent artery increases and may reach a maximum value as high as 30%.[36] However, following the creation of large denuded surfaces in arteries without branch points, re-endothelialization often stops prior to complete coverage, leaving areas persistently devoid of endothelium. Endothelial cell ingrowth over rat aortas following balloon de-endothelialization injury occurs largely from intercostal arteries.[37] However, the same injury in a rat carotid artery, devoid of branches, results in more limited re-endothelialization.[24] In humans, this situation occurs in the case of implanted vascular grafts whose composition or construction is such that transinterstitial capillary ingrowth is limited. Pannus ingrowth stops 1 to 2 cm from either anastomosis with either Dacron or ePTFE.

Endothelial cells growing into a wounded region, or onto a graft surface, undergo phenotypic modulation, and produce a variety of bioactive substances which may modulate graft healing. Among them are growth factors which stimulate smooth muscle cell and fibroblast proliferation and endothelial cell expression of glycosaminoglycans which may inhibit smooth muscle cell proliferation. The release of smooth muscle cell mitogens from endothelial cells was first reported by Gajdusek,[38] and subsequently found by DiCorleto[39] to represent PDGF production. Endothelial cells in culture constitutively secrete PDGF at a rate independent of cell cycling. By contrast, endothelial cell exposure to phorbol esters or endotoxin increases their PDGF production. This suggests the possibility that chronic endothelial cell injury, as one may postulate, occurs in a peri-anastomotic zone, and may increase the rate of synthesis of PDGF by endothelial cells. In addition to PDGF, endothelial cells also produce at least one other significant mitogen for smooth muscle cells and fibroblasts: connective tissue growth factor (CTGF).[40] CTGF may account for up to 70% of the mitogenic activity secreted by endothelial cells.

Endothelial cell biology is highly modulated by local hemodynamic and biomechanical characteristics. Endothelial cells in culture align themselves in the direction of flow. In areas of disturbed flow, such as at flow dividers including bifurcations and anastomoses, endothelial cells frequently take on rounded, less aligned shapes. Laminar flow in vitro induces cell alignment without cell cycling, whereas turbulent flow results in an increased DNA synthesis without cell alignment.[41] Fluctuating shear stress, often the case in the region of an anastomosis, may result in increased endothelial cell pinocytosis.[42] This may lead to an increased transendothelial transport of macromolecules in the area of the anastomosis with subsequent influence on peri-anastomotic pseudointimal hyperplasia. Thus, the highly "abnormal" biomechanics, seen in many currently available vascular graft materials, and the disordered hemodynamics induced by the presence of an anastomosis, may greatly affect endothelial cell biology and influence intimal proliferation and thrombogenicity.

The regulation of smooth muscle cell migration and proliferation across anastomoses likely involves both stimulatory and inhibitory factors produced by platelets, neutrophils, macrophages, endothelial cells, and smooth muscle cells themselves as well as local hemodynamic and biomechanical parameters. Under quiescent conditions, the mitotic index of arterial smooth muscle cells is quite low, with a tritiated thymidine incorporation in culture of only 0.16% over 7 hours.[43] However, following injury, both smooth muscle cell migration and proliferation are increased. Clowes and Schwartz[44] have demonstrated these to be separable phenomena. Following the de-endothelialization of a rat carotid artery, migrating smooth muscle cells not undergoing proliferation comprise the bulk of the response, but a subset of cells do enter the S phase of DNA synthesis. The regulation of this response is still unclear, but it is critical to our ultimate control of

the processes of pseudointimal hyperplasia and restenosis. Following the clinical implantation of vascular grafts, it is specifically the region covered by endothelium (the para-anastomotic region) that maintains chronically elevated rates of smooth muscle cell proliferation. Proliferating smooth muscle cells undergo an ultrastructural phenotypical alteration resulting in a synthetic phenotype, and the cells produce large amounts of collagen and extracellular matrix components. Cyclic deformation of smooth muscle cells in vitro causes them to increase synthesis of collagen, hyaluronate, and chondroitin sulfate.[45]

Vascular smooth muscle cells are known to produce a variety of growth modulating substances including PDGF, FGF, TGF-β, and the cytokines IL-1 and TNF-α. Smooth muscle cells cultured from human carotid artery atherosclerotic plaques have been shown to express high levels of PDGF A chain message.[46] Both Dacron and ePTFE grafts implanted into canine models, and later explanted and placed in culture for 72 hours, have been shown by radioreceptor assay to release PDGF.[47,48] Although these studies did not definitely identify the cells expressing PDGF, it is thought by the authors to be predominantly endothelial cells and quite likely the subendothelial smooth muscle cells as well. As previously mentioned, Clowes and his colleagues at the University of Washington have demonstrated that widely expanded 60 μ internodal distance ePTFE grafts in baboons occur via a transinterstitial capillary ingrowth resulting in early endothelialization (Figure 2).[13] They have further shown that aspects of this healing process may be mediated by the production of PDGF by ingrowing endothelium and smooth muscle cells within the neointima.[49] However, this suggestion of a role in vivo for PDGF still requires additional proof.

The role of FGF-2 in vascular healing in vivo has recently been supported by research from Lindner and Reidy.[50] Rat carotid artery balloon de-endothelialization injury, followed by the intravenous administration of an anti-FGF-2 antibody, resulted in an 80% to 90% reduction in the first wave of smooth muscle cell proliferation, whereas the administration of a recombinant FGF-2 significantly stimulated smooth muscle cell proliferation. Macrophages, endothelial cells, and smooth muscle cells can all synthesize FGF-2, and may do so in response either to surgical injury or the presence of vascular graft materials.

Characteristics of Grafts

Both the chemical composition and the construction of a vascular graft influence its healing and its functional efficacy.

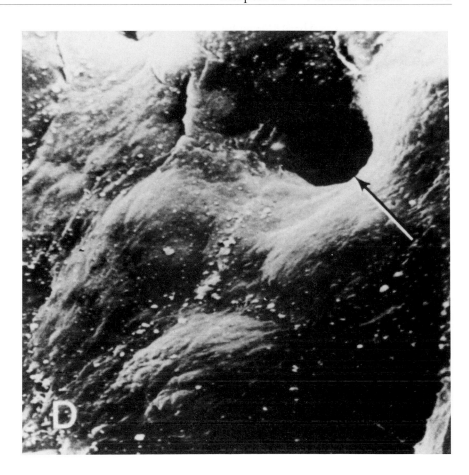

Figure 2. Magnified view of 2-week 60 μ internodal distance ePTFE graft in baboon showing a capillary orifice (**arrow**). (Reproduced with permission from Clowes AW, Kirkman TR, Reidy MA: *Am J Path* 123:220, 1986.)

Composition

As described above, the composition of a prosthetic material significantly impacts upon the relative adsorption of different proteins from the circulation onto the biomaterial surface, and this in turn has ramifications on all later aspects of graft healing. For example, ePTFE may be less prone to complement activation than is Dacron.[10] Dacron may be more potent than resorbable lactide/glycolide copolymers in activating macrophages to release TGF-β,[35] while the latter may more strongly activate macrophages to produce FGF-2.[51] Fluorocarbons, such as are found in ePTFE, may induce less platelet adhesion as compared to polyester materials such as Dacron.

Porosity

Pioneering research concerning graft porosity was done by Wesolowski[52] who favored high porosity to encourage transinterstitial ingrowth and incorporation into the surrounding tissues. Disadvantages of this approach include the need for preclotting, which is not desirable in emergency situations, such as a ruptured aneurysm or in a coagulopathic patient. More extensive calcification may develop within the incorporating

tissues. Any woven or knitted graft with a water porosity greater than 300 mL to 400 mL/cm²/min at 120 mm Hg requires preclotting. Although many preclotting protocols have been espoused, most surgeons simply instill fresh whole blood into the graft lumen and allot adequate time for this blood to coagulate. Intraluminal thrombus is then removed prior to graft implantation. This requires 3 to 10 minutes of additional operating time, unless this process is carried out by a member of the operating team simultaneous with other aspects of the surgical procedure. Woven grafts have a tighter construction than do knitted grafts, with woven Dacron generally displaying water porosities of 100 mL to 500 mL/cm²/min compared to knitted Dacron generally having water porosities around 1200 mL/cm²/min. Although Wesolowski has clearly shown the impact of porosity on graft healing, Sottiurai[53] could demonstrate no significant difference in pseudointima formation in dogs, within the range of porosities in commonly used grafts.

The issue of graft incorporation is of more than theoretical concern. A poorly incorporated graft, as may be seen at the lower limits of water porosity, may result in a thin friable outer capsule poorly adherent to the prosthetic material; this results in chronic movement within the tissues and transudation of serum through the prosthetic wall into the space between the graft and the outer capsule, and yields a chronic perigraft hematoma or seroma, both of which may be prone to infection. Currently used grafts, however, do not promote a transinterstitial ingrowth of fibroblasts, smooth muscle cells, or capillaries, and the inner capsule is composed primarily of a compacted fibrin coagulum.

Textile grafts may incorporate a velour where loops of yarn are extruded perpendicular to the surface. An external velour permits more extensive incorporation of the graft into the surrounding tissue and, thus, diminishes the likelihood of perigraft seroma formation. An inner velour makes preclotting easier and enhances inner capsule attachment to the graft.

Graft porosity may be relevant in the issue of inner capsule healing within ePTFE grafts as well. As discussed above, Clowes[13] reported that ePTFE grafts constructed with a 60 μ or 90 μ internodal distance and implanted into baboons resulted in transinterstitial capillary ingrowth with endothelialization of the lumen, but this was not seen with 30 μ internodal distance ePTFE grafts such as those used clinically. Those grafts constructed with a 90 μ internodal distance, however, yielded focal areas of endothelial cell loss at late time periods, not seen in similar 60 μ internodal distance ePTFE grafts.

Durability

Graft durability has long been considered an essential characteristic for an ideal vascular prosthesis. Although the expected life span of many elderly patients with clinically significant atherosclerotic disease may be short, in many instances, grafts are implanted into patients whose expected life span is quite long. However, hemodynamic stresses on the biomaterial wall as well as modification of the material by exposure to body fluids may result in graft dilatation. Both woven Dacron and ePTFE have withstood the test of time vis-a-vis durability. Knitted Dacron is more prone to graft dilatation and, on average, dilates 10% when initially exposed to arterial pressure and 25% over time.[54] On occasion, much greater degrees of dilatation have been reported.[55] However, the degree of dilatation does not seem to be related to graft complications, and knitted Dacron grafts have an excellent track record in large diameter, high flow implant situations.

By contrast, late biodegradation resulting in aneurysmal dilatation has been a problem encountered by many biologic grafts. The modified bovine arterial graft is no longer in common use largely because of its 3% to 6% incidence of aneurysmal dilatation 2 years following implantation.[56,57] The negatively charged glutaraldehyde tanned bovine graft is a modification of the original bovine heterograft and has been reported to have both excellent long-term patency and a diminished tendency toward biodegradation and aneurysmal dilatation,[58] but sufficient corroborating data have yet to be reported.

The human umbilical vein graft has been in use for infrainguinal reconstructions with excellent patency data reported by Dardik.[59] However, he found by B-mode imaging aneurysms in 36% and dilation in 21% of the grafts at 5 years. Thirty-one human umbilical vein grafts were explanted after 24 hours to 5 years postimplantation and analyzed by Guidoin.[60] The grafts were fragile and easily delaminated. These adverse changes may be a function of the methods for cross-linking collagen in the graft wall, and new methods for processing biologic grafts, currently being studied in a number of laboratories, may resolve these problems. The tendency toward biodegradation may reflect proteolytic digestion, and in vitro exposure of prepared grafts to collagenase may be a useful test of potential aneurysmal degeneration.[61]

Flexibility

Flexibility allows a graft to maintain its contour and to bend without kinking. The presence of an external support surrounding a graft promotes both kink resistance and crush resistance. The former may be desirable when a graft crosses a joint such as the knee, whereas the latter may be important when grafts are placed extra-anatomically, such as in an axillofemoral bypass in which the long stretch of subcutaneously placed graft may theoretically be crushed when a patient lies on his or her side. However, there are very little data to support the need for such an external support in terms of either kink resistance or crush resistance. Gupta[62] implanted both ringed and nonringed ePTFE grafts into 122 patients in the femoral-popliteal position in a randomized prospective study. The study failed to demonstrate any significant difference in patency rates, suggesting no clinically significant advantage in adding this form of kink resistance. Another study[63] evaluated distal perfusion, specifically ankle and calf pressures, 2 to 7 months following implantation of axillofemoral grafts without rings. There was no significant difference with the patients lying either supine or on the side of the graft.

Kink resistance can also be enhanced by crimping a textile prosthesis. The application of the crimp improves the handling characteristics of the graft by providing a more circular end to construct the anastomosis. However, the clinical advantage of the enhanced kink resistance provided by a crimp likely is minimal due to the early development of fibroplasia surrounding most grafts. In addition, the crimp provides a com-

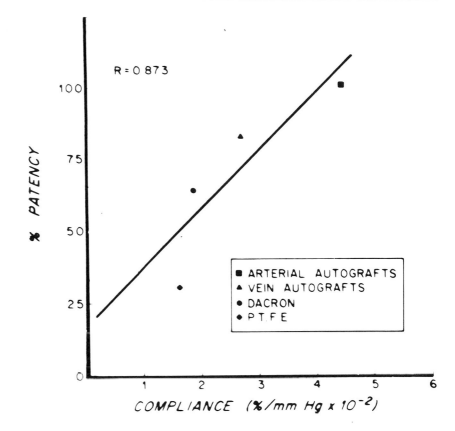

R = 0.873

% PATENCY

COMPLIANCE (%/mm Hg x 10⁻²)

- ARTERIAL AUTOGRAFTS
- ▲ VEIN AUTOGRAFTS
- DACRON
- ◆ P.T.F.E

Figure 3. Linear regression analysis of compliance versus patency. (Reproduced with permission from Abbott WM, Cambria RP: Control of physical characteristics (elasticity and compliance) of vascular grafts. In: Stanley JC (ed). *Biologic and Synthetic Vascular Prostheses.* New York: Grune & Stratton; 189, 1982.)

plex flow surface with concavities that can alter laminar flow and cause thicker inner capsule formation.

Compliance

The issue of graft wall compliance remains controversial. Abbott[64] has demonstrated a direct relationship between compliance and patency among clinically available vascular prostheses (Figure 3). Noncompliant materials do not exhibit elastic recoil during diastole and, thus, diastolic prograde flow is diminished. At the anastomoses between relatively compliant arteries and incompliant grafts, flow disruption may occur. This compliance mismatch has been postulated to play a role in the development of anastomotic pseudointimal hyperplasia. The area of the anastomosis is exceedingly complex and it is difficult to separate one variable from another. The issue becomes yet more complicated when one considers the relatively inelastic nature of the arteries of atherosclerotic patients. Research aimed at the development of elastomeric biomaterials to diminish this compliance mismatch has been disappointing to date due to the fibroplasia developing around biomaterials following their implantation, which results in a progressive diminution in the compliance of the prosthesis/tissue complex over time.

Modes of Graft Failure

As a rule of thumb, immediate failure of vascular grafts usually reflects an error in surgical judgment or technique. Failure occurring in the first month following implantation is most commonly a function of inadequate thromboresistance of the surface for the flow rate imposed by the distal resistance. Graft failure occurring from 6 months to 3 years following implantation is most commonly a function of anastomotic pseudointimal hyperplasia, while later failures reflect progression of distal atherosclerosis. Therefore, the two common intrinsic causes of graft failure are thrombogenicity and intimal hyperplasia.

Thrombogenicity

As outlined above, graft composition and construction parameters modulate the initial differential adsorption of proteins onto the blood-contacting surface, and this in turn significantly impacts on platelet deposition and thrombogenicity. Platelet adhesion is greatly increased by the presence of RGD sequence-containing proteins such as fibrinogen. Pretreating prosthetic materials to alter protein adhesion is a process known as surface passivation. Experimental surface passivation methods have included the use of lipophilic materials to bind albumin,[65] plasma polymerization of fluorocarbons,[66] immobilization of anti-coagulant or fibrinolytic substances,[67,68] and endothe-lial cell seeding.[69] Although in vitro and animal experi-ments often show decreased platelet deposition onto these surfaces, clinical benefit in terms of improved patency has not been demonstrated.

Local hemodynamics also significantly affect platelet deposition. Expanded PTFE grafts exposed to flowing nonanticoagulated blood at shear rates ranging from 106 sec^{-1} to 1690 sec^{-1} demonstrate greater plate-let deposition at higher shear rates.[70] By contrast, persistent exposure to high shear rates results in an apparent increased platelet dislodgement and micro-embolization.

Biomechanics of the prosthetic wall similarly in-fluence platelet deposition. Relatively noncompliant vascular grafts demonstrate a diminution of prograde flow during diastole due to the absence of elastic recoil found in normal arteries. In the extreme case, flow reversal may occur. This results in a decreased shear rate at the interface, but a prolonged particle residence time. Increased particle residence time is also seen with turbulent or complex nonlaminar flow, as in the areas of flow separation at bifurcations. Such flow sep-aration is also encountered in the concavities of crimped grafts and results in greater fibrin and platelet deposition within these recesses.

Surface thrombogenicity of Dacron is often con-sidered to be greater than that of ePTFE. Data from Callow[71] support this belief. [111]Indium-labeled plate-lets were infused 1 hour after implantation of Dacron and ePTFE grafts into baboon arteries and subsequent platelet deposition was measured by gamma imaging. Platelet accumulation on Dacron surfaces began al-most immediately and peaked after 1 to 2 hours, whereas ePTFE grafts accumulated smaller numbers of platelets. However, these data do not necessarily lead one to conclude that ePTFE grafts should perform better in clinical implants. There is inconclusive docu-mentation that early platelet deposition directly corre-lates with long-term graft patency. In addition, quanti-tative analyses of platelet adhesion do not necessarily reflect progressive platelet thrombus thickening. Tran-sient platelet deposition may be followed by platelet desquamation with no significant clinical consequence.

Platelet deposition and activation by prostheses continues chronically. Fifty-cm-long Dacron pros-theses implanted as canine carotid to distal aorta by-pass grafts produced elevated rates of thromboxane B$_2$ concentration along the length of the graft as late as 1 year following implantation.[6] Implanted prostheses also have an effect in inducing a systemic activation of platelets. Shoenfeld[72] demonstrated increased platelet deposition on ePTFE grafts placed distal to Dacron grafts in baboons. This systemic activation of platelets by proximally placed biomaterials suggests the poten-tial for platelet/material interactions to affect both dis-tal atherogenesis and pseudointimal hyperplasia at the distal anastomosis.

Clinical studies by Wakefield[73] have corroborated the animal data on long-term platelet activation by im-planted biomaterials. Dacron and ePTFE aortic inter-position grafts were studied after 1 week, 3 months, and 6 months by a combination of gamma imaging and plasma beta thromboglobulin and platelet factor 4 mea-surements, these being indices of platelet activation and release. No differences in thromboreactivity or platelet release were found between the two materials at 1 week. After 3 months, Dacron and ePTFE yielded 87% and 47% (p < 0.005) respectively greater platelet adhesion than the iliac artery control, and corre-sponded to differences in both beta thromboglobulin and platelet factor 4 concentrations. However, the dif-ferences did not persist at 6 months.

Interpretation of thrombogenicity data collected from either ex vivo models or in vivo animal studies is difficult and cannot necessarily be applied to the clin-ical situation. In most animals, grafts heal with an en-dothelialized surface, which may enhance thrombore-sistance, and this does not occur in currently available vascular grafts implanted into humans. In addition, in most animal models, grafts are implanted into normal arteries perfused with pulsatile flow under high pres-sure. Thus, the hemodynamics of circulation through the graft may not mimic those seen in patients with arterial disease characterized by irregular surfaces and calcified low compliance arteries.

Anastomotic Pseudointimal Hyperplasia

Pannus ingrowth of smooth muscle cells and endo-thelial cells from the adjacent artery is a function of both cell migration and proliferation and extracellular matrix deposition. It can be considered a normal com-ponent of graft healing. Under "normal" circum-stances, however, this progressive accumulation of cells and deposition of matrix stops prior to the devel-opment of luminal stenosis. The mechanism for cessa-tion of cell migration, proliferation, and extracellular matrix production is unexplained. All forms of vascular injury, including graft implantation, angioplasty, end-arterectomy, atherectomy, etc., result in the complex interactions described above, and these interactions may cross the line from "normal healing" to the estab-lishment of intimal hyperplasia. Clinically significant intimal hyperplasia occurs in 30% to 50% of percutane-ous coronary and superficial femoral artery angioplas-ties, 20% of carotid endarterectomies, 10% to 20% of femoral-distal vein grafts, and 10% to 30% of coronary vein grafts.[74] The incidence is higher in prosthetic grafts, due to both the presence of a foreign body, which incites a persistent chronic inflammatory and foreign body response, and the alterations in hemodynamics induced by the prosthesis/tissue complex. Both Dacron and ePTFE are prone to the development of the anastomotic pseudointimal hyperplasia lesion and probably to a similar degree. A quantitative and qualitative analysis of this lesion, following implantation of both Dacron and ePTFE grafts into a canine carotid artery model, demonstrated a significantly greater degree of lesion formation at the distal anastomosis, but without any significant difference between the two biomaterials.[12]

As discussed above, persistent platelet deposition onto and activation by the prosthetic surface may induce a persistently elevated release of platelet products, such as PDGF and TGF-β, which may primarily affect the distal (downstream) anastomosis. Systemic platelet activation, as has been shown by Shoenfeld,[72] may affect pseudointimal hyperplasia at the proximal anastomosis. However, the role of these platelet products in the development of intimal hyperplasia in vivo remains speculative. The use of antiplatelet agents, including aspirin and dipyridamole, has resulted in a slight improvement in patency rates of vein grafts implanted into the coronary circulation.[75,76] By contrast, such benefit has not been conclusively demonstrated for bypasses of peripheral arteries.

In the area adjacent to the anastomosis, endothelial cells and smooth muscle cells undergo cytoskeletal reorganization, enter the cell cycle and divide, and their daughter cells migrate onto the highly abnormal surface of the prosthesis/tissue complex. Endothelial cells in this region have been shown to have a persistently elevated rate of turnover, despite the lack of progressive migration onto the graft surface.[77] Injured endothelium has been shown by DiCorleto[39] to release increased amounts of PDGF in vitro. As discussed above, the implantation of widely expanded 60 μ internodal distance ePTFE grafts into baboons results in endothelialization of the surface.[49] In this neointima, PDGF A chain message and protein are detected primarily in the endothelium and in the immediately subjacent smooth muscle cell population. Although smooth muscle cell proliferation is generally a hallmark of endothelial denuding injury, in the situation of implanted vascular grafts, it is precisely the area covered by endothelium, the area of pannus ingrowth, in which muscle cell proliferation is greatest. This suggests the possible role of endothelial stimulatory products in the pathophysiology of anastomotic pseudointimal hyperplasia.

Compliance mismatch at the anastomosis has been postulated as etiologic in the development of intimal hyperplasia. Such a compliance mismatch may theoretically result in high frequency vibration, endothelial dysfunction, plasma insudation, local platelet deposi-tion, and monocyte recruitment to the subendothelial space of the peri-anastomotic region. This may, in turn, induce the release of growth factors from the various cell types. Intimal hyperplasia may also result from excessive or prolonged extracellular matrix deposition. Smooth muscle cells in the area of pannus ingrowth are ultrastructurally altered to a secretory phenotype and synthesize increased amounts of collagen and extracellular matrix components.[78] Cyclic stretch in vitro also increases smooth muscle cell production of collagen.[79] The possible role of the macrophage in intimal hyperplasia is suggested by studies documenting the ability of biomaterials including Dacron and lactide/glycolide copolymers to activate macrophages to release both FGF-2 and TGF-β.[35,51]

Current Vascular Grafts

The superior patency rates of large diameter aortoiliac reconstructions, as compared to infrainguinal reconstructions, are a function of their decreased distal resistance and increased blood flow. The discrepancy in patency rates among infrainguinal reconstructions, compared to autogenous saphenous vein versus clinically available vascular prostheses, is multifactorial and reflects differences in prosthetic composition, construction, biomechanical characteristics, and thrombogenicity.

Aortic Grafts

Large diameter vascular grafts used to replace the aortoiliac system have high flow rates and patency has been reported to be as high as 95% at 5 years.[80] If one considers only those patients undergoing aortoiliac or aortofemoral bypass with an occluded superficial femoral artery, this increased distal resistance causes a significant diminution in 5-year patency rates. The bulk of these procedures have been performed with a variety of Dacron prostheses, with knitted grafts displaying better handling characteristics and tissue incorporation than woven grafts, but at a cost of requiring preclotting.

Knitted Dacron prostheses coated with albumin, gelatin, or collagen are currently available for clinical use. The protein coating was initially applied to decrease implantation porosity and thus the need for preclotting, yet permit tissue ingrowth and inner and outer capsule incorporation after resorption of the applied substance. However, the applied protein may theoretically yield some degree of surface passivation by altering the relative deposition of proteins from those which promote platelet adhesion (such as the family of RGD-containing proteins) to those with less platelet adhesive properties.

Attempts at surface passivation by applied albumin have dated back to the early 1970s. However, albumin desorption in the face of the fluid shear field following restitution of circulation led to the more recent development of sophisticated methods for optimizing surface affinity for albumin.[65,81–83] Notable among these methods is the alkylation of the surface to enhance albumin deposition which may both decrease platelet adhesion and biomaterial-induced complement activation. The covalent binding of [16]C or [18]C alkyl groups to polymer surfaces increases albumin adsorption through hydrophobic interactions.[65] Other methods for optimizing albumin adsorption to textile surfaces have been studied, including the use of plasma discharge technology,[81,82] and the application of thin polymer films with high albumin affinity to polymer surfaces.[83] These modalities of derivatization of surfaces to optimize albumin adsorption are currently experimental and their clinical efficacy is unknown. Currently available Dacron prostheses to which albumin, gelatin, or collagen have been preadsorbed do not rely on these experimental surface modification techniques.

The rate of resorption of the applied sealant is critically important. While a low implantation porosity is desirable in diminishing transinterstitial hemorrhage, a relatively rapid resorption may be required for tissue incorporation. The rate of albumin resorption is dependent upon the method of cross-linking. When evaluated in canine thoracic aortic implants, grafts treated with albumin cross-linked either by 1.6% glutaraldehyde or by carbodiimide resulted in more extensive penetration of surrounding outer capsule tissues into and through the graft interstices as compared to those treated with 2.5% glutaraldehyde.[84] This is consistent with the slower rate of albumin resorption following exposure to the higher concentration of glutaraldehyde. Cziperle[85] implanted albumin coated Vasculour II Dacron grafts (CR Bard) into canine aortoiliac positions and found no demonstrable differences in healing characteristics in these grafts as compared to otherwise identical, but uncoated preclotted Dacron grafts. Immunoperoxidase staining demonstrated near total resorption of the albumin by 1 month following implantation.

Kottke-Marchant[86] evaluated the surface passivation properties of albumin coated Dacron grafts using an in vitro perfusion system with a battery of tests to measure platelet and neutrophil interactions with the grafts. There was a significant decrease in circulating platelet count in the untreated Dacron group compared to the albumin impregnated group. This correlated with significant increases in indices of platelet activation, including platelet factor 4 and beta thromboglobulin release. Total circulating leukocyte concentration similarly decreased in the control, untreated Dacron group.

Theoretical concern exists as to the potential immunogenicity of glutaraldehyde cross-linked albumin impregnated onto Dacron. Merhi[87] placed disks of albumin coated and uncoated Dacron grafts into mouse peritoneal cavities and serially quantitated T-cell and T-cell subsets (helper, suppressor, and Ia-bearing T-lymphocytes) as a function of time following implantation. No differences were seen in the two graft types and the authors concluded that albumin impregnation elicited no significant immunologic reactions.

A clinical trial evaluated 123 albumin impregnated Dacron aortoiliac grafts implanted into 120 patients.[88] At an average follow-up of 8.2 months, primary patency rate was 93% and secondary patency was 98%. While these data appear promising, this study was not a randomized prospective analysis and extrapolation of these data to the small diameter vascular graft environment is not possible.

Gelatin impregnated grafts recently became available for clinical use. In vitro biodegradation studies on gelatin, or soluble collagen, impregnated Dacron grafts demonstrated complete resorption by hydrolysis after 8 days, or by trypsin after 6.5 days. In vitro thrombogenicity experimentation, demonstrated on scanning electron microscopy, significantly decreased platelet deposition and activation as compared to the similar uncoated Dacron controls.[89] Short-term animal implantation studies revealed substantial gelatin resorption by 5 days, little or no gelatin remaining after 10 days, and no demonstrable difference in the histology of graft healing as compared to similar uncoated Dacron grafts.

As was the case in albumin impregnated grafts, the rate of gelatin resorption is likely important in the modulation of tissue ingrowth. Analysis of minimally cross-linked gelatin impregnated Dacron grafts implanted into dogs, either between the right ventricle and pulmonary artery, or between the aortic arch and the descending aorta, demonstrated at 6 months a well-adherent inner capsule with incorporation of a fibrous outer capsule.[90] By contrast, similar analysis of glutaraldehyde cross-linked insoluble collagen grafts (as opposed to gelatin) showed poor adhesion between pseudointima and prosthetic surface. It is more likely that these differences are an effect of cross-linking technique as opposed to the difference between soluble and insoluble collagen. Gelatin impregnated Dacron grafts cross-linked with isocyanate and implanted into canine femoral arteries revealed a diminished foreign body reaction to the gelatin with histologic evidence suggesting a possible increase in capillary ingrowth into the inner capsules.[91]

In a prospective clinical study,[92] gelatin impregnated aortic grafts (Gelseal, Vascutek) were implanted in 100 consecutive patients and followed for up to 57 months. These grafts were impervious to blood at implantation and demonstrated a 99% cumulative patency rate.

Dacron grafts impregnated with bovine insoluble collagen are also currently clinically available (Hemashield, Meadox Medicals). Early prototypes of the collagen impregnated graft were evaluated for surface thrombogenicity and graft healing.[93] These grafts were treated with bovine skin collagen minimally cross-linked with formaldehyde vapor. When implanted into canine infrarenal aortas, explants after 3, 6, and 9 months showed no difference in histologic analysis as compared to similar untreated Dacron grafts. Guidoin[94] compared the histologic reactions to Dacron grafts pretreated with collagen either weakly cross-linked with formaldehyde vapors or more strongly cross-linked with glutaraldehyde. Although both were impervious to blood at implantation, the former preparation resulted in a more rapid resorption of the collagen. Following explantation from canine thoracic aortas after 4 hours to 6 months, the former group showed a significantly enhanced neointima incorporation histologically. The more strongly cross-linked collagen impregnated grafts retained their collagen after 6 months of implantation.

The concern over immunogenicity of bovine collagen impregnated grafts was evaluated in a prospective randomized clinical trial comparing the collagen impregnated Hemashield graft with a similar untreated control Dacron graft.[95] Humoral and cell-mediated immune responses were both analyzed, the former by enzyme-linked immunosorbent assay (ELISA) techniques and the latter by a lymphocyte proliferation response to the collagen. Results indicated that a small subgroup of patients (5 of 68) seroconverted in response to bovine type I collagen, but no patient displayed evidence of cell-mediated immune reactivity. Thus, bovine collagen impregnated grafts may be weakly activating of a humoral response, but probably with minimal, if any, clinical consequence.

The primary clinical advantage of albumin, gelatin, or collagen impregnated grafts for use in aortoiliac reconstructions lies in the lack of preclotting requirements due to the low implantation porosity. The effects of the applied protein on graft healing clinically may be of lesser concern in this high flow situation. However, the application of these prostheses to small vessel reconstructions has not been thoroughly evaluated clinically and their clinical efficacy for these indications remains unknown.

Besides Dacron, aortic ePTFE grafts are now commercially available. These ePTFE aortic grafts were implanted by Corson[96] into 241 patients with a mean follow-up of 26 months. No graft thromboses or dilatation were reported and the only complication was a single graft infection. Although long-term experience with aortic ePTFE grafts has been small, it is likely that the results in this large diameter, high flow situation will be equivalent to those reported for Dacron. However, a recent prospective randomized trial found greater complications in the ePTFE group resulting in more reoperations and suggested a preferential use of Dacron for aortic bifurcation grafting.[97]

Femoral-Popliteal/Tibial Grafts

In contrast to aortic grafts, the long-term patency rates in small diameter, low flow, high resistance femoral-popliteal and femoral-tibial bypasses are significantly worse. As distal resistance increases, flow rate through the graft decreases and the relative advantage of autogenous saphenous vein becomes more apparent. A multi-institutional randomized prospective study[98] involving 845 infrainguinal bypass operations evaluated the differences in patency rates between autogenous saphenous vein and ePTFE in the femoral-popliteal and in the infrapopliteal positions (Figures 4 and 5). For femoral-popliteal bypasses, life table primary patency rates showed ePTFE grafts to parallel the patency rate of saphenous vein grafts through 2 years, but then decrease significantly at 4 years (47% versus 68% with saphenous vein, p < 0.025). When one compares primary patency at 4 years for infrapopliteal bypass grafts, ePTFE was significantly worse than saphenous vein (12% versus 49%, p < 0.001).

Prendiville[99] reviewed 114 above-knee ePTFE bypasses done in patients with claudication and found a 5-year primary patency rate of 70% in patients with two to three vessel arteriographic runoff, as compared to 30% in patients with zero to one vessel runoff. It may, thus, be logical to preferentially use ePTFE for above-knee femoral-popliteal bypasses for patients either with a relatively short anticipated life span (5 years or less) and/or for patients with two to three vessel runoff by arteriography. By contrast, Whittemore[100] found a 5-year patency rate of above-knee femoral-popliteal ePTFE bypass grafts to not be significantly greater than below-knee reconstructions, and thus recommend a preferential use of autogenous saphenous vein for all infrainguinal reconstructions. Based on a 10-year retrospective study, Quiñones-Baldrich[101] concluded that the role for ePTFE above the knee is important whereas for infrapopliteal reconstructions, it is very limited.

Although numerous older clinical studies have suggested the superiority of ePTFE over Dacron for infrainguinal reconstructions, a provocative retrospective review recently found better results with a knitted nonvelour Dacron graft compared to ePTFE for femoral-popliteal procedures.[102] The 5-year patency for Dacron was 48% versus 27% for ePTFE (p = 0.0096). New prospective comparisons are under way.

The glutaraldehyde-stabilized human umbilical

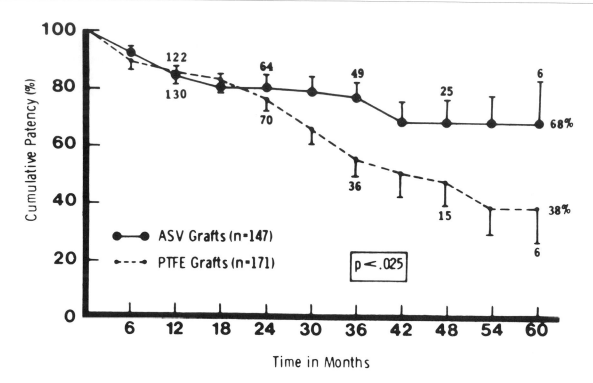

Figure 4. Cumulative life-table primary patency rates for all randomized bypasses performed to popliteal arteries with autologous saphenous vein (ASV) and PTFE grafts. **Number with each point** indicates number of patent grafts observed for that length of time. Standard error of each point is shown. (Reproduced with permission from Reference 98.)

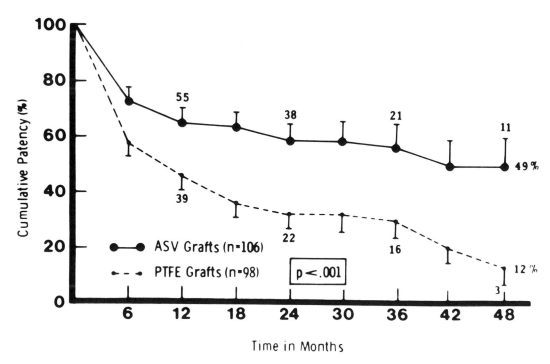

Figure 5. Cumulative life-table primary patency rates for all randomized bypasses performed to infrapopliteal arteries with autologous saphenous vein (ASV) and PTFE grafts. **Number with each point** indicates number of grafts observed to be patent for that length of time. Standard error of each point is shown. (Reproduced with permission from Reference 98.)

vein graft has been used since 1975 for infrainguinal reconstructions. Dardik's review of 907 lower limb bypasses in 799 limbs demonstrated a cumulative patency rate at 61 to 72 months of 53% for femoral-popliteal grafts (n = 90), 26% for femoral-tibial bypass grafts (n = 28), and 28% for femoral-peroneal bypass grafts (n = 12).[59] While these data suggest this biologic graft to be superior to ePTFE, not all reports have corroborated this. In addition, as mentioned earlier, biologic grafts have been problematic in the area of late biodegradation and aneurysmal dilatation. Therefore, Dardik concluded that this graft is an acceptable alternative when autologous saphenous vein is absent or inadequate, and in patients with a relatively limited life expectancy.[59,103]

Another alternative to autogenous saphenous vein is homologous vein. Early vein homografts had poor patency rates largely because of inadequate preservation techniques and immunologic barriers. Ochsner[104] found better graft survival in ABO-matched recipients, suggesting the importance of immunologic barriers in vein transplantation. Tice[105] demonstrated an improvement in patency when saphenous homografts were cryopreserved. Many laboratories have investigated methods of optimizing cryopreservation techniques. With these improved preservation techniques, several small clinical series have been recently reported.

Sellke[106] described six patients who underwent femoral-tibial reconstruction with cryopreserved saphenous vein homografts. Cryopreservation technique was optimal and included 10% dimethyl sulfoxide (DMSO) with freezing at a rate of 1°C/minute to -40°C, followed by a rate of 5°C/minute to -80°C, and then storage in liquid nitrogen at −196°C. Five of the six bypasses were performed on ABO-matched patients with the sixth O-positive patient receiving a vein from a B-positive blood group donor. Only two of the six grafts were patent at 18 to 20 months, with failure modes including distal anastomotic stenoses and both early and late thromboses. Edwards[107] reported on 13 cryopreserved saphenous vein homografts in ABO-compatible patients. At the time of the report, seven of the 13 grafts remained patent at 2 to 10 months following surgery. The other six grafts all occluded within 4 months of implantation. Fugitani[108] used cryopreserved saphenous vein homografts in 10 lower extremity arterial reconstructions. At a mean follow-up of 9.5 months, one patient died at 5 weeks with a patent graft, two grafts occluded with patency restored by thrombectomy in one, and the remaining seven remained patent. Harris[109] implanted 25 grafts to infrapopliteal arteries in 24 patients and reported a secondary patency of only 36% at 1 year. Walker[110] had similar results with 39 grafts, three in below-knee femoral-popliteal, 35 in femoral-tibial, and one in femoral-pedal reconstruction. Primary graft patency was 56% at 3 months

and 28% at 1 year. These experiences indicate that further work is required to improve cryopreservation techniques, maximize endothelial and smooth muscle cell viability, and minimize the antigenicity of the vein without a concomitant alteration in endothelial cell function.

Experimental Biohybrid Prostheses

The application of a biologic substance to a synthetic prosthesis results in a biohybrid. The Dacron grafts coated with albumin, gelatin, or collagen discussed earlier are biohybrids. Endothelial cell seeding of a synthetic graft would make it a biohybrid. Experimental biohybrids include synthetics to which antibiotics, anticoagulant and fibrinolytic agents, or chemotactic and mitogenic substances have been applied.

Antimicrobial Agents

Synthetic materials impregnated with antimicrobial agents to reduce their infectivity have been under investigation since the early 1970s. Although relatively uncommon, graft infections are often catastrophic and often result in loss of limb or life. Graft infections may occur from late bacteremia or from early perioperative bacterial inoculation. Early postoperative graft infections may result either from a break in sterile technique or from colonization from concomitant infections, as may occur in patients with infected ulcers, cellulitis, or lymphangitis. Perioperative inoculation of the graft with the skin organism *Staphylococcus epidermidis* may result in a delayed clinical infection months to years following surgery. This organism secretes a biofilm which adheres to the prosthetic surface yielding a low-grade inflammatory reaction.[111] A prosthesis impregnated with an antibiotic may theoretically be relatively resistant to either early graft infection or delayed infection secondary to perioperative *S. epidermidis* inoculation of the foreign material. Resistance to infection due to late bacteremia, however, would likely not be affected by impregnation with antibiotics. LePort[112] demonstrated that transient bacteremia, induced by injection of *Staphylococcus aureus* intravenously at varying times following the implantation of Dacron grafts into canine thoracoabdominal aortas, resulted in progressively less colonization of the prosthetic material with time, suggesting that the retention by the prosthetic surface of the impregnated antibiotic need not persist indefinitely to have a beneficial effect. Six months after implantation, virtually no colonization was demonstrated. However, it must be recognized that the more extensive tissue ingrowth which occurs in this canine model, as compared to the human, may render it more protective against graft infection due to bacteremia than one would expect in the clinical setting.

Endothelial cell seeding of ePTFE grafts was reported to decrease the propensity for graft infection from circulating bacteria 4 to 8 weeks following implantation.[113] However, a later study[114] failed to show this increased resistance to infection when bacteria were inoculated at 45 weeks after implantation. This apparent paradox probably is explained by the development of the neointima in the unseeded control ePTFE grafts which occurs to a greater extent in dogs than in humans.

Many studies have been reported in which various antibiotics have been combined by a variety of methods to either Dacron or ePTFE surfaces and evaluated either in vitro or in animal models as to their ability to resist colonization or infection. Greco[115,116] has developed methods of applying surfactant treatments to either Dacron or ePTFE surfaces to which anionic antibiotics including penicillins and cephalosporins can be noncovalently bound. Dacron grafts treated with tridodecylmethylammonium chloride and oxacillin were more resistent to infection from injected *S. aureus* compared to untreated Dacron grafts in a canine model. Haverich[117] applied gentamicin to Dacron grafts with fibrin glue and implanted the grafts into the aorta of pigs after direct contamination with *S. aureus*. Upon explantation at 1 week, all of the untreated grafts were infected while half of the treated grafts were sterile. Colburn and Moore[118] bonded rifampin to Dacron grafts using collagen and used them for in situ replacement of previously infected (with *S. aureus*) untreated Dacron grafts in canine aortas. With 2 weeks of supplemental cephalosporin administration, there was a significant reduction in graft colonization compared to control.

These encouraging results may not be directly extrapolated to humans due to species differences in graft healing and resistance to *Staphylococcus* infection. However, Torsello and his colleagues[119] recently reported their early experience with gelatin sealed Dacron grafts soaked in rifampin for in situ replacement of infected grafts in five patients. After a follow-up of at least 6 months, all grafts were patent without signs of reinfection.

Although the above data are difficult to interpret, clinical trials are under way and biohybrids may become useful in the prevention and treatment of graft infections. The catastrophic effect of graft infections is such that even a small benefit from the applied antibiotic would be of great clinical value.

Anticoagulant Substances

Extensive investigation of methods of affixing antithrombotic, anticoagulant, and fibrinolytic agents to biomaterial surfaces has produced an improvement in surface thrombogenicity of grafts implanted into animal models. However, the lack of a suitable animal model for evaluating clinical surface thromboresistance makes extrapolation of data difficult. Heparin immobilization onto polyurethane and polydimethylsiloxane surfaces has been extensively evaluated by Park.[120] Heparin immobilized onto polyurethane using polyethylene oxide spacers yielded an improved patency when implanted into canine aortas with a thinner protein layer containing less fibrinogen at the blood-contacting surface. However, fibrinolytic and coagulation pathways in dogs bear marked differences from those in humans. Forrester[121] developed a method of affixing urokinase to ePTFE surfaces using tridodecylmethylammonium chloride as a surfactant. Dichek[122] has successfully transfected endothelial cells with the gene for tissue plasminogen activator such that the cells overexpressed this fibrinolytic agent. These cells can then be seeded onto prosthetic surfaces. Extensive animal studies of thrombogenicity of surfaces using either of these techniques are still pending.

Growth Factors

Stimulation of transinterstitial capillary ingrowth through a prosthetic wall, resulting in an enhanced spontaneous endothelialization of the blood-contacting surface, may theoretically be achieved through the impregnation of synthetic biomaterials with endothelial mitogens. Our laboratory has developed a method of impregnating porous synthetic materials including 60 μ internodal distance ePTFE grafts with a fibrin glue suspension containing FGF-1 and heparin. This preparation results in a 13% retention of FGF on the surface following 1 week in circulation, diminishing to 4% after 1 month. Implantation of these FGF impregnated ePTFE grafts into canine models results in extensive transinterstitial capillary ingrowth and a significant increase in endothelial cell proliferation, with complete confluence by 28 days (Figure 6).[17] Evaluation of thoracoabdominal aortic implants of these FGF-treated ePTFE grafts shows no persistence in subendothelial cellular proliferation when evaluated by cross-sectional autoradiography at 20 weeks and no intimal hyperplasia. Further investigation needs to be performed prior to clinical application, but the use of endothelial cell mitogens on prosthetic surfaces, either to stimulate spontaneous endothelialization or to speed the development of confluence of seeded endothelial cells, may show promise.

Bioresorbable Synthetic Grafts

One of the basic tenets in the design of novel biomaterials intended for implantation as vascular re-

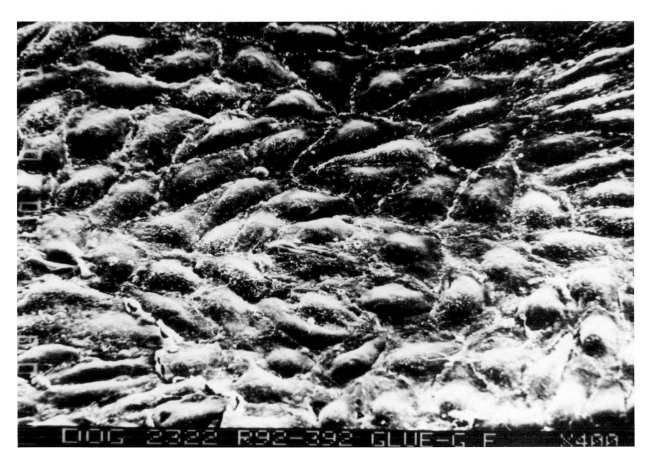

Figure 6. Scanning electron micrograph of the blood-contacting surface of an ePTFE graft impregnated with fibrin glue containing heparin and FGF-1 implanted into a canine aortoiliac system, showing a confluent cobblestone endothelialized surface. (Original magnification × 400.)

placements has been that the material be permanent and minimally modified by the host. However, recent studies have demonstrated that different biomaterials can differentially stimulate or inhibit aspects of vascular healing. Theoretically, a biomaterial might be capable of stimulating rapid and extensive ingrowth of tissue with adequate load bearing to resist dilatation and include cellular components with desirable physiologic characteristics. That material itself might no longer be necessary following tissue ingrowth and, in fact, as a foreign body which might perpetuate an inflammatory process and be amenable to bacterial infection, might be disadvantageous. Recent studies have demonstrated that at least one family of bioresorbable materials, the lactide/glycolide family of copolymers, might be capable of stimulating such ingrowth and thereby have clinical efficacy.

Early studies demonstrated that vascular prostheses woven from yarns of the bioresorbable polyglycolic acid (PGA) yielded a significantly more cellular and thicker tissue ingrowth when implanted into New Zealand white rabbit aortas as compared to nearly

identically woven Dacron prostheses.[10,31,32] In a series of related experiments, a variety of lactide/glycolide copolymers differing in the rate of resorption were evaluated, and the rate of tissue ingrowth was seen to always parallel the kinetics of macrophage-mediated prosthetic resorption.[10,15] Ex vivo mechanical studies of regenerated aortas showed a slight increase in dynamic radial compliance following implantation, and a resistance to fatigue or bursting at up to 6000 mm Hg peak systolic and 2000 mm Hg mean pressures.[123]

If the rate of tissue ingrowth is sufficiently rapid and occurs prior to a significant loss of strength of the resorbable material, the risk of aneurysmal dilatation is minimized. In most reported animal series investigating this family of bioresorbable prostheses, the incidence of aneurysmal dilatation has been less than 5% when followed for 1 year. However, the theoretical concern over aneurysmal degeneration in any biologic prosthesis must be considered. In the case of bioresorbable materials, three possible ways exist to prevent such dilatation. The bioresorbable material may be compounded with a nonresorbable material which

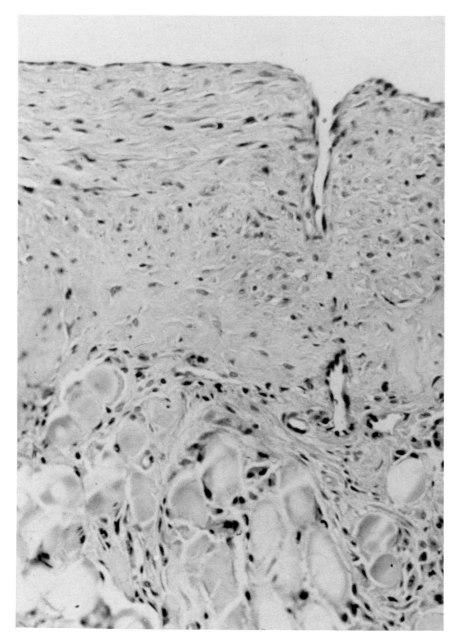

Figure 7. Midportion of PDS specimen at 2 months showing capillary invasion of the inner capsule and communication with the luminal surface. The endothelial-like cellular luminal surface appears to be continuous with the capillary wall. (Hematoxylin and eosin, original magnification × 180.)

would remain behind as a mechanical strut. Secondly, two or more resorbable materials can be combined such that the more rapidly resorbed material elicits the tissue ingrowth, while the more slowly resorbed material remains temporarily in place. Thirdly, growth-promoting substances, such as growth factors and chemoattractants, can be applied to the biomaterial prior to its implantation. All three of these concepts have been described.

Woven and knitted vascular prostheses of com- pound yarns containing both resorbable materials, PGA, polyglactin 910, or polydioxanone (PDS), and a nonresorbable material, Dacron or polypropylene, have been studied.[124-126] The effect of the presence of as little as 20% Dacron in the yarn was to significantly inhibit and delay the ingrowth of tissue into the inner capsule, an effect not seen in the relatively more inert polypropylene. Bicomponent bioresorbable vascular grafts containing 74% PG910 and 26% PDS interposed into New Zealand white rabbit aortas and explanted through 12 months had a 100% patency rate with no aneurysms and only 3% stenoses.[125] The kinetics of inner capsule thickening was midway between that in response to the more rapidly resorbed (PG910) and the more slowly resorbed (PDS) components.[127]

The source of ingrowing tissue following implantation of bioresorbable materials appears to be a transinterstitial ingrowth from the surrounding tissue bed.[15,16] For example, a compound prosthesis in which the resorbable material is placed in the center between two Dacron ends elicits an extensive ingrowth into the center portion, while the inner capsule within the Dacron remains a fibrin coagulum. The ingrowing tissue is very vascular, with areas of capillary communication with the blood-contacting surface (Figure 7).

Confirmatory data have been published by Wildevuur in the Netherlands and Galletti at Brown University. Wildevuur and van der Lei have extensively published on a compound polyurethane/poly-L-lactic acid graft implanted into rat models with promising results.[128,129] Galletti has developed methods of chemically modifying lactide/glycolide copolymers to prolong their functional life and to decrease the rate of strength diminution following implantation.[130]

Tissue ingrowth following implantation of these grafts appears to be mediated by chemoattractant and mitogenic substances, including FGF-2, produced by macrophages interacting with the bioresorbable materials.[51] Macrophages, cultured in vitro in the presence of polyglactin, release into the media more mitogenic activity when tested against quiescent smooth muscle cells, endothelial cells, and fibroblasts, as compared to similar macrophages cultured in the presence of Dacron. The mitogenic activity is blocked by approximately 50% following preincubation of the conditioned media with a neutralizing anti-FGF-2 antibody, and the media shows immunoreactivity with an anti-FGF-2 antibody when evaluated by Western blotting techniques.[35,131]

The potential clinical efficacy of totally or partially bioresorbable prostheses remains an open question. The in vitro and animal studies appear promising, but the slower healing characteristics displayed by humans, as well as differences in macrophage physiology among species, may impact upon the potential efficacy of this family of materials.

References

1. Voorhees AB, Jaretzki A, Blakemore AH: The use of tubes constructed from Vinyon N cloth in bridging arterial defects. *Ann Surg* 135:332, 1952.
2. Andrade JD, Hlady V: Plasma protein adsorption: the big twelve. *Ann NY Acad Sci* 516:158, 1987.
3. Vroman L: Methods of investigating protein interaction on artificial and natural surfaces. *Ann NY Acad Sci* 516: 300, 1987.
4. Roohk HV, Pick J, Hill R, et al: Kinetics of fibrinogen and platelet adherence to biomaterials. *Trans Am Soc Artif Intern Organs* 22:1, 1976.
5. Shepard AD, Gelfand JA, Callow AD, et al: Complement activation by synthetic vascular prostheses. *J Vasc Surg* 1:829, 1984.
6. Ito RK, Rosenblatt MS, Contreras MA, et al: Monitoring platelet interactions with prosthetic graft implants in a canine model. *Trans Am Soc Artif Intern Organs* 36:M175, 1990.
7. McCollum CN, Kester RC, Rajah SM, et al: Arterial graft maturation: the duration of thrombotic activity in Dacron aortobifemoral grafts measured by platelet and fibrinogen kinetics. *Br J Surg* 68:61, 1981.
8. Stratton JR, Thiele BL, Ritchie JL: Platelet deposition on Dacron aortic bifurcation grafts in man: quantitation with indium-111 platelet imaging. *Circulation* 66:1287, 1982.
9. Stratton JR, Thiele BL, Richie JL: Natural history of platelet deposition on Dacron aortic bifurcation grafts in the first year after implantation. *Am J Cardiol* 52: 371, 1983.
10. Lackie JM, DeBono D: Interactions of neutrophil granulocytes and endothelium in vitro. *Microvasc Res* 13: 107, 1977.
11. DiCorleto PE, De La Motte CA: Characterization of the adhesion of the human monocytic cell line U-937 to cultured endothelial cells. *J Clin Invest* 75:1153, 1985.
12. Clowes AW, Gown AM, Hanson SR, et al: Mechanisms of arterial graft failure. *Am J Pathol* 118:43, 1985.
13. Clowes AW, Kirkman TR, Reidy MA: Mechanisms of arterial graft healing. *Am J Path* 123:220, 1986.
14. Kohler T, Stratton JR, Kirkman TR, et al: Conventional versus high-porosity polytetrafluoroethylene grafts: clinical evaluation. *Surgery* 112:901, 1992.
15. Greisler HP, Ellinger J, Schwarcz TH, et al: Arterial regeneration over polydioxanone prostheses in the rabbit. *Arch Surg* 122:715, 1987.
16. Greisler HP, Dennis JW, Endean ED, et al: Derivation of neointima of vascular grafts. *Circulation* 78:16, 1988.
17. Greisler HP, Cziperle DJ, Kim DU, et al: Enhanced endothelialization of expanded polytetrafluoroethylene grafts by fibroblast growth factor type I pretreatment. *Surgery* 112:244, 1992.
18. Gray JL, Zenni GC, Ellinger J, et al: Fibroblast growth factor-1 (FGF-1) immobilization increases endothelialization without intimal hyperplasia in canine 30-cm ePTFE grafts. *Surg Forum* 44:394, 1993.
19. Bradshaw RA, Rubin JS: Polypeptide growth factors: some structural and mechanistic considerations. *J Supramol Struct* 14:183, 1980.
20. Bowen-Pope DF, Malpass TW, Foster DM, et al: Platelet-derived growth factor in vivo: levels, activity, and rate of clearance. *Blood* 64:458, 1984.
21. Heldin C-H, Ronnstrand L: Characterization of the receptor for platelet-derived growth factor on human fibroblasts: demonstration of an intimate relationship with a 185,000-dalton substrate for the platelet-derived growth factor-stimulated kinase. *J Biol Chem* 258: 10054, 1983.
22. Habenicht AJR, Glomset JA, King WC, et al: Early changes in phosphatidylinositol and arachidonic acid metabolism in quiescent Swiss 3T3 cells stimulated to divide by platelet-derived growth factor. *J Biol Chem* 256:12329, 1981.
23. Habenicht AJR, Goerig M, Grulich J, et al: Human platelet-derived growth factor stimulates prostaglandin

synthesis by activation and by rapid de novo synthesis of cyclooxygenase. *J Clin Invest* 75:1381, 1985.

24. Reidy MA, Clowes AW, Schwartz SM: Endothelial regeneration. V. Inhibition of endothelial regrowth in arteries of rat and rabbit. *Lab Invest* 49:569, 1983.

25. Fingerle J, Johnson R, Clowes AW, et al: Role of platelets in smooth muscle cell proliferation and migration after vascular injury in rat carotid artery. *Proc Natl Acad Sci USA* 86:8412, 1989.

26. Ferns GAA, Raines EW, Sprugel KH, et al: Inhibition of neointimal smooth muscle accumulation after angioplasty by an antibody to PDGF. *Science* 253:1129, 1991.

27. Jawien A, Bowen-Pope DF, Lindner V, et al: Platelet-derived growth factor promotes smooth muscle migration and intimal thickening in a rat model of balloon angioplasty. *J Clin Invest* 89:507, 1992.

28. Hosein B, Bianco C: Monocyte receptors for fibronectin characterized by a monoclonal antibody that interferes with receptor activity. *J Exp Med* 112:157, 1985.

29. Shimokado K, Raines EW, Madtes DK, et al: A significant part of macrophage-derived growth factor consists of at least two forms of PDGF. *Cell* 43:277, 1985.

30. Baird A, Mormede P, Bohlen P: Immunoreactive fibroblast growth factor in cells of peritoneal exudate suggests its identity with macrophage-derived growth factor. *Biochem Biophys Res Comm* 126:358, 1985.

31. Greisler HP: Arterial regeneration over absorbable prostheses. *Arch Surg* 117:1425, 1982.

32. Greisler HP, Kim DU, Price JB, et al: Arterial regenerative activity after prosthetic implantation. *Arch Surg* 120:315, 1985.

33. Greisler HP, Petsikas D, Lam TM, et al: Kinetics of cell proliferation as a function of vascular graft material. *J Biomed Mater Res* 27:955, 1993.

34. Greisler HP, Ellinger J, Henderson SC, et al: The effects of an atherogenic diet on macrophage/biomaterial interaction. *J Vasc Surg* 14:10, 1991.

35. Petsikas D, Cziperle DJ, Lam TM, et al: Dacron-induced TGF-β release from macrophages: effects on graft healing. *Surg Forum* 42:326, 1991.

36. Schwartz SM, Benditt EP: Aortic endothelial cell replication. I. Effects of age and hypertension in the rat. *Circ Res* 41:248, 1977.

37. Haudenschild CC, Schwartz SM: Endothelial regeneration. II. Restitution of endothelial continuity. *Lab Invest* 41:407, 1979.

38. Gajdusek CM, DiCorleto PE, Ross R, et al: An endothelial cell derived growth factor. *J Cell Biol* 85:467, 1980.

39. DiCorleto PE, Bowen-Pope DF: Cultured endothelial cells produce a platelet-derived growth factor-like protein. *Proc Natl Acad Sci USA* 80:1919, 1983.

40. Bradham DM, Igarashi A, Potter RL, et al: Connective tissue growth factor: a Cysteine-rich mitogen secreted by human vascular endothelial cells is related to the SRC-induced immediate early gene product CEF-10. *J Cell Biol* 114:1285, 1991.

41. Davies PF, Remuzzi A, Gordon EJ, et al: Turbulent fluid shear stress induces vascular endothelial cell turnover in vitro. *Proc Natl Acad Sci USA* 83:2114, 1986.

42. Davies PF, Dewey CF Jr, Bussolari SR, et al: Influence of hemodynamic forces on vascular endothelial function: in vitro studies of shear stress and pinocytosis in bovine aortic endothelial cells. *J Clin Invest* 73:1121, 1984.

43. Webster WS, Bishop SP, Geer JC: Experimental aortic intimal thickening, part 1 (morphology and source of intimal cells). *Am J Path* 76:245, 1974.

44. Clowes AW, Schwartz SM: Significance of quiescent smooth muscle cell migration in the injured rat carotid artery. *Circ Res* 56:139, 1985.

45. Leung DYM, Glagov S, Mathews MB: Cyclic stretching stimulates synthesis of matrix components by arterial smooth muscle cells in vitro. *Science* 191:475, 1976.

46. Libby P, Warner SJC, Salomon RN, et al: Production of platelet-derived growth factor-like mitogen by smooth muscle cells from human atheroma. *N Engl J Med* 318:1493, 1988.

47. Kaufman BR, DeLuca DJ, Folsom DL, et al: Elevated platelet-derived growth factor production by aortic grafts implanted on a long-term basis in a canine model. *J Vasc Surg* 15:806, 1992.

48. Margolin DA, Kaufman BR, DeLuca DJ, et al: Increased platelet-derived growth factor production and intimal thickening during healing of Dacron grafts in a canine model. *J Vasc Surg* 17:858, 1993.

49. Golden MA, Au YPT, Kirkman TR, et al: Platelet-derived growth factor activity and mRNA expression in healing vascular grafts in baboons. *J Clin Invest* 87:406, 1991.

50. Lindner V, Reidy MA: Proliferation of smooth muscle cells after vascular injury is inhibited by an antibody against basic fibroblast growth factor. *Proc Natl Acad Sci USA* 88:3739, 1991.

51. Greisler HP, Henderson SC, Lam TM: Basic fibroblast growth factor production in vitro by macrophages exposed to Dacron and polyglactin 910. *J Biomater Sci Polym Ed* 4:415, 1993.

52. Wesolowski SA, Fries CC, Karlson KE, et al: Porosity: primary determinant of ultimate fate of synthetic vascular grafts. *Surgery* 50:91, 1961.

53. Sottiurai VS, Lim Sue S, Hsu MK, et al: Pseudointima formation in woven and knitted dacron grafts. *J Cardiovasc Surg* 30:808, 1989.

54. Blumenberg RM, Gelfand ML, Barton EA, et al: Clinical significance of aortic graft dilation. *J Vasc Surg* 14:175, 1991.

55. Nunn DB, Carter MM, Donohue MT, et al: Postoperative dilatation of knitted Dacron aortic bifurcation graft. *J Vasc Surg* 12:291, 1990.

56. Rosenberg N, Thompson JE, Keshishian JM, et al: The modified bovine arterial graft. *Arch Surg* 111:222, 1976.

57. Dale WA, Lewis MB: Further experiences with bovine arterial grafts. *Surgery* 80:711, 1976.

58. Sawyer PN, Stanczewski B, Mistry FD: Current appraisal of negatively charged glutaraldehyde-tanned graft. In: Stanley JC (ed). *Biologic and Synthetic Vascular Prostheses*. New York: Grune & Stratton; 467, 1982.

59. Dardik H, Miller N, Dardik A, et al: A decade of experience with the glutaraldehyde-tanned human umbilical cord vein graft for revascularization of the lower limb. *J Vasc Surg* 7:336, 1988.

60. Guidoin R, Gagnon Y, Roy P-E, et al: Pathologic features of surgically excised human umbilical vein grafts. *J Vasc Surg* 3:146, 1986.

61. Hamilton G, Megerman J, L'Italien GJ, et al: Prediction of aneurysm formation in vascular grafts of biologic origin. *J Vasc Surg* 7:400, 1988.

62. Gupta SK, Veith FJ, Kram HB, et al: Prospective, randomized comparison of ringed and nonringed polytetrafluoroethylene femoropopliteal bypass grafts: a preliminary report. *J Vasc Surg* 13:162, 1991.

63. Jarowenko MV, Buchbinder D, Shah DM: Effect of external pressure on axillofemoral bypass grafts. *Ann Surg* 193:274, 1981.

64. Abbott WM, Cambria RP: Control of physical characteristics (elasticity and compliance) of vascular grafts. In: Stanley JC (ed). *Biologic and Synthetic Vascular Prostheses.* New York: Grune & Stratton; 189, 1982.

65. Munro MS, Eberhart RC, Maki NJ, et al: Thromboresistant alkyl derivatized polyurethanes. *J Am Soc Artif Intern Organs* 6:65, 1983.

66. Yeh Y-S, Iriyama Y, Matsuzawa Y, et al: Blood compatibility of surfaces modified by plasma polymerization. *J Biomed Mater Res* 22:795, 1988.

67. Kim SW, Freijen J: Surface modification of polymers for improved blood compatibility. In: Williams D (ed). *CRC Critical Reviews in Biocompatibility.* Boca Raton, FL: CRC Press; 229, 1985.

68. Josefowicz M, Josefonvicz J: New approaches to anticoagulation: heparin-like biomaterials. *J Am Soc Artif Intern Organs* 8:218, 1985.

69. Herring, MB: Endothelial cell seeding. *J Vasc Surg* 13:731, 1991.

70. Badimon L, Badimon JJ, Turitto VT, et al: Thrombosis: studies under flow conditions. *Ann NY Acad Sci* 516:527, 1987.

71. Callow AD, Connolly R, O'Donnell TF Jr, et al: Platelet-arterial synthetic graft interaction and its modification. *Arch Surg* 117:1447, 1982.

72. Shoenfeld NA, Connolly R, Ramberg K, et al: The systemic activation of platelets by Dacron grafts. *Surg Gynec Obstet* 166:454, 1988.

73. Wakefield TW, Shulkin BL, Fellows EP, et al: Platelet reactivity in human aortic grafts: a prospective, randomized midterm study of platelet adherence and release products in Dacron and polytetrafluoroethylene conduits. *J Vasc Surg* 9:234, 1989.

74. Clowes AW, Reidy MA: Prevention of stenosis after vascular reconstruction: pharmacologic control of intimal hyperplasia—a review. *J Vasc Surg* 13:885, 1991.

75. Chesebro JH, Clements IP, Fuster V, et al: Effect of dipyridamole and aspirin on late vein-graft patency after coronary bypass operations. *N Engl J Med* 310:209, 1984.

76. Goldman S, Copeland J, Moritz T, et al: Saphenous vein graft patency 1 year after coronary artery bypass surgery and effects of antiplatelet therapy. *Circulation* 80:1190, 1989.

77. Campbell GR, Campbell JH: Recent advances in molecular pathology. *Experiment Mol Path* 42:139, 1985.

78. Sumpio BE, Banes AJ, Johnson G: Enhanced collagen production by smooth muscle cells during mechanical stretching. *Arch Surg* 123:1233, 1988.

79. Cantelmo NL, Quist WC, LoGerfo FW: Quantitative analysis of anastomotic intimal hyperplasia in paired Dacron and PTFE grafts. *J Cardiovasc Surg* 30:910, 1989.

80. Moore WS, Cafferata HT, Hall AD, et al: In defense of grafts across the inguinal ligament: an evaluation of early and late results of aorto-femoral bypass grafts. *Ann Surg* 168:207, 1968.

81. Sipehia R, Chawla AS: Albuminated polymer surfaces for biomedical applications. *Biomater Med Dev Artif Organs* 10:229, 1982.

82. Kiaei D, Hoffman AS, Horbett TA: Tight binding of albumin to glow discharge treated polymers. *J Biomater Sci Polym Ed* 4:35, 1992.

83. Ishikawa Y, Sasakawa S, Takase M, et al: Effect of albumin immobilization by plasma polymerization on platelet reactivity. *Thromb Res* 35:193, 1984.

84. Ben-Slimane S, Guidoin R, Merhi Y, et al: In vivo eval-

85. Cziperle DJ, Joyce KA, Tattersall CW, et al: Albumin coated vascular grafts: albumin resorption and tissue reactions. *J Cardiovasc Surg* 33:407, 1992.

86. Kottke-Marchant K, Anderson JM, Umemura Y, et al: Effect of albumin coating on the in vitro blood compatibility of Dacron arterial prostheses. *Biomater* 10:147, 1989.

87. Merhi Y, Roy R, Guidoin R, et al: Cellular reactions to polyester arterial prostheses impregnated with cross-linked albumin: in vivo studies in mice. *Biomater* 10:56, 1989.

88. Banchereau A, Rudondy P, Gournier J-P, et al: The albumin-coated knitted Dacron aortic prosthesis: a clinical study. *Ann Vasc Surg* 4:138, 1990.

89. Drury JK, Ashton TR, Cunningham JD, et al: Experimental and clinical experience with a gelatin impregnated Dacron prosthesis. *Ann Vasc Surg* 1:542, 1987.

90. Jonas RA, Ziemer G, Schoen FJ, et al: A new sealant for knitted Dacron prostheses: minimally cross-linked gelatin. *J Vasc Surg* 7:414, 1988.

91. Bordenave L, Caix J, Basse-Cathalinat B, et al: Experimental evaluation of a gelatin-coated polyester graft used as an arterial substitute. *Biomater* 10:235, 1989.

92. Reid DB, Pollock JG: A prospective study of 100 gelatin-sealed aortic grafts. *Ann Vasc Surg* 5:320, 1991.

93. Quinones-Baldrich WJ, Moore WS, Ziomet S, et al: Development of a ''leak-proof'' knitted Dacron vascular prosthesis. *J Vasc Surg* 3:895, 1986.

94. Guidoin R, Marceau D, Couture J, et al: Collagen coatings as biological sealants for textile arterial prostheses. *Biomater* 10:156, 1989.

95. The Canadian Multicenter Hemashield Study Group: Immunologic response to collagen-impregnated vascular grafts: a randomized prospective study. *J Vasc Surg* 12:741, 1990.

96. Corson JD, Baranlewski IIM, Shah DM, et al: Large diameter expanded polytetrafluoroethylene grafts for infrarenal aortic aneurysm surgery. *J Cardiovasc Surg* 31:702, 1990.

97. Polterauer P, Prager M, Hölzenbein T, et al: Dacron versus polytetrafluoroethylene for Y-aortic bifurcation grafts: a six-year prospective, randomized trial. *Surgery* 111:626, 1992.

98. Veith FJ, Gupta SK, Ascer E, et al: Six-year prospective multicenter randomized comparison of autologous saphenous vein and expanded polytetrafluoroethylene grafts in infrainguinal arterial reconstructions. *J Vasc Surg* 3:104, 1986.

99. Prendiville EJ, Yeager A, O'Donnell TF Jr, et al: Long-term results with the above-knee popliteal expanded polytetrafluoroethylene graft. *J Vasc Surg* 11:517, 1990.

100. Whittemore AD, Kent KC, Donaldson MC, et al: What is the proper role of polytetrafluoroethylene grafts in infrainguinal reconstruction? *J Vasc Surg* 10:299, 1989.

101. Quiñones-Baldrich JW, Prego AA, Ucelay-Gomez R, et al: Long-term results of infrainguinal revascularization with polytetrafluoroethylene: a ten-year experience. *J Vasc Surg* 16:209, 1992.

102. Pevec WC, Darling RC, L'Italien GJ, et al: Femoropopliteal reconstruction with knitted, nonvelour Dacron versus expanded polytetrafluoroethylene. *J Vasc Surg* 16:60, 1992.

103. Miyata T, Tada Y, Takagi A, et al: A clinicopathologic

study of aneurysm formation of glutaraldehyde-tanned human umbilical vein grafts. *J Vasc Surg* 10:605, 1989.

104. Ochsner JL, DeCamp PT, Leonard GL: Experience with fresh venous allografts as an arterial substitute. *Ann Surg* 173:933, 1971.

105. Tice DA, Zerbino V: Clinical experience with preserved human allografts for vascular reconstruction. *Surgery* 72:260, 1972.

106. Sellke FW, Meng RC, Rossi NP: Cryopreserved saphenous vein homografts for femoral-distal vascular reconstruction. *J Cardiovasc Surg* 30:836, 1989.

107. Edwards WH: Alternate sources of autogenous or homologous venous tissue. *Surg Rounds* 8(16):41–54, 1989.

108. Fugitani RM, Bassiouny HS, Gewertz BL, et al: Cryopreserved saphenous vein allogenic homografts: an alternative conduit in lower extremity arterial reconstruction in infected fields. *J Vasc Surg* 15:519, 1992.

109. Harris RW, Schneider PA, Andros G, et al: Allograft vein bypass: is it an acceptable alternative for infrapopliteal revascularization? *J Vasc Surg* 18:553, 1993.

110. Walker PJ, Mitchell RS, McFadden PM, et al: Early experience with cryopreserved saphenous vein allografts as a conduit for complex limb-salvage procedures. *J Vasc Surg* 18:561, 1993.

111. Bergamini TM, Bandyk DF, Govostis D, et al: Infection of vascular prostheses caused by bacterial biofilms. *J Vasc Surg* 7:21, 1988.

112. LePort C, Goeau-Brissonniere O, Lebrault C, et al: Experimental colonization of a polyester vascular graft with Staphylococcus aureus: a quantitative and morphologic study. *J Vasc Surg* 8:1, 1988.

113. Birinyi LK, Douville EC, Lewis AS, et al: Increased resistance to bacteremic graft infection after endothelial cell seeding. *J Vasc Surg* 5:193, 1987.

114. Keller JD, Falk J, Bjornson HS, et al: Bacterial infectibility of chronically implanted endothelial cell-seeded expanded polytetrafluoroethylene vascular grafts. *J Vasc Surg* 7:524, 1988.

115. Greco RS, Harvey RA: The role of antibiotic bonding in the prevention of vascular prosthetic infections. *Ann Surg* 195:168, 1982.

116. Shue WB, Worosilo SC, Donetz AP, et al: Prevention of vascular prosthetic infection with an antibiotic-bonded Dacron graft. *J Vasc Surg* 8:600, 1988.

117. Haverich A, Hirt S, Karck M, et al: Prevention of graft infection by bonding of gentamicin to Dacron prostheses. *J Vasc Surg* 15:187, 1992.

118. Colburn MD, Moore WS, Chvapil M, et al: Use of an antibiotic-bonded graft for in situ reconstruction after prosthetic graft infections. *J Vasc Surg* 16:651, 1992.

119. Torsello G, Sandmann W, Gehrt A, et al: In situ replacement of infected vascular prostheses with rifampin-soaked vascular grafts: early results. *J Vasc Surg* 17:768, 1993.

120. Park KD, Okano T, Jojiri C, et al: Heparin immobilization onto segmented polyurethane urea surface: effect of hydrophilic spacers. *J Biomed Mater Res* 22:977. 1988.

121. Forrester RI, Bernath F: Analysis of urokinase immobilization on the polytetrafluoroethylene vascular prosthesis. *Am J Surg* 156:130, 1988.

122. Newman KD, Nguyen N, Dichek DA: Quantification of vascular graft seeding by use of computer-assisted image analysis and genetically modified endothelial cells. *J Vasc Surg* 14:140, 1991.

123. Greisler HP, Kim DU, Dennis JW, et al: Compound polyglactin 910/polypropylene small vessel prostheses. *J Vasc Surg* 5:572, 1987.

124. Greisler HP, Endean ED, Klosak JJ, et al: Polyglactin 910/polydioxanone bicomponent totally resorbable vascular prostheses. *J Vasc Surg* 7:697, 1988.

125. Greisler HP, Schwarcz TH, Ellinger J, et al: Dacron inhibition of arterial regenerative activities. *J Vasc Surg* 3:747, 1986.

126. Greisler HP, Tattersall CW, Klosak JJ, et al: Partially bioresorbable vascular grafts in dogs. *Surgery* 110:645, 1991.

127. Greisler HP, Petsikas D, Lam TM, et al: Kinetics of cell proliferation as a function of vascular graft material. *J Biomed Mater Res* 27:955, 1993.

128. van der Lei B, Nieuwenhuis P, Molenaar I, et al: Long-term biologic fate of neoarteries regenerated in microporous, compliant, biodegradable, small-caliber vascular grafts in rats. *Surgery* 101:459, 1987.

129. Yue X, van der Lei B, Schakenraad JM, et al: Smooth muscle cell seeding in biodegradable grafts in rats: a new method to enhance the process of arterial wall regeneration. *Surgery* 103:206, 1988.

130. Galletti PM, Aebischer P, Sasken HF, et al: Experience with fully bioresorbable aortic grafts in the dog. *Surgery* 103:231, 1988.

131. Greisler HP, Dennis JW, Endean ED, et al: Macrophage/biomaterial interactions: the stimulation of endothelialization. *J Vasc Surg* 9:588, 1989.

CHAPTER 26

Statistics for the Vascular Surgeon

Sushil K. Gupta, MD; Nissage Cadet, MD
Frank J. Veith, MD

A review of any recent surgical or vascular surgery journal will show that statistical methods are being used more frequently to present research and clinical data. Statistical methods commonly used to analyze data presented in journal articles ought to be understood by both the scientist, investigator, and the practicing clinician. Some of the statistical methods reported in the current journals (Mantel-Haenszel test and Mann-Whitney U test)[1,2] are known to only a handful of vascular surgeons, since several researchers use the help of professional statisticians for analysis of their data. In addition, incorrect analysis methods and reports have been known to escape publishing editors and hence may lead to erroneous conclusions. About 42% to 78% of original publications in critical reviews of selected medical journals have been reported to contain inappropriate data analysis.[3] Therefore, basic knowledge of biostatistics is of the utmost importance for practicing clinicians if they wish to keep abreast with the rapid explosion of new tests, diagnostic tools, and procedures.

The purpose of this chapter is twofold: first, to provide readers with a working knowledge of some of the most frequently used statistical methods, so that they might undertake some of the simpler analyses themselves; and second, to equip them with an adequate understanding of some of the more complex statistical methods, so that they can use this knowledge when reading and analyzing another researcher's data. It would be an impossible in this chapter to present a detailed analysis of all the statistical methods. Hence, areas that may require further study are appropriately referenced to some of the standard textbooks.[4–7]

Fundamental Concepts

Sample Versus Population

Any set of individuals or objects having some common observable characteristics constitutes a population. Any subset of a population is a sample from that population. The target population is the population under investigation. However, the sample taken from the target population may differ from the target population. This is known as error in sampling.

There are many factors that introduce error in sampling, and knowledge of these factors is essential to minimize sample. The sample size, represented by the letter "n," is the total number of observations in the sample. A sample may be any size, ranging from n = 1 to n = entire target population. Within practical limits, the larger the sample size and the closer to the target population size, the chances of error due to sampling are less and the precision is greater in estimating population parameters.

Random Sampling

In a random sample, every observation has an equal and independent chance of being selected. Selection of one member of the population has no effect on the selection of another member. This method of choosing a sample is an important factor in limiting bias. If confounded effects are to be avoided, the control and treatment group must be similar with respect to any characteristics that could affect the result (age, sex, race, general health, etc.) Investigators use var-

From *The Basic Science of Vascular Disease*. Edited by Sidawy AN, Sumpio BE, and DePalma RG. Armonk, NY: Futura Publishing Company, Inc.; © 1997.

ious methods to ensure a nonsubjective random selection, for example, coded cards in a shuffled deck, last digit of a social security number, or a hospital chart number, etc. Perhaps the best method of random sampling is by utilizing preprinted or computer generated random number tables. Sometimes random sampling may not be possible; then it becomes particularly important to check for the imbalance between study groups. If an imbalance does exist, statistical analysis should be performed to determine its potential for affecting the results.

Descriptive Versus Inferential

Statistics can be defined as the scientific process of collecting, organizing, analyzing, and interpreting data. The study of statistics can be divided into two branches: descriptive and inferential statistics. The descriptive branch of statistics deals with those methods that are used to present the data in a more understandable and simpler form, whereas inferential statistics, which is the most important branch, permits us to go beyond the original data and draw inferences and generalizations concerning the population from which the data have been sampled.

Descriptive Statistics

Data Collection

Data scales are various forms in which the data are presented. *Nominal scale* is the simplest form of data collections. Numbers are arbitrarily assigned for classification of characteristics without any regard for ordering or ranking. For example:

1. Diabetic foot ulcers
2. Ischemic foot ulcers

Ordinal scale defines a predetermined order to denote rank. Questionnaires are usually designed on an ordinal scale, and there is usually no consistent difference between ranks. For example, a clinical description of claudication:

0 = asymptomatic

1 = mild claudication

2 = moderate claudication

3 = severe claudication

In contrast to ordinal scales, *interval scales* have units of equal magnitude to describe predetermined order, but with an arbitrary zero point. A *ratio scale* is an interval scale that has a meaningful 0 point on the scale.[8]

Table 1
Example of Frequency Distribution by Age for 479 Patients Who Underwent Femoropopliteal Bypasses

Class Age in Years	Frequency Number of Patients	% Frequency Percent
20–29	4	0.83
30–39	12	2.5
40–49	55	11.48
50–59	89	15.58
60–69	125	26.10
70–79	112	23.38
80–89	70	14.61
90–99	12	2.50

Frequency Distribution

Once data is collected, it often becomes necessary to reveal how the data is distributed, whether it represents either large or small values which are spread evenly, unevenly, or clumped together. This information is given by frequency distributions. Frequency distribution includes measures of central tendency and variability. This distribution is shown by a table consisting of a series of predetermined classes or categories (such as age intervals) and their frequency of occurrence (Table 1). This display provides the most convenient format for summarizing and presenting the data. For example, the ages of 479 patients who underwent femoropopliteal bypasses at an institution can be presented in a frequency distribution table.

There are generally two considerations in constructing frequency distributions: the number of class intervals and the range of values contained in each class. In general, the rules that should be followed in making these decisions are :

1. The number of classes should be between 5 and 20.
2. The minimum and maximum values of the data must be accommodated in the lowest and highest classes.
3. Overlapping of class intervals should be avoided.
4. Whenever possible, class intervals of equal length should be selected.

Histogram

Frequency distributions can be presented in several appealing graphic formats, one of which is a histogram. (Figure 1A) The units of measurements are plotted on the horizontal scale (X axis), and the frequencies in each class are plotted on the vertical scale (Y axis).

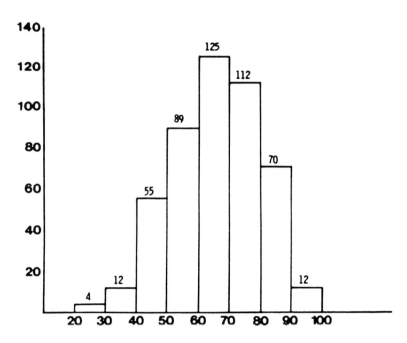

Figure 1A. Frequency distribution histogram for data presented in Table 1.

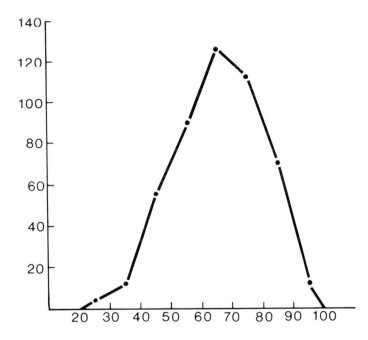

Figure 1B. Frequency polygon for data presented in Table 1.

Each rectangle constructed consists of a base equal to the class interval and height equal to the frequency in that class. (Figure 1B)

Frequency Polygon

Although less commonly used than histogram distribution, frequency polygons provide a useful method for comparing two sets of data on the same graph. To draw a frequency polygon, one simply connects the midpoints of the top of the successive bars of the histograms.

Location: Measures of Central Tendency

Arithmetic Mean

The mean is the most common measure of central tendency (often referred to as average). It is the sum of all observations divided by the number of observations.

$$(\text{mean})\overline{x} = \sum x/n$$

where x is the value of each observation and n is the number of observations. For example, for the group of values, $-2, 0, 2, 4, 6$ (n = 5), the mean is calculated as:

$$\bar{x}(\text{mean}) = -2 + 0 + 2 + 4 + 6 = 10/5 = 2$$

The mean can be calculated for interval and ratio scale data, but generally it is misleading for ordinal scale data. The mean is usually affected by outliers, which are extreme values of a data distribution.

Median

Since the arithmetic mean can be influenced to a great extent by extreme values, median or the "middle most" observation may be a better measure of central tendency. Median is the observation lying exactly in the center or 50th percentile when all values have been rank ordered from the lowest to the highest. One half the observations are above it and one half are below it. It is easy to calculate the median when the number of observations is an odd number. For example, the median of the values 2, 5, 7, 12, and 45 is 7. If the data consists of even numbers of observations, the median is calculated as the average of the two middle items in the data set. Thus, the median of 2, 5, *7, 9*, 12, and 45 is (7 + 9)/2 = 8. Whenever a mean or median is reported, a measure of deviation associated with it should also be reported to enable the reader to visualize the data.

Mode

Mode is defined as the value that occurs most often or with the highest frequency. For example, in the data set: 3, 5, *7, 7*, 13, 17, 21, the mode is *7* since this value occurs twice.

Location: Quartiles, Deciles, and Percentiles

The quartiles of a distribution are defined as values that divide data into four equal parts. Thus, the first quartile, Q_1, is a value below which lie one quarter of the data, while three quarters of the data fall below Q_3, the third quartile. Q_2, the second quartile, is the same as the median—a value below which one half the data fall.

Deciles are values that divide the distribution in 10 equal parts. For example, D_3, the third decile, is a value under which lie 30% of the data.

Percentiles are values that divide the distribution in 100 equal parts. For example, the 15th percentile, P_{15}, is the value that exceeds the lowest 15% of the data, and P_{85} is the 85th percentile or the value that is exceeded by only the highest 15% of the data.

Measure of Variability or Spread

Measures of variation provide information concerning the extent to which the data is dispersed or spread out. It is a measure that will be large if the observations are farther apart from the mean and small if the observations are closely grouped around the mean.

Minimum and Maximum and Range

Minimum and maximum denote the smallest and the largest values in a data set, and the range is defined as the interval between the highest and the lowest values within a data group (maximum minus the minimum.) Some authors use the 25th to 75th interquartile range instead of range. However, range many not provide sufficient information about dispersion of the data, and it usually increases as more observations are added. It also may be greatly influenced by outliers.

Mean Deviation

The range has limitations because it employs the two extreme observations and neglects all the information regarding variations of the remaining observations. The mean deviation is the sum and average of the deviation of observations from the mean (x − x.) At first glance, this may seem to be good measures for the purpose of variability. As shown in Table 2, column C, however, these are always zero; hence, the mean deviation cannot be a useful statistical measure.

Variance

If the deviation of observations from the mean is squared first, as shown in Table 2, column D, and then the mean is calculated, the result is a significant statistical measure known as variance or s^2. (other symbols

Table 2
Example of Calculation of Variance and Standard Deviation

(A) Values	(B) Mean	(C) Deviation	(D) Deviation Square
−2	2	−4	16
0	2	−2	4
2	2	0	0
4	2	2	16
6	2	4	40

Sum = 0
Mean = 0

Table 3
Statistical Symbols

Symbol	Mean
n =	Number of observations
x =	Observation
x̄ =	Mean of sample
μ =	Mean of population
s^2 =	Variance of sample
δ^2 =	Variance of population
s = SD	Standard deviation of sample
δ =	Standard deviation of population
SEM = SEx	Standard error of mean
z =	Critical ratio
r =	Pearson product moment correlation
t =	Critical statistic for *t*-test
df =	Degrees of freedom

that are frequently used in statistical textbooks are shown in Table 3.) Thus, the definition of variance is the average of the sum of squares of deviation from the mean.

$$s^2 = \sum (x - \overline{x})^2/(n - 1)$$

and using data from Table 2,

$$s^2 = (16 \mid 4 \mid 0 \mid 4 \mid 16)/(5 \quad 1) = 40/4 = 10$$

Note that in calculating the variance, the denominator used is (n − 1) and not n. This change is made to avoid the problem of underestimation of variance in a smaller sample size since for most samples, the variance of a sample (s^2) will be less than the variance of the target population (δ^2) (3).

Standard Deviation

As we noted in calculating the variance, the deviations from the mean were squared. However, squared units are not meaningful. Therefore, if we take the square root of the average value variance (s^2), the result is known as standard deviation(s) (Table 2). Thus,

$$s = \sqrt{s^2} = \sqrt{\sigma} (x - \overline{x})^2/(n - 1)$$

again, using Table 2 data,

$$s(SD) = s^2 = 10 = 3.16$$

In practice, to simplify calculations, this formula can be written as:

$$s = \sqrt{\frac{\text{sum of squares} - \text{square of sum}/n}{n - 1}}$$

$$s = \sqrt{\frac{\sum x^2 - (\sum x)^{1/2}}{n - 1}}$$

Standard deviation is the most frequently used measure of variation. It provides an estimate of the degree of variability of individual data points about the sample mean. As such, it is considered to be a descriptive statistic. It is used most appropriately when the data being analyzed is normally distributed, and is applicable to interval or ratio scale data.

Distribution Curves

Normal Distribution/Bimodal Distribution

Once data is collected and organized into a distribution table, it can be illustrated by means of a histogram or bar graph. Histograms are approximate pictures of the mathematical way of describing the distribution of collected data. The frequency distribution table can be converted by creation of a curve to a smooth curve graphic format, which is a more accurate representation of the distribution. This smooth curve is called the distribution or probability curve. The distribution curve can have different shapes. When the shape is symmetrical, bell shaped, it is said to define a "normal distribution" or normal probability curve.

A normal distribution curve (symmetrical, bell shaped) is illustrated in Figure 2. As shown, (mean of population) μ + δ (standard deviation) includes approximately 68% of all observations, μ + 2δ includes 95% of all observations, and μ ± 3δ includes almost all of the distribution (99.7%). Bimodal distributions have two peaks or means with high frequency level.

Kurtosis

Kurtosis is a measure of relative peakedness or flatness of the curve. Normal distribution has a kurtosis of zero. A positive value means that the curve is more peaked (narrow), and a negative value means that it is flatter (Figure 3).[5]

Outlier

When a value is clearly dissimilar to the other observation (whether it is too high or too low, too big or too small) it is termed an outlier. When outliers are included in the calculation of descriptive statistics, the

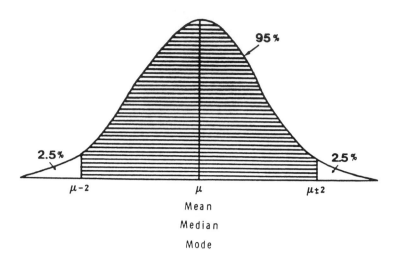

Figure 2. Bell-shaped curve of normal distribution showing that 95% of the distribution lies between μ (mean) $\pm$ 2δ (standard deviation).

mean and standard deviation do not provide an accurate description of the set of data.

Skewness

In a biologic distribution of data, it is almost impossible to find a symmetrical, bell-shaped curve. Furthermore, the mean and the standard deviation may not always provide sufficient information about the population. Two distributions could have identical means and standard deviations,[7] but differ significantly in appearance. Skewness is a measure of deviation from the symmetry. It is zero when the distribution is a complete, symmetrical, bell-shaped curve. A positive value denotes a curve skewed to the right with most observations clustered to the left of mean and the extreme values falling to the right (Figure 3). A right skewed curve is frequently encountered in laboratory data since there are no negative values.[5]

When the data is highly skewed, or when extreme outliers are represented, the median is a better measure of central tendency. Variability is best described by range and percentiles.

Inferential Statistics

Inferential statistics use methods to estimate unknown population parameters from sample observations that permit generalizations about the population from which the sample is drawn.

Standard Error of Mean

When dealing with large populations, it may not be possible to calculate population mean (μ) and standard deviation of the population (δ). Sample mean and standard deviation (x and s) may be used to estimate μ and δ. If several different random samples are drawn from the population, different $\bar{x}$ and s (random variables) can be obtained for each of the samples. This variation in the means of sample can be estimated by calculating the standard deviation of the sample means. This standard deviation of sample means is known as standard error of mean (SE) and is calculated by SEM or Se$\bar{x}$ = SD/n, where SD is the standard deviation of individual values in the sample and n is the count of values in the sample. The lower the value of standard error of mean, the smaller the chance of sampling errors. SE$\bar{x}$ decreases with larger sample sizes. With samples of sufficient size, 95% of all sample means are within two standard errors of the population mean. Therefore, 95% confidence interval (CI) can be calculated as 95% CI = $\bar{x}$ $\pm$ 2 $\times$ SEM.

Confidence Intervals

Confidence Interval (CI) is a range of values which is likely to be representative of the population parameters from which the sample came. It would be impossible to study all members of a population. Therefore, a representative sample of the population is studied. The confidence interval is the calculated interval of all plausible values from the mean and the SEM of the population which will give, for example, 95% confidence that the interval is truly representative of the population under study. It is notable that the CI is an inferential statistic, which only conveys the effects of sampling variations and is not appropriate for descriptive data.

Significance Tests

A test of significance is a statistical procedure by which one determines the degree to which collected data is consistent with a specific hypothesis under investigation. The purpose of a significance test is to determine that the observed results could not be ex-

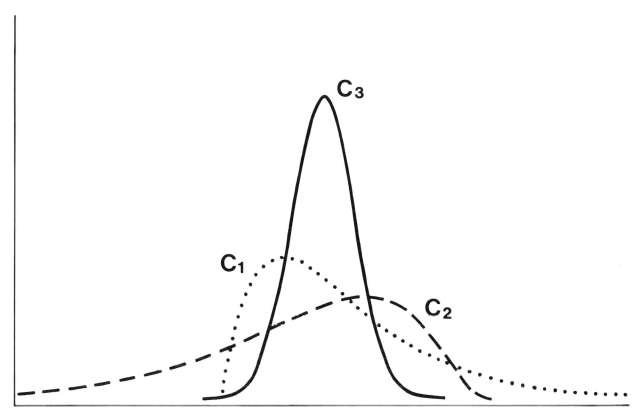

Figure 3. Probability curves illustrating right C_1 and left C_2 skewed distributions, and a positive kurtotic distribution C_3.

plained by random variation or chance alone. The term "statistically significant," is understood to mean that a test of significance or a statistical procedure has been applied to the collected data. Statistical significance does not necessarily imply clinical significance.

Hypothesis Testing

Statistical inference involves testing hypothesis about population parameters. A statistical hypothesis is an assumption made about a parameter of one or more populations. Underlying all statistical tests is a "null hypothesis." This hypothesis states that there is no difference in the target and sample populations, or two sample populations or two variables. In other words, the null hypothesis is consistent with the idea that the observed differences are simply a result of random variation in the data. The null hypothesis can be accepted or rejected. To decide whether it is accepted or rejected, a test statistic is computed and compared with a set of critical values in a statistical table. When the test statistics exceed the critical value, the null hypothesis is rejected and differences in the two variables can be declared statistically significant. If the null hypothesis is rejected, then the alternative hypothesis is accepted.

Error of Hypothesis Testing

The significance level—the risk of rejecting the null hypothesis when it is really true—is known as type I error or α error. The β error, or type II error, is defined as the chance of failure to reject a hypothesis that is false. In hypothesis testing, type I error is usually considered more serious. It is generally accepted in the medical literature that it is safe to reject a null hypothesis when there is less than a 5% chance of being wrong.

Statistical Power and Sample Size

Often it is difficult to specify how many subjects (or patients) are required to participate in a study, clinical trial, or experiment. The sample size is of paramount importance when embarking upon any study. The larger the sample size, the closer it reflects the population under investigation; but, it is impractical in many situations to increase the sample size either because of logistics, expense, and time constraints. Therefore, sample size will always be an approximation. The calculation depends on the objective of the study, the proposed method of analysis, the significance level of the report, and the magnitude of the difference the investigator wants to detect.

Failure to reject the null hypothesis when it is false is a type II error or β. The statistical power is the probability of not making a type II error, therefore $(1 - \beta.)$ Statistical power is also the ability to detect differences between groups when it exists. Although it is often ignored, statistical power is significant, especially when study between two groups (for example, clinical trials between two drugs) yield no statistical significance. In this instance, interpretation is difficult. There is a close relationship between the sample size and the power of the statistical test. As sample size increases, so does the power.

In summary, the required sample size is affected by the significance level, the power, and the magnitude of the difference.

P Value

P values indicate the probability that the difference observed between the control group and treatment group has occurred by chance alone.

For example, the specific meaning of the statement P < 0.05 is that the observed difference or a more extreme difference between the compared groups of variables would have occurred by chance alone only 5% of the time. Conversely, this means that there is a 95% probability that the observed difference is the result of the report or study. P values are a way of reporting the result of statistical tests. They do not define the statistical importance of the result. They imply little about the magnitude of the difference present between values or groups. P values depend on assumptions about the data, i.e., test statistics, null hypothesis, and alternate hypothesis. Therefore, P values can be misleading and are best used when they are reported with descriptive information regarding the study result.

Commonly, researchers state the smallest level at which the sample results are accepted as significant. Most researchers use 5% (or P < .05) as the lowest level for determining the statistical significance.

One-Tail Versus Two-Tail Test

In circumstances in which the true mean of the population being tested can only be above the sample mean, investigators may decide to use only a one-tail test of significance. In these instances, the negative or lower value has no meaning, and only when the test values are higher than the null hypothesis value will the hypothesis be rejected. For example, if the investigator was solely studying improvements in ankle systolic pressures following successful vascular reconstructions, the one-tail test may be used to test the level of significance. In the two-tail test, both the higher and lower values (either

above or below the population value) could result in rejection of the null hypothesis. The two-tail test is the test used in most situations. Ideally, the decision to use either the one-tail or the two-tail test should be made before the data is collected.

Student's t-Test

The student t-test is the most commonly used statistical method reported in the medical literature. It is used to accept or reject the null hypothesis and it is based upon three major assumptions:

1. Populations from which the samples were drawn are normally distributed.
2. The population's variances are equal or nearly equal.
3. The observations made within the sample are independent.

The t-test is calculated from the means, standard deviations, and variances of the data. If the data does not meet these assumptions, then the t-test is not the appropriate method to use. It is best used when single comparison is being made between two groups.

Inference on Means

In cases in which the δ (SD of the population) is known, the critical ration (z) for the null hypothesis can be calculated by:

$$z = \frac{\bar{x} - \mu O}{\delta / \sqrt{n}}$$

Paired where μO = expected population mean.

However, if δ is unknown, which is frequently the case, s (the sample SD) can be substituted as an estimate of δ. If sample size is large (>30), this substitution is reliable. For a smaller sample size, however, the substitution of s for δ requires a statistical correction. This correction is provided by use of a t-distribution, which is a set of theoretical probability distributions resembling normal distribution. In situations in which δ is not known and the sample size is small (<30), the above formula can be written as:

$$t_{n-1} = \frac{x - \mu O}{s / \sqrt{n}}$$

where t is the critical statistic, n − 1 is the degree of freedom (df), and μO is the expected population mean. To test this hypothesis, the critical value obtained by the above calculation is looked up against a standard t-distribution table under the corresponding df (n − 1) and the level of significance is estimated. For example, the national mean hospital stay following below-knee amputation is 45 days. In hospital "A," 10 patients undergoing below-knee amputations have a mean stay of 57 days ± 15 SD (s). Substituting the appropriate values in the above formula, we can calculate the critical ratio for t:

$$t_{n-1} = \frac{x - \mu O}{s/n} = \frac{57 - 45}{15/10} = \frac{12}{15/3.16} = 2.53.$$

A standard t-distribution table reveals that the critical ratio for a 5% significance level is 2.26 (two-tail) for 9 df. Since 2.53 is higher than 2.26, the null hypothesis (that there is no difference in the national mean hospital stay value and those for hospital "A") can be rejected. Hence, there is a significant difference in the hospital "A" mean stay for below-knee amputation patients as compared to the national mean stay, and the significance level is less than 5% (P < .05).

Comparison of Means

Most medical observations are, by nature, comparative. Therefore, comparison of means is one of the most commonly encountered modes of statistical analyses. In general, there are two samples of populations with two sets of values for means, $\bar{x}_1$ and $\bar{x}_2$, and two standard deviations, s_1 and s_2. The target population values are denoted by μ_1 and μ_2 (means) and δ_1 (standard deviations).

Paired Samples

In paired samples, each observation in one sample has one and only one matching observation in the other sample. Observations between samples are dependent upon one another. The simplest example of such pairing occurs when the sample population acts as its own control, i.e., before and after treatment. In Table 4, the values for 10 sample pairs of ankle systolic pressures before and after transluminal angioplasty are presented. To calculate the t statistic, the following interim values are needed-mean of the difference between the two populations and standard deviation of the difference. The following formula then is applied:

$$t_{n-1} = \frac{d - O}{Sd/\sqrt{n}}$$

(where d = mean of difference; S_d = SD of difference). substituting data from Table 4,

$$\text{t-test of } t_9 = \frac{18.8}{12.90/\sqrt{10}} = 4.60$$

from T table (one tail, 9 df) = P = < .005

Table 4
Example of Calculation of t-Test in Paired Samples

Patient No.	Before TLA a	After TLA b	Difference c (b − a)	Square of Difference (c)2
1	70	95	25	625
2	65	85	20	400
3	47	68	21	441
4	67	76	9	81
5	31	66	35	1225
6	29	56	27	729
7	68	57	− 11	121
8	49	61	12	144
9	37	65	28	784
10	51	73	22	484

Sum of difference = 188
Mean of difference (d) = 18.8
Sum of squares = 5034
(Sum)2/n = (188)2/10 − 3534
SD Standard deviation(s) = $\frac{5034 - 3534}{10 - 1}$ = 12.90

Unpaired Samples

t-Test for comparison of two independent means: in many situations the samples do not contain paired samples, but instead, independent observations from the control and test populations. For example, when one administers a placebo for a control group and a vasodilating agent for a treatment group, the results from each group is completely independent from one another. In these instances, the number of test observations may not be the same as the number of control observations. The following formula is used to calculate the t-test statistic:

$$t_{(n1 + n2 - 2)} = \frac{(\bar{x}_1 - \bar{x}_2)}{\sqrt{s2 \left(\frac{1}{n_1} + \frac{1}{n_2} \right)}}$$

where:

$$s^2 = \frac{\sum (x_1 - \bar{x}_1)^2 + \sum (x_2 - \bar{x}_2)^2}{n_1 + n_2 - 2)}$$

and:

n_1 = number in sample one

n_2 = number in sample two

x_1 = mean of sample one

x_2 = mean of sample two

s^2 = pool estimate of common variance.

Inference on Proportions

Chi-Square Test

A great deal of data gathered in medicine is numerical (count of different variables) and binary in nature (mutually exclusive pairs such as pass/fail, dead/alive, yes/no, etc.). Chi-square is the most frequently performed test for comparison of data arising from such pairs, although it can be extended to the comparison of multiple proportions. The chi-square test is applicable only to actual numbers counted and not to the percentages or ratios. Its use is appropriate for nominal data scale. Observation within each sample or group must be independent from each other. The sum of observed frequency must equal observed frequency.

The most frequently encountered situation (comparing the survival of patients in two different treatment protocols—group 1 and group 2) is summarized in a 2 × 2 table in Table 5. The general formula for calculation of chi-square is:

$$x^2 = \frac{\sum (O - E)^2}{E}$$

where:

O = observed count in category

E = expected count for that category if the null hypothesis is true.

Substituting data in Table 5, chi-square can be calculated:

$$\frac{\sum (O - E)^2}{E}$$

$$= (6.8)^2 \times \frac{1}{44.2} + \frac{1}{45.8} + \frac{1}{10.8} + \frac{1}{11.2}$$

$$= 46.2 \times .226 = 10.4$$

Expected count is calculated by formulating a null hypothesis that there is no difference between the two groups. Hence, as shown in Table 5, the number of patients expected to be alive in group A is 55 × (90/112) = 44.2. The expected counts for the other three values can be calculated by the same method or by subtracting the known values from the row or column totals (Table 5). Another curious mathematical phenomenon seen is that O − E) for each category is the same number, i.e., (51 − 44.2) = 6.8 and (39 − 45.8) = 6.8, etc. This knowledge can be used to simplify the chi-square formula shown in Table 5. A limitation in the use of chi-square is that none of the expected values can be less than 5. Furthermore, a continuity correction must be made in the calculation for most small samples. This correction is called "Yates' correction" and is shown below.

$$\frac{\sum ([(O - E] - \frac{1}{2})^2}{E}$$

$$= (6.8 - 5)^2 \times \frac{1}{44.2} + \frac{1}{45.8} + \frac{1}{10.8} + \frac{1}{11.2}$$

$$= 39.69 \times .226 = 8.96$$

The chi-square value obtained is looked up against a standard table under appropriate df, and the level of significance is derived. Degree of freedom is calculated as numbers of rows 1 × number of columns − 1. Most tables are 2 × 2, and, hence, the df is 1. For 2 × 3 tables, the df would be (1 × 2) or 2. The equation depicted below, shows an equation that may be easier to use when calculating chi-square.

Table 5
Example of Calculation of Chi-Square Test

		Group 1		Group 2		Total
Alive	A	51	C	39	(A + C)	90
Dead	B	4	D	18	(B + D)	22
Total	(A + B)	55	(C + D)	57	n =	112
Exp. Alive	A	44.2	C	45.8		90
Exp. Dead	B	10.8	D	11.2		22
		55		57		112

$$\frac{(AD - BD) - n/2)^2 n}{(A + B)(A + C)(B + D)(C + D)}$$

$$= \frac{(51 \times 18 - 4 \times 39) - 112/2)^2 \times 112}{(55)(90)(22)(57)}$$

$$= 8.96$$

Note that the results of the calculation in both the Yates correction and the chi-square are the same.

Fisher's Exact Test

In instances in which the observed frequencies are small (total number of observations, n < 50, or the expected frequency in either cell is <5), Yate's modification of chi-square is unreliable. In these cases, the probability that the two groups are equal can be calculated by using Fisher's exact test probability tables.[4]

Regression and Correlation

Regression

It is of interest to examine the effects some variables have on others in a number of situations. Two principal types of variables can be distinguished: independent and dependent. Independent variables are those that can be fixed in advance (controls) or are only observed, but not altered. Generally, one is interested in the way independent variables affect dependent variables. That is, the dependent variable is a function of the independent variable.[9] This functional relationship between two variables is called regression analysis.

The least square method is a formula for calculations to estimate the regression analysis. The equation for the regression line is called a regression equation. An example of a simple linear regression equation is:

$$Y = a + bx$$

where y is the dependent variable, x is the independent variable, a is the intercept, and b is the slope of the line. The regression line is a unique line so that the sum of squared deviations of each observed point from the line is minimum. Figure 4 shows a classic example described by Pearson and Lee in 1903 to estimate the relationship of a father's height (x or independent variable) on son's height (y or dependent variable). The straight line in the figure shows that there is a regression of son's height towards the average and the slope of the line (b) is the coefficient of regression.[10]

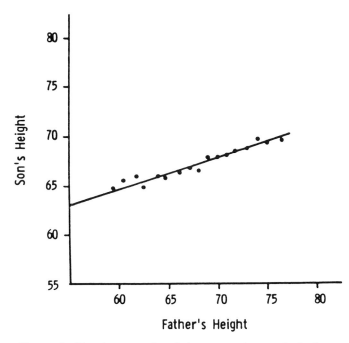

Figure 4. Classic example of the regression analysis from Pearson and Lee[8] showing the relationship of father's height to son's height.

Correlation

In regression analysis, there is a set of independent variables that affect the outcome of a dependent variable, but in correlation analysis both the variables are random. In simple terms, correlation means any kind of association or interdependence between sets of data. Correlation analysis provides a mathematical way of measuring the degree of association between two independent variables. The measurement of correlation usually lies between perfect negative (-1) and perfect positive ($+1$) and if there is no association whatsoever, the value is close to 0. This measurement of correlation is called correlation coefficient (r). It is a numerical value describing the strength of the relationship. A frequently used method to calculate the correlation coefficient is the Pearson product moment correlation (r).

$$r = \delta\, xy \quad \text{or} \quad \frac{\sum xy - \sum xy - (\sum x)(\sum y)/n}{\delta\, x\, \delta\, y (SDx)(SDy)}$$

where $\delta\, xy$ is the covariance of x and y and $\delta\, x$ and $\delta\, y$ are the standard deviations of x and y.

Nonparametric Methods or Distribution-Free Methods

Statistical methods for testing hypothesis can be divided in two broad classes: parametric tests and non-

Table 6
Example of Calculation of Signed Rank Test (Wilcoxon)*

Difference:	−25	−20	−20	−9	−35	−27	11	−12	−28	−22
Rank	7	4	5	1	10	8	2	3	9	6

Sum of + Ranks = 2
P Value = <0.01

* Values are ranked irrespective of the signs, and then the sum of rank of the + and the − values is obtained.

parametric tests or distribution-free tests. Those which require normal or near-normal distribution assumption are called parametric tests; for example, student t-tests, Fisher's correlation, and regression analysis. They are applied to most interval or ratio scales whose data collection are from samples of a normally distributed population, whereas nonparametric tests are useful when the data does not conform to the standard statistical methods that assume a particular parametric frequency distribution of the population. In fact, these tests can be applied irrespective of the distribution. However, nonparametric tests have less power than the corresponding parametric tests. Therefore, for samples with near normal distributions, it is better to use parametric than nonparametric methods.[11] The most frequently used nonparametric methods are signed rank test, Wilcoxon rank sum test, Mann Whitney U test, and Kruskal-Wallis test.

Signed Rank Test (Wilcoxon)

This test is designed to compare two groups in paired sample and is an analog of the paired t-test. The null hypothesis for the test states that the median difference between the pairs is zero. To calculate the signed rank test, the differences are ranked in order of their values from the lowest to the highest irrespective of + or − signs. The sums of positive ranks and nega-

tive ranks then are calculated and the P value looked up against a standard table. Table 6 shows a typical calculation that is based on the data in Table 4.

Wilcoxon Rank Sum Test

This method of comparing two unmatched samples is analogous to the t-test for unpaired samples. An example of this calculation is shown in Table 7, and the P value is looked up against a standard table.

Mann-Whitney U Test

This is another nonparametric procedure for testing the difference between two independent samples. It is analogous to the t-test. The Mann-Whitney test can be used as a one tail or two tail test. Therefore, it is similar to the Wilcoxon Rank Sum Test. This test is based on the assignment of ranks to the two groups of measures. The sum of ranks for the two groups can be compared by calculating the U statistic. The calculations of the U statistics will vary with the sample size.

Kruskal-Wallis Test

This test is an extension of the Wilcoxon test. It is applied in situations in which there are more than

Table 7
Wilcoxon Rank Sum Test

Values from Group A* =					21	24	24	30	23	22	27	28	25
Values from Group B* =					29	33	22	31	28	38	29	24	29
Order	21	22	22	23	24	24	24	25	27	28	28	29	29	29
Rank	1	2½	2½	4	6	6	8	9	9	10½	10½	13	13	13
Order	30	31	33	38
Rank	15	16	17	18

Sum of Group A Ranks (underlined) = 62
Sum of Group B Ranks   = 109
P Value from Rank Sum Tables   = P > .05

two sets of measurements, thus comparing three or more unmatched random samples of measurements.

Life-Table Analysis

This method is also known as the actuarial survival method. The life-table method of presenting data is one of the most important statistical analyses used by vascular surgeons. This method is applicable to the results obtained by any vascular reconstructive procedure, or to the use of grafts where a series of patients is followed for a long period of time to an end point of patient survival, graft survival, or limb survival. The untoward events or end points may affect some or all of the patients at different intervals from the time the patients entered the study (usually the date the procedure was performed). An example of a typical-life table calculation is shown in Table 8, section A.[3,12,13]

In Figure 5, the solid line shows a graphic representation of the life-table data in Table 8A. The data represents the graft patency of saphenous vein above-knee femoropopliteal bypasses performed during a randomized trial comparing saphenous vein and polytetrafluoroethylene (PTFE), grafts.[14] Note that the X axis represents interval periods or months since operation, and the Y axis represents the cumulative life-table patency rates. The numbers on top of the curve represent the number of patients at risk at the start of that interval. Alternatively, one can use vertical bar lines on the curve to show one standard error above and below the curve point. The methods for calculating and presenting the life-table data conform to the recommendations made by the SVS/ISCVS Ad Hoc Committee on Reporting Standards.[15] It was also recommended that data be omitted or highlighted when the standard error exceeds 10% to indicate poor reliability of estimates beyond that point, because the number of patients contributing to the curve decreases with time and, thus, makes it less reliable. Complete life-table analysis should be submitted in table form to allow analysis even if patency rates are also graphically illustrated. In the graphic form, the curve p ideally should be joined in a stepwise fashion.[16]

In spite of all the advantages of life-table analysis, it is noteworthy to mention that this is not a standard test.

In an effort to precisely define and make life-table reports uniform, the Ad Hoc Committee on Reporting Standards published the following guidelines. Life-table analysis should include the following columns in the life table: intervals in months, number at risk at the start of the period, number failed during the period, number withdrawn because of death or loss to follow-up, interval patency, cumulative patency, and standard error.[12]

Report of patency rates may be subject to biased reporting. It is important to define patency rate and differentiate primary from secondary patency. Primary patency refers to a graft which has remained open according to objective, documented tests with no procedure performed on it. If, on the other hand, any procedure such as thrombolysis, thrombectomy, or transluminal angioplasty is performed on the graft itself, or above or below the graft in order to prevent eventual graft failure, it is considered secondary patency.[12]

Therefore, to avoid biased results, it is incumbent upon the investigator to clearly describe procedures, sampling, patients lost to follow-up, withdrawals, and other factors that may influence outcome.

Kaplan–Meier Curve

The methodology described above is based on Berkson and Gage,[9] and Cutler and Ederer.[10] Since patients are followed at regular intervals, it is the most appropriate method for vascular surgeons to use; survival or patency times are grouped into intervals, and the number of events in each period is recorded. However, the accuracy may be affected by the frequency at which the patients are being studied. In studies involving terminal illness such as cancer where the end point is death (which can be definitely pinpointed in contrast to graft closure that may have occurred at any time between the last visit and the current visit), researchers use the Kaplan-Meier estimate of survival.[17] The calculations are similar to those for the cumulative life-table method with one exception—the failures are recorded at the precise point that they occur and curve values are calculated at each point of "failure."

Log Rank Test or Mantel–Haenszel Test

In vascular surgery, it is frequently necessary to compare the cumulative life-table rates of two groups based on a certain factor (comparison of two grafts, comparison of results between two surgical groups, etc.) For example, in Table 8A and B, the results of saphenous vein and PTFE femoropopliteal bypasses performed to above-knee popliteal arteries are shown. Upon casual observation, it appears that the 48-month life-table patency of 61% in saphenous vein grafts is far superior to the 38% rate achieved in PTFE grafts. To determine if there is a difference between the two groups however, one has to perform the log rank test. Calculation of the log rank test (shown in Table 8C) involves calculating the chi-square for each interval line by presenting a null hypothesis that there are no two different groups.[18,19] The expected failure rate of group A at each interval is then calculated (as previ-

Table 8

Example of Calculation of Cumulative Life-Table and Log Rank Test

		A							B			C		
	a Int.	b No. Risk	c "Fail"	d "Pass"	e Int. Pat.	f Cum. Pat.	g SE	h No. Risk	i "Fail"	j Cum. Pat.	k A + B Risk	l A + B Fail	m Expect "A"
1	0–30 days	85	4	8	95.0	100	0	91	7	100	176	11	5.3
2	1–6 mos	73	2	8	97.1	95.0	2.3	77	3	92	150	5	2.4
3	6–12 mos	63	6	10	89.3	92.3	2.9	57	3	87.5	120	9	4.7
4	13–18 mos	47	3	7	93.3	82.7	4.3	48	3	83.6	95	6	3.0
5	19–24 mos	37	0	6	100	77.4	5.3	36	3	77.8	73	3	1.5
6	25–30 mos	31	1	5	96.4	77.4	6.0	24	1	69.2	55	2	1.1
7	31–36 mos	25	1	8	95.1	74.1	6.7	19	2	66.3	44	3	1.7
8	37–42 mos	16	2	5	85.4	70.3	7.6	10	2	58.1	26	4	2.5
9	43–48 mos	9	0	1	100	60.8	9.4	6	1	37.5	15	1	0.6
Totals		19 O_A						25 O_B				44 Expect "B"	22.8 E_A 21.2 E_B

Chi-square

$$\frac{(O_A - E_A)^2}{E_A} + \frac{(O_B - E_B)^2}{E_B} = \frac{(19 - 22.8)^2}{22.8} + \frac{(25 - 21.2)^2}{21.2} = \frac{(3.8)^2}{22.8} + \frac{(3.8)^2}{21.2} = .649 + .702 = 1.351$$

$P < 0.25$

where

Col. a = Interval period—Time elapsed since surgery for any onset point). The number of patients that have end points (fail or pass) falling in each of the intervals is counted.

Col. b = Number at risk—The first line shows the total number of patients entered in the study and, hence, who were at risk at zero period. Each subsequent line has numbers that are at risk at the beginning of that period. These are calculated as follows: number at risk in previous period—(number "failed" + number "passed" [see Col. d] in that period).

Col. c = Numbers "failing"—Numbers meeting the adverse end point (failed, closed, or died, depending upon what is being studied) during that period. This is calculated by Date Fail–Date Onset and incrementing the count by one for each patient failing in that interval. For example, if a patient has surgery on 01/01/80 and his graft closes on 04/15/82, then the "fail" count in the interval 25 to 30 months (line 6) is increased by one.

Col. d = For the sake of simplicity, all patients that leave the study for any cause other than the adverse endpoint (hence, "pass") are counted in each interval based on (Date Leaving Study) minus (Date Onset).
There are several reasons why a patient drops out of the study with a "pass" label. If only the graft patency is being studied, all the patients dying with their graft patent have left the study with "good outcome" at Date of Death minus Date Onset interval. Some patients drop out of the study because they can no longer be followed (e.g., they may have moved), therefore, their status on the closing day of the study is unknown. The period of observations for these patients is from time of onset to date last seen. The third group of patients that are included in Col. d are those that are withdrawn from the study on the last day of the study based on the length of follow-up. Obviously, operations for all patients entering the study are not performed on the same day; hence, those patients who have been operated on most recently have the shortest follow-up and dropout of life-table calculations in the early intervals, and the patients who entered the study in the beginning of the study have the longest follow-up.

Col. e = Interval patency—This calculation requires some explanation. For calculation of interval patency, an assumption is made that the patients leaving the study with a "pass" label are all withdrawn precisely at the mid-point of the interval range. Hence, it is assumed that during the half of the interval they were followed, they were subject to only half the chance of failure of the entire interval. Hence, interval patency = number failed (number at risk—½ total "pass"). Therefore,

$$\text{Col. e} = \left(100 - \left(\frac{c}{b - (d/2)}\right) \times 100\right)$$

Col. f = Cumulative patency—For the first line, the cumulative life-table patency is always 100% for the first period, since the probability of the graft being patent at insertion is 100%. Cumulative patencies for the subsequent periods are calculated by

$$\text{Col. f} = \frac{\text{interval patency* } \times \text{ cumulative patency*}}{100}$$

(* From the previous line)
Hence, line 2 (1–6 months), cumulative patency, in Table 8 is calculated as $95 \times 100 = \underline{95.0}$.

Col. g = Standard error—The formula for calculating the standard error of life-table at each interval is

$$L \sqrt{(1 - L)/n}$$

where L = cumulative patency rate and n = number of patients at risk.
Thus, standard error of the second interval in Table 8A is

$$.95 \sqrt{(1 - .95)/85} = .023 \text{ or } 2.3\%$$

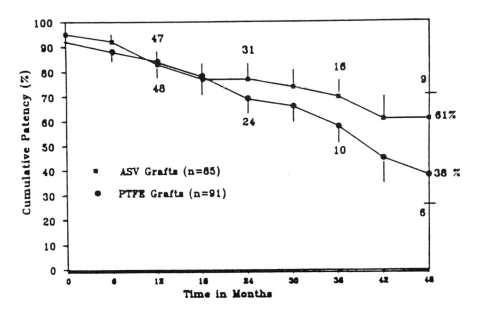

Figure 5. Example of life-table patency rates showing comparison of saphenous vein and PTFE grafts to above-knee femoropopliteal bypass grafts.

ously shown in calculating chi-square) by the following (Table 8C, column m) formula:

$$\frac{\text{Combined Failure } (A + B)(\text{col. l})}{\text{Combined At Risk } (A + B)(\text{col. k})}$$

$$\times \text{ No. at Risk for A (col. b)}$$

Hence, line 1 = 11/176 × 85 = 5.3 is the expected failure rate for 0 to 30 days. The total expected failure rate for group A (if there was no difference in the two groups) is 22.85 and (44 − 22.85) = 21.15 for group B. The chi-square calculation is shown in Table 8, and the P value is looked up against a standard chi-square and is less than 0.25. Hence, the null hypothesis that there is no difference in the patency rates of the two groups cannot be rejected. The graph in Figure 5 shows that the curves for the two groups are almost identical except for the last few months, and the standard error is quite large in these last intervals, thus, confirming the conclusion reached by the log rank test.

Meta-Analysis

Since Glass[20,21] introduced the term Meta-analysis in the mid 1970s, the medical literature has seen an increased use of the meta-analytic method in many reports, especially in controlled clinical trials.[20]

Meta-analysis (or overview analysis) is a quantitative summary of multiple studies with the aim to reach a generalized conclusion. This new technique makes it possible to study trends in a particular research topic and to detect differences in outcome between reports. The goals of meta-analysis are:

1. To increase the statistical power.
2. To resolve uncertainty when similar studies report conflicting results.
3. To improve estimates of size of effect.
4. To elucidate or clarify problems from individuals studies.
5. To pose and answer new questions about individual studies.

This overview analytical method is most valuable for cumulative analysis of new treatment versus old treatment, especially when their effect is less pronounced, but real difference or benefit indeed exists. The techniques of meta-analysis in controlled, randomized trials have been well described.[22–24]

First, a comprehensive literature search is compiled, with systematic analysis of each study followed by selection of authors. After comparative analysis of multiple studies, results are then combined using standard statistical formula to draw conclusions. The most commonly used statistical formula is the Mantel-Haenszel test.[25]

Although meta-analysis uses formal statistical techniques to analyze and summarize results of combined studies, it is not an exact statistical science. The pitfalls include[26,27]:

1. Study design and design differences between studies.

Table 9
"Gold Test"

		+		−		
New +	A	50	B	5		
Test −	C	50	D	195	(A + B)	55
Total	(A + C)	100	(B + D)	200	(C + D)	245

2. The literature search may not be extensive enough.
3. Choice of reports and authors may result in selection bias.
4. Appropriate combination of reports and studies.
5. Application of results and statistical method.
6. Valid conclusions.

Evaluation of a New Diagnostic Test

Before a new diagnostic test is widely used, it is essential to evaluate its performance for reliability and accuracy especially in relation to a more conventional pre-existing gold standard test. With the advent of new diagnostic noninvasive machines appearing in vascular laboratories, these principles are particularly applicable (28, 29). Frequently, the new noninvasive test is compared to the conventional invasive angiography or venography.

The calculation of different parameters is shown in Table 9.

Reliability

The reliability of a method is its ability to provide the same answer in repeated observations.

Sensitivity

The sensitivity of a test is the ability of the test to diagnose disease when disease is present. In Table 9, there are 100 positive diagnoses by the gold test; however, the new test diagnosed only 50 of these. Hence, the sensitivity is number tested positive over total with condition:

$$\frac{A}{A + C} = \frac{50}{100} = 50\%.$$

Specificity

The ability of a test to indicate no disease when disease does not exist is the specificity. In the example

in Table 9, patients were found to have no disease by the gold standard and 195 no disease by the new test. Hence, the specificity is the number tested negative over total with conditions:

$$\frac{D}{B + D} = \frac{195}{200} = 98\%$$

False-Positive

These are cases that were negative by the gold standard, but were found to be positive by the new test divided by the total number of positive results:

$$\frac{B}{A + B} = \frac{5}{55} = 9\%$$

False-Negative

This refers to cases that were positive by the gold standard test, but were found to be negative by the new test divided by the total number of negative results:

$$\frac{C}{C + D} = \frac{5}{245} = 20\%$$

Positive Predictive Values

The percentage of patients found positive by the new test who were also found positive by the "gold standard" test is the positive predictive value. In all likelihood a positive result denotes the presence of disease:

$$\frac{A}{A + B} = \frac{50}{55} = 91\%$$

Negative Predictive Values

The percentage of patients that were found negative by the new test and were also found negative by the gold standard test is called the negative predictive value. In all likelihood, a negative test denotes the absence of disease:

$$\frac{D}{C + D} = \frac{195}{245} = 80\%$$

Overall Accuracy

The percentage of patients correctly predicted to be either positive or negative divided by the total number of patients is the overall accuracy:

$$\frac{A + D}{A + B + C + D} = \frac{245}{300} = 82\%$$

Receiver Operating Characteristic Curve

Accuracy as calculated above is not very descriptive because it does not reflect important critical parameters such as sensitivity and specificity. In comparing and/or choosing a test, the distribution and the severity of the disease play important roles. Therefore, choosing a very sensitive test is imperative when considering a lethal disease. On the other hand, a test with high specificity is preferable when confronted with a benign but nonetheless treatable disease. The relationship between important parameters, sensitivity, specificity, positive and negative predictive values, and prevalence is best understood by the receiver operating curve (ROC). The ROC curve relates the degree of positivity of the test to the presence or absence of the trait in the gold standard. To plot the ROC curves, the specificity and sensitivity are plotted with different diagnostic measurements of the test.[30]

In Figure 6, ROC curves are generated with regard to sensitivity and specificity of a given test. The sensitivity of the test at point A is 95% and its specificity is 65%. The downward slope of the curve indicates the increase in specificity at the expense of sensitivity. Yet, with the same test, the sensitivity and specificity can be changed as long as the criteria for the test can be manipulated. A different ROC curve can be obtained if the criteria are changed, for example the A[1] curve in Figure 6. Hence, a family of curves is necessary to document the accuracy of a given test when different criteria are used. In clinical practice, two or more tests are usually compared because together they improve the accuracy of proving the presence or absence of disease.

Use of Microcomputers

The advances of technology and the proliferation of microcomputers have made many statistical formu-

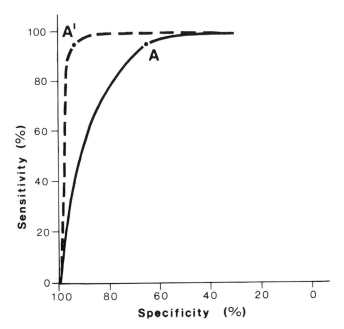

Figure 6. Receiver operator curve illustrating varying relationships between sensitivity and specificity depending on prevalence.

lae easier, more accessible and manageable. The statistical software packages such as SPSS/PC, SASS can carry out many, if not all, of the most commonly used statistical methods. The operation of the software packages are well described in several text books and manuals.[31–33]

Generally, the easier statistical calculations can be performed by a hand-held calculator. Mainframe computers are used for more complex statistical methods. However, the spreadsheet programs which allow microcomputers to emulate an accounting pad of rows and columns that can be linked by mathematical formulas (Microsoft Excel, Lotus 1-2-3®) support a large number of mathematical and statistical functions: count, sum, mean, min., maximum, SD, and variance. These functions can be combined with other mathematical and logical functions to set up templates in the program that allow repeated statistical analysis with differing data values. Templates can be developed for the following commonly used statistics: mean, s2, SD, SEM, chi-square, t-test, paired t-test, coefficient of correlation, regression analysis, and the log rank test. A template also can be designed for the evaluation of any new test to calculate the specificity, sensitivity, false-positive, false-negative, accuracy, positive predictive value, and negative predictive value. Furthermore, any number of templates for other statistical tests can be created as long as the statistical calculation is based on mathematical formulas. Simple graphic representation of data also can be obtained immediately. These statistical templates can save innumerable hours in analysis of research results.

In many instances, it is easier and more reliable to use a computer for statistical calculations Applications of formulae and computations may be so tedious that errors are almost inevitable if they are done manually. Computers can carry out many formulae and calculate statistical data, but the analysis remains the domain and the responsibility of the investigator. If calculations violate rules and assumptions, the outcome will be misleading.

References

1. Dalsing MC, White JV, Yao JST, et al: Infrapopliteal bypass for established gangrene of the forefoot or toes. *J Vasc Surg* 2:669, 1985.
2. Cohen JR, Perry MO, Hariri R, et al: Aortic collagenase activity as affected by laparotomy cecal resection, aortic mobilization, and aortotomy in rats. *J Vasc Surg* 1:562, 1994.
3. Colton T: *Statistics in Medicine.* Boston: Little, Brown & Co., 1974.
4. Matthews DE, Farewell VT: *Using and Understanding Medical Statistics.* Basel: Switzerland, S. Karger; 1985.
5. Nie NH, Hull CH, Jenkins JG, et al: *Statistical Package for the Social Sciences.* 2nd Ed. New York: McGraw-Hill, Inc., 1970.
6. Broyles RW, Lay CM: *Statistics in Health Adminisration.* Vol 1, *Basic Concepts and Applications.* Germantown, MD: Aspen Systems Corp., 1979.
7. O'Brien PC, Shampo MA: Statistics for clinicians. 1. Descriptive statistics. *Mayo Clinic Proc* 56:47, 1981.
8. Gaddis ML, Gaddis GM: Introduction to Biostatistics. Basic Concepts-Parts 1. *Annals of Emer Med.* 19:1, 1990.
9. Rimm A, et al: *Basic Biostatistics in Medicine and Epidemiology.* New York: Appleton-Century Crofts, 1980.
10. Pearson K, Lee A: On the laws of inheritance in man 1. Inheritance of physical characters. *Biometrika* 2:357, 1903.
11. Shott Susan: Statistics for Health Professionals. New York: WB Saunders Co.; 1990.
12. Berkson J, Gage RP: Calculation of survival rates for cancer. *Proc Staff Meet Mayo Clin* 25:270, 1950.
13. Cutler SJ, Ederer F: Maximum utilization of the life-table method in analyzing survival. *J Chron Dis* 8:699, 1958.
14. Veith FJ, Gupta SK, Ascer E, et al: Six-year prospective multicenter randomized comparison of autologous saphenous vein (ASV) and expanded polytetrafluoroethylene (PTFE) grafts in infrainguinal arterial reconstructions. *J Vasc Surg* 3:104, 1986.
15. Rutherford RB, Flanigan DP, Gupta SK, et al: Suggested standards for reports dealing with lower extremity ischemia. *J Vasc Surg* 4:8, 1986.
16. Underwood CJ, Faragher EB, Charlesworth D: The uses and abuses of life-table methods in vascular surgery. *Br J Surg* 71:495, 1984.
17. Kaplan EL, Meier P: Nonparametric estimation from incomplete observations. *J Am Statist Ass* 53:457, 1958.
18. Peto R, Pike MC, Armitage P, et al: Design and analysis of randomized clinical trials requiring prolonged observation of each patient. I. Introduction and design. *Br J Cancer* 34:585, 1976.
19. Peto R, Pike MC, Armitage P, et al: Design and analysis of randomized clinical trials requiring prolonged observation of each patient. II. Analysis and examples. *Br J Cancer* 35:1, 1977.
20. Glass GV: Primary, Secondary and meta analysis of research. *Educ Res* 6:3–8, 1976.
21. Glass GV: Integrating findings: the meta analysis of research. *Rev Res Educ* 5:351–379, 1977.
22. Ellenberg SS: Meta analysis the quantitative approach to research review. *Seminar Oncology* 14(5):472–481, 1988.
23. Schell CL, Rate RJ. Meta Analysis: A tool for medical and scientific discoveries. *Bulletin Med Library Assoc* 80(3):219, 1992.
24. Rosenthal R: Meta analysis: A Review. *Psychosom Med* 53(3):247–271, 1991.
25. Manzel N, Haensel W: Statistical Aspects of the analysis of data from retrospective studies of disease. *J Natl Cancer Inst* 22:719–748, 1959.
26. Thompson, Pocok SJ: "Can meta analyses be trusted? *Lancet* 338(8775):1127–1130, 1992.
27. Kassierer JP: Clinical trials and meta analysis: what do they do for us? *N Engl J Med* 327(4):273–274, 1992.
28. Lambeth A: Statistics in the vascular laboratory. *Bruit* VI:47, 1982.
29. Hayes AC: Calculation and implication of accuracy measurements. *Bruit* IX:178, 1985.
30. Johnston KW, Haynes RB, Douville Y, et al: Accuracy of carotid Doppler peak frequency analysis: Results determined by Receiver operating characteristic curves and likelihood ratios. *J Vasc Surg* 2:515, 1985.
31. Norusis MJ: *The SPSS Guide to Data Analysis for SPSS/PC +.* Chicago: SPSS, 1988.
32. Norusis MJ: *SPSS/PC + V3.0 Base Manual for the IBM PC/XT/AT and PS/2.* Chicago: SPSS, 1989.
33. Norusis MJ: *SPSS/PC + Advanced Statistics V3.0 for the IBM PC/XT/AT and PS/2.* Chicago: SPSS, 1989.

III

The Science of Selected Titles:

Physiology and Pathophysiology

CHAPTER 27

Aneurysmal Disease
of the
Abdominal Aorta

M. David Tilson, MD; Anita K. Gregory, MD
Anil P. Hingorani, MD

Introduction

The abdominal aortic aneurysm (AAA) continues to be a significant cause of morbidity and mortality, ranking fifteenth as a leading cause of death in the United States.[1] Despite accurate methods of detection and effective surgical therapy prior to rupture, a recent population-based study suggests that the mortality rate remains high for this disease entity in a country with sophisticated medical care.[2] The etiology of the AAA has historically been attributed to atherosclerotic degeneration of the aorta. However, the overall incidence of aortic aneurysms has been steadily increasing despite a general decline in the incidence of atherosclerosis.[3] Although AAAs show gross and microscopic evidence of atheromatous disease, the exact role of atherosclerosis in their pathogenesis has become controversial. Many investigations over the past decade have documented various histologic, genetic, biochemical, and epidemiologic differences between patients with aneurysms and those with atherosclerosis.

Incidence

The increased incidence of this disease was well documented by Melton et al in a population-based study published in 1984.[3] A sevenfold increase was seen between 1951 and 1980, which cannot be entirely explained by increasing longevity of the population. The increased prevalence of aortic aneurysmal disease is both age and sex specific. Of 45838 patients studied at autopsy between 1958 and 1986, aneurysms were found in 4300/100000 men and 2100/100000 women, making the mean age-standardized incidence 4.7% and 3.0% among men and women, respectively.[4] The prevalence among men appeared to climb rapidly after the age of 55 to a peak of 5.9% at age 80; and among women a peak of 4.5% was seen above age 90. In a similar study compiled from mortality statistics in England and Wales, deaths due to aneurysms were uncommon below age 55, and a tenfold increase then occurred among men as they progressed from ages 55 to 64 to ages 85 and older.[5]

AAAs are more common in males than in females, with deaths due to aneurysm in the United States Caucasian population occurring in a male:female ratio of 4 to 1.[6] A similar ratio was found in a defined region in Australia, where all deaths and hospital admissions due to AAAs were reviewed.[7] The male:female ratio, however, declines with age. Collin reported that the male:female ratio of 11 at ages 60 to 64 declined to 3 at ages 85 to 89.[8] In addition to the substantial male predominance of aneurysm disease, a racial difference also exists. AAAs are more common among whites than blacks, with males having a threefold higher incidence than black males or females. Black males, black females, and white females share approximately equal incidence.[9]

The results of published data are often difficult to compare and interpret because of a lack of standardization regarding the exact definition of an aneurysm. Most surgical textbooks define AAA as a permanent "dilatation" of the aorta, but often do not distinctly specify what criteria are used for dilatation. Measurement of the external diameter of the aorta is now relatively accurate using ultrasonography, but there is little agreement as to which diameter is most important: anteroposterior (AP); transverse, a mean of AP and transverse; or simply the maximum in any plane.[10] Some studies have implied that the AP diameter may be a better predictor of subsequent aneurysm rupture than the transverse diameter[11]; however, others have suggested that the ratio of the infrarenal to suprarenal diameter may be an even better indicator of rupture risk than actual size.[12] DeWeese and others have suggested that ratio of the aneurysm diameter to the transverse diameter of the third lumbar vertebral body, as an index of patient body size, accurately predicts rupture risk.[13]

Collin reviewed several possible definitions in 1990.[10] They included: 1) an aortic diameter of at least 4 cm; 2) a mean normal aortic diameter, plus two standard deviations; 3) a diameter which is one and a half times that of the suprarenal aorta; and 4) an infrarenal aorta with a diameter 0.5 cm greater than that of the suprarenal aorta. Each of these has inherent weaknesses and pitfalls addressed in the analysis. Collin concluded that a diameter of either 4 cm or greater, or 0.5 cm greater than that of the suprarenal aorta, is the best operational definition.

To address the imprecision in AAA nomenclature and inconsistencies in reporting standards, the Joint Councils of the Society for Vascular Surgery and the North American Chapter of the International Society for Cardiovascular Surgery appointed an ad hoc committee to formulate some guidelines. The suggested standards for reporting on arterial aneurysms were published in 1991. An aneurysm was defined as a permanent, localized (i.e., focal) dilatation of an artery and having at least a 50% increase in diameter compared to the expected normal diameter of the artery.[14] Additional standards for classification, etiology, risk factors, histologic features, and clinicopathologic manifestations of aneurysm disease were suggested. Adoption of these proposed standards would lead to a more unified body of literature which could further scientific investigation and clinical understanding of this complex disease.

The overall prevalence of aneurysm disease in the community has been difficult to assess, as aneurysms were often missed or falsely diagnosed on physical examination alone. Ultrasound screening of the general population is the simplest, relatively accurate method for determining overall prevalence. Many screening studies have been published to date, but they are difficult to compare as most have been restricted to specific age, sex, or possible risk groups. The screening program published by Collin et al of a large population of males 65 to 74 years of age estimates the overall prevalence of abdominal aneurysms (either >4 cm or 0.5 cm greater than the suprarenal aorta) to be approximately 2%.[15] Ultrasound screening of first-degree relatives of patients with AAAs showed a prevalence of 25% of men and 6.9% of women over age 55.[16] Collin found that 29% of 17 brothers of AAA probands, who were examined by ultrasound, had an AAA.[17] Bengtsson et al found similarly high rates of aneurysm disease in the siblings and offspring of patients with AAAs.[18,19] These data strongly support ultrasonographic screening of high-risk individuals, particularly elderly siblings of those patients with documented aneurysms.

Risk Factors

Historically, studies of aneurysm risk factors paralleled those of atherosclerotic disease, since aneurysms were, and still are, considered by some to be a manifestation of atherosclerosis. One of the earliest references to atherosclerosis as the cause of aortic aneurysm disease comes from Scarpa's 1804 *Treatise on the Anatomy, Pathology, and Surgical Treatment of Aneurism*. He stated, "Of all the possible causes capable of producing the rupture in any part of the proper coats of the aorta, especially the internal, I have great reason to believe, that the slow morbid, ulcerated, steatomatous, fungous, squamous degeneration of the internal coat of the artery, has a share in it much more frequently, than violent exertions of the whole body, violent blows, or an increased impulse of the heart."[20] Interestingly, he described atherosclerotic plaque before the term "atherosclerosis" was coined.

Factors which place one at risk for the development of aortic aneurysms overlap with those for atherosclerosis, although the pathophysiologic mechanisms may not be the same. The two most common risk factors are smoking and hypertension. A large prospective longitudinal study which commenced in the 1950s demonstrated a strong correlation between smoking, hypertension, or both, and the development of AAAs.[21] A more recent study by Reed et al has confirmed these findings.[22] Smoking is remarkably common among patients with AAAs; two large series revealed an incidence of approximately 85%.[23,24] A similarly high incidence of hypertension (approximately 60%) was documented by Cronenwett and co-workers.[11] Although hypertension and smoking are statistically associated with aortic aneurysms, there is a sizable group of patients in whom neither risk factor is present.[25] Elevated serum cholesterol has been postulated to play a role in the pathogenesis of aneurysm disease, but the Whitehall study found no correlation between serum cholesterol level and risk of death from an AAA.[26] The incidence of atherosclerosis in arterial beds other than the aorta is also high among aneurysm patients. Coronary artery disease is present in 33% to 68%,[11,27] cerebrovascular disease in 20%,[11] and symptomatic lower extremity occlusive disease in 25%.[11] Thus, it appears that atherosclerosis, hypertension, and smoking are associated with aortic aneurysm disease; however, their precise contribution to its development is unclear.

A causal relationship between atherosclerotic risk factors and the development of AAAs was proposed by Reed et al in 1992.[22] They concluded that the risk factors for aortic atherosclerosis itself are necessary elements in the causal pathway of aneurysm formation. Two arguments were presented to support their view. First, the conventional atherosclerotic risk factors of hypertension, smoking, and hypercholesterolemia were associated with an increased incidence of AAA. Second, autopsy review of aneurysm specimens showed that a significant percentage of the aortic wall was affected by raised atherosclerotic lesions.

Alternative explanations have been proposed for some of these observations.[78] Hypertension could promote aneurysm formation due to elevated mechanical stresses alone. These forces may stress the structural integrity of the aortic wall, in addition to their other effects of stimulating the proliferation of smooth muscle cells (SMCs) that leads to atherosclerotic plaque formation. Similarly, as a separate mechanism from its effects as an SMC mitogen, cigarette smoking blocks the active site of α1–antitrypsin, which may promote the destruction of the aortic matrix by endogenous proteases.[29] Hypercholesterolemia may arise from diets which include tropical oils, which tend to produce a panarterial inflammatory infiltrate in animal models. This inflammatory component may play a separate and significant role in aneurysm development.[30] Also, it has recently been proposed that it is not atherosclerosis itself, but rather regression of this disease, which is essential for aneurysm formation.[31] The finding of raised atherosclerotic lesions on autopsy examination is not unique to atherosclerotic aneurysms; these lesions are seen in syphilitic aneurysms and poststenotic dilatations as well. Flow disturbances created by the geometry of an aneurysmal dilatation include turbulence, boundary layer separation, and reversal of flow,[32] all of which are associated with atherosclerotic degeneration. Finally, the notion that atherosclerosis "causes" aneurysms does not take into account numerous recent scientific advances, which suggest that aneurysm disease has unique genetic and biochemical determinants.

Genetics

From the first report of three brothers who suffered rupture of an AAA,[33] the familial tendency for developing this disease and its consequences have been investigated and more precisely defined. A genetic basis for aneurysm disease was postulated by Tilson and Dang in 1981. They noted the familial predisposition, preponderance of male over female patients, and possible parallels to the aneurysm-prone Blotchy mouse model among human aneurysm patients.[34] In 1984, three reports of familial clustering of aneurysm disease were published,[35-37] suggesting that a positive family history may be a significant risk factor in the development of AAAs. A subsequent study, with a control group of probands with atherosclerotic disease of the abdominal aorta, carried out by Johansen and Koepsell, demonstrated an 11.6-fold increased risk of developing an aneurysm among first-degree relatives of the AAA probands versus atherosclerotic controls.[38] Cole has shown a similar positive history of an affected first-degree relative (11%), and has documented a very high incidence of the disease (69%) among families where the mother was affected.[39]

Tilson and Seashore first attempted to identify a predominant pattern of inheritance in 1984.[36] Some pedigrees were consistent with X-linked inheritance, but others suggested autosomal dominant or multifactorial mechanisms. From ultrasound screening, it is known that 20% to 30% of male siblings of a given proband will be positive for an AAA.[15-17] It has been speculated that the true lifetime incidence in a sibling surviving to old age may approach 50%, which would be compatible with a single dominant gene pattern.[40] Mathematical models and extensive genetic analyses, however, have led to other interpretations. Powell and Greenhalgh concluded that the development of familial aneurysms was due to multifactorial inheritance with a genetic component of 70%.[41] The most extensive genetic analysis reported to date proposes a single recessive gene at an autosomal major locus.[42]

Is Abdominal Aortic Aneurysm a Unique Clinical Entity?

There have been several other challenges to the traditional theory of the "atherosclerotic" AAA. As early as 1978, Martin noted distinct differences between those patients with atherosclerotic occlusive disease and those with aneurysmal disease.[43] These included incidence of coronary artery disease, peripheral vascular disease, lipid profiles, and Rh factors. Tilson and Stansel also noted marked differences among the patient population with aneurysm disease and that with occlusive disease.[44] Patients with aneurysms are more likely to be male and older; they are less likely to have claudication, limb-threatening ischemia, or late graft failure. Because of these observations and the emergence of theories of AAA genetics, there has been a renewed interest in the histopathology and biochemistry of aneurysm disease.

Histology

Sumner et al were the first to report significant changes in the protein matrix components of aneurysm walls.[45] They found that the contents of elastin and collagen were decreased in the aortic walls of those patients with aneurysms, compared to control and atherosclerotic aortas. Extensive destruction of the elastin matrix in the media of aneurysms has been confirmed in histochemical studies.[46] In contrast, the media is usually better preserved in atherosclerotic occlusive disease, and it is the intima which is primarily altered by cellular proliferation and accumulation of extracellular matrix (ECM) components.[47] White has recently confirmed the substantial loss of medial elastin in aneurysms and has also shown that elastin depletion is essentially complete at early stages of aneurysm development.[48] This loss of medial elastin appears not to have a major effect on the overall mechanical strength of the aortic wall. One may speculate that ongoing destruction, synthesis, and reorganization of adventitial collagen is more important in the progression of aneurysmal dilatation and subsequent rupture.

Another prominent histologic feature in aneurysm disease is an inflammatory infiltrate of mononuclear cells at the junction between the adventitia and the media. In a review of 156 aortic specimens, Beckman documented in over two thirds a notable inflammatory cell infiltrate.[49] Immunophenotypic analysis by Koch et al has demonstrated T lymphocytes in the aneurysmal adventitia (with an elevated T helper to T suppressor cell ratio), B lymphocytes, and macrophages.[30] Whereas macrophages are present in both aneurysmal and occlusive aortas, T lymphocytes are less frequently seen in the adventitia of normal or occlusive vessels.[48] Lymphocytes are known to secrete gamma interferon, tumor necrosis factor-α (TNF-α), and interleukin-2 (IL-2), which increase macrophage proteolytic activity and, therefore, may be important in the pathogenesis of aneurysm disease.[50] Macrophages are a potential source of matrix metalloproteases (MMPs) and various cytokines as well. By analogy to the term "tumor-infiltrating lymphocytes," we are calling these macrophages the "AAA infiltrating macrophages" or AIM cells, and the lymphocytes we are calling "AAA infiltrating lymphocytes" or AIL cells. These immune cells may be intimately involved in the destruction of the aortic matrix. Elevated levels of immunoglobulins have also been seen in aneurysmal tissue as Russell bodies and also by Western blot analysis.[51]

The mesenchymal cells of the aorta may also play a significant role in aneurysm development. The SMCs in the adventitia of inflammatory aneurysms have been found to have abundant rough endoplasmic reticulum by transmission electron microscopy.[52] These SMCs may be involved with matrix deposition and the production of the enzymes responsible for its destruction.[53,54] The exact roles of each cell type, and how they interact with the matrix, each other, and fibroblasts, is not yet understood in detail; however, these interactions are a field of active research.

Experimental Models

Spontaneous Animal Models

Spontaneous aortic aneurysms occur consistently in the Blotchy mouse due to a genetic defect at the mottled locus on the X chromosome.[55] The mutation causes decreased intestinal absorption of copper and subsequent systemic copper deficiency, which decreases the activity of a copper-dependent enzyme, lysyl oxidase, which is essential for collagen and elastin cross-linking.[56,57] Decreased tensile strength of skin and development of aortic aneurysms are manifestations of the deficiency in cross-linking of the matrix components.[58] This deficiency apparently parallels the sex-linked disorder in humans, Menke's kinky hair syndrome, in which altered intestinal absorption of copper leads to progressive neurologic impairment and arterial abnormalities.[59,60]

The progression of aneurysm formation in the Blotchy mouse has been studied histologically and graded with respect to integrity and content of elastin fibers, ground substance, number and organization of fibroblasts, degree and nature of inflammatory cell infiltrates, and miscellaneous features such as angiogenesis, hemorrhage, lipid, iron, calcium, and mucopolysaccharide content. By 21 days of age, early degenerative changes are seen in the elastic fibers of the media.[61] The majority of Blotchy mice develop aneurysms by 4 months of age, and all have aneurysms by 6 months of age.[62] Ruptures occur at stress points; the three most common being the supravalvular ascending aorta and arch, the proximal descending aorta, and at the diaphragmatic hiatus.[62]

Spontaneous aneurysms also occur in certain strains of the turkey (for example, the Broad-Breasted Bronze), known to have hypertension and early formation of atheromatous plaques. These factors may contribute to the development of aneurysms.[63] Most aneurysms occur in the abdominal aorta, where poor supply of nutrients to the media at this level is the proposed mechanism of dilation and rupture.[64] Medial degeneration at the level of the aortic ring is responsible for spontaneously occurring aneurysms in the stallion as well.[65]

Pharmacologic Models

Most pharmacologic models of aneurysm disease are induced by lathyrism. The most common lathyrogen is {-aminoproprionitrile (BAPN), which has been studied extensively in turkeys and rats. This compound interrupts normal connective tissue protein cross-links by inactivating lysyl oxidase. The formation of lysine-derived aldehydes is inhibited,[66] resulting in weakened arterial walls, ectatic vessels, aortic dissections, aneurysm formation, and rupture.

Corticosteroids have also been used to induce aortic aneurysms or rupture in hamsters and mice. It was noted that hamsters treated with steroids during transplantation research protocols often died with massive intrathoracic or intraperitoneal hemorrhage.[67] Pathologic examination revealed that these animals had sustained aortic rupture. These findings led to clinical investigations, whereby aortic aneurysms and subsequent rupture were produced in hamsters over time depending on the corticosteroid dose used.[68] The heterozygous female Blotchy mouse was used by Reilly and coworkers to study the effects of steroids on aneurysm progression. Hydrocortisone was administered via drinking water in a concentration of 0.45 mg/mL. Aortic rupture was induced in 90% of these heterozygous females (which are usually resistant to aneurysm formation) within 2 weeks.[69] The mean aortic diameter was measured in normal C57BL6 mice who ingested hydrocortisone in similar doses. Aortic ectasia was seen even in these normal laboratory mice. Steroids are known to impair wound healing, reduce inflammation, and decrease protein and collagen synthesis, but the precise mechanism by which aneurysms are promoted is unknown. Steroids also cause salt retention and hypertension, yet no increase in blood pressure was seen in the hamster model of aneurysm rupture.[67] There is no known steroid effect on the expression of the major tissue inhibitor of matrix metalloproteinases (TIMP), and steroids actually decrease the expression of collagenase in fibroblasts in vitro,[70] so that the mechanism of aneurysm formation and rupture is yet to be elucidated.

Dietary Models

Dietary models of aneurysm disease have been based on the fact that copper is a necessary trace element for the activity of lysyl oxidase.[71] Pigs fed copper-deficient diets appear to be particularly prone to the development of aneurysms.[72] Tilson first proposed in 1981 that copper deficiency may be important in the pathogenesis of human aortic aneurysms.[73] Subsequently, other studies reported normal or even elevated hepatic and skin copper levels,[74,75] suggesting that the pathogenesis of aneurysm disease in humans is not comparable to the animal models which feature copper deficiency and reduced lysyl oxidase-dependent cross-linking.

Atherogenic diets have been used in an attempt to induce experimental aneurysms in animal models; however, true aneurysms are infrequent. Strickland reported only one aneurysm among 730 squirrel monkeys who were fed atherogenic diets.[76] Regression of atherosclerosis in dogs was associated with a unique form of aneurysm development, chiefly small "punched out" saccular lesions.[77] More recently, Zarins reported that 13% of cynomolgus monkeys developed aneurysms after being fed diets containing 25% peanut oil.[78] However, the criteria which were used to define aneurysms in this study were not clearly stated. In a subsequent study, animals placed on a regression diet following a period of hypercholesterolemia were noted to have a twofold increase in the area of the internal elastic lamella corresponding to a 38% increase in aortic diameter.[31] These results were based on six animals, of which one developed a large fusiform AAA. Whether or not the regression of atherosclerosis in humans contributes to aneurysm formation is presently an interesting, but unresolved question.

"Surgical" Models

The "surgical" models of aneurysm disease are due to iatrogenic destruction of the media and/or adventitia. Toxic substances such as acetrizoate can be introduced by intramedial injection.[79] The introduction of elastase has induced aneurysms in ex vivo infusion.[80] Dobrin found that elastase infusion resulted in dilatation, and infusion with collagenase resulted in rupture. Tilson et al made additional interpretations of this data, suggesting that the collagen must fail along with the elastin to get dilatation that approaches aneurysmal dimensions.[81]

An in vivo rat model has also been developed in which aneurysms were induced by perfusing an isolated segment of abdominal aorta with pancreatic elastase.[82] Aneurysm formation in vivo was associated with a marked inflammatory cell infiltrate comprised primarily of macrophages and T lymphocytes.[83] Recent work in our laboratory, using infusion of pancreatic elastase into an isolated segment of rat aorta, confirmed a significant inflammatory infiltrate during the evolution of AAAs in this model, along with a pattern of induction of endogenous proteinases.[84] Another surgical model of aneurysm formation occured in aortic allografts.[85] Transplantation of infrarenal segments from Wistar Kyoto (WKY) rats into spontaneously hypertensive rats (SHRs) resulted in dilation and/or aneurysm formation in at least two thirds of the specimens within a brief period of time. In contrast, SHR aortic allografts placed into WKY recipients remained isodiametric. Aortic allografts across the major histocompatibility barrier have also been studied in Brown-Norway and Lewis inbred rats. In this model, immunosuppression with cyclosporine (CsA) was explored as a means of preventing arterial allograft rejection and failure.[86] Aneurysmal dilatation was significantly reduced or prevented with all CsA regimens.

Role of Hemodynamics

The contribution of mechanical flow characteristics or hemodynamic factors to aneurysm development is also under investigation. It is known that the geometric changes of aneurysmal dilatation cause flow disturbances with boundary layer separation and reversal of flow.[32] These conditions contribute to the development of atherosclerosis and may potentiate aneurysm formation. Hemodynamic changes such as these are also seen in poststenotic dilatations.[87] Halsted first described a poststenotic dilatation in 1918 in a patient who developed a subclavian artery aneurysm distal to a stenosis caused by a cervical rib.[88] Poststenotic dilatations beyond coarctations are also well known. It is interesting that these lesions may become calcified and atherosclerotic,[89] even in young people without atherosclerotic risk factors.

The mechanisms of this type of aneurysmal dilatation were later studied by Roach and others.[87,90,91] Factors which have been postulated as initiators of poststenotic dilatation include elevated lateral wall pressures, abnormal shear stress, turbulence, and vibratory forces. Acceleration of flow past a stenotic segment creates an increase in the lateral wall pressures, as predicted by Bernoulli's principle. Endothelial cells which are exposed to abnormal pressures and shear stress can secrete vasoactive substances and other enzymatic factors which could promote matrix remodeling and vessel dilatation. In fact, increased collagenase activity of aortic tissue distal to a stenosis has been shown in the cynomolgus monkey.[92]

Asymmetrical flow patterns within the aorta are also felt to contribute to aneurysm development. The infrarenal aorta was examined by ultrasound in 329 World War II amputees and 702 other veterans who were similarly matched for age and arteriosclerotic risk factors. AAAs were found in 5.8% of the amputees compared with 1.1% of the nonamputees.[93] The asymmetrical flow pattern at the aortic bifurcation, as a consequence of unilateral flow reduction after leg amputation, was felt to be the principal cause of late aneurysmal degeneration of the aorta in this population.

Disparity in size or surface characteristics be-

tween a native artery and graft material causes compliance mismatch and turbulence, which can contribute to anastomotic aneurysms. Aneurysm formation is a reported complication of almost every prosthetic graft material used in vascular surgical procedures.[94] Bovine heterografts and human umbilical vein grafts, despite circumferential Dacron mesh reinforcement, have shown significant aneurysmal degeneration.[95] Similarly, venous autografts sometimes become aneurysmal, especially when used to bypass the popliteal artery in patients with an underlying predisposition to aneurysm disease. When used in extremity arterial reconstruction, the saphenous vein has a reported 4% incidence of aneurysm formation.[96]

Aspects of Material Failure in Abdominal Aortic Aneurysm Disease

Aneurysms are felt to occur secondary to the breakdown of the tensile strength of abdominal aorta in the face of systemic blood pressure. Several mechanical factors may play roles in this dilatation. The arterial pressure wave is transformed as it is transmitted from the aortic valve to the femoral arteries because of three factors. First, the aorta tapers in diameter as it travels from the supradiaphragmatic area to the subdiaphragmatic area. As it progresses distally, the aorta becomes stiffer with an increased ratio of collagen to elastin.[97,98] Third, the pressure wave reflects off the peripheral arteries to add to the incoming pressure wave. As atherosclerosis builds up in the ostia of the peripheral arteries, the reflected pressure wave theoretically increases. The combination of geometry, decreased compliance, and increased reflected pressure waves augments the arterial pressure in the abdominal aorta.

On the other hand, the abdominal aorta has a decreased margin of safety to handle the increasing load. The media of the aorta has minimal vasa vasorum.[99] Therefore, intima and media depend on diffusion from the lumen. This may render this zone susceptible to injury and may decrease the potential for repair. Furthermore, as atherosclerosis builds in the subendothelial region, diffusion may become increasingly impaired.

Elastin is arranged in layers between the SMCs to form lamellar units. The number of lamellar units is a function of the load carried by the arterial wall. A linear relationship prevails throughout mammalian species, except in the human abdominal aorta where there are fewer lamellar units than would be expected based upon the load that the abdominal aorta bears.[99] This may be one of the reasons why the abdominal aorta is the most frequent site of aneurysm formation. Thus, the abdominal aorta may have decreased strength, increased load, and decreased potential to recover from injury.

Biochemistry

Collagen

Dobrin isolated dog common carotid and human iliac arteries to study the effects of collagenase and elastase on the formation of aneurysms.[100] The tissue treated with collagenase dilated, became more compliant, and ruptured. Based on these studies, collagen was felt to have an important role in the tensile strength of the vessels.

The family of collagens is composed of more than 19 different kinds of collagen (Table 1).[101-104] Collagen is the most abundant protein in mammals and makes up about 30% of the protein content. Collagen is involved with early development, organogenesis, cell attachment, chemotaxis, platelet aggregation, and filtration through basement membranes. Collagen is felt to be the ECM protein that plays the dominant role in maintaining the structural integrity of tissues. Tissues rich in collagen include bone, skin, tendon, cartilage,

Table 1
Collagen Types and the Location of Their Genes on Human Chromosomes

Type	Constituent Chains	Gene	Chromosome	Occurrence
I	α_1(I)	COL1A1	17q21.3-q22	ubiquitous
	α_2(I)	COL1A2	7q21.3-q22	
II	α(II)	COL2A1	12q13-q14	cartilage, vitreous humor
III	α_1(III)	COL3A1	2q24.3-q31	As type I
IV	α_1(IV)	COL4A1	13q34	basement membrane
	α_2(IV)	COL4A2	13q34	
	α_3(IV)	COL4A3	2q35-q37	
	α_4(IV)	COL4A4	2q35-q37	
	α_5(IV)	COL4A5	Xq22	
V	α_1(V)	COL5A1	9q34.2-q34.3	interstitial tissue
	α_2(V)	COL5A2	2q24.3-q31	
	α_3(V)	COL5A3		
VI	α_1(VI)	COL6A1	21q22.3	soft tissue
	α_2(VI)	COL6A2	21q22.3	
	α_3(VI)	COL6A3	2q37	
VII	α_1(VII)	COL7A1	3p21	Anchoring fibrils
VIII	α_1(VIII)	COL8A1	3q12-q13.1	endothelium, mesenchyme
	α_2(VIII)	COL8A2	1p32.3-p34.3	
IX	α_1(IX)	COL9A1	6q12-q14	cartilage, vitreous humor
	α_2(IX)	COL9A2		
	α_3(IX)	COL9A3		
X	α_1(X)	COL10A1	6q13-q14	hypertrophic cartilage
XI	α_1(XI)	COL11A1	1p21	cartilage, vitreous humor
	α_2(XI)	COL11A2	6p21.2	
	α_3(XI)*	COL2A1*	12q13-q14	
XII	α_1(XII)	COL12A1	6	many tissues
XIII	α_1(XIII)	COL13A1	10q22	many tissues
XIV	α_1(XIV)	COL14A1		skin, tendon
XV	α_1(XV)	COL15A1	9q21-22	many tissues
XVI	α_1(XVI)	COL16A1	1p34-35	fibroblasts, keratinocytes
XVII	α_1(XVII)**	COL17A1	10q24.3	skin hemidesmosomes
XVIII	α_1(XVIII)	COL18A1		liver, kidney
Y	α_1(Y)***	D6S228E	6q12-q14	Rhabdomyosarcoma cells

* α_3(XI) is a post-translational variant of α_1(II); * also known as the 180 kDa bullous pemphigoid antigen; *** Only preliminarily characterized.
(Adapted with permission from Reference 105.)

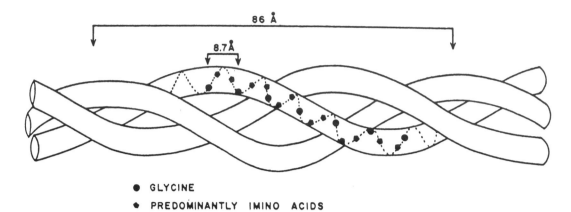

Figure 1. Collagen triple helix. The individual α chains are left-handed helices. The chains are, in turn, coiled around each other following a right-handed twist. (Reproduced with permission from Reference 118.)

ligaments, and vascular walls. Different tissues have varying amounts of each type of collagen.

The collagens are divided into four classes. Class I (collagen types I, II, III, V, and XI) forms long, uninterrupted collagenous domains that form fibrils and, therefore, is called the fibrillar collagens. Type I is the most abundant in humans. Class II collagen (collagen types IX and XII) does not form supramolecular aggregates alone, but participates in the formation of fibrils by adhering to the surface of filbrillar collagen. The third class (types IV, VI, VII, and X) forms supramolecular assemblies, independently. The last class includes various other types not able to be classified in the other groups.

These collagens can have various types of domains. All collagens are made up 3-α chains.[105] Each individual chain is made up a left-handed helix (Figure 1). The chains, in turn, are coiled around each other following a right-handed twist. Some collagens contain noncollagenous domains, in addition to the actual collagenous domains. Other collagens form sheets that make up basement membranes or laterally aggregated antiparallel dimers such as in anchoring fibrils. Finally, some collagens have tertiary forms that are globular domains interspersed between the α helices.

The hallmark of every type of collagen is a unique protein structure that consists of highly repetitive sequences of amino acids in the format Gly-X-Y, where the amino acid in the X position is frequently proline and the amino acid in the Y position is frequently hydroxyproline. This allows a regular pattern of the amino acids, helical formation of the molecules, and stable cross-linking between fibrils and, thus, maintains the tensile strength of collagen.[106,107]

The smallest amino acid, glycine, is essential in every third amino acid, as it occupies the restricted space in the center of the triple helix. Glycine is the only amino acid that fits into this position without disruption of the helices of collagen.[108] If a mutation changes this glycine, it would result in an interruption in the triple helix with changes in the stability of collagen.[109–117] Many mutations have been described in the primary sequence of the collagens (Table 2). Each mutation is associated with a disease process, with a change in the stability of collagen.

The study of these mutations is based on the understanding of the genetics and the synthesis of collagen. Many of the exons of the collagen gene are 54 base pairs in length and are separated by large introns, suggesting a common ancestral gene for collagens was assembled by multiple duplications of a single genetic unit. After transcription, the mRNA is spliced in the nucleus and then translated by the ribosome. As the peptide is being formed, some lysines and prolines are hydroxylated. Some of these hydroxylysine groups go on to be glycosylated. After certain cysteine residues are juxtaposed to allow formation of the disulfide bridges between the peptide chains, the triple helix forms between three chains to form procollagen (Figure 2). Procollagen is then packaged by the Golgi apparatus to form secretory vesicles which fuse with the cytoplasmic membrane for extrusion to take place (Figures 3 and 4).

Important extracellular events start with the extrusion. Lysyl oxidase deaminates lysine and hydroxylysine residues to form aldehydes. Lysyl oxidase is irreversible inhibited by {-aminopropionitrile. Formation of the aldehyde groups allows the formation of cross-links which are important for the structural integrity of collagen. The nonhelical amino and carboxyl extension of the procollagen molecule are cleaved, and the collagen molecules spontaneously aggregate into microfibrils composed of a quarter-staggered array of the collagen molecules by a process of nucleated growth (Figure 5). These microfibrils are cross-linked to form the collagen fibers. The collagen fiber itself

Table 2
Disease in Which Mutations in Collagen Genes or Deficiencies in the Activities of Post-Translational Enzymes of Collagen Synthesis Have Been Demonstrated

Disease	Gene or Enzyme
Osteogenesis imperfecta	COL1A1; COL1A2
Ehlers-Danlos syndrome type VIIA	COL1A1
Ehlers-Danlos syndrome type VIIB	COL1A2
Marfan's syndrome	COL1A2*
Osteoporosis	COL1A1; COL1A2
Achondrogenesis	COL2A1
Hypochondrogenesis	COL2A1
Spondyloepiphyseal dysplasia	COL2A1
Stickler syndrome	COL2A1
Osteoarthrosis	COL2A1; Col9A1**
Ehlers-Danlos syndrome type IV	COL3A1
Aortic aneurysms	COL3A1***
Alport syndrome	COL4A5
Epidermolysis bullosa, dystrophic forms	COL7A1
Spondylometaphseal dyplasia	COL10A1**
Ehlers-Danlos syndrome type VI	Lysyl hydroxylase
Ehlers-Danlos syndrome type VIIC	Procollagen N-proteinase
Ehlers-Danlos syndrome type IX	Lysl oxidase****
Menkes syndrome	Lysyl oxidase****

* In exceptional cases; >95% of Marfan's patients have a mutation in the gene for fibrillin on chromosome 15.

** Demonstrated so far only in transgenic mice.

*** In a small subset.

**** Secondary to an abnormality in copper metabolism.

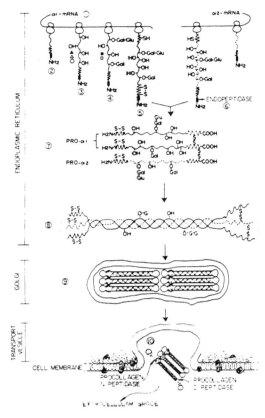

Figure 3. Summary of events in the biosynthesis of collagen: 1) synthesis of mRNAs; 2) translation of mRNA; 3) hydroxylation of proline and lysine residues; 4) glycosylation of hydroxylysine; 5) removal of N-terminal signal peptide; 6) release of completed α chains from ribosomes; 7) formation of disulfide cross-links; 8) folding of molecule to form triple helix; 9) packaging of procollagen into vessicles; and 10) extrusion of procollagen and removal of terminal extensions. (Reproduced with permission from Reference 118.)

TYPE I PROCOLLAGEN

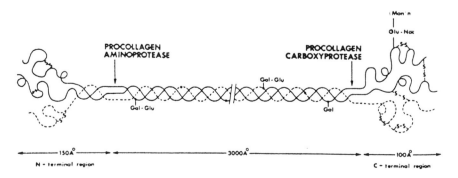

Figure 2. Procollagen molecule with its nonhelical extensions. (Reproduced with permission from Reference 118.)

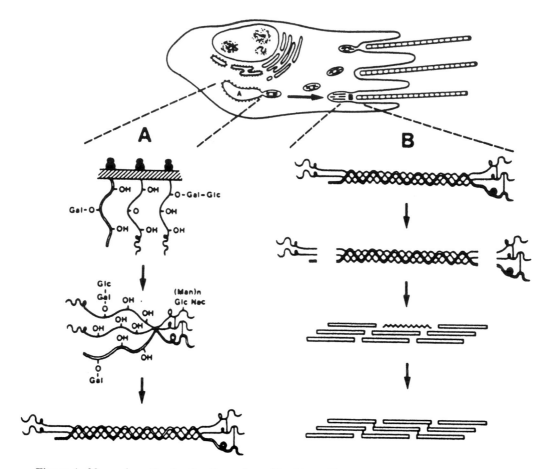

Figure 4. Normal synthesis of collagen by a fibroblast. The events depicted include synthesis of pro-α chains (**left**) by ribosomes, post-translational hydroxylations and glycosylations, folding into a triple helix, proteolytic cleavage of terminal extensions to form collagen, and self-assembly of fibrils by nucleated growth with covalent cross-linking of fibrils. (Reproduced with permission from Reference 108.)

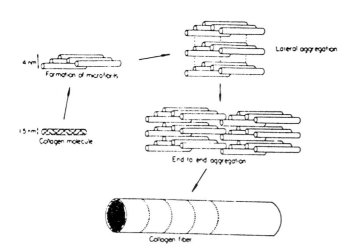

Figure 5. Formation of microfibril and aggregation to form fibers. (Reproduced with permission from Reference 118.)

most often is an assembly of two or more types of collagen, depending on the type of tissue it is making up.[118]

In the aorta, two thirds of the collagen is type I,[119] and it is mostly in the adventitial layer. The metabolism of collagen in normal tissue is a balance between degradation and biosynthesis.[97] If the balance between degradation and production were upset, this might contribute to the weakening of the aortic wall.

After Sumner et al reported a decrease in collagen and elastin contents of AAA in autopsy specimens,[45] other studies have shown a more variable content of collagen with some reporting normal or high levels.[119,120] An increase may not be entirely unexpected, as the cells of the connective tissue matrix have a substantial potential for the synthesis of new collagen. However, these cells may not be able to synthesize new collagen with the intricate fibrillar structure or the mature cross-linking needed to maintain the strength and the normal diameter of the abdominal aorta.

Elastin

In an ex vivo model of human iliac arteries,[100] the vessels treated with elastase dilated and became stiffer. Elastin is felt to contribute elastic recoil to the aorta, and it is mostly found in the media.

Elastin is a 74 kDa molecule. It is extremely insoluble and is characterized by its lysine cross-links.[121] High elastin content is found in skin, ligaments, lung, and the wall of arteries. The amino acid sequence of elastin is one third glycine and approximately 11% proline.[122] It has very little hydroxyproline and no hydroxylysine. It is rich in nonpolar amino acids such as alanine, valine, leucine, and isoleucine.[123,124] The half-life of elastin is estimated to be 70 years.[125] This stability may be due to high number of cross-links of elastin.[126] Elastin is characterized by its rapid extensibility to two to three times its resting length and its recoil.

The biochemistry of elastogenesis is poorly understood in comparison to that of collagen. There is a large amount of formation of elastin in late fetal life, which is complete by the first decade of life. Elastin is produced by SMCs, chondroblasts, mesothelial cells, fibroblasts, and myofibroblasts. Elastin undergoes little intracellular post-transcriptional modifications. Since elastin has no glycosylation to act as intracellular trafficking signals, a receptor seems to specifically bind to elastin intracellularly to "chaperone" the elastin molecule to the cell surface.

Elastin is laid as amorphous clumps on a microfibrillar scaffold. As the precursor form tropoelastin is laid down onto the microfibrills, cross-links formed by lysyl oxidase allow the clumps to coalesce to form the final product of elastin.

The marked decrease of elastin in AAAs on histology and biochemical assays is felt to be evidence that the degradation of elastin also plays a significant role in the pathogenesis of AAAs.[46,51,127–131] Although the recent work of Baxter has questioned whether there is conservation of the disrupted elastin, considering the total mass of an AAA,[131] there have been numerous studies focused on the elastases as a contributing cause of AAAs.

Other Matrix Components

Laminin, glycosaminoglycans, proteoglycans, and fibronectin may also play a role in aneurysm formation, perhaps by involvement with aspects of resistance to inflammation, or perhaps, by significant variations in primary structure. The aortic matrix was long felt to be an inert framework. More recently, it has become appreciated that the matrix macromolecules play a central role in the remodeling, degradation, and formation of new connective tissue. Some evidence suggests that after injury, the matrix releases basic fibroblast growth factor (bFGF) causing cell proliferation.[132] The matrix also may serve as a roadmap for inflammatory cells as they are being attracted to injury, by serving as binding sites for specific receptors of inflammatory cells.[132]

Proteases

Elastases

In 1982, Busuttil reported elevated elastase activity in the walls of AAAs.[133] Cannon and Read attributed this to a serine protease. They detected elevated serum elastolytic activity in patients with AAAs who smoked. They found elevated activity of the granules in the peripheral neutrophils and attributed it to leukocyte elastase.[134] Dubick et al also implicated a serine protease, based on the finding that the activity was inhibited by the serine protease inhibitor phenyl methyl sulfonyl fluoride (PMSF). This research group proposed that it was pancreatic elastase, based on immunoreactivity to an antibody to pancreatic elastase.[128] Cohen et al found the highest release of elastolytic activity from cultured SMCs of the aorta in response to elastin degradation products in AAA patients. They found the activity to be inhibited by PMSF and attributed it to a serine protease, perhaps a smooth muscle elastase.[135]

However, studies starting with Brown et al suggested a nonserine protease based on a failure of inhibition with PMSF.[136] A specific leucocyte elastase assay with substrate pyro-glutamine proline valine p-nitro-anilide and S2484 failed to show any activity. Both pancreatic and leucocyte elastase hydrolyze fluoresceinated elastin, but this elastase did not. The activity was inhibited with EDTA (ethylenediamine tetraacetic acid) which suggested a metalloprotease. There was moderate inhibition with antipain and leupeptin, which are thiol protease inhibitors, and moderate inhibition with pepstatin, a carboxyl enzyme inhibitor. Thus, the protease was found to have characteristics of thiol, carboxyl, and metalloenzymes. Campa found that the elastase did not cross-react with antibody to leucocyte elastase, and confirmed the inhibition with EDTA.[129]

Reilly confirmed inhibition with EDTA in an experiment to study the degradation of intact elastin in frozen section by the elastase.[137] This protease then was found to bind with recombinant tissue inhibitor of metaloprotease (TIMP) allowing partial purification. An antibody to matrix metalloprotease 9 (MMP 9) reacts with the partially purified activity by immunoblotting technique and immunoprecipitates the enzymatic activity.[138] As MMP 9 has been shown to have

Table 3

Name	Size kDa	Degrades
MMP 1		
(type I collagenase)	42	I, II, III collagen
(interstitial collagenase)		
(vertebral collagenase)		
MMP 2		
(human 72 kDa gelatinase)	66	IV, V, VII collagen
(72 kDa gelatinase)		
(type IV collagenase)		
MMP 3		
(stromelysin)	48	proteoglycans, Laminin, fibronectin,
(proteoglycanase)		III, IV, V collagen, gelatins
(transin)		
(procollagen-activating factor)		
MMP 7		
(pump-1)	19	gelatins, fibronectin
(small metalloproteinase of uterus)		
(putative MMP 1)		
MMP 8		
(pmn collagenase)	65	I, II, III collagen
MMP 9		
(human 92 kDa gelatinase)	84	IV, V collagen, gelatins
(type IV collagenase)		
(gelatinase type B)		
MMP 10		
(human stromelysin 2)	47	III, IV, V collagen, fibronectin, gelatins
(transin 2)		

A summary of the MMPs and their common names.
(Adapted with permission from References 141 and 226.)

elastolytic activity in other studies,[139,140] we believe that MMP 9 is an excellent candidate for being an important elastase of AAA disease.

The MMPs are a group of proteases found in the matrix of connective tissue. They digest collagen, elastin, fibronectin, laminins, and proteoglycans.[141] They are felt to be important in the constant remodeling of tissue matrix. Each is associated with zinc and has highly conserved areas of amino acid sequence. They have also been called the "matrixins." Table 3 shows some of the known MMPs and their common names.

MMP 3 has been found to activate the precursor forms of MMP 1 and MMP 9.[142,143] This may have important consequences for a special role for activated MMP 3 in activating other members of the MMP family.

Two specific inhibitors have been found to exist for the MMPs. TIMP1 is 29 kDa while TIMP2 is approximately 20 kDa.[144,145] TIMPs are heavily glycosylated proteins with 30% of the molecular weight being attributed to carbohydrate.[146] Of note, TIMP has been found to be secreted in complexes with the MMPs.[147]

Collagenases

In 1980, Busuttil demonstrated increased collagenase activity in AAA samples.[133] Menashi found the collagenolytic activity was elevated in ruptured AAA tissue or explant cultures, but detected none in unruptured AAA tissue.[120] Another study found no detectable collagenase.[148] One group felt that the activity was increased, but the enzyme was not extractable.[149] On the other hand, Vine and Powell reported the detection of collagenase by C-14 collagen assay and by specific antibody in the extracts of AAA tissue.[150] Some of the differences in results may have arisen because the collagenase may be bound to its inhibitor, thereby masking its detection.

Recent work in our laboratory has focused on this issue of whether collagenase (MMP 1) is present. After running the extracted proteins from AAA specimens on PAGE (polyacrylamide gel electrophoresis) and equalizing for protein loads, immunoblotting was performed under nonreducing and reducing conditions to detect the enzyme in its complex forms and isoforms.

Antibody to MMP 1 reacts strongly with bands corresponding to the expected molecular forms of MMP 1, with low levels in controls.[151]

Plasmin

Plasmin may also be involved with the cascade of the development of aneurysms. In other recent studies, we have detected plasmin by immunoblotting techniques in AAA tissue.[151A] Plasmin degrades ECM and activates MMP 9, MMP 3, and MMP 1.[152] Thus, it could also play a central role in the development of AAA. Anidjar et al have shown that plasmin and macrophages infused together into the aortas of rats resulted in aneurysm formation.[82] However, infusion of neither macrophages nor plasmin alone resulted in aneurysms. The development of these aneurysms was accompanied by a dense inflammatory infiltrate consisting of mostly macrophages and lymphocytes.[153]

Tissue plasminogen activator (tPA) has also been found to be elevated in AAAs compared to that of aorto-occlusive disease.[154] tPA is produced by arterial smooth muscle and has the additional property of inducing secretion of MMP 9 by macrophages.[155]

Inhibitors of Proteases

While some investigators have postulated that overactivity of the proteolytic enzymes, such as the elastases and the collagenases, may play an important role in the development of aneurysms, others have suggested that there may be a failure of proteolytic inhibitors contributing to the breakdown of matrix proteins. Cohen proposed that there may be an imbalance between serine elastase and its inhibitor, α-1 antitrypsin. A decreased ratio of α-1 antitrypsin to elastase was found in AAA patients, as compared to that of normal or aorto-occlusive patients. Patients with ruptured aneurysms had the lowest ratio.[156,157]

Smoking is a risk factor for the development of AAAs. There is data suggesting that smoking methylates α-1 antitrypsin and, thereby, inactivates the enzyme.[158] Serum elastase activity is higher in AAA patients who smoke when compared to nonsmoking AAA patients and patients with aorto-occlusive disease.[159] The activity of α-1 antitrypsin inhibitor seems to be increased in AAA patients versus that of aorto-occlusive disease patients.[160] One of the more significant risk factors found for AAA rupture is the degree of chronic obstructive pulmonary disease (COPD) in patients.[161] Perhaps, the same enzymatic processes occurring in these patients' lungs resulting in the COPD may be also influencing the integrity of the connective tissue of the aortic wall.

Cohen et al looked at the α-1 antitrypsin phenotypes of 47 patients with AAAs. They found the MZ phenotype to occur significantly more often in AAA patients than would be expected in the general population. The MZ phenotype is associated with 65% reduction in the normal inhibitory capacity of serum. Perhaps this may represent a genetic predisposition of AAA patients to have lower levels of α-1 antitrypsin activity.[162] However, a separate study did not confirm these results and, therefore, the question remains open.[163]

Our research group has found that AAA patients may have a relative deficiency of TIMP.[164] This deficiency may allow MMPs to digest more structural proteins, resulting in weakening of the aortic wall. DNA sequencing of the TIMP gene in six patients with AAAs revealed that two patients had an identical point mutation at codon 101.[164] However, as this was in the third position of the codon, the amino acid was conserved. This limited study, to date, did not establish any abnormality of TIMP1 expression. Further investigation may yet demonstrate that TIMP1 or TIMP2 may be involved with an imbalance between the proteinases and their inhibitors.

The genes controlling production and remodeling of the macromolecules of the matrix may also play an important role in the development of aneurysms. They may be involved with permitting either a genetic predisposition or a biochemical milieu that would contribute to the failure of the integrity of the connective tissue matrix. Studies cited earlier in this chapter suggesting a hereditary predisposition for the development of AAAs would implicate these genes.

Some studies have looked at properties of DNA and RNA involved in the production of collagen in AAA patients. As yet, no structural mutations or evidence for decreased expression of the transcribed mRNAs has been found to help explain the weakening of collagen in the ECM in a large portion of AAA patients.[108,165] Other studies of the genes controlling proteinases and their inhibitors have not revealed how they may be involved with the development of AAAs.[166] Other possibilities include a genetic influence that exposes the immune system to an abnormal antigen as an initial insult or an abnormal response of the immune response to this antigen. Studies are ongoing to define the putative "AAA gene(s)."

Cellular Pathophysiology of Matrix Destruction

Investigation of the proteases has led to studies of their cellular origins. SMCs in the media and fibroblasts in the adventitia produce ECM.[167–172] Other studies show that they may also be involved with the production and regulation of the proteases involved with the breakdown of the matrix.[151,173] Marshall et al showed that mesothelial cells produced both metalloproteinases and TIMP.[174] Cohen suggested that the SMCs were producing the elastase of interest.[175] In a sheep model, Il-1{ (interleukin-1{) stimulated aortic explants to produce stromelysin, gelatinase, collagenase, and TIMP. This response was increased with TNF-α. Because of the fastidious growth requirements of these cells, the authors felt that these were SMCs.[176] Another study found that monolayers of mesenchymal cells from explants of thoracic aorta produced MMP 1 in response to platelet-derived growth factor (PDGF).[54] The authors felt that based on the "hill and valley" morphology, these cells were SMCs. Preliminary data from our lab also suggests that both mesenchymal cells and endothelial cells may be sources of MMP 1 in the adventitia.[176A]

Macrophages are abundant in the cellular infiltrate of aneurysm walls,[30,49,51,177] and may play a central role in the sequence of events in the pathogenesis of aneurysms. Preliminary work from our lab (and previous work from others) suggest that the AIM cells may produce cytokines, superoxide radicals, and a myriad of proteases including the metalloproteases.[178–180] The macrophages play a pivotal role in modulating the turnover of matrix by secretion of proteases, such as elastases and collagenases,[181,182] and by the production of cytokines. The Il-1 and TNF released by macrophages may alter the expression of SMC genes for collagenase and TIMP.[183] Both Il-1{ and TNF-α have been found to be released by cells cultured from AAA tissue (unpublished data). In addition, the secreted products of cultured aortic macrophages stimulate medial explants of AAA patients to produce six times the control level of collagenase.[184] The products released by the macrophages may degrade the ECM, stimulate lymphocytes, amplify the response of lymphocytes, and continue the inflammatory cycle.

Brophy et al found large amounts of plasma cells and Russell bodies in the walls of AAAs.[51] Macrophage Fc receptors regulate secretion of proteinases by receptor-specific mechanisms.[185] Furthermore, in the Anidjar/Dobrin model of aneurysms after infusion of the aorta with elastase, we have also found deposition of immunoglobulin on the elastic lamina of the aorta.[186] These findings implicate a possible immune response in the development of AAAs.

Elastin degradation products (EDPs) are highly chemotactic.[187] As elastin is broken down by elastases released by the macrophages and/or the mesenchymal cells, the EDPs released would theoretically attract more macrophages, which would release more cytokines and proteinases. This notion would help link the proteolytic process to the immune response in the overall picture of AAA development.

Cytokines also play a role in the maintenance and repair of the connective tissue matrix. They could play a role in the activation and proliferation of inflammatory cells and communication between the cells. For example, TNF-α and Il-1{ are secreted by macrophages and T cells. They function to activate macrophages and mesenchymal cells to produce MMPs.[188,189] Il-1 increases collagen synthesis.[190] TNF-α is cytotoxic and inhibits the growth of SMC.[191] Transforming growth factor-β (TGF-{) has been shown to upregulate TIMP, downregulate MMP 1 and MMP 3,[192] and increase secretion of elastin.[193] TGF-{ is one of the more potent stimulators of collagen synthesis.[172,190,194,195] Gamma interferon inhibits smooth muscle proliferation[196,197] and may decrease collagen synthesis.[198–200] Il-1 and TGF-{ upregulate their own gene expression, which may serve as another important positive feedback loop.[201] The mechanism by which these cytokines may play a role in inflammation of the aortic matrix is under investigation.

A new set of molecules called the integrins and intracellular adhesion molecules (ICAMs) have been proposed to play a significant role in inflammation and remodeling of connective tissue matrix. ICAM levels are increased in endothelial cell tissue culture when exposed to Il-1{ and TNF-α.[202] The integrins are transmembrane glycoproteins which act as receptors for inflammatory cells.[203] They bind to endothelial adhesion molecules and the ECM macromolecules to result in the adhesion of inflammatory cells to the endothelium, proliferation, locomotion, and cell differentiation.[204] These adhesion molecules may have a crucial role in the immune phase of aneurysm development, other connective tissue inflammatory states, and tumor metastasis.[205]

It is possible to develop a hypothetical schema of the interactions of the immune system and the proteolytic processes involved with the pathogenesis of AAAs. An initial insult on the matrix, influenced by a genetic predisposition, may result in degradation of some structural proteins. The destruction of these proteins could lead to weakening of the aortic matrix, and products of the degradation would trigger further inflammation. An immune response would intensify the degradation of the ECM, with the production of more proteases and cytokines. The system would continue to propagate itself without the negative feedback loop seen in normal biologic systems (Figure 6).

Inflammatory Aneurysms

It is still uncertain whether the inflammatory aneurysm is the "tail-end" of the normal distribution of the spectrum of inflammation seen in all AAAs, or whether it is a truly unique disease entity. Inflammatory aneurysms (IAAAs) are characterized by a dense, fibrotic,

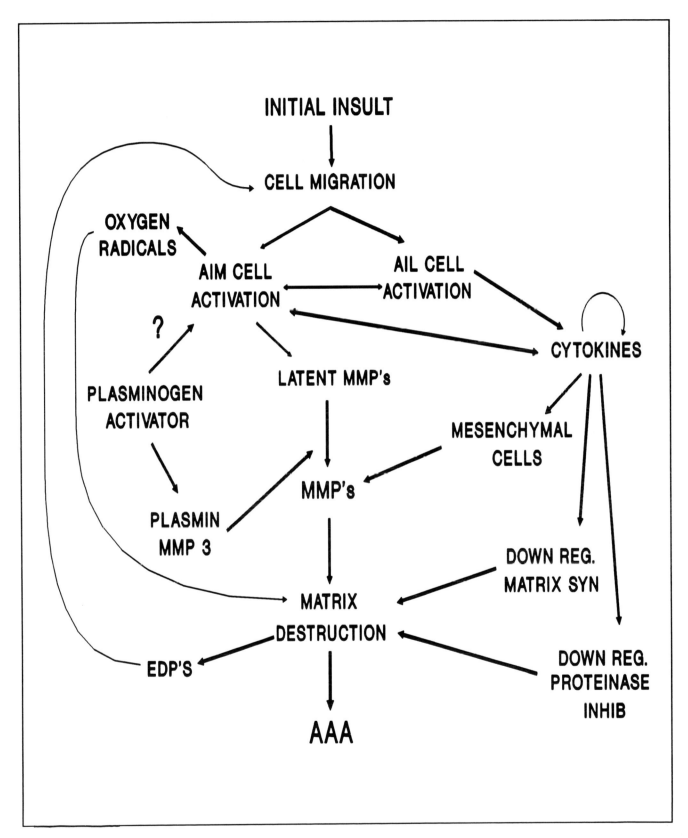

Figure 6. A summary of the pathogenesis of AAA.

glistening inflammatory infiltrate surrounding the aorta that, at times, involves the ureters, duodenum, or inferior vena cava.[127,206] They develop excessive mural thickening, often sparing the posterior wall. IAAAs may make up as much as 7.2% of AAAs as noted in one recent series.[207] Again, the types of cells seen by immunohistochemistry are the macrophages, B cells, and the T cells, with sparse edematous amorphous fibrillary elastin in the adventitia.[208] The inflammatory infiltrate of IAAAs seems more pronounced than that of AAAs with more B cells and macrophages.[30] The cause of these aneurysms is unclear. One interesting possibility is the liberation from the attacked matrix of some particular EDP or cytokine with intense angiogenic properties.

Molecular Basis of Aneurysm Disease

By analogy to osteogenesis imperfecta and forms of Ehlers-Danlos, it may be expected that different mutations will be found to correlate with different phenotypic variations of AAA disease. There have recently been significant new developments with respect to understanding the molecular basis of Marfan's syndrome, a connective tissue disorder involving the skeleton, eyes, and cardiovascular system.[209,210] A microfibrillary protein called fibrillin was discovered by Sakai in 1986, and an abnormality of fibrillin has now been found in Marfan's patients. A combination of "classic" and "reverse" genetics has lead to the discovery of fibrillin as the biochemical basis of Marfan's.

The classic approach is to begin with a candidate protein and to pursue it to the gene level, while the reverse approach is to start with genomic DNA of members of affected families. One then studies the segregation of different chromosomes with the phenotype by analysis of marker restriction fragment length polymorphisms within the family. Eventually, the long arm of chromosome 15 was assigned the Marfan gene using the reverse approach in several Finnish families.[211] Along the classic line, in 1990, an abnormality of fibrillin in skin and cultured fibroblasts from Marfan's syndrome was found,[212] and the gene was mapped to the same chromosome.[213] Dietz then reported an identical point mutation in the fibrillin gene in two Marfan's patients, changing the codon for arginine at residue 239 to glycine.[209]

Kontussarri et al defined the first mutation cosegregating with the aneurysm phenotype in a family with AAAs.[214] A point mutation in the procollagen III gene at position 691 changes a glycine to arginine. This results in a thermally unstable collagen with a decrease in the melting point. Changing from a small amino acid to a larger amino acid may interfere with the triple helical structure of the collagen and lead to instability.

However, two of the patients ruptured their aneurysms at young ages, which is atypical of the common form of AAAs. On follow-up sonography of three family members with the mutation, one 16-year-old boy developed an early aortic aneurysm.[108] This family may be come to be viewed as a Ehlers-Danlos IV variant.[215]

Based on this study and the syndromes of Ehlers-Danlos where there are hereditary mutations of collagen synthesis, others have tried to determine if other mutations of collagen may contribute to the pathogenesis of AAAs. One study has examined the cultures of skin fibroblasts of 14 patients with AAAs.[216] Two of the patients were found to have an elevated collagen type I:III ratio. One of the patients had decreased amounts of intracellular procollagen III. The other patient had altered thermal stability of collagen, suggesting a change in the amino acid sequence.

DNA sequencing was performed on 54 patients with AAAs using PCR (polymerase chain reaction).[165] Two mutations of the procollagen III gene were found. In one patient, the change of a threonine for a proline was felt not to be a cause of destabilization of the collagen since 6 of 14 threonines are also in the third position of the Gly-X-Y sequence of collagen.[217] In addition, threonine and proline have been exchanged during the evolution of collagen.[218]

The second patient had a point mutation with a change of glycine to an arginine at amino acid number 136. The patient was an 18–year-old with a dissection of the entire aorta and generalized fibromuscular dysplasia. Three siblings with the same mutation are unaffected as of yet. This finding may be more relevant to the understanding of aortic dissection in non-Marfanoid patients than to the common pattern of AAA disease with clusters of older brothers.

Powell et al found an association of AAAs with one of the alleles for haptoglobin on chromosome 16. The gene product of this allele appears to promote the activity of a serine elastase in vitro and may be another mechanism for amplifying the initial insult to the matrix of the aorta.[219] However, this result has not been confirmed so far in a separate study by Webster.[163]

Potential for Intervention Based on Pathophysiology

Pieces of the puzzle to understand the sequence or cascade of events for the development of AAAs are slowly falling into place. Each of these steps presents an opportunity to slow or halt the cycle of inflammation leading to degradation of proteins, weakening of the matrix, and more inflammation. Theoretically, some interventions could lead to stabilization of the connective tissue matrix or perhaps prevent the disease entirely, in patients who may be defined in the future as genetically susceptible.

For example, propranolol appears to reduce the incidence of AAA formation in the BAPN-treated turkey model by some property other than its effect on blood pressure and pulse.[220] Propranolol also decreases the rate of aneurysm formation and may stabilize connective tissue in the Blotchy mouse model.[221] It has been proposed that the effect of propranolol is a direct stimulus promoting the cross-links of collagen, thereby increasing the stability of connective tissue matrix.[222-226]

If the gene for the initial susceptibility to formation of AAAs were found, perhaps screening for the gene could result in identification of a high-risk population where intervention would lead to the greatest impact on the progression of the disease. If inflammation is found to be a fundamental pathophysiologic feature of aneurysms, anti-inflammatory medications may help slow the progression of the disease. If the inciting cause of the original inflammation were characterized, perhaps early intervention may lead to halting the cycle of degradation of the ECM. Now, as the elements of the sequence are being understood, each step poses an opportunity to intervene in the progression of the process.

Acknowledgment: Special acknowledgment to Madeline Vitale for expert technical assistance.

References

1. Silverberg E, Boring CC, Squires TS: Cancer statistics 1990. *Cancer J Clin* 40:9–26, 1990.
2. Bengtsson H, Bergqvist D: Ruptured abdominal aortic aneurysm: a population-based study. *J Vasc Surg* 18:74–80, 1993.
3. Melton L, Bickerstaff L, Hollier L, et al: Changing incidence of abdominal aortic aneurysms: a population-based study. *Am J Epidemiol* 120:379–386, 1984.
4. Bengtsson H, Bergqvist D, Sternby NH: Increasing prevalence of abdominal aortic aneurysms: a necropsy study. *Eur J Surg* 158:19–23, 1992.
5. Fowkes FGR, MacIntyre CA, Ruckley CV: Increasing incidence of aortic aneurysms in England and Wales. *Br Med J* 298:33–35, 1989.
6. Lillienfeld DE, Gunderson PD, Sprafka JM, et al: The epidemiology of abdominal aortic aneurysms: mortality trends in the United States 1951–1980. *Arteriosclerosis* 7:637–643, 1987.
7. Castleden WM, Mercer JC, and members of the West Australian Vascular Service: Abdominal aortic aneurysms in Western Australia: descriptive epidemiology and patterns of rupture. *Br J Surg* 72:109–112, 1985.
8. Collin J: The epidemiology of abdominal aortic aneurysms. *Br J Hosp Med* July 64–67, 1988.
9. Johnson G, Avery A, McDougal G, et al: Aneurysms of the abdominal aorta: incidence in blacks and whites in North Carolina. *Arch Surg* 120:1138–1140, 1985.
10. Collin J: A proposal for a precise definition of abdominal aortic aneurysm: a personal view. *J Cardiovasc Surg* 31:168–169, 1990.
11. Cronenwett J, Murphy T, Zelnock G, et al: Actuarial analysis of variables associated with rupture of small abdominal aortic aneurysms. *Surgery* 98:472–483, 1985.
12. Sterpetti AV, Schultz RD. Feldhaus RJ et al: Factors influencing enlargement rate of small abdominal aortic aneurysms. *J Surg Res* 43:211–219, 1987.
13. Ouriel K, Green RM, Donayre C, et al: An evaluation of new methods of expressing aortic aneurysm size: relationship to rupture. *J Vasc Surg* 15(1):12–20, 1992.
14. Johnston KW, Rutherford RB, Tilson MD, et al: Suggested standards for reporting on arterial aneurysms. *J Vasc Surg* 13:452–458, 1991.
15. Collin J, Araujo L, Walton J, Lindsell D: Oxford screening programme for abdominal aortic aneurysm in men aged 65–74 years. *Lancet* 2:613–615, 1988.
16. Webster MW, Ferrell RE, St. Jean PL, et al: Ultrasound screening of first-degree relatives of patients with an abdominal aortic aneurysm. *J Vasc Surg* 13:9–14, 1991.
17. Collin J, Walton J: Is abdominal aortic aneurysm familial? *Br Med J* August 19, 299:493, 1989.
18. Bengtsson H, Sonesson B, Lanne T, et al: Prevalence of abdominal aortic aneurysm in the offspring of patients dying from aneurysm rupture. *Br J Surg* 82:1142–1143, 1992.
19. Bengtsson H, Norrgard O, Angquist KA, Eckberg O, Obereg L, Bergqvist D: Ultrasonographic screening of the abdominal aorta among siblings of patients with abdominal aortic aneurysms. *Br J Surg* 76:589–591, 1989.
20. Scarpa A: *Treatise on the Anatomy, Pathology, and Surgical Treatment of Aneurism, With Engravings.* Translated from the Italian by John Henry Wishart. Edinburgh: FRCS, 1808.
21. Hammond E, Garfield L: Coronary heart disease, stroke, and aortic aneurysm. *Arch Environ Health* 19:167–189, 1969.
22. Reed D, Reed C, Stemmermann G, Haysashi T: Are aortic aneurysms caused by atherosclerosis? *Circulation* 85:205–211, 1992.
23. Darling III RC, Brewster DC, Darling RC, et al: Are familial abdominal aortic aneurysms different? *J Vasc Surg* 10:39–43, 1989.
24. Johnston KW, Scobli KT: Multicenter prospective study of nonruptured abdominal aortic aneurysms. I. Population and operative management. *J Vasc Surg* 7:69–81, 1988.
25. Reilly JM, Tilson MD: Incidence and etiology of abdominal aortic aneurysms. *Surg Clin N Am*, 69:705–711, 1989.
26. Strachan DP: Predictors of death from aortic aneurysm among middle-aged men: the Whitehall study. *Br J Surg* 78:401–404, 1991.
27. Norrgard O, Anguist KA, Dahlen G: High concentrations of Lp(a) lipoproteins in serum are common among patients with abdominal aortic aneurysms. *Int Angiol* 7:46–49, 1987.
28. Tilson MD: Aortic aneurysms and atherosclerosis (editorial). *Circulation* 85:378–379, 1992.
29. Cohen JR, Sarfati I, Ratner L, Tilson MD: Alpha-1 antitrypsin phenotypes in patients with abdominal aortic aneurysms. *J Surg Res* 49:319–321, 1991.
30. Koch AE, Haines GK, Rizzo RJ: Human abdominal aortic aneurysms: immunophenotypic analysis suggesting an immune-mediated response. *Am J Pathol* 137:1199–1219, 1990.
31. Zarins CK, Xu C, Glagov S: Aneurysmal enlargement of the aorta during regression of experimental atherosclerosis. *J Vasc Surg* 15:90–101, 1992.

32. Scherer PW: Flow in an axisymmetrical glass model aneurysm. *J Biomech* 6:695–700, 1973.
33. Clifton M: Familial abdominal aortic aneurysms. *Br J Surg* 64:765–766, 1977.
34. Tilson MD, Dang C: Generalized arteriomegaly: a possible predisposition to the formation of abdominal aortic aneurysms. *Arch Surg* 16:1030, 1981.
35. Norrgard O, Rais O, Angquist KA: Familial occurrence of abdominal aortic aneurysms. *Surgery* 95:650–656, 1984.
36. Tilson MD, Seashore MR: Human genetics of abdominal aortic aneurysm. *Surg Gynecol Obstet* 15:129, 1984.
37. Tilson MD, Seashore MR: Fifty families with abdominal aortic aneurysms in two or more first-order relatives. *Am J Surg* 147:551–553, 1984.
38. Johansen K, Koepsell T: Familial tendency for abdominal aortic aneurysms. *JAMA* 256:1934–1936, 1986.
39. Cole CW, Barber GG, Bouchard AG, et al: Abdominal aortic aneurysm: consequences of a positive family history. *Can J Surg* 32:117–120, 1988.
40. Tilson MD, Gandhi RH, Rutherford RB: Arterial aneurysms: etiologic considerations. In: *Vascular Surgery*. 4th ed. Philadelphia: WB Saunders, Co.; 253–264, 1995.
41. Powell JT, Greenhalgh RM: Multifactorial inheritance of abdominal aortic aneurysm. *Eur J Vasc Surg* 1:29–31, 1987.
42. Majmunder PP, St. Jean PL, Rerrell RE, et al: On the inheritance of abdominal aortic aneurysm. *Am J Hum Genetics* 48:164–170, 1991.
43. Martin P: On abdominal aortic aneurysms. *J Cardiovasc Surg* 19:597–598, 1978.
44. Tilson MD, Stansel HC: Differences in results for aneurysms vs. occlusive disease after bifurcation grafts: results of 100 elective grafts. *Arch Surgery* 115:1173–1175, 1980.
45. Sumner DS, Hokanson DE, Strandness DE: Stress-strain characteristics and collagen-elastin content of abdominal aortic aneurysms. *Surg Gynecol Obstet* 130:459–466, 1970.
46. Tilson MD: Histochemistry of aortic elastin in patient with nonspecific aortic aneurysmal disease. *Arch Surg* 123:503–505, 1988.
47. Zarins CK, Glagov S: Aneurysms and obstructive plaques: differing local responses to atherosclerosis. In: Bergan JJ, Yao JST (eds). *Aneurysms: Diagnosis and Treatment.* New York: Grune and Stratton, Inc; 61–82, 1981.
48. White JV, Haas K, Phillips S, Comerota AJ: Adventitial elastolysis is a primary event in aneurysm formation. *J Vasc Surg* 17(2):371–381, 1993.
49. Beckman EN: Plasma cell infiltrates in abdominal aortic aneurysm. *Amer J Clin Path* 85:21–24, 1986.
50. Jonasson L, Holm J, Skalli O: Regional accumulation of T cells, macrophages, and smooth muscle cells in the human atherosclerotic plaque. *Arteriosclerosis* 6:131–138, 1986.
51. Brophy CM, Reilly JM, Smith GJW, Tilson MD: The role of inflammation in nonspecific abdominal aortic aneurysm disease. *Ann Vasc Surg* 5:229–233, 1991.
52. Pasquinelli G, et al: An immunohistochemical study of inflammatory abdominal aortic aneurysms. *J Submic Cytol Pathol* 25(1):103–112, 1993.
53. Evans CH, Georgescu HI, Lin CS, et al: Inducible synthesis of collagenase by cells of aortic origin. *J Surg Res* 51:399–404, 1991.
54. Yanagi H, Sasaguri Y, Sugama K, Morimatsu M, Nagase H: Production of tissue collagenase (matrix metalloproteinase 1) by human aortic smooth muscle cells in response to platelet-derived growth factor. *Atherosclerosis* 3:207–216, 1991.
55. Rowe DW, McGoodwin EB, Martin GR, et al: A sex-linked defect in the cross-linking of collagen and elastin associated with the mottled locus in mice. *J Exp Med* 139:180–192, 1974.
56. Hunt DM: Primary defect in copper transport underlies mottled mutants in the mouse. *Nature* 249:852, 1974.
57. Rowe DW, McGoodwin EB, Martin GR, Grahn D: Decreased lysyl oxidase activity in the aneurysm-prone mottled mouse. *J Biol Chem* 252:939, 1977.
58. Elefteriades J, Panjabi MJ, Tilson MD: Reduced tensile strength of skin from the spontaneously aneurysm-prone Blotchy mouse. *Surg Forum* 33:58–60, 1982.
59. Danks DM, Campbell PE, Walker-Smith G, et al: Menkes' kinky-hair syndrome. *Lancet* 1:1100, 1972.
60. Danks DM, Campbell PE, Stevens PJ, et al: Menke's kinky hair syndrome: an inherited defect in copper absorption with widespread effects. *Pediatrics* 50:188–201, 1972.
61. Brophy CM, Tilson JE, Braverman IM, Tilson MD: Age of onset, pattern of distribution, and histology of aneurysm development in a genetically predisposed mouse model. *J Vasc Surg* 8:45–48, 1988.
62. Andrews EJ, White WJ, Bullock LP: Spontaneous aortic aneurysms in Blotchy mice. *Am J Pathol* 78:199, 1975.
63. Gresham GA, Howard AN: Aortic rupture in the turkey. *J Atheroscl Res* 1:75–80, 1961.
64. Neumann F, Ungar H: Cystic medial degeneration of the aorta in poultry. *J Comp Pathol* 82:147–150, 1972.
65. Rooney JR, Prickett ME, Crowe MW: Aortic ring ruptures in stallions. *Pathol Vet* 4:268–274, 1967.
66. Siegel EC, Martin GR: Collagen crosslinking: enzymatic formation of lysine-derived aldehydes and the production of cross-linked components. *J Biol Chem* 245:1653–1658, 1970.
67. Frenkel JK, Rasmussen P, Smith OD: Synergism of cortisol and desoxycorticosterone in the production of dissecting aneurysms in hamsters. *Fed Proc* 18:477, 1959.
68. Frenkel JK: Dissecting aneurysms of the aorta and pancreatic islet hyperplasia with diabetes in corticosteroid and chlorthiazide treated hamsters. *Prog Exp Tumor Res* 16:300, 1972.
69. Reilly JM, Brophy CM, Tilson MD: Hydrocortisone rapidly induces aortic rupture in a genetically susceptible mouse. *Arch Surg* 125:707–709, 1990.
70. Clarck SD, Kobayashi DK, Welgus HG: Regulation of the expression of tissue inhibitor of metalloproteinases and collagenase by retinoids and glucocorticoids in human fibroblasts. *J Clin Inv* 80:1280, 1987.
71. Carnes WH: Role of copper in connective tissue metabolism. *Fed Proc* 40:995–1000, 1971.
72. Coulson WF, Carnes WH: Cardiovascular studies on copper-deficient swine. *Am J Path* 43:945–954, 1963.
73. Tilson MD: Decreased hepatic copper levels: a possible chemical marker for the pathogenesis of aortic aneurysms in man. *Arch Surg* 117:1212–1213, 1982.
74. Senapati A, Carsson L, Fletcher C, et al: Is tissue copper deficiency associated with abdominal aortic aneurysms? *Br J Surg* 72:352–353, 1985.
75. Alston J, Fody E, Counch L, et al: A prospective study of hepatic and skin copper levels in patients with abdominal aortic aneurysms. *Surg Forum* 24:466–468, 1983.
76. Strickland HL, Bond MG: Aneurysms in a large colony

of squirrel monkeys (Samimi sciureus). *Lab Anim Sci* 33:589–592, 1983.

77. DePalma R, Koletsky S, Bullon E, et al: Failure of regression of atherosclerosis in dogs with moderate cholesterolemia. *Atherosclerosis* 27:297–310, 1977.

78. Zarins CK, Glagov S, Vesselinovitch D, Wissler RW: Aneurysm formation in experimental atherosclerosis: relations to plaque evolution. *J Vasc Surg* 12:246–256, 1990.

79. Economou SG, Taylor CB, Beattie EJ, Davis CB: Persistent experimental aortic aneurysms in dogs. *Surgery* 47:21, 1960.

80. Dobrin PB, Baker WH, Gley WC: Elastolytic and collagenolytic studies of arteries: implications for the mechanical properties of arteries. *Arch Surg* 119:405–409, 1984.

81. Tilson MD, Elefteriades J, Brophy CM: Tensile strength and collagen in abdominal aortic aneurysms. In: Greenhalgh RM, Mannick JA (ed). *The Cause and Management of Aneurysms*. Philadelphia, WB Saunders; 97–104, 1990.

82. Anidjar S, Salzmann JL, Gentric D, Lagneau P, Camilleri JP, Michel JB: Elastase induced experimental aneurysms in rats. *Circulation* 82:973–981, 1990.

83. Anidjar S, Dobrin PB, Chejfec G: Progressive enlargement of experimental aortic aneurysms is associated with infiltration of inflammatory cells. *J Cardiovasc Surg* 32(suppl):39–40, 1991.

84. Nackman GB, Halpern V, Gandhi R, et al: Induction of endogenous proteinases and alterations of extracellular matrix in a rat model of aortic aneurysm formation. *Surg Forum* 43:348–350, 1992.

85. Petersen MJ, Abbott WM, H'Doubler PB: Hemodynamics and aneurysm development in vascular allografts. Proceedings Eastern Vascular Society, Seventh Annual Meeting (abstr) 66, 1993.

86. Schmitz-Rixen T, Megerman J, Colvin RB, et al: Immunosuppressive treatment of aortic allografts. *J Vasc Surg* 7:82–92, 1988.

87. Roach MR: Hemodynamic factors in arterial stenosis and poststenotic dilation. In: Stehbens WE (ed). *Hemodynamics and the Blood Vessel Wall* Springfield, IL: Charles C. Thomas; 104–110, 1979.

88. Halsted WS: Cylindrical dilatation of the common carotid artery following partial occlusion of the innominate and ligation of the subclavian. *Surg Gyn Obstet* 27:547, 1918.

89. Rob CG, Eastcott HHG, Owen K: The reconstruction of arteries. *Br J Surg* 43:449–466, 1956.

90. Boughner DR, Roach MR: Effect of low frequency vibration on the arterial wall. *Circ Res* 29:136–144, 1971.

91. Rodbard S, Ikeda K, Montes M: An analysis of the mechanisms of poststenotic dilatation. *Angiol* 18:348–367, 1967.

92. Zarins CK, Runyon-Hass A, Zatina MA, et al: Increased collagenase activity in early aneurysmal dilatation. *J Vasc Surg* 3:238, 1986.

93. Vollamr JF, Paes E, Pauschinger P, Henze E, Friesch A: Aortic aneurysm as late sequelae of above-knee amputation. *Lancet* 2(8667):834–835, 1989.

94. Edward WS: Arterial grafts: past, present, and future. *Arch Surg* 113:1225, 1978.

95. Karkow WS, Cranley JJ, Cranley RD, et al: Extended study of aneurysms formation in umbilical vein grafts. *J Vasc Surg* 4:486, 1986.

96. Szilagyi EE, Elliot JP, Hageman JH, et al: Biologic fate of autogenous vein implants as arterial substitutes. *Ann Surg* 178:232, 1973.

97. Harkness MLR, Harkness RD, McDonald DA: The collagen and elastin content of the arterial wall in the dog. *Proc R Soc Lond* (B) 146:231–240, 1971.

98. McDonald DA: Blood Flow in Arteries. Baltimore: Williams & Wilkins; 90, 1974.

99. Wolinsky H, Glagov S: Comparison of abdominal and thoracic aortic medial structure in mammals: deviation of man from the usual pattern. *Circ Res* 29:677–686, 1969.

100. Dobrin PB: Pathophysiology and pathogenesis of aortic aneurysms: current concepts. *Surg Clin North Am* 69(4):687–702, 1989.

101. Prockop DJ, Kivirikko KI: Heritable diseases of collagen. *New Eng J Med* 311:376–386, 1984.

102. Piez KA: Molecular and aggregate structures of collagens. In: Piez KA, Reddi AH (eds). *Extracellular Matrix Biochemistry*. New York: Elsevier, Science Publishing Co., Inc.; 1–40, 1984.

103. Fleischmajer R, et al: Biology, chemistry, and pathology of collagen. *Ann of NY Acad Sci* 460:1, 1985.

104. Prockop DJ: Mutations that alter the primary structure of type I collagen: the perils of a system for generating large structures by the principle of nucleated growth. *J Biol Chem* 265:15349–52, 1990.

105. Kivirikko KI: Collagens and their abnormalities in a wide spectrum of disease. Ann Med 25:113–126, 1993.

106. Prockop DJ, Kivirikko KI: Heritable disease of collagen. *N Eng J Med* 311:376–386, 1984.

107. Piez KA: Molecular and aggregate structures of collagens. In: Piez KA, Reddi AH (eds). *Extracellular Matrix Biochemistry*. New York: Elsevier; Science Publishing Co., Inc. 1–40, 1984.

108. Prockop DJ: Mutations in collagen genes as a cause of connective tissue diseases. *N Eng J Med* 326(8):540–546, 1992.

109. Mayne R, Burgeson RE (eds). *Structure and Function of Collagen Types*. Orlando: Academic Press, Inc.; 1987.

110. Burgeson RE: New collagens, new concepts. *Ann Rev Cell Biol* 4:551–577, 1988.

111. Fleishmajer R, Olsen B, Kuhn K Eds: Structure, molecular biology, and pathology of collagen. *Ann NY Acad Sci* 580:1–592, 1990.

112. Vuorio E, de Crombugghe B: The family of collagen genes. *Annu Rev Biochem* 59:837–872, 1990.

113. Ramirez F, di Liberto M: Complex and diversified regulatory programs control the expression of vertebrate collagen genes. *FASEB J* 4:1616–1623, 1990.

114. Shaw LM, Olsen BR: FACIT collagens: diverse molecular bridges in extracellular matrices. *Trends Biochem Sci* 16:191–194, 1991.

115. van der Rest M, Garrone R: Collagen family of proteins. *FASEB J* 5:2814–2823, 1991.

116. Royce PM, Steinmann B (eds). *Connective Tissue and its Heritable Disorders: Molecular, Genetic, and Medical Aspects*. New York: Wiley-Liss, 181–184, 1992.

117. Prockop DJ: Mutations that alter the primary structure of type I collagen: the perils of a system for generating large structures by the principle of nucleated growth. *J Biol Chem* 265:15349–15352, 1990.

118. Burgeson RE, Nimni ME: Basic science and pathology: collagen types molecular structure and tissue distribution. *Clin Orthop* 282:250–272, 1992.

119. Rizzo RJ, McCarthy WJ, Dixit SN, Lilly MP, Shevely VP, Flinn WR: Collagen types and matrix protein con-

tent in human abdominal aortic aneurysms. *J Vasc Surg* 10:365–373, 1989.

120. Menashi S, Campa JS, Greenhalgh RM, et al: Collagen in abdominal aortic aneurysm: typing, content, and degradation. *J Vasc Surg* 6:578–582, 1987.

121. White A, et al: Connective tissue. In: *Principles of Biochemistry* 1978. 6th Ed. 110.

122. Schultz RM: Proteins II: Physiologic Proteins. In: Devlin RM (ed). *Textbook of biochemistry with clinical correlations*. second edition pp 111.

123. Partridge SM: Elastin. *Adv Prot Chem* 17:277–302, 1962.

124. Franzblau C: *Comp Biochem* 26c:659–712, 1971.

125. Rucker RB, Tinker D: Structure and metabolism of arterial elastin. *Int Rev Exp Pathol* 17:1–46, 1977.

126. Lefevre M, Rucker RB: Aorta elastin turnover in normal and hypercholesterolemic Japanese quail. *Biochim Biophys Acta* 630:519–529, 1980.

127. Arums DV: The spectrum of chronic periaortitis. *Histopathol* 16:423–431, 1990.

128. Dubick MA, Hunter GC, Perez-Lizano E, Mar G, Geokas MC: Assessment of the role of pancreatic Proteases in human abdominal aortic aneurysms and occlusive disease. *Clin Chem Acta* 177:1–10, 1988.

129. Campa JS, Greenhalgh RM, Powell JT: Elastin degradation in abdominal aortic aneurysms. *Atherosclerosis* 65:13–21, 1987.

130. Brophy CM, Smith GJW, Tilson MD: Pathology of Nonspecific Abdominal Aortic Aneurysm Disease. In: CB Ernst and JC Stanley (eds). *Current Therapy in Vascular Surgery* 2nd Ed. Philadelphia: BC Decker Inc.; 238–241, 1991.

131. Baxter BT, McGee GS, Shively VP: Elastin content, cross-links, and mRNA in normal and aneurysmal human aorta. *J Vasc Surg* 16:192–200, 1992.

132. Skerrett PJ: "Matrix Algebra" heals life's wounds. *Science* 252:1064–1066, 1991.

133. Busuttil RW, Abou-Zamzam AM, Machleder HI: Collagenase activity of the human aorta: a comparison of patients with and without abdominal aortic aneurysms. *Arch Surg* 115:1373–1378, 1980.

134. Cannon DJ, Read RC: Blood elastolytic activity in patients with aortic aneurysm. *Ann Thorac Surg* 34:10–15, 1982.

135. Cohen JR, Mandell C, Wise L: Characterization of human aortic elastase found in patients with abdominal aortic aneurysms. *Surg Gynecol Obstet* 165:301–304, 1987.

136. Brown SL, Backstrom B, Busuttil FW: A new serum proteolytic enzyme in aneurysm pathogenesis. *J Vas Surg* 2:393–399, 1982.

137. Reilly JM, Brophy CM, Tilson MD: Characterization of an elastase from aneurysmal aorta which degrades intact aortic elastin. *Ann Vasc Surg* 6:499–502, 1992.

138. Newman KM, Malon AM, Shin R, et al: Matrix metalloproteinases in abdominal aortic aneurysm disease. *FASEB J* 6:A1914, 1992.

139. Senior RM, Griffin GL, Fliszar CJ, Shapiro SD, Goldberg GL, Welgus HG: Human 92- and 72-kilodalton type IV collagenases are elastases. *J Biol Chem* 266:7870–7875, 1991.

140. Murphy G, Cockett MI, Ward RV, Docherty AJP: Matrix metalloproteinase degradation of elastin, type IV collagen, and proteoglycan. *Biochem J* 277:277–279, 1991.

141. Matrisian LM: Metalloproteinases and their inhibitor in matrix remodeling. *Trends in Genet* 6(4):121–125, 1990.

142. Woessner Jr. JF: Matrix metalloproteinases and their inhibitors in connective tissue remodeling. *FASEB J* 5:2145–2154, 1991.

143. Chin J, Murphy G, Werb Z: Stromelysin, a connective tissue-degrading metalloproteinase secreted by stimulated rabbit synovial cells in parallel with collagenase. *J Biol Chem* 260:12367–12376, 1985.

144. Stetler-Stevenson WG, Krutzsch HC, Liotta LA: Tissue inhibitor of metalloproteinase (TIMP-2): a new member of the metalloproteinase inhibitor family. *J Biol Chem* 264:17274–17278, 1989.

145. De Clerck YA, Yean TD, Ratzkin BJ, Lu HS, Langley KE: Purification and characterization of two related but distinct metalloproteinase inhibitors secreted by bovine aortic endothelial cells. *J Biol Chem* 264:17445–17453, 1989.

146. Cawston TE: Proteins inhibitors of metallo-Proteases. In: Barret AJ, Salvesen G (eds). *Proteinase Inhibitors*. Amsterdam: Elsevier Science Publishing, Co., Inc.; 589–610, 1986.

147. Goldberg GI, Strongin A, Collier IE, Genrich LT, Mahmer BL: Interaction of 92-kDa Type IV collagenase with the tissue inhibitor of metalloproteinases prevents dimerization, complex formation with interstitial collagenase, and activation of the proenzyme with stromelysin. *J Biol Chem* 267:4583–4591, 1992.

148. Herron GS, Unemori E, Wong M, et al: Connective tissue proteinases and inhibitors in abdominal aortic aneurysms. *Arterioscler Thromb* 11:1667–1677, 1991.

149. Webster MW, McAuley CE, Steed DL, Miller DD, Evans CH: Collagen stability and collagenolytic activity in the normal and aneurysmal human abdominal aorta. *Am J Surg* 161:635–638, 1991.

150. Vine N, Powell JT: Metalloproteinases in degenerative aortic disease. *Clin Sci* 81:233–239, 1991.

151. Irizarry E, Newman KM, Gandhi RH, et al: Demonstration of interstitial collagenase in abdominal aortic aneurysm disease. *J Surg Res* 54:571–574, 1993.

151A. Jean-Claude J, Newman KM, Li H, Tilson MD: Possible key role for plasmin in the pathogenesis of abdominal aortic aneurysms. *Surgery* 116:472–478, 1994.

152. He C, Wilhelm SM, Pentland AP: Tissue cooperation in a proteolytic cascade activating human interstitial collagenase. *Proc Natl Acad Sci USA* 86:2632–2636, 1989.

153. Anidjar S, Dobrin PB, Eichorst M, et al: Correlation of inflammatory infiltrate with the enlargement of experimental aortic aneurysm. *J Vasc Surg* 16:139–147, 1992.

154. Reilly JM, Sicard GA, Lucore CL: Differential expression of plasminogen activators in abdominal aneurysm and occlusive disease. *Circulation* 86(4)(suppl I):I306, 1992.

155. Tryggvason K, Huhtala P. Tuuttila A, et al: Structure and expression of type IV collagenase genes. *Cell Differ Develop* 32:307–312, 1990.

156. Cohen JR, Mandell C, Margolis I, Chang J, Wise L: Altered aortic protease and antiprotease activity in patients with ruptured abdominal aortic aneurysms. *Surg Gyn Obstet* 164:355–358, 1987.

157. Cohen JR, Mandell C, Chang JB, Wise L: Elastin metabolism of the infrarenal aorta. *J Vasc Surg* 7:210–214, 1988.

158. Cohen AB, James HL. Reduction of the elastase inhibitory capacity of alpha-one antitrypsin by peroxides in cigarette smoke. *Lung Res* 1:225–237, 1980.

159. Cannon DJ, Read RC: Blood Elastolytic activity in pa-

tients with aortic aneurysm. *Ann Thoracic Surg* 34: 10–15, 1982.

160. Powell JT, Muller BR, Greenhalgh RM: Acute phase proteins in patients with abdominal aortic aneurysms. *J Cardiovasc Surg* 28:528–530, 1987.

161. Cronenwett JL, Sargent SK, Wall MH, et al: Variables that affect the expansion rate and outcome of small abdominal aortic aneurysms. *J Vasc Surg* 11:260–269, 1990.

162. Cohen JR, Sarfati I, Ratner L, Tilson DM: Alpha-one antitrypsin phenotypes in patients with abdominal aortic aneurysms. *J Sur Res* 49:319–321, 1990.

163. St. Jean PL, Ferrall RE, Majumder PP, Steed DL, Webster MW: Abdominal aortic aneurysm (AAA) association with alpha-1 antitrypsin, haptoglobin, and type III colagen. *J Cardiovasc Surg* 32:38, 1991.

164. Tilson MD, Reilly JM, Brophy CM, Webster EL, Barnett TR: Expression and sequence of the gene for tissue inhibitor of metalloproteinases (TIMP-1) in patients with abdominal aortic aneurysms. *JVS.* (In press.)

165. Tromp G, et al: Sequencing of cDNA from 50 unrelated patients reveals that mutations in the triple-helical domain of type III procollagen are an infrequent cause of aortic aneurysms. *J Clin Invest* 91:2539–2545, 1993.

166. Brophy CM, Marks WH, Reilly JM, Tilson MD: Decreased tissue inhibitor of metalloproteinases (TIMP) in abdominal aortic aneurysm tissue: a preliminary report. *J Surg Res* 50:653–657, 1991.

167. Harvey W, Amlot PL: Collagen production by human mesothelial cells in vitro. *J Pathol* 139:337–347, 1983.

168. Stylianou EL, Jenner A, Davies M, Coles GA, Williams JD: Isolation, culture, and characterization of human peritoneal mesothelial cells. *Kidney Int* 37:1563–1570, 1990.

169. Ross R, Klebanoff SJ: The smooth muscle cell: I. In vivo synthesis of connective tissue proteins. *J Cell Biol* 50:159–171, 1971.

170. Ross R: Connective tissue cells, cell proliferation and synthesis of extracellular matrix-A review. *Phil Trans R Soc Lond* 271:247–259, 1975.

171. Muir LW, Bornstein P, Ross R: A presumptive subunit of elastic fiber microfibrils secreted by arterial smooth muscle cells in culture. *Eur J Biochem* 64:105–114, 1976.

172. Burke JM, Balian G, Ross R, Bornstein P: Synthesis of types I and III procollagen and collagen by monkey aortic smooth muscle cells in vitro. *Biochemistry* 16: 3242–3249, 1977.

173. Clark IM, Cawston TE: Fragments of human fibroblast collagenase: purification and characterization. *Biochem J* 263:201–206, 1989.

174. Marshall BC, Santana A, Xu QP, et al: Metalloproteinases and tissue inhibitor of metalloproteinases in mesothelial cells: cellular differentiation influences expression. *J Clin Invest* 91:1792–1799, 1993.

175. Cohen JR, Sarfati I, Danna D, Wise L: Smooth muscle cell elastase, atherosclerosis and abdominal aortic aneurysms. *Ann Surg* 216:327–330, 1992.

176. Evans CH, Georgescu HI, Lin CW, Mendelow D, Steed DL, Webster MW: Inducible synthesis of collagenase by cells of aortic origin. *J Surg Res* 51:399–404, 1991.

176A. Newman KM, Jean-Claude J, Li H, et al: Cellular localization of matrix metalloproteinases in the abdominal aortic aneurysm wall. *J Vasc Surg* 20:814–820, 1994.

177. Pearce WH, Koch A, Haines GK, Mesh C, Parikh D, Yao JST: Cellular components and immune response in abdominal aortic aneurysms. *Surg Forum* 42:328–330, 1991.

178. Hartung HP, Kladetzky RG, Hennerici M: Chemically modified low density lipoproteins as inducers of enzyme release from macrophages. *FEBS Lett* 186: 211–214, 1985.

179. Rouis M, Nigon F, Lafuma C: Expression of elastase activity by human monocyte-macrophage is modulated by cellular cholesterol content, inflammatory mediators and phorbol myristate acetate. *Arteriosclerosis* 10: 246–255, 1990.

180. Werb Z, Banda MJ, Jones PA: Degradation of connective tissue matrices by macrophages. I. Proteolysis of elastin, glycoproteins, and collagen by proteinases isolated from macrophages. *J Exp Med Nov* 152: 1340–1357, 1980.

181. Welgus HG, Campbell EJ, Bar-Shavit Z, Senior RM, Teitelbaum SL: Human alveolar macrophages produce a fibroblast-like collagenase and collagenase inhibitor. *J Clin Invest* 76:219–224, 1985.

182. Sandhaus RA, McCarthy KM, Musson RS, Henson PM: Elastolytic proteinases of the human macrophage. *Chest* 83(suppl):60–62, 1983.

183. Nolan KD, Mesh CL, Shively VP, Pearce WH, Chisholm RL, Yao JST: Cytokines modulate matrix metalloprotease and TIMP gene expression. *Surg Forum* 43: 346–348, 1992.

184. Powell J, Greenhalgh RM: Cellular, enzymatic, and genetic factors in the pathogenesis of abdominal aortic aneurysms. *J Vasc Surg* 9:297–304, 1989.

185. Takemura R, Werb Z: Regulation of elastase and plasminogen activator secretion in resident and inflammatory macrophages for the Fc domain in immunoglobulin G. *J Exp Med* 159:152–178, 1984.

186. Halpern V, Nackman GB, Gandhi RH: Irizarry E, Scholes JV, Ramey WG, Tilson MD. The elastase infusion model of experimental aortic aneurysms: II. Quantitative analysis of the inflammatory cell response. *JVS.* (In press.)

187. Senior RM, Griffin GL, Mecham RP: Chemotactic activity of elastin derived peptides. *J Clin Invest* 66: 859–862, 1980.

188. Page RC: The role of inflammatory mediators in the pathogenesis of periodontal disease. *Peridontal Res* 26(3 Pt 2):230–242, 1991.

189. Brenner DA, et al: Prolonged activation of *jun* and collagenase genes by TNF-alpha. *Nature* 337:661–663, 1989.

190. Amento EP, Ehsani N, Palmer H, Libby P: Cytokines and growth factors positively and negatively regulate interstitial collagen gene expression in human vascular smooth muscle cells. *Arterioscler Thromb* 11(5): 1223–1230, 1991.

191. Hansson GK, Jonasson S, Seifert PS, Stemme S: Immune mechanisms in atherosclerosis. *Arteriosclerosis* 9:567–578, 1989.

192. Edwards DR, Murphy G, Reynolds JJ: Whitham SE, Docherty JP, Angel P, Heath JK. Transforming growth factor beta modulates the expressin of collagenase and metalloproteinase inhibitor. *J Eur Mole Biol Org* 6: 1899–1904, 1987.

193. McGowan S: Influences of endogenous and exogenous TGF-B on elastin in lung fibroblasts and aortic smooth muscle cells. *Am J Physiol* 263:L257–263, 1992.

194. Strepp MA, Kindy MS, Franzblau C, Sonenshein GE: Complex regulation of collagen gene expression in cul-

tured bovine aortic smooth muscle cells. *J Biol Chem* 261:6542–6547, 1986.

195. Liau G, Chan LM: Regulation of extracellular matrix RNA levels in cultures smooth muscle cells: relationship to cellular quiescence. *J Biol Chem* 264:1–6, 1989.

196. Hansson GK, Jonasson L, Holm J, Clowes MK, Clowes A: Gamma-Interferon regulates vascular smooth muscle proliferation and Ia expression in vivo and in vitro. *Circ Res* 63:712–719, 1988.

197. Warner SJC, Friedman GB, Libby P: Immune interferon inhibits proliferation and induces 2′, 5′-oligoadenylate synthetase gene expression in human vascular smooth muscle cells. *J Clin Invest* 83:1174–1182, 1989.

198. Hansson GK, Jonasson L, Holm J, Clowes MM, Clowes AW: Gamma interferon regulates vascular smooth muscle proliferation and Ia antigen expression in vivo and in vitro. *Circ Res* 63:712–719, 1988.

199. Amento EP, Bhan AK, McCullagh KG, Drane SM: Influences of gamma interferon on synovial fibroblast-like cells: Ia induction and inhibition of collagen synthesis. *J Clin Invest* 76:837–848, 1985.

200. Granstein RD, Murphy GF, Margolis RJ, Byrne MH, Amento EP: Gamma interferon inhibits collagen synthesis in vivo in the mouse. *J Clin Invest* 64:5–15, 1987.

201. Van Obberghen-Schilling E, Roche NS, Flanders KC, Sporn MB, Roberts AB: Transforming growth factor beta 1 positively regulates its own expression in normal and transformed cells. *J Biol Chem* 263:7741–7746, 1988.

202. Dustin ML, Rothlein R, Bhan AK, et al: Induction by Il-1 and gamma interferon: tissue distribution, biochemistry, and function of a natural adherence molecule (ICAM-1). *J Immunol* 137(1):245–254, 1986.

203. Madri J, et al. Endothelial cell-extracellular matrix interaction: Matrixins-as a modulator of cell function. In: Simonescu N, Simonescu M, (eds). *Endothelial Cell Biology*. New York: Plenum Publishing; 167, 1988.

204. Travis J: Biotech gets a grip on cell adhesion. *Science* 260:906–908, 1993.

205. Pearce WH, Koch A, Haines GK, Mesh C, Parikh D, Yao JST: Cellular components and immune response in abdominal aortic aneurysms. *Surg Forum* 42:328–330, 1991.

206. Sterpetti AV, Hunter WJ, Feldhaus RJ, et al: Inflammatory aneurysms of the abdominal aorta: incidence, pathologic, and etiologic considerations. *J Vasc Surg* 9:643–650, 1989.

207. Moosa HH, Peitzman AAB, Steed DL, Julian TB, Jarrett F, Webster MW: Inflammatory aneurysms of the abdominal aorta. *Arch Surg* 124:673–675, 1989.

208. Stella A, Gargiula M, Pasquinelli G, et al: The cellular component in the parietal infiltrate of inflammatory abdominal aortic aneurysms (IAAA). *Eur J Vasc Surg* 5:65–70, 1991.

209. Dietz HC, Cutting GR, Pyeritz RE, et al: Marfan syndrome caused by a recurrent de novo missense mutation in the fibrillin gene. *Nature* 352:337–339, 1991.

210. Cotran RS, Kumar V, Robbins SL (eds). *Robbin's*

Pathologic Basis of Disease. 5th ed. Philadelphia: WB Saunders, Co.; 132–133, 1994.

211. Kainulainen K, Pulkkinen L, Savolainen A, Kaitila I, Peltonen L: Location on chromosome 15 of the gene defect causing Marfan syndrome. *N Engl J Med* 323:935–939, 1990.

212. Hollister DW, Godfrey M, Sakai LY, Pyeritz RE: Immunohistologic abnormalities of the microfibrillar-fiber system in the Marfan syndrome. *N Engl J Med* 323:152–159, 1990.

213. Lee B, Godfrey M, Vitale E, et al: Linkage of Marfan syndrome and a phenotypically related disorder to two different fibrillin genes. *Nature* 352:330–334, 1991.

214. Kontusaari S, Tromp G, Kuivaniemi H, et al: A mutation in the gene for type III Procollagen (COL3A1) in a family with aortic aneurysms. *J Clin Invest* 86:1465–1473, 1990.

215. Tilson MD: Commentary on "Multiple aneurysms in a young man," by A Nemers and C Dzinich. *Postgraduate Vasc Surg* 2:14–16, 1991.

216. Deak SB, Ricotta JJ, Mariani TJ, et al: The role of abnormal type III colagen in the development of common aneurysms. *J Vasc Surg* 15:926–927, 1992.

217. Ala-Kokko LS, Kontusaari S, Baldwin C, Kievaniemi H, Prockop DJ: Structure of cDNA clones coding for the entire prepro-alpha-I (III) chain of human type III procollagen: differences in protein structure from type I procollagen and conservation of codon preferences. *Biochem J* 260:509–516, 1989.

218. Sanger F, Nicklen S, Coulson AR: DNA sequencing with chain-terminating inhibitors. *Proc Natl Acad Sci USA* 74:5463–5467, 1977.

219. Powell JT, Bashir A, Dawson S, Vine N, et al: Genetic variation on chromosome 16 is associated with abdominal aortic aneurysm. *Clin Sci* 78:13–16, 1990.

220. Simpson CF, Kling JM, Palemer RF: The use of propranolol for the protection of turkeys from the development of beta-aminoproprionitrile induced aortic rupture. *Angiology* 19:414, 1968.

221. Brophy CE, Tilson JE, Tilson MD: Propranolol delays the formation of aortic aneurysms in the male Blotchy mouse. *J Surg Res* 44:687–689, 1988.

222. Boucek RJ, Gunia-Smith Z, Noble NL, Simpson CF: Modulation by propranolol of the lysyl cross-links in aortic elastin and collagen of the aneurysm-prone turkey. *Biochem Pharmacol* 32:275, 1983.

223. Harty RF: Sclerosing peritonitis and propranolol. *Arch Int Med* 138:1424, 1978.

224. Tilson MD: Propranolol versus placebo for small abdominal aortic aneurysms. *J Vascular Surgery* 15:872–873, 1992.

225. Reilly JM, Tilson MD: The effects of pharmacologic agents on aortic aneurysm disease. In: FJ Veith (ed). *Current Critical Problems in Vascular Surgery*, St. Louis: Quality Medical Publishing, Inc.; 222–226, 1990.

226. Woessner Jr. JF: Matrix metalloproteinases and their inhibitors in connective tissue remodeling. *FASEB J* 5:2145–2154, 1991.

CHAPTER 28

Cerebral Blood Flow

George H. Meier, MD

Introduction

The importance of the brain to life is exemplified by the protection and consideration that evolution has provided to maintain its function under adverse circumstances. While blood flow in other vascular beds may be compromised, the body attempts at all costs to maintain perfusion to the brain. In addition, the brain is encased in a rigid, protective shell, and is the only organ in the body offered such security. Thus, the physiology of cerebral blood flow (CBF) is unique to this organ and is influenced greatly by the special mechanisms designed to maintain its function and viability.

In the evolutionary course leading to *Homo sapiens*, the greatest change in skeletal dimensions was in the size of the cranial vault. The earliest human fossil remains are those of pre-Neanderthal man, *Homo erectus*, which demonstrate clearly a primitive vascular pattern with diminished brain volume, particularly in the anterior fossa.[1] As the cranial capacity expanded, so did the blood supply. This increase in blood supply was associated with an increase in vascular complexity and the necessary control systems. The development of the modern human brain, therefore, resulted not only from an increase in total brain volume, but also from an increase in cerebral vasculature and blood flow as well. With this increase in blood flow, regulatory mechanisms also became more complex.

Anatomically, CBF is maintained by four main arteries, as well as numerous collateral vessels. Anteriorly, the internal carotid arteries provide the bulk of the blood flow to the cerebral hemispheres under normal circumstances. Posteriorly, the paired vertebral arteries provide blood flow to the cerebellum via the basilar artery and its branches. The blood flow from all sources is redistributed in the Circle of Willis, surrounding the pituitary gland at the base of the brain. This redistribution allows significant extracranial obstruction to remain compensated, avoiding hypoperfusion to any given brain segment. With surgical manipulation of the vascular supply, perfusion often remains normal in spite of significant alteration of inflow, such as seen with carotid clamping for endarterectomy. Nonetheless, developmental abnormalities involving the Circle of Willis are quite common, at least 50% being abnormal in autopsy studies.[2] The vessels arising from the circle vary in length and diameter,[3] which serves to alter the pathway and resistance of collateral flow. Therefore, while the Circle of Willis is an important anatomic mechanism for collateral flow, its variability prevents complete reliance on its presence for compensation. Much of the clinical work being done today on ischemic cerebrovascular disease represents an effort to define the collateralization via the Circle of Willis and its adequacy. In those patients without adequate collateral compensation, direct anatomic revascularization may provide more benefit than in those patients with an intact, functioning Circle of Willis. The clinical dilemma is predicting the given pattern of blood flow in the Circle of Willis in any individual patient and, therefore, the risk of cerebral hypoperfusion based on regional maldistribution of blood flow.

Regulation of Cerebral Blood Flow

The brain is unique in its relative demand for constant blood flow, averaging about 750 cc/min or about 15% of the resting cardiac output. This correlates with a normal regional cerebral blood flow (rCBF) of about 50 to 55 mL per 100 g of brain tissue per minute. In the event of hypotension, the brain maintains its perfusion until such time as systemic blood flow is critically lim-

From *The Basic Science of Vascular Disease.* Edited by Sidawy AN, Sumpio BE, and DePalma RG. Armonk, NY: Futura Publishing Company, Inc.; © 1997.

ited. The need for continuous delivery of both oxygen and glucose underlies the necessity of this constant blood flow. Glucose remains the sole energy substrate for brain metabolism, with more than 95% of its energy requirements coming from oxidation of glucose to water and carbon dioxide. There are minimal reserves of glucose and glycogen within the brain and, therefore, a constant supply of glucose and oxygen is essential to prevent reduction in tissue adenosine triphosphate (ATP). If the oxygen supply is interrupted by stopping blood flow, tissue ATP in the brain reduces to zero within 7 minutes.[4]

Oxygen consumption by the brain is regulated within fairly narrow limits, varying only a few percent from the baseline level of 3.5 mL of oxygen per 100 g of brain tissue per minute. If the blood flow to the brain becomes insufficient to supply this required amount, the resultant hypoxia induces vasodilatation to increase local blood flow. This compensation is critical to prevent a reduction of tissue pO_2 below 20 mm Hg, a point at which coma can result. Since baseline levels of brain parenchymal pO_2 are between 35 and 40 mm Hg, maintenance of oxygen delivery is critical for normal activity.

While the maintenance of CBF is essential, its regulation is an inherently complex interaction of both neuronal and local vascular effects. In addition, there are fundamental mechanisms for maintaining large vessel tone which contribute to control of distal vascular bed blood flow.[5] The combination of all of these mechanisms is what we refer to as cerebral autoregulation, although each piece of the whole represents a form of autoregulation in and of itself. In the remainder of this discussion, the term autoregulation will represent the regulation of normal CBF as a whole.

Mechanical Effects On Cerebral Blood Flow

The brain is unique in that it is encased in a solid container. Any increase in cerebral blood volume can fundamentally affect the intracranial pressure (ICP) within the container and, therefore, the blood flow. In other vascular beds, blood flow is determined by the pressure gradient from arterial to venous circulations. In the brain, the venous circulation is maintained at a pressure slightly above ICP and the critical value determining CBF is the cerebral perfusion pressure, defined as the difference between the arterial pressure and the highest of the venous pressure or the ICP. With experimentally-induced intracranial hypertension, venous pressure rises in parallel with the ICP, remaining about 3 to 5 mm Hg higher than the ICP.[6] Usually, the cerebral perfusion pressure is approximated by the difference between the intra-arterial pressure and the ICP. While venous capillary pressure in the intracra-

nial venules is above ICP, a short distance away in the internal jugular vein the pressure remains low, often only a few mm Hg above atmospheric pressure. Venous drainage is never dependent on extracranial physiology, and remains normal even in extremes of congestive heart failure and venous hypertension. Under normal physiologic circumstances, a change in cerebral perfusion pressure between the limits of 50 to 130 mm Hg produces no change in CBF (Figure 1).[7–10] The fact that constant flow is maintained despite an increase in perfusion pressure implies that the cerebrovascular bed produces rapid changes in resistance, with a resultant reduction in the caliber of the principle resistance vessels. This has been confirmed with direct observation of the pial arteries.[11–13] In contrast to the vascular supply in the remainder of the body, the larger arteries of the brain often serve as functional resistance vessels.[14] This tends to lower the systemic arterial pressure seen by the cerebral arterioles and, therefore, limit increases in ICP.

While autoregulation seems to have upper and lower limits in any given individual, changes can occur in these limits under certain circumstances. For example, long-standing arterial hypertension can result in an increased cerebral perfusion pressure without any increase in CBF.[15] The increase in cerebral vascular resistance in hypertensive patients upwardly adjusts the range over which autoregulation is maintained, allowing the complete range of blood pressures seen in the daily life of the individual to remain compensated for under normal circumstances. This upward adaptation of CBF autoregulation is appropriate normally, but under certain circumstances can result in decompensation of blood flow. In these subjects, the threshold level of cerebral perfusion pressure at which cerebral ischemia begins to develop is also shifted upward; there-

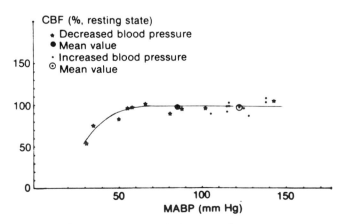

Figure 1. Pressure autoregulation. Hemispheric mean flows during changes in blood pressure. (Reproduced with permission from Olesen J: Quantitative evaluation of normal and pathologic cerebral blood flow regulation to perfusion pressure. *Arch Neurol* 28:143–152, 1979.)

fore, cerebral ischemia may occur at an arterial pressure much higher than that seen in normotensive individuals (Figure 1). This has important ramifications in those situations where induction of relative hypotension may be beneficial. In those circumstances, autoregulation may be lost in hypertensive patients and cerebral ischemia may result. Similarly, the occasional abrupt changes in blood pressure associated with changes in antihypertensive medications may temporarily lower the systemic blood pressure below the lower limit of autoregulation in the severely hypertensive patient. While autoregulation will adjust to the lower set point over time, the rapid change may transiently remain uncompensated, allowing cerebral hypoperfusion to occur. Finally, the use of general anesthesia with relative hypotension in an otherwise compensated, poorly controlled hypertensive patient may increase the risk of cerebral ischemia in carotid surgery, lending theoretical benefit to regional anesthesia in this procedure.

Lowering ICP under circumstances where it may be abnormally elevated will result in improved blood flow and restoration of autoregulation to normal. This is particularly important in situations where ICP may be elevated secondary to trauma or ischemia. In those circumstances, the reduction of ICP by normal clinical measures may be sufficient to dramatically improve blood flow. This also applies to the spinal cord, as is seen in the repair of thoracoabdominal aneurysms. An increase in ICP may diminish spinal cord blood flow in spite of adequate arterial perfusion pressures. Therefore, measures to reduce cerebral spinal fluid (CSF) pressure in thoracoabdominal aneurysm surgery may be important in maintaining blood flow to the thoracic spinal cord.

Neurogenic Coupling Mechanisms in Cerebral Blood Flow

The brain is composed of neurons and support cells with the neuronal tissue representing about 40% of the brain volume. Neuronal mass has ramifications in virtually every area of brain metabolism and physiology. The number of substances excreted by these neuronal dendrites seems limitless. Nonetheless, for years it has been known that CBF in any given region changes with the neuronal activity of that region. For example, the use of a hand for a simple motor task results in an immediate increase in blood flow in the motor cortex on the opposite side of the brain. Similarly, light stimulation to the eye or simply reading can increase blood flow in the occipital cortex. The mechanisms responsible for these increases in blood flow and the associated metabolic coupling of blood flow remain poorly defined.

Perhaps the most overwhelming advance in our knowledge of the regulation of CBF came with the discovery of nitric oxide (NO) synthetase in virtually all tissues of the body. The ubiquity of NO vasodilatation has been exemplified by its high concentration within the brain and cerebral circulation.[16] The discovery that NO is produced by active neurons[17,18] has led to a hypothesis that this could be the long-sought coupling agent between brain activity and CBF. NO, previously known as endothelial-derived relaxing factor (EDRF), is extensively distributed in the circulatory system as a local autoregulator of blood flow. In addition to its direct role, it appears that certain neurons are specialized for secretion of NO.[19] This, therefore, results in an increase in blood flow locally with cerebral activity in those neurons. In addition, NO appears to be released with activation of receptors for the excitatory amino acid n-methyl-d-aspartate (NMDA). Topical NMDA has been shown to produce vasodilatation in pial arteries that can be blocked by inhibiting NO synthetase.[20] This and other evidence suggests that NO plays a strong role in mediating increases in local blood flow during increases in neuronal activity.

Other factors appear to play a significant role as well. Both angiotensin and vasopressin have a significant role in the regulation of vascular resistance in cerebral arteries and the latter appears to also have a significant role in the production of CSF.[21,22] Prostaglandins have also been implicated in these pathways,[23] but they have proven to be variable from one animal species to the next.[24,25] This variability argues against a fundamental role in cerebral autoregulation, but does suggest that there is some role played by the interaction of prostaglandins with other regulatory systems.

Local Effects on Cerebral Blood Flow

As with any other system, the metabolism of local tissues results in altered regulation of blood flow. In the brain, this is carried to a higher level as a result of the greater demand for stable blood flow within the cerebral system. Perhaps the most potent mechanism for regulating local CBF is that associated with an increase in arterial pCO_2. The increase in local carbon dioxide concentration results in increasing CBF which serves to remove carbon dioxide from the system. This also helps to regulate the acidity of the brain tissues, since carbon dioxide is at equilibrium with tissue pH via carbonic acid. Blood flow changes induced by increases in arterial pCO_2 begin within 2 minutes and reach stability over about 12 minutes.[26] It should be noted that alterations in blood pH secondary to metabolic alkalosis or acidosis have very little influence on CBF.[27] Prolonged changes in arterial pCO_2 lead to chronic adaptation after the first 36 hours.[27]

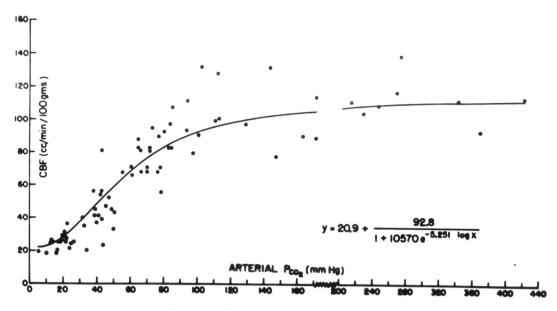

Figure 2. Carbon dioxide autoregulation.

Carbon dioxide reactivity can be impaired by physical insults such as trauma or surgery.[28,29] This can also occur with surgical manipulation of extracranial vessels,[30,31] by atherosclerosis,[32] and by arterial hypotension. With tissue injury, all normal regulatory mechanisms seem to be altered and CBF may paradoxically fall with elevation of arterial pCO_2.[33]

At an arterial pCO_2 above 70 mm Hg, maximum vasodilatation has occurred and no further increase in CBF will occur (Figure 2). The mechanism responsible for this vasodilatation in response to pCO_2 seems to

be, once again, the formation of NO. Experimentally blocking NO synthesis results in obliteration of CBF responses to elevated pCO_2.[34] There is some controversy about the role of NO in the response to acidosis by the cerebral vasculature, but this appears to be attenuated as well by NO blockade.[35]

Oxygen reactivity, on the other hand, results in an increase in CBF when arterial pO_2 falls below 50 mm Hg (Figure 3). This reactivity is abolished by severe hypoglycemia, suggesting that lactic acid production by anaerobic glycolysis may be partially responsible

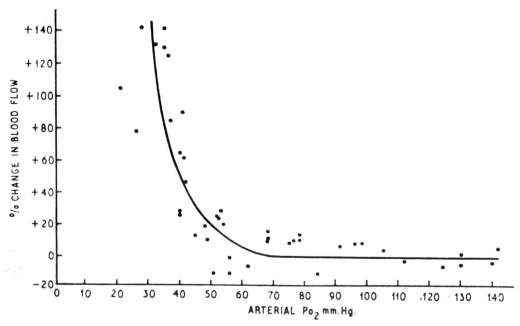

Figure 3. Oxygen autoregulation.

for the rise in CBF that accompanies hypoxia.[36] The association between cerebral inflow and hydrogen ion activity can be variable, with CBF rising in spite of insignificant changes in hydrogen ion concentration. Therefore, this mechanism does not clearly initiate increased CBF in response to hypoxia. It also appears that NO synthetase blockade has no effect on hypoxic responses of CBF.[37] This implies that a different mechanism is responsible, again suggesting a metabolic response perhaps secondary to intracellular acidosis.

As body temperature falls, cerebral metabolism decreases as well, although it never disappears completely. In general, CBF and metabolism decrease about 7% per degree Celsius.[38] While no data exist to document that reductions in hypothermia-induced CBF exactly parallels reduction in cerebral metabolism, it is generally accepted that blood flow to metabolic coupling persists in hypothermia. The reduced CBF requirements in hypothermia are clinically utilized to limit ischemic risk in hypothermic cardiac arrest for otherwise impossible cerebral vascular interventions.

While many systemic changes occur with aging that decrease the compensation in many organ systems, no direct decrease in cerebral autoregulation occurs in the absence of previously discussed mechanisms. Aging is associated with a higher incidence of hypertension and the associated shift in the autoregulation curve to higher pressures. Similarly, atherosclerotic vascular disease involving the cranial vessels may limit collateral compensation and result in global reduction of CBF. Finally, cerebral metabolism decreases with age, resulting in decreases in CBF proportional to metabolic changes. No independent change specific to aging is apparent in any study of CBF.

Methods for Evaluating Cerebral Blood Flow

The assessment of CBF, either segmental or absolute, requires analysis of both the arterial and venous circulations to the brain. The complexity of these vascular systems makes isolation of blood flow difficult, and measurement is often dependent on the methods used. In all CBF research, the methodology forces many assumptions upon the data generated. Knowledge of the method of CBF assessment, therefore, requires critical analysis relative to the conclusions of the research.

Methods of CBF assessment fall into the two broad categories of experimental and clinical methods. While the distinction is at best artificial, it serves to differentiate those methods useful in basic animal research from those appropriate in human clinical research settings.

Experimental Methods

Pial Artery Diameter

In the simplest assessment technique, CBF is correlated with changes in pial artery diameter. After surgical exposure, this technique uses direct television microscopy imaging[39] to determine the responsiveness of pial vessels to topically applied agents.[40,41] Recent refinements add the use of pulsed Doppler velocity measurements[42,43] to allow direct assessment of changes in pial arterial flow as well. This technique is accurate and reproducible. The major limitation in this technique results from the vessel preparation itself. Surgical manipulation of the site of microscopic observation results in local trauma and changes in vasospastic responses. These changes may irreversibly affect the results of observations on these vessels. Regional blood flow cannot be determined using this technique, since only a single area of regional blood flow is visualized in a given experimental preparation. Differential blood flow assessment is not feasible.

Hydrogen Diffusion

Since its introduction in 1964,[44] hydrogen diffusion has been the most commonly used experimental technique for the assessment of rCBF. In spite of its wide application, there remains little standardization of measurements and little correlation with other techniques of CBF measurement. Since no commercial source of hydrogen clearance equipment is available, blood flow laboratories have designed and constructed electrodes and amplifiers unique to their institution. This lack of standardization is the main drawback to this technique, which remains invaluable in measuring CBF.

Hydrogen diffusion relies on the use of inspired hydrogen gas as a tracer to assess regional blood flow. A platinum electrode is inserted into the cortex of the experimental animal and driven to a positive voltage relative to a reference electrode (normally Ag/AgCl). This oxidizes all hydrogen molecules near the electrode according to the equation:

$$H_2 \rightarrow 2H^+ + 2e^-$$

The diffusion of hydrogen into the region sampled by the electrode results in the production of a current flow, which reaches a maximum with tissue saturation. The rate of saturation is determined by blood flow alone and is independent of hydrogen gas concentration, allowing assessment of rCBF. This technique has the advantages of allowing repetitive measurements of rCBF at intervals as short as 15 minutes.

Hydrogen clearance samples approximately a 3 mm³ volume surrounding the platinum wire electrode. In most cases, sampling of gray and white matter simultaneously results in a biexponential clearance of hydrogen tracer, as is seen with most diffusion techniques. A number of problems can distort these measurements. For instance, the design of the hydrogen gas circuit used to introduce the tracer gas into the anesthesia equipment must be carefully engineered to limit recirculation of gases once hydrogen injection is stopped. If not, then the recirculation and washout of hydrogen gas will decay over a variable interval, resulting in significant errors in measurement. A second problem arises from the edema surrounding the electrode. If the local tissue trauma is excessive, then the measurements may be abnormal or nonlinear. Since the design and use of hydrogen diffusion is a difficult and time-consuming endeavor, readers interested in employing hydrogen clearance are referred to a more complete description of this experimental technique and its problems.[45]

Radioactive Microspheres

The use of radioactively labeled microspheres was introduced in 1947[46] and has since undergone significant evolution. In this technique, spheres made of styrene or other substances are injected into a central portion of the arterial circulation and their distribution in the brain is determined by gamma scintillation counting. Once the microspheres are distributed in the capillary bed, detection is accomplished by gamma scintillation counting of the brain tissue being examined. The determination of relative blood flow is then simple, dividing the counts in the tissue being examined (per gram wet weight) by the total counts injected.

There remain several areas of concern for this technique. First, artifacts can be introduced in several ways:

1. Mixing: if the spheres do not become adequately mixed with the blood, then the maldistribution will lead to errors.

2. Tissue trapping: calculation of blood flow is based on first pass trapping of microspheres. Any deviation or significant arteriovenous shunting will introduce bias.

3. Cardiovascular effects: if injection of microspheres into the central circulation alters cardiac performance in any way, then the introduction of the microspheres will lead to errors.

The determination of absolute perfusion volume requires calibration relative to a "standard" perfusion. The easiest method of providing a standard is the calibrated withdrawal of blood during the injection of microspheres. For example, a calibrated pump that withdraws 100 cc/min allows scintillation counting of the reference blood relative to that of a given tissue sample. The ratios between the sample tissue and the reference blood can then be corrected to the reference perfusion (100 cc/min). In this manner, absolute tissue perfusion can be measured.

In general, CBF measurements are performed with 15 μ carbonized microspheres, attempting to deliver about 400 microspheres per gram of brain tissue. Estimates suggest that this number of microspheres blocks about 0.01% of the cerebral capillaries per single blood flow evaluation.[47] The major variability in blood flow measurement appears to be the differences between experimental animals, often exceeding 15%.[48] Examples of dog CBF calculated by the microsphere technique are seen in Figure 4. These techniques are not applicable in humans, since capillary obliteration may be permanent. The use of degradable albumin microspheres with external counting has been tested in humans and appears feasible.[49]

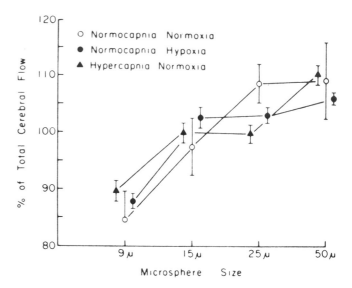

Figure 4. Measurement of cerebral blood flow in dogs, using microspheres. Effect of microsphere size on total cerebral blood flow. (Reproduced with permission from Marcus ML: Total and regional cerebral blood flow measurement with 7-, 10-, 15-, 25-, and 50-μm microspheres. *J Appl Physiol* 40: 501–507, 1976.)

Laser-Doppler

The application of laser technology to cutaneous blood flow measurements began in the early 1970s when laser light was first used to measure skin blood flow velocity.[50] This application relies on the measurement of the frequency shift in laser light reflected from the moving red blood cells in skin or other superficial capillaries such as the surface of the brain. The frequency shift of the laser light can then be analyzed to determine an average blood velocity in the capillary bed underlying the probe. Typical sampling volumes for the probes are approximately 0.5 mm³ at a depth of less than 1 mm. In addition to the average velocity underlying the probe, the reflectance of light from the underlying tissue provides an indication of blood volume in the capillary bed. The combination of this blood volume and average velocity allows a flow-equivalent value (flux) to be calculated. The laser-Doppler waveforms on normal skin have three major characteristics: 1) pulse waves which coincide with the cardiac cycle; 2) preserved diastolic blood flow above a zero baseline; and 3) vasomotor waves that occur four to six times per minute.[51] Similar patterns occur in other tissues as well, reflecting capillary vasomotor stability independent of the end organ being evaluated.

In the brain, rhythmical variations in the regional cortical blood flow have been reported during intraoperative assessment.[52,53] Recent experimental study has defined the baseline cerebral vasomotion in anesthetized rats.[54] At baseline, cerebral capillary circulation exhibits vasomotion with a frequency of 8 to 10 cycles per minute at an amplitude of 5% to 10% of baseline blood flow. As the cerebral perfusion pressure decreases below 50 mm Hg, frequency and amplitude of the vasomotion decreases as well. Similarly, the amplitude and frequency of vasomotion decreases in association with increases in pCO₂. The results of this experimental study suggest that the frequency of vasomotion is correlated with wall tension and cellular pH, while amplitude is best correlated with decreased tissue oxygen delivery.

The flexibility of laser-Doppler flowmetry (LDF) lies in the ability of modern fiberoptics to deliver and return the incident laser light through a variety of instruments. One such benefit is the ability to deliver laser Doppler light intracranially via a burr hole in the skull. This technique allows the monitoring of regional cortical blood flow in comatose patients in a continuous fashion at the bedside.[55,56] Further refinements of this technique may broaden the applicability of bedside intracranial blood flow monitoring.

A novel new application of laser-Doppler technology is the measurement of optic disk blood flow by reflecting laser light off the retina introduced through the lens.[57] This provides an indirect assessment of intracranial blood flow by assessing the flow delivered to the optic nerve. In anesthetized experimental animals, rapid changes in blood flow can be monitored while administering drugs or gases without altering local autoregulation by surgically manipulating the local environment. These results are analogous to pial artery diameter measurements without the associated surgical manipulation.

While LDF is a relatively new technique for measurement of CBF, some correlations with more established techniques do exist.[58] Hydrogen clearance studies show a strong correlation with cerebral perfusion measurements derived from laser-Doppler studies.[52] Some researchers are beginning to use this modality in lieu of more conventional techniques for blood flow correlations.[59] As more experience with this technique is accrued, LDF may supplant some of the more traditional techniques for experimental and clinical measurement of rCBF.

Clinical Methods

Duplex Ultrasound

Duplex ultrasound is a technique well known to anyone involved in cerebrovascular diagnosis. Nonetheless, the application of this technique to CBF measurement is limited by numerous obstacles. First, the measurement of rCBF velocities in the larger intracranial vessels is limited by the inability of conventional ultrasound to effectively penetrate the cranial bone. Extracranial blood vessels, particularly the carotid, are, therefore, the mainstay of duplex ultrasound. Second, multiple vessels provide blood flow to the brain and these cannot be monitored simultaneously for changes or redistribution of CBF. Changes in the flow within a single vessel may not accurately reflect the changes in total CBF. Finally, the regional distribution of extracranial atherosclerotic disease can be well defined by duplex ultrasonography, but the pattern of CBF associated with this disease is difficult to define. The main advantage of duplex ultrasound in cerebral circulation is the diagnosis of extracranial stenotic lesions at risk for embolization to the distal circulation with resultant stroke. The delineation of global ischemia is much more difficult and is better assessed by examination of the intracranial vessels nearer the point of critical flow limitation.

Transcranial Ultrasound

Until 1982, the inability to direct ultrasound energy through the cranium limited the usefulness of this technology. In that year, the first successful attempt at ultrasonographic insonation of the intracranial vessels was reported using defined anatomic "windows" and low frequency pulsed ultrasound.[60] Since that introduction, numerous clinical uses have been developed for this technology. The transcranial Doppler (TCD) technique remains an investigational tool, allowing assessment of Circle of Willis blood flow under a variety of clinical and experimental situations.

Technique

TCD utilizes a 2 MHz ultrasound probe focused by a plastic lens. The low frequency of this modality allows greater tissue penetration than the more common 5 to 10 MHz probes associated with conventional ultrasound. As in all ultrasound blood flow measurements, the erythrocyte in flowing blood reflects the ultrasound beam, producing a Doppler shift. This shift then allows a velocity to be calculated based on the angle of insonation relative to the flowing blood. Pulsed or gated ultrasound signals allow the depth of insonation to be adjusted by changing the time between emitted signal and sampling. Therefore, the depth of the artery, as well as the velocity of flow, can be measured within the Circle of Willis.

Three transcranial ultrasound windows are commonly employed: a transtemporal window through the temporalis bone, a transorbital window over the eye, and a suboccipital window at the posterior base of the skull. These windows allow specific sampling of the vessels at the base of the skull, assessing both the direction and velocity of flow within the intracranial vessels. Identification of intracranial vessels relies on the insonation depth, the direction of flow, the velocities detected, the location of the probe, the ability to trace the vessel, and other factors. Operator experience is critical to the success of these measurements.

Applications

The use of TCD data is limited by the relative nature of the velocities generated. Normal reference ranges for flow velocities have been published.[61-63] Nonetheless, many factors affect the velocity measurements, including the patient's pCO_2[61] and hematocrit.[64] The relationship between CBF and Circle of Willis flow velocities remains unclear in any given individual. In spite of these problems, relative changes in blood flow velocity seem to correlate well with relative changes in rCBF.[65,66] Some recent studies suggest that increases in middle cerebral flow velocity may not be associated with an increase in CBF during exercise[67] and head-down tilt.[68]

A subcommittee of the American Academy of Neurology has published a position paper outlining the clinical uses of TCD[69] (Table I). The most clinically useful indication is for defining the collateral flow pathways in the Circle of Willis. If an extracranial arterial stenosis or occlusion is present, then its collateral flow can come from a number of sources. TCD reliably defines the contributions and their relative velocities with a high sensitivity.[70,71]

Experimentally, the use of TCD relies on its ability to measure arterial blood flow continuously, often in response to changing physiology. This has led to the use of TCD for intraoperative monitoring of middle cerebral artery blood flow during extracranial carotid artery surgery.[72,73] Virtually any physiologic alteration in CBF can be monitored continuously using TCD. Most of the use of TCD for continuous CBF monitoring involves an anesthetized subject and the changes in physiology associated with general anesthesia. This continuous assessment of CBF remains the major experimental utility of TCD.

Xenon Clearance

The use of the Fick principle in measuring CBF relies on the use of a soluble agent as an indicator of diffusion rate and, therefore, rCBF. This concept advanced dramatically in the 1960s with the use of radioisotopes for in vivo assessment of rCBF.[74-76] Since then, numerous improvements have been made to the technique, allowing for more refined assessments.

The most commonly used diffusible tracer is the noble gas [133]xenon (Xe). This agent can be introduced through multiple routes to determine blood flow. Its initial use was by intracarotid (IC) injection. While this technique greatly enhanced our knowledge of cerebral physiology, it is more invasive than usually acceptable and has been replaced by inhalational or intravenous (IV) techniques. These noninvasive methods of [133]Xe

---

Table 1
Clinical Uses of Transcranial Doppler

Established Indications for Transcranial Doppler Ultrasound

Detecting severe stenosis (>65%) in the major basal intracranial arteries.

Assessing patterns and extent of collateral circulation in patients with known stenosis or occlusion.

Evaluating and following vasospasm.

Detecting arteriovenous malformations and their flow patterns.

Assessing suspected brain death.

Investigational Indications for Transcranial Doppler Ultrasound

Assessing patients with migraine.

Monitoring during cerebrovascular and cardiovascular procedures.

Evaluating dilated vasculopathies (i.e., fusiform aneurysms).

Assessing autoregulation, physiologic, and pharmacologic cerebrovascular responses.

Evaluating vasculopathy in children (sickle cell, neurofibromatosis, etc.).

introduction allow adequate measurements of regional perfusion, particularly using newer methods of detection. However, the technique of delivery of the ^{133}Xe isotope is important to the imaging that results. The IV technique is essentially the same in terms of kinetics and distribution as the inhalation technique preferred by many centers. While the IV technique is less invasive than IC injection, the distribution of radioactivity is generalized not only to the opposite hemisphere, but also to the scalp and face. In addition, the duration of tracer injection is greatly prolonged, making analysis of the exponential decay used to determine blood flow more prone to error. Advocates of this technique accept the need for repeated measurements in order to increase the reliability of the data.

The inhalation of Xe gas has greatly simplified the delivery of isotope for imaging. Nonetheless, one should note that the limitation in inhaled Xe gas concentration results in a lower signal-to-noise ratio than would be otherwise expected. Xe was investigated in the 1950s as an anesthetic agent secondary to its effects on the central nervous system (CNS). At 50% inhaled concentration, Xe causes sedation and induces bronchospasm. The most common concentrations used for inhalational studies are 25% to 30%, and minimal respiratory or CNS effects are seen.[77]

As the method of ^{133}Xe injection has changed, so has the detection of it within the tissues. Initially, sodium iodide detectors were used singly to measure local CBF. As the technique became more widespread, the number of detectors has increased. Most two-dimensional systems incorporate 16 paired detectors over the two hemispheres. Now three-dimensional reconstruction of CBF is possible by computed tomographic (CT) analysis. Many conventional CT scanners are easily modified for the detection of CBF using Xe clearance. Improvements in detectors have compensated for the technical difficulties resulting from the use of less invasive injection techniques.

Analysis of the Xe washout is generally complicated and best derived from computerized techniques. For a complete report, the interested reader is referred to a more basic discussion.[78] The presence of both gray and white matter in the brain results in a biexponential washout curve, consistent with two compartments of blood flow as is seen in other forms of diffusion-based measurement. Numerous corrections must be applied to the specific technique being used and the resultant technique validated. In the case of Xe CT, validation of blood flow data has been shown with radioactive microspheres.[79,80] Similar correlations are available in most active areas of CBF research.

Single Photon Emission Cerebral Tomography

Recent advances in nuclear medicine have resulted in the development of techniques and tracers for imaging rCBF. One such technique is single photon emission cerebral tomography (SPECT), where qualitative blood flow abnormalities can be accurately defined. An early useful isotope is N-isopropyl-^{123}I-p-iodoamphetamine (IMP) which is highly lipophilic and readily crosses the blood-brain barrier (BBB) with complete extraction in a single pass through the cerebral circulation.[81] Newer techniques yield similar results using ^{99m}Technicium compounds which are cheaper and easier to handle.[82,83]

The imaging in SPECT is done either with a multidetector or rotating gamma camera system. Since the latter is readily available in most major centers, it is the more commonly used technique. In general, the studies are qualitative rather than quantitative indicators of CBF. Areas of hyper- or hypoperfusion are readily detected visually without further analysis. For quantitative information, a more detailed analysis is needed.[82]

The clinical utility of SPECT lies in that period where abnormalities of CBF have not yet developed to be detectable by other means, such as radiologic CT scanning or magnetic resonance imaging (MRI). Generally, conventional CT scans cannot detect ischemic cerebral events for the first 48 hours. SPECT can easily demonstrate blood flow abnormalities associated with ischemic events during this period. Similarly, hyperperfusion syndromes as are occasionally seen after cerebral revascularization are also readily detected by SPECT. The use of SPECT is, thus, limited currently to a very specific set of circumstances not readily addressed by other techniques of CBF assessment.

Magnetic Resonance Techniques

Nuclear magnetic resonance has been a fundamental tool in chemistry and physics for the past 40 years. Only recently has the technology been developed to allow the computerized analysis and reconstructions necessary for imaging in three dimensions. Clinical experience with MRI is, therefore, limited to the past 10 years in this rapidly evolving technique.

Fundamentally, MRI relies on the radiofrequency analysis of unpaired protons (usually hydrogen) exposed to pulsed magnetic field gradients. When these unpaired protons are placed in an external magnetic field, they tend to align themselves along the axis of the magnetic field. When a radiofrequency pulse is applied, a secondary magnetic field is created which tips the axis away from the main magnetic field. The rotation of these magnetic dipoles generates a radiofrequency signal whose frequency is dependent on the strength of the magnetic field. By varying the magnetic gradient in defined ways, spatial orientation in three dimensions can be determined. In addition, the magnetic gradients can be varied in any plane, allowing reconstruction of the radiofrequency signal in any two-dimensional plane. A more complete explanation of the technique is impossible in this space and, therefore, the interested reader is referred to recent reviews for a more rigorous discussion.[84-86]

In the simplest analysis, image reconstruction can be done, analyzing for the presence of the hydrogen nucleus and its relaxation. Since most of the tissues in the body (except bone) are composed of 65% to 80% water, an image based on signal strength alone might provide limited anatomic detail between adjacent tissues. This difficulty led to the development of techniques to allow variation in contrast between adjacent tissues. Two time constants have been exploited to provide contrast: T1, the time of realignment with the external magnetic field; and T2, the time of decay for the transverse magnetic pulse. The time between radiofrequency pulses, the strength of radiofrequency pulse, and the delay prior to signal detection can, thus, be varied to allow alteration of contrast in adjacent tissues. In any given image sequence, contrast can be varied repeatedly, allowing increased sensitivity to varying tissue structure for any given region. This, combined with the ability to generate magnetic gradients in any direction, allows maximum resolution of tissue differences.

Basic MRI presents the paramagnetic spin data as a reconstructed map of signal intensity. The contrast is varied according to the two time constants, yielding different resolutions in any given region. MRI is currently the standard for imaging in the CNS, as well as other anatomic locations. The maximum resolution is limited to about 1 mm; nonetheless, work continues on MRI microscopy,[87-89] and magnetic resonance (MR) images of large single cells have been published[90] suggesting that this limit may improve with further research.

Magnetic Resonance Angiography

In an effort to provide better blood flow data, MRI has been modified to examine the patterns of blood flow directly, visually representing the MR data similar to an angiogram. In order to allow vessel reconstruction, the most common technique, referred to as the "bright blood" technique, provides saturation pulses in the plane of imaging, allowing inflowing blood which has not been saturated to remain bright. By stacking multiple thin slices on top of each other, a two- or three-dimensional reconstruction can be made to provide an anatomic outline similar to an angiogram. One of the limitations in this technique is the artifact introduced by this stacking process: if the scanned segments are not carefully aligned, there will be an artifact generated

by the misalignment. These limitations appear to be better addressed by the three-dimensional technique.[91-93]

The magnetic resonance angiography (MRA) signal strength does not require injection of contrast, but relies on the flow of blood to provide the contrast necessary for the image. Nonetheless, multiple other mechanisms can induce the loss of MRA signal. The most common is the loss of flow associated with a stenosis, resulting from the slowing of blood before and after a stenosis. At slow flow rates, the blood becomes saturated and does not flow quickly enough to bring high signal blood into the segment being studied. In this setting, a stenosis may appear to be a complete occlusion, overestimating the degree of stenosis. Similarly, turbulent flow around the area of a stenosis may cause signal dropout from the summation of multiple vectors to a net vector of zero. This effect can occur in normal individuals in areas of flow separation and reversal such as at the carotid bifurcation.

MRA is applicable to the assessment of CBF in two general areas: the great vessels in the neck and the Circle of Willis. The course of the great vessels from the arch to the brain provides three separate areas with varying ability of visualization. Clearly, the greatest effort in MRA has been expended in the visualization of the carotid and vertebral vessels in the midneck. This region provides the least tortuosity, the largest vessels, the highest flow velocities and, therefore, the easiest view by MRA. At the origin of the great vessels, the direction of flow can be variable, making judgement of stenosis difficult.[94] Intracranially, the tortuosity of normal vessels makes MRA less useful although visualization of the Circle of Willis, particularly the basilar artery, is quite good.[95] Similarly, experience with MRA suggests that it will play an important role in the evaluation of intracranial arteriovenous malformations, aneurysms, large vessel occlusive disease, and dural sinus thrombosis.[96] This area is expected to be one in which MRA may rapidly replace conventional angiography, since brain scanning can be combined with arterial anatomic studies in a single test using MRA.

A new and emerging technology in MR involves the use of gated phase shift data to determine the direction and velocity of blood flow.[97,98] These data are analogous to those derived from Doppler ultrasound, and will ultimately provide physiologic data to corroborate stenosis severity in the future. This technology is still in its infancy, but may improve future MR data by providing a correlation between anatomic and physiologic data (Figure 5). Currently, a large number of cardiac cycles are required to obtain these data and the spatial resolution is the same as conventional MR (about 1 mm). Ultimately, the advantage of this technique will be the lack of limitations commonly seen

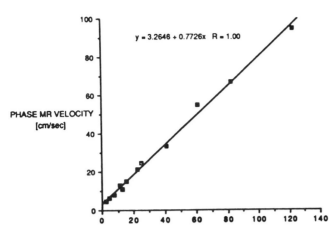

Figure 5. Magnetic resonance (MR) phase-shift flow assessment. Correlation of Doppler and phase-shift MR in vivo. (Reproduced with permission from Reference 95.)

with ultrasound, namely overlying bone, gas, or vessel calcification. Extension of these data to plaque may allow the differentiation of thrombus from flowing blood as has been previously shown with conventional MR.[99]

The future of MRA remains bright, with numerous areas of active research and development. The use of MR contrast agents will soon become a clinical reality. These agents improve the contrast between tissue and blood, potentially altering the sensitivity of MR to flowing blood.[100] The most commonly used media are those containing gadolinium or other paramagnetic metal ions (manganese, iron, copper, or chromium); the second type of contrast agents are those which induce a local magnetic field gradient, the most common being magnetite.[101,102] Both types of agent allow improved signal from any compartment containing the contrast. In the brain, the BBB is normally impermeable to these agents. In patients with disruption of the BBB, the contrast may enhance local cerebral imaging and indicate pathologic changes. Otherwise, the enhancement is limited to the blood stream, allowing improved MRA imaging.

Magnetic Resonance Spectroscopy

The application of NMR techniques to live animal phosphate spectroscopy was first demonstrated in 1980 by Ackerman.[103] Since then, extensive work has been done in an effort to improve the utility of this spectroscopic technique, particularly relative to cerebral ischemia.[104] Currently, clinical application of magnetic resonance spectroscopy (MRS) is limited to ^{31}P and ^{1}H. The most common measurements allow assessment of the ratio of ATP, adenosine dephosphate (ADP), and inorganic phosphate. Changes in the ratio of these fractions represent the energy state of the tissue and, therefore, its function. In addition, since the inorganic phosphate is in equilibrium as expressed by:

$$H^+ + HPO_4^{2-} \rightleftharpoons H_2PO_4^-$$

the ratio of hydrogen ion (and therefore pH) can be determined from the inorganic phosphate peak, since the peak represents a resonance between the two types. Thus, the position of this peak relative to the high energy phosphate peaks determines the pH of the region. While some problems exist,[105,106] this technique remains valuable in evaluating metabolic state.

The difficulty of the technique lies in the inability to quantify any of the spectral components, only ratios of metabolites. Therefore, the greatest use of this technique has been in the ratios of phosphorus metabolites. Hydrogen metabolites overlap strongly, and are often obscured next to the signal from the nuclei in water molecules. Some experimental work has been done with other imaging nuclei including ^{23}Na,[107] ^{13}C labeled glucose,[108] and ^{19}F.[109,110] Further research is needed before these may be routinely applied to physiologic studies.

In CBF, the focus of MRA spectroscopy has been the local changes in tissue milieu associated with stroke. Strokes occur when a single artery is obstructed, depriving the region of its oxygenated blood supply. This results in a rapid decrease in high energy phosphates, and a resultant acidosis at the ischemic focus.[111] Phosphorus NMR has confirmed the loss of high energy phosphates, as well as the lactate accumulation and acidosis.[112] As the stroke injury matures, the pH of the tissue in the ischemic focus changes from acidotic to alkalotic, a fact that has been confirmed in experimental stroke models[113-115] as well as by in vivo studies using MR spectroscopy.[116] The physiology behind this flip-flop of pH is unclear, although it may result from intrinsic cellular buffering of pH.

Perfusion/Diffusion MRI

Perhaps the most active area of cerebral MR research is in the area of quantification of organ blood flow. Many rapid scanning techniques in conjunction with intravascular contrast agents have shown promise in quantitating volume flow.[117-119] Areas of abnormal brain parenchyma have been demonstrated to be perfused at a different rate than normal brain.[117,120] Nonetheless, the clinical significance of these findings and their application to patient care remain undefined.

The addition of gradient pulses to some MRI sequences allows the signal from rapidly moving protons to be reduced.[121,122] Regions with rapidly moving water protons appear dark in the images, while slower regions appear bright. This allows both perfusion and diffusion to be estimated, although some controversy exists as to how these flow parameters relate to more traditional techniques.[123] Diffusion weighted images have been shown to be very sensitive to infarcted brain tissue.[124,125] In fact, diffusion weighted images appear to become abnormal early in acute stroke, often within 1 hour. Further evaluation of this unique technique should be forthcoming in the near future.

Positron Emission Tomography

While many indirect and direct techniques have been developed for the assessment of CBF and metabolism, none has exhibited the promise that positron emission tomography (PET) has in CBF and function. Although this technique is limited by its complexity, expense, and restricted availability, it holds the promise of a new understanding of cerebral function and metabolism in the future. Currently, PET is being applied mainly to the study of rCBF. In the future, its value will most likely be related to the diagnosis of cerebral disease states based on functional and metabolic differences of tissues.

PET requires the use of a radiotracer which decays by releasing a positron, a small particle of the same mass as an electron, but with opposite charge. The positron so emitted travels through the tissue until it encounters an electron, resulting in the destruction of both particles and the release of two gamma photons which travel in opposite directions. Detection of positron release is by capturing these gamma photons, with elimination of background noise by requiring the near-simultaneous detection of these photons by detectors on opposite sides of the positron annihilation. Typically, this is done by electronic coincidence circuits that record a signal only when the two photons arrive on opposite sides within a very short time interval (usually 5 to 20 nsec). The construction of PET scanners combines detectors, coincidence circuits, and computer processing for image reconstruction to produce usable images.

The radiotracers used for PET are unique to this technique. Generally, these are divided into two groups: first, radioisotopes of normal biologic molecules (^{11}C, ^{13}N, ^{15}O); and second, nonbiologic elements that can be used to radiolabel biologic molecules (^{18}F, ^{68}Ga, ^{75}Br). Positron emitting radionuclides have short half-lives which allow them to be used recurrently without adverse effect. Nonetheless, the short half-life also requires that a cyclotron be available on site to produce the positron emitters needed for a diagnostic study. Synthesis of biomolecules incorporating short-lived radiotracers requires great expertise[126] and must be performed rapidly with high levels of purity.

Finally, PET imaging requires that a defined mathematical relationship exist between the radiotracer molecule and the physiologic process being evaluated. This relationship should include uptake, diffusion across the BBB, washout, metabolism, and recirculation of tracer and active metabolites to allow accurate assessment of the underlying physiology. From this, the concentration of radiotracer detected can predict the physiologic state of the region in question.

The earliest and most widely utilized PET technique is that designed for rCBF measurement. Most models of CBF assessment are based on a model of in vivo inert, diffusible flow tracers developed by Kety and his colleagues[127,128] using the Fick principle. In the most common method, inhaled $C^{15}O_2$ is delivered at a constant rate. Similarly, $H_2^{15}O$ may be used as a steady infusion.[129] After about 10 minutes, the steady state is reached and CBF is determined by the ratio of tracer detected in the brain by PET to that in the arterial system as determined by blood sampling. This technique is limited at high flows by the nonlinearity of radiotracer uptake.[130,131]

Numerous other tracers for blood flow and metabolism have been devised for use with PET. An area of active interest currently is the use of acetazolamide to increase regional blood flow and provide a provocative "stress" test for the cerebral circulation.[132] This remains an area of active investigation and early work has clearly demonstrated that rCBF is a poor indicator of the functional or metabolic state of the surrounding tissue.[133]

Clinical Research Areas in Cerebral Blood Flow

Pharmacologic Effects

Obviously, many drugs have a fundamental effect on CBF and its regulation. Most drugs that affect the cerebral circulation do so by altering cerebral vasomotor tone. In these cases, changes in cerebral vascular tone can be determined in animals by the direct observation of the response of cerebral blood vessels to topical application of the drug in question. The side effects of the experimental preparation on cerebral vasomotor tone result in inconsistencies based on the model used, the dosage of drug, and the route and rate of administration. Therefore, any discussion of drug effects on CBF are by necessity limited in their applicability to a given clinical setting.

In discussing the pharmacologic effects of various substances, the concept of the BBB is of fundamental importance. It arose from the work of early investigators who demonstrated that certain protein-bound substances and pharmacologically active compounds readily entered most organs, but did not cross into the brain. This barrier serves as a boundary that restricts diffusion across the capillary basement membrane. Histologically, this barrier is composed of endothelial and arachnoid tissue joined by tight intracellular junctions, which restrict diffusion. While some limited pinocytosis is present at this level, cross-cellular transport is minimal.[134] The BBB appears to be primarily a vascular one, since no restriction of entry is seen when compounds are injected directly into the CSF.

The diffusion characteristics across the BBB are determined by the type of molecule, as well as the CBF. Small molecules such as sugars are readily diffusible across the BBB and the only limitation to their delivery to the brain tissue is the CBF. Other molecules such as electrolytes and large molecules depend on the characteristics of the BBB itself as the rate limiting step for diffusion into the brain parenchyma. In addition, the characteristics of the BBB are not uniform throughout the brain, with some areas such as the pineal gland, the hypothalamus, and the area postrema having limited barrier function.

The BBB is altered by a number of injurious stimuli, resulting in variable permeability, either diffusely through the brain or regionally in limited areas. Perhaps the most common stimulus that results in altered BBB permeability is an increase in perfusion pressure. This can occur as a result of systemic hypertension, regional hypertension induced by hypercapnia, or seizure-induced regional hypertension.[135] Some evidence also exists that the barrier can be disrupted by high osmotic gradients.[136] Of note, the BBB is relatively resistant to ischemic disruption.[137] Changes in BBB permeability occur only after significant injury occurs to the surrounding brain parenchyma, associated with irreversible cytologic changes.[138]

In the remainder of this chapter, the relevant pharmacology will be discussed in conjunction with the topic of that section. Specific pharmacologic issues are generally beyond the scope of this chapter and the interested reader is referred elsewhere.[139]

Anesthesia

A special category of pharmacologic agents are the drugs commonly used to induce general anesthesia. While each of these agents has a specific pharmacology associated with it, there are several general concepts which are important to this class of drugs. In all cases, it can be quite difficult to distinguish between the direct effect of the anesthetic and secondary effects related to changes in metabolism, blood pressure, arterial blood gas, and modification of cerebral autoregulation. While the remainder of the cerebral regulation issues are discussed in earlier sections, the modification of cerebral autoregulation is unique to anesthetic agents.

Generally, any anesthetic agent which produces cerebral vasodilation can result in the loss of autoregulation. In fact, a given drug's ability to produce cerebral vasodilation correlates well with its potency in modifying cerebral autoregulation. At high anesthetic doses, particularly with volatile anesthetic agents, autoregulation can be completely lost. At this point, CBF is completely dependent on the cerebral perfusion pressure. This effect is best illustrated in Figure 6. In the conscious patient, cerebral autoregulation occurs over a wide range of blood pressure, maintaining a constant CBF at varying perfusion pressures. As the anesthetic dose is increased, the plateau phase of cerebral autoregulation decreases until at high doses, CBF is directly proportional to the cerebral perfusion pressure. While this has obvious clinical consequences for the neurosurgical patient, it is equally as important in a research setting where CBF is being evaluated. Therefore, any experimental evaluation of CBF has the added variable of anesthesia to confound the measurements derived. In addition, any attempt to control for the effects of anesthetic agents are contaminated by the use of multiple agents in combination for most forms of acceptable clinical anesthesia. In many models of CBF assessment, a standardized method of anesthesia is imperative to minimize additional variability in the data collected.

While some anesthetic agents confer a generalized change in CBF, others generate regional flow disturbances. An excellent example of this concept is ketamine anesthesia. Ketamine is a unique drug that generates a ''dissociative'' state; the individual is awake, but dissociated from sensory input including noxious stimulation. This class of anesthetic agent is of limited use in human adults secondary to dysphoria after anes-

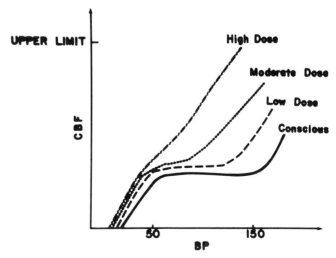

Figure 6. Effects of anesthesia on autoregulation. Schematic representation of the effect of a progressively increasing dose of a volatile anesthetic agent on cerebral blood flow (CBF) autoregulation. (Reproduced with permission from Reference 148.)

thesia, but can be used effectively in children and animals. CBF studies in animals demonstrate increases in limbic and brainstem blood flow associated with simultaneous decreases in somatosensory and auditory regional perfusion.[140] This pattern correlates well with the clinical effects seen in this type of anesthesia and is representative of the changes induced by specific anesthetic agents. Any specific rCBF measurement may, therefore, be altered by the anesthetic agent and the dosage used. Similar regional variability has been demonstrated with barbiturates.[141]

Several general concepts relative to anesthetic agents can be stated; specific changes associated with an anesthetic technique are more difficult to define. Volatile inhalational anesthetics, such as halothane and enflurane, are potent cerebral vasodilators, uniformly increasing CBF acutely. Nonetheless, CBF returns to control levels with these agents under steady state conditions.[142] The modification or loss of pressure autoregulation with these agents at high doses was previously discussed.

NO is a widely used gaseous anesthetic commonly used in combination with other anesthetics. When used with thiopental induction, little change in CBF occurs.[143] Without the use of adjunctive anesthetic agents, an increase in CBF is seen.[144,145] This variability in CBF responses is noted in much of the literature associated with anesthetic agents. Narcotic agents are variable in the changes induced in CBF, with the same agent often associated with increased, decreased, or unchanged CBF in different models. Barbiturates cause a relatively uniform decrease in CBF and metabolism.[146,147] For a more complete review of anesthetic agents and CBF, the interested reader is referred to appropriate references.[148,149]

Neonatal Cerebral Blood Flow

Abnormalities in regulation of CBF in premature neonates has been long recognized as a significant problem in preterm delivery. Two basic lesions are defined in this high-risk group: hypoxic-ischemic encephalopathy and intracranial hemorrhage. Hypoxic injury is seen at all gestational ages equally, while intracranial bleeding is increased in preterm infants. Both of these lesions appear to be increased in infants with impairment of CBF or cerebral autoregulation.[150] Most brain lesions appear early in life, usually within the first few days.[151-153] During this period, premature infants experience significant variations in cerebral perfusion due to a myriad of complications. With these changes, cerebral ischemia can easily occur, as has been demonstrated with asphyxia,[154] hyperventilation,[155] septicemia,[156] and anemic states.[151] As one would expect, intracranial hemorrhage is increased by those states

which would normally result in hyperperfusion such as hypoxia, hypercapnia, or uncontrolled hypertension.[157-159]

In normal brain, CBF is regulated by changes in regional metabolic demand. Neonatal brain has few synaptic connections and low neuronal demand. Therefore, rCBF in infants is diminished (10 to 20 mL/100 gm/min), about one third that of adults.[160,161] The regulation of neonatal blood flow is similar to adults with increases in CBF associated with hypoxia, hypercapnia, and metabolic changes. While regulation of glucose delivery is an attractive concept for neonatal brain in particular, the evidence for this mechanism is contradictory.[162-164] No clear mechanism for the proposed response to hypoglycemia has been defined, although catecholamines have been implicated.[165]

Abnormal states of autoregulation often provide the first evidence of brain damage in neonates. Specifically, the absence of a hypercapnic or hypoxic response is an indicator of severe cerebrovascular pathology and subsequent evidence of brain damage.[166,167] At present, no method of reliably detecting impaired neonatal autoregulation exists. Current recommendations consist of maintaining normal arterial blood pressure, avoiding abrupt changes in blood flow, and avoiding conditions associated with impaired autoregulation (hypoxia, hypercapnia, hypoglycemia).[168] Recently, postural responses in CBF have been shown to be an indicator of mature cerebral autoregulation in neonates.[169] If reliable prediction of immature autoregulation were available, the promise of early detection and prevention of neonatal cerebral complications may become feasible, since several protection schemes have been proposed for the high-risk neonate.[170,171] Clearly, neonatal CBF research remains active with clear, clinical benefits for the advancement of knowledge concerning CBF changes in the perinatal period.

Cerebral Blood Flow in Altitude Sickness

Altitude sickness is a syndrome of headache, anorexia, lassitude, insomnia, and, rarely, cerebral or pulmonary edema seen in humans exposed to high altitudes of over 3,000 meters. The true incidence of altitude sickness remains unknown,[172] but occurs in a majority of climbers on major mountains.[173] Despite its frequency, little is known concerning the pathophysiology of this syndrome. After a period of acclimatization, the altitude sickness resolves spontaneously, although in rare cases returning to a lower altitude may be required to treat severe complications.

The physiologic changes of altitude sickness center on the relative hypoxia at altitude. This results in an increased hypoxic respiratory drive and a resultant hypocapnea. In healthy subjects, arterial pCO_2 can decrease to 20 mm Hg or less. CBF measurements have been performed using a variety of techniques with varying results, although significant increases in CBF appear to occur.[174–176] These data are consistent with the presumed changes associated with hypoxic autoregulation, but are opposite those normally seen with hypocapnea. As further evidence of the necessity of hypoxia, some investigators have noted that supplemental oxygen may prevent altitude sickness.[177] More importantly, inhaled carbon dioxide can rapidly reverse the symptoms of altitude sickness,[174,178,179] while the recommended therapeutic use of acetazolamide reverses the symptoms more slowly.[180] The focus of future research centers on the effects of carbon dioxide on altitude sickness, particularly relative to regional autoregulation.

Cerebral Blood Flow Following Cardiac Arrest

The consequences of cardiopulmonary arrest are well documented, with fewer than 10% of all CPR attempts outside of an ICU setting resulting in survival with normal cerebral function.[181–183] The suboptimal outcome of CPR results primarily from the loss of CBF with the development of subsequent reperfusion injury and necrosis. While CPR guidelines for cerebral resuscitation were first proposed in 1961,[184] the limited success seems to result not from ineffective CPR, but from delayed application of CPR[181,185] and preexisting disease.[186] Nonetheless, research into improving cerebral outcome after cardiopulmonary arrest has produced steady advances since its inception.

Perhaps the first effort to improve cerebral perfusion and recovery centers on the early utilization of CPR. Reducing arrest time by teaching CPR to laypersons is feasible and clinically effective.[181,187,188] The maximum duration of normothermic cardiopulmonary arrest with complete cerebral recovery is 4 or 5 minutes.[189,190] It has been estimated that 100,000 additional lives could be saved in the United States each year if the interval for cerebral recovery could be extended to 10 minutes.[191]

The cause of cardiopulmonary arrest determines the rapidity of cerebral ischemia. Instantaneous circulatory arrest occurs with cardiac arrhythmias, while primary pulmonary arrest results in the gradual onset of circulatory insufficiency over several minutes. With hypovolemic shock or hypoxemia, the development of cerebral hypoperfusion may be hours in developing. Therefore, any model of cardiopulmonary arrest must be specific as to the mechanism of arrest so that the duration of cerebral hypoperfusion can be accurately defined.

As previously discussed, normal brain autoregulation maintains a CBF of about 50 mL/100 g brain/minute, with cerebral perfusion pressures between 50 and 150 mm Hg. At cerebral perfusion pressures less than 50 mm Hg in adults, CBF is compromised. Incomplete ischemia with cerebral perfusion pressures less than 30 mm Hg threatens cerebral viability[192,193] as does a decrease in CBF to less than 15 mL/100 g/minute.[194] In addition, low CBF (10% to 20% of normal) seems to be better tolerated than no flow,[195] although very low flow ($\leq$ 10%) seems to be worse than no flow.[196]

When complete, sudden circulatory arrest occurs, loss of brain O_2 stores occurs within 10 to 20 seconds[197] associated with loss of consciousness.[198] The 5-minute limit to no flow cerebral ischemia is supported by data that glucose and cerebral ATP stores are depleted over the same time course.[199,200] Similarly, membrane ion pumps appear to be completely arrested within 3 to 5 minutes of no flow ischemia.[197,201] In spite of this metabolic evidence of irreversible changes, occasional survival with normal cerebral function is seen after prolonged normothermic arrest in animals[202,203] and humans.[204] Obviously, many factors may explain these discrepancies, probably unique to the individuals involved.

Numerous metabolic changes occur with the onset of complete cerebral ischemia. Many of these result in changes in perfusion on resumption of flow and set up the brain for reperfusion injury. Cerebral lactate accumulation from anaerobic brain metabolism seems to correlate with increased evidence of brain damage.[205–207] Similarly, significant calcium shifts,[208] increases in free fatty acids,[209] and increases in extracellular excitatory amino acids (glutamate and aspartate)[210–214] are seen. How these metabolic alterations relate to the events following reperfusion are unclear and remain to be defined.

With reperfusion after prolonged ischemia, a cerebral postresuscitation syndrome occurs with four basic components: 1) perfusion failure; 2) reoxygenation; 3) extracerebral derangements; and 4) blood abnormalities.[215] Changes indicative of permanent neurologic deficits are first seen at about 24 hours on light microscopy.[196,216–219] These changes are scattered throughout the brain although certain regions seem to be more vulnerable, particularly the hippocampus, the neocortex, and the cerebellum.

Perfusion failure after prolonged anoxia begins as no-reflow in multiple areas of the brain almost immediately.[220–222] With time, this no-reflow phenomenon seems to be overcome with normotensive or hypertensive reperfusion.[220,221,223] The second phase of perfusion failure is transient global reactive hyperemia which lasts 15 to 30 minutes.[224–226] At about 30 minutes postreperfusion, global hypoperfusion develops and lasts from 2 to 12 hours with a significant mismatch between O_2 delivery and O_2 uptake.[223–225,227] The cause of this hypoperfusion remains unclear although vasospasm,[223] edema,[228,229] and blood aggregates[230,231] have all been implicated. Finally, a stable perfusion state develops about 20 hours after injury, which is determined by the severity of the ischemic insult.

The second component of cerebral postresuscitation syndrome, reoxygenation, is an essential part of recovery in reversible cerebral ischemia. Nonetheless, this mechanism seems to be responsible for irreversible reperfusion injury in many areas secondary to free radical generation and lipid peroxidation of membranes.[232–236] Mechanisms for amelioration of reoxygenation injury center on prevention of free radical generation or quenching of them once formed. The optimal pO_2 for reperfusion remains to be determined.[237]

Extracerebral derangements clearly worsen cerebral outcome.[238,239] The most often affected organ is the heart, with recurrent ventricular fibrillation[240] or cardiopulmonary failure[238] being most common. Cardiac arrest in previously healthy animals seems to result in reduction of cardiac output at any given perfusion pressure.[241,242] No convincing evidence exists for a central toxic effect from postischemic viscera.[243]

The final component of cerebral postresuscitation syndrome is blood abnormalities. An early derangement is the accumulation of polymorphonuclear leukocytes and macrophages as a component of reperfusion injury.[230,231,244] Indeed, reperfusion injury in other systems can be prevented by elimination of white blood cells from the reperfusate.[245] Large vessel thrombosis does not usually occur during 20 minutes of no flow.[246]

The experimental study in animal models of prolonged cardiopulmonary arrest requires aggressive ICU management after a standard ischemic insult in order to demonstrate neurologic complications.[247,248] All acceptable models are in large animals, since many small animals tend to spontaneously defibrillate.[191] Recently, an acceptable arrest model has been developed in the rat.[249] Nonetheless, lower animal models are limited by obvious differences in cerebral capabilities.

Several areas provide promise in cerebral resuscitation. In dog models, early hypertension for 1 to 5 minutes after reperfusion eliminated no-reflow[223] and provided improved outcome.[250] This effect is further enhanced by hemodilution,[223] although hemodilution alone has an uncertain effect on outcome.[250,251] In humans, induced hypertension postarrest has not been studied. Clinically, a systolic pressure of 200 mm Hg has been recommended for 1 to 5 minutes after arrest.[191]

The most consistent mechanism for cerebral protection seems to be induced or accidental hypothermia. This results presumably from the decreases in cerebral metabolism associated with decreased tissue temperature. Moderate hypothermia to 30°C induced prior to circulatory arrest protects the brain for up to 20 minutes.[252,253] Deeper hypothermia protects the brain longer,[254,255] but also increases cardiac arrhythmias or asystole. The prolonged ischemia tolerated after cold water drowning[256] results from the fact that circulation stops slowly over several minutes, allowing deep tissue cooling to occur before circulatory arrest. Normothermic drowning does not exhibit any improvement in survival over other methods of asphyxial arrest.[257] The use of hypothermia induced after arrest is more controversial, with limited benefits experimentally[258] or clinically.[259]

Another technique for reducing cerebral metabolism is induced barbiturate coma. While this has been an attractive technique clinically, the results of a multicenter clinical study were negative.[260] Nonetheless, in this study patients with long arrest times or CPR demonstrated a trend toward better cerebral outcome. Subsequent studies have given mixed results.[261–263]

Since significant calcium shifts occur after cerebral ischemia, efforts to block cerebral calcium channels have been undertaken to improve postischemia cerebral recovery. Two calcium entry blockers have been studied: lidoflazine and nimodipine. Both have shown benefit in experimental studies.[264,265] Nevertheless, clinical trials of both drugs have failed to show overall improvement in cerebral outcome.[240,266] Further studies of newer calcium channel blockers are ongoing.

Future approaches for further evaluation center on two main areas. First, various postischemia cocktails have been tested to reduce reoxygenation injury.[232,237,267–269] These appear promising,[270–274] although a consistent result remains elusive. Second, reduction of increased postarrest excitatory neurotransmitters may decrease cerebral metabolism and improve oxygen delivery.[275,276] These and other approaches will, hopefully, provide improved cerebral protection with prolonged ischemia.

Head Trauma and Cerebral Blood Flow

When force is applied to the head, protection is afforded by the enveloping shell of bone known as the skull. Two forms of injury can occur to the underlying brain tissue, depending on the protection afforded by the rigid shell. If the skull is breached, then the injury to the underlying brain results from direct trauma such as from depressed skull fragments or direct brain laceration. This type of injury is focal and limited, and tends not to result in progressive brain dysfunction. More commonly, if the rigid skull remains intact, then deceleration injury can occur when the brain comes in contact with the inner table of the cranial vault. Often, this results in a second, contrecoup injury when the rebounding brain contacts the opposite side of the skull and suffers a smaller, second deceleration injury. The resultant brain injury is a contusion, composed of intra-parenchymal hemorrhage interposed among preserved tissue. This type of inertial injury is a shearing injury, which causes diffuse axonal damage.[277] After the initial injury, further derangements in brain function develop secondary to regional ischemia or hypoxia.[278] Often the two types of injury coexist, resulting from the direct force imparting an acceleration or deceleration to the underlying brain parenchyma.

In animal models, the immediate response to brain injury is an increase in arterial blood pressure with an associated rise in ICP, temporary apnea, and flattening of the EEG.[279] These rapid changes tend to resolve in about 1 minute, but apnea is often seen as a prolonged response in otherwise stable patients.[280] No data are available to corroborate these early changes in humans.

ICP begins to rise in the majority of patients with head injury, exceeding 40 mm Hg in about 10%.[278] Often, this is secondary to an increased cerebral blood volume from vasodilatation, particularly in children.[281] As autoregulation is frequently lost in head injuries,[281,282] the CBF is uncoupled from metabolism and varies directly with cerebral perfusion pressure. In addition, brain injury is often focal, with regional differences in local tissue pressure,[283] resulting in similar differences in perfusion.

If hypotension is present from other injuries, the associated decrease in cerebral perfusion pressure may generate additional ischemic injury. Many different types of injury are associated with vasospasm, and the restoration of global perfusion to normal may not restore rCBF in all areas.[278] Studies of the brains from consecutive patients with fatal, blunt head injury demonstrate obvious ischemic brain damage in 91%, with a varied distribution.[284]

Normal cerebral autoregulation results in vasodilation and an increased ICP associated with hypoxia or hypercarbia. Any reduction in cerebral perfusion may then increase ischemia, resulting in further increases in ICP. These "plateau waves" of ICP may reach 50 to 100 mm Hg and last for minutes.[285] These changes in CBF are variable; about half of all patients with severe head injury develop diffuse hyperemia in excess of metabolic demands.[282] The common thread behind these changes is the loss of cerebral autoregulation. In comatose patients with apparently intact autoregulation, decreased CBF results from preserved metabolic flow coupling.

As the injury matures, almost all patients with severe head injury develop capillary leakage and resultant vasogenic cerebral edema. This may develop as early as 30 minutes after injury,[286] but is maximal between the third and seventh days.[287] The ICP returns

to normal in 10 to 14 days if recovery occurs. Nonetheless, restoration of the BBB may not be complete for months after injury.[287]

Experimental Models of Head Injury

Since human studies of head injury are by default observational, much of the knowledge concerning changes in CBF associated with head injury are derived from animal studies. Four main models of cerebral trauma have evolved in experimental study. First, Gennarelli[288] developed a nonimpact controlled acceleration device which delivers motion of the head in a single plane. Using this model, Gennarelli showed that sagittal acceleration produced higher ICP elevation than did coronal acceleration.[288]

A second experimental model for head injury is the impact acceleration model developed by Nilsson.[289] In this model, an impact of 7 to 9 m/sec is used to impart a standard trauma in rats. Injury is followed by an increased metabolic rate and increased neuronal activity. Within minutes, this transient increase was associated with an increase in CBF, followed minutes later by a 30% to 40% decrease.[289] Normalization of CBF then occurs over 20 to 30 minutes. A late decrease in brain metabolism was seen, correlating with the severity of the injury.

In 1976, Sullivan and colleagues developed a fluid percussion model in cats.[290] In this model, cerebral blood volume is increased,[291] but CBF remains unchanged.[292] Similar changes have been noted in the fourth model, the Remington stunner model in cats.[293,294] The challenge of this experimental work remains the definition of the injury and the correlation and explanation of the variety of changes seen. For now, the changes noted are model-dependent and generalizations await further experimental study.

Atherosclerotic Cerebrovascular Disease

Atherosclerotic disease involving the cerebral circulation is a common condition in Western societies, making this disease process the third leading cause of death in the U.S.[4,295] The pattern of disease is familiar to anyone dealing with cerebrovascular conditions, with relative sparing of the intracranial vessels and significant involvement of the large extracranial arteries.[296,297] In contrast to other organ systems, the large cerebral vessels play an important role in the regulation of CBF.[298] Therefore, large vessel atherosclerosis may be more important to the disruption of CBF than in most organ systems. Flow can be limited in the cerebral circulation by two mechanisms: local restriction of flow by embolic occlusion, or a more generalized ischemia secondary to medium-sized arterial thrombosis.

While the embolic origin of cerebrovascular events is now widely accepted, the original impetus for extracranial arterial revascularization was the presence of hemodynamically significant carotid artery disease.[299,300] The premise of this etiology for cerebral ischemia was that the extracranial lesion was flow limiting, resulting in hypoperfusion and, therefore, transient ischemia. In what proved to be a defining experiment, Kendall and Marshall demonstrated that controlled hypotension in patients with documented transient ischemic attacks could not reproduce their transient ischemia.[301] These clinical findings were confirmed by others,[302] ending the hemodynamic theory for cerebrovascular events.

A relationship between hemodynamics and embolic events is clearly present, although not obvious at first review. The association of embolic events with intraplaque hemorrhage is well documented,[303-306] as is the association of intraplaque hemorrhage with increased severity of stenosis.[307] Therefore, the major relationship between degree of stenosis and symptoms is the common association of both with intraplaque hemorrhage. As the stenotic atherosclerotic lesion progresses, it often does so by developing intraplaque hemorrhage; with the development of intraplaque hemorrhage, ulceration and symptoms become more common.

In spite of these clinical observations, the hemodynamic theory remains of interest in certain clinical settings. First, even embolic events will at some point disrupt hemodynamics, although these changes will be in the periphery at the arteriolar level. Second, the ill-defined entity of global hemispheric ischemia is clearly a hemodynamic issue and seems to be increasing in incidence as more patients with diffuse atherosclerosis are surviving into advanced age. Thus, hemodynamics remain an issue relative to intracranial pathology and diffuse extracranial occlusive disease.

As previously discussed, large vessel abnormalities are partially compensated for by the collateral pathways at the base of the brain, commonly referred to as the Circle of Willis. In spite of its well-documented function in humans, the collateral pathways are often incomplete.[3,308] As a result, the collateral circulation function in any given patient remains undefined. Newer methods of assessing cerebral collateral flow and hemodynamic compensation have shown that the degree of stenosis in an extracranial atherosclerotic blood vessel is a poor indicator of collateral reserve.[309,310] Many investigators feel that newer techniques for assessment of collateral flow will play an increasingly important role in determining the adequacy of collateral pathways in individual patients and, therefore, the necessity for cerebral revascularization.

Some authors have gone so far as to propose that the concept of a hemodynamically significant degree of extracranial carotid stenosis be abandoned in favor of a regional assessment of collateral reserve.[311] This approach again negates the issue of ulceration and symptoms, both of which have a dramatic influence on the natural history of extracranial cerebrovascular disease.

Three types of stroke occur in humans: ischemic, hemorrhagic, or lacunar. Hypertension is a significant risk factor in stroke, particularly the lacunar or hemorrhagic type.[312] A cerebral hemorrhage has the characteristics of a mass lesion of the brain, although regional blood flow abnormalities may be present within the areas surrounding the hemorrhage. Lacunes are small areas of injury in the internal capsule of the brain, sometimes related to Charcot-Bouchard aneurysms which may rupture or occlude with thrombus. These are the lesions most commonly associated with hypertension. Ischemic stroke is the most common and may be further subdivided into embolic or thrombotic etiologies. Embolic stroke can occur secondary to any source for emboli, originating anywhere from the heart to the extracranial arterial tree. In general, the most consistently associated area for embolic events is the extracranial carotid artery. It is in this area that platelet aggregation occurs most frequently and fibrinous debris is deposited, providing an origin for cerebrovascular events.

When atherosclerotic lesions lead to platelet aggregation, vasoactive substances are released which may have profound effects on downstream vasomotor tone. These substances include serotonin, ADP, and thromboxane[313,314] these may contribute to the development of downstream vasospasm, particularly in arteries with underlying arteriosclerosis.[315,316] In these experimental studies, serotonin and thromboxane had minimal vasoconstrictor effects in large arteries of normal monkeys, but produced a marked increase in resistance in the large arteries of atherosclerotic monkeys.[315] Similar results have been seen in a hypercholesterolemic pig model, where basilar artery endothelial-dependent relaxation is impaired while vasoconstriction is enhanced.[317] The etiology behind this enhanced vasoconstrictor response in atherosclerotic arteries remains undefined.

The completion of an atherosclerotic stenosis by thrombosis and occlusion results in dramatic changes in distribution of blood flow. The more peripheral the occlusion occurs, the more significant the regional hemodynamic changes. The extent of the ischemic injury depends on the effectiveness of the regional collateral blood flow. Hemodynamically significant decreases in perfusion pressure associated with internal carotid occlusions do not produce decreases in regional blood flow.[318] In contrast, more distal occlusion of the middle cerebral artery sharply reduces perfusion pressure and blood flow, resulting in ischemia.[319,320] Normal pial artery pressures of 55 to 60 mm Hg are reduced by middle cerebral artery occlusion to 8 mm Hg after 15 minutes of occlusion and increase only modestly to 16 mm Hg over the next 2 hours.[320] Nonetheless, in this model small increases in perfusion pressure are associated with significant increases in local blood flow and electrocortical activity.

In the larger vessels, reduction in distal blood flow is normally seen only when about a 75% reduction in arterial cross-sectional area occurs. Similar changes are seen in cat middle cerebral arteries where a reduction from 700 μM to 200 μM is required to reduce local blood flow.[321] As is seen in other experimental models, when distal middle cerebral artery pressure fell below 35 mm Hg, blood flow was also decreased.[321]

Acute cerebrovascular occlusion produces a central focus of ischemia, with a continuum between the severely ischemic core and the normal peripheral brain.[322] In humans, neurologic function is preserved in areas where regional blood flow is greater than 19 mL/100 g/min; evidence of cerebral infarction by CT scan is seen in areas where the regional blood flow is less than 15 mL/100 g/min.[323,324] Autoregulation is compromised at the decreased perfusion pressures seen around an acute infarction and reduction in blood pressure secondary to hemodynamic instability will further compromise blood flow. It is significant that up to 60% of patients will have instability of cardiac output in the first 24 hours following acute stroke.[325] The result is that extension of infarction is a common occurrence, resulting from further hemodynamic instability.

Following cerebrovascular occlusion, the complications associated with reperfusion are present, since spontaneous lysis of thrombus can occur. With the reperfusion of ischemic brain parenchyma, many of the changes seen after cardiac arrest occur, as discussed earlier in this chapter. With irreversible ischemia, there is an initial increase in perfusion, followed by a decrease over the ensuing hours or days. These changes are seen with ischemia of any sort and are not specific for ischemic stroke.

The major focus of research in reversal of acute stroke lies in the use of thrombolysis to remove cerebrovascular occlusions and, thereby, limit the damage associated with the regional ischemia. Experimental models of acute stroke allow accurate assessment of the reduction in infarct volume associated with thrombolytic therapy. These models in both rabbits[326] and rats[327] have demonstrated a benefit in the reduction of infarct volume. In the rat model assessed by cerebral angiography, one third of all animals receiving thrombolytic therapy had a reduction in infarct size with no hemorrhagic complications.[327] In the rabbit model, the incidence of hemorrhagic complications was increased with streptokinase, but not with tissue plasminogen activator (tPA).[328] While the clinical application of these findings is just beginning to become apparent, thrombolysis in acute stroke will remain an active area of both clinical and basic science investigation for the indefinite future.

Future Directions

The future of cerebrovascular and CBF research centers on the cellular and molecular mechanisms behind cerebral ischemia and blood flow regulation. Clearly, the definition of NO as EDRF has completed a significant segment of the puzzle, but the effects of this remarkable substance are only now beginning to be defined. A significant area of future cerebrovascular research lies in the definition of the role of NO in reperfusion injury and cerebral vasospasm. The pathophysiology of autoregulation and the role of vasodilators will provide new insights into the regional regulation of CBF.

The role of new technology in defining CBF changes remains an area of great promise for future research. The advances in PET imaging have provided new insights into CBF in a number of disease states. Similarly, the evolution of MR technology and computer processing has led to innovative methods of imaging CBF with new advances occurring regularly. These technologies hold great promise for further advances.

Perhaps the greatest advances are those yet to be imagined. The future of this area of research is ensured by both the complexity and the mystique associated with the brain. The mystery surrounding the brain and its function will remain a motivating force for continuous advances in our knowledge of its physiology and function.

References

1. de Lumley MA: Meningeal vascularization of preneanderthal man. In: G. Salamon (ed). *Advances in Cerebral Angiography*. Berlin: Springer-Verlag; 115–121, 1975.
2. Alpers BJ, Berry RG, Paddison RM: Anatomical studies of the circle of Willis in normal brain. *Arch Neurol Psychiatry* 81:409–422, 1959.
3. Kameth S: Observation of the length and diameter of vessels forming the circle of Willis. *J Anat* 133:419–423, 1981.
4. Siesjo BK: Cerebral circulation and metabolism. *J Neurosurg* 60:883–908, 1984.
5. Faraci FM, Heistad DD: Regulation of large cerebral arteries and cerebral microvascular pressure. *Circ Res* 66:8–17, 1990.
6. Yada K, Nakagawa Y, Tsuru M: Circulatory disturbance of the venous system during experimental intracranial hypertension. *J Neurosurg* 39:723–729, 1973.
7. Harper AM: Autoregulation of cerebral blood flow: influence of the arterial blood pressure on the blood flow

through the cerebral cortex. *J Neurol Neurosurg Psychiatry* 29:398–403, 1966.

8. Lassen NA: Cerebral blood flow and oxygen consumption in man. *Physiol Rev* 39:183–238, 1959.

9. Rapela CE, Green HD: Autoregulation of canine cerebral blood flow. *Circ Res* 15(suppl 1):205–212, 1964.

10. Schneider M: Critical blood pressure in the cerebral circulation. In: Schade JP, McMenemy WH (eds). *Selective Vulnerability of the Brain in Hypoxaemia*. Oxford: Blackwell Scientific; 7–20, 1963.

11. Fog M: Cerebral circulation: the reaction of the pial arteries to a fall in blood pressure. *Arch Neurol Psychiatry* 37:351–364, 1937.

12. Fog M: Cerebral circulation: II. Reaction of pial arteries to increase in blood pressure. *Arch Neurol Psychiatry* 41:260–278, 1939.

13. Forbes HS, Cobb SS: Vasomotor control of cerebral vessels. *Brain* 61:221–233, 1938.

14. Faraci FM, Heistad DD: Regulation of cerebral blood vessels by humoral and endothelium-dependent mechanisms: update on humoral regulation of vascular tone. *Hypertension* 17:917–922, 1991.

15. Strandgaard S, Jones JV, MacKenzie ET, Harper AM: Upper limit of cerebral blood flow autoregulation in experimental renovascular hypertension in the baboon. *Circ Res* 37:164–167, 1975.

16. Edelman GM, Gally JA: Nitric oxide: linking space and time in the brain. *PNAS* 89:11651–11652, 1992.

17. Snyder SH: Nitric oxide: first in a new class of neurotransmitters. *Science* 257:494–496, 1992.

18. Iadecola C: Regulation of the cerebral microcirculation during neural activity: is nitric oxide the missing link? *Trends Neurosci* 16:206–214, 1993.

19. Ma L: Evidence for nitric oxide-generator cells in the brain. Bull Tokyo Med Den Univ, 40:125–134, 1993.

20. Faraci FM, Breese KR: Nitric oxide mediates vasodilatation in the response to activation of N-methyl-D-aspartate receptors in brain. *Circ Res* 72:476–480, 1993.

21. Faraci FM, Mayhan WG, Farrell WJ, Heistad DD: Humoral regulation of blood flow to the choroid plexus: role of arginine vasopressin. *Circ Res* 63:373–379, 1988.

22. Faraci FM, Mayhan WG, Heistad DD: Effect of vasopressin on production of cerebrospinal fluid: possible role of vasopressin (V_1)-receptors. *Am J Physiol* 258: R94–R98, 1990.

23. Pickard JD, MacKenzie ET: Inhibition of prostaglandin synthesis and the response of baboon cerebral circulation to carbon dioxide. *Nature* 245:187–188, 1973.

24. Jackson EK, Gerkens JF, Symon L, et al: Prostaglandin biosynthesis does not participate in hypercapnia-induced cerebral vasodilatation in the dog. *J Pharmacol Exp Ther* 226:486–492, 1983.

25. Siesjo BK, Nilsson B: Prostaglandins and the cerebral circulation. *Adv Prostaglandin Thromboxane Leukot Res* 10:367–380, 1982.

26. Raper AJ, Kontos HA, Patterson JL: Response of pial precapillary vessels to changes in arterial carbon dioxide tension. *Circ Res* 28:518–523, 1971.

27. Harper AM, Bell RA: The effect of metabolic acidosis and alkalosis on the blood flow through the cerebral cortex. *J Neurol Neurosurg Psychiatry* 26:341–344, 1963.

28. Lewelt W, Jenkins LW, Miller JD: Effects of experimental fluid percussion injury of the brain on cerebrovascular reactivity to hypoxia and hypercapnia. *J Neurosurg* 56:332–333, 1982.

29. Saunders ML, Miller JD, Stablein D, Allen G: The ef-

fects of graded experimental trauma on cerebral blood flow and responsiveness to CO_2. *J Neurosurg* 51:18–26, 1979.

30. Bell Ba, Foubister GC, Neto NGF, Miller JD: Effect of experimental common carotid arteriotomy on cerebral blood flow in rats. *Neurosurgery* 16:332–326, 1985.

31. Jennett WB, Miller JD, Harper AM: *Effects of Carotid Artery Surgery on Cerebral Blood Flow*. Amsterdam: Excerpta Medica; 1976.

32. Heistad DD, Marcus ML, Piegors DJ, Armstrong ML: Regulation of cerebral blood flow in atherosclerotic monkeys. *Am J Physiol* 239:H539–H544, 1980.

33. Cold GE: Cerebral blood flow in acute head injury: the regulation of cerebral blood flow and metabolism during the acute phase of head injury, and its significance for therapy. *Acta Neurochir* S49:1-64, 1990.

34. Buchanan JE, Phillis JW: The role of nitric oxide in the regulation of cerebral blood flow. *Brain Res* 610: 248–255, 1993.

35. Niwa K, Lindaer U, Villringer A, Dirnagl U: Blockade of nitric oxide synthesis in rats strongly attenuates the CBF response to extracellular acidosis. *J Cereb Blood Flow Metab* 13:535–539, 1993.

36. Thomas D, Crockard A: Cerebral metabolism and blood flow. In: Crockard A, Hayward R, Hoff JT (eds). *Neurosurgery: The Scientific Basis of Clinical Practice*. Oxford: Blackwell Scientific; 223–39, 1985.

37. Kozniewska E, Oseka M, Stys T: Effects of endothelium-derived nitric oxide on cerebral circulation during normoxia and hypoxia in the rat. *J Cereb Blood Flow Metab* 12:311–317, 1992.

38. Rosomoff HL, Holaday DA: Cerebral blood flow and cerebral oxygen consumption during hypothermia. *Am J Physiol* 179:85–92, 1954.

39. Baez S: Recording of microvascular dimensions with an image splitter television microscope. *J Appl Physiol* 21:299–301, 1966.

40. Kontos HA, Raper AJ, Patterson J: Analysis of vasoreactivity of local pH, pCO_2, and bicarbonate on pial vessels. *Stroke* 8:358–360, 1977.

41. Wei EP, Ellis EF, Kontos HA: Role of prostaglandins in pial arteriolar response to CO_2 and hypoxia. *Am J Physiol* 238:H226–H230, 1980.

42. Marcus ML, Busija DW, Bischof CJ, et al: Method for measurement of cerebral blood flow. *Fed Proc* 40: 2306–2310, 1981.

43. Busija DW, Heistad DD, Marcus ML: Continuous measurement of cerebral blood flow in anesthetized cats and dogs. *Am J Physiol* 241:H228–H234, 1981.

44. Auklund K, Bower BF, Berliner RW: Measurement of local blood flow with hydrogen gas. *Circ Res* 14: 164–187, 1964.

45. Farrar JK: Hydrogen clearance technique: In:Wood JH (ed). *Cerebral Blood Flow*. New York: McGraw-Hill; 275–87, 1987.

46. Prinzmetal M, Simkin B, Bergman HC, Kruger HE: Studies on the coronary circulation. II. The collateral circulation of the normal human heart by coronary perfusion with radioactive erythrocytes and glass spheres. *Am Heart J* 33:420–442, 1947.

47. Heistad DD, Marcus ML, Busija DW: Measurement of cerebral blood flow in experimental animals with microspheres: applications of the method. In: Passunneau JV (ed). *Cerebral Metabolism and Neural Function*. Baltimore: Williams & Wilkins; 1980.

48. Dole WP, Jackson DL, Rosenblatt JI, Thompson WL: Relative error and variability in blood flow measure-

ments with radiolabeled microspheres. *Am J Physiol* 243:371–378, 1982.

49. Rhodes BA, Zolle I, Buchanan JW, Wagner HN: Radioactive albumin microspheres for studies of the pulmonary circulation. *Radiology* 1969;92:1453–1460.

50. Morikawa S, Lanz O, Johnson CC: Laser-Doppler measurements of localized pulsatile fluid velocity. *IEEE Trans Biomed Eng* 18:416–420, 1991.

51. Karanfilian RG, Lynch TG, Zirul VT, et al: The value of laser Doppler velocimetry and transcutaneous oxygen tension determination in predicting healing of ischemic forefoot ulcerations and amputations in diabetic and nondiabetic patients. *J Vasc Surg* 4:511–516, 1986.

52. Arbit E, Diresta GR, Bedford RF, et al: Intraoperative measurement of cerebral and tumor blood flow with laser Doppler flowmetry. *Neurosurgery* 24:166–170, 1989.

53. Rosenblum BR, Bonner RF, Oldfield EH: Intraoperative measurement of cortical blood flow adjacent to cerebral AVM using laser Doppler velocimetry. *J Neurosurg* 66:396–399, 1987.

54. Morita-Tsuzuki T, Bouskela E, Hardebo JE: Vasomotion in the rat cerebral microcirculation recorded by laser-Doppler flowmetry. *Acta Physiol Scand* 146:431–439, 1992.

55. Meyerson BA, Gunasekera L, Linderoth B, et al: Bedside monitoring of regional cortical blood flow in comatose patients using laser Doppler flowmetry. *Neurosurgery* 29:750–755, 1991.

56. Muir JK, Boerschel M, Ellis EF: Continuous monitoring of posttraumatic cerebral blood flow using laser-Doppler flowmetry. *J Neurotrauma* 9:355–362, 1992.

57. Riva CE, Harino S, Petrig BL, Shonat RD: Laser Doppler flowmetry in the optic nerve. *Exp Eye Res* 55:499–506, 1992.

58. Bolognese P, Miller JI, Heger IM, et al: Laser-Doppler flowmetry in neurosurgery. *J Neurosurg Anesthesiol* 5:151–158, 1993.

59. Kloiber O, Miyazawa T, Hoehn-Berlage M, Hossmann KA: Simultaneous ^{31}P NMR spectroscopy and laser Doppler flowmetry of rat brain during global ischemia and reperfusion. *NMR in Biomedicine* 6:144–152, 1993.

60. Aaslid R, Markwalder TM, Nornes H: Noninvasive transcranial Doppler recording of flow velocity in basal cerebral arteries. *J Neurosurg* 57:769–774, 1982.

61. Arnolds BJ, von Reutern GM: Transcranial Doppler sonography: examination technique and normal reference values. *Ultrasound Med Biol* 12:115–123, 1986.

62. Hennerici M, Rautenberg W, Sitzer G, Schwartz A: Transcranial Doppler ultrasound for the assessment of intracranial flow velocity. Part 1: examination technique and normal values. *Surg Neurol* 27:439–448, 1987.

63. Vriens EM, Kraaier V, Musbach M, Wieneke GH, van Huffelen AC: Transcranial pulsed Doppler measurements of blood velocity in the middle cerebral artery: reference values at rest and during hyperventilation in healthy volunteers in relation to age and sex. *Ultrasound Med Biol* 15:1–8, 1989.

64. Brass LM, Pavlakis SG, DeVivo D, Piomelli S, Mohr JP: Transcranial Doppler measurements of the middle cerebral artery: effect of hematocrit. *Stroke* 19:1466–1469, 1988.

65. Ringelstein EB, Sievers C, Ecker S, et al: Noninvasive assessment of CO_2-induced cerebral vasomotor response in normal individuals and patients with internal carotid artery occlusions. *Stroke* 19:963–969, 1988.

66. Ringlestein EB, Van Eyck S, Mertens I: Evaluation of cerebral vasomotor reactivity by various vasodilating stimuli: comparison of CO_2 to acetazolamide. *J Cereb Blood Flow Metab* 12:162–168, 1992.

67. Madsen PL, Sperling BK, Warming T, et al: Middle cerebral artery blood velocity and cerebral blood flow and O_2 uptake during dynamic exeicse. *J Applied Physiol* 74:245–250, 1993.

68. Frey MA, Mader TH, Bagian JP, Charles JB, Meehan RT: Cerebral blood velocity and other cardiovascular responses to 2 day head-down tilt. *J Applied Physiol* 74:319–325, 1993.

69. American Academy of Neurology, Therapeutics, and Technology Assessment Subcommittee. Assessment: transcranial Doppler. *Neurology* 40:680–681, 1990.

70. Lindegaard KF, Bakke SJ, Gromlimund P, et al: Assessment of intracranial hemodynamics in carotid artery disease by transcranial Doppler ultrasound. *J Neurosurg* 63:890–898, 1985.

71. Grolimund P, Seiler RW, Aaslid R, Huber P, Zurbruegg H: Evaluation of cerebrovascular disease by combined extracranial and transcranial Doppler sonography: experience in 1,039 patients. *Stroke* 18:1018–1024, 1987.

72. Halsey JH, McDowell HA, Gelmon S, Morawetz RB: Blood velocity in the middle cerebral artery and regional cerebral blood flow during carotid endarterectomy. *Stroke* 20:53–58, 1989.

73. Schroeder T: Hemodynamic significance of internal carotid artery disease. *Acta Neurol Scand* 77:353–372, 1988.

74. Lassen NA, Ingvar DH: Regional cerebral blood flow in man. *Arch Neurol* 9:615–622, 1963.

75. Agnoli A, Principe M, Priori AM, Bozzao L, Fieschi C: Measurements of rCBF by intravenous injection of 133-Xenon. In: M. Brock, Fieschi C, Ingvar DH, Lassen NA, Schurmann K, (eds). *Cerebral Blood Flow.* Berlin: Springer-Verlag;31–34, 1969.

76. Mallet BL, Veall N: Investigation of cerebral blood flow in hypertension, using radioactive-xenon inhalation and extracranial recording. *Lancet* 1:1081–1082, 1963.

77. Latchaw RE, Yonas H, Pentheny SL, Gur D: Adverse reactions to xenon-enhanced CT cerebral blood flow determination. *Radiology* 163:251–254, 1987.

78. Jaggi JL, Obrist WD: Regional cerebral blood flow determination by $^{133}Xenon$ clearance. In: Wood JH, (ed). *Cerebral Blood Flow.* New York: McGraw-Hill; 1987.

79. Gur D, Yonas H, Jackson DL, et al: Simultaneous measurements of cerebral blood flow by the xenon/CT method and the microsphere method: a comparison. *Invest Radiol* 20:672–677, 1985.

80. Fatouros PP, Wist AO, Kishore PR, et al: Xenon/computed tomography cerebral blood flow measurements: methods and accuracy. *Inves Radiol* 22:705–712, 1987.

81. Winchell HS, Horst WD, Braun L, et al: N-isopropyl-^{123}l-*p*-iodoamphetamine: single-pass brain uptake and washout; binding to brain synaptosomes; and localization in dog and monkey brains. *J Nucl Med* 21:947–952, 1980.

82. Ell PJ, Hocknell JML, Jarritt PH, et al: A Tc-99m-labelled radiotracer for the investigation of cerebral vascular disease. *Nucl Med Commun* 6:437–441, 1985.

83. Holmes RA, Chaplin SB, Royston KG, et al: Cerebral uptake and retention of Tc-99m-hexamethylpropyleneamine oxine (Tc-99m-HMPAO). *Nucl Med Commun* 6:443–447, 1985.

84. Horowitz AL: *MRI Physics for Physicians.* New York: Springer-Verlag; 1989.

85. Morris PG: *Nuclear Magnetic Resonance Imaging in Medicine and Biology.* Oxford: Clarendon; 1986.

86. Valk J, MacLean C, Alara PR: *Basic Principles of Nuclear Magnetic Resonance Imaging.* Amsterdam: Elsevier; 1985.

87. Suddarth SA, Johnson GA: Three-dimensional MR microscopy with large arrays. *Magn Reson Med* 18:132–141, 1991.

88. Eccles CD, Callaghan PT: High-resolution imaging: the NMR microscope. *J Magn Reson* 68:393–398, 1986.

89. Johnson GA, Thompson MB, Gewoalt SL, Hayes CE: Nuclear magnetic resonance imaging at microscopic resolution. *J Magn Reson* 68:129–137, 1986.

90. Aguayo JB, Blackband SJ, Schoeniger J, et al: Nuclear magnetic resonance imaging of a single cell. *Nature* 322:190–191, 1986.

91. Keller P, Drayer B, Fram E, et al: MR angiography with two-dimensional acquisition and three-dimensional display: work in progress. *Radiology* 173:527–532, 1989.

92. Masaryk TJ, Modic MT, Ruggieri PM: Three-dimensional (volume) gradient-echo imaging or the carotid bifurcation: preliminary clinical experience. *Radiology* 171:801–806, 1989.

93. Dumoulin C, Cline HE, Souza S, et al: Three-dimensional time-of-flight magnetic resonance angiography using spin saturation. *Magn Reson Med* 11:35–46, 1989.

94. Anderson C, Saloner D, Fortner S, Lee R: Dedicated coil for carotid MR angiography. *Radiology* 176:868–872, 1990.

95. Tsuruda JS, Saloner D, Anderson C: Noninvasive evaluation of cerebral ischemia: trends for the 1990s. *Circulation* 83:(suppl I)176–189, 1991.

96. Ruggieri PM, Masaryk TJ, Ross JS, Modic MT: Intracranial magnetic resonance imaging. *Invest Radiol* 27:S33–39, 1992.

97. Meier D, Maier S, Boesigner P: Quantitative flow measurements on phantoms and on blood vessels with MR. *Magn Reson Med* 8:25–34, 1988.

98. Detre JA, Leigh JS, Williams DS, Koretsky AP: Perfusion imaging: magnetic resonance in medicine, 23:37–45, 1992.

99. Pan X, Rapp JH, Harris HW, et al: Identification of aortic thrombus by magnetic resonance imaging. *J Vasc Surg* 9:801–805, 1989.

100. Lauffer RB: Magnetic resonance contrast media: principles and progress. *Magn Reson Q* 6:65–84, 1990.

101. Stark DD, Weissleder R, Elizondo G, et al: Superparamagnetic iron oxide: clinical application as a contrast agent for MR imaging of the liver. *Radiology* 168:297–301, 1988.

102. Weissleder R, Elizondo G, Wittenberg J, et al: Ultrasmall superparamagnetic iron oxide: characterization of a new class of contrast agents for MR. *Radiology* 175:489–493, 1990.

103. Ackerman JJH, Grove TH, Wong GG, et al: Mapping of metabolites in whole animals by ^{31}P NMR using surface coils. *Nature* 283:167–170, 1980.

104. Welch KMA, Levine SR, Martin G, et al: Magnetic resonance spectroscopy in cerebral ischemia. *Neurologic Clinics* 10:1–29, 1992.

105. Gadian DG, Radda GK, Richard RE, et al: ^{31}P NMR in living tissue: the road from a promising to an important tool in biology. In: Shulman RG (ed). *Biological Applications of Magnetic Resonance.* New York: Academic Press, Inc.; 463–535, 1970.

106. Jacobson L, Cohen JS: Improved technique for investigation of cell metabolism by ^{31}P NMR spectroscopy. *Biosci Rep* 1:141–150, 1981.

107. Maudsley AA, Hilal SK: Biologic aspects of sodium-23 imaging. *Br Med Bull* 40:165–166, 1984.

108. Mason GF, Behar KL, Rothman DL, Shulman RG: NMR determination of intracerebral glucose concentration and transport kinetics in rat brain. *J Cereb Blood Flow Metab* 12:448–455, 1992.

109. Ewing JR, Branch CA, Helpern JA, et al: Cerebral blood flow measured by NMR indicator dilution in cats. *Stroke* 20:259–267, 1989.

110. van Zijl, Ligeti L, Sinnwell T, et al: Measurement of cerebral blood flow by volume-selective ^{19}F NMR spectroscopy. *Magn Reson Med* 16:489–495, 1990.

111. Michenfelder JD, Theye RA: The effects of anesthesia and hypothermia on canine cerebral ATP and lactate during anoxia produced by decapitation. *Anesthesiology* 33:430, 1979.

112. Levine SR, Helpern JA, Welch KM, et al: Human focal cerebral ischemia: evaluation of brain pH and energy metabolism with P^{31} NMR spectroscopy. *Radiology* 185:537–544, 1992.

113. Kogure K, Busto R, Schwartzman RJ, et al: The dissociation of cerebral blood flow, metabolism, and function in the early stages of developing cerebral infarction. *Ann Neurol* 8:278–290, 1980.

114. Mabe H, Blomqvist P, Siesjo BK: Intracellular pH in the brain following transient ischemia. *J Cereb Blood Flow Metab* 3:109–114, 1983.

115. Welch KM, Levine SR, Martin G, et al: Magnetic resonance spectroscopy in cerebral ischemia. *Neurol Clin* 10:1–29, 1992.

116. Welch KM, Levine SR, Helpern JA: Pathophysiological correlates of cerebral ischemia: the significance of cellular acid-base shifts. *Funct Neurol* 5:21–31, 1990.

117. Edelman RR, Mattle HP, Atkinson DJ, et al: Cerebral blood flow: assessment with dynamic contrast-enhanced T2* weighted MR imaging at 1.5 T. *Radiology* 176:211–220, 1990.

118. Gore JC, Majumdar S: Measurement of tissue blood flow using intravascular relaxation agents and magnetic resonance imaging. *Magn Reson Med* 14:242–8, 1990.

119. Kent TA, Quast MJ, Kaplan BJ, et al: Assessment of a superparamagnetic iron oxide (AMI-25) as a brain contrast agent. *Magn Reson Med* 13:434–443, 1990.

120. Rosen BR, Belliveau JW, Vevea JM, Brady TJ: Perfusion imaging with NMR contrast agents. *Magn Reson Med* 14:249–265, 1990.

121. Le Bihan D, Breton E, Lallemand D, et al: MR imaging of intravoxel incoherent motions: applications to diffusion and perfusion in neurologic disorders. *Radiology* 161:401–407, 1986.

122. Turner R, Le Bihan D, Maier J, et al: Echo-planar imaging of intravoxel incoherent motion. *Radiology* 177:407–414, 1990.

123. Henkelman RM: Does IVIM measure classic perfusion? *Magn Reson Med* 16:470–475, 1990.

124. Mintorovitch J, Moseley ME, Chileuitt L, et al: Comparison of diffusion- and T2-weighted MRI for the early detection of cerebral ischemia and reperfusion in rats. *Magn Reson Med* 18:39–50, 1991.

125. Moseley ME, Kucharczyk J, Mintorovitch J, et al: Diffusion-weighted MR imaging of acute stroke: correlation with T2-weighted and magnetic susceptibility-enhanced MR imaging in cats. *Am J Neuroradiol* 11:423–429, 1990.

126. Wolf A: Special characteristics and potential for radio-

pharmaceuticals for positron emission tomography. *Semin Nucl Med* 11:2–12, 1981.

127. Kety SS: Measurement of local blood flow by the exchange of an inert diffusible substance. *Methods Med Res* 8:228–236, 1979.

128. Landau WM, Freygang WH, Rowland LP, et al: The local circulation of the living brain: values in the unanesthetized and anesthetized cat. *Tran Am Neurol Assoc* 80:125–129, 1955.

129. Jones SC, Greenberg JH, Dann R, et al: Cerebral blood flow with the continuous infusion of oxygen-15-labelled water. *J Cereb Blood Flow Metab* 5:566–575, 1985.

130. Jones SC, Greenberg JH, Reivich M: Error analysis for the determination of cerebral blood flow with the continuous inhalation of ^{15}O-labelled carbon dioxide and positron emission tomography. *J Comput Assist Tomogr* 6:116–124, 1982.

131. Lammertsma AA, Heather JD, Jones T, et al: A statistical study of the steady-state technique for measuring regional cerebral blood flow and oxygen utilization using ^{15}O. *J Comput Assist Tomogr* 6:566–573, 1982.

132. Yonas H, Smith HA, Durham SR, et al: Increased stroke risk predicted by compromised cerebral blood flow reactivity. *J Neurosurg* 79:483–489, 1993.

133. Powers WJ, Raichle ME: Positron emission tomography and its application to the study of cerebrovascular disease in man. *Stroke* 16:361–376, 1985.

134. Reese TS, Karnovsky MJ: Final structural localization of a blood-brain barrier to exogenous peroxidase. *J Cell Biol* 34:207–217, 1967.

135. Johannson B, Nilson B: The pathophysiology of the blood brain barrier dysfunction induced by severe hypercapnia and by epileptic brain activity. *Acta Neuropathologica* 38:153–158, 1977.

136. Rapaport SI, Hori M, Klatzo I: Testing of a hypothesis for osmotic opening of the blood brain barrier. *Am J Physiol* 223:323–331, 1972.

137. Goodale RL, Goetzman B, Visscher MB: Hypoxic and codoacetic acid and alveolocapillary barrier permeability to albumin. *Am J Physiol* 219:1226–1230, 1970.

138. Siesjo BK, Ljundggren B: Cerebral energy reserves after prolonged hypoxia and ischemia. *Arch Neurol* 29:400–407, 1973.

139. Goodman LS, Gilman A: *The Pharmacological Basis of Therapeutics*, 5th Ed. New York: MacMillan; 1975.

140. Crosby G, Crane AM, Sokoloff L: Local changes in cerebral glucose utilization during ketamine anesthesia. *Anesthesiology* 56:437–443, 1982.

141. Landau WM, Freygang WH, Rowland LP, et al: The local circulation of the living brain, values in the unanesthetized and anesthetized cat. *Trans Am Neurol Assoc* 80:125–132, 1955.

142. Albrecht RF, Miletich DJ, Madala LR: Normalization of cerebral blood flow during prolonged halothane anesthesia. *Anesthesiology* 58:26–31, 1983.

143. Phirman JR, Shapiro HM: Modification of nitrous oxide induced intracranial hypertension by prior induction of anesthesia. *Anesthesiology* 46:150–151, 1977.

144. Pelligrino DA, Miletich DJ, Hoffman WE, et al: Nitrous oxide markedly increases cerebral cortical metabolic rate and blood flow in the goat. *Anesthesiology* 60:405–412, 1984.

145. Sakabe T, Kuramoto T, Kumagae S, et al: Cerebral effects of nitrous oxide in the dog. *Anesthesiology* 48:195–200, 1978.

146. Sokoloff L: The action of drugs on the cerebral circulation. *Pharmacol Rev* 11:1–22, 1959.

147. Lassen NA: Cerebral blood flow and oxygen consumption in man. *Physiol Rev* 39:183–238, 1959.

148. Shapiro HM: Anesthesia effects upon cerebral blood flow, cerebral metabolism, electroencephalogram, and evoked potentials. In: Miller RD (ed). *Anesthesia*. New York: Churchill Livingstone, Inc.; 1249–1288, 1986.

149. Stoelting RK, Dierdorf SF: Diseases of the nervous system. In: Stoelting RK, Dierdorf SF (eds). *Anesthesia and Co-existing Disease*, 3rd Ed. New York: Churchill Livingstone, Inc.; 181–196, 1993.

150. Young RSK, Hernandez MJ, Yagel SK: Selective reduction of blood flow to white matter during hypotension in newborn dogs: a possible mechanism of periventricular leucomalacia. *Ann Neurol* 12:445–448, 1982.

151. Trounce JQ, Shaw DE, Levene MI, Rutter N: Clinical risk factors and periventricular leucomalacia. *Arch Dis Child* 63:17–22, 1988.

152. McDonald MM, Koops BL, Johnson ML, et al: Timing and antecedents of intracranial hemorrhage in the newborn. *Pediatrics* 74:32–36, 1984.

153. De Crespigny L, Mackay R, Murton LJ, et al: Timing of neonatal cerebroventricular hemorrhage with ultrasound. *Arch Dis Child* 57:231–233, 1982.

154. Volpe JJ, Herscovitch P, Perlman JM, et al: Positron emission tomography in the asphyxiated term newborn: parasagittal impairment of cerebral blood flow. *Ann Neurol* 17:287–296, 1985.

155. Greisen G, Munck H, Lou H: Severe hypocarbia in preterm infants and neurodevelopmental deficit. *Acta Paediatr Scand* 76:401–404, 1987.

156. Young RSK, Yagel SK, Towfighi J: Systemic and neuropathologic effects of *E. Coli* endotoxin in neonatal dogs. *Pediatr Res* 17:349–353, 1983.

157. Cooke RWI: Factors associated with periventricular hemorrhage in very low birthweight infants. *Arch Dis Child* 56:425–431, 1981.

158. Volpe JJ: Intraventricular hemorrhage in the premature infant: current concepts. Part I. *Ann Neurol* 25:3–11, 1989.

159. Volpe JJ: Intraventricular hemorrhage in the premature infant: current concepts. Part 2. *Ann Neurol* 25:109–116, 1989.

160. Altman DI, Powers WJ, Perlman JM, et al: Cerebral blood flow requirement for brain viability in newborn infants is lower than adults. *Ann Neurol* 24:218–226, 1988.

161. Greisen G: Cerebral blood flow in infants during the first week of life. *Acta Paediatr Scand* 75:43–51, 1986.

162. Hernandes MJ, Vannucci RC, Salcedo A, Brennan RW: Cerebral blood flow and metabolism during hypoglycemia in newborn dogs. *J Neurochem* 35:622–628, 1980.

163. Sieber FE, Derrer SA, Suadek CD, Traystman RJ: Effect of hypoglycemia on cerebral metabolism and carbon dioxide reactivity. *Am J Physiol* 256:H697–706, 1989.

164. Bryan RM, Hollinger BR, Keefer KA, Page RB: Regional cerebral and neural lobe blood flow during insulin-induced hypoglycemia in unanesthetized rats. *J Cereb Blood Flow Metab* 7:96–102, 1987.

165. Pryds O, Christensen NJ, Friis-Hansen B: Increased CBF and plasma epinephrine in hypoglycemic, preterm infants. *Pediatrics* 85:172–176, 1990.

166. Pryds M, Greisen G, Lou H, Friis-Hansen B: Vasoparalysis is associated with brain damage in asphyxiated term infants. *J Pediatr* 117:119–125, 1990.

167. Raemakers VT, Cassaer P: Defective regulation of cere-

bral oxygen transport after severe birth asphyxia. *Dev Med Child Neurol* 32:556–562, 1990.

168. Pryds O: Control of cerebral circulation in the high-risk neonate. *An Neurol* 30:321–329, 1991.

169. Anthony MY, Evans DH, Levene MI: Neonatal cerebral blood flow velocity responses to changes in posture. *Arch Dis Childhood* 69:304–308, 1993.

170. Meldrum B: Protection against ischaemic neuronal damage by drugs acting on excitatory neurotransmission. *Cerebrovasc Brain Metab Res* 2:27–57, 1990.

171. Vannucci RC: Current and potentially new management strategies for perinatal hypoxic-ischemic encephalopathy. *Pediatrics* 85:961–968, 1990.

172. Hamilton AJ, Cymmerman A, Black PM: High altitude cerebral edema. *Neurosurgery* 19:841–849, 1986.

173. Singh I, Khanna K, Srivastava MC, et al: Acute mountain sickness. *N Engl J Med* 280:175–184, 1969.

174. Jensen JB, Wright AD, Lassen NA, et al: Cerebral blood flow in acute mountain sickness. *J Appl Physiol* 69:430–433, 1990.

175. Otis SM, Rossman ME, Schneider MD, et al: Relationship of cerebral blood flow regulation to acute mountain sickness. *J Ultrasound Med* 8:143–148, 1989.

176. Houston CS, Dickinson J: Cerebral form of high altitude illness. *Lancet* 2:758–761, 1975.

177. Roy SB, Guleria JS, Khanna PK, et al: Immediate circulatory response to high altitude hypoxia in man. *Nature* 217:1177–1178, 1968.

178. Harvey TC, Raichle MH, Winterborn MH, et al: Effect of carbon dioxide in acute mountain sickness: a rediscovery. *Lancet* 2:639–641, 1988.

179. Kety SS, Schmidt CF: The effects of altered arterial tensions of carbon dioxide and oxygen on cerebral blood flow and cerebral oxygen consumption of normal young men. *J Clin Invest* 27:484–492, 1948.

180. Lassen NA, Friberg AL, Kastrup J, et al: Effects of acetazolamide on cerebral blood flow and brain tissue oxygenation. *Postgrad Med J* 63:185–187, 1987.

181. Eisenberg MS, Horwood BT, Cummins RO, et al: Cardiac arrest and resuscitation: a tale of 29 cities. *Ann Emerg Med* 19:179–186, 1990.

182. Levy DE, Caronna JJ, Singer BH, et al: Predicting outcome from hypoxic-ischemic coma. *JAMA* 253:1420–1426, 1985.

183. Longstreth WT, Invi TS, Cobb LA, et al: Neurologic recovery after out of hospital cardiac arrest. *Ann Intern Med* 98:588–592, 1983.

184. Safer P: International symposium on resuscitation: controversial aspects in *Anesthesiology Monograph and Resuscitation Series,* Vol. 1 Heidelberg: Springer-Verlag, Inc.; 1963.

185. Cummins RO, Ornato JP, Thies WH, et al: Improving survival from sudden cardiac arrest: the "Chain of Survival" concept. *Circulation* 83:1832–1847, 1991.

186. Safer P, Bircher N: *Cardiopulmonary Cerebral Resuscitation: Guidelines by the World Federation of Societies of Anesthesiologists,* 3rd Ed. Philadelphia: WB Saunders, Co.; 1988.

187. Safer P, Berkebile P, Scott MA, et al: Education research on life-supporting first aid and CPR self-training Systems. *Crit Care Med* 9:403–440, 1981.

188. Winchell SW, Safer P: Teaching and testing lay and paramedical personnel in cardiopulmonary resuscitation. *Anesth Analg* 45:441–449, 1966.

189. Heymans C: Survival and revival of nervous tissue after arrest of the circulation. *Physiol Rev* 30:375–392, 1950.

190. Cole SL, Corday E: Four-minute limit for cardiac resuscitation. *JAMA* 161:1454–1458, 1956.

191. Safar P: Cerebral resuscitation after cardiac arrest: research initiatives and future directions. *Ann Emerg Med* 22:324–349, 1993.

192. Bar-Joseph G, Safar P, Saito R, et al: Monkey model of severe volume-controlled hemorrhagic shock with resuscitation to outcome. *Resuscitation* 22:27–43, 1991.

193. Kovach AGB, Sandor P: Cerebral blood flow and brain function during hypotension and shock. *Annu Rev Physiol* 38:571–596, 1976.

194. Symon L: Flow thresholds in brain ischemia and the effects of drugs. *Br J Anesth* 57:34–43, 1985.

195. Steen PA, Michenfelder JD, Milde JH: Incomplete versus complete cerebral ischemia: improved outcome with a minimal blood flow. *Ann Neurol* 6:389–398, 1979.

196. Siesjo BK: Mechanisms of ischemic brain damage. *Crit Care Med* 16:954–963, 1988.

197. Siesjo BK: Cell damage in the brain: a speculative hypothesis. *J Cereb Blood Flow Metab* 1:155–185, 1981.

198. Rossen R, Cabat H, Anderson JP: Acute arrest of cerebral circulation in man. *Arch Neurol* 50:510–528, 1943.

199. Michenfelder JK, Theye RA: The effects of anesthesia and hypothermia on canine cerebral ATP and lactate during anoxia produced by decapitation. *Anesthesiology* 33:430–439, 1970.

200. Kramer RS, Sanders AP, Lesage AM, et al: The effect of profound hypothermia on preservation of cerebral ATP content during circulatory arrest. *J Thorac Cardiovasc Surg* 56:699–709, 1968.

201. Astrup J, Rehncrona S, Siesjo BK: The increase in extracellular potassium concentration in the ischemic brain in relation to the preischemic functional activity and cerebral metabolic rate. *Brain Res* 199:161–74, 1980.

202. Negovsky VA: Neurological aspects of reanimatology. *Anaesthesiol Reanim* 15:337–341, 1990.

203. Safer P: Resuscitation from clinical death: pathophysiologic limits and therapeutic potentials. *Crit Care Med* 16:923–941, 1988.

204. Breivik H, Safer P, Sands P, et al: Clinical feasibility trials of barbiturate therapy after cardiac arrest. *Crit Care Med* 6:228–244, 1978.

205. Ginsberg MD, Welsch FA, Budd WW: Deleterious effect of glucose pretreatment on recovery from diffuse cerebral ischemia in the cat. *Stroke* 11:347–354, 1980.

206. Rehncrona S, Rosen I, Siesjo BK: Excessive cellular acidosis: an important mechanism of neuronal damage in the brain? *Acta Physiol Scand* 110:425–427, 1980.

207. Siemkowicz E, Hansen AJ: Clinical restitution following cerebral ischemia in hypo-, normo-, and hyperglycemic rats. *Acta Neurol Scand* 58:1–8, 1978.

208. Miller RJ: Multiple calcium channels and neuronal function. *Science* 235:46–52, 1987.

209. Bazan NG: Effects of ischemia and electroconvulsive shock on free fatty acid pool in the brain. *Biochem Biophys Acta* 218:1–10, 1970.

210. Benveniste H: The excitotoxine hypotheses in relation to cerebral ischemia. *Cerebrovasc Brain Metab Rev* 3:213–245, 1991.

211. Globus MYT, Ginsberg MD, Busto R: Excitotoxic index: a biochemical marker of selective vulnerability. *Neurosci Lett* 127:39–42, 1991.

212. Hendrickx HHL, Safer P, Baer BP, et al: Brain lactate and alanine-glutamate ratios during and after asphyxia in rats. *Resuscitation* 12:129–140, 1984.

213. Rothman SW, Olney JW: Glutamate and the pathophys-

iology of hypoxic-ischemic brain damage. *Ann Neurol* 19:105–111, 1986.

214. Meldrum B: Possible therapeutic applications of antagonists of excitatory amino acid neurotransmitters. *Clin Sci* 68:113–122, 1975.

215. Safer P: Cerebral resuscitation after cardiac arrest: a review. *Circulation* 74(suppl IV):IV138–153, 1986.

216. Vaagenes P, Safer P, Diven W, et al: Brain enzyme levels in CSF after cardiac arrest and resuscitation in dogs: markers of damage and predictors of outcome. *J Cereb Blood Flow Metab* 8:262–275, 1988.

217. Nemoto EM, Bleyaert AL, Stezoski SW, et al: Global brain ischemia: a reproducible monkey model. *Stroke* 8:558–564, 1977.

218. Garcia JH, Lossinsky AS, Kauffman FC, et al: Neuronal ischemic injury: light microscopy, ultrastructure, and biochemistry. *Acta Neuropathol* (Berl) 43:85–95, 1978.

219. Brierley JB, Meldrum BS, Brown AW: The threshold and neuropathology of cerebral "anoxic-ischemic" cell change. *Arch Neurol* 29:367–374, 1973.

220. Fischer EG, Ames A: Studies on mechanisms of impairment of cerebral circulation following ischemia: effect of hemodilution and perfusion pressure. *Stroke* 3:538–542, 1972.

221. Nemoto EM, Erdman NW, Strong E, et al: Regional brain pO_2 after global ischemia in monkeys: evidence for regional differences in critical perfusion pressures. *Stroke* 10:44–52, 1979.

22. Ames A, Wright RL, Kowada M, et al: Cerebral ischemia. II. The no-reflow phenomenon. *Am J Pathol* 52:437–453, 1968.

223. Leonov Y, Sterz F, Safer P, et al: Hypertension with hemodilution prevents multifocal cerebral hypoperfusion after cardiac arrest in dogs. *Stroke* 23:45–53, 1992.

224. Snyder JV, Nemoto EM, Carroll RG, et al: Global ischemia in dogs: intracranial pressures, brain blood flow, and metabolism. *Stroke* 6:21–27, 1975.

225. Lind B, Snyder J, Safer P: Total brain ischemia in dogs: cerebral physiologic and metabolic changes after 15 minutes of circulatory arrest. *Resuscitation* 4:97–113, 1975.

226. Haggendal E, Lofgren J, Nilsson NJ, et al: Prolonged cerebral hyperemia after periods of increased cerebrospinal fluid pressure in dogs. *Acta Physiol Scand* 79:272–279, 1970.

227. Kofke WA, Nemoto EM, Hossmann KA, et al: Monkey brain blood flow and metabolism after global brain ischemia and post-insult thiopental therapy. *Stroke* 10:554–560, 1979.

228. Klatzo I: Brain edema following brain ischaemia and the influence of therapy. *Br J Anaesth* 57:18–22, 1985.

229. Dietrich WD, Halley M, Valdes I: Interrelationships between increased vascular permeability and acute neuronal damage following temperature-controlled brain ischemia in rats. *Acta Neuropathol* 81:615–625, 1991.

230. Kochanek PM, Hallenbeck JM: Polymorphonuclear leukocytes and monocyte-macrophages in the pathogenesis of cerebral ischemia and stroke: a review. *Stroke* 23:1367–1375, 1992.

231. Hossmann V, Hossmann KA, Takagi S: Effect of intravascular platelet aggregation on blood recirculation following prolonged ischemia of the cat brain. *J Neurol* 22:159–170, 1980.

232. Traystman RJ, Kirsch JR, Koehler RC: Oxygen radical mechanisms of brain injury following ischemia and reperfusion. *J Appl Physiol* 71:1185–1195, 1991.

233. McCord JM: Oxygen derived free radicals in postischemic tissue injury. *N Engl J Med* 312:159–163, 1985.

234. Babbs CP: Role of iron ions in the genesis of reperfusion injury following successful cardiopulmonary resuscitation: preliminary data and a biochemical hypothesis. *An Emerg Med* 14:777–783, 1985.

235. Fridovich I: Superoxide radical: an endogenous toxicant. *Annu Rev Pharmacol Toxicol* 23:239–257, 1983.

236. Demopoulous HB, Flamm ES, Pietronigro DD, et al: The free radical pathology and the microcirculation in major central nervous system disorders. *Acta Physiol Scand* 492(suppl):91–119, 1980.

237. Cerchiari EL, Hoel TM, Safer P, et al: Protective effects of combined superoxide dismutase and desferoxamine on recovery of cerebral blood flow and function after cardiac arrest in dogs. *Stroke* 18:869–878, 1987.

238. Smith J, Penninckx JJ, Kampschulte S, et al: Need for oxygen enrichment in myocardial infarction, shock and following cardiac arrest. *Acta Anaesthesiol Scand* (suppl 29):127–145, 1968.

239. Jennings RB, Reimer KA, Steenbergen C: Complete global myocardial ischemia in dogs. *Crit Care Med* 16:988–996, 1988.

240. Brain Resuscitation Clinical Trial II Study Group: A randomized clinical study of a calcium-entry blocker (lidoflazine) in the treatment of comatose survivors of cardiac arrest. *N Engl J Med* 324:1225–1231, 1991.

241. Cerchiari EL, Safer P, Klein E, et al: Cardiovascular function and neurologic outcome after cardiac arrest in dogs: the cardiovascular post-resuscitation syndrome. *Resuscitation* 25:119–136, 1993.

242. Kampschulte S, Smith J, Safer P: Oxygen transport after cardiopulmonary resuscitation. *Anaesthesiol Reanim* 30:95–101, 1969.

243. Stertz F, Safer P, Diven W, et al: Detoxification with hemabsorption after cardiac arrest does not improve neurologic recovery: review and outcome study in dogs. *Resuscitation* 25:137–160, 1993.

244. Baethmann A, Maier-Hauff K, Kempsk O, et al: Mediators of brain edema and secondary brain damage. *Crit Care Med* 16:972–978, 1988.

245. Rubin B, Tittley J, Chang G, et al: A clinically applicable method for long-term salvage of postischemic skeletal muscle. *J Vasc Surg* 13:58–68, 1991.

246. Furchgott RF, Vanhoutte PM: Endothelium derived relaxing and contracting factors. *FASEB J* 3:2007–2018, 1989.

247. Brown CG, Werman HA, Davis EA, et al: Comparative effect of graded doses of epinephrine on regional blood flow during CPR in a swine model. *Ann Emerg Med* 15:1138–1144, 1986.

248. Sterz F, Safer P, Tisheman S, et al: Mild hypothermic cardiopulmonary resuscitation improves outcome after prolonged cardiac arrest in dogs. *Crit Care Med* 19:379–389, 1991.

249. Katz L, Sim KM, Radovsky A, et al: Asphyxial cardiac arrest survival model in rats with quantitative brain histopathological evaluation (abstr). *Ann Emerg Med* 21:633, 1992.

250. Sterz F, Leonov Y, Safer P, et al: Hypertension with or without hemodilution after cardiac arrest in dogs. *Stroke* 21:1178–1184, 1990.

251. Lin SR, O'Connor MJ, Fischer HW, et al: The effect of combined dextran and streptokinase on cerebral function and blood flow after cardiac arrest: an experimental study on the dog. *Invest Radiol* 13:490–498, 1978.

252. Rosomoff HL: Protective effects of hypothermia against pathologic processes of the nervous system. *Ann NY Acad Sci* 80:475–486, 1959.

253. Bigelow WG, Lindsay WK, Greenwood WF: Hypothermia: its possible role in cardiac surgery. *Ann Surg* 132:849–866, 1950.

254. Tisherman SA, Safer P, Radovsky A, et al: Therapeutic deep hypothermic arrest in dogs: a resuscitation modality for hemorrhagic shock with 'irreparable' injury. *J Trauma* 30:836–847, 1990.

255. White RJ: Hypothermic preservation and transplantation of the brain. *Resuscitation* 4:197–210, 1975.

256. Frumin MJ, Epstein RM, Cohen G: Apneic oxygenation in man. *Anesthesiology* 20:789–798, 1959.

257. Frates RC: Analysis of predictive factors in the assessment of warm-water near-drowning in children. *Am J Dis Child* 135:1006–1008, 1981.

258. Wolfe KB: Effect of hypothermia on cerebral damage resulting from cardiac arrest. *Am J Cardiol* 6:809, 1960.

259. Benson DW, Williams GR, Spencer FC, et al: The use of hypothermia after cardiac arrest. *Anesth Analg* 38:423–428, 1958.

260. Brain Resuscitation Clinical Trial I Study Group: Randomized clinical study of thiopental loading in comatose survivors of cardiac arrest. *N Engl J Med* 314:397–403, 1986.

261. Grisvold SE, Safer P, Hendrickx HHL, et al: Thiopental treatment after global brain ischemia in pigtail monkeys. *Anesthesiology* 60:88–96, 1984.

262. Koch KA, Jackson DL, Schmiedl M, et al: Effect of thiopental therapy on cerebral blood flow after total cerebral ischemia. *Crit Care Med* 12:90–95, 1984.

263. Todd MM, Hindman B, Warner DS: Barbiturate protection and cardiac surgery: a different result. *Anesthesiology* 74:402–405, 1991.

264. Vaagenes P, Cantadore R, Safe P, et al: Amelioration of brain damage by lidoflazine after prolonged ventricular fibrillation cardiac arrest in dogs. *Crit Care Med* 12:846–855, 1984.

265. Steen PA, Grisvold SE, Milde JH, et al: Nimodipine improves outcome when given after complete cerebral ischemia in primates. *Anesthesiology* 62:406–414, 1985.

266. Roine RO, Kaste M, Kinnamen A, et al: Nimodipine after resuscitation from out-of-hospital ventricular fibrillation: a placebo-controlled, double-blind randomized trial. *JAMA* 264:3171–3177, 1990.

267. Ernster L: Biochemistry of reoxygenation injury. *Crit Care Med* 16:947–953, 1991.

268. White BC, Nayini NR, Krause GS, et al: Effect of biochemical markers of brain injury on therapy with desferoxamine or superoxide dismutase following cardiac arrest. *Am J Emerg Med* 6:569–576, 1988.

269. Forsman M, Fleischer JE, Milde JH, et al: Superoxide dismutase and catalase failed to improve neurologic outcome after complete cerebral ischemia in the dog. *Acta Anaesthesiol Scand* 32:152–155, 1988.

270. Eddy L, Hurvitz R, Hochstein P: A protective role for ascorbate in induced ischemic arrest associated with cardiopulmonary bypass. *J Appl Cardiol* 5:409–414, 1990.

271. Imaizumi S, Woolworth V, Fishman RA, et al: Liposome-entrapped superoxide dismutase reduces cerebral infarction in cerebral ischemia in rats. *Stroke* 21:1312–1317, 1990.

272. White CW, Jackson JH, Abuchowski A, et al: Polyethylene glycol-attached antioxidant enzymes decrease pulmonary oxygen toxicity in tats. *J Appl Physiol* 66:584–590, 1989.

273. Babbs CF: Role of iron ions in the genesis of reperfusion injury following successful cardiopulmonary resuscitation: preliminary data and a biochemical hypothesis. *Ann Emerg Med* 14:777–783, 1985.

274. Weisman HF, Bartow T, Leppo MK, et al: Soluble human complement receptor type 1: *in-vivo* inhibitor of complement suppressing post-ischemic myocardial inflammation and necrosis. *Science* 249:146–151, 1990.

275. Buchan AM, Xue D, Huang ZG, et al: Delayed AMPA receptor blockade reduces cerebral infarction induced by focal ischemia. *Neuroreport* 2:473–476, 1991.

276. Mosinger JL, Price MT, Bai HY, et al: Blockade of both NMDA and non-NMDA receptors is required for optimal protection against ischemic neuronal degradation in in-vivo adult mammalian retina. *Exp Neurol* 113:10–17, 1991.

277. Ommaya AK, Gennarelli TA: Cerebral concussion and traumatic unconsciousness: correlation of experimental and clinical observations on blunt head injuries. *Brain* 97:633–654, 1974.

278. Miller JD: Head injury and brain ischemia: implications for therapy. *Br J Anaesth* 57:120–130, 1985.

279. Sullivan HG, Martinez J, Becker DP, et al: Fluid-percussion model of mechanical brain injury in the cat. *J Neurosurg* 45:520–534, 1976.

280. Levine JE, Becker DP, Chun T: Reversal of incipient brain death from head-injury apnea at the scene of accidents (letter). *N Eng J Med* 301:109, 1979.

281. Bruce DA: Cerebrovascular dynamics following brain insults. In: James HE, Anas NG, Perkin RM, (eds). *Brain Insults in Infants and Children: Pathophysiology and Management*. Orlando: Grune & Stratton, Inc.; 83–88, 1985.

282. Obrist WD, Langfitt TW, Jaggi JL, et al: Cerebral blood flow and metabolism in comatose patients with acute head injury: relationship to intracranial hypertension. *J Neurosurg* 61:241–253, 1984.

283. Weaver DD, Winn HR, Jane JA: Differential intracranial pressure in patients with unilateral mass lesions. *J Neurosurg* 56:660–665, 1982.

284. Graham DI, Adams JH, Doyle D: Ischaemic brain damage in fatal non-missile head injuries. *J Neurol Sci* 39:213–234, 1978.

285. Rosner MJ, Coley IB: Cerebral perfusion pressure, intracranial pressure, and head elevation. *J Neurosurg* 65:636–641, 1986.

286. Tornheim PA, McLaurin RL: Acute changes in regional brain water content following experimental closed head injury. *J Neurosurg* 55:407–413, 1981.

287. Cao M, Lisheng H, Shouzheng S: Resolution of brain edema in severe brain injury at controlled high and low intracranial pressures. *J Neurosurg* 61:707–712, 1984.

288. Gennarelli TA: Head injury in man and experimental animals: clinical aspects. *Acta Neurochir,* 32(suppl):1–13, 1983.

289. Nilsson B, Nordstrom CH: Experimental head injury in the rat. Part 3: cerebral blood flow and oxygen consumption after concussive impact acceleration. *J Neurosurg* 47:262–273, 1977.

290. Sullivan HG, Martinez J, Becker DP, et al: Fluid percussion model of mechanical brain injury in the cat. *J Neurosurg* 45:520–534, 1975.

291. Duckrow RB, LaManna JC, Rosenthal M, Levasseur JE: Oxidative metabolic activity of the cerebral cortex

after fluid-percussion head injury in the cat. *J Neurosurg* 54:607–614, 1981.

292. DeWitt DS, Wei EP, Lutz H, et al: Effects of fluid-percussion brain injury on regional cerebral blood flow and pial arteriolar diameter. *J Neurosurg* 64:787–794, 1986.

293. Tornheim PA, McLaurin RL: Acute changes in regional brain water content following experimental closed head injury. *J Neurosurg* 55:407–413, 1981.

294. Tornhein PA, Liwnicz BH, Hirsch CS, et al: Acute response to blunt head trauma: experimental model and gross pathology. *J Neurosurg* 59:431–438, 1983.

295. Kuller LH, Cook LP, Friedman GD: Survey of stroke epidemiology studies. *Stroke* 3:579–585, 1972.

296. Taylor CB, Cox GE, Manalo-Estrella P, Southworth J: Atherosclerosis in rhesus monkeys. II. Arterial lesions associated with hypercholesterolemia induced by dietary fat and cholesterol. *Arch Pathol* 74:16–34, 1962.

297. Solberg LA, Eggar DA: Localization and sequence of development of atherosclerotic lesions in the carotid and vertebral arteries. *Circulation* 43:711–724, 1971.

298. Faraci FM, Heistad DD: Regulation of large cerebral arteries and cerebral microvascular pressure. *Circ Res* 66:8–17, 1990.

299. Crawford ES, DeBakey ME, Blaisdell FW, et al: Hemodynamic alterations in patients with cerebral arterial insufficiency before and after operation. *Surgery* 48:76–94, 1960.

300. Hohf RP: The clinical evaluation and surgery of internal carotid insufficiency. *Surg Clin North Am* 47:1:71–89, 1967.

301. Kendall RE, Marshall J: Role of hypertension in the genesis of transient focal cerebral ischemic attacks. *Br Med J* 2:344–348, 1963.

302. Fazekas JF, Alman RW: The role of hypotension in transitory focal cerebral ischemia. *Am J Med Sci* 248:567–570, 1964.

303. Imparato AM, Riles TS, Mintzer R, Baumann FG: The importance of hemorrhage in the relationship between gross morphologic characteristics and cerebral symptoms in 376 carotid artery plaques. *Ann Surg* 197:195–203, 1983.

304. Lusby RJ, Ferrell LD, Ehrenfeld WK, et al: Carotid Plaque hemorrhage: its role in production of cerebral ischemia. *Arch Surg* 117:1479–1488, 1982.

305. Fryer JA, Myers PC, Appleberg M: Carotid intraplaque hemorrhage: the significance of neovascularity. *J Vasc Surg* 6:341–349, 1987.

306. Persson AV, Robichaux WT, Silverman M: The natural history of carotid plaque development. *Arch Surg* 118:1048–1052, 1983.

307. Theile BL, Strandness DE: Distribution of intracranial and extracranial arterial lesions in patients with symptomatic cerebrovascular disease. In: Bernstein EF (ed) *Vascular Diagnosis*. 4th Ed. St. Louis: C. V. Mosby, Inc.; 302–307, 1993.

308. Powers WJ, Press GW, Grubb RL, et al: The effect of hemodynamically significant carotid artery disease on the hemodynamic status of the cerebral circulation. *Ann Intern Med* 106:27–35, 1987.

309. Russell D, Dybevold S, Kjartansson O, et al: Cerebral vasoreactivity and blood flow before and 3 months after carotid endarterectomy. *Stroke* 21:1029–1032, 1990.

310. Levine RL, Rozental JM, Nickles RJ: Blood flow asymmetry in carotid occlusive disease. *Angiology* 43:100–109, 1992.

311. Powers WJ: Cerebral hemodynamics in ischemic cerebrovascular disease. *Ann Neurol* 29:231–240, 1991.

312. Strandgaard S, Paulson OB: Hypertensive disease and the cerebral circulation. In: Laragh JH, Brenner BM (eds). *Hypertension: Pathophysiology, Diagnosis, and Management*. New York: Raven Press; 399–416, 1990.

313. Zucker MB, Nachmias VT: Platelet activation. *Arteriosclerosis* 5:2–18, 1985.

314. Vanhoutte PM, Houston DS: Platelets, endothelium, and vasospasm. *Circulation* 72:728–734, 1985.

315. Heistad DD, Breese K, Armstrong ML: Cerebral vasoconstrictor responses to serotonin after dietary treatment of atherosclerosis: implications for transient ischemic attacks. *Stroke* 18:1068–1073, 1987.

316. Heistad DD, Armstrong ML, Marcus ML, et al: Augmented responses to vasoconstrictor stimuli in hypercholesterolemic and atherosclerotic monkeys. *Circ Res* 54:711–8, 1984.

317. Shimokawa H, Kim P, Vanhoutte PM: Endothelium-dependent relaxation to aggregating platelets in isolated basilar arteries of control and hypercholesterolemic pigs. *Circ Res* 63:604–612, 1988.

318. Faraci FM, Williams JK, Breese KR, et al: Atherosclerosis potentiates constrictor responses of cerebral and ocular blood vessels thromboxane in monkeys. *Stroke* 20:242–247, 1989.

319. Schmidt-Kastner R, Hossmann KA, Ophoff BG: Pial artery pressure after one hour of global ischemia. *J Cereb Blood Flow Metab* 7:109–117, 1987.

320. Shima T, Hossmann KA, Date H: Pial arterial pressure in cats following middle cerebral artery occlusion. *Stroke* 14:713–719, 1983.

321. Date H, Hossmann KA, Shima T: Effect of middle cerebral artery compression on pial artery pressure, blood flow, and electrophysiological function of cerebral cortex of cat. J Cereb Blood Flow Metab 4:593–598, 1983.

322. Astrup J, Siesjo BK, Symon L: Thresholds in cerebral ischaemia: the ischaemic penumbra. *Stroke* 12:723–725, 1981.

323. Power WJ, Grubb RL, Darriet D, et al: Cerebral blood flow and cerebral metabolic rate of oxygen requirements for cerebral function and viability in humans. *J Cereb Blood Flow Metab* 5:600–608, 1985.

324. Bell BA, Symon L, Branston NM: CBF and time thresholds for the formation of ischemic cerebral edema and the effects of reperfusion in baboons. *J Neurosurg* 62:31–46, 1985.

325. Mikolich JR, Jacobs WC, Fletcher GF: Cardiac arrhythmias in patients with acute cerebrovascular accidents. *JAMA* 246:1314–1317, 1981.

326. Benes V, Zabramski JM, Boston M, et al: Effect of intra-arterial tissue plasminogen activator and urokinase on autologous arterial emboli in the cerebral circulation of rabbits. *Stroke* 21:1594–1599, 1990.

327. Overgaard K, Sereghy T, Boysen G, et al: Reduction of infarct volume by thrombolysis with rt-PA in an embolic rat stroke model. *Scand J Clin Lab Invest* 53:383–393, 1993.

328. Lyden PD, Madden KP, Clark WM, et al: Incidence of cerebral hemorrhage after treatment with tissue plasminogen activator or streptokinase following embolic stroke in rabbits. *Stroke* 21:1589–1593, 1990.

CHAPTER 29

Basic Science of Renovascular Hypertension

David L. Robaczewski, MD; Richard H. Dean, MD

Introduction and Historical Perspective

The importance of the kidney in hypertension was first recognized by Richard Bright when he described the association between left ventricular hypertrophy and contracted kidneys in 1827. By 1836, Bright had reported the association of albuminuria, cardiac hypertrophy, shrunken kidneys, and hardness of the pulse.[1] His impact on the understanding of the cause of hypertension is unparalleled. For much of the nineteenth century, the medical community blindly accepted the premise that all causes of hypertension emanated from the kidney. This perception was augmented when in 1898 Tigerstedt and Bergman suggested the presence of a pressor substance in the kidney. In their experiments, a crude saline extract derived from rabbit kidneys was shown to increase the blood pressure when injected into other rabbits. They termed the uncharacterized chemical in the kidney extract renin. Their observations remained controversial and only a matter of curiosity for over three decades. Goldblatt provided more support for the concept that a renal hormonal mechanism could induce hypertension.

By the late 1920s and early 1930s, the association between hypertension and arteriolar nephrosclerosis was widely recognized. What was not agreed on was the order of occurrence. Did hypertension cause arteriolar nephrosclerosis or did primary arteriolar nephrosclerosis produce the hypertension? Goldblatt et al[2] reasoned that arteriolar nephrosclerosis was the equivalent of millions of tiny vascular clamps limiting inflow into the glomerulus. Since placement of such microscopic clamps was impossible, they concluded that constriction of the main renal artery would serve the same purpose of reducing flow to the glomeruli. Their observation that hypertension developed after placement of the clamp seemed to confirm what they suspected: arteriolar nephrosclerosis produced hypertension.[2] However, they did not expect to find the dissipation of hypertension that occurred when they subsequently removed the occluding clamp. These events constituted the beginning of our understanding of renovascular hypertension (RVH).

In 1939, cooperative studies in the laboratories of Irvin Page in the United States and Braun-Menendez in Argentina led to the characterization of renin as a proteolytic enzyme and the discovery of a rapidly acting, potent, pressor byproduct. This was followed by the structural characterization of angiotensin I (AI), angiotensin-converting enzyme, and angiotensin II (AII) by Skeggs and Lentz in the 1950s. By the end of that decade, Cook localized renin production to the juxtaglomerular apparatus, while the rapid conversion of AI to AII during its passage through the lungs was demonstrated by Ng and Vane in the late 1960s. Subsequent research has resulted in identification and manipulation of the renin gene, angiotensin-converting enzyme inhibitors, angiotensin receptors, active metabolic byproducts of angiotensin, and discovery of local renin-angiotensin systems.[3]

Sixty years of thorough laboratory investigation allowed the characterization of the mechanisms responsible for RVH, and led to new methods of medical and surgical intervention. Clinical application of these

From *The Basic Science of Vascular Disease*. Edited by Sidawy AN, Sumpio BE, and DePalma RG. Armonk, NY: Futura Publishing Company, Inc.; © 1997.

discoveries has significantly improved diagnostic capabilities and overall patient management. The renin-angiotensin system is responsible for the hypertensive response seen with renal artery disease. The physiologic effects of the renin-angiotensin system influence renal, cardiovascular, neural, adrenal, and microcirculatory function. Controversy still exists, however, concerning many of the basic considerations of cause, diagnosis, and management of RVH and ischemic nephropathy. Complicating the incomplete understanding and debatable issues of renal control of blood pressure and pathophysiology of RVH are prevalent misconceptions regarding anatomy and the importance of properly performed diagnostic studies. Intuitively, restoration of blood flow to the chronically ischemic kidney should correct the hormonal overactivity and result in normalization of blood pressure and renal function. Unfortunately, this is frequently not the case.[4–7] The pathophysiologic mechanisms that limit the success of reperfusion are incompletely characterized. After reviewing the basics of renal anatomy, physiology, and angiotensin metabolism, this chapter presents the physiologic mechanisms associated with RVH and basic considerations referable to the clinical management of renovascular disease.

Anatomy of the Renal Vasculature

Knowledge of basic anatomy and an understanding of the potential for anatomic variation is paramount to the surgeon as well as the scientific investigator. For centuries, anatomists have been fascinated by the renal vessels and their propensity for variation. Leonardo da Vinci (circa 1510) and Vesalius (circa 1543) sketched the common anatomic arrangement of the renal vessels. Bartolommeo Eustachius in 1552 made a detailed set of anatomic plates recording a wide range of variation and multiplicity in both renal arteries and veins (Figure 1).

Twentieth-century anatomists and surgeons became interested in renal vascular anomalies and variations due to the everbroadening surgical frontier, and the increasing need for renal and retroperitoneal surgical exposures. Rupert in 1913[8] and 1915[9] reported that multiplicity was commonplace in the renal arteries and in the right renal veins, while multiples of the left renal vein were extremely rare. Based on the relative frequency of renal arterial and venous variants, he warned that if surgical misadventure and dangerous hemorrhage were to be avoided, anomalies of the renal vessels should be expected and looked for.

Arterial Anatomy

Although most anatomic descriptions show one renal artery supplying each kidney, cumulative au-

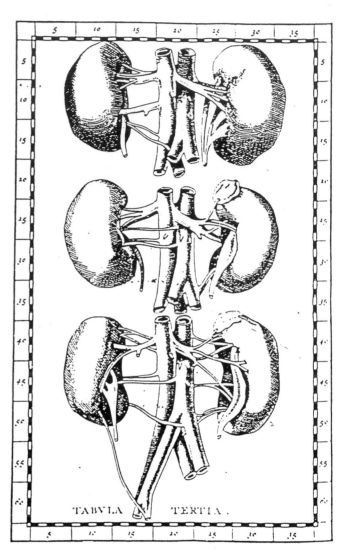

Figure 1. Bartolommeo Eustachius (1524–1574) was the first to engrave anatomic figures on copper plates. This is one example of his finely detailed plates, demonstrating some of the many possible anatomic arrangements of the renal vessels. Although these plates were completed in 1552, they remained hidden in the Vatican library and unpublished until 1714.

topsy series have shown that more than a total of two renal arteries were present in 59% of the autopsied individuals, and that 37% of kidneys were supplied by more than one renal artery.[8,10–12] Multiple renal arteries occur with equal frequency on either side.[13,14] As many as five separate renal arteries supplying a single kidney have been reported.[12] Though the renal artery usually originates from the aorta at the level of the upper part of the second lumbar vertebra, it may originate as high as T-11 and as low as the external iliac artery.[13,14] These variations in normal anatomy are of critical importance, for inadvertent ligation of an "aberrantly" arising renal artery can lead to severe hypertension, as well as sacrifice of renal parenchymal function (Figure 2).

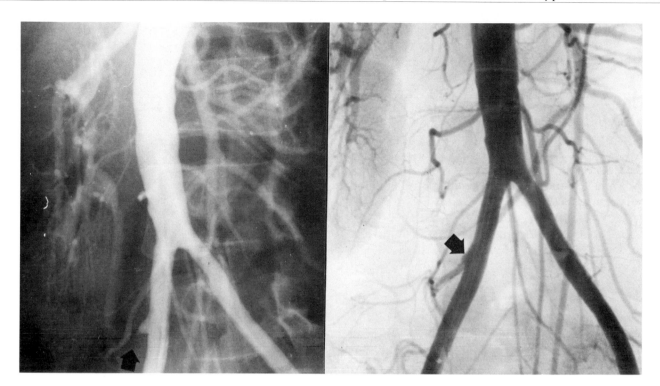

Figure 2. Patient referred with severe postoperative hypertension. Exploration for a pelvic mass had been performed at an outside hospital with the only finding being a pelvic kidney. Arteriograms obtained after the patient's arrival demonstrated the ligated stump of a lower pole renal artery, originating from the common iliac artery. Severe hypertension and lower pole infarction occurred as a consequence of this anatomic misunderstanding, necessitating heminephrectomy.

Another clinically important consideration is the course traversed by the renal arteries on their route to the kidney. Normally, the renal arteries lie posterior to the renal vein on the left, and posterior to the vena cava and renal vein on the right. A relatively frequent aberrant pathway exists when a large lower pole right renal artery is present. In such cases, the vessel originates from the anterior aorta and courses anterior to the vena cava on its way to the kidney; it can easily be traumatized during dissection of the anterior vena cava if its presence is not appreciated.

In the presence of main renal artery occlusive disease and renal ischemia, the development of collateral circulation becomes important for the maintenance of viable and functional parenchyma. Abrams and Cornell evaluated the collateral circulation of ischemic kidneys and found the lumbar, internal iliac, gonadal, and inferior adrenal arteries to be important in providing such blood flow.[15] In particular, the first three lumbar arteries appear to be very important origins of collateral circulation. Of these, the third lumbar artery most commonly serves as the significant source of perfusion. The course of blood flow from these collateral sources to the ischemic parenchyma is usually via superior and inferior capsular, suprarenal, and ureteric branches (Figure 3).

Venous Anatomy

Multiplicity of the renal veins is less common than with the arteries. In cadaver studies, right renal vein multiples were present in 11% to 27% of the specimens examined, while left renal vein multiples were present in only 1% to 3%.[9–11] The left renal vein has several extrarenal tributaries with common variability in the number and size of these nonrenal branches. The adrenal and gonadal veins seldom enter the right renal vein, but enter the left renal vein in nearly 100% of specimens. Additionally, one to two lumbar tributaries enter the posterior left renal vein in over 50% of the specimens.[11,16–20] The average number of nonrenal tributaries of the left renal vein is four (range 2 to 7) with the remainder of the extrarenal tributaries being capsular, ureteral, and duplicate branches. Almost all of the extrarenal venous tributaries enter the left renal vein in the middle third of its trunk (Figure 4).[20] Interestingly, a renal vein hiatus may exist in 2% to 4% of specimens through which the gonadal artery may pass.[11] This is more commonly seen on the left side. A persistent left inferior vena cava of variable size is found in 3% of cadaver specimens.[18] Of left renal veins, 1% to 3% are retroaortic in position while a circumaortic variant,

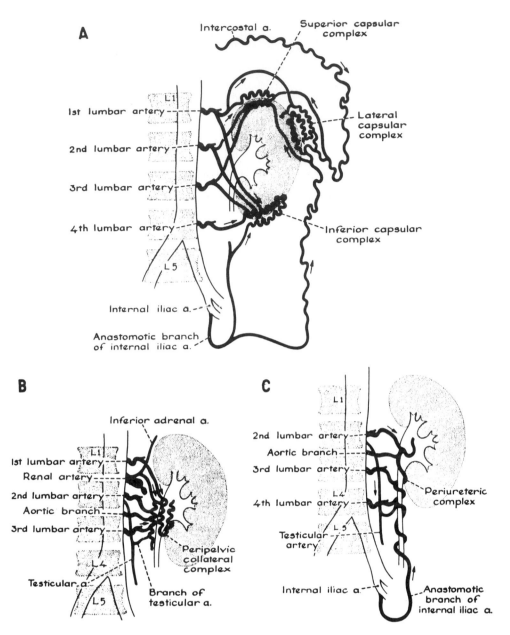

Figure 3. A. The first four lumbar arteries along with branches of the intercostals and the internal iliac artery contribute to the capsular circulation of the kidney. The lateral capsular complex represents a continuation of the superior capsular distribution. **B.** The aorta, first three lumbar, and testicular or ovarian arteries contribute to the anastomoses around the renal pelvis. **C.** The most common single collateral source to the ureter is from the internal iliac artery. The second to fourth lumbar, testicular, and direct aortic branches also contribute to this important area. (Reproduced with permission from Reference 18.)

with one branch anterior and one branch posterior to the aorta, is seen in 6% of cadaver specimens.[11,17,18]

The clinical pertinence of the multiple nonrenal venous channels that enter the midportion of the left renal vein is significant. First, unless the frequent variations and multiple nonrenal venous branches are recognized, the risk of inadvertent trauma to the nonrenal branches during dissection of this area is increased.[21,22] Second, since the multiple nonrenal branches offer an alternate pathway for renal venous effluent through collateral systems on the left, this vessel can be divided in its proximal portion without significantly affecting renal outflow.[22-24] This is of special value in the occasional patient who requires extensive exposure of the juxtarenal aorta for management of high aneurysms or occlusive disease. Finally, knowledge of venous trunk and tributary anatomy is very important in renal venous renin sampling, since the

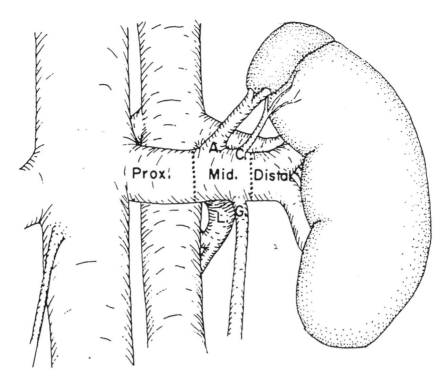

Figure 4. The left renal vein with the common number and variety of extrarenal tributaries. The proximal trunk is branchless and is the optimal site for vein division when this is necessary. The midportion of the left renal vein is the point of entry of the major tributaries. The distal vein trunk is relatively branchless and is the proper site for renal vein renin sampling. A = adrenal; C = capsular; G = gonadal; L = lumbar.

validity of this test depends upon the purity of the renal venous effluent. False-negative determinations are more likely to occur if the sampling catheter tip is near the entry points of the major extrarenal tributaries, causing an admixture of renal and systemic blood to be obtained.[20,25–27] It is, therefore, important to advance the sampling catheter tip beyond the middle zone of the left renal vein to avoid sampling of nonrenal blood for renin determination.

Physiology of the Renin-Angiotensin System

The metabolic process responsible for RVH is complex and continues to be investigated. The major components of this process are the renin-angiotensin system, the sympathetic nervous system, and vasoactive hormones. Though these components have global influences, they especially effect renal, cardiovascular, central nervous, and adrenal functions. In the classic two-kidney, one-clip Goldblatt model, renal perfusion pressure and glomerular filtration are reduced by the critical renal artery stenosis. The renin-angiotensin system becomes activated by tubuloglomerular, sympathetic, and renal baroreceptor mechanisms. These

mechanisms induce production of the proteolytic enzyme, renin. This rate-limiting enzyme initiates the cascade of angiotensin peptides responsible for the changes associated with the renin-angiotensin system. This hormonal system can be viewed in short- and long-term clinical settings. With regard to short-term decreases in renal perfusion pressure, such as in hypovolemia, this system reestablishes "normal" rates of renal blood flow and glomerular filtration by increasing blood pressure, sodium retention, and enhancing behavior activities associated with thirst. In long-term disease processes, such as renovascular occlusive disease, renal blood flow and glomerular filtration are chronically decreased, resulting in sustained activation of the renin-angiotensin system. This chronic activation of the renin-angiotensin system is responsible for the dangerous elevations in blood pressure associated with RVH.

In this enzyme cascade, renin cleaves AI from plasma angiotensinogen. Hemodynamically inactive AI is then metabolized by angiotensin-converting enzyme to produce the potent vasoconstrictor, AII. AII increases systemic arterial pressure by increasing vascular resistance, and enhancing salt and water conservation. These activities are accomplished through its influence on the renal, cardiovascular, central nervous, and adrenal systems. Our understanding of the renin-angiotensin system has been markedly changed by new gene technology. With these techniques, the capacity to produce the components of the renin-angiotensin system have been found in these four organ systems.[28] The activity of these tissue renin-angiotensin systems is regulated by various factors. This has led to new hypotheses regarding the mechanisms that maintain RVH. Contemporary schemes incorporate the classic systemic renin-angiotensin system as the developmental phase of hypertension. This relates to the fact that immediately following critical renal artery stenosis plasma renin activity, AII levels and systemic arterial pressure increase. These changes are completely reversed by early revascularization or administration of angiotensin-converting enzyme inhibitors.[29,30] After this initiating phase, the salt and water conserving actions of the renin-angiotensin system gradually become more important in the maintenance of hypertension. Chronic hypertension and elevated AII levels upregulate the production of angiotensin peptides by local integrated renin-angiotensin systems of the kidney, cardiovascular, adrenal, and central nervous systems. Eventually, these tissue renin-angiotensin systems gain a prominent position in the maintenance of renovascular hypertension.[31]

Renin

As mentioned, renin is a proteolytic enzyme that is produced and released from the juxtaglomerular apparatus. Specialized vascular smooth muscle cells (SMCs) of the afferent and efferent arterioles, and juxtaglomerular cells, are the sites of production and storage. Stimuli for renin production and secretion include tubuloglomerular feedback, hyponatremia, renal baroreceptors, prostaglandin I2, AII, and postganglionic sympathetic nerves. Once produced, renin is stored in granules or is released into the plasma. Renin enzymatically cleaves a plasma alpha-2-globulin, angiotensinogen, to produce AI. Metabolism and clearance of renin occur in the liver. Interestingly, renin production is not limited to the afferent arterioles. In fact, renin is present in the plasma of nephrectomized patients. The sources of this renin are many and include the vascular endothelium. This discovery of specific tissue renin-angiotensin systems has led to reevaluation of the factors involved in the development and maintenance of RVH.

Angiotensin Peptides

Angiotensinogen is an alpha-2-globulin abundantly produced by the liver and secreted in the plasma. Recently, the vascular endothelium of the brain, heart, adrenal glands, and kidneys has also been found to produce this substrate. For all of these organ beds, gene expression and substrate production increases in the presence of AII and chronic hypertension.[32-34] The byproduct of this substrate, AI, has no significant vasoactivity. However, it may influence renal tubular function.[35] Angiotensin metabolism continues as angiotensin-converting enzyme removes two amino acids from the carboxyl end of AI to form the potent vasoconstrictor, AII. Though the traditional description of the renin-angiotensin system limits angiotensin-converting enzyme activity to the pulmonary circulation, it is accepted that angiotensin-converting enzyme is produced and enzymatically active in many vascular endothelial cells. Angiotensin-converting enzyme production also increases under the influence of hypertension and AII. Pharmacologic inhibitors of this enzyme block the activities associated with AII. These agents have had a major impact on the clinical management of hypertension and our understanding of the renin-angiotensin system. Their development has led to the identification of new angiotensin peptides, angiotensin receptor subtypes, and their specific tissue activities. To appreciate the physiologic importance of converting enzyme inhibitors, it is necessary to understand the activities of AI, AII, their metabolites, and different receptor subtypes.

The major metabolites of angiotensinogen are shown in Figure 5. Beside angiotensin-converting enzyme, several other AI and AII processing enzymes exist. They produce the heptapeptides angiotensin-(1–7) from AI and AIII from AII. The activities of the major angiotensinogen metabolites are included in Table 1. The octapeptide, AII, has numerous effects in many organ systems. As with other endothelial hormones, AII acts through specific cell surface receptors to produce its effects.[36] The carboxy terminus, phenylalanine, is thought to mediate binding to the receptor associated with vasoconstriction. Thus far, two angiotensin receptor subtypes have been identified. The angiotensin type 1 receptor is the best characterized. It is given credit for mediating the vasoconstricting properties of AII. This receptor activates a G-protein/phospholipase apparatus to increase intracellular inositol triphosphate and diacylglycerol. The resulting increase in intracellular calcium triggers the contractile mechanisms in vascular smooth muscle and mesangial cells. Systemic blockade of this receptor results in a pharmacologic pattern similar to angiotensin-converting enzyme inhibition.[36,37] Of note, the specific angiotensin type 1 receptor blocker Losartan (DuP 753) is undergoing clinical trials for treatment of hypertension. Though the angiotensin type 2 receptor is incompletely characterized, it is known to mediate physiologic activities in several organs. The activities associated with type 2 receptors include natriuresis and vasodilation. The

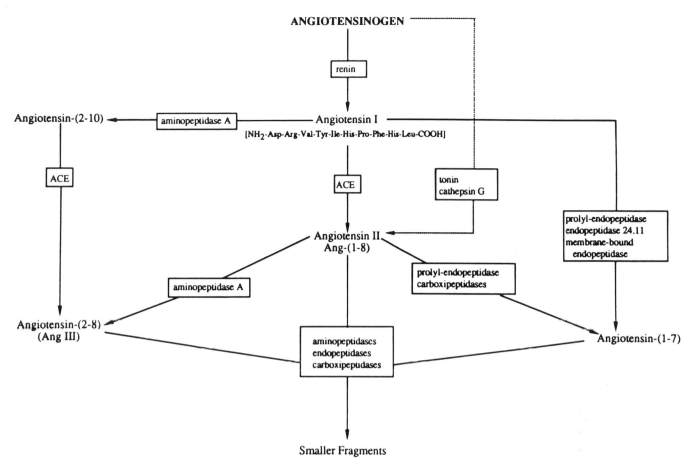

Figure 5. Schematic outline of alternate enzymatic cascades participating in generation of biologically active angiotensin peptides in tissues. Putative pathways contributing to formation of angiotensin-(1–7) are based on data obtained by this laboratory. (Reproduced with permission from Reference 91.)

specific blocking agents for this receptor are known as CGP42112A and PD123177. The existence of other receptors is highly likely from studies of specific angiotensin type 1 and angiotensin type 2 receptor antagonists.[38]

Renal Function and the Renin–Angiotensin System

An understanding of basic renal physiology is needed to appreciate the mechanisms responsible for

Table 1
The Renal Actions of Angiotensin Peptides

Specific Renal Response	Angiotensinogen Metabolite	Receptor Subtype Mediating Effect
1. Proximal Tubular Ion Transport	1. Ang I*, Ang II & Ang-(1–7)	1. AT1/AT2
2. Afferent/Efferent Arteriolar Constriction	2. Ang II	2. AT1
3. Inhibition of Renin Release	3. Ang II	3. AT1
4. Increased Mesangial Tone	4. Ang II	4. AT1

Description of the physiologic activities of angiotensin-(1–7) [Ang-(1–7)], angiotensin II [Ang II], angiotensin III [Ang III], and the two main angiotensin receptor subtypes in the kidney. *Most likely, angiotensin I is metabolized locally to form angiotensin II. Locally produced angiotensin II then directly influences tubular function.

RVH. Although a complete discussion of normal renal physiology is beyond the scope of this text, a brief overview of the main components of renal function is included to enhance understanding of the pathophysiology of the renin-angiotensin system and related hypertension.[39,40]

The regulation of extracellular fluid and electrolyte balance is dependent upon the delivery of adequate blood volume to the kidney and efficient filtration, reabsorption, secretion, and excretion by the nephron. Under normal physiologic conditions, the kidneys receive 25% of cardiac output. Though this amount far exceeds the minimal metabolic needs of the individual renal cell, the high flow is necessary for adequate systemic homeostasis. Based on a 5 L/min cardiac output and a hematocrit of 45 mL/dL, approximately 900 L of plasma flow through the kidneys each day. Normally, the kidneys filter 20% of this plasma, or 180 L, into the tubular system, where appropriate fluid balance is achieved through reabsorption and waste is excreted. When one considers that the normal 24-hour urine output for a 70 kg man is less than 1.8 L, the impressiveness of the reabsorption and excretion ability of the renal system becomes apparent. The major structures responsible for this process are the glomerulus, Bowman's capsule, tubular system, and collecting ducts. Among their many areas of physiologic activity, angiotensin peptides have been found to have significant influence on renal hemodynamics and tubular function.

The Nephron and Angiotensin Peptides

The functional unit of the renal system is the nephron. Each human kidney contains an estimated one million nephrons. The starting point for each nephron is the glomerulus. The glomerulus is made up of the glomerular capillary tuft and the Bowman's capsule. The significance of this configuration exists in the interface of these two structures. Three layers make up this interface: the fenestrated glomerular capillary endothelium, the basement membrane, and the mesangial cells of the Bowman's capsule. Each mesangial cell contains contractile filaments and extends numerous foot processes to partially envelope adjacent glomerular capillary loops. The relationship between these interfacing cells is dynamic. An increase in the tone of the mesangial cells diminishes the glomerular filtration surface area, while a decrease in tone allows for increased filtration across the glomerular capillaries. The dynamic anatomy of the fenestrated capillaries and the mesangial cells is under the influence of numerous compounds, especially angiotensin peptides. Mathematically, the relationship was expressed by Starling as the filtration coefficient (Kf). In Starling's equation, opposing capillary and tubular hydrostatic and oncotic

forces also directly determine the glomerular filtration rate. In addition to these cellular components, negatively charged glycosaminoglycans of the basement membrane serve to repel passage of similarly charged molecules and proteins of varying size. Finally, intrarenal regulatory mechanisms control the amount of blood delivered to the glomerulus and the degree of filtration of plasma into the tubular system. Thus, the glomerulus has a unique design that results in the ultrafiltration of the plasma from blood. Once this has occurred, the ultrafiltrate passes from Bowman's capsule to the proximal tubule. For the purposes of this discussion, the mechanisms of sodium, potassium, and water reabsorption will primarily be reviewed.

The tubular system of the nephron has several specialized areas that serve to reabsorb water and electrolytes into the circulation and concentrate the urine (Figure 6). As mentioned, this process results in the reabsorption of approximately 99% of the sodium and water from the glomerular ultrafiltrate. The proximal tubule is the first specialized segment of the nephron encountered by the ultrafiltrate. Reabsorption of electrolytes from the tubular fluid occurs both by active transport and passive back-diffusion. The sodium ion is reabsorbed in the early proximal tubule by its cotransportation with organic solutes and bicarbonate through an active transport mechanism. Similarly, sodium is actively transported in the late proximal tubule in linkage with chloride transport. Prior to entering the descending loop of Henle, approximately two thirds of the ultrafiltrate is reabsorbed from the tubular system. Furthermore, since water freely follows this movement of solutes and ions, the tubular fluid is iso-osmotic to plasma as it enters the loop of Henle. The tubular cells of the loop of Henle vary in permeability to sodium and water depending on their location in the loop. The descending loop of Henle is permeable to water, but relatively impermeable to sodium and chloride, while the ascending loop of Henle is impermeable to water, but relatively impermeable to sodium and chloride. The thick ascending loop of Henle is impermeable to water, but actively transports Na^+, K^+, and Cl^- via a $Na^+/K^+/2Cl^-$-ATPase pump. The vasa recta approximate the tubules throughout their descent into the medullary interstitium. This medullary tubule/capillary design results in countercurrent multiplication and exchange mechanisms which produce a medullary osmotic gradient that can regulate urine osmolarity from 50 to 1200 mOsm. Urea concentrations assist in the development of this medullary osmotic gradient. The rates of ultrafiltrate flow through this segment of the tubular system, and blood flow through the corresponding vasa recta determine the concentration of the medullary and papillary interstitium and thus the tubular fluid. When fluid passes slowly through the tubular system during periods of low glomerular filtration rates

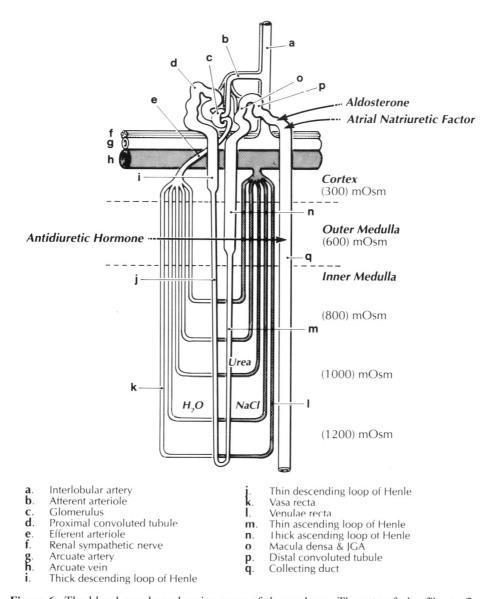

a. Interlobular artery
b. Afferent arteriole
c. Glomerulus
d. Proximal convoluted tubule
e. Efferent arteriole
f. Renal sympathetic nerve
g. Arcuate artery
h. Arcuate vein
i. Thick descending loop of Henle
j. Thin descending loop of Henle
k. Vasa recta
l. Venulae recta
m. Thin ascending loop of Henle
n. Thick ascending loop of Henle
o. Macula densa & JGA
p. Distal convoluted tubule
q. Collecting duct

Figure 6. The blood supply and major areas of the nephron. The rate of ultrafiltrate flow through the nephron is dependent on RBF and GFR. During periods of low renal perfusion, such as renal artery stenosis, the tubular flow rate decreases. The combination of low tubular flow, decreased medullary blood flow, and decreased medullary interstitial pressure leads to countercurrent multiplication of the medullary osmotic gradient. This results in the production of urine that is concentrated with respect to waste products, while relatively dilute with respect to NaCl. The sites of activity of aldosterone, antidiuretic hormone, and atrial natriuretic factor are also displayed.

(GFR), reabsorption is optimized and allows for significant countercurrent multiplication of the osmotic gradient of the medullary interstitium. This results in the delivery of a dilute tubular fluid, in terms of NaCl, to the thick ascending loop of Henle, and thus the macula densa. When fluid passes rapidly through the tubular system during periods of high GFR, reabsorption is diminished. The countercurrent multiplier is not able to produce a significant medullary osmotic gradient, resulting in delivery of increasing amounts of sodium and chloride to the thick ascending loop of Henle and

macula densa. When blood flow is increased through the vasa recta, countercurrent exchange washes solute out of the medullary interstitium resulting in diminished tubular reabsorption. When blood flow through the vasa recta is slow, as in states of hypoperfusion, the medullary osmotic gradient increases to 1200 mOsm allowing for maximal reabsorption of tubular fluid. Distal tubular reabsorption of sodium is also active. In the distal tubule, sodium is actively reabsorbed under the control of aldosterone. During this final segment, remaining tubular sodium reabsorption is under the control of aldosterone and atrial natriuretic factor (ANF). Aldosterone serves to facilitate nearly complete reabsorption of sodium in this segment, while ANF enhances sodium excretion. Antidiuretic hormone, secreted by the posterior pituitary in response to plasma osmotic stimuli and angiotensin peptides, acts in the late distal convoluted tubules and collecting ducts to enhance passive reabsorption of water. This diminishes free water clearance. High levels of antidiuretic hormone result in hyperosmotic urine formation, while low levels, as in the syndrome of inappropriate antidiuretic hormone, result in dilute, hyposmotic urine. Of the approximately 25,000 mEq of sodium filtered daily, only 50 to 200 mEq is ultimately excreted through urination. The production and release of aldosterone and antidiuretic hormone is directly stimulated by angiotensin peptides. These adrenal and pituitary compounds are of primary importance in facilitating the sodium retention and increased intravascular volume that is associated with RVH.

Filtered potassium is almost totally reabsorbed in the proximal tubule and the loop of Henle. However, reabsorption of this ion is influenced by the electronegatively of the tubular fluid, the intracellular concentration of potassium, and the presence of aldosterone. The influence of these factors is seen mostly in the distal tubules and early collecting ducts where potassium is passively secreted into the tubular lumen. Under normal physiologic conditions, the degree of distal potassium secretion is in balance with hydrogen ion excretion and is dependent on the pH of the tubular fluid. In the case of metabolic acidosis, hydrogen ion concentrations in the distal tubule become elevated and potassium secretion diminished. The opposite is true in metabolic alkalosis. In that situation, hydrogen ions are reabsorbed to compensate for the systemic alkalosis, while potassium is secreted to maintain anion and cation balance in the distal tubular fluid. In the case of RVH, the increased aldosterone activity results in selective potassium wasting by the distal convoluted tubule and enhanced sodium reabsorption. These processes are responsible for the transportation of nearly all of the potassium measured in the final urine product. The effects of aldosterone on potassium excretion in patients with RVH are clinically relevant. In fact, this patient population is commonly found to have spontaneous hypokalemia that is not associated with diuretic usage.[41]

In addition to their arteriolar and glomerular effects, angiotensin peptides directly influence tubular reabsorption (Table 1). In fact, the influence of AII on proximal tubular sodium reabsorption is dose-dependent by in vivo micropuncture studies. The specific ability of AII to augment sodium reabsorption by the proximal tubule has been localized to the luminal sodium/hydrogen exchange pump.[42] However, the influence of AII on basolateral sodium/bicarbonate cotransport mechanisms remains unresolved. Though AI has been associated with increased sodium reabsorption in the proximal tubule, it is more likely that AII is being generated by local angiotensin-converting enzymes. The finding that angiotensin-converting enzyme inhibitors diminish the sodium reabsorption associated with these angiotensin peptides lends support to this hypothesis.[42]

As in other organ systems, intrarenal angiotensin activity is dependent on receptor-mediated mechanisms that likely vary between species. The locations of various angiotensin peptides and receptor subtypes in normal and chronically ischemic human kidneys have recently been described by Diz and coworkers.[43] Using receptor autoradiography, the densities of the two known receptors have been characterized in the renal circulation and the nephron. These findings point to a significant intrarenal influence of angiotensin peptides. In the normal kidney, angiotensin activity is highest in the large preglomerular arteries. Activity sequentially decreases in the glomeruli and tubulointerstitial areas of the cortex (Figure 7). Regarding specific angiotensin receptor subtypes, type 1 receptors predominate in the glomerulus and the efferent arteriole. Mesangial cells also have mostly type 1 receptor populations. Type 2 receptors, on the other hand, predominate in the large preglomerular arteries. In the tubulointerstitial areas of the renal cortex, the respective mixture of type 1 and 2 receptors was found to be 60% and 40%, respectively. The functional impact of this configuration relates to the ability of angiotensin peptides to regulate vascular tone, mesangial tone, the filtration fraction, and tubular function. While AII is able to interact with both receptor subtypes, angiotensin-(1–7) interacts with type 2 receptors. Activation of type 2 receptors decreases tone in the larger preglomerular vessels, thus enhancing blood flow to the preglomerular vessels. On the other hand, stimulation of type 1 receptors in the glomeruli and postglomerular vessels by AII is associated with vasoconstriction. Vasoconstriction is greatest in the postglomerular arterioles. The combination of increased flow through the larger preglomerular arteries and increased resistance in the postglomerular arterioles produces higher glomerular hydrostatic pressure and leads to an increase in the filtration fraction. Regarding tubular function, type 1 receptors are associated with increased sodium reabsorption, while type 2 receptors augment natriuresis. The ability of angiotensin-(1–7) to reduce preglomerular resistance and tubular sodium reabsorption may be partly a result of their ability to stimulate local release of prostacyclin.[38]

Interestingly, the densities of these receptor populations change in patients with critical renovascular occlusive disease.[43] This may impact on angiotensin pep-

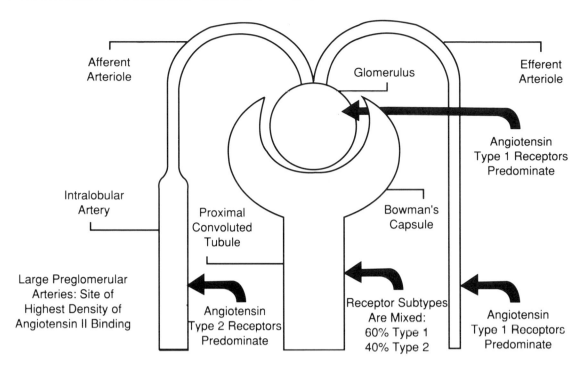

Figure 7. Angiotensin receptor subtypes in the nonischemic human kidney. This diagram illustrates the relative predominance of different angiotensin receptor populations in the renal circulation and proximal tubule. While angiotensin II is able to activate both receptor subtypes, angiotensin-(1–7) only activates type 2 receptors. Type 1 receptors are associated with vasoconstriction and increased tubular reabsorption of sodium. Type 2 receptors are associated with vasodilation and natriuresis. (Adapted with permission from Reference 43.)

tide influence on renal hemodynamics and tubular function in this setting. When comparing normal and ischemic human kidneys, our laboratory demonstrated that the number of receptors in large preglomerular and glomerular vessels decreased by 50% to 60% in ischemic kidneys, while the number of receptors in the tubules increased by 65%. The ratio of type 1 and type 2 receptors in these areas was also altered by RVH. In particular, the ratio of type 1 and type 2 receptors increased in large preglomerular arteries, while it decreased in the glomeruli and tubules. The functional significance of these changes remains to be proven.

Finally, renovascular disease in the atherosclerotic age group frequently includes a variable amount of arteriolar disease at the glomerular level. In these patients, and in nephron units experiencing extreme ischemia, the excretory functional responses to impaired perfusion may be less physiologic, and the capacity to hyperconcentrate urine may be lost. Since such events are not uniform among all units, a spectrum of changes within the kidney may be present, thus further masking the clarity of the normal kidney's response to impaired perfusion.

Mechanisms of Renal Autoregulation

The kidneys have two major mechanisms of autoregulation: tubuloglomerular feedback, and a myogenic vascular response. External regulatory control occurs through multiple vasoactive and natriuretic substances, and the sympathetic nervous system. Data from several different animal models suggest that these regulatory mechanisms have various complex interactions,[44–46] which occur at many levels including the vascular smooth muscle, glomerular mesangium, tubular system, and vascular endothelium. Importantly, these regulatory mechanisms are of primary importance in the development and maintenance of RVH.

The Myogenic Mechanism and Angiotensin Peptides

The renal microcirculation has a unique design that controls blood flow into the glomeruli, the degree of plasma ultrafiltration, and the degree of reabsorption from the tubules.[39,40,47,48] Glomerular blood flow has been shown to be tightly regulated between 80 and 180 mm Hg. Critical components of the microcirculatory design include the afferent arterioles, the glomeruli, the efferent arterioles, the peritubular capillaries and vasa recta, and the vascular endothelium. In this design, the pattern of resistor (aa) capillary bed resistor (ea) capillary bed in close approximation to the tubular apparatus helps account for the unique autoregulatory abilities of the kidneys and allows for multiple regulation patterns.[49] The baseline tone of the resistors is altered in response to variations in blood pressure, neural activity and vasoactive hormones. In such a scheme, baroreceptors in the renal arteries alter sympathetic output to the renal circulation and tubules. This directly effects renal blood flow (RBF), GFR, and tubular reabsorption. The two major opposing vasoactive hormones thought to be responsible for myogenic autoregulation are nitric oxide (NO) and AII.[50–56] Endothelial-derived relaxing factors, particularly NO, have a tonic relaxing effect on the afferent and efferent arterioles and is associated with increased natriuresis. According to Romero et al, NO production and release from endothelial cells throughout the renal circulation increases with perfusion pressure between 80 and 180 mm Hg. Prostacyclin production, on the other hand, increases when perfusion pressure drops below these levels of renal autoregulation.[50] This configuration augments diuresis during times of high renal perfusion pressure, while maintaining tubular oxygen delivery and excretion of systemic waste when renal perfusion is low.

The precision of this control mechanism can be appreciated by reviewing the effects of isolated resistor changes.[39] Multiple combinations of resistor tones occur in various physiologic conditions resulting in precision autoregulation. In the face of critical renal artery stenosis, AII directly increases the tone of the afferent and efferent arterioles. Interestingly, the tone of the efferent arteriole increases more in this setting. This augments glomerular hydrostatic pressures, and thus glomerular filtration. This increase in the filtration fraction helps maintain delivery of systemic waste products to the tubules in the face of low renal perfusion pressures. While the filtration fraction increases in this setting, medullary blood flow and interstitial pressure decrease. This configuration enhances the countercurrent multiplication mechanism and tubular reabsorption of sodium and free water. Since the kidney interprets the condition of renal artery stenosis as hypovolemia, these forces act to increase intravascular volume. The reproducibility of such excretion patterns led to the development of split renal function studies. Such studies are used to confirm the functional significance of a renovascular lesion.

Regulation of regional blood flow in the kidney also impacts on reabsorption of the tubular fluid. Under normal circumstances, more than 90% of renal blood flow is distributed to the renal cortex. The remainder of blood flow is distributed to the outer and inner medulla. The gradation of flow in these areas is such that the outer medulla receives the bulk of medullary blood flow, and the inner tissues receive progressively less flow. Medullary blood flow dynamics are influenced by the relatively long, small caliber vasa

recta, increased viscosity of medullary blood, hormonal activity of the vasa recta endothelium, and renal sympathetic nerve activity. Finally, the pattern of regional renal blood flow has a direct impact on the countercurrent multiplier mechanism of the renal medulla. In renovascular hypertension, AII diminishes blood flow to the medulla by increasing efferent arteriolar tone.

Tubuloglomerular Feedback and Angiotensin Peptides

In this mechanism of autoregulation, the contents of tubular fluid influence glomerular blood flow. The unique anatomy of the glomerulus and its associated tubule allows for this feedback mechanism (Figure 8). The distal end of the thick ascending loop of Henle lies beside its glomerulus of origin. This anatomic entity is known as the juxtaglomerular apparatus. It includes the macula densa of the thick ascending loop of Henle, the afferent and efferent arterioles, and the mesangial cells. The cells of the macula densa are able to detect the concentration of NaCl of the local tubular fluid. $Na^+/K^+/2Cl^-$ cotransport pumps, long known to exist in the thick ascending loop of Henle, have been identified in the macula densa and likely play an important role in the assessment of NaCl levels.[44,45] As mentioned, the concentration of NaCl at the thick ascending loop of Henle is determined by the tubular flow rate. The macula densa accurately translates the tubular flow rate from the salt concentration and alters afferent and efferent arteriole resistance as needed to maintain normal distal tubular salt delivery. Though both arterioles are affected by this mechanism, the afferent arteriole is the primary site of autoregulation. The effect on afferent and efferent arteriole resistance is accomplished via local intercellular mechanisms and systemic release of renin. Locally active renin-angiotensin systems may also influence this aspect of autoregulation.[38,43] Adenosine byproducts from $Na^+/K^+/2Cl^-$ cotransport pump ATP metabolism is thought to drive the vasoconstriction of the arterioles.[44] This mechanism may also alter GFR through direct effects on the mesangial cell tone and, thus the filtration surface area.

Under normal conditions, solute reabsorption from the more proximal nephron produces tubular fluid that has a lower NaCl concentration relative to plasma when it arrives at the distal thick ascending loop of Henle. During periods of low GFR, as in hemorrhagic shock or critical renal artery stenosis, the decreased tubular flow results in maximal reabsorption of solute and hence fluid with low NaCl concentrations. Because less work is performed by the $Na^+/K^+/2Cl^-$ cotransport pump, the macula densa is able to sense the low NaCl concentrations. This results in decreased

a. Thick Ascending Loop of Henle
b. Macula Densa
c. Juxtaglomerular Cells
d. Afferent Arteriole
e. Efferent Arteriole
f. Glomerular Capillary
g. Mesangial Cell
h. Bowman's Space
i. Proximal Convoluted Tubule
j. Renal Sympathetic Nerves

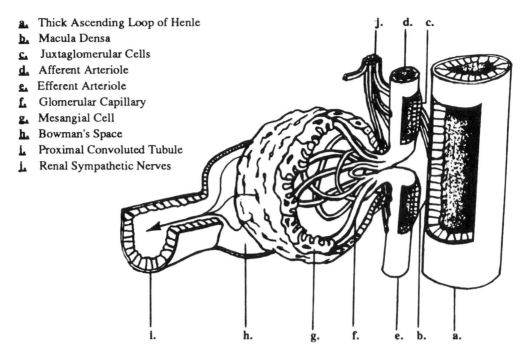

Figure 8. The juxtaglomerular apparatus and tubuloglomerular feedback. The open section of the distal thick ascending loop of Henle reveals the cells of the macula densa, while similar sections of the afferent and efferent arterioles reveal the renin producing juxtaglomerular cells. The macula densa estimates the tubular flow rate from distal NaCl concentrations. When NaCl is low (renal blood flow [RBF] and glomerular filtration rate [GFR]) afferent and efferent arteriole resistance decreases, while renin secretion increases. When NaCl is high (RBF and GFR) arteriole resistance increases while renin secretion decreases. The afferent arteriole is the primary site of autoregulation. Arteriolar constriction is likely facilitated by adenosine byproducts of macula densa sodium/potassium/chloride pump metabolism. Locally produced angiotensin II (AII) decreases the sensitivity of the afferent and efferent arterioles to tubuloglomerular feedback. Thus, in the setting of renal ischemia, local AII helps maintain increased glomerular tone, tubular sodium reabsorption, and juxtaglomerular renin release.

local adenosine production, decreased afferent arteriolar resistance, and increased renin production and secretion. The exact mechanism of increased renin production is unresolved. Renin causes the production of AII. AII increases systemic blood pressure through various effects on several organ systems, including the cardiovascular, central and autonomic nervous, and adrenal and renal systems. Under otherwise normal circumstances, these systemic actions restore renal plasma flow, GFR, and distal NaCl delivery to normal levels. During periods of increased tubular flow and distal NaCl delivery, the macula densa increases afferent arteriole resistance to decrease RBF and GFR. Usually, this mechanism allows for fine control of renal plasma flow and GFR. However, in pathologic situations such as critical renal artery stenosis, the change in afferent arteriolar resistance does not adequately correct tubular flow and distal NaCl delivery. This results in chronic activation of the renin-angiotensin system, and renovascular hypertension may activate local angiotensin peptide production. As mentioned, AII

also has direct local renal effects. In addition to its effect on sodium reabsorption by the proximal tubule, AII has been found to decrease the sensitivity of the afferent and efferent arterioles to tubuloglomerular feedback. In other words, tone in these vessels remains high despite the influence of the macula densa. This serves in tandem with its other effects to enhance tubular sodium reabsorption, while maintaining renin release by the juxtaglomerular cells. Thus, a locally active renal renin-angiotensin system may exacerbate the increased volume status and hypertension associated with critical renovascular occlusive disease.[28] This becomes important clinically when one considers the deleterious impact of angiotensin-converting enzyme inhibitors in patients with renal artery stenosis. By blocking local AII effects on efferent arteriolar tone, angiotensin-converting enzyme inhibitors lower the filtration fraction, and thus the ability of the kidneys to excrete systemic waste (Figure 9). The clinical result is an increase in plasma creatinine, urea nitrogen levels, and renal insufficiency. This deleterious intrarenal

A. Normal

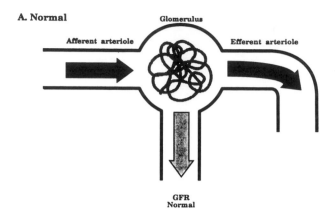

B. Renal Artery Stenosis

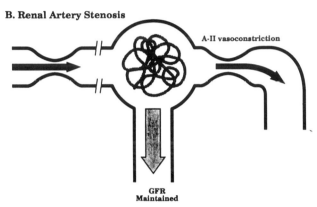

C. Renal Artery Stenosis plus Captopril

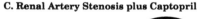
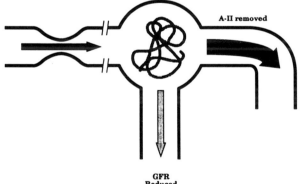

Figure 9. Schematic figure of the effect of captopril on renal function. A = Normal; B = RAS; C = RAS plus captopril. (Reproduced with permission from Reference 58.)

effect on GFR is likely more significant than the decrease in the systemic arterial pressure also induced by these inhibitors.[43,57,58]

Vascular Endothelial Substances

Increasing attention has been given to the effects of vascular endothelial substances on the renal microcirculation and autoregulation. These substances interact with both myogenic and tubuloglomerular feedback mechanisms. Changes in vascular shear stress induce production and release of different vasoactive substances by the endothelial cells. In general, hormones induce vasodilation or constriction. NO and endogenous AII are now considered the most likely determinants of myogenic renal autoregulation.[50–53] Importantly, these are not the only vasoactive hormones that influence normal and pathologic renal function. In addition to their direct vascular effects, these compounds have regulatory effects on endothelial production and release of prostaglandins, thromboxanes, and other vasoactive hormones. The other recognized vasoactive hormones influencing renal hemodynamics and function are endothelin, thromboxane A_2, prostaglandins, platelet activating factor, and ANF. All of these, have profound influences on the renal microcirculation and mesangium (Table 2). Their opposing actions influence the tone of the renal circulation and, thus, RPF, GFR, and natriuresis.[59] Furthermore, their production, secretion, and activity are directly influenced by the renin-angiotensin system. In the setting of renovascular occlusive disease, several physiologic factors work together to enhance renal hemodynamics and filtration, despite low perfusion pressures. Specifically, the local intrarenal levels of AII, endothelin 1, thromboxane A_2, prostaglandin I2, and prostaglandin E2 are elevated in ischemic kidneys.[38,43,60–63] AII and endothelin 1 increase efferent arteriolar resistance, mesangial cell tone, and reabsorption of sodium by the tubules.[64–66] Thromboxane A_2 increases resistance of the afferent arteriole, and likely has direct effects on sodium reabsorption as well.[61,67,68] Though prostacyclin does not exert a tonic influence on the vasculature during normal circumstances, it maintains RBF during states of low renal perfusion pressure.[50,59,69,70] This is in contradistinction to the vasodilating activity of NO, which has basal effects on autoregulation and increases activity during states of high renal perfusion pressure. This eicosanoid, like NO, selectively dilates the afferent arteriole.[51,52,55] Recently, our laboratory has shown that AII and angiotensin-(1–7) directly increase prostaglandin release from human renal arteries. During low flow states, such as main renal artery occlusion, it is likely that angiotensin peptides increase the release of prostacyclin. In the presence of selective efferent arteriolar constriction from AII and endothelin 1, the resulting resistor pattern attempts to maintain GFR by increasing the filtration fraction. Finally, AII stimulates production and release of ANF by the heart. The balance of these compounds determines the overall effect on renal function. Thus, their activities are an important consideration in the pathophysiology of RVH.[71]

Renal Nerves and Function Regulation

The autonomic nervous system plays an important role in the modulation of renal function in states of

Table 2
Vasoactive Hormones that Interact With the Angiotensin Peptides and Influence Renal Hemodynamics and Tubular Function

Vasoactive Hormone	Mechanism of Action	Effect on Arteriole Tone	Effect on Mesangial Tone	Medullary Blood Flow	Natriuretic Effect
Angiotensin II (Ang II)	AT1 Receptor/ Phospholipase/ ITP & Diacyl glycerol→ ↑ cellular Ca+ +	↑ ↑ AA tone ↑ ↑ ↑ EA tone ↑ Filtration %	↑ Tone/ ↓ GFSA	Decreased	Decreased
Endothelin 1 (ET 1)	ET Receptor/ Phospholipase/ ITP & Diacyl glycerol→ ↑ cellular Ca+ +	↑ AA tone ↑ ↑ ↑ EA tone ↑ Filtration %	↑ Tone/ ↓ GFSA	Decreased	Decreased
Thromboxane A2 (TXA$_2$)	TXA2 Receptor/ Phospholipase/ ITP & Diacyl glycerol→ ↑ cellular Ca+ +	↑ ↑ AA tone ↑ EA tone	↑ Tone/ ↓ GFSA	Decreased	Decreased
Nitric Oxide (NO)	Diffuses through cell membrane then ↑ cyclic GMP	↓ ↓ AA tone ↓ ↓ ↓ EA tone	↓ Tone/ ↑ GFSA	Increased	Increased
Prostacyclin/ Prostaglandin E2 (PGI$_2$/PGE$_2$)	PGI2 Receptor then ↑ cyclic AMP **(PGI2)**	↓ ↓ AA tone ↓ EA tone **(PGI2)**	↓ Tone/ ↑ GFSA	Increased **(PGI2)**	Increased **(PGE2)**
Atrial Natriuretic Factor (ANF)	ANF Receptor/ then ↑ cyclic GMP	↓ AA tone ↓ EA tone	↓ Tone/ ↑ GFSA	Increased	Increased

AA = Afferent Arteriole; EA = Efferent Arteriole; GFSA = Glomerular Filtration Surface Area; ITP = Inositol Triphosphate; GMP = Guanosine Monophosphate; AMP = Adenosine Monophosphate

normotension and hypertension. The sympathetic nervous system innervates both the renal microvascular and tubular structures. Major vascular structures directly innervated by adrenergic nerves include the afferent and efferent arterioles. Tubular structures so influenced, in descending magnitude of innervation, include the thick ascending loop of Henle, the juxtaglomerular apparatus, the distal convoluted tubules, and the proximal tubules. Renal sympathetic nerves regulate renal sodium excretion, RBF, GFR, and renin secretion rate through alpha-1-adrenergic receptors in the vessels and tubules, and alpha-1-receptors in the juxtaglomerular apparatus.[72] Renal sympathetic nerve

activity varies with afferent stimulation from renal vascular baroreceptors, ureteral mechanoreceptors, and pelvic chemoreceptors. Additionally, renal sympathetic tone is influenced by the degree of sympathetic response to stressful stimuli.[31] Interestingly, the input from one kidney modulates function of the other and is termed the reno-renal reflex. Afferent input from ureteral mechanoreceptors is increased with obstruction, and results in decreased ipsilateral and increased contralateral natriuresis. Increased sodium concentration detected by renal pelvic chemoreceptors results in a similar situation. According to DiBona,[72] graded frequency of efferent nerve stimulation results in variable effects on renal function. With increasing stimulation, renal function parameters are affected in the following order: 1) renin secretion rate is increased; 2) sodium and water reabsorption increases; and 3) GFR and RBF are decreased. Baroreceptor stimuli influence the sensitivity of juxtaglomerular apparatus renin production. With increased baroreceptor stimulation during states of hypotension, renin secretion is augmented. The opposite occurs during states of high renal artery pressure and low baroreceptor stimulation.

It is likely that renal nerve activity contributes to RVH. Studies by Kopp and Buckley-Bleiler have shown that the reno-renal reflex is directly affected in two-kidney, one-clip RVH.[73] In this setting, efferent renal nerve activity is increased. Denervation of the unclipped kidney results in an ipsilateral increase in sodium excretion and GFR, while clipped kidney denervation results in bilateral natriuresis and increased GFR.[31] Additionally, selective afferent denervation of the clipped kidney results in decreased hypothalamic norepinephrine stores, decreased peripheral sympathetic nerve activity, and reduced arterial pressure. With regard to renovascular hypertension, AII directly increases central and renal sympathetic nerve activity.

Tissue Renin-Angiotensin Systems

Since Bright observed the association between renal disease and cardiac hypertrophy in 1827, multidisciplinary investigations of angiotensin peptides have led to a new appreciation of the scope of their systemic effects and the identification of locally integrated tissue renin-angiotensin systems. The activities of these local systems are summarized in Table 3.

Angiotensin Peptides and the Cardiovascular System

Patients with renovascular occlusive disease commonly have concurrent cardiac and peripheral vascular disease. As renovascular hypertension develops and becomes severe, the risk of cardiovascular morbidity and mortality increases. Much of this increased risk is due to the adverse effects of angiotensin peptides on preload, afterload, cardiac contractility, systemic vascular resistance, coronary vasoconstriction, and heart rate.

Angiotensin peptides, especially AII, influence the metabolic activities of endothelial and vascular

Table 3
Actions of Angiotensin Peptides and Receptor Subtypes in Major Organ Systems

Organ System Involved	Specific Tissue Response	Angiotensinogen Metabolite	Receptor Subtype Mediating Effect
Blood Vessels and Vascular Smooth Muscle Cells	1. Vasoconstriction	1. Ang II & Ang III	1. AT1
	2. Mitogenesis/Hypertrophy	2. Ang II	2. AT1
	3. Angiogenesis	3. Ang II	3. AT1/AT2
	4. Intimal Hyperplasia	4. Ang II	4. AT1
	5. Endothelial PG Release	5. Ang II	5. AT2
	6. Vasodilation	6. Ang-(1–7)	6. Undetermined
Myocardium	1. Positive Inotrope	1. Ang II	1. AT1
	2. Hypertrophy	2. Ang II	2. AT1
	3. Stimulation of Atrial Natriuretic Release	3. Ang II	3. Undetermined
	4. Coronary Vasoconstriction	4. Ang-(1–7)	4. Undetermined
Central Nervous System	1. Arginine Vasopressor (ADH) Release	1. Ang-(1–7), Ang II & Ang III	1. AT1
	2. Thirst/Drinking	2. Ang II & Ang III	2. AT1
	3. Baroreceptor	3. Ang-(1–7), Ang II & Ang III	3. AT1/AT2
Sympathetic Actions	4. Potentiation of Norepinephrine Release From Nerve Terminal	4. Ang II & Ang III	4. AT1
Adrenal Cortex	1. Aldosterone Release	1. Ang II & Ang III	1. AT1
	2. Corticotropin Release	2. Ang II & Ang III	2. AT1
Medulla	3. Catecholamine Release	3. Ang II	3. AT1

Description of the physiologic activities of angiotensin-(1–7) [Ang-(1–7)], angiotensin II [Ang II], angiotensin III [Ang III], and the two main angiotensin receptor subtypes in several organ systems.

SMCs.[74–78] Acutely, stimulation of AI receptors effects an increase in intracellular calcium and vasoconstriction. Over increased periods of exposure, AII induces hypertrophy of the SMCs.[79,80] This is related to its ability to upregulate the activity of several different sodium pumps and, thus, elevate intracellular sodium concentrations. In vascular SMCs, these higher sodium concentrations induce compensatory increases in intracellular calcium. In the chronic setting, increased sodium and calcium concentrations exaggerate the response to constricting stimuli such as catecholamines, while attenuating the response to endothelium-dependent dilating hormones such as NO, prostacyclin, and acetylcholine.[80] Additionally, angiotensin peptides increase the number of these sodium/potassium pumps by stimulating their genetic expression. Krug and Berk[80] have observed that increased gene expression and cellular hypertrophy occurs within 24 hours of AII exposure. As noted, angiotensin peptides also upregulate endothelial expression of angiotensin-converting enzyme, AI, endothelin 1, and eicosanoids. Finally, AII increases smooth muscle proliferation by inducing production of transforming growth factor 2 and platelet-derived growth factors.[81,82] This influence at the gene level is likely responsible for the changes in arterial structure and reactivity that are associated with renovascular hypertension.[78] Recent investigations have found that not all angiotensin peptides induce the above changes in vascular SMCs or systemic vascular resistance. In particular, angiotensin-(1–7) is associated with vasodilation. The vasodilator activity of this peptide is a result of its direct actions on the vascular smooth muscle and its ability to induce the release of vasodilator prostaglandins. Its actions are thought to be accomplished through an angiotensin receptor other than types 1 and 2.[83,84]

After the introduction of angiotensin-converting enzyme inhibitors to clinical practice, physicians observed a dramatic effectiveness in the management of heart failure. Subsequent laboratory investigation found that the myocardium is also influenced by a local, active renin-angiotensin system. The ability to express angiotensinogen, renin, AI, angiotensin-converting enzyme, and AII is present in the atria and ventricles.[74] Additionally, angiotensin receptors have been identified in the myocardium, coronary arteries, and cardiac sympathetic nerves. Several investigators have demonstrated that angiotensin peptides have positive inotrope activity, stimulate release of ANF, and induce myocyte hypertrophy.[74,85–87] AII exerts its cardiac effects by activating phospholipase enzyme cascades and by inhibiting cyclic AMP accumulation. Increased myocardial production of angiotensin peptides is associated with pressure overload-induced and post-infarction cardiac hypertrophy. Underscoring the autonomous activity of the cardiac renin-angiotensin system in this setting is the observation that simultaneous increases in angiotensin peptide production does not occur in other vascular beds.[74] Angiotensin peptides exert positive inotropic and chronotropic influences on the myocardium, increase coronary artery tone, and stimulate the release of ANF. The positive inotropic activity is thought to be related to its influence on intracellular and transmembrane conductance. Because AII increases the height and duration of the plateau phase of the cardiac action potential with corresponding increases in myocardial tension, the slow inward calcium channels are thought to be the main site of its inotropic influence. According to Lindpainter and Ganten,[74] the sinoatrial and atrioventricular nodes have high densities of angiotensin receptors. When coupled with their influence on adrenomedullary secretion of catecholamines and cardiac sympathetic and vagal nerve activity, the potential of the renin-angiotensin system to modulate inotropic and chronotropic activity in the healthy heart can be appreciated. In the setting of congestive heart failure and myocardial ischemia, angiotensin peptides worsen coronary blood flow and diminish myocardial function. By increasing afterload and coronary artery tone, these peptides increase myocardial demand and wall tension while diminishing diastolic coronary perfusion.

Angiotensin-converting enzyme successfully blocks these effects in the diseased myocardium, while decreasing preload and afterload.[88,89] In addition, angiotensin-converting enzyme inhibition results in increased production of angiotensin-(1–7) and decreased metabolism of bradykinin. Angiotensin-converting enzyme, also referred to as kininase II, is responsible for the inactivation of bradykinin. When this enzyme is blocked, the vasodilator activity of bradykinin is maintained while the activity of angiotensin-(1–7) is increased. As mentioned, these hormones stimulate the production and release of the vasodilators, NO, and prostaglandins. The cumulative effect is a considerable impact on systemic vascular resistance and cardiac function. Thus, angiotensin-converting enzyme may effect systemic blood pressure by altering the balance of opposing vasoactive hormone systems.[90]

Angiotensin Peptides and the Central Nervous System

The central nervous system also has been shown to respond to and produce angiotensin peptides.[91] Angiotensin peptide production and receptor populations are concentrated in areas of the medulla, hypothalamus, and pituitary that are responsible for central blood pressure control.[92] Specifically, AII is able to enhance both peripheral and central neural activity. By directly increasing norepinephrine secretion from nerve terminals and simultaneously inhibiting its reuptake from the synapse, AII increases peripheral sympathetic nerve activity.[91-94] Centrally, angiotensin peptides influence the activity of the baroreceptor reflex, vagal tone, sympathetic tone, and hormone release from the pituitary gland. Regarding its effect on baroreceptor activity, AII prevents the reflex bradycardia usually associated with systemic hypertension.[91] The specific site in the medulla where this occurs is one of the major centers for vagal efferent activity, the nucleus of the tractus solitarus. It appears that plasma angiotensin peptides are able to infiltrate the blood-brain barrier at a site directly dorsal to the nucleus of the tractus solitarius called the area postrema. Additionally, astrocytes in this area are able to produce angiotensin peptides. These peptides reduce vagal efferent activity from the nucleus of the tractus solitarius that would otherwise decrease the heart rate in the face of systemic arterial hypertension.[72,95] Since systemic pressure is a consequence of cardiac stroke volume, heart rate, and systemic vascular resistance, the activity of angiotensin peptides on the baroreceptor reflex supports its cardiovascular effects to increase systemic arterial blood pressure.[96,97]

In addition to diminishing baroreceptor activity, angiotensin peptides enhance activity of sympathetic outflow from vasomotor centers. These centers are responsible for the sympathetic efferent activity to the renal nerves, peripheral vasculature, and the adrenal medulla. Finally, angiotensin peptides act in the hypothalamus to increase thirst-related behavior, and in the pituitary, to increase release of antidiuretic hormone (vasopressin) and adrenocorticotropic hormone.[93] All of these activities can be diminished or blocked by angiotensin-converting enzyme inhibitors or specific angiotensin receptor blockers. Due to their ability to modulate these central and peripheral neural activities, angiotensin peptides are also considered neurotransmitters.[93,94]

Adrenal Effects

Angiotensin peptides influence both the cortex and medulla of the adrenal gland. In the medulla, both epinephrine and norepinephrine production and release are increased by AII.[98] AII accomplishes this action directly by stimulation of the medullary cells and indirectly by increasing central nervous system sympathetic output. The resulting increase in plasma catecholamines enhances the vasoconstricting and inotropic effects of AII. In the adrenal cortex, AII and AIII are equally able to increase production of aldosterone by cells in the zona glomerulosa. By increasing adrenocorticotropic hormone secretion by the anterior pituitary, angiotensin peptides indirectly augment aldosterone and cortisol production. Aldosterone enhances sodium reabsorption and potassium excretion by the distal convoluted tubules. Nishimura and colleagues have shown the adrenals also have local integrated renin-angiotensin systems that are able to produce angiotensin peptides.[28] Although local production has not been found to alter systemic levels, it does have the ability to act in a paracrine fashion to influence adrenal cortical and medullary activity.

Pathologic Considerations

RVH can be produced by several underlying conditions of the renal vasculature. In essence, any underlying condition that disturbs perfusion to the nephron unit can activate the renin-angiotensin system and lead to RVH.

Atherosclerosis

Among the causes of RVH, atherosclerotic occlusion of the renal artery is most common, accounting for about 70% of cases. A long history of hypertension is not uncommon in patients with atherosclerosis and RVH. It is probable that the primary, or essential, hypertension in these patients serves to accelerate the growth of atherosclerosis. Frequently, however, this group has a long history of mild, easily controlled hypertension upon which is superimposed the more severe secondary renovascular form. A potential etiologic factor predisposing the renal artery to involvement by atherosclerosis is the presence of the splanchnic plexus of nerves encasing the origin of the renal arteries. In the process of mobilization of the renal artery, its origin is always firmly encased in a sheath of neural tissue that creates a firm fixation point. Like the fixation of the popliteal artery by the adductor hiatus and of the celiac axis by the median arcuate ligament, this fixation of the renal artery origin probably accelerates atherosclerosis at this site and leads to occlusion more frequently than at other bifurcation points not similarly affected by extreme fixation. Finally, diffuse involvement of the distal renal artery by intrarenal arteriolar atherosclerosis may also produce RVH. Frequently found in conjunction with extrarenal occlusions, the clinical pertinence of such intrarenal disease is variable. When severe, it leads to destruction of the nephron unit and an irretrievable, nonfunctioning kidney. Nevertheless, the juxtaglomerular network of blood pressure control may still be viable and produce RVH even when no excretory function remains.

Pathologically, there is nothing peculiar to the atherosclerosis of a renal artery. The pathogenesis parallels that of atherosclerotic lesions elsewhere, with cho-

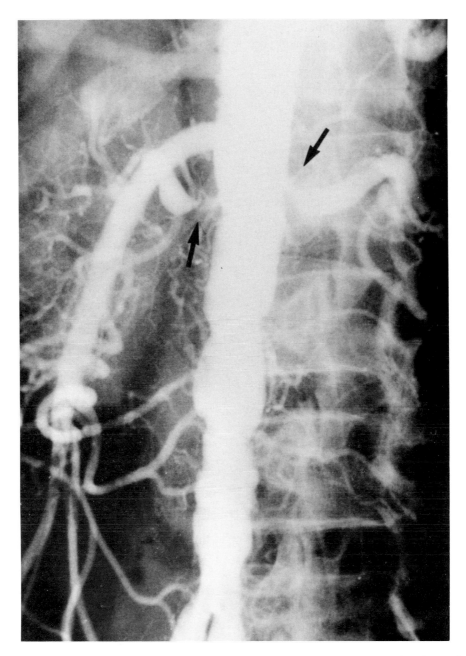

Figure 10. Arteriogram of a patient with severe hypertension, demonstrating the typical angiographic appearance of atherosclerotic renal arterial occlusive disease. Two right renal arteries and the single left renal artery are all severely affected. The aortorenal orifice and proximal arterial trunk is the common site of heaviest atheromatous deposit.

lesterol-rich lipid deposition and intimal thickening. This "atheroma" later may undergo central degeneration and even calcification. They typically occur at or near the renal artery ostium (Figure 10), are most commonly found on the left, and account for about 70% of cases of RVH. Often, there is arteriographic evidence of asymptomatic, simultaneous involvement of the abdominal aorta and its bifurcation. Occasionally, the renal artery stenosis is only one manifestation of severe end-stage generalized atherosclerosis.

Fibromuscular Dysplasia

Fibromuscular dysplastic lesions account for about 25% of all causes of renovascular disease. Although categorized under a single term, these lesions represent an array of histologic patterns and are produced by no single underlying malady. Generally, they are subcategorized according to their angiographic appearance and the layer of arterial wall that is predominantly affected. In this manner, they can be divided into intimal dysplasia, medial hyperplasia, medial dysplasia, and perimedial dysplasia.

Although many theories have been explored to explain the presence of fibrodysplastic renal artery lesion, no single explanation is adequate. The finding of the medial and perimedial varieties primarily in women suggests hormonal influences. Proof of specific hormonal influences, however, is lacking.[99,100] Similarly, the common finding of fibrodysplastic lesions in ptotic kidneys has led to the suggestion that the lesions might be a consequence of the stretching of the vessel wall.[101] Alternatively, mural ischemia secondary to inadequate nutrient vasa vasorum in the renal artery wall has been suggested as an etiologic factor.[102] Although one or all of these factors may be etiologically important, their pertinence remains speculative.

Intimal Dysplasia

Intimal lesions are uncommon and account for about 5% of all fibrodysplastic lesions. Primarily found in children, without sex predilection, the lesion appears as a short, smooth, concentric narrowing of the main renal artery. Histologically, it is composed of an accumulation of irregularly positioned subendothelial mesenchymal cells with a relatively normal appearing medial and adventitial layer.

Like other varieties of fibromuscular dysplasia, the cause of intimal dysplasia is unknown. Its intimal location and occurrence in the young suggests a developmental anomaly or consequence of an intrauterine event.

Medial Hyperplasia

Although frequently misused to describe all fibrodysplastic lesions, fibromuscular hyperplasia of the medial layer is the least common variety and accounts for less than 1% of all fibrodysplastic lesions. Histologically characterized by the presence of well organized yet excessive amounts of medial SMCs, it appears angiographically as an isolated, single, mural, concentric narrowing of the renal artery. It is found primarily in females during their third and fourth decade and appears to be a progressive lesion that is capable of rapid development. The cause of medial hyperplasia is unknown.

Medial Fibrodysplasia

Medial fibrodysplasia with microaneurysms is by far the most common variety of fibromuscular dysplasia and accounts for over 85% of dysplastic lesions of the renal artery. It is seen almost exclusively in women. Although usually identified in the fourth or fifth decade, we have found it in a patient in her ninth decade (Figure 11). The cause of medial fibrodysplasia with microaneurysm is unknown, yet it appears to be a systemic arteriopathy. In contrast to the other varieties of fibromuscular dysplasia, medial fibrodysplasia is also found in the carotid and iliac arteries. Nevertheless, lesions in these extrarenal locations are very uncommon compared with the frequency of renal artery involvement.

Angiographically, medial dysplasia usually appears as a "string of beads," with sites of web-like stenoses alternating with small fusiform or saccular appearing aneurysms of the renal artery. It usually involves the distal third of the main renal artery, but commonly extends into the proximal portion of the first level of branches.

The histologic appearance of medial fibrodys-

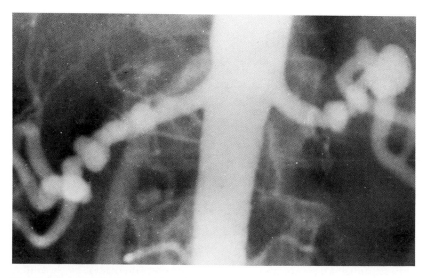

Figure 11. Arteriogram demonstrating the typical "string of beads" appearance of medial fibrodysplasia. The intraluminal webs are interspersed with mural aneurysms.

plasia includes sites of fibrous connective tissue accumulation within the media, creating the appearance of clefts. Adjoining these sites are areas of disruption of the internal elastic lamina, thinning of the medial layer, and formation of microaneurysms. The adventitial layer appears normal.

A subcategory of medial dysplasia—namely, medial dysplasia with dissection—may represent the same underlying pathologic condition, with disruption of the intimal layers that leads to an acute dissection instead of progressive microaneurysm development. Any hypothesis, however, is conjectural, for the cause of any of the varieties is not known.

Perimedial (Subadventitial) Fibrodysplasia

Accounting for about 10% of renal artery fibrodysplastic lesions, perimedial fibrodysplasia is predominantly found in women in their fourth and fifth decade. Although angiographically similar to medial dysplasia, with multiple, focal stenoses of the involved portion, there are no microaneurysms. Histologically, the vessel wall has an accumulation of elastic tissue in the border between the media and adventitia at the sites of stenosis, with the intimal layer appearing normal.

Developmental Lesions

Congenital or developmental lesions of the renal vasculature are a common source of hypertension in children. Although frequently classified as fibrodysplastic lesions when identified in later childhood, most of these lesions are developmental in origin. In contrast to fibromuscular dysplasia, most developmental lesions are ostial in location, have no sex predilection, and are frequently bilateral. They are often associated with congenital narrowing of the juxtarenal aorta, or may be a component of hypoplasia or atresia of the abdominal aorta. In one series,[103] nearly 80% of abdominal aortic coarctation also involved the renal arteries. Histologically, these lesions may appear intimal in location, but usually are associated with narrowing of the entire vessel and suggest a lack of normal growth of that segment.

The cause of developmental renal artery lesions is unknown, yet several hypotheses have been suggested. Maycock[104] proposed that faulty or unequal fusion of the two omphalomesenteric arteries or dorsal aortas might lead to obliteration or loss of one of them, with a resulting coarctate segment. When occurring early and extensively in embryologic life, aortic atresia might be produced. Alternatively, if limited to the juxtarenal area and if partial maturation occurred prior to developmental arrest, stenosis primarily affecting the renal artery ostium might be created. Certainly, some lesions identified in later childhood appear to represent failure of growth of an arterial segment.

Uncommon Lesions

A number of infrequently seen causes of renovascular disease may produce RVH. Rarely, neurofibromatosis may be associated with renal artery stenosis and RVH. Flynn and Buchanan[105] reviewed the literature and found 52 cases of renal vascular lesions in patients with neurofibromatosis; 64% of the patients were male, and 71% of combined patients were less than 20 years old. Characteristically, lesions involve the origin of the renal artery. Histologic study, however, may show no difference from ordinary fibromuscular dysplasia. Abrams[106] has stated that there does not appear to be any overgrowth of neural tissue within the arterial wall. The classification of lesions as secondary to neurofibromatosis requires that other nonvascular manifestations of that disease be present.

Finally, previous irradiation,[107] previous renal artery trauma,[108] nonspecific arteritis (Takayasu's arteritis),[109] renal artery aneurysm,[110] arteriovenous fistulas,[111] spontaneous dissection,[112] renal artery emboli,[113] and stenosis of the renal artery in transplanted kidneys[114] have been recorded as rare causes of renal artery stenosis and RVH.

Diagnostic Studies

Screening Studies for Renovascular Occlusive Disease

A number of screening diagnostic studies have been advocated for the recognition of RVH. The role of such studies is to determine the anatomic presence of renovascular disease, as well as its functional significance. Historically, screening techniques were limited to the rapid sequence intravenous pyelogram, peripheral plasma renin assays, plasma renin activity in response to angiotensin-converting enzyme inhibitors, and isotope renography. Theoretically, each of these techniques should adequately screen for RVH; however, clinical application has not proven any of them to be optimal screening tests. Recent advances in imaging and computer technology have led to the development of more reliable screening techniques. Despite these advances, most screening methods for functional renovascular disease are plagued by operator-dependent variability. Currently, intravenous digital subtraction angiography, renal duplex ultrasonography, and isotope renography are employed as initial screening tests for RVH.

Rapid Sequence Excretory Pyelogram

Many physicians still rely on the rapid sequence intravenous pyelogram (IVP) alone to screen patients for the presence of significant renal arterial lesions and resultant hypertension. The findings suggestive of the presence of RVH are: unilateral delay in caliceal appearance time; difference in renal length of 1.5 cm or more, compared with the contralateral kidney; hyperconcentration of the contrast medium on late films; ureteral notching secondary to increased size and tortuosity of the ureteral artery; and defect in the renal silhouette, suggestive of segmental renal infarction. In 122 proven cases of RVH, only 69%, in our experience, had a positive IVP using the above criteria.[115] The fact that half of the false-negative results were in patients with bilateral lesions explains in part the high incidence of false-negative results, but does not negate the fact that if one is relying on this screening test to detect RVH, many cases will be missed. In fact, the group in which the rapid sequence pyelogram has the most popularity as the definitive screening tool is the pediatric hypertensive population. Review of the results of this study in our center revealed that it was positive in only 42% of 21 children with RVH.[107]

Although we do not believe that the rapid sequence IVP should be used as the sole screening test for the detection of RVH, it is important in the evaluation of associated lesions of the genitourinary tract. Furthermore, if positive preoperatively, it is a simple examination that gives valuable information in postoperative assessment of the revascularization. A normal postoperative pyelogram is very reassuring.

Peripheral Plasma Renin Assays

Since RVH is frequently maintained by an increased release of renin from the ischemic kidney, identification of increased circulating levels of renin activity in the peripheral venous blood is used in many centers as a screening test for RVH.[116] Although the simplicity of obtaining a peripheral venous sample that might exclude the majority of the hypertensive population from further intensive investigation has obvious appeal, many factors affect the accuracy of this determination. Under strict conditions of controlled sodium intake (13.5 mmol/day), with blood samplings taken between 8 and 9 A.M. after 12 hours of recumbence and no antihypertensive drugs given for the previous 2 to 3 weeks, Cohen and associates[117] found that some 40% of patients with true RVH may have peripheral plasma renin activity within normal limits. Several investigators have shown that severe sodium restriction (100 mmol/day) and the upright posture for 4 hours prior to the study produce an excessive response in plasma

renin activity in patients with RVH.[118,119] An acute sodium depletion test with furosemide also has been introduced to decrease the time involved in using low sodium diets. Despite enthusiasm for this change in methodology, Genest and associates have noted paradoxically lower renin values in peripheral blood 3 hours after furosemide (40 mg) administration than in the control period in as many as 15 of 60 patients studied.[120]

The time involved in establishing sodium balance in a calculated sodium diet, the frequent inability to discontinue antihypertensive medications for prolonged periods, and the variability of peripheral renin assays (even when these requirements are met) make such assays too inaccurate for use as a screening tool on which to base a decision regarding further evaluation. Furthermore, when one considers that most physicians do not follow the strict control criteria in preparing the patient for this study, its results seem to be even less reliable.

Comparison of baseline plasma renin activity to postcaptopril plasma renin activity is the next logical step in this screening method. Unfortunately, the same pitfalls apply to this study method. A recent prospective evaluation of this technique at Duke University confirmed the inadequacy of this screening method. In their study, captopril stimulated peripheral renin activity had a positive predictive value of only 38% with a negative predictive value of 92%.[121]

Renal Duplex Ultrasonography

Advances in ultrasonography in the 1980s have led to the development of an accurate and noninvasive method of screening for renovascular occlusive disease. With the combination of a B-scan image and fast Fourier transform analysis of renal arterial and aortic Doppler shift signals, the sensitivity and specificity of ultrasonography was significantly improved (Figure 12).[122–124] In these studies, the peak systolic velocities of the renal arteries and aorta were compared. From these findings, Taylor et al[124] defined the criteria for critical renal artery occlusive disease using the renal aortic ratio in which a renal artery lesion greater than 60% was associated with a ratio greater than 3.5. Additionally, findings of no associated Doppler shift was consistent with renal artery occlusion. Using this method, Taylor et al were able to predict renovascular disease with 84% sensitivity and 97% specificity.[124] Subsequent work by Hansen et al[125] prospectively confirmed the validity of this screening tool when comported to angiography. In this study, renal duplex ultrasonography had a sensitivity of 93%, a specificity of 98%, and a negative predictive value of 94% in patients with single renal arteries. A retrospective evaluation of Hansen's et al data revealed that a main renal artery

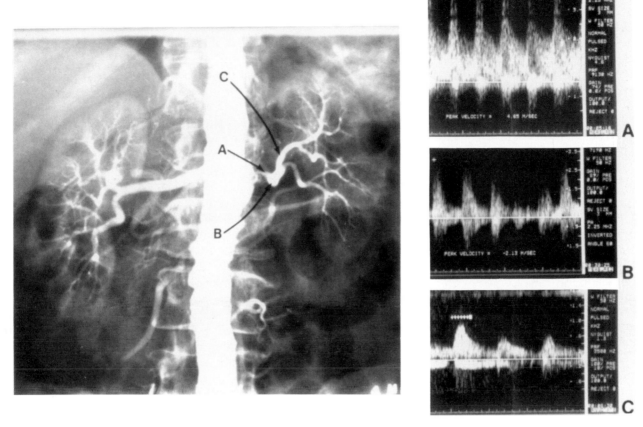

Figure 12. Use of duplex scanning in renovascular hypertension. An aortogram of this patient's renal artery disease demonstrates the sites of renal artery interrogation. The flow velocities by duplex are highest at the site of the most significant stenosis (**A**) and return to normal velocities within just a few centimeters (**C**). Failure to obtain such a thorough study can lead to false negative results.

peak systolic velocity 2 m/sec was equally able to predict critical renal artery stenosis (60%) as a renal aortic ratio of 3.5.[125] Hudspeth et al later confirmed this finding in a prospective study evaluating long-term renal artery graft patency.[126]

With regard to the utility of renal duplex ultrasonography in determining the functional significance of a renal artery stenosis, it remains an inadequate tool. Although Norris et al[122] have demonstrated an inverse relationship between serum creatinine and renal artery cnd diastolic resistance in a canine model utilizing microsphere embolization of the kidney, similar predictive patterns have not been consistently reproduced in clinical studies.

Although the results of these studies show renal duplex to exceed the abilities of other screening techniques, there are limitations to this study. Significantly, this study requires an experienced and skilled technician who is able to completely interrogate the renal artery from its origin to the renal hilum. Failure to achieve such a complete sampling will result in false-negative studies. Finally, similar to intravenous digital

subtraction angiography, renal duplex is unable to detect most multiple renal arteries. Because this study is accurate, noninvasive, does not expose the kidneys to nephrotoxic agents, is relatively inexpensive, and can be performed in an outpatient setting, it serves as the screening method of choice at our institution.

Renal Arteriography

Both aortography and selective renal arteriography using multiple projections are necessary to adequately examine the entire renal artery.[127] As is shown in Figure 7, the proximal third of the left renal artery usually courses anteriorly, the middle third transversely, and the distal third posteriorly, whereas the right renal artery pursues a more consistent posterior course. Lesions in portions of the renal artery, which are coursing anteriorly or posteriorly, are frequently not seen or may appear insignificant in an anteroposterior (AP) aortogram. Oblique aortography or oblique selective renal arteriography will project these portions of the vessels in profile and identify the stenosis. Figure 7 shows how the delicate septal lesions of fibromuscular dysplasia may be unrecognizable or appear insignificant in the AP projection, whereas, in the oblique projection, their true severity is demonstrated.

A common cause of false-positive angiography is the creation of renal artery spasm at the tip of the angiography catheter. In most cases, this phenomenon is easily recognized when the area in question is studied on the flush AP or oblique aortogram. Occasionally, however, instillation of a vasodilator and repeat study after repositioning the catheter may be necessary to distinguish it from a true renal artery stenosis.

Through the introduction of computer assisted intravenous digital subtraction angiography, one can now obtain anatomic definition of the renal vasculature as an outpatient screening procedure. A recent prospective study evaluating the validity of this screening method demonstrated IV digital subtraction angiography to have a sensitivity of 100% and a specificity of 71% when compared to standard aortography.[121] In this technique, 40 mL of contrast are required for adequate visualization of the arterial anatomy. Currently, IV digital subtraction angiography does not identify fibromuscular dysplastic lesions or multiple renal arteries with accuracy, and it frequently provides a picture that underestimates the severity of atherosclerotic lesions. Positive studies are usually followed up with conventional angiography and, thus another contrast load. Unfortunately, further technologic refinements are required before this study can replace conventional intra-arterial angiography.

When subtraction angiography is used with arterial cannulation and intra-arterial injection, the amount of contrast material required for visualization of arterial segments is dramatically reduced. Abdominal aortography of archaontography can be performed with as little as 6 mL of dye. This is of tremendous value when both cerebral and renal vascular beds require assessment. In such patients, simultaneous evaluation of these segments can be performed without concern for the permissible limits of contrast volume injected. Similarly, it is of great value in the azotemic patient, since the nephrotoxicity of contrast material is dose-related. By using the digital subtraction technique, the risk of contrast medium-induced deterioration in renal function can be effectively minimized.

Functional Studies

Once a significant renovascular lesion has been identified, the functional significance of the lesion should be proven before one proceeds with revascularization. Functional significance refers to the likelihood that revascularization of the ischemic kidney will

reverse the secondary hypertension and ischemic nephropathy. Renal vein renin assays (RVRA) and split renal function studies have served as the mainstays of functional evaluation. Over the past decade, isotope renography has been increasingly utilized to assess both the presence of an anatomic lesion and to evaluate its functional significance. Unfortunately, as with the screening studies for anatomic lesions, studies used to assess the functional significance of renovascular lesions suffer from operator-dependent variability.

Isotope Renography

The isotopic renogram has had wide popularity as a screening tool for the diagnosis of RVH. Based on the kidney's management of Hippuran (Mallinckrodt) labeled with 131Iodine, isotope renography gives a measure of both renal perfusion and excretory function. Initial use of this study has showed it to parallel the rapid sequence IVP in its unacceptable incidence of false-normal sequence IVP in its unacceptable incidence of false-normal interpretation. Recent advances with the gamma scintillation camera and improved techniques of computer assisted mathematical derivations have led to a resurgence of its popularity. The addition of 99mTc-DMSA and 99mTc-DPTA to the study allows calculation of percent differential renal excretory function from the individual kidneys. An ACE inhibitor challenge appears to improve both the sensitivity and specificity of renography in diagnosing RVH (Figure 13).[128,129] Finally, the recent introduction of mercaptoacetyltriglycine (MAG3) has improved the imaging quality of renal scans over those employing orthoiodohippurate.[128] Despite the increased popularity of renography, with and without captopril challenge, recent reports continue to show a significant variability in its usefulness as a single effective screening test for critical, correctable renovascular lesions.[41,119,129–131]

There are many sources of error in the interpretation of the isotope urogram. Since the uptake slope is made up of a combination of the rate of isotope appearance in the kidney and, to a lesser degree, the early phase of excretion from the kidney, those kidneys with poor excretory function or high peripheral resistance to flow may have abnormal appearance slopes without an actual occlusion to renal inflow. Similarly, since the primary method of interpretation is a comparison of the isotope uptake and its disappearance between the two kidneys, these sources of error can be magnified in patients with bilateral renal artery lesions. Nevertheless, we find isotopic renography to be a valuable non-invasive method to follow renal function sequentially and to identify deterioration in functioning renal parenchyma.

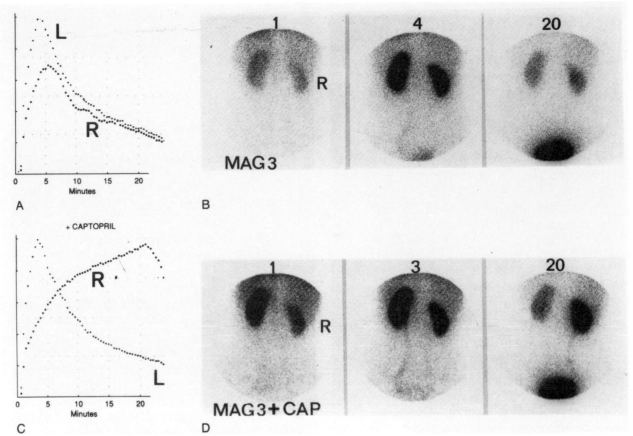

Figure 13. A 99mTc-MAG3 study showing grade 1 on the baseline study, turning into a grade 2 during captopril renography. Data obtained from a 33-year-old woman with a right-sided stenosis. During the baseline study (**A**) the curves follow a symmetrical course with a peak in the 5th minute. The sequential images (**B**) show a smaller kidney on the right side. The start of the excretion in the renal pelvis is not clearly visualized; there is indication of radioactivity in the bladder in the 4th minute. In the 20th minute, there is no retention of activity in the kidneys. The captopril study (**C**) gives a normal shape of the curve on the left; on the right, the maximum height is reached much later, followed by a slight fall. The sequential images (**D**) show the left ureter in the 3rd minute, whereas the right ureter is not distinctly visible until the 20th minute. (Reproduced with permission from Reference 128.)

In order to improve the consistency of captopril renography examinations, a consensus statement has been formulated by hypertension clinicians and nuclear medicine physicians.[57,132] As an initial step, physicians and institutions are encouraged to minimize operator variability by standardizing local techniques. With regard to the evaluation of the scintigraphic images, analysis should include kidney size, renal perfusion, and excretory capacity. A standard grading system has been proposed for evaluating time activity curves (Table 4). In this grading system, the upslope and excretory phases are compared before and after captopril challenge. Captopril-stimulated changes in time activity curves are labeled as low, intermediate, and high probability of renal artery stenosis. This grading scheme is illustrated in Tables 4 and 5. It remains to be seen whether standardization of techniques and

Table 4
Proposed Grading System for the Renogram

Grade 0	Normal
Grade 1	Mild delay in upslope, maximal activity, T_{max} ($6 \leq T_{max} \leq 11$), or excretory phase
Grade 2	A. Delay in upslope and T_{max} *with* evidence of an excretory phase
	B. Delay in upslope and T_{max} *without* evidence of an excretory phase
Grade 3	Marked reduction or absence of uptake

Table 5
Patient Preparation for Renal Vein Renin
Assays

Long-term salt restriction (2-gm/day sodium diet)
Discontinue all antihypertensive drugs except diuretics for at least 5 days prior to study
Oral furosemide (40 mg) diuresis night before the study
NPO for 8 hours prior to study
Strictly flat bed-rest for 4 hours before and during study
Prestudy sedation with IM diazepam (Valium, 5 mg)

grading will result in more consistent predicting of renovascular disease.

Renal Vein Renin Assays

When an obstructive lesion is found by renal arteriography, its functional significance should be evaluated. Most centers rely solely on RVRAs to establish the diagnosis of RVH. The unfortunate consequence of this trend is that one must presume that all patients with RVH will have lateralizing RVRAs.

The effect of antihypertensive medications and unrestricted sodium intake on renin release, and thus on the RVRA, is widely recognized. Many antihypertensive medications, especially those that function through beta-adrenergic blockade, suppress renin output and can lead to false nonlaterlization of RVRA. Most common of the beta-blockers in use today is propranolol. Before one can consider that there is no drug interference in the release of renin, all such medications must be withheld for at least 5 days prior to the measurement of RVRA. Similar effects on renin levels are seen when sodium intake is not restricted. For this reason, the patient should be on no more than a 2 g/day sodium diet for at least 2 weeks prior to the study. The preparation of patients for RVRA in our center is summarized in Table 5.

The technical aspects of performing RVRA as a potential source of error cannot be overemphasized. Since the left renal vein contains not only renal venous effluent but also adrenal, gonadal, and lumbar venous effluent, misplacement of the venous catheter into the origin of one of the nonrenal branches of sampling in the proximal renal vein, where a mixture from these other sources is present, may dilute the renin activity coming from the kidney. This will lead to erroneously low measurements of renin activity and produce a false interpretation of RVRA.

The time of sampling the two renal veins for renin

activity is also a potential source of error in RVRA. In studies performed with a single catheter, several minutes may elapse between sampling the two renal veins as the catheter is switched from one side to the other. Furthermore, manipulation of the catheter and the patient's discomfort may affect renin release. It is not surprising, therefore, that when the single catheter is used, both false-positive and false-negative RVR ratios are frequent. Studies in our center have shown that in patients with normal arteriograms in whom RVRA was performed with the single catheter technique, 24% had RVR ratios in excess of 1.5 to 1.0. Whelton and associates[133] also found false-positive ratios (>1.5) in 22% of patients with normal arteriograms. Similarly, only 79% of a group of 39 patients in our center who were cured of hypertension by unilateral operation (proven RVH) had an RVR ratio in excess of 1.5 when studied by the single catheter technique.[134]

For these reasons, we now use simultaneous bilateral catheters, collect three sets of samples, and consider the test positive only if two of three sets lateralize to one side. This methodology has minimized false-positive and false-negative determinations. Our most recent data suggest that this method will be positive in excess of 90% when RVH is secondary to unilateral renovascular disease.

Several methods of stimulating renin release have been suggested over the past 15 years. These include tilting the patient to the upright posture during the study, and stimulation with IV nitroprusside. Although all of these methods increase renin release, they also increase the incidence of false-positive determinations and reduce the reliability of RVRA to unacceptable levels.

Vaughn et al[135] stressed the importance of expressing RVRA in relation to the systemic renin activity, rather than simply evaluating the ratio of renin activity between the two renal veins. In patients with RVH secondary to unilateral renal artery stenosis, one should find hypersecretion of renin from the ischemic kidney and suppression of renin secretion from the normal kidney. With the application of this hypothesis, Stanley and Fry[136] have shown a statistically significant difference in the renal systemic renin indices in patients who were totally cured of RVH by operation, when compared with those who had only improvement. Although this method has appeal as a predictor of the extent of benefit, its value in patients with bilateral renal artery lesions is limited. Since both lesions may be producing RVH, both this method and RVR ratios have reduced validity as predictors of response to operation. In addition, the risk of hypertension is more directly related to its severity than to its absolute presence or absence. If one bases the decision for operative management solely on whether absolute cure is to be expected, many patients who would receive the benefit of a reduction in severity of hypertension to a mild, easily controlled level would be excluded from consideration as operative candidates. Therefore, this method of RVRA interpretation should be considered only as an additional predictive tool, not an alternative to the evaluation of RVR ratios.

RVRAs also may be spuriously unrevealing in patients with accessory or segmental renal artery stenosis if renal venous sampling is limited to the main renal vein. Since recognition of renin hypersecretion depends on sampling the ischemic area of the kidneys, selective segmental venous sampling must be done in these patients. When segmental sampling is required, the renin activity from the segment sampled is compared with the simultaneously collected contralateral main renal vein sample to calculate the RVR ratio.

Split Renal Function Studies

Examination of individual kidney function was the first clinically applicable test available for identifying the functional significance of renal artery stenoses in hypertensive patients. Although only indirectly related to the pathogenesis of secondary hypertension, the ischemic kidney has certain characteristic alterations in its handling of water and solute loads. Split renal function studies compare individual kidneys to identify these changes and, thereby, predict the functional significance of renal stenoses.

Split renal function studies are performed according to the method of Stamey[137] with certain modifications.[138] Owing to the necessity of ureteral catheterization and large volume challenge, they are not performed in young children or elderly patients with clinically significant congestive heart failure.

Adequate urine flow (at least 2 mL/min) must be present for the correct interpretation of split renal function studies. With a lesser diuresis, water reabsorption from the normal kidney may mask the differential increase in water reabsorption from the involved kidney and prevent an accurate interpretation. Urinary leakage around the ureteral catheters also results in falsely low urine flow rates. Unless recognized, this can lead to false-positive interpretations based on low urine flows. Indigo carmine may be injected through the ureteral catheters, and the ureteral orifices examined for leakage prior to removing the cystoscope.

Different methods of performing split renal function studies have led to several criteria of interpretation. Howard's and Connor's[139] original criteria for a positive test included a reduction in urine volume from the affected side of at least 40% coupled with a reduction in sodium concentration of at least 15%, or a 50% increase in creatinine concentration, as compared with the uninvolved kidney. The "classic" criteria for a pos-

itive Stamey test in the presence of main renal artery occlusion consisted of at least a 3 to 1 difference in urine flow rates on the affected side and 100% increase in the concentration of para-amino hippuric acid (PAH) on the affected side. Howard and Connor[139,140] repeatedly pointed out that osmotic diuresis as used in Stamey's method renders "urinary sodium concentration worthless for interpretation." In interpretating the Howard portion of the test, we rely solely on urine volume and creatinine concentration changes.

In a review of the early Vanderbilt experience with split renal function studies, we found the classic criteria of interpretation too rigid. Therefore, we redefined the criteria for positive split renal function studies and considered the result positive if there was consistent lateralization to the involved side in each of the three collection periods, with a decrease in urine volume and increase in creatinine and PAH concentrations. Using these criteria for interpretation, the incidence of false-negative results was reduced to 8%.

Conclusion

Our understanding of the events responsible for the development and maintenance of RVH has increased dramatically over the past 60 years. Despite this, the renin-angiotensin system remains incompletely understood. Though once seen as a purely systemic hormonal mechanism responsible for hypertension, the presence and significant activities of renal, cardiovascular, central nervous, and adrenal renin-angiotensin systems are widely recognized. In addition to being responsible for many of the pathophysiologic changes observed in RVH, these local systems likely have baseline tonic influence on the functions of these organ systems. Research in this area has yielded potent antihypertensive agents such as angiotensin-converting enzyme inhibitors and angiotensin receptor blockers. These agents have dramatically improved our ability to manage disease states such as essential hypertension and congestive heart failure. No similar medical therapy has been effective in treating RVH. On the contrary, angiotensin-converting enzyme inhibitors have actually been shown to increase the development of renal insufficiency in patients with critical renal artery stenosis. Importantly, research findings have improved our ability to determine which patients will benefit from revascularization or removal of chronically ischemic kidneys. Examples of these diagnostic advances include assessment of renal vein renin levels and captopril renography. Centers experienced in the management of RVH have reported significant improvement or total cure of hypertension in 90% to 98% of patients.[4-7] The hypertension and renal function responses to intervention appear dichotomous.

Improved hypertension does not ensure improved renal function. In fact, nearly one third of patients with disease caused by atherosclerosis continue to have some measure of renal dysfunction after intervention.[6,7,141-144] Although the reasons for this are unknown, the function of vascular endothelial cells in the diseased kidney may be important. Disturbances in such opposing local vasoactive hormones as AII and NO may impact on renal resistance and tubular function.[52,53] Additionally, the ability of the kidney to produce and systemically release such recently identified compounds as platelet activating factor and medullipin may influence both renal function and the reversal of systemic hypertension after reperfusion.[145-147] Moreover, a reperfusion injury may impact on all of these variables.[148,149] It is hoped that ongoing research in these areas will improve our ability to cure patients with RVH. In the future, discoveries relating to organ specific renin-angiotensin systems will hopefully improve our understanding of and ability to treat other cardiovascular and neurologic disease processes.

References

1. Bright R: Cases and observations illustrative of renal disease accompanied with secretion of albuminous urine. *Guy's Hosp Rep* 1:339, 1836.
2. Goldblatt H, Lynch J, Hanzal RF, et al: Persistent elevation of systolic blood pressure by means of renal ischemia. *J Exp Med* 59:347, 1934.
3. Peart WS: Evolution of renin. *Hypertension* 18(suppl III):100–108, 1991.
4. Dean RH: Renovascular hypertension. In: WS Moore (ed). *Vascular Surgery: A Comprehensive Review*. New York: Grune & Stratton, Inc.; 561–592, 1986.
5. Dean RH, Keyser JE III, Dupont WD, et al: Aortic and renal vascular disease: factors affecting the value of combined procedures. *Ann Surg* 200:336–344, 1984.
6. Stanley JC, Ernst CB, Fry WJ: *Renovascular Hypertension*. Philadelphia: WB Saunders, Co.; 363–371, 1984.
7. Dean RH: Renovascular hypertension. In: *Current Problems in Surgery*. Vol. 22. Chicago: Mosby-Year Book, Inc.; 1985.
8. Rupert R: Irregular kidney vessels in fifty cadavers. *Surg Gynecol Obstet* 17:580, 1913.
9. Rupert R: Further study of irregular kidney vessels in one hundred eighteen cadavers. *Surg Gynecol Obstet* 21:471, 1915.
10. Anson BJ, Richardson GA, Minear WL: Variation in the number and arrangement of the renal vessels. *J Urol* 36:211, 1936.
11. Pick JW, Anson BJ: The renal vascular pedicle: an anatomical study of 430 body halves. *J Urol* 44:411, 1940.
12. Weinstein BR, Countiss EH, Derbes VJ: The renal vessels in 203 cadavers. *Urol Cutan Rev* 44:137, 1940.
13. Schultz RD: Collateral circulation of the kidney. In: DE Strandness, Jr (ed). *Collateral Circulation in Clinical Surgery*. Philadelphia: WB Saunders, Co.; 1969.
14. Clemente CD (ed). *Anatomy of the Human Body*. 30th Am Ed. Philadelphia: Lea & Febiger; 746, 1985.
15. Abrams HL, Cornell SH: Patterns of collateral flow in renal ischemia. *Radiology* 84:1001–1012, 1965.
16. Fagarasanu I: Recherches Anatomiques Sur la Veine Rénale Gauche et Ses Collatérales: Leurs Rapports Avec la Pathogénie du Variococéle Essentiel et Des Varices du Ligament Large. *Ann Anat Pathol* (Paris) 15:9, 1938.
17. Davis RA, Milloy FJ, Anson BJ: Lumbar, renal, and associated parietal and visceral veins based upon a study of 100 specimens. *Surg Gynecol Obstet* 107:1, 1958.
18. Anson BJ, Daseler EH: Common variations in renal anatomy affecting blood supply, form, and topography. *Surg Gynecol Obstet* 112:439, 1961.
19. Milloy FJ, Anson BJ, Cauldwell EW: Variations in the inferior caval veins and in their renal and lumbar communications. *Surg Gynecol Obstet* 115:131, 1962.
20. Meacham PW, Hollifield JW, Burko H, et al: Predictable variation of plasma renin activity within the human left renal vein, and correlation with an anatomic study of the left renal venous tributaries. *Surg Forum* 31:220, 1980.
21. Brener BJ, Darling RC, Frederick PL, et al: Major venous anomalies complicating abdominal aortic surgery. *Arch Surg* 108:159, 1974.
22. Royster TS, Lacey L, Marks RA: Abdominal aortic surgery and the left renal vein. *Am J Surg* 127:552, 1974.
23. James EC, Fedde CW, Khuri NT, et al: Division of the left renal vein: a safe surgical adjunct. *Surgery* 83:151, 1978.
24. Neal HS, Shearburn EW: Division of the left renal vein as an adjunct to resection of abdominal aortic aneurysms. *Am J Surg* 113:763, 1967.
25. Poutasse EF, Marks LS, Wisoff CP, et al: Renal vein renin determinations in hypertension: falsely negative tests. *J Urol* 110:371, 1973.
26. Paster SB, Adams DF, Abrams HL: Errors in renal vein renin collections. *AJR* 122:804, 1974.
27. Chuang VP, Mena CE, Hoskins PA: Congenital anomalies of the left renal vein: angiographic consideration. *Br J Surg* 47:214, 1974.
28. Nishimura M, Brosnihan KB, Ferrario CM, et al: Tissue renin-angiotensin systems in renal hypertension. *Hypertension* 20:158–167, 1992.
29. Masaki Z, Ferrario CM, Bumpus FM: Effects of SQ 20,881 on the intact kidney of dogs with two-kidney, one clip hypertension. *Hypertension* 2:649–656, 1980.
30. Martinez-Maldonado M: Pathophysiology of renovascular hypertension. *Hypertension* 17:708–719, 1991.
31. Masaki Z, Ferrario CM, Khosla MC, et al: The course of arterial pressure and the effect of sar1-thr8-angiotensin II in a new model of two-kidney hypertension in conscious dogs. *Clin Sci Mol Med* 52:1–8, 1977.
32. Ganten D, Lindpainter K, Mullins J, et al: Gentic basis of hypertension: the renin-angiotensin paradigm. *Hypertension* 18(suppl III):109–114, 1991.
33. Jeunemaitre X, Soubrier F, Corvol P, et al: Molecular basis of human hypertension: role of angiotensinogen. *Cell* 71:169–180, 1992.
34. Gomez RA, Chevalier RL, Peach MJ, et al: Molecular biology of the renal renin-angiotensin system. *Kid Int* 38(suppl 30):S18-S23, 1990.
35. Mitchell KD, Braam B, Navar LG: Hypertensinogenic mechanisms mediated by renal actions of renin-angiotensin system. *Hypertension* 19(suppl I):18–27, 1992.
36. Timmermans PBMWM, Benfield P, Smith RD, et al: Angiotensin II receptors and functional correlates. *Am J Hypertens* 5:221S-235S, 1992.
37. Timmermans PBMWM, Carini DJ, Johnson AL, et al:

Angiotensin II receptor antagonists: from discovery to antihypertensive drugs. *Hypertension* 18(suppl III): 136–142, 1991.

38. Goldfarb DA, Diz DI, Novick AC, et al: Characterization of angiotensin subtypes in human kidney and renal carcinoma. *J Urol* (In press.)

39. Valtin H: Renal Function: *Mechanisms Preserving Fluid and Solute Balance in Health.* 2nd Ed. Boston: Little, Brown; 1983.

40. Berne RM, Levy MN: *Physiology.* 2nd Ed. Washington, DC: Mosby-Year Book, Inc.; 741–745, 1988.

41. Vidt DG: The diagnosis of renin vascular hypertension: a clinicians viewpoint. *Am J Hypertens* 4:663S-668S, 1991.

42. Saccomani G, Mitchell KD, Navar LG: Angiotensin II stimulation of Na^+H^+exchange in proximal tubular cells. *Am J Physiol* 258:F1188-F1195, 1990.

43. Diz DI, Goldfarb DA, Novick AC, et al: Parallel changes in receptors sensitive to angiotensin-(1–7) and AT2 antagonists in human kidneys with renal artery disease. *Hypertension* 21:528, 1993.

44. Holstein-Rathlou NH: Dynamic aspects of the tubuloglomerular feedback mechanism. *Danish Med Bull* 39(2): 134–154, 1992.

45. Briggs JP, Schnermann J: The tubuloglomerular feedback mechanism: functional and biochemical aspects. *Ann Rev Physiol* 49:251–273, 1987.

46. Aukland K, Øien AH: Renal autoregulation: models combining tubuloglomerular feedback and myogenic response. *Am J Physiol* 252:F768-F783, 1987.

47. Guyton AC: Kidneys and fluids in pressure regulation: small volume but large pressure changes. *Hypertension* 19(suppl I).2–8, 1992.

48. Granger JP: Pressure natriuresis: role of interstitial hydrostatic pressure. *Hypertension* 19(suppl I):9–17, 1992.

49. Beeuwkes R, Brenner BM: The renal circulation. In: Brenner BM, Rector, Jr FC (eds). *The Kidney.* 2nd Ed. Philadelphia: WB Saunders, Co.; 1981.

50. Romero JC, Lahera V, Biondi ML, et al: Role of the endothelium-dependent relaxing factor nitric oxide on renal function. *J Am Soc Nephrol* 2:1371–1387, 1992.

51. Sigmon DH, Carretaro OA, Beierwaltes WH: Plasma renin activity and the renal response to nitric oxide synthesis inhibition. *J Am Soc Nephrol* 3:1288–1294, 1992.

52. Sigmon DH, Carretero OA, Beierwaltes WH: Angiotensin dependence of endothelium-mediated renal hemodynamics. *Hypertension* 20:643–650, 1992.

53. Salazar FJ, Romero JC, Quesada T, et al: Renal effects of prolonged synthesis inhibition of endothelium-derived nitric oxide. *Hypertension* 20:113–117, 1992.

54. Zatz R, De Nucci G: Effects of acute nitric oxide inhibition on rat glomerular microcirculation. *Am J Physiol* 261:F360-F363, 1991.

55. Ito S, Johnson CS, Carretero OA, et al: Endothelium-derived relaxing factor modulates endothelin action in afferent arterioles. *Hypertension* 17:1052–1056, 1991.

56. Salom MG, Lahera V, Romero JC, et al: Blockade of pressure natriuresis induced by inhibition of renal synthesis of nitric oxide in dogs. *Am J Physiol* 262:F718-F722, 1992.

57. Nally VJ Jr, Black HR: State of the art review: captopril renography—pathophysiological considerations and clinical observations. *Sem Nucl Med* 22(2):85–97, 1992.

58. Nally VJ Jr: Renal physiology of renovascular hypertension: implications for captopril-stimulated renography. *Am J Hypertens* 4(12pt2):669S-674S, 1991.

59. Henrich WL: The endothelium: a key regulator of vascular tone. *Am J Med Sci* 302(5):319–328, 1991.

60. Katušic ZS, Shepherd JT: Endothelium-derived vasoactive factors. II. Endothelium-dependent contraction. *Hypertension* (suppl III):86–92, 1991.

61. Ballermann BJ, Marsden PA: Endothelium-derived vasoactive mediators and renal glomerular function. *Clin Invest Med* 14(6):508–517, 1991.

62. Shepherd JT, Katušic ZS: Endothelium-derived vasoactive factors. I. Endothelium-dependent relaxation. *Hypertension* (suppl III):76–85, 1991.

63. Dohi Y, Lüscher TF: Endothelin in hypertensive resistance arteries: intraluminal and extraluminal dysfunction. *Hypertension* 18:543–549, 1991.

64. López-Farré A, Gómez-Garre D, López-Novoa JM, et al: Renal effects and mesangial cell contraction induced by endothelin are mediated by PAF. *Kid Int* 39(4): 624–630, 1991.

65. Hirata Y, Matsuoka H, Sugimoto T, et al: Role of endothelium-derived relaxing factor in endothelin-induced renal vasoconstriction. *J Cardiovasc Pharmacol* 17(suppl 7):S169-S171, 1991.

66. Kohno M, Yasunari K, Takeos T, et al: Plasma immunoreactive endothelin in essential hypertension. *Am J Med* 88:614–618, 1990.

67. Remuzzi G, Fitzgerald GA, Patrino C, et al: Thromboxane synthesis and action with the kidney. *Kid Int* 41: 1483–1493, 1992.

68. Anggard EE: The regulatory functions of the endothelium. *Jap J Pharmacol* 58(suppl 2):200P-206P, 1992.

69. Smith WL: Prostanoid biosynthesis and mechanisms of action. *Am J Physiol* 263:F181-F191, 1992.

70. McGiff JC, Carroll MA, Escalante B: Arachidonate metabolites and kinins in blood pressure regulation. *Hypertension* 18(suppl III):150–157, 1991.

71. Cooke JP: Endothelium-derived factors and peripheral vascular disease. *Cardiol Clin* 22(3).3–17, 1992.

72. DiBona GF: Sympathetic neural control of the kidney in hypertension. *Hypertension* 19(suppl I):28–35, 1992.

73. Kopp UC, Buckley-Bleiler RL: Impaired renorenal reflexes in two-kidney, one clip hypertensive rats. *Hypertension* 14:445–452, 1989.

74. Lindpainter K, Ganten D: The cardiac renin-angiotensin system: an appraisal of present experimental and clinical evidence. *Circ Res* 68:905–921, 1991.

75. Bumpus FM: Angiotensin I and II: some early observations made at the Cleveland Clinic Foundation and recent discoveries relative to angiotensin II formation in human heart. *Hypertension* 18(suppl 37):S51-S55, 1991.

76. Lever AF, Lyall F, Folkow B, et al: Angiotensin II, vascular structure, and blood pressure. *Kid Int* 41(suppl 37):S51-S55, 1992.

77. Gohlke P, Bünning P, Unger T: Distribution and metabolism of angiotensin I and II in the blood vessel wall. *Hypertension* 20:151–157, 1992.

78. Shiota N, Miyazaki M, Okunishi H: Increase of angiotensin converting enzyme gene expression in the hypertensive aorta. *Hypertension* 20:168–174, 1992.

79. Rakugi H, Jacob HJ, Pratt RE, et al: Vascular injury induces angiotensin gene expression in the media and neointima. *Circulation* 87:283–290, 1993.

80. Krug LM, Berk BC: Na^+, K^+, adenosine triphosphate regulation in hypertrophied vascular smooth muscle cells. *Hypertension* 20:144–150, 1992.

81. Dzau VJ, Gibbons GH: Endothelium and growth factors in vascular remodeling of hypertension. *Hypertension* 18(suppl III):115–121, 1991.

82. Bohr DF, Dominiczak AF, Webb RC: Pathophysiology of the vasculature in hypertension. *Hypertension* 18(suppl III):69–75, 1991.

83. Benter IF, Diz DI, Ferrario CM: Cardiovascular actions of angiotensin-(1–7). *Peptides* 14:679–684, 1993.

84. Jaiswal N, Diz DI, Ferrario CM, et al: Stimulation of endothelial cell prostaglandin production by angiotensin peptides: characterization of receptors. *Hypertension* 19(suppl II):49–55, 1992.

85. Focaccio A, Volpe M, Chiariello M, et al: Angiotensin II directly stimulates release of atrial natriuretic factor in isolated rabbit hearts. *Circulation* 87:192–198, 1993.

86. Sarzani R, Arnaldi G, Chobanian AV, et al: Effects of hypertension and aging on platelet-derived growth factor and platelet-derived growth factor receptor expression in rat aorta and heart. *Hypertension* 18(suppl III): 93–99, 1991.

87. Sunga PS, Rabkin SW: Angiotensin II-induced protein phosphorylation in the hypertrophic heart of the Dahl rat. *Hypertension* 20:633–642, 1992.

88. Ondetti MA: Angiotensin converting enzyme inhibitors: an overview. *Hypertension* 18(suppl III):134–135, 1991.

89. Hirooka Y, Imaizumi T, Takeshita A, et al: Captopril improves impaired endothelium-dependent vasodilation in hypertensive patients. *Hypertension* 20:175–180, 1992.

90. Campbell DJ, Kladis A, Duncan AM: Bradykinin peptides in kidney, blood, and other tissues of the rat. *Hypertension* 21:155–165, 1993.

91. Ferrario CM, Barnes KL, Santos RAS, et al: Pathways of angiotensin formation and function in the brain. *Hypertension* 15(suppl I):13–19, 1990.

92. Barnes KL, Diz DI, Ferrario CM: Functional interactions between angiotensin II and substance P in the dorsal medulla. *Hypertension* 17:1121–1126, 1991.

93. Ferrario CM, Brosnihan KB, Tallant EA, et al: Angiotensin-(1–7): a new hormone of the angiotensin system. *Hypertension* 18(suppl III):126–133, 1991.

94. Diz DI, Pirro NT: Differential actions of angiotensin II and angiotensin-(1–7) on transmitter release. *Hypertension* 19(suppl II):41–48, 1992.

95. Ferrario CM, Jaiswal N, Schiavone MT, et al: Hypertensive mechanisms and converting enzyme inhibitors. *Clin Cardiol* 14(suppl IV):56–62, 1991.

96. Reid IA: Interactions between angiotensin II, sympathetic nervous system, and baroreceptor reflexes in regulation of blood pressure. *Am J Physiol* 262:E763-E778, 1992.

97. Kumagai H, Averill DB, Ferrario CM, et al: Role of nitric oxide and angiotensin II in the regulation of sympathetic nerve activity in spontaneously hypertensive rats. *Hypertension* 21:476–484, 1993.

98. Williams GH, Hollenberg NK: Functional derangements in the regulation of aldosterone secretion in hypertension. *Hypertension* 18(suppl III):143–149, 1991.

99. Stanley JC, Graham LM: Renovascular hypertension. In: Miller DC, Roon AJ (eds). *Diagnosis and Management of Peripheral Vascular Disease*. Menlo Park, NJ: Addison-Wesley; 231, 1981.

100. Stanley JC, Gewertz BL, Bove EL, et al: Arterial fibrodysplasia: histopathologic character and current etiologic concepts. *Arch Surg* 110:561, 1975.

101. Kaufman JJ, Maxwell MH: Upright aortography in the study of nephroptosis, stenotic lesions of the renal artery, and hypertension. *Surgery* 53:736, 1963.

102. Sottiurai VS, Fry WJ, Stanley JC: Ultrastructural characteristics of experimental arterial medial fibrodysplasia induced by vasa vasorum occlusion. *J Surg Res* 24:169, 1978.

103. Graham LM, Zelenock GB, Erlandson EE, et al: Abdominal aortic coarctation and segmental hypoplasia. *Surgery* 86:519, 1979.

104. Maycock WD: Congenital stenosis of the abdominal aorta. *Am Heart J* 13:633, 1937.

105. Flynn MP, Buchanan JB: Neurofibromatosis, hypertension, and renal artery aneurysms. *South Med J* 73:618, 1980.

106. Abrams J: Renovascular hypertension in the pediatric patient. *Arch Surg* 107:692, 1933.

107. Lawson JD, Boerth RK, Foster JH, et al: Diagnosis and management of renovascular hypertension in children. *Arch Surg* 112:1307, 1977.

108. Stables DP, Fouche RF, de Villiers van Niekerk JPD, et al: Traumatic renal artery occlusion: twenty-one cases. *J Urol* 115:229, 1976.

109. Lande A: Takayasu's arteritis and congenital coarctation of the descending thoracic and abdominal aorta: a critical review. *AJR* 127:227, 1966.

110. Stanley JC, Rhodes EL, Gewertz BL, et al: Renal artery aneurysms: significance of macroaneurysms exclusive of dissections and fibrodysplastic mural dilations. *Arch Surg* 100:1327, 1975.

111. Bosnick MA: Radiographic manifestations of massive arteriovenous fistula in renal carcinoma. *Radiology* 85: 454, 1965.

112. Smith BM, Holcomb GW III, Richie RE, et al: Renal artery dissection. *Ann Surg* 200:134, 1984.

113. Lacombe M: Surgical versus medical treatment of renal artery embolism. *J Cardiovasc Surg* 18:281, 1977.

114. Ricotta JJ, Schaff HV, Williams GM, et al: Renal artery stenosis following transplantation: etiology, diagnosis, and prevention. *Surgery* 84:595, 1978.

115. Foster JH, Dean RH, Pinkerton JA, et al: Ten years experience with the surgical management of renovascular hypertension. *Ann Surg* 177:755, 1973.

116. Laragh JH, Case DB: The renin system for understanding and managing renovascular hypertensions. In: Bergan JJ, Yao JST (eds). *Surgery of the Aorta and its Body Branches*. New York: Grune & Stratton, Inc.; 339–354, 1979.

117. Cohen EL, Rovner DR, Conn JW: Postural augmentation of plasma renin activity: importance in diagnosis of renovascular hypertension. *JAMA* 197:973, 1966.

118. Hunt JC: Diagnosis of renovascular hypertension. *Bull NY Acad Med* 45:877, 1969.

119. Nielson JB, Nerstrom JG, Jacobsen JG, et al: The postural plasma renin response in renovascular hypertension. *Acta Med Scand* 189:213, 1971.

120. Genest J, Boucher R, Rojo-Ortega JM, et al: Renovascular hypertension. In: Genest J, Koiw E, Kuchel O (eds). *Hypertension*. New York: McGraw-Hill; 815, 1977.

121. Svetkey LP, Bollinger RR, Klotman PE, et al: Prospective analysis of strategies for diagnosing renovascular hypertension. *Hypertension* 14:247–257, 1989.

122. Norris CS, Pfeiffer JS, Barnes RW, et al: Noninvasive evaluation of renal artery stenosis and renovascular disease. *J Vasc Surg* 1:192–201, 1984.

123. Kohler TR, Zierler RE, Martin RL, et al: Noninvasive diagnosis of renal artery stenosis by ultrasonic duplex scanning. *J Vasc Surg* 4:450–456, 1986.

124. Taylor DC, Kettler MD, Moneta GL, et al: Duplex ultrasound scanning in the diagnosis of renal artery steno-

sis: a prospective evaluation. *J Vasc Surg* 7:363–369, 1988.

125. Hansen KJ, Tribble RW, Dean RH, et al: Renal duplex sonography: evaluation of clinical utility. *J Vasc Surg* 12:227–236, 1990.

126. Hudspeth DA, Hansen KJ, Dean RH, et al: Renal duplex sonography after treatment of renovascular disease. *J Vasc Surg* 18:381–390, 1993.

127. Dean RH, Burko H, Wilson JP, et al: Deceptive patterns of renal artery stenosis. *Surgery* 76:872, 1974.

128. Oei HY: Captopril renography: early observations and diagnostic criteria. *Am J Hypertens* 4:678S–684S, 1991.

129. McLean AG, Hilson AJW, Sweny P, et al: Screening for renovascular disease with captopril-enhanced renography. *Nephrol Dial Transplant* 7:211–215, 1992.

130. Meier GH, Sumpio B, Gusberg RJ, et al: Captopril renal scintigraphy: a new standard for predicting outcome after renal revascularization. *J Vasc Surg* 17:280–287, 1993.

131. Setaro JF, Chen CC, Black HR, et al: Captopril renography in the diagnosis of renal artery stenosis and the prediction of improvement with revascularization. *Am J Hypertens* 4:698S–705S, 1991.

132. Nally JV Jr, Chen CC, Sfakianakis G, et al: Diagnostic criteria of renovascular hypertension with captopril renography: a consensus statement. *Am J Hypertens* 4: 749S–752S, 1991.

133. Whelton PK, Harrington DP, Russel RP, et al: Renal vein renin activity: a prospective study of sampling techniques and methods of interpretation. *Johns Hopkins Med J* 141:112, 1977.

134. Dean RH, Foster JH: Criteria for the diagnosis of renovascular hypertension. *Surgery* 74:926, 1973.

135. Vaughn ED, Buhler FR, Larach JH, et al: Renovascular hypertension: renin measurements to indicate hypersecretion and contralateral suppression, estimate renal plasma flow, and score for surgical curability. *Am J Med* 55:402, 1973.

136. Stanley JC, Fry WJ: Surgical treatment of renovascular hypertension. *Arch Surg* 112:291, 1977.

137. Stamey TA: *Renovascular Hypertension*. Baltimore: Williams & Wilkins; 1963.

138. Dean RH, Rhamy RK: Split renal function studies in renovascular hypertension. In: Ernst CB, Fry WJ, Stanley JC (eds). *Renovascular Hypertension*. Philadelphia: WB Saunders, Co.; 135, 1984.

139. Howard JE, Connor TB: Hypertension produced by unilateral renal disease. *Arch Intern Med* 109:8, 1962.

140. Howard JE: Hypertension as related to renal ischemia. *Circulation* 29:657, 1964.

141. Stanley JC: Renal artery stenosis and hypertension. In: Brewster DC (ed). *Common Problems in Vascular Surgery*. Chicago: Mosby-Year Book, Inc.; 187–195, 1989.

142. Hansen KJ, Metropol SH, Dean RH, et al: Management of renovascular hypertension in the elderly population. *J Vasc Surg* 10(3):266–273, 1989.

143. Dean RH, Tribble RW, Hansen KJ, et al: Evolution of renal insufficiency in ischemic nephropathy. *Ann Surg* 213(5):446–455, 1991.

144. Hansen KJ, Plonk GW Jr, Dean RH, et al: Contemporary surgical management of renovascular disease. *J Vasc Surg* 16(3):319–330, 1992.

145. Sušic D: The role of the renal medulla in blood pressure control. *Am J Med Sci* 295:234–240, 1988.

146. Göthberg G, Karlström G: Physiological effects of the humoral renomedullary antihypertensive system. *Am J Hypertens* 4:569S–574S, 1991.

147. Muirhead EE, Brooks B, Pitcock JA, et al: Medullipin system: generation of medullipin II by isolated kidney-liver perfusion. *Hypertension* 18(suppl III):158–163, 1991.

148. Perry MO: Ischemia/reperfusion syndromes: clinical relevance. In: *Ischemia, Reperfusion and Organ Dysfunction/Research Initiatives in Vascular Disease*. February, 3–7, 1993.

149. Granger DN, Villareal D: Mechanisms of reperfusion-induced microvascular dysfunction. In: *Ischemia, Reperfusion and Organ Dysfunction/Research Initiatives in Vascular Disease*. February 7–11, 1993.

CHAPTER 30

Basic Mechanisms in Mesenteric Ischemia

Amy C. Sisley, MD; Michael J. Tullis, MD
Elizabeth T. Clark, MD; Bruce L. Gewertz, MD

Introduction

Acute mesenteric ischemia may result from acute arterial emboli, in situ thrombosis of a preexistent arterial lesion, primary vasoconstriction ("nonocclusive" ischemia), or venous thrombosis. The continued high mortality of these syndromes reflects the too frequent delays in diagnosis, and the difficulties in accurately identifying patients at risk prior to catastrophic events. While future efforts to improve outcomes must address these important clinical issues, it is equally clear that the care of these patients is advanced by better understanding of normal circulatory regulation and those pathophysiologic mechanisms which accompany reductions in splanchnic blood flow. This discussion will begin with these mechanisms, and then focus on the processes of hypoxic cell death and reperfusion injury as they apply to the intestine. Finally, we will consider potential new treatments which may extend the tolerance of the tissue to ischemia and/or reperfusion.

Anatomy and Regulation of Mesenteric Blood Flow

Vascular Anatomy

The principal arterial blood supply to the human gut is derived from three vessels arising from the abdominal aorta. The celiac artery and its branches supply the stomach, liver, spleen, and a portion of the pancreas and proximal duodenum. The superior mesenteric artery (SMA) supplies the remaining pancreas and duodenum as well as the entire small bowel and approximately two thirds of the transverse colon. The distal colon and proximal rectum is perfused via the inferior mesenteric artery (IMA).

The intestinal microcirculation consists of an extensive network of intramural arteries located in the deep submucosal plexus. The arterial supply to the villi is provided by eccentrically located vessels, which nourish the villus tip and arterioles from adjacent crypts which supply the base.[1] In conscious, resting mammals, blood flow in the SMA ranges from 12 to 15 mL/min/kg. Some controversy exists as to the distribution of intestinal blood flow (IBF) throughout the gut; flow is thought to be either similar throughout the regions of the duodenum, jejunum, and ileum (approximately 75 mL/min/100 gm tissue), or preferentially increased in the jejunum (23% of total) and ileum (40% of total). In the jejunum, villi receive 75% of mucosal flow with 25% of IBF directed to the crypts. Corresponding values for the values for the ileum are 66% and 34%.[2] There is agreement that mucosal blood flow exceeds that of muscular flow by a factor of three to four. Estimates of blood volume in anesthetized mammals range from 8.6 to 18 mL/100 gm with average vascular compliance of 2.19 mL/kg/mm Hg.[2]

The intestines are protected from ischemia to a great extent by the abundant collateral circulation between the celiac artery, SMA, and IMA. The main communications between the celiac and SMA are the gastroduodenal artery and the superior and inferior pancreaticoduodenal arteries. These collaterals are illustrated in Figure 1. A marginal artery located at the mesenteric border of the left colon and a more centrally

From *The Basic Science of Vascular Disease*. Edited by Sidawy AN, Sumpio BE, and DePalma RG. Armonk, NY: Futura Publishing Company, Inc.; © 1997.

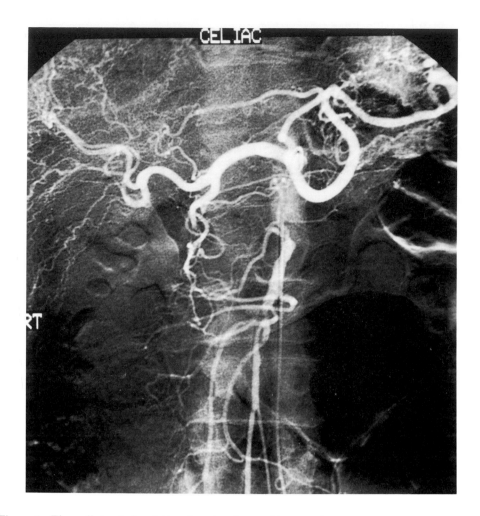

Figure 1. The collateral circulation that develops with stenosis or occlusion of the superior mesenteric artery (SMA) is illustrated in this angiogram. The gastroduodenal superior and inferior pancreaticoduodenal arteries enlarge and reconstitute flow through the SMA.

located vessel (within the mesentery) comprise the major collaterals between the SMA and IMA. Finally, the IMA has arterial communications with the middle and inferior rectal arteries via branches of the internal iliac arteries.[3]

Although extensive in the mature mesenteric circulation, collateral blood supply is poorly developed early in life. In one study of neonatal piglets, acute SMA occlusion was accompanied by little, if any, collateral flow to the small intestine. In contrast, following arterial occlusion in 1-day- and 1-month-old piglets, flow was maintained at 25% and 70% of normal values.[4] Collaterals appear to function most effectively in the absence of vasoactive substances. In one experimental study of adjacent canine jejunal segments, collateral flow to an ischemic region was decreased by both vasodilators (due to dilatation of the nonischemic bed) and vasoconstrictors (due to constriction of the ischemic bed).[5]

Intrinsic Control of the Circulation

There are two prevailing theories of intrinsic control which are used to explain various intestinal vasoregulatory phenomena. The ''metabolic theory'' supposes a local control system of vascular smooth muscle tone which maintains a balance between oxygen supply and demand. When a shortage of oxygen occurs, anaerobic metabolites accumulate within the tissue. These substances produce relaxation of arteriolar tone and/ or precapillary sphincters which both restores blood flow and augments oxygen extraction. Overabundance of tissue oxygen results in vasoconstriction and decreased capillary density. In short, the metabolic theory contends that oxygen delivery, as opposed to blood flow, is the controlled variable.

In the alternate ''myogenic theory,'' arteriolar tension receptors modulate vascular smooth muscle tone in response to changes in transmural pressure.

According to the law of Laplace (tension = pressure × radius), any transient increases in transmural pressure associated with increases in flow would induce vaso-constriction and subsequent normalization of blood flow. Similarly, decreases in pressure and flow initiate vasodilation, again returning flow to baseline.[6]

Depending on the specific conditions, myogenic or metabolic control mechanisms may predominate. The best example of metabolic control is the well-described relationship between oxygen uptake ($\dot{V}O_2$) and blood flow. Different experimental models consistently show that $\dot{V}O_2$ remains constant over a wide range of blood flows (40 to 70 mL/min/100 gm tissue) and progressively decreases only at flows below 40 mL/min/100 gm. At this "critical point," the major compensatory mechanisms of greater oxygen extraction and increased capillary filtration coefficient are exhausted and tissue oxygenation falls.[7-10]

We attempted to define these relationships in isolated segments of human small bowel obtained at organ harvest. We perfused human small intestine with an ex vivo circuit which allowed precise manipulation of blood flow and perfusion pressure. We began perfusion with an autologous blood solution through an extracorporeal membrane oxygenation circuit. Arterial and venous blood gases were measured at varying flow rates while maintaining a constant hematocrit. Arterial and venous oxygen content, arteriovenous oxygen difference, and oxygen consumption were then calculated. The "critical" flow rate in denervated human intestine (30 mL/min/100 gm) was similar to that found in canine and feline intestine, but lower than that of rodent species. At blood flows greater than 30 mL/min/100 gm, oxygen consumption by human small intestine was flow-independent (1.7 mL/min/100 gm) and oxygen extraction was inversely related to flow. Below this flow rate, oxygen extraction could not increase further (maximal A-$\dot{V}O_2$ diff 6.6 vol%), and oxygen consumption became flow-dependent.[11]

Pressure:flow autoregulation, the ability of the intestinal vasculature to adjust its resistance in response to changes in perfusion pressure, is another example of intrinsic regulation. This phenomenon has been consistently demonstrated in various experimental models, although its power can be compromised by changes in extrinsic innervation and circulating vaso-active substances. For example, in a denervated rat preparation, systemic arterial pressure was maintained constant while the SMA perfusion pressure was progressively reduced. IBF was within normal limits until a perfusion pressure of approximately 70 mm Hg was reached (the pressure:flow autoregulatory limit) at which time flow progressively decreased (Figures 2A and 2B). Oxygen extraction progressively increased below this perfusion pressure such that $\dot{V}O_2$ was preserved until the point of maximal A-$\dot{V}O_2$ difference

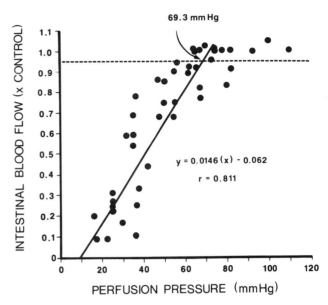

Figure 2A. Pressure:flow autoregulation is the ability of the intestinal vasculature to adjust its resistance in response to changes in perfusion pressure. Below the autoregulatory limit (about 70 mm Hg), reduction in pressure is accompanied by decreased intestinal blood flow.

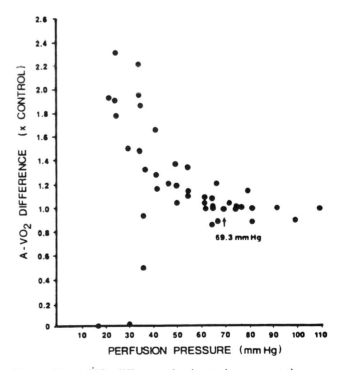

Figure 2B. A-$\dot{V}O_2$ difference begins to increase at the pressure:flow autoregulatory limit.

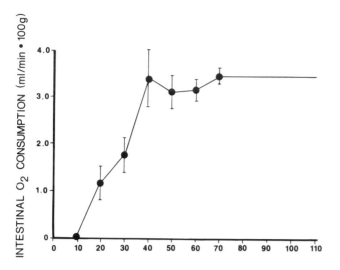

Figure 3. Intestinal oxygen consumption is maintained beyond the limit of pressure:flow autoregulation as a result of increased A-$\dot{V}O_2$. Once pressure decreased below the ability of the gut to increase A-$\dot{V}O_2$ difference ("critical limit"), $\dot{V}O_2$ decreases along with IBF.

(about 30 mm Hg), after which $\dot{V}O_2$ progressively decreased (Figure 3). In other experiments in anesthetized dogs, in whom the systemic baroreceptor reflex was eliminated, autoregulation maintained flow within 5% of control for perfusion pressures between 85 to 125 mm Hg. The phenomenon was influenced by the metabolic state of the gut; "superregulation" (increased flow) was seen in fed dogs, whereas there was less effective autoregulation in fasted dogs.[12] Locally active substances, such as histamine and adenosine, also appear to be important in autoregulation. In swine, histamine 1 (H1) and adenosine receptor blockade abolished and attenuated IBF autoregulation, respectively.[13] Pressure:flow autoregulation is not grossly impaired by ischemia and reperfusion (Figure 4A), or intravenous infusion of digoxin (Figure 4B) which does have effects on vascular reactivity in other perfusion beds.[14]

Acute venous hypertension is a well-studied experimental perturbation which results in increased vascular resistance and decreased blood flow in the stomach, small intestine, and colon.[16] While this finding is most consistent with the myogenic theory of regulation, there are variations to this response which may

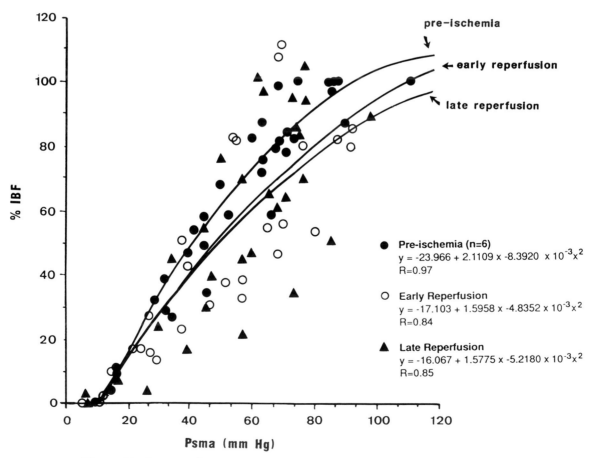

Pre-ischemia (n=6)
$$y = -23.966 + 2.1109\,x - 8.3920 \times 10^{-3}x^2$$
$$R=0.97$$

Early Reperfusion
$$y = -17.103 + 1.5958\,x - 4.8352 \times 10^{-3}x^2$$
$$R=0.84$$

Late Reperfusion
$$y = -16.067 + 1.5775\,x - 5.2180 \times 10^{-3}x^2$$
$$R=0.85$$

Figure 4A. Pressure:flow autoregulation is not altered by ischemia/reperfusion.

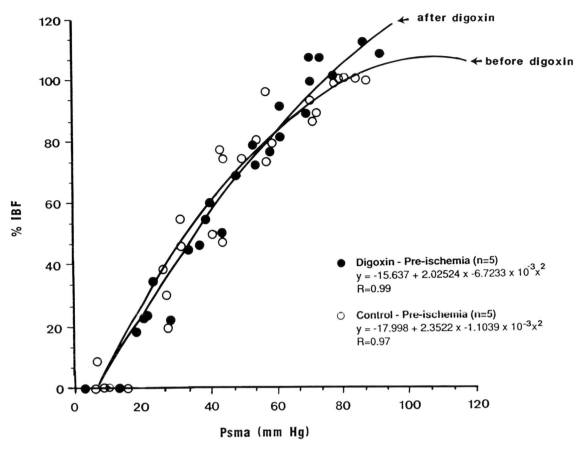

Figure 4B. Pressure flow autoregulation is not altered by intravenous digoxin infusion.

be of some physiologic significance. For example, dogs given a luminal food source or intra-arterial dinitrophenol (a drug which induces hypermetabolic state) showed reduction or reversal of the vasoconstriction elicited by acute venous hypertension.[16] In contrast, chronic digitalis administration appears to exacerbate the myogenic response to acute venous hypertension. Chronic venoconstriction, with decreased splanchnic venous capacitance, appears to be the mechanism.[17]

An accentuated myogenic response may be of clinical importance when patients with chronic mesenteric arterial occlusions are revascularized and normal perfusion pressure re-established. Gewertz and Zarins reported three patients who demonstrated intramural edema of the gut and symptoms of continued intestinal ischemia in the postoperative period despite patent reconstructions.[18] Angiograms revealed diffuse mesenteric vasospasm; conservative treatment including bowel rest, vasodilators, and calcium channel blocking agents resulted in complete and permanent remission of symptoms (Figure 5).

While the origin of this syndrome is unknown, these findings clearly reflect an inability of the intestinal microcirculation to prevent the accumulation of absorbed fluid within the interstitium of the gut. This may represent failure of capillary "derecruitment" after reinstitution of luxuriant blood flow. In support of this hypothesis, it is well-known that the density of perfused capillaries increases in the intestine in response to both feeding (metabolic hyperemia) and local hypoxia (reactive hyperemia).[19,20] Since one would suppose that the capillary bed distal to a superior mesenteric artery occlusion would be maximally dilated, it is understandable that the sudden restoration of high pressure perfusion would be poorly tolerated. The tendency to local edema would be perioperatively exacerbated by progressive dilution of local plasma oncotic pressure caused by increased absorption of infused crystalloid.

The vasospasm of medium-sized vessels could, therefore, be construed as an adaptive response to "protect" the maximally dilated capillary bed. Vasoconstriction would be mediated by the myogenic mechanisms intrinsic to vascular smooth muscle. Since these distal vessels would have been chronically exposed to low perfusion pressures, they would be exquisitely sensitive and respond disproportionately to even slight increases in pressure.

Alterations in hematocrit and PO_2 also have an effect on intrinsic flow regulation. In isolated canine

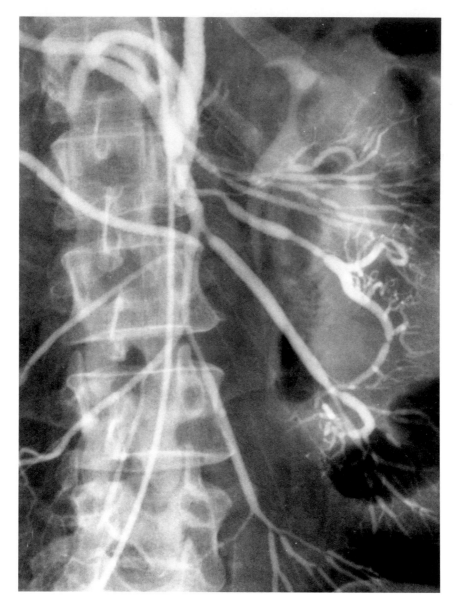

Figure 5. Selective arteriogram 1 week after revascularization demonstrates vasospasm in the distribution of the superior mesenteric artery. Note characteristic tapering at branch points.

intestinal loops perfused at a constant pressure, there is a linear relationship between decreasing hematocrit and increasing intestinal blood flow. Oxygen extraction exhibits a parabolic function to changing hematocrit, with maximum $\dot{V}O_2$ occurring when the hematocrit is approximately 50%.[21] Intraluminal solutes increase this optimal hematocrit. The same relationship between decreasing hematocrit and increasing IBF was seen in a rat model, where IBF increased nearly twofold as hematocrit was reduced from 41% to 17% (Table). At profound reductions in hematocrit, mucosal oxygen delivery in the stomach and intestine is compromised, probably secondary to countercurrent

shunting of the microcirculation.[22] Decreased arterial oxygen content, unassociated with changes in carrying capacity, also increases IBF.[23]

Other Vasoregulatory Phenomena

Reactive hyperemia is the hemodynamic response of intestinal vasculature to the sudden correction of arterial occlusion. The intensity and duration of the hyperemic response increases with increasing times of flow interruption. In denervated feline intestine, hyperemia following release of acute arterial occlusion

Table 1
Effect of Hematocrit of Hemodynamics and Metabolism

		Intestinal Blood Flow (mL/min·100 gm)	Oxygen Consumption (mL/min·100 gm)
Hct_1	40.5 ± 0.8	77.5 ± 9.8*	2.91 ± 0.33
Hct_2	23.5 ± 2.5	125.4 ± 16.1	2.96 ± 0.19
Hct_3	17.2 ± 2.5	132.15 ± 15*	2.61 ± 0.11
		*P < 0.01	NS

was associated with a decrease in A-$\dot{V}O_2$ difference.[24] However, if flow was held constant after reperfusion, there was an increase in A-$\dot{V}O_2$ difference. The hyperemic response reflects a powerful drive to repay an "oxygen debt" by whatever mechanisms are available. Interestingly, in some experimental conditions, venous occlusion results in a greater reperfusion oxygen debt than that seen with arterial occlusion.

The predictable mesenteric vasodilatation following a meal is termed postprandial hyperemia. Cephalic influences are dominant primarily and impact on changes in the mesenteric circulation during ingestion, while changes during digestion are locally determined by the amount and character of food in the gut and the actions of gastrointestinal hormones. The regional distribution of the incremental increase in mesenteric blood flow has been quantitated using microspheres. Food ingestion is associated with initial sympathetic-mediated vasoconstriction, followed by increases in mesenteric blood flow and vasodilation that are maximal at 60 minutes after food intake. In conscious baboons studied 1 hour after eating, mean mesenteric blood flow nearly doubled.[25] Atropine attenuated the response, implicating a cholenergic mechanism. In conscious fed dogs, there were no changes in systemic hemodynamics at the same time that substantial increases in flow to the pancreas, duodenum, and jejunum were noted.[26] The increased flow was largely distributed to the mucosal/submucosal layer; laser Doppler demonstrated a reduction of flow to the muscularis/serosa of 10% and an increase of about 40% to the mucosa.[27] Regional differences were also noted, with more modest vasodilation in the distal gut segments (ileum and colon).

The exact mechanism responsible for postprandial hyperemia remains unclear. Luminal bile seems to be important in combination with other nutrients. Although luminal bile concentrations as high as 33% of that seen in the gallbladder do not increase IBF when alone, bile seems to be a required cofactor for the vasodilation seen with luminal instillation of oleic acid, caproic acid, and amino acids.[28] Intraluminal glucose, which increases mucosal blood flow by itself, has an even greater effect when bile is added.

The role of gastrointestinal hormones in postprandial hyperemia is less clear; at concentrations calculated to match postprandial levels, intra-arterial secretin, cholecystokinin, or neurotensin have little, if any, effect on IBF.[29] Increasing flow in experimental preparations requires concentrations 100 times greater than those seen in physiologic conditions. Other local vasodilators and neurogenic mechanisms are certainly involved. Blocking the histamine H1 receptor has been shown to attenuate the increase in blood flow and oxygen uptake after feeding.[30] In a rat model, both capsaicin (a neurotoxin which depletes afferent C-fibers of peptide transmitters) and lidocaine abolished the oleic acid/bile-induced increase in blood flow when they were topically applied to the mucosa.[31] Furthermore, there was a marked attenuation in hyperemia when antiserum to vasoactive intestinal peptide (VIP) was administered prior to oleic acid/bile instillation. Since there was no change seen with administration of hexamethonium (ganglionic blockade), atropine (cholenergic blockade), or reserpine (chemical sympathectomy), it appears that postprandial hyperemia involves those primary afferent nerve fibers of the gut which release VIP and other locally active peptides. Prostaglandins have also been implicated in this process; cyclooxygenase inhibitors have been shown to augment postprandial hyperemia while arachnidonic acid inhibits the increases in IBF.[32]

Extrinsic Control

Extrinsic regulation of mesenteric blood flow via neural and hormonal mechanisms allows redistribution of circulating blood volume with changing activities and in times of stress. Extrinsic neurovascular control is primarily through the sympathetic splanchnic nerves which are noradrenergic. The arteries of the gut are innervated primarily by perivascular nerves which penetrate the gut wall. There is also an extensive submucosal nervous plexus. In contrast, there are very few nerves supplying lymphatics and veins in the gut.[33] In canine experiments, direct electrical stimulation of the thoracic splanchnic nerves decreased splanchnic blood volume by nearly half, with much of the reduction occurring within the first 30 seconds.[34] During a 2-minute hemorrhage, 54% of the bled volume was mobilized from the splanchnic bed, presumably through the carotid sinus reflex.

Although sympathetic stimulation initially results in vasoconstriction, continued stimulation results in a reproducible partial recovery of blood flow known as "autoregulatory escape." It is thought that reductions in local blood flow lead to local acidosis which selectively inhibits the postjunctional alpha 2-receptor response to norepinephrine.[35–37]. There is also evidence that adenosine accumulation is involved.[38] Consistent with the higher metabolic rate of the mucosa, this region exhibits a greater propensity for autoregulatory escape than the muscularis.[39]

Circulating vasoactive compounds are also important extrinsic regulators of mesenteric flow. Norepinephrine, angiotensin II, and vasopressin are adrenergic vasoconstrictors which uniformly produce decreases in both IBF and $\dot{V}O_2$. In contrast, epinephrine produces variable responses in flow and $\dot{V}O_2$ depending on dose.[40] Angiotensin II receptors have been identified in rat mesenteric arteries and exhibit a high affinity at physiologic levels.[41] In dogs, angiotensin II receptor antagonists administered in association with hemorrhage attenuated the decrease in IBF without systemic effects, indicating a local mechanism of action.[42]

Intestinal Ischemia and Reperfusion

When the intestine experiences acute reductions in blood flow, tissue injury results from both the hypoxia incurred during flow interruption and the deleterious effects of reperfusion. Ischemic injury is a consequence of a complicated sequence of cellular events which reflect the basal metabolic rate of the tissue, as well as the duration of flow interruption. Reperfusion injury is mediated principally by neutrophils and oxygen free radicals and may occur following even brief periods of ischemia. In practice, ischemia is usually heterogeneous due to the extensive collateral flow present in the intestine, as well as the local vascular autoregulatory factors described above. As a consequence, blood flow is rarely reduced to zero and reflow may be intermittent or incomplete. Nonetheless, since ischemia and reperfusion injuries are mediated by different processes, they will be considered separately in our discussion.

Ischemia

General Observations

Intestinal ischemia results in a spectrum of function and morphologic alterations, which range from minor changes in mucosal permeability to transmural necrosis. The earliest changes, noted at 10 to 30 minutes of ischemia, are increases in the fluid layer between the cells and the basement membrane.[43] The villus tips then begin to slough followed by submucosal bleeding and an increase in both vascular and mucosal permeability. Tissue damage progresses sequentially from the lumen (villus tips) outward, ultimately resulting in transmural necrosis.

In animal models, the outcome of an episode of intestinal ischemia reflects both the severity of the flow disturbance and its duration. Ischemic injury is likely if flow is completely interrupted for even a short period of time (15 minutes) whereas less severe flow reductions are tolerated for longer periods of time prior to injury (Figure 6). Experimentally, it has been demonstrated that increasing the basal metabolic rate of intestinal tissue by the administration of intravenous glucagon results in a shift of this ischemic threshold; that is, when exposed to a comparable duration and severity of ischemia, intestine with an increased metabolic rate suffers a greater degree of histologic injury than intestine with a normal metabolic rate.[44]

The role of neutrophils (PMN) in low flow intestinal ischemia has also been evaluated. It was found that in a severe blood flow reduction, filtering PMN had no beneficial effects. However, at moderate reductions in flow (30 mL/min/100 gm), filtering of PMN resulted in a reduction of ischemic damage. This implies that restriction of PMN to ischemic intestine may extend the tolerance of marginally perfused but still viable tissue.[45]

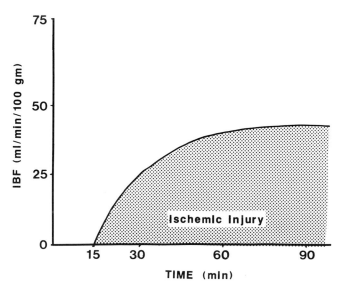

Figure 6. Schematic illustrating the concept of an "ischemic threshold" (**shaded area**) that relates mucosal injury to both blood flow and duration of ischemia. Mucosal injury requires some finite time of flow interruption and may not occur at all if perfusion is maintained above an arbitrary limit.

Cellular Events

New technologies enabling the direct study of cellular processes in isolated cells have elucidated some of the biochemical events associated with hypoxic cellular death. Mitochondrial dysfunction leading to depletion of cellular ATP appears to be the critical factor, initiating a cascade of events which ultimately results in hypoxic injury.[46] The depletion of ATP results in loss of ionic homeostasis, changes in both membrane fluidity and permeability, as well as an increase in degradative processes mediated by the activation of proteases and lipases.

Over the past several years, attention has focused on alterations in mitochondrial calcium homeostasis as important indicators of progressive hypoxic injury; a rise in cytosolic calcium appears to be an initiating factor in cell surface bleb formation. These blebs grow and coalesce until one to three large terminal blebs remain. Ultimately, one of the terminal blebs ruptures, marking the transition from reversible to irreversible injury.

Although there is much support for this hypothesis, contradictory evidence has been developed. In particular, some recent studies failed to demonstrate a rise in intracellular calcium levels until long after irreversible injury was evident.[47] Aw and colleagues studied the mitochondrial calcium flux driven by differences in membrane potential and pH.[48] They demonstrated that ischemic mitochondria have an intrinsic adaptive mechanism which maintains calcium homeostasis. During early hypoxia, ionic gradients are maintained by some nonenergy-dependent inhibition of ion movement across the inner mitochondrial membrane, rather than an energy-dependent process requiring ATP from glycolysis. A better understanding of the role of calcium has been achieved through the use of multiparameter digitized video microscopy (MDVM). This technique allows measurement of cytosolic calcium and sodium, mitochondrial membrane potential, pH, and membrane fluidity of single cells. Using MDVM, Lemasters et al observed no increase in cytosolic free calcium with hypoxia, even though they did observe terminal bleb formation.[49] Taken together, these recent data tend to refute the notion that the loss of mitochondrial calcium homeostasis is a final common pathway to cell death.

An alternative hypothesis as to the sequence of hypoxic cell death implies a protective effect of intracellular acidosis. Using a fluorescent probe and MDVM, Gores et al demonstrated that intracellular pH dropped by more than one full point during hypoxia.[50] After 40 to 50 minutes, intracellular pH began to rise with rapid leakage of fluorescent probe and subsequent cell death. Those manipulations which maintained intracellular acidosis also prolonged cell survival, while manipulations which prevented acidosis from developing accelerated cell death. They proposed that intracellular acidosis depresses the activity of the critical degradative enzymes (primarily proteases and phospholipases) which are activated during ATP depletion. These enzymes damage the cytoskeleton, resulting in an increase in membrane permeability and leakage of hydrogen ions from the cell. Once hydrogen ions begin to leak, a positive feedback loop is created in which an increase in intracellular pH results in less suppression of the degradative enzymes with further leakage of hydrogen ion.

The protective effect of intracellular acidosis carries implications for reperfusion injury as well, since the abrupt rise in pH with reoxygenation may accentuate cell damage. Currin et al demonstrated that on reperfusion of ischemic rat hepatocytes, the sudden increase in pH precipitated cell killing.[51] Cellular injury was avoided if pH was slowly increased after reoxygenation. These data have important clinical implications since reperfusate pH can be readily manipulated.

Another potential mechanism of hypoxic cellular injury is the formation of reactive oxygen species (ROS) during hypoxia. ROS generation may occur in hypoxic tissue during the period when the level of molecular oxygen is declining, but still present in sufficient amounts to interact with a reduced mitochondrial respiratory chain.[52] The exact role of ROS in ischemic injury is still incompletely understood and is likely to be less critical than in reperfusion injury.

Reperfusion Injury

While it is clear that re-establishment of blood flow is essential to prevent the death of ischemic tissue, intestinal reperfusion results in an additional tissue injury. Parks and Granger demonstrated that the mucosal injury observed after 3 hours of ischemia followed by 1 hour of reperfusion was more severe than the injury observed after 4 hours of ischemia alone.[53] Clark and Gewertz showed that intermittent episodes of ischemia and reperfusion resulted in a significantly worse histologic injury than a comparable time of continuous ischemia.[54]

Such reperfusion injury is due at least in part to the cytotoxic effect of reactive oxygen species. Grogaard placed the oxygen free radical generating system of xanthine oxidase and hypoxanthine in the lumen of small intestine and observed a histologic injury equivalent to 1 hour of ischemia followed by reperfusion.[55] Amelioration of injury has been demonstrated with xanthine oxidase inhibitors and free radical scavengers, as well as by decreasing the oxygen content of the reperfusate.[56,57] This lends support to the notion that ROS generated on reintroduction of oxygenated blood initiate and, in part, mediate intestinal reperfusion injury.

Formation of Reactive Oxygen Species

Generation of ROS in biologic systems during ischemia/reperfusion can occur by at least three mechanisms: a) by redox reactions of low molecular weight compounds; b) as byproducts of enzyme substrate reactions; c) following activation and degranulation of inflammatory cells.

a) Redox reactions

When molecular oxygen (O_2) accepts one electron, a superoxide anion radical (O_2^-) is generated.

$$O_2 + e^- \rightarrow O_2^-$$

While the superoxide radical is relatively nonreactive, it acts as a precursor to more reactive free radical species such as the hydroxyl radical ($OH\bullet$). First, H_2O_2 is formed either as a result of a double reduction of O_2, or as a dismutation product of O_2^-:

$$2O_2^- + 2H \rightarrow H_2O_2 + O_2$$

The hydroxyl radical is then formed on reduction of H_2O_2 by O_2^- in the Haber-Weiss reaction:

$$O_2^- + H_2O_2 \rightarrow O_2 + HO^- + OH\bullet$$

Under most biologic conditions, the classic Haber-Weiss reaction occurs much too slowly to account for significant generation of $OH\bullet$; however, the reaction rate is greatly increased in the presence of metal catalysts such as Fe^{3+}. First, trace metals are reduced by O_2^-. The reduced metal then reacts with H_2O_2 to produce $OH\bullet$, regenerating the oxidized metal in the process.

$$O_2^- + Fe^{3+} \rightarrow Fe^{2+} + O_2$$

$$Fe^{2+} + H_2O_2 \rightarrow Fe^{3+} + OH^- + OH\bullet$$

This modification of the Haber-Weiss reaction, known as the Fenton reaction, may be an important biologic pathway of $OH\bullet$ generation, since the intestinal mucosa is a rich source of Fe^{3+}. Furthermore, it has been shown experimentally that pretreatment with either deferoxamine (an iron chelator), or apotransferrin (an iron binding protein), results in a significant attenuation of the increased microvascular permeability associated with reperfusion injury.[58]

b) Enzyme-substrate reactions

Another important source of ROS in postischemic tissue is the hypoxanthine-xanthine oxidase system (Figure 7). During ischemia, ATP is sequentially metabolized to hypoxanthine. At the same time, xanthine dehydrogenase (XDH) is proteolytically converted to xanthine oxidase (XO).[59] While XDH uses NAD^+ as its electron acceptor, XO, the form of the enzyme predominating in ischemic tissue, uses molecular oxygen as its electron acceptor. On reperfusion, XO catalyzes the conversion of hypoxanthine to uric acid, generating O_2^- and H_2O_2 in the process.

The critical importance of the hypoxanthine-xanthine oxidase system in intestinal reperfusion injury is supported by experimental evidence demonstrating that allopurinol, a competitive inhibitor of XO, attenuates both the mucosal lesions and the increased vascular permeability associated with reperfusion.[60] Other less specific XO inhibitors such as oxypurinol, pterin aldehyde, and soybean trypsin inhibitor have also been shown to attenuate reperfusion injury.[61]

c) Activation/degranulation of inflammatory cells

ROS produced by neutrophils are also important mediators of tissue injury. When PMN are stimulated, they exhibit a respiratory burst characterized by increased oxygen consumption. More than 90% of the consumed O_2 can be attributed to the generation of O_2^-, which is catalyzed by NADPH oxidase, an enzyme localized within the plasma membrane of phagocytes.[62,63] The O_2^- then undergoes spontaneous dismutation to H_2O_2. Myeloperoxidase (MPO), an enzyme found within the lysosomal granules of PMN, then catalyses the formation of hypochlorous acid (HOCl) from H_2O_2.

Mechanisms of ROS Cell and Tissue Injury

ROS cause lipid peroxidation of cell membranes and organelles resulting in alteration of membrane function and structural integrity. Peroxidation of biomembranes has been shown to modify the affinity of the active sites for $Na^\pm K^\pm$ ATPase resulting in decreased availability of energy for transmembrane transport processes.[64] Peroxidized cell membranes do not maintain ionic gradients leading to an influx of Na^+ and Ca^{++} and an efflux of K^+. As noted above, accumulation of intracellular Ca^{++} is associated with activation of a number of enzymes such as phospholipase and protein kinase, resulting in further changes in cell membrane composition. Lipid peroxides can cause protein depolymerization directly and are capable of acting as intermediates in the transfer of electrons to other molecules. Neutrophil-derived N-chloromines damage proteins by interacting with cysteine and tyrosine residues. In addition, they oxidize sufhydryls and damage cytochromes and heme proteins.[65,66]

The structural matrix of tissue is directly damaged by ROS. H_2O_2 has been shown to promote the hydroly-

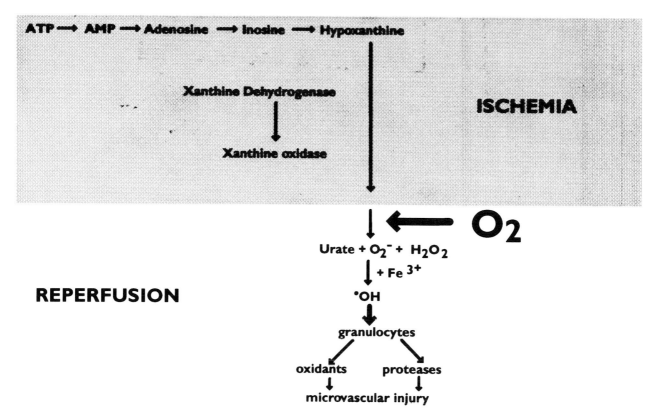

Figure 7. Xanthine oxidase, oxidants, and granulocytes play central roles in the generation of ischemia-reperfusion-induced microvascular injury.

sis of basement membrane. O_2 can depolymerize hyaluranate as well as damage the proteoglycans of collagen and cartilage.[67] It is the degradation of basement membrane by ROS which contributes to the uniform increases in both vascular and mucosal permeability observed in reperfusion injury.[68]

Polymorphonuclear Leukocytes in Reperfusion Injury

While there is general agreement that ROS initiate reperfusion injury, recent experimental evidence implicates PMN as the primary mediators of the actual tissue damage. The importance of PMN in reperfusion injury is illustrated by numerous experiments in which neutrophil depletion, accomplished by either antineutrophil serum or neutrophil filters, resulted in amelioration of the increased vascular permeability and mucosal lesions associated with reperfusion injury[69].

In order for neutrophils to participate in the reperfusion phenomenon, they must be attracted to the site of postischemic tissue, adhere to the microvascular endothelium, and migrate through the vessel wall to infiltrate the tissue. Experimental evidence indicates that XO-generated ROS are involved in the recruitment of PMN to postischemic tissue. XO inhibitors and free

radical scavengers have been shown to decrease both the number of PMN in reperfused tissue and the associated reperfusion injury.[70,71] Zimmerman and Granger have postulated that PMN are attracted by a two-step mechanism.[59] First, ROM activate phospholipase A_2 in the endothelial cell membrane. Phospholipase A_2 activation leads to the formation of leukotriene B_4 (LTB₄) and platelet-activating factor (PAF), both potent chemoattractants for PMN. In support of this theory, it has been demonstrated that LTB₄ and PAF levels increased dramatically on reperfusion of ischemic intestine in both canine and feline models.[72,73] In addition, PMN infiltration of reperfused tissue was significantly decreased in animals treated with either an LTB₄ or PAF receptor antagonist.[59]

Neutrophil binding to the vascular endothelium is mediated by a glycoprotein adhesion complex on the PMN known as CD11-CD18, as well as by endothelial-based adhesion complexes (ELAM and ICAM). The use of monoclonal antibodies against the CD11-CD18 complex (MoAb 60.3) inhibits adherence of PMN to the microvascular endothelium. It also results in a decrease in observed reperfusion injury equivalent to that obtained with neutrophil depletion.[69]

ROS derived from XO promote leukocyte adherence as demonstrated by the fact that XO inhibitors significantly decrease the number of adherent PMN in reperfused tissue.[71] In addition, the neutrophil-derived ROS, H_2O_2, and monochlorlamine have been shown to promote PMN adherence by upregulation of the CD11-CD18 complex.[66]

Activated PMN also release a number of proteases (collagenase, elastase, gelatinase) which promote PMN migration and infiltration into reperfused tissue. Pretreatment of animals with elastase inhibitors prevented the infiltration of reperfused intestinal mucosa by PMN, implying that neutrophil-derived enzymes are necessary for PMN migration through the vascular wall.[74]

The adhesion of neutrophils to endothelial cells is a complex function which is currently of great research interest. Investigations are focused on both the endothelial receptors themselves, as well as the cytokines which modify their expression.

Two endothelial cell membrane receptors are believed to play a central role in both the activation of neutrophils and release of cytokines.[75] Intercellular adhesion molecule (ICAM-1), with a molecular weight of 76–114 kDa, is basally expressed on endothelial cells. Expression is increased in response to cytokines. Endothelial-leukocyte adhesion molecule (ELAM-1, or E-selectin) is a 115 kDa selectin that is not expressed basally on cell surfaces, but is present once cells are stimulated with cytokines.

The time course of surface expression of these receptors was characterized by McEver et al in 1991.[76] ICAM-1 shows a plateau of maximal expression at 8 hours following stimulation with cytokine, while ELAM-1 expression peaks at 4 hours and then returns to baseline (Figure 8).

As our understanding of the relationship between endothelial cells and circulating leukocytes continues to evolve, two other receptors are currently being studied. VCAM (vascular cell adhesion molecule), first cloned in 1989, is a cytokine-induced protein on endothelial cells that binds lymphocytes. VCAM is involved in the adhesion of leukocytes to endothelial cells, especially following activation by interleukin-1 (IL-1) or tumor necrosis factor (TNF). Another receptor, PECAM (platelet-endothelial cell adhesion molecule), is constitutively expressed on cultured human umbilical vein endothelial cells (HUVEC) and recently has been more specifically localized to endothelial cell junctions. While it has close homology to other vascular cell adhesion molecules, the role of PECAM is, as yet, undefined.[75]

Interleukin-1 alpha (IL-1 alpha) has been shown to promote leukocyte adhesiveness by inducing expression of ICAM-1 and ELAM-1.[77,78] IL-1 belongs to a group of cytokines with overlapping biologic properties which include IL-1, IL-6, and TNF. These all share the ability to stimulate lymphocytes, augment cell proliferation, and effect gene expression for several proteins. Recently, the naturally occurring IL-1 receptor antagonist (IL-1RA) has been cloned, and is shown to block the triggering of IL-1 receptors without agonist effects.[79] The ability to block IL-1 activity has many clinical implications, specifically in the treatment of tissues at risk from IR.

Recent Laboratory Efforts

Our recent studies have been aimed at identifying a more objective and reproducible method of quantitating the effects of hypoxia and reoxygenation on cultured endothelial cells. By concentrating on the cellular mechanisms, we hoped to identify therapeutic manipulations which will modify the course of local ischemia-reperfusion injury and distant organ damage.

Preliminary work in our laboratory with flow cytometry confirmed stable expression of ICAM-1 on unstimulated HUVEC, although there is some diminution of receptor expression after three passages. There is minimal basal expression of ELAM-1 on unstimulated HUVEC through passage three with a moderate increase in ELAM-1 in subsequent passages. As a consequence of these observations, all experimental work has involved cells in passages one to three.

Viability studies were undertaken to determine a hypoxic insult which would not cause massive cell death. Cell viability was quantitated using trypan blue exclusion as a measure of cell membrane integrity. Confluent monolayers of HUVEC on 60 mm culture dishes were exposed to varying periods of hypoxia after exchange of media with oxygen-depleted M-199 via nitrogen bubbling. Viability was then assessed with 0.4% trypan blue after cells were harvested using 500

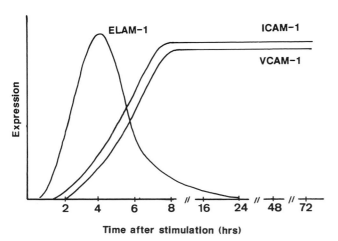

Figure 8. Expression of endothelial cell receptors following cytokine stimulation. (Reproduced with permission from Reference 76.)

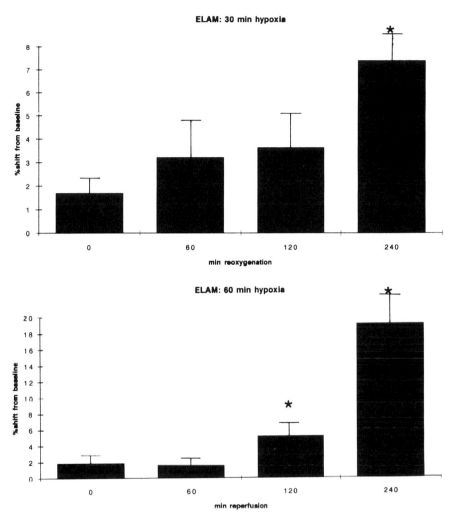

Figure 9. Increases in ELAM expression in human umbilical vein endothelial cells with I/R.

ul 0.1% collagenase and 0.25% EDTA. LD_{50} was determined to occur at 150 min hypoxia.

We next exposed HUVEC to hypoxia and reoxygenation (HR) using an incubator chamber purged of oxygen with 100% nitrogen and reoxygenated after either 30 or 60 minutes. We demonstrated signficiant increases in ELAM expression as early as 120 minutes after reoxygenation. While there was a similar trend toward increased ICAM expression, these results did not achieve statistical significance (Figure 9).

We then contrasted the effects of the cytokine IL-1 with those of hypoxia. We first documented increased expression of ICAM-1 and ELAM-1 on HUVEC incubated with 5 ng/mL IL-1, with time courses consistent with work by McEver. Interestingly, when we used hypoxia as a stimulus for expression we demonstrated different times of peak expression. There were two peaks of ELAM-1 expression (90 minutes and 4 hours), while ICAM-1 expression increased at 120 minutes. Although these different time courses suggested that the mechanisms of upregulation

in response to IL-1 and hypoxia are different, addition of an IL-1 receptor antagonist eliminated the expected increases in expression of both receptors following 60 minutes of hypoxia (Figure 10). Hence, it is clear from the work to date that IL-1 is involved in some way in the response of ICAM-1 and ELAM-1 to hypoxia.

Finally, to correlate these ex vivo findings with ischemia-reperfusion (IR) phenomena in vivo, HUVEC were exposed to venous effluent from reperfused human small intestinal segments. Venous effluents were obtained at various time periods during reperfusion (T1:1–10 min, T2:11–20 min, T3:21–35 min, T4:36–50 min, T5:51–65 min) and were incubated with HUVEC for 4 hours. We demonstrated increases in both ICAM-1 and ELAM-1, with ELAM-1 upregulation exceeding that of ICAM-1 (Figure 11). This upregulation of endothelial cell membrane receptors by effluent from reperfused human intestine is a novel finding which is consistent with the known involvement of PMN in local reperfusion phenomena (Figure 12).

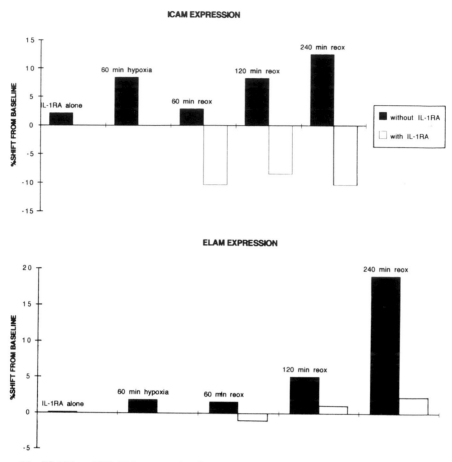

Figure 10. ICAM and ELAM expression in response to hypoxia reoxygenation and IL-1 RA.

To further our ultimate goal of applying these treatment strategies to patients, it was necessary to test these hypotheses in a clinically relevant model of human IR injury. Human small bowel segments were obtained at the time of routine organ harvest for transplantation. Tissue was transported to the laboratory in iced Belzer solution, rewarmed, and perfused on an ex vivo circuit with autologous oxygenated blood. Viability was confirmed by serosal hyperemia, return of peristalsis, and the demonstration of both satisfactory oxygen consumption and appropriate relationships between blood flow and oxygen uptake.

Attention was then focused on identifying an objective method of quantifying reperfusion injury. Such a marker was needed, 1) to delineate which factors influence the extent of injury, and 2) to determine the efficacy of protective interventions. The mucosal enzyme alkaline phosphatase appeared to be such a marker. Dudeja and Brasitus have recently demonstrated specific inactivation of this enzyme when isolated rat small intestinal brush border membranes were exposed to a reactive oxygen species (ROS) in vitro.[80] This was presumably due to direct action of ROS on the exposed metal binding sites of this enzyme.

Alkaline phosphatase enzyme activity was quantitated in mucosal scrapings following ischemia and reperfusion of isolated human small bowel segments. Enzyme specific activity was significantly decreased in reperfused segments compared to nonreperfused tissues; it was noted that alkaline phosphatase activity was markedly reduced much before any histologic degradation was evident. Importantly, there was no change in enzyme activity even with prolonged warm ischemia, indicating that the decrease in alkaline phosphatase activity was specifically associated with reperfusion.[81] Finally, the decrease in alkaline phosphatase activity seen with IR was attenuated when human intestinal segments were reperfused with leukocyte-poor blood (Figure 13).[87]

To determine if this marker would allow quantitative assessments of reperfusion injury, small bowel harvested from 12 canines was subjected to 60 minutes ischemia followed by 60 minutes reperfusion with oxygenated ($PO_2 > 100$) or deoxygenated ($PO_2 < 50$) autologous blood. While alkaline phosphatase activity was decreased in both reperfusion groups, reperfusion with oxygenated blood resulted in a significantly greater decrease in enzyme activity than reperfusion with deoxy-

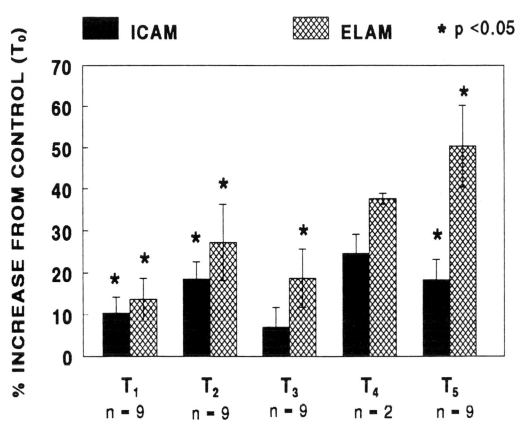

Figure 11. Increased ICAM and ELAM expression with venous effluent from ischemic, then reperfused human bowel.

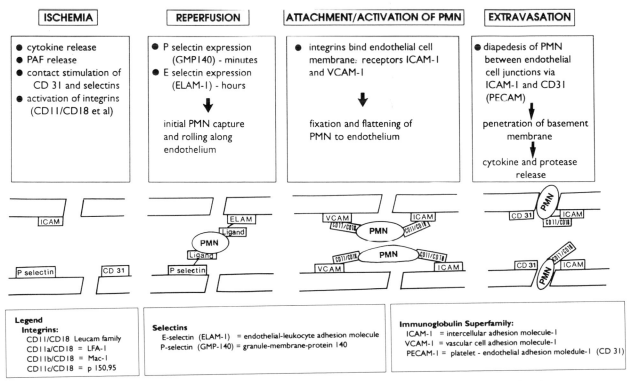

Figure 12. A reperfusion cascade is initiated when ROS are generated on reintroduction of oxygen in ischemic tissue. ROS are directly cytotoxic, promote PMN adherence and activation, and facilitate PMN infiltration and tissue injury.

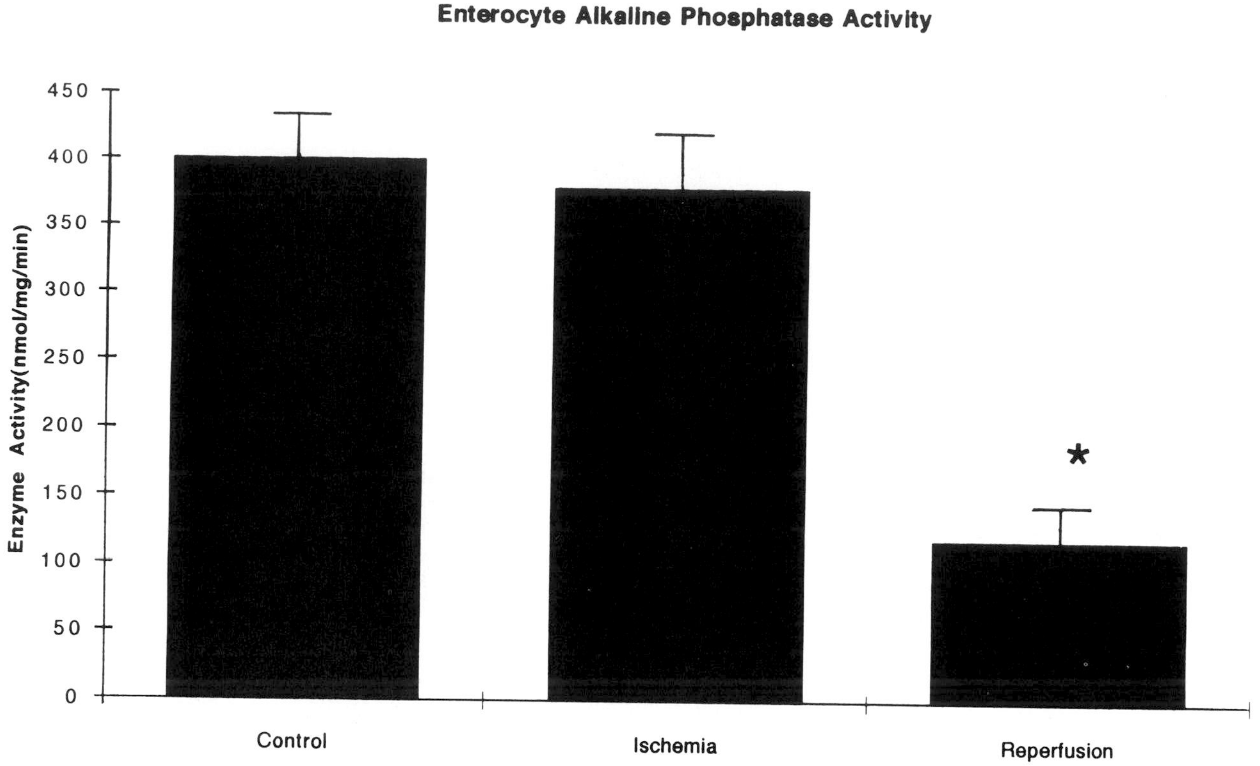

Enterocyte Alkaline Phosphatase Activity

Figure 13. Decreases in alkaline phosphatase activity are specifically associated with reperfusion in human bowel segments.

genated blood (Figure 14).[83] Enzyme activity did not decrease with ischemia alone. Evaluation of other brush border membrane enzyme activities (sucrase, maltase, GGTP, and leucine aminopeptidase) revealed no significant changes in ischemic versus reperfused bowel. Thus, from all experiments to date, we conclude that mucosal alkaline phosphatase is a specific marker of reperfusion injury in humans as well as common experimental models which will allow quantitative evaluation of therapeutic interventions in the clinical setting.

New Approaches to Treatment of Ischemia-Reperfusion

While some details have yet to be elucidated, the large body of evidence obtained to date describes a reperfusion cascade initiated when ROS are generated on reintroduction of oxygen in ischemic tissue. These ROS act directly as cytotoxic agents, as well as indirectly as attractants and promoters of PMN adherence. PMN themselves release ROS which further attract and promote leukocyte adherence. Once adherent and activated, PMN infiltrate the interstitium, elaborating a variety of cytotoxic substances including ROS and proteases, which culminate in the tissue damage associated with reperfusion.

Based on these mechanisms of I/R injury, a number of clinical treatment strategies have been advocated. These include changes in the nature of the reperfusate, alterations in the adherence or activation of PMN, and the administration of pharmocologic "scavengers" of reactive oxygen species.

Reperfusate modifications would appear to be easily implemented at the time of restoration of blood flow. Reduction in oxygen content toward that seen in venous blood (PO_2 = 40–50 mm Hg), reduction in pH, and filtration of reperfusate PMN have shown consistent benefit in a wide range of experimental models. These approaches have been recently applied to myocardial reperfusion after cardiopulmonary bypass.

Reduction in the adherence of PMN can be accomplished by systemic blockade of the principal neutrophil-based adhesion molecules (CD11-CD18). Theoretically, this approach may adversely impact resistance to infectious agents, mimicking the rare congenital disorder of leukocyte adhesion molecule deficiency syndrome. A more targeted strategy would be directed against the endothelial cell receptors in only the organ of interest. Monoclonal antibodies to ICAM-1 and ELAM-1 are available and appear to have a rapid enough onset of action to be used clinically. Yet another option would be the administration of antibodies

Enterocyte Alkaline Phosphatase Activity

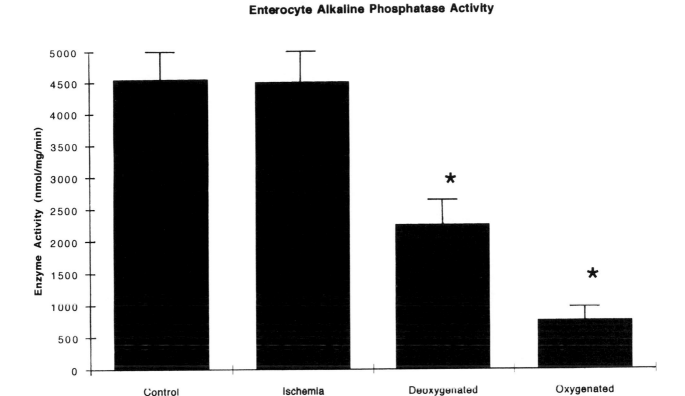

Figure 14. Reperfusion with deoxygenated blood moderates decreases in alkaline phosphatase.

to cytokines known to be involved in endothelial cell receptor upregulation (TNF, IL-1, PAF).

Finally, the use of various compounds which neutralize ROS directly, or reduce their generation through binding heavy metals such as iron, have long been advocated in I/R. Unfortunately, clinical application of these agents has not been particularly successful to date due, perhaps, to the fact that enzymes and ROS derived from activated neutrophils within the interstitium are not easily neutralized by agents delivered intravascularly.

Regardless of the limited role for such protective strategies in current practice, it is reasonable to expect increased application of some or all of these strategies in the near future. This trend will be accentuated by the continued improvements in our understanding of the basic mechanisms involved in intestinal ischemia and reperfusion.

References

1. Casley-Smith JR, Gannon BJ: Intestinal microcirculation: spatial organization and fine structure. In: Shephard AP, Granger DN (eds). *Physiology of the Intestinal Circulation.* New York: Raven Press; 9–31, 1984.

2. Donald DE: Splanchnic circulation. In: Sheperd JT, Abboud FM, Geiger SR (eds). *Handbook of Physiology: The Cardiovascular System.* vol III. Baltimore, MD: Williams & Wilkins; 219–240, 1983.

3. Kornblith PL, Boley SJ, Whitehouse BS: Anatomy of the splanchnic circulation. *Surg Clin North Am* 72(1): 1–30, 1992.

4. Crissenger KD, Granger DN: Characterization of intestinal collateral blood flow in the developing piglet. *Pediatr Res* 24(4):473–476, 1988.

5. Bulkley GB, Womack WA, Downey JM, Kvietys PR, Granger DN: Collateral blood flow in segmental intestinal ischemia: effects of vasoactive agents. *Surgery* 100: 157–167, 1986.

6. Granger DN, Richardson PDI, Kvietys PR, Mortillaro NA: Intestinal blood flow. *Gastroenterology* 78: 837–863, 1980.

7. Granger DN, Kvietys PR, Perry MA: Role of exchange vessels in the regulation of intestinal oxygenation. *Am J Physiol* 242:G570-G574, 1982.

8. Nowicki PT, Hansen NB, Menke JA: Intestinal blood flow and oxygen uptake in the neonatal piglet during reduced perfusion pressure. *Am J Physiol* 252:G190-G194, 1987.

9. Bulkley GB, Kvietys PR, Perry MA, Granger DN: Effects of cardiac tamponade on colonic blood flow and oxygenation. *Am J Physiol* 244:G604-G612, 1983.

10. Granger DN, Granger HJ: Systems analysis of intestinal hemodynamics and oxygenation. *Am J Physiol* 245: G786-G795, 1983.

11. Mesh CL, Gewertz BL: The effect of hemodilution on blood flow regulation in normal and postischemic intestine. *J Surg Res* 48:183–189, 1990.

12. Norris CP, Barnes GE, Smith EE, Granger HJ: Autoregulation of superior mesenteric flow in fasted and fed dogs. *Am J Physiol* 237:H174-H177, 1979.

13. Buckley NM, Diamants J, Frasier ID, Owusu K: Histamine or adenosine blockade alters intestinal blood flow autoregulation in swine. *Am J Physiol* 254:G156-G161, 1988.

14. Moawad J, Malago M, Gewertz BL: Intestinal blood flow regulation after ischemia. *FASEB J* 5(6):7913, 1991.

15. Johnson PC: Myogenic and venous-arteriolar responses in intestinal circulation. Shepard AP, Granger DN (eds). *Physiology of the Intestinal Circulation.* New York: Raven Press; 49–60, 1984.

16. Granger DN, Norris CP: Intrinsic regulation of intestinal oxygenation in the anesthetized dog. *Am J Physiol* 238: H836-H843, 1980.

17. Kim EH, Gewertz BL: Chronic digitalis administration alters mesenteric vascular reactivity. *J Vasc Res* 43: 183–189, 1990.

18. Gewertz BL, Zarins CK: Postoperative vasospasm after antegrade mesenteric revascularization: a report of three cases. *J Vasc Surg* 14:382–385, 1991.

19. Pawlik WW, Fondacaro JD, Jacobson ED: Metabolic hyperemia in canine gut. *Am J Physiol* 239:G12-G17, 1980.

20. Sheperd AP: Intestinal capillary blood flow during metabolic hyperemia. *Am J Physiol* 237:E548–554, 1979.

21. Shepard AP, Riedel GL: Optimal hematocrit for oxygenation of canine intestine. *Circ Res* 51(2):233–240, 1982.

22. Kiel JW, Reidel GL, Shepard AP: Effects of hemodilution on gastric and intestinal oxygenation. *Am J Physiol* 256:H171-H178, 1989.

23. Shepard AP: Intestinal oxygen consumption and 86Rb extraction during arterial hypoxia. *Am J Physiol* 234: E248-E251, 1978.

24. Mortillaro NA, Granger HJ: Reactive hyperemia and oxygen extraction in the feline small intestine. *Circ Res* 41: 859–865, 1977.

25. Vatner SF, Patrick TA, Higgins CB, Franklin D: Regional circulatory adjustments to eating and digestion in conscious unrestrained primates. *J Appl Physiol* 36: 524–529, 1974.

26. Gallavan RH, Chou CC, Kvietys PR, Sit SP: Regional blood flow during digestion in the conscious dog. *Am J Physiol* 238:H220-H225, 1980.

27. Shepard AP, Riedel GL: Laser-Doppler blood flowmetry of intestinal mucosa hyperemia induced by glucose and bile. *Am J Physiol* 248:G393-G397, 1985.

28. Kvietys PR, Gallavan RH, Chou CC: Contribution of bile to postprandial intestinal hyperemia. *Am J Physiol* 238:G284-G288, 1980.

29. Premen AJ, Kvietys PR, Granger DN: Postprandial regulation of intestinal blood flow: role of gastrointestinal hormones. *Am J Physiol* 249:G250-G255, 1985.

30. Chou CC, Siregar H: Role of histamine H_1 − and H_2 − receptors in postprandial intestinal circulation and oxygen consumption. *Acta Physiol Scan* 74(3–5):277–283, 1989.

31. Rozsa Z, Jacobson ED: Capsaicin-sensitive nerves are involved in bile-oleate induced intestinal hyperemia. *Am J Physiol* 256:G476-G481, 1989.

32. Proctor KG: Differential effects of cyclooxygenase inhibitors on absorptive hyperemia. *Am J Physiol* 249: H755-H762, 1985.

33. Furness JB, Costa M: Types of nerves in the enteric nervous system. *Neuroscience* 5:1–19, 1980.

34. Brooksby GA, Donald DE: Dynamic changes in splanchnic blood flow and blood volume in dogs during activation of sympathetic nerves. *Circ Res* 24(3):227–238, 1971.

35. Chen LQ, Shepard AP: Role of H^+ and alpha 2-receptors in escape from sympathetic vasoconstriction. *Am J Physiol* 261:H868-H873, 1991.

36. Chen LQ, Riedel GL, Shepard AP: Norepinephrine release during autoregulatory escape: effects of alpha 2-receptor blockade. *Am J Physiol* 260:H400-H408, 1991.

37. Biber B, Lundgren O, Svanik J: Studies on the intestinal vasodilatation observed after mechanical stimulation of the mucosa of the gut. *Acta Physiol Scan* 82:177–190, 1971.

38. Crissenger KD, Kvietys PR, Granger DN: Autoregulatory escape from norepinephrine infusion: roles of adenosine and histamine. *Am J Physiol* 254:G560-G565, 1988.

39. Shepard AP, Riedel GL: Intramural distribution of intestinal blood flow during sympathetic stimulation. *Am J Physiol* 255:H1091-H1095, 1988.

40. Kvietys PR, Granger DN: Vasoactive agents and splanchnic oxygen uptake. *Am J Physiol* 243:G1-G9, 1982.

41. Gunther S, Gimbrone MA, Alexander RW: Identification and characterization of the high affinity vascular angiotensin II receptor in rat mesenteric artery. *Circ Res* 47(2):278–286, 1980.

42. Suvannapura A, Levens NR: Local control of mesenteric blood flow by the renin-angiotensin system. *Am J Physiol* 255:G267-G274, 1988.

43. Patel A, Kaleya RN, Dammartano RJ: Pathophysiology of mesenteric ischemia. *Surg Clin North Am* 72(1): 31–41, 1992.

44. Clark ET, Gewertz BL: Glucagon potentiates intestinal reperfusion injury. *J Vasc Surg* 2:270–277, 1990.

45. Malago M, Noda S, Gewertz B: Role of neutrophils in low flow intestinal ischemia. *FASEB J* 6(5):5138, 1992.

46. Kehrer JP, Jones DP, Lemasters JJ, Farber JL, Jaeschke H: Mechanisms of hypoxic cell injury. *Toxicol Appl Pharmacol* 106:165–178, 1990.

47. Nieminen AL, Gores GJ, Wray BE, Tanaka Y, Herman B, Lemasters, JJ: Calcium dependence of bleb formation and cell death in hepatocytes. *Cell Calcium* 9:237–246, 1988.

48. Aw TY, Andersson BS, Jones DP: Suppression of mitochondrial respiratory function after short-term anoxia. *Am J Physiol* 252:C362-C368, 1987.

49. Lemasters JJ, DiGuiseppi J, Nieminen AL, Herman B: Blebbing free Ca^{++} and mitochondrial membrane potential preceding cell death in hepatocytes. *Nature* (London) 325:78–81, 1987.

50. Gores GJ, Nieminen AL, Fleishman KE, Dawson TL, Herman B, Lemasters JJ: Extracellular acidosis delays onset of cell death in ATP-depleted hepatocytes. *Am J Physiol* 255:C315-C322, 1988.

51. Currin RT, Gores GJ, Thurman RG, Lemaster JJ: Protection by acidic pH against anoxic injury in perfused rat liver: evidence for a "pH paradox". *FASEB J* 3: A626, 1989.

52. Raeder L, Siems W, Mueller M, Gerber G: Formation of activated oxygen in the hypoxic liver. *Cell Biochem Funct* 3:289–296, 1985.

53. Parks DA, Granger DN: Contributions of ischemia and reperfusion to mucosal lesion formation. *Am J Physiol* 250 (13):G749–753, 1986.

54. Clark ET, Gewertz BL: Intermittent ischemia potentiates intestinal reperfusion injury. *J Vasc Surg* 13: 601–606, 1991.

55. Grogaard B, Parks DA, Granger DN, McCord JN, Folsberg JO: Effects of ischemia and oxygen radicals on mucosal albumin clearance in intestine. *Am J Physiol* 242(5): G448–454, 1982.

56. Korthius RJ, Smith JK, Carden DL: Hypoxic reperfusion attenuates postischemic microvascular injury. *Am J Physiol* 256:H315, 1989.

57. Clark ET, Gewertz BL: Limiting oxygen delivery attenuates intestinal reperfusion injury. *Surg Res* 53:485–489, 1992.

58. Hernandez LA, Grisham MB, Granger DN: A role for iron in oxidant-mediated ischemic injury to intestinal microvasculature. *Am J Physiol* 253:649, 1987.

59. Zimmerman BJ, Granger DN: Reperfusion injury. *Surg Clin North Am* 72(1):65–83, 1992.

60. Parks DA, Granger DN: Ischemia induced vascular changes: role of xanthine oxidase and hydroxyl radicals. *Am J Physiol* 245:G285–289, 1983.

61. Parks DA, Granger DN, Bulkley GB: Soybean trypsin inhibitor attenuates ischemic injury to the feline small intestine. *Gastroenterology* 89:6, 1985.

62. Dahinden CA, Fehr J, Hugli T: Role of cell surface contact in the kinetics of superoxide production by granulocytes. *J Clin Invest* 72:113–121, 1983.

63. Klebanoff SJ: Oxygen metabolism and the toxic properties of phagocytes. *Ann Intern Med* 93:480–489, 1980.

64. Mishra OP, Delivoria Papadopoulos M, Cahillane G, Wagerle LC: Lipid peroxidation as the mechanism of modification of the affinity of the Na^+, K^+-ATPase active sites for ATP, K^+, Na^+, and strophanthidin in vitro. *Neurochem Res* 14(9):845–851, 1989.

65. Grisham MB, Jefferson MM, Melton DF, Thomas EL: Chlorination of endogenous amines by isolated neutrophils: ammonia-dependent bactericidal, cytotoxic, and cytolytic activities of the chloramines. *J Biol Chem* 259: 10404–10413, 1984.

66. Granger DN, Hernandez LA, Grisham MB: Reactive oxygen metabolites: mediators of cell injury in the digestive system. *Viewpoints Dig Dis* 18:13, 1986.

67. Freeman BA, Crapo JD: Biology of disease: free radicals and tissue injury. *Lab Invest* 47:412–426, 1982.

68. Klebanoff SJ: The iron-H_2O_2-iodide cytotoxic system. *J Exp Med* 156:1262–1267, 1982.

69. Hernandez LA, Grisham MB, Twohig B: Role of neutrophils in ischemia-reperfusion-induced microvascular injury. *Am J Physiol* 253:H699, 1987.

70. Zimmerman BJ, Grisham MB, Granger DN: Role of oxidants in ischemia/reperfusion-induced granulocyte infiltration. *Am J Physiol* 258:G185, 1990.

71. Suzuki M, Inauen W, Kvietys PR: Superoxide mediates reperfusion induced leukocyte endothelial cell interaction. *Am J Physiol* 257:H1740, 1989.

72. Kubes P, Suzuki M, Granger DN: Platelet-activating factor-induced microvascular dysfunction: role of adherent leukocytes. *Am J Physiol* 258(21):G158, 1990.

73. Otamiri T, Lindahl M, Tagesson C: Phospholipase A_2 inhibition prevents mucosal damage associated with small intestinal ischemia in rats. *Gut* 29:489, 1988.

74. Zimmerman BJ, Granger DN: Reperfusion-induced leukocyte infiltration: role of elastase. *Am J Physiol* 259: H390-H394, 1990.

75. Benton LD, Khan BA, Greco RS: Integrins, adhesion molecules, and surgical research. *Surg Gynecol Obstet* 177:311–327, 1993.

76. McEver RP: Selectins: novel receptors that mediate leukocyte adhesion during inflammation. *Thromb Haemost* 65:223–228, 1991.

77. Bochner BS, Luscinskas FW, Schleimer RP, et al: Adhesion of human basophils, eosinophils, and neutrophils to interluekin-1-activated human vascular endothelial cells: contributions of endothelial cell adhesion molecules. *J Exp Med* 173:1553–1556, 1991.

78. Edjana E, Breviario F, Mantovani A, et al: Modulation of endothelial cell functions by different molecular species of interleukin-1. *Blood* 69(2):695–699, 1987.

79. Dinarello CA: Interleukin-1 and interleukin-1 antagonism. *Blood* 77(8):1627–1652, 1991.

80. Dudeja PK, Brasitus TA: Inactivation of rat small intestinal brush-border membrane alkaline phosphatase by oxygen free radicals. *Gastroenterology* 105 357–366, 1993.

81. Sisley AC, Gewertz BL, Harig J: Membrane transport in assessment of intestinal ischemia. *Physiologist* 35:A-24, 1992.

82. Sisley AC, Harig JM, Gewertz BL: Neutrophil depletion attentuates human intestinal reperfusion injury. *J Surg Res* 192–196, 1994.

83. Sisley AC, Gewertz BL: Alkaline phosphatase in the human enterocyte is a specific marker of reperfusion injury. *FASEB J* 7(3):A658, 1993.

CHAPTER 31

Hemodynamic Basis of Portal Hypertension

Richard J. Gusberg, MD

Introduction

What is Portal Hypertension?

The liver is a complex organ with varied metabolic functions and a dual blood supply. Under normal conditions, the liver receives about 25% of the cardiac output. Portal flow accounts for about two thirds of the total hepatic blood flow and 50% of the oxygen supply; the balance of blood and oxygen are supplied by the hepatic artery. The pressure in the portal vein is 2 to 6 mm Hg; the pressure in the hepatic artery is systemic. In this context, hepatic physiology and function are closely linked to both splanchnic and systemic hemodynamics. While the high oxygen demand of the metabolically active liver renders it particularly sensitive to oxygen deprivation, structural changes within the liver can secondarily affect the way in which blood and oxygen are delivered to the hepatocytes. When such structural changes result in increased resistance to portal flow, portal hypertension develops.

Portal hypertension is a common and lethal complication of chronic, progressive liver disease. The fibrosis associated with cirrhosis results in increased intrahepatic resistance and can produce profound splanchnic and systemic hemodynamic abnormalities. As the portal pressure increases, portal-systemic collaterals develop, provide partial decompression, and exert a major influence on the splanchnic vascular response to portal hypertension. This collateralization underlies the development of the two most significant complications of portal hypertension: hemorrhage from gastroesophageal varices, and portal-systemic encephalopathy. Furthermore, portal hypertension is accompanied by a hyperdynamic circulatory state characterized by an increase in both regional and systemic blood flows, intestinal and peripheral vasodilatation, and a decrease in arterial pressure. This high output-low resistance state is the systemic context in which the regional complications of portal hypertension develop.

Since the portal venous system has no valves, pressures in the portal vein and the varices are usually equivalent.[1] At 12 mm Hg portal pressure, varices develop and this represents the threshold above which they bleed. There is, however, no correlation between the severity of portal hypertension and either variceal size or the initial risk of hemorrhage[2,3]; however, the degree of pressure elevation appears predictive of recurrent bleeding.[4] This latter correlation exists for both late and early recurrent hemorrhage.[5]

What Are Varices and Why Do They Bleed?

Varices are thought to develop when elevated portal venous pressure increases the wall stress and causes an expansion of the venous bed. Juhl et al studied the effects of partial portal vein stenosis (in a rabbit) on the mechanical and morphologic characteristics of the esophageal and mesenteric veins.[6] The elevated portal pressure appeared to be a primary determinant of media thickness, but not of lumen diameter. Isolated reduction in esophageal venous flow reduced the

From *The Basic Science of Vascular Disease.* Edited by Sidawy AN, Sumpio BE, and DePalma RG. Armonk, NY: Futura Publishing Company, Inc.; © 1997.

lumen diameter of the varices. Changes in vascular morphology have been shown in other systems to be flow-related. As portal-systemic collaterals develop in response to changes in intra- and extrahepatic resistance, the size and development of gastroesophageal varices appear to be the consequence of increases in both portal pressure and azygous blood flow.

While the presence of collaterals and varices are the consequence of elevated portal pressure, the factors that predispose to variceal hemorrhage remain ill defined. Since only about one third of portal hypertensive patients with documented varices ever bleed from them, defining and controlling the risk factors should have important implications for the prophylactic and overall management of these patients. Garcia-Tsao et al, using hepatic vein catheterization to study 93 alcoholic cirrhotics with variceal hemorrhage, found several factors that correlated with the occurrence of bleeding: 1) a wedged hepatic vein pressure gradient (HVPG)—an accurate reflection of corrected sinusoidal pressure and portal pressure in alcoholic cirrhosis—of 12 mm Hg; 2) the HVPG was significantly higher in those who bled than in those who did not; 3) large varices were more likely to bleed than small ones (even with equivalent HVPGs, consistent with the law of Laplace).[7]

In studies using latex tubes of various diameters and thicknesses, distended with increasing pressure until rupture occurred, Polio and Groszmann concluded that thin-walled, large diameter varices are mostly likely to rupture and thick-walled, small diameter varices are the least likely.[3]

It appears that multiple hemodynamic and morphologic factors (pressure, flow, diameter, wall thickness) contribute to both the development of varices and the risk of variceal rupture with hemorrhage in patients with portal hypertension. Further studies are needed to define the conditions that promote these hemodynamic and morphologic changes.

What Characterizes the Portal-Systemic Collaterals?

An extensive network of portal-systemic collaterals develops, presumably, in a decompressive response to the hypertensive portal circulation. While the vascular resistance of the portal hypertensive collateral bed is higher than the portal resistance associated with a normal liver, it is lower than that of the portal hypertensive cirrhotic liver.[8,9] Despite the importance of this collateral network in defining the hemodynamic and clinical consequences of portal hypertension, the factors that initiate and modulate its development are poorly understood. It is known that this marked collateral development results in a pro-

gressive decrease in prograde portal flow, depriving the liver of both oxygen and splanchnic-derived hepatotrophic humoral factors. In fact, these collaterals may carry most of the portal flow[10] and exert a dominant influence on splanchnic and systemic hemodynamics.

These portal-systemic collaterals have been clearly identified and well described in both animal models and humans. Most studies that have attempted to elucidate the pharmacologic and mechanical characteristics of the portal system have been indirect and inconclusive. There has been little direct information regarding the terminal collateral venules. Are these collaterals a reflection of new vessel formation, or the opening of preexisting vascular channels? What might be the role of this large population of endothelial cells in modulating collateral progression and flow?

A number of studies have focused on the humoral control and hemodynamic characteristics of this collateral bed. Using an in situ portal-systemic collateral perfusion model developed in portal hypertensive rats, Mosca et al studied the hemodynamic stages of collateral development, the vascular reactivity to naturally occurring vasoconstrictors, and the possible regulatory role of nitric oxide (NO).[11]

Recent work has attempted to clarify the factors that modulate the development and progression of the portal-systemic collaterals. The rapid dilatation of this vascular bed appears to be both a passive response to the increased pressure, as well as a response to other humoral and hemodynamic stimuli. The identification of these factors and the elucidation of their role would enhance the understanding of the hemodynamic context in which portal hypertension develops and is maintained. Such an understanding should also form a more rational basis for the treatment of the complications of portal hypertension.

Chapter Objectives

In this chapter, the recent advances in portal hypertension research are described in the context of their clinical implications. The research reviewed focuses on intrahepatic and extrahepatic events, and splanchnic and systemic responses. In studies that range from human to animal to molecular, significant recent progress has been made in elucidating the pathophysiology and complications of portal hypertension. These studies have begun to define the broad spectrum of responses that characterize the portal hypertensive state:

1. Intrahepatic structural changes and their hemodynamic consequences.
2. Extrahepatic hemodynamic changes (splanchnic and systemic):

a) The development and control of portal-systemic collaterals (including the gastroesophageal varices).

b) The "hyperdynamic state" (including the roles of vasodilators, vasoconstrictor inhibition, and plasma volume expansion).

c) Flow relationships between the hepatic artery and portal vein.

3. The effect of the hypertensive and "hyperdynamic" splanchnic system on both the liver and other organs (e.g., heart and gastrointestinal tract); the response to hemorrhage.

4. Overview: pathophysiology, clinical implications.

The Questions

Research in portal hypertension has focused primarily on the associated morphologic and hemodynamic derangements: what intrahepatic and extrahepatic events, particularly in patients with cirrhosis, predispose to the development of portal hypertension and gastroesophageal varices? What are the systemic and splanchnic hemodynamic manifestations of portal hypertension? What is the role of collateralization in decompressing the hypertensive portal system and what controls it? What are the relative influences of resistance and inflow in initiating and sustaining the portal hypertensive state? What characterizes and modulates the hyperdynamic circulation? What are the implications of these hemodynamic alterations relative to both treatment alternatives and prognosis?

In this chapter, we review the advances in research that have provided some answers to these questions.

Portal Hypertension and Variceal Bleeding

Pathophysiologic Overview

Resistance

Portal pressure, like all pressure, is generated by an interaction between flow and resistance. Pressure changes occur in direct proportion to changes in flow or resistance. The factors that define resistance (described by Poiseuille's law) are viscosity, vessel length, and vessel radius.

Under normal conditions, the liver is the primary source of resistance to portal flow. Intrahepatic resistance is normally low; in this setting, large increases in splanchnic blood flow result in little change in portal pressure. As cirrhosis progressively disrupts the nor-

mal hepatic architecture, however, changes in intrahepatic resistance are presumed to follow.[12] Early pathologic observations suggested that the diffuse hepatic fibrosis seen in cirrhosis was associated with constriction of the intrahepatic venous vasculature causing increased portal vascular resistance and portal hypertension.[12,13] Subsequent studies focused on intrahepatic vascular compression by regenerating nodules.[14,15] Since the hepatic venules are considered more vulnerable to extrinsic compression than the portal tributaries, the primary site of increased portal vascular resistance has been thought to be postsinusoidal.[16] While this concept may be valid in alcoholic cirrhosis, it cannot fully explain the increased resistance and portal hypertension associated with presinusoidal obstructive lesions and noncirrhotic liver disease.

Several studies have attempted to define more specifically the relationship between hepatic ultrastructural morphologic changes and portal hemodynamics. Collagen deposition within the space of Disse[17] has been postulated as a cause of sinusoidal compression and increased portal vascular resistance; in alcoholics, the degree of collagenization has been correlated with sinusoidal and portal pressure elevation.[18]

Progressive fibrosis, as well as inflammatory and occlusive changes affecting the hepatic veins, has been described in alcoholics with and without cirrhosis, and these changes have been reported to correlate with the degree of portal hypertension.[19,20]

Several other factors may contribute to increased intrahepatic resistance in cirrhosis associated with portal hypertension: 1) sympathetic venous tone has been shown to modulate portal pressure; and clonidine, an inhibitor of sympathetic activity, causes a specific decrease in portal pressure that is independent of systemic hemodynamic changes[21]; 2) myofibroblast proliferation adjacent to sinusoids and terminal hepatic venules in cirrhosis appears to correlate with vascular resistance, with the enhanced contractile state associated with an increase in both resistance and portal pressure[21]; 3) hepatocyte enlargement, a response to a variety of toxic and metabolic hepatic insults, could lead to sinusoidal compression with a secondary increase in intrahepatic resistance and portal hypertension.[22]

While the resistance changes associated with portal hypertension are incompletely defined, it is clear that the sites and mechanisms of the increase in intrahepatic resistance are diverse. It is also clear that the source of the increased resistance to portal flow in cirrhotic portal hypertension may be prehepatic as well as intrahepatic. Recent studies have suggested that the maintenance of portal hypertension depends as well on an increased resistance in the portal-systemic collateral network.[23,24]

What Are the Relative Roles of Resistance and Flow Changes?

In essence, the initiation and maintenance of portal hypertension associated with cirrhosis is a result of the cumulative effects of the resistance and flow changes, both intra- and extrahepatic, that characterize patients with chronic, progressive liver disease. Controversy persists regarding the relative contributions to the elevated portal pressure of increased portal venous resistance and the increased splanchnic blood flow. Two theories have framed this controversy: the "backward flow" and "forward flow" theories.

The "backward flow" theory is supported by evidence suggesting that portal hypertension is initiated and sustained by an increased resistance to portal flow that results from morphologic and hemodynamic changes within the liver and the collateral circulation. While decreased portal flow has been reported in patients with portal hypertension, most portal hypertensive patients have increased portal flow and an extensive network of relatively low-resistance, portal-systemic collaterals that incompletely decompress the portal system.

The maintenance of the portal hypertensive state appears to be best explained by the "forward flow" theory, with its emphasis on increased splanchnic blood flow. Much of the current investigation of the hemodynamics of portal hypertension has focused on the elucidation of this "hyperdynamic state."

What Is the Hyperdynamic Circulation?

The hyperdynamic circulation associated with portal hypertension is characterized by increased cardiac output, decreased peripheral resistance, and increased splanchnic blood flow. While the initiation of the portal pressure increase appears to be the consequence of an increase in resistance, the maintenance of portal hypertension is assumed to be dependent on the hyperdynamic state. In this forward flow theory, supported by observations in both animal models and portal hypertensive patients, there is peripheral vasodilatation and splanchnic hyperemia.[8,25,26]

While the hyperdynamic systemic circulation associated with cirrhosis has been recognized for some time, the associated splanchnic hemodynamic alterations have only recently been elucidated. Because of challenges posed by studying portal hypertension in humans, most of the current understanding of this dynamic and complex state has come from questions addressed in animal models. The most widely studied and hemodynamically relevant animal model is the rat with a high-grade portal vein stenosis.[25] In this model, a tightly constricting tie is placed around the main portal vein and the manifestations of portal hypertension are apparent within 24 hours and are well developed by 72 hours. Also, the acute and chronic changes in splanchnic and systemic hemodynamics have been characterized using radioactive microsphere techniques.[27] The portal hypertensive rats have greater than 95% portal-systemic shunting with a 60% increase in portal venous inflow, a 50% decrease in splanchnic arteriolar resistance, a 50% elevation in cardiac index, and a 60% decrease in total peripheral resistance. Blood flow to the extrasplanchnic organs (other than the kidneys in which blood flows increase by 40%) insignificantly changes. Similar findings have been confirmed in rats with carbon tetrachloride cirrhosis[28] and dogs with biliary cirrhosis.[29]

In the immediate changes seen following portal vein constriction in the rat model, portal hypertension appears to develop primarily as a consequence of increased resistance. As portal resistance and portal pressure rise, portal venous inflow falls. By the eighth day, however, significant hemodynamic changes have occurred with the development of widespread portal-systemic shunting, a decrease in portal resistance, and an increase in portal flow.[26] In this model (and perhaps relevant to the portal hypertension that accompanies human cirrhosis), the portal pressure rise appears to be initiated by an increase in resistance, while the portal hypertension is maintained by a subsequent increase in portal venous flow. This high-flow splanchnic circulation, with its regional and systemic correlates, characterizes the "hyperdynamic state."

Hyperdynamic State: What Are the Pathophysiologic Mechanisms?

Two mechanisms have been proposed to explain the hyperdynamic circulation associated with chronic portal hypertension: 1) an increase in circulating vasodilators; and 2) a reduced responsiveness to endogenous vasoconstrictors.[30] In addition, an expanded plasma volume has been postulated as an important precondition for the expression and maintenance of this state.

Vasodilators: The Role of Glucagon

In cross-perfusion studies done in control and portal hypertensive rats, Groszmann and Atterbury demonstrated a role for circulating humoral factors in the splanchnic hyperemia.[31] The endogenous source of these splanchnic-derived vasoactive substances is presumed to be either the small intestine or the endothelial cells of the mesenteric or portal vasculature. Increased levels of circulating vasodilators might result from both extensive portal-system shunting as well as reduced hepatic elimination. In this context, a variety of agents have been investigated.

Using the portal vein constricted rat model, Benoit et al developed an in situ, blood-perfused, small intestinal preparation to characterize the hemodynamic effects of portal hypertension[32] and the role of neural, metabolic, and humoral factors in modulating the hyperemic response. The vagus nerves, responsible for some vasodilator reflexes of intestinal origin, appeared to exert no controlling influence; the hyperemia was unaltered following their transection.

Is the hyperemic response a reflection of the release of vasodilators generated by metabolically active tissues? In the portal hypertensive rats, there was no increase in intestinal oxygen consumption, making it unlikely that local metabolic factors produce the hyperemia associated with chronic portal hypertension.

Increased circulating levels of glucagon, known to be a potent vasodilator in the intestine and kidney, have been reported in humans and animals with cirrhosis.[33,34] These studies have documented an increased pancreatic secretion of glucagon in patients with cirrhosis, perhaps promoted by the extensive portal-systemic shunting. Furthermore, portacaval shunts done in normal animals produce changes in splanchnic hemodynamics similar to those seen in chronic portal hypertension. This suggests that splanchnic-derived vasodilators, normally metabolized by the liver, accumulate in the systemic circulation as they escape first pass hepatic degradation. Since the portal-vein constricted portal hypertensive rat has greater than 90% portal-systemic shunting, it seems likely that plasma glucagon levels would be elevated in these animals and might significantly affect systemic and splanchnic hemodynamics. In this model, plasma glucagon levels are three times controls. In studies in which the intestine of normal rats was cross-perfused with arterial blood from portal hypertensive rats (achieving plasma glucagon levels comparable to those detected in donor blood), the total vascular resistance fell by about 20%. Based on these observations, Benoit et al concluded that the vasoactivity associated with the elevated plasma glucagon levels accounted for a significant proportion of the decreased mesenteric vascular resistance produced by portal vein constriction.[32]

The role of glucagon as a mediator of the splanchnic hyperemia has been supported further by studies in which highly specific glucagon antiserum was administered to portal hypertensive (portal vein stenosed) rats.[35] Regional blood flows were measured using radioactive microspheres and the reference-sample method. While the glucagon antiserum had no significant effect on the gastrointestinal blood flow of controlled rats, portal venous blood flow was reduced by approximately 30% in the portal hypertensive rats. Based on these observations, it was proposed that the elevated circulating level of plasma glucagon, seen in portal hypertensive patients, accounts for about one third of the splanchnic hyperemia and is, therefore, partly responsible for the maintenance of portal hypertension.

Silva et al studied the hemodynamic effects of glucagon in portal hypertensive and control subjects.[36] Patients with cirrhosis and portal hypertension had significantly higher plasma glucagon levels than noncirrhotic controls and demonstrated a decreased hemodynamic response to glucose administration. Despite the blunted response to glucose, there were significant increases in both portal pressure and azygous blood flow (a reflection of portal-systemic collateral flow), findings consistent with a glucagon-modulated contribution to both the splanchnic vasodilatation and the elevated portal pressure seen in cirrhosis.

The resistance to the systemic effects of glucagon suggests a down-regulation of vascular glucagon receptors in these patients. The exact mechanisms by which glucagon exerts its effects on the splanchnic circulation have, however, been incompletely defined. In part, the increase in portal blood flow can be explained by its known direct stimulation of precapillary vasodilatation.[37] In addition, this splanchnic vasodilatation could be a reflection of a glucagon promoted vascular unresponsiveness to circulating vasoconstrictors.[38,39]

Hyperdynamic State: What Defines the Decreased Vasoconstrictor Response and the Role of Vasodilators?

In normal and portal hypertensive (portal vein constriction) rats, Joh et al studied the intestinal microvascular sensitivity to norepinephrine.[40] Using a video microscope, the diameters of first, second, or third order arterioles and the arteriolar erythrocyte velocity were measured and arteriolar blood flow was calculated. Dose response curves were constructed relating the change in arteriolar diameter and blood flow to norepinephrine concentration. In this prehepatic, chronic portal hypertensive model, there was a loss of vascular responsiveness to norepinephrine localized to the terminal-most arterioles of the intestinal submucosa.

Although this altered vascular response to vasoconstrictors appears to be well documented, its molecular basis is poorly understood. While down-regulation of receptors has been a postulated mechanism,[41] this theory cannot account for the site-specific decrease in splanchnic vascular responsiveness identified in portal hypertension. Faber[42] has documented differences in adrenergic receptor populations between large and small arterioles in skeletal muscle; the site-specific reduction in α adrenergic responsiveness in the portal hypertensive splanchnic circulation could reflect a selective inactivation of the α 2-receptors on the arteriolar smooth muscle cells (SMCs).

Alternatively, hemodynamic factors might promote this altered vasoconstrictor responsiveness. Tesfamarian and Cohen[43] noted an inhibition of adrenergic vasoconstriction in response to endothelial shear stress in isolated rabbit carotid arteries. They suggested that endothelial-derived relaxants mediated this reduced responsiveness. While Joh et al were unable to confirm increased shear rates in the splanchnic circulation of portal hypertension rats,[40] the role of the endothelium and its mechanoreceptors in modulating the hyperdynamic circulation in portal hypertension merits clarification.

A third possible explanation for the impaired vasoconstrictor response lies in the role of elevated circulating vasodilators. Pizcueta et al, studying portal hypertensive and normotensive hyperglucagonemic rats, found comparably impaired vascular sensitivity to norepinephrine in both groups. They linked the elevated circulating vasodilators to the decreased vasoconstrictor response, and suggested that glucagon played a significant mediating role in the hyperdynamic, portal hypertension state.[44] Furthermore, microcirculation studies in portal hypertensive rats confirmed a glucagon-induced attenuation of the vasoconstrictor response in the terminal arterioles.[40]

While glucagon levels are clearly elevated in cirrhotic portal hypertension, with convincing evidence linking this elevated circulating vasodilator to the impaired vasoconstrictor response, the hemodynamic alterations in the hypertensive splanchnic circulation may well represent a nonspecific response to a variety of endogenous vasodilators. Glucagon is known to induce vasodilatation via adenosine 3',5'-cyclic monophosphate-mediated events. Other substances, however, with different mechanisms of action (i.e., nitroprusside) have been shown to mimic glucose-induced vasodilatation and lend support to the view that a variety of vasodilators may be important mediators of the hemodynamic changes observed in chronic portal hypertension.

In studies done in portal hypertensive rabbits, Wu et al evaluated the role of the prostaglandin system in ameliorating the splanchnic vascular response to an angiotensin II (AII) infusion. Using a Doppler flow probe to measure superior mesenteric artery and systemic resistance, they studied normal and portal hypertensive rabbits after cyclooxygenase blockade and during continuous prostacyclin infusion. The normal, expected AII-induced increase in mesenteric resistance was blunted in the portal hypertensive animals.[45] This could be explained by either a decrease in AII receptors or the competitive influence of elevated circulating vasodilators. Prostacyclin, a potent mesen-

teric vasodilator, has been shown to be elevated in the portal blood of portal hypertensive rabbits, and cyclooxygenase blockade can decrease the portal pressure.[46,47] Wu et al demonstrated that prostacyclin will directly decrease the normal splanchnic response to AII and that cyclooxygenase blockade will dramatically improve the blunted response to AII seen in the portal hypertensive rabbits.[45] In this model, prostacyclin appeared to mediate the altered vasoconstrictor response, further supporting the modulating role of circulating vasodilators.

The role of prostaglandins in the hyperdynamic circulation of portal hypertension has also been studied in patients with cirrhosis of the liver.[48] Bruix et al found that prostaglandin inhibition with indomethacin resulted in an amelioration of the hyperdynamic state by significantly reducing cardiac output, increasing peripheral vascular resistance, and decreasing both hepatic blood flow and portal pressure. Their results suggested that endogenous prostaglandins contribute to both the splanchnic and systemic hemodynamic changes that characterize these patients. Prior studies in animals, demonstrating splanchnic vasoconstriction in response to prostaglandin inhibition by indomethacin,[49] lend further support to the vasoactive role of prostanoids in cirrhosis.

Adenosine, a vasoactive purine nucleoside, has also been implicated as a potential modulator of portal hypertensive hemodynamics. The data are, however, conflicting. Adenosine is known to regulate microcirculatory blood flow by interacting with purine receptors to elicit vascular smooth muscle relaxation or to attenuate catecholamine-induced vasoconstriction.[50,51] Enhanced adenosine triphosphate (ATP) degradation, resulting in adenosine release, occurs in association with tissue hypoxia when oxygen demand exceeds supply. In alcoholic liver disease, increased adenosine release might result from ATP degradation associated with mitochondrial damage.[52,53] It has been proposed that hepatocellular injury with the release of adenosine could contribute to the increased splanchnic and systemic vasodilatation observed in portal hypertension. In contrast, MacMathuna et al, studying patients with alcoholic liver disease, used adenosine receptor blockade by theophylline to assess the effect of adenosine on splanchnic and systemic hemodynamics. Based on their observations, they concluded that, while adenosine might enhance systemic vasodilatation in cirrhosis, it appeared to have no effect on splanchnic vasoreactivity or portal pressure.[54]

Serum bile acids, elevated in portal hypertension and known to have vasodilator properties, have been postulated as mediators of the hyperdynamic circulation. Genecin et al, studying portal hypertensive rats gavaged with bile acid-lowering cholestyramine, found no amelioration of the hyperdynamic state. They concluded that bile acids were elevated because of the extensive portal-systemic shunting, but exerted no hemodynamic influence on the hyperdynamic state.[55]

The hemodynamic alterations, now well characterized in both animal models and humans with chronic portal hypertension, appear to be the consequence of both increased circulating vasodilators and decreased responsiveness to endogenous vasoconstrictors. These changes clearly affect both the systemic and splanchnic circulations.

What Is the Role of the Sympathetic Nervous System?

Sympathetic nervous activity, as reflected by plasma catecholamines, increases with the progression of liver disease.[56] Despite these raised catecholamine levels, however, reduced vascular reactivity to vasoconstrictors has been observed repeatedly in both portal hypertensive animals and patients with cirrhosis. Despite these observations, the precise role of the sympathetic nervous system in the pathogenesis of the hyperdynamic circulation is uncertain. Abergel et al, attempting to clarify this role, studied rats with portal hypertension, with and without associated cirrhosis, in which all neurologic control was eliminated by pithing.[57] Whereas the hyperdynamic circulation reverted toward normal in the pithed portal hypertensive noncirrhotic rats, the hyperdynamic circulation persisted in the cirrhotic rats following removal of the sympathetic nervous system. Pithing reduced portal pressure in both groups. While sympathetic activity is clearly relevant to the hemodynamic changes seen in portal hypertension, nonneurogenic factors exert significant control. Clearly, the pathogenesis of arterial vasodilatation in chronic liver disease is multifactorial.

Nitric Oxide

The splanchnic vascular bed, site of the major portal hemodynamic alterations, includes a large population of endothelial cells. As recent investigation has emphasized the biologic activity of these cells, attention has focused on the vasoactive role of a variety of endothelial-produced substances.

In attempting to define the factors that modulate the hyperdynamic, hypertensive portal circulation (and the inhibition of the vasoconstrictor response), recent studies have addressed the role of endothelium-derived relaxing factor (EDRF) including NO. EDRF has recently been shown to cause relaxation of isolated blood vessels[58] and NO accounts for most of its biologic activity.[59] Furthermore, EDRF inhibition has been shown to augment vasoconstrictor activity in both large vessels[60] and arterioles.[61]

NO is synthesized from the guanidine nitrogen of L-arginine and molecular oxygen; this synthesis can be inhibited by L-arginine analogs such as NG-monomethyl L-arginine.[62] NO is produced in endothelial cells (as well as macrophages and neutrophils) by NO synthases. There are two types of NO synthases: the constitutive form that accounts for a rapid, transient calcium-dependent production of EDRF/NO by the endothelial cells (in response to a variety of physiologic stimuli); and the inducible form, associated with the slow onset of calcium-independent NO synthesis in inflammatory cells (in response to bacterial endotoxins and cytokines, including those in endothelial cells and hepatocytes).[59,62]

In animals, agonist-induced NO release from vascular endothelium causes peripheral vasodilatation, a drop in blood pressure, and tachycardia.[117,118] These effects are, however, short-lived. Porcine aortic endothelial cells in culture have been found to express a second, inducible long-acting NO synthase similar to the inducible enzyme found in activated macrophages.[119] Incubation of vascular rings with endotoxin or cytokines results in induction of NO synthase in both endothelial and SMCs and leads to both vasorelaxation and attenuated vasoconstrictor responsiveness.[120]

In this context, Lee et al studied the role of NO in mediating the hyporesponsiveness to vasoconstrictors in portal hypertension. In studies done in the partial portal vein ligated rat model, they constructed dose-response curves to methoxamine, an α adrenoceptor antagonist, with and without N-nitro-L-arginine (NNA), a specific inhibitor of NO synthesis.[63] They demonstrated a decreased vascular responsiveness to methoxamine in portal hypertensive rats which was reversed by blockade of NO. Since NNA has no direct effect on vascular smooth muscle, NNA-stimulated vasoconstriction appears to be the result of its inhibition of NO synthesis. These data support an important role for NO in mediating the arterial vasodilatation associated with portal hypertension.

In studies using a model of in vitro perfused mesenteric resistance vessels in portal hypertensive (portal vein ligated) rats, Sieber and Groszmann demonstrated vascular hyporesponsiveness to norepinephrine, arginine vasopressin, and potassium chloride.[64] This hyporesponsiveness was receptor-independent, unaffected by circulating vasodilators, and reversed by NO synthesis blockade. They postulated that locally-released NO, exerting its vasodilator effect, mediated the reduced vascular response to methoxamine in portal hypertensive rats.[65] Since NO acts only locally,[66] the possibility that NO might exert both a regional and systemic influence on the vasodilatation in portal hypertension implies a widespread induction of NO synthase in patients with chronic liver disease. While further clarifying research is required, its production and vasodilatory effect would appear to exert an important influence on vascular tone in both portal and extraportal vascular tissues.

Iwata et al, attempting to further define the mediating role of NO, used NNA to block the action of endogenous NO in portal vein stenosed rats. In contrast to Sieber and Groszmann, they concluded that NO played an unimportant role in the hemodynamic circulation associated with portal hypertension.[67] In their studies, NNA significantly reduced splanchnic blood flow in both normal and portal hypertensive rats, and the percent reduction of portal venous inflow following NNA administration was lower in the portal hypertensive than in the control rats. In this model, however, the portal vein stenosed rats remained moderately hyperdynamic, despite what appeared to be potent NO blockade.

Pizcueta, in studies that confirmed Sieber's observations, found that competitive inhibition of NO synthase by NG-monomethyl-L-arginine (NMMA) resulted in amelioration of the hyperdynamic portal hypertensive circulation by normalizing arterial blood pressure, cardiac output, and both splanchnic and peripheral resistances.[44] NMMA-induced splanchnic vasoconstriction resulted in decreased portal venous inflow but no significant reduction in portal pressure, seeming to reflect the relevance of both arterial vasoconstriction and venoconstriction in the extensive portal-systemic collateral circulation. Furthermore, when NMMA-treated portal hypertensive rats were pretreated with arginine (the precursor of NO) these effects of NMMA were reversed, supporting the role of NO in the development of the hemodynamic changes.

Based on present evidence, NO appears to play a significant modulating role in the hemodynamic changes of portal hypertension. Whether the vasoactivity of NO in this setting reflects enhanced synthesis, decreased metabolism, or increased vascular sensitivity to this potent vasodilator is not yet known.

It has been postulated that endotoxemia in cirrhosis, produced as a consequence of portal-systemic shunting and decreased clearance by hepatic macrophages, could provide a continuous stimulus for NO synthase induction in endothelial cells, vascular smooth muscle, lung, and liver.[68] High circulating levels of endotoxin have been found in cirrhotic patients with and without clinical evidence of infection.[121] Vallance and Moncada have proposed that this endotoxemia induces NO synthase either directly or indirectly (via cytokines), and that the increased NO synthesis and release mediates the hyperdynamic circulation.[122] This postulated increase in enzyme activity has not, however, been confirmed. Furthermore, while the

splanchnic response to NO in chronic liver disease might have a deleterious effect, the NO influence on basal vascular tone may be important in sustaining normal perfusion in extrasplanchnic vascular beds.

What Is the Relationship of Plasma Volume to the Hyperdynamic Circulation?

While vasodilatation underlies the splanchnic and systemic hemodynamic changes seen in portal hypertension, the role of plasma volume expansion has been less well studied. In both humans and animals, vasodilators reduce vascular resistance, while causing an increased vascular capacitance and relative hypovolemia. This results in either a decrease or no change in cardiac output. Patients with chronic liver disease and portal hypertension generally have an expanded plasma volume. In the portal vein stenosis rat model, Genecin et al examined the role of plasma volume expansion in the development of the hyperdynamic circulation.[69] They found that sodium restriction prevented the plasma volume expansion in the portal hypertensive rats, and resulted in a significant amelioration of the hyperdynamic circulation by reducing both splanchnic and systemic blood flows. The decrease in splanchnic flow caused a marked drop in portal pressure, emphasizing the importance of the hyperdynamic state in maintaining the portal hypertension.

To define the temporal relationships between these volume and hemodynamic changes, Colombato et al sequentially measured volume and hemodynamic parameters from Day 1 to Day 4 following partial portal vein ligation in rats. Peripheral vasodilatation was the initial hemodynamic change in the development of the hyperdynamic circulation and preceded plasma volume expansion.[70] In this model, peripheral vasodilatation develops without an increase in cardiac output. Once the plasma volume expands, splanchnic blood flow and cardiac output increase.

Based on these observations, it would appear that an expanded plasma volume may be an important precondition for the development of the hyperdynamic circulation and the maintenance of the portal hypertension.

What Are the Normal Regulatory Factors in the Hepatic-Portal Circulation?

What Is the Impact of Cirrhosis and Portal Hypertension?

Hepatic perfusion is regulated primarily by changes in resistance: hepatic arterial vascular resistance which regulates hepatic arterial flow; the resistance of the preportal vascular bed which determines inflow into the portal veins; and the intrahepatic portal vascular resistance. The regulation of and relative resistances to hepatic arterial and portal venous flow determine total hepatic blood flow and the nutrient and oxygen supply to the liver. The hemodynamic interrelationships between the portal venous and hepatic arterial beds may have significant implications with regard to both hepatic perfusion and prognosis in patients with altered portal-hepatic hemodynamics.

Under normal conditions, the high pressure, well-oxygenated arterial blood mixes within the hepatic sinusoids with the lower pressure, less well-oxygenated, nutrient-rich portal blood. In addition to the obvious relevance of hepatic blood flow to splanchnic hemodynamics, this high volume-high flow hepatic circulation, receiving about 25% of the cardiac output, plays a central role in cardiovascular homeostasis.

Microcirculation

The microvascular unit of the liver is the acinus, which represents a cluster of parenchymal cells oriented around terminal branches of the hepatic arteriole and portal venule.[71] The one-way sinusoidal flow precludes any direct influence in the regulation of hepatic arterial resistance from humoral factors in the venous drainage from the hepatic parenchyma. In this context, hepatocytes are incapable of regulating hepatic artery flow in response to metabolic requirements.

Microsphere injection studies have confirmed the uniform distribution within the liver of portal and arterial blood flow.[72] Neither increased venous pressure, decreased portal flow, nor increased resistance (by norepinephrine infusion) results in flow redistribution within the liver.[73,74]

Hepatic Blood Flow and Its Control

The portal circulation is responsible for most of the hepatic blood flow. While interrelationships exist between the hepatic arterial and portal venous beds, the importance of pressure-flow autoregulation in the control of the hepatic circulation is unclear. The role of hepatic arterial autoregulation appears small and portal autoregulation does not occur.[59] This absence of pressure-flow portal autoregulation suggests that the principle regulatory determinants of portal flow are outflow from the spleen and intestine, rather than intrahepatic portal resistance. In an effort to maintain a constant total hepatic blood flow, a compensatory relationship appears to exist between the hepatic arterial and portal venous flows. Humoral substances released from the gastrointestinal tract can attain portal venous concentrations sufficient to exert a vasoregulatory influence

on hepatic arterial blood flow. Furthermore, factors released from hepatocytes could have effects on either systemic hemodynamics or intravascular volume that could influence liver blood flow indirectly.[75] Such compensatory responses might serve to maintain hepatic perfusion in some patients with chronic liver disease.

While maximal activation of intrahepatic resistance sites can markedly raise portal pressure, portal venous flows are unaltered. Since the liver cannot directly control portal venous flow, intrahepatic flow regulation occurs via the hepatic artery.[76] Though reduced portal venous blood flow results in hepatic arterial dilatation, the mechanism by which this occurs is poorly defined; it appears to be neither metabolic (reduced oxygen supply) nor myogenic (related to reduced portal pressure or mechanical stretch of SMCs). Lautt found that reducing the hepatic oxygen supply by isovolumic hemodilution, resulting in decreased oxygen content in both the inflow and outflow vessels, caused no dilatation of the hepatic artery.[77] Furthermore, when hepatic metabolic needs and oxygen demands rise (as with chronic alcohol ingestion), the oxygen extraction by the liver is markedly increased, but there is no hepatic arterial dilatation.[78]

The intrinsic regulation of hepatic arterial flow appears to be dictated partly by an arterial autoregulatory mechanism (constriction in response to a rise in arterial pressure) and mostly by compensatory responses to portal flow (hepatic artery dilatation as the portal blood flow is reduced, constriction as portal flow increases). Adenosine has been postulated as an important, though unconfirmed, mediator of these hepatic arterial responses.[78] A reciprocal alteration in portal flow or resistance in response to changes in hepatic arterial perfusion has been inconsistently demonstrated.

The extrinsic, humoral regulation of hepatic arterial hemodynamics is less well understood. Though a variety of splanchnic-derived vasoactive peptides and hormones can be found in portal blood, none has been shown to play a regulatory role in controlling hepatic arterial flow.

In cirrhotic patients, the hepatic arterial bed is hypertrophied and carries a much higher proportion of the total hepatic blood flow.[124] In addition, as a result of the alterations in intrahepatic architecture and their effects on the sinusoids, the autoregulatory mechanisms by which arterial pressure is dissipated in the sinusoidal system is attenuated.[17] In this setting, any decrease in portal pressure that might follow a reduction in portal venous flow could be abolished by minor increases in hepatic artery flow.

This interface between intrahepatic and extrahepatic events, and the interrelationships between the portal venous and hepatic arterial circulations, define the portal-hepatic vascular bed as well as the context in which any hemodynamic changes occur.

Hepatic Artery: Portal Vein Interactions

Hepatic perfusion is clearly a consequence of arterial-portal flows and interactions, and these relationships have an impact on the development, maintenance, and prognosis of portal hypertension. Total occlusion of one reduces the vascular resistance of the other by about 20%.[75,79] It has been clearly demonstrated that a decrease in portal venous flow and pressure is accompanied by a compensatory increase in hepatic artery flow.[80,81] Groszmann et al, in normal dogs, produced a consistent drop in sinusoidal pressure following partial occlusion of the superior mesenteric artery; furthermore, a decrease in portal venous flow resulted in hepatic arterial dilatation.[82]

Kock et al, studying the interrelationships between portal venous and hepatic arterial blood flow in normal dogs, demonstrated an increase in hepatic arterial flow and a 25% decrease in arterial resistance in response to a reduction in portal inflow. Unlike previous studies, hepatic artery occlusion produced no change in portal flow or pressure. Postocclusion reactive hyperemia was detected in the hepatic arterial bed, but not in the portal. These studies were consistent with autoregulation of the hepatic arterial circulation in contrast to what appeared to be a passive portal flow response.[83] Mathie confirmed this hepatic arterial response to portal vein occlusion in dogs with denervated livers or hepatic arteries, concluding that there was no neurogenic component in the initiation or modulation of this response.[84]

Inconsistencies among previous studies may be attributable to species and preparation differences in the wide variety of experimental models used. Attempting to limit these variables, Kawasaki et al used the radioactive microsphere technique (a well-established method of comparing regional blood flows) to study the relationship between portal and hepatic arterial flows in awake and unrestrained male Sprague-Dawley rats (a well-studied species). This model eliminated the variable, but significant effect on splanchnic and systemic hemodynamics of different anesthetic agents. They described a range of responses: ethanol, glucagon, and prostacyclin increased portal, but not hepatic arterial flow; vasopressin, acute partial portal vein ligation, and hypoxia decreased portal blood flow and increased hepatic artery flow; acute hepatic artery ligation increased portal flow and decreased hepatic artery flow.[85] In all instances, blood flow responses were accompanied by the expected resistance changes in the portal tributaries and hepatic arterial bed. These data are consistent with the concept that hepatic arterial

blood flow is regulated by hepatic arterial resistance, and that portal blood flow is regulated mainly by extrahepatic portal tributary resistance (localized in the mesenteric, splenic, and gastric beds). Lautt et al, studying anesthetized cats, suggested that the compensatory response occurs only following changes in portal vein flow: an increase in hepatic artery flow in response to a decrease in portal flow with compensatory increases in portal blood flow observed only inconsistently, following decreases in hepatic arterial flow.[88,89] While Lautt has proposed the adenosine-mediated buffer response as the mechanism that underlies the hepatic arterial response to decreases in portal flow (76), Verma-Ansil et al have contradictory data in chronic, partial portal vein ligated rats, with no evidence of an adenosine-mediated compensatory increase in hepatic arterial flow.[123]

Despite multiple observations in animal models and humans, these relationships and responses remain incompletely defined and controversial. While reciprocal resistance and flow changes in the portal and hepatic arterial beds have been postulated as a mechanism for maintaining a constant total hepatic blood flow,[86,87] this explanation appears to be incomplete. In response to different stimuli and under different conditions, the portal and hepatic arterial vascular beds may react either reciprocally or independently. Clearly, no one unifying concept can account for all observed patterns of response.

These different and sometimes independent resistance responses in the portal and hepatic arterial circulations could reflect a difference in type or density of receptors. Furthermore, the response might vary depending upon whether the modulating influences are neurogenic, pharmacologic, humoral, mechanical, or metabolic. Based on current available evidence, it appears that the portal and arterial regulatory mechanisms permit both reciprocal and independent changes. In addition, while compensatory changes tend to maintain total hepatic blood flow at normal or baseline levels, these levels are not consistently or predictably maintained.

The implications of these observations in cirrhotic patients are uncertain, particularly in the context of treatment interventions that may alter portal hemodynamics. Under normal circumstances, the liver regulates portal pressure, but not portal flow. In cirrhosis, a significant amount of portal and hepatic arterial blood bypasses the sinusoids as a result of intrahepatic shunting.[90,91] It must be presumed that with this decreased sinusoidal contact, there is less autoregulation of the liver blood flow. With increased intrahepatic shunting, the expected hepatic arterial response to a decrease in portal flow or pressure would likely be less.

Kessler et al, studying cirrhotic patients, demonstrated an unpredictable hepatic arterial response to portal decompression. In some patients, a decrease in portal flow resulted in a significant increase in hepatic artery flow, often maintaining the portal venous pressure constant. In others, no such compensatory hepatic arterial response occurred. This alteration in the portal vein-hepatic artery interaction presumably reflects both a disruption of autoregulation, as well as anatomic changes in the hepatic microcirculation.[90,92] The capacity of the hepatic arterial circulation to compensate for loss of portal blood flow has been postulated as a factor predictive of outcome following portal decompression.

Burchell et al have documented significant increases in hepatic artery flow following portacaval shunts in patients with cirrhosis and portal hypertension.[93] In a group of 47 patients, the immediate postshunt increase in hepatic artery flow correlated directly with hospital mortality, the incidence of encephalopathy, and long-term survival. They attributed the alterations in hepatic arterial compensation to the degree of encasement and constriction of hepatic arterioles by intrahepatic fibrosis.

While our understanding of these interrelationships has improved, sustained or predictable hemodynamic responses following portal decompression have not been consistently demonstrated. It is conceivable that with newer, noninvasive methods of delineating the portal-hepatic circulations, relevant hemodynamic classification and reliable outcome prediction will become possible.

Portal Hypertension: The Extrahepatic Responses

Cardiac and Systemic Hemodynamics

The extrasplanchnic hemodynamic alterations that characterize chronic portal hypertension include a hyperdynamic circulation with increased cardiac output and decreased total peripheral resistance, portal-systemic shunting, increased flow to the kidneys and skeletal muscle, and decreased mean arterial pressure. The increased splanchnic blood flow, presumed to be a reflection of both altered vascular responsiveness to vasoconstrictors and the vasodilator influence of humoral factors, appears to be important in maintaining the portal hypertensive state.

It has been postulated that pressure mechanoreceptors may play a role in the cardiac and systemic hemodynamic changes reflecting disorders in baroreflex function. Tilt test studies in cirrhotic patients have suggested disorders in baroreceptor function reflected by impaired tachycardic and peripheral resistance responses, attenuation of the normal skin and skeletal muscle flow responses to cold stress, as well

as a reduction in the vasodilator and tachycardic responses to psychogenic stress.[94–96] The ability of the adrenergic nervous system to maintain arterial pressure also appears to be compromised in cirrhosis.[97]

In an effort to clarify some of these responses, Battarbee et al studied heart rate and mean arterial pressure responses in conscious, unrestrained portal vein constricted, portal hypertensive rats.[98] Using pulsed Doppler flowmetry in chronically instrumented animals, they documented a reduction in reflex tachycardia and the skeletal muscle baroreflex responses to nitroprusside-induced hypotension. In these portal hypertensive animals with a lower mean arterial pressure and higher basal heart rate, they found a 70% attenuation in pressure sensitivity to phenylephrine and more pronounced bradycardic responses to increases in mean arterial pressure. Evaluating conductance responses in various vascular beds, they concluded that the accentuation of both the bradycardic response and the baroreflex-mediated diminution in sympathetic tone affecting both the skeletal muscle and renovascular beds were responsible for some of the altered extrasplanchnic hemodynamics and decreased pressor sensitivity observed in these portal hypertensive animals.[99] These responses closely resembled those seen in cirrhotic patients, seeming to confirm the validity and relevance of this animal model of prehepatic portal hypertension.

In further studies focused on cardiac performance in portal vein constricted rats, Batterbee and Zavecz used a model of spontaneously beating atria and paced right ventricular strips to investigate the effects of chronic portal hypertension on heart rate and cardiac contraction.[100] In this portal hypertensive animal with extensive portal-systemic collaterals, they documented impaired basal myocardial contractility and a decrease in both the chronotropic and inotropic responsiveness to the beta adrenoreceptor agonist isoproterenol. Previous studies, demonstrating an alteration in the chronotropic and peripheral resistance reflex response to hypotension, failed to clarify the site of impairment.[98] In this study, the attenuated cardiovascular response to hypotension and the changes in reflex-mediated tachycardia appeared to be explained in part by a diminished cardiac responsiveness to pressor agonists. These observations in a noncirrhotic portal hypertensive model suggest both a systemic role for mediating factors, similar to that seen in the splanchnic circulation, as well as the hemodynamic and humoral impact on the systemic circulation of the portal-systemic collaterals.

Gastrointestinal Effects

Chronic portal hypertension also has an effect on gastric physiology and function. Portal hypertensive gastropathy has been identified as an important cause of gastrointestinal hemorrhage in portal hypertensive patients; the portal hypertensive gastric mucosa has distinct microvascular abnormalities and an increased susceptibility to injury.[101,102]

Microvascular changes marked by decreased radius and increased wall thickness have been described in hypertensive portal vessels.[102,103] This appears to be an attempt in these initially thin-walled, but progressively congested and hypertensive veins to maintain a constant wall tension and limit increases in wall stress. The splanchnic vascular response to chronically elevated portal pressure includes both portal-systemic collateralization and structural changes in the microvasculature. Though the collateral circulation develops in response to portal venous outflow obstruction associated with increased intrahepatic vascular resistance, the resistance in the collateral bed is both lower than in the hypertensive portal-hepatic bed and higher than that of the normal liver.[21] This high flow, high resistance splanchnic bed has been referred to as hyperdynamic congestion.[104]

Portal hypertensive gastropathy is a late complication of portal hypertension,[105] developing at a time when the portal-systemic collaterals are well-established and extensive. The vascular abnormality identified in the stomach in humans is characterized by dilated and tortuous submucosal veins and capillaries. Tarnawski et al, studying the rat gastric microvasculature 5 days following partial portal vein constriction, demonstrated an increased endothelial cytoplasmic area and thickened capillary basement membrane, both resulting in reduced capillary luminal area. Based on these observations, in contrast to those in chronic portal hypertension in humans, they postulated gastric mucosal hypoperfusion as the factor predisposing to mucosal injury.[102]

It has been suggested that these studies, done relatively early after portal vein constriction, might not reflect the stable microcirculatory changes seen in chronic portal hypertension.[106] In rats studied 15 days following induction of portal hypertension, the gastric submucosal vessels had large lumens and thin walls, similar to the changes seen in chronic human portal hypertension.[106] Furthermore, in observations made in human cirrhotics, studied by reflectance spectrophotometry and laser-Doppler flowmetry during endoscopy, increased gastric perfusion without congestion characterized patients with portal hypertensive gastropathy.[107] This is consistent with structural abnormalities identified in the advanced stages of portal hypertension in both rats and humans, inconsistent with increased mucosal sensitivity on an ischemic basis.

As in other vascular beds, structural adaptation of blood vessels is dictated by hemodynamic imperatives, and changes in flow and pressure. The gastric mucosa

in portal hypertension is clearly more susceptible to injury and hemorrhage. The vascular changes are a response to the altered portal hemodynamics.

Portal Hypertension

The Response to Hemorrhage and Resuscitation

An expanded plasma volume appears to play a role in the chronic maintenance of portal hypertension.[69] Furthermore, it has been shown that volume expansion in patients with established portal hypertension may further increase the portal pressure and precipitate variceal hemorrhage.[108–110] Conversely, volume depletion will lower portal pressure.[111] Since portal hypertension appears to be regulated by factors that modulate both portal resistance and portal blood flow, any evaluation of the impact of volume changes on portal pressure must focus on volume-related changes in both resistance and flow. An enhanced understanding of these interrelationships between volume and hemodynamics might further clarify the pathophysiology of portal hypertension and have important therapeutic implications.

Kravetz et al, using the anesthetized portal vein constricted portal hypertensive rat model, studied splanchnic and systemic hemodynamic changes during hemorrhage and blood volume resuscitation.[112] Controlled hemorrhage produced a significant drop in arterial pressure, portal pressure, and portal venous inflow. Following blood reinfusion, however, while arterial pressure and portal flow returned to control values, the portal pressure increased by approximately 20% above baseline. This postresuscitation pressure rise was accompanied, and apparently explained, by a significant increase in portal-collateral resistance. They postulated that this resistance increase was mediated by vasoconstrictors released during hemorrhage. Furthermore, it has been shown that portal veins subjected to chronically elevated pressures have a thickened muscular layer, and demonstrate a contractile force in response to vasoconstrictors that is more pronounced than that seen in portal veins from normal rats.[103]

The hemodynamic responses to hemorrhage and resuscitation have also been studied in portal hypertensive rats with carbon tetrachloride-induced cirrhosis.[113] In this model, the cirrhosis results in only mild portal-systemic shunting. In an effort to define the role of these collaterals in controlling the response to changes in intravascular volume, cirrhotic rats were studied with and without partial portal vein constriction (a maneuver that significantly increases the portal-systemic shunting). Portal and arterial pressure were measured directly, and cardiac output, regional blood flows, and portal-systemic shunting were determined using radioactive microspheres. In the portal hypertensive animals with significant shunting, posthemorrhage resuscitation resulted in portal pressures that were significantly elevated above baseline. In contrast, in animals with low degrees of shunting, posthemorrhage volume resuscitation produced no significant alteration in splanchnic or systemic hemodynamics. These experiments appeared to confirm the importance of the extent of portal-systemic shunting in mediating the splanchnic hemodynamic response to acute changes in intravascular volume associated with portal hypertension. In this model, the increase in portal pressure associated with blood volume resuscitation could be explained by a significant, documented increase in portal vascular resistance, since there were no significant changes in either portal flow or systemic hemodynamics.

These observations are in contrast to those of Koshy et al who studied the effects of hemorrhage and volume expansion in portal-systemic collateral resistance in conscious rats with total portal vein occlusion and 100% shunts.[114] In this model, a similar postresuscitation rise in portal pressure was observed, but was associated with increased portal blood flow and decreased collateral vascular resistance.

The discrepancy in these studies has not been reconciled, although the model differences and the effects of anesthesia on mechanisms that regulate resistance have been cited as a partial explanation.

It is clear, however, that the splanchnic circulation is a dynamic, multiple-modulated system. Just as a variety of humoral factors mediate the splanchnic response to cirrhosis and portal hypertension, alterations in systemic hemodynamics and intravascular volume may exert a significant influence on the portal circulation.

Pathophysiology of Portal Hypertension

Overview and Clinical Implications

Disturbances in splanchnic and systemic hemodynamics often complicate the course of patients with cirrhosis, and the extent of hemodynamic abnormalities correlates with prognosis.[115] While a hyperdynamic circulation (with a high heart rate and cardiac output, and low mean arterial pressure and systemic vascular resistance) characterizes the portal hypertensive state, the exact mechanisms underlying these cardiovascular changes remain incompletely understood. Resistance to vasoconstriction—supported by observations demonstrating peripheral vasodilatation despite increased sympathetic tone, high concentrations of circulating norepinephrine, and activation of the renin-angiotensin system—is a consistent finding.[116,121] The excess production of the vasodilators glucagon and prostacyclin has been confirmed in many models and appears to play a significant modulating role.

NO, a vasodilator synthesized from L-arginine, is central to the maintenance of vascular tone in the normal liver, and may be the dominant modulator of the hyperdynamic response associated with portal hypertension. Its hemodynamic effects are consistent with the regional and systemic alterations seen in advanced portal hypertension. Endotoxemia-induced NO synthesis, as proposed by Moncada, might be the principal mediator of the hyperdynamic circulation in cirrhotic patients.

Portal hypertension and its clinical consequences are a reflection of the hemodynamic derangements associated with chronic liver disease. As we better understand the hemodynamic basis of portal hypertension, we should be able to better predict the hemodynamic impact of its various treatments. Whether the approach to the patient with variceal hemorrhage is pharmacologic, intrahepatic or extrahepatic shunts, or transplantation, the clinical outcome will be dictated to a significant extent by the effect of the treatment on regional and systemic hemodynamics.

Particularly over the past decade, the pathophysiology of the portal hypertensive state has been extensively investigated. Hemodynamic factors predisposing to variceal hemorrhage have been identified. The splanchnic and systemic responses to cirrhosis and portal hypertension have been characterized. Attention has been focused on the hyperdynamic circulation, and many of the controlling mechanisms and mediators have been elucidated. While short- and long-term prognoses have been linked to the severity of the hemodynamic derangements, hemodynamic staging of patients with portal hypertension has been both unreliable and elusive. With improved understanding of the pathophysiology and the advent of noninvasive technologies that can delineate both splanchnic and systemic hemodynamics, outcome prediction based on hemodynamic classification should become more feasible. Furthermore, with improved hemodynamic categorization of patients and identification of the factors that modulate the hemodynamic alterations, selective therapy—individualized for each hemodynamic stage—might improve the management and prognosis of these challenging and high-risk patients.

References

1. Dawson J, Gertsch P, Mosimann F, et al: Endoscopic variceal pressure measurements: response to isosorbide dinitrate. *Gut* 26:843–847, 1985.

2. Lebrec D, DeFleury P, Rueff B, et al: Portal hypertension, size of oesophageal varices, and risk of gastrointestinal bleeding in alcoholic cirrhosis. *Gastroenterology* 79:1139–1144, 1980.

3. Polio J, Groszmann R: Haemodynamic factors involved in the development and rupture of oesophageal varices: a pathophysiologic approach to treatment. *Semin Liver Dis* 6:318–329, 1986.

4. Adamsons R, Butt K, Dennis D, et al: Prognostic significance of portal pressure with bleeding esophageal varices. *Surg Gynecol Obstet* 145:353–357, 1977.

5. Ready J, Robertson A, Goff J, Rector W: Assessment of the risk of bleeding from esophageal varices by continuous monitoring of portal pressure. *Gastroenterology* 100:1403–1408, 1991.

6. Juhl C, Jensen L, Mulvany M: Time course of development of changes in the structure and reactivity of small veins from portal hypertensive rabbits. *Clin Sci* 77: 205–211, 1989.

7. Garcia-Tsao G, Groszmann R, Fisher R, Conn H, Atterbury C, Glickman M: Portal pressure, presence of gastroesophageal varices, and variceal bleeding. *Hepatology* 5:419–424, 1985.

8. Benoit J, Womack W, Hernandez L: "Forward" and "backward" flow mechanisms of portal hypertension: relative contributions in the rat model of portal vein stenosis. *Gastroenterology* 89:1092–1096, 1985.

9. Sikuler E, Groszmann R: Interaction of flow and resistance in maintenance of portal hypertension in a rat model. *Am J Physiol* 250:G205–G212, 1986.

10. Reichen J: Liver function and pharmacological considerations in the pathogenesis and treatment of portal hypertension. *Hepatology* 11:1006–1028, 1990.

11. Mosca P, Lee F-Y, Kaumann A, Groszmann R: Pharmacology of portal-systemic collaterals in portal hypertensive rats: role of endothelium. *Am J Physiol* 262: G544–G550, 1992.

12. McIndoe A: Vascular lesions of portal cirrhosis. *Arch Pathol* 5:23–40, 1928.

13. Whipple A: The problem of portal hypertension in relation to hepatosplenopathies. *Ann Surg* 122:449–475, 1945.

14. Kelty R, Bagenstoss A, Butt H: The relation of the regenerated liver nodule to the vascular bed in cirrhosis. *Gastroenterology* 15:285–295, 1950.

15. Popper H, Elias H, Petty D: Vascular patterns of the cirrhotic liver. *Am J Clin Pathol* 22:717–732, 1952.

16. Baldus W, Hoffbauer F: Vascular changes in the cirrhotic liver as studied by the injection technique. *Am J Dig Dis* 8:689–692, 1963.

17. Schaffner F, Popper H: Capillarization of the hepatic sinusoids in man. *Gastroenterology* 44:239–251, 1963.

18. Orrego H, Blendis L, Crossley I, et al: Correlation of intrahepatic pressure with collagen in the Disse space and hepatomegaly in humans and in the rat. *Gastroenterology* 80:546–556, 1981.

19. Miyakawa H, Shinji I, Leo M, et al: Pathogenesis of pre-cirrhotic portal hypertension in alcohol-fed baboons. *Gastroenterology* 88:143–150, 1985.

20. Goodman Z, Ishar K: Occlusive venous lesions in alcoholic liver disease. *Gastroenterology* 83:786–796, 1982.

21. Bhathal P, Grossman H: Contractile fibroblasts in the pathogenesis of cirrhotic portal hypertension (abstr). *Hepatology* 2:155, 1982.

22. Blendis L, Orrego H, Crossley I, et al: The role of hepatocyte enlargement in hepatic pressure in cirrhotic and noncirrhotic alcoholic liver disease. *Hepatology* 2: 539–546, 1982.

23. Zimmon D, Kessler R: Effect of portal venous blood flow diversion on portal pressure. *J Clin Invest* 65: 1388–1397, 1980.

24. Moreno A, Burchell A, Rousselot L, et al: Portal blood flow in cirrhosis of the liver. *J Clin Invest* 46:436–445, 1967.

25. Vorobioff J, Bredfeldt J, Groszmann R: Hyperdynamic circulation in portal hypertensive rat model: a primary factor for maintenance of chronic portal hypertension. *Am J Physiol* 244:G52–G57, 1983.

26. Sikuler E, Kravetz D, Groszmann R: Evolution of portal hypertension and mechanisms involved in its maintenance in a rat model. *Am J Physiol* 248:G618–G625, 1985.

27. Chojkier M, Groszmann R: Measurement of portal-systemic shunting in the rat by using gamma-labeled microspheres. *Am J Physiol* 240:G371–G375, 1981.

28. Vorobioff J, Bredfeldt J, Groszmann R: Increased blood flow through the portal system in cirrhotic rats. *Gastroenterology* 87:1120–1126, 1984.

29. Bosch J, Enriquez R, Groszmann R, Storer E: Chronic bile duct ligation in the dog: hemodynamic characterization of a portal hypertensive model. *Hepatology* 3: 1002–1007, 1983.

30. Kiel J, Pitts V, Benoit J, Grange D, Shepherd A: Reduced vascular sensitivity to norepinephrine in portal hypertensive rats. *Am J Physiol* 248:G192–G195, 1985.

31. Groszmann R, Atterbury C: Portal hypertension: classification and pathogenesis. *Semin Liver Dis* 2:177–186, 1982.

32. Benoit J, Barrowman J, Harper S, Kvietys P, Granger D: Role of humoral factors in the intestinal hyperemia associated with chronic portal hypertension. *Am J Physiol* 247:G486–G493, 1984.

33. Marco J, Diego J, Villanueva M, Diaz-Fierras M, Valverda G, Segoria J: Elevated plasma glucagon levels in cirrhosis of the liver. *N Engl J Med* 289:239–242, 1973.

34. Sherwin R, Hoshi P, Hendler R, Felig P, Conn H: Hyperglucagonemia in Laënnec's cirrhosis: the role of portal-systemic shunting. *N Engl J Med* 290:239–242, 1974.

35. Benoit J, Zimmerman B, Premen A, Go V, Granger D: Role of glucagon in the splanchnic hyperemia of chronic portal hypertension. *Am J Physiol* 251:G674–G677, 1986.

36. Silva G, Navasa M, Bosch J, et al: Hemodynamic effects of glucagon in portal hypertension. *Hepatology* 11:668–673, 1990.

37. Chou C, Mangino M, Sawmiller D: Gastrointestinal hormones and intestinal blood flow. In: Shepherd A, Granger D (eds). *Physiology of the Intestinal Circulation*. New York: Raven Press; 121–130, 1984.

38. Kitano S, Koyanagi N, Sugimuchi K, Kobayashi M, Inokuchi K: Mucosal blood flow and modified vascular responses to norepinephrine in the stomach of rats with liver cirrhosis. *Eur Surg Res* 10:221–230, 1982.

39. Richardson P, Withrington P: Glucagon inhibition of hepatic arterial responses to hepatic nerve stimulation. *Am J Physiol* 233:H647–H654, 1977.

40. Joh T, Granger D, Benoit J: Intestinal microvascular responsiveness to norepinephrine in chronic portal hypertension. *Am J Physiol* 260:H1135–H1143, 1991.

41. Murray B, Paller P: Decreased pressor reactivity to angiotensin II in cirrhotic rats: evidence for a post-receptor defect in angiotensin action. *Circ Res* 57:424–431, 1985.

42. Faber J: In situ analysis of alpha-adrenoceptor on arteriolar and venular smooth muscle in rat skeletal muscle microcirculation. *Circ Res* 62:37–50, 1988.

43. Tesfamarian B, Cohen R: Inhibition of adrenergic vasoconstriction by endothelial shear stress. *Circ Res* 63:720–725, 1988.

44. Pizcueta M, Pique J, Bosch J, Whittle B, Moncada S: Nitric oxide and hyperdynamic circulation in portal hypertension. *Br J Pharmacol* 105:184–190, 1992.

45. Wu Y, Li S, Campbell K, Sitzmann J: Modulation of splanchnic vascular sensitivity to angiotensin II. *Surgery* 110:162–168, 1991.

46. Sitzmann J, Bulkley G, Mitchell M, Campbell K: Role of prostacyclin in the splanchnic hyperemia contributing to portal hypertension. *Ann Surg* 209:322–327, 1989.

47. Hamilton G, Phing R, Hutton R, Dandora P, Hobbs R: The relationship between prostacyclin activity and pressure in the portal vein. *Hepatology* 2:236–242, 1982.

48. Bruix J, Bosch J, Kravetz D, Rodes RMJ: Effects of prostaglandin inhibition on systemic and hepatic hemodynamics in patients with cirrhosis of the liver. *Gastroenterology* 88:430–435, 1985.

49. Novak J, Wenninalm A: Influence of indomethacin and prostaglandin E1 on total and regional blood flow in man. *Acta Physiol Scand* 102:484–491, 1978.

50. Berne R: Criteria for the involvement of adenosine in the regulation of blood flow. In: Paton D (ed). *Methods in Adenosine Research.* New York: Plenum Press; 1986.

51. Sparks H, Gorman M: Adenosine in the local regulation of blood flow: current controversies. In: Gerback E, Becker B (eds). *Topics and Perspectives in Adenosine Research.* Heidelberg: Springer-Verlag; 1987.

52. Miyamoto K, French S: Hepatic adenine nucleotide metabolism measured in vivo in rats fed ethanol and a high-fat low protein diet. *Hepatology* 8:52–60, 1988.

53. Arai M, Leo M, Nakamo M, et al: Biochemical and morphological alterations of baboon hepatic mitochondria after chronic ethanol consumption. *Hepatology* 4:165–174, 1984.

54. MacMathuna P, Vlavianos P, Wendon J, et al: Role of adenosine in the hemodynamic disturbances of cirrhosis and portal hypertension. *Hepatology* 12:852, 1990.

55. Genecin P, Polio J, Colombato L, Ferraioli G, Reuben A, Groszmann R: Bile acids do not mediate the hyperdynamic circulation in portal hypertensive rats. *Am J Physiol* 259:G21–G25, 1990.

56. Henriksen J, Ring-Larsen H, Kanstrup I, et al: Splanchnic and renal elimination and release of catecholamine in cirrhosis: evidence of enhanced sympathetic nervous activity in patients with decompensated cirrhosis. *Gut* 25:1034–1043, 1984.

57. Abergel A, Braillon A, Gaudin C, Kleber G, Lebrec D: Persistence of a hyperdynamic circulation in cirrhotic rats following removal of the sympathetic nervous system. *Gastroenterology* 102:656–660, 1992.

58. Furchgott R, Vanhoutte P: Endothelium-derived relaxing and contracting factors. *FASEB J* 3:2007–2018, 1989.

59. Palmer R, Ferrige A, Moncada S: Nitric oxide release accounts for the biological activity of endothelium-derived relaxing factor. *Nature* 327:524–526, 1987.

60. Vanhoutte P, Rubanyi G, Miller V, Houston D: Modulation of vascular smooth muscle contraction by the endothelium. *Annu Rev Physiol* 48:307–320, 1986.

61. Ito S, Johnson C, Carretero O: Modulation of angiotensin II-induced vasoconstriction by endothelium-derived relaxing factor in the isolated microperfused rabbit afferent arteriole. *J Clin Invest* 87:1656–1663, 1991.

62. Nathan C: Nitric oxide as a secretory product of mammalian cells. *FASEB J* 6:3051–3064, 1992.

63. Lee F-Y, Albillos A, Colombato L, Groszmann R: The role of nitric oxide in the vascular hyporesponsiveness to methoxamine in portal hypertensive rats. *Hepatology* 16:1043–1048, 1992.

64. Sieber C, Groszmann R: In vitro hyporeactivity to methoxamine in portal hypertensive rats: reversal by nitric oxide blockade. *Am J Physiol* 262:G996–G1001, 1992.

65. Sieber C, Groszmann R: Nitric oxide mediates hyporeactivity to vasopressors in mesenteric vessels of portal hypertensive rats. *Gastroenterology* 103:235–239, 1992.

66. Moncada S, Palmer R, Higgs E: Biosynthesis of nitric oxide from L-arginine: a pathway for the regulation of cell function and communication. *Biochem Pharmacol* 38:1709–1715, 1989.

67. Iwata F, Joh T, Kawai T, Itoh M: Role of EDRF in splanchnic blood flow of normal and chronic portal hypertensive rats. *Am J Physiol* 263:G149–G154, 1992.

68. Vallance P, Moncada S: Hyperdynamic circulation in cirrhosis: a role for nitric oxide. *Lancet* 337:776–778, 1991.

69. Genecin P, Polio J, Groszmann R: Na restriction blunts expansion of plasma volume and ameliorates hyperdynamic circulation in portal hypertension. *Am J Physiol* 259:G498–G503, 1990.

70. Colombato L, Abillos A, Groszmann R: Temporal relationship of peripheral vasodilation, plasma volume expansion and the hyperdynamic circulatory state in portal-hypertensive rats. *Hepatology* 15:323–328, 1991.

71. Rappaport A: The microcirculatory hepatic unit. *Microvasc Res* 6:212–228, 1973.

72. Greenway C, Oshiro G: Intrahepatic distribution of portal and hepatic arterial blood flows in anaesthetized cats and dogs and the effects of portal occlusion, raised venous pressure and histamine. *J Physiol* 227:473–485, 1972.

73. Gumucio D: Functional and anatomic heterogeneity in the liver acinus: impact on transport. *Am J Physiol* 244:G578–G582, 1983.

74. Greenway C, Oshiro G: Comparison of the effects of hepatic nerve stimulation on arterial flow, distribution of arterial and portal flows and blood content in the livers of anaesthetized cats and dogs. *J Physiol* 227:487–501, 1972.

75. Richardson P, Withrington P: Pressure-flow relationships and the effects of noradrenaline and isoprenaline on the simultaneously-perfused hepatic arterial and portal venous vascular beds of the dog. *J Physiol London:* 282, 1978.

76. Lautt W, Greenway C: Conceptual review of the hepatic vascular bed. *Hepatology* 7:952–963, 1987.

77. Lautt W: Relationship between hepatic blood flow and overall metabolism: the hepatic arterial buffer. *Fed Proc* 42:1662–1666, 1983.

78. Bredfeldt J, Riley E, Groszmann R: Compensatory mechanism in response to an elevated hepatic oxygen consumption in chronic ethanol-fed rats. *Am J Physiol* 248:G507–G511, 1985.

79. Hanson K, Johnson P: Local control of hepatic arterial and portal venous flow in the dog. *Am J Physiol* 211:712–720, 1966.

80. Ternberg J, Butcher H: Blood flow relation between artery and portal vein. *Science* 150:1030–1031, 1965.

81. Cohn R, Kountz S: Factors influencing control of arterial circulation in the liver of the dog. *Am J Physiol* 205:1260–1264, 1963.

82. Groszmann R, Blei A, Kniaz J, et al: Portal pressure reduction induced by partial mechanical obstruction of the superior mesenteric artery in the anesthesized dog. *Gastroenterology* 75:187–192, 1978.

83. Kock N, Hahnloser P, Roding B, Schenk W: Interaction between portal venous and hepatic arterial blood flow: an experimental study in the dog. *Surgery* 72:414–419, 1972.

84. Mathie R, Lam P, Harper A, Blumgart L: The hepatic arterial blood flow response to portal vein occlusion in the dog: the effect of hepatic denervation. *Eur J Physiol* 386:77–83, 1980.

85. Kawasaki T, Carmichael F, Saldiva V, Roldan L, Orrego H: Relationship between portal venous and hepatic arterial blood flows: spectrum of response. *Am J Physiol* 259:G1010–G1018, 1990.

86. Richardson P, Withrington P: Liver blood flow. I. Intrinsic and nervous control of liver blood flow. *Gastroenterology* 81:159–173, 1981.

87. Soskin S, Essex H, Herrick J, Mann F: The mechanisms of the regulation of the blood sugar by the liver. *Am J Physiol* 124:558–567, 1938.

88. Greenway C, Lautt W: Hepatic circulation. Soc AP (ed). In: *Handbook of Physiology. The Gastrointestinal System: Motility and Circulation.* Vol 1. Bethesda, MD: 1519–1564, 1989.

89. Lautt W, D'Almeida M, McQuaker J, D'Aleo L: Impact of the arterial buffer response on splanchnic vascular responses to intravenous adenosine, isoproterenol, and glucagon. *Can J Physiol Pharmacol* 66:807–813, 1988.

90. Groszmann R, Kravetz D, Parysow O: Intrahepatic arterio-venous shunting in cirrhosis of the liver. *Gastroenterology* 72:201–204, 1977.

91. Groszmann R, Kotelanski B, Cohn J, et al: Quantitative assessment of portal-systemic shunting from the splenic and mesenteric beds in alcoholic liver diseases. *Am J Med* 53:715–722, 1972.

92. Kessler R, Tice D, Zimmon D: Autoregulation of portal pressure in man. *Surgical Forum* 22:351–352, 1971.

93. Burchell A, Moreno A, Panke W, et al: Hepatic artery flow improvement after portacaval shunt. *Ann Surg* 184:289–302, 1976.

94. Bernardi M, Trevisani F, Santini C, Zoli G, Baraldini M: Impairment of blood pressure control in patients with liver cirrhosis during tilting: study on adrenergic and renin-angiotensin systems. *Digestion* 25:124–130, 1982.

95. Lunzer M, Newman S, Sherlock S: Skeletal muscle blood flow and neurovascular reactivity in liver disease. *Gut* 14:354–359, 1973.

96. Lunzer M, Newman S, Bernard A, Manghani K, Sherlock S, Ginsburg J: Impaired cardiovascular responsiveness in liver disease. *Lancet* 2:282–385, 1975.

97. Bernardi M, Trevisani F, Santini C, et al: Plasma norepinephrine, weak neurotransmitters, and renin activity during active tilting in liver cirrhosis: relationship with cardiovascular homeostasis and renal function. *Hepatology* 3:56–64, 1983.

98. Battarbee H, Farrar G, Spears R: Responses to hypotension in conscious rats with chronic portal venous hypertension. *Am J Physiol* 259:G48–G55, 1990.

99. Battarbee H, Farrar G, Spears R: Pressor responses in conscious rats with chronic portal venous hypertension. *Am J Physiol* 257:G773–G781, 1989.

100. Battarbee H, Zavecz J: Cardiac performance in the portal vein stenosed rat. *Am J Physiol* 263:G181–G185, 1992.

101. Sarfeh I, Tarnawski A, Malki A, Mason G, Mach T, Ivey K: Portal hypertension and gastric mucosal injury in rats. *Gastroenterology* 84:987–993, 1983.

102. Tarnawski A, Sarfeh I, Stachura J, et al: Microvascular abnormalities of the portal hypertensive gastric mucosa. *Hepatology* 8:1488–1494, 1988.

103. Johansson B: Structural and functional changes in rat portal veins after experimental portal hypertension. *Acta Physiol Scand* 98:381–383, 1976.

104. Groszmann R, Colombato L: Gastric vascular changes in portal hypertension. *Hepatology* 8:1708–1710, 1988.

105. McCormack T, Sims J, Eyre-Brook I, et al: Gastric lesions in portal hypertension: inflammatory gastritis or congestive gastropathy? *Gut* 26, 1985.

106. Albillos A, Colombato L, Enriquez R, Ng O, Sikuler E, Groszmann R: Sequence of morphological and hemodynamic changes in gastric microvessels in portal hypertension. *Gastroenterology* 102:2060–2070, 1992.

107. Panes J, Bordas J, Pique J, et al: Increased gastric mucosal perfusion in cirrhotic patients with portal hypertensive gastropathy. *Gastroenterology* 103:1875–1882, 1992.

108. Boyer J, Chatterjee C, Iber F, Basut A: Effect of plasma-volume expansion on portal hypertension. *N Engl J Med* 275:750–755, 1966.

109. Zimmon D, Kessler R: The portal pressure-blood volume relationship in cirrhosis. *Gut* 15:99–101, 1974.

110. Wilkinson P, Sherlock S: Effect of repeated albumin infusions in patients with cirrhosis. *Lancet* ii:1125–1129, 1962.

111. Kessler R, Santoni E, Tice D, Zimmon D: Effect of lymph drainage on portal pressure and bleeding esophageal varices. *Gastroenterology* 56:538–547, 1969.

112. Kravetz D, Sikuler E, Groszmann R: Splanchnic and systemic hemodynamics in portal hypertensive rats during hemorrhage and blood volume restitution. *Gastroenterology* 90:1232–1240, 1986.

113. Kravetz D, Bosch J, Arderiu M, Pizcueta M, Rodes J: Hemodynamic effects of blood volume restitution following a hemorrhage in rats with portal hypertension due to cirrhosis of the liver: influence of the extent of portal-systemic shunting. *Hepatology* 9:808–814, 1989.

114. Koshy A, Sekiyama T, Cereda J, Hadengue A, Girod C, Lebrec D: Effects of haemorrhage and volume expansion on portal-systemic collateral vascular resistance in conscious portal hypertensive rats. *Clin Sci* 78:193–197, 1990.

115. Bosch J, Gines P, Arroyo V, Nasara M, Rodes J: Hepatic and systemic hemodynamics and the neurohumoral systems in cirrhosis. In: Epstein M (ed). *The Kidney in Liver Disease.* Baltimore: Williams and Wilkins: 286–305, 1988.

116. Bendtsen F, Henriksen J, Sorensen T, Christensen N: Effect of oral propranolol on circulating catecholamine in cirrhosis: relationship of severity of liver disease and splanchnic hemodynamics. *J Hepatol* 10:198–204, 1990.

117. Rees D, Palmer R, Moncada S: The role of endothelium-derived nitric oxide in the regulation of blood pressure. *Proc Natl Acad Sci USA* 86:3375–3378, 1989.

118. Aisaka K, Gross S, Griffith O, Levi R: L-arginine avail-

ability determines the duration of acetylcholine-induced systemic vasodilatation in vivo. *Biochem Biophys Res Commun* 163:710–717, 1989.

119. Radlomski M, Palmer R, Moncada S: Glucocorticoids inhibit the expression of an inducible, but not constitutive, nitric oxide synthase in vascular endothelial cells. *Proc Natl Acad Sci USA* 87:10043–10047, 1990.

120. Rees D, Cellek S, Palmer R, Moncada S: Dexamethasone prevents the induction of endotoxin by a nitric oxide synthase and the associated effects on vascular tone: an insight into endotoxin shock. *Biochem Biophys Res Commun* 173:541–547, 1990.

121. Lumsden A, Henderson J, Kutner M: Endotoxin levels measured by a chromogenic assay in portal, hepatic, and peripheral blood in patients with cirrhosis. *Hepatology* 8:232–236, 1988.

122. Vallance P, Moncada S: Hyperdynamic circulation in cirrhosis: a role for nitric oxide? *Lancet* 337:776–778, 1991.

123. Verma-Ansil B, Carmichael F, Saldivia V, Varghese G, Orrego H: Effect of ethanol on splanchnic hemodynamics in awake and unrestrained rats with portal hypertension. *Hepatology* 10:946–952, 1989.

124. Hales MR, Allen JS, Hall EM: Injection corrosion studies of normal and cirrhotic livers. *Am J Pathol* 35:909–941, 1959.

CHAPTER 32

Anatomy and Physiology of Normal Erection:

Pathogenesis of Impotence

Ralph G. DePalma, MD

Introduction

During the last fifteen years, our understanding of the mechanisms of normal erection has increased considerably.[1,2] Since impotence is associated with aortoiliac disease and erection is a dramatic vascular event, it was initially believed that impotence was due mainly to arterial insufficiency with aging and that progressive arterial occlusion caused loss of the erectile capacity. Treatment efforts were first directed to procedures aimed at increasing corpus cavernosal blood flow.[3] However, it was soon recognized that several neurovascular factors interacted in a complex manner to cause normal penile erection. While failure of erection is almost always a dysfunctional vascular phenomenon, a variety of mechanisms lead to vasculogenic impotence, and other nonvascular causes of impotence are often dominant.

Penile erection follows a neurally-mediated arterial inflow increase into the corpus cavernosum, along with a reduction or cessation of venous outflow. New experimental findings[4] support the hypothesis that nitric oxide (NO), an endothelially-derived relaxant factor, is involved in the nonadrenergic, noncholinergic neurotransmission that leads to cavernous smooth muscle relaxation required for penile erection. The primacy of smooth muscle relaxation in enhancing arterial inflow, as well as producing relative venous outflow reduction, is key to understanding erectile physiology.

Vascular surgeons have long been interested in Leriche's[5] observation, in 1923, that erectile failure was often the first signal of aortoiliac atherosclosis. They subsequently observed that aortoiliac reconstruction, itself, might provoke sexual dysfunction not present preoperatively. Techniques to avoid neural damage and to maintain internal iliac flow were developed[6] to prevent this outcome and also to treat this problem when possible. Considerable work has been done by urologists[2,7] and also by vascular surgeons in venous interruption for cavernosal leakage[8,9] and arterial reconstruction[10,11] as therapy for the chief complaint of impotence. Impotence is a complex phenomenon. The ultimate expression of erectile failure relates to multiple, interacting factors in many cases; in certain cases, however, a single and discrete vascular etiology might offer a prospect for correction.

General Causes of Impotence

Clinical conditions causing impotence provide a basis for understanding erectile physiology. In generic terms, these include neurogenic and vasculogenic disorders, endocrine abnormalities, psychic causes, and probably factors ascribed to aging. In the author's experience of screening over 1000 men during the past decade, the complaint of impotence is most commonly associated with diabetes and antihypertensive agents. Impotence, often neurogenic and sometimes vasculogenic, follows operations on the prostate or distal rectal

From *The Basic Science of Vascular Disease.* Edited by Sidawy AN, Sumpio BE, and DePalma RG. Armonk, NY: Futura Publishing Company, Inc.; © 1997.

Table 1
Factors in Vasculogenic Impotence

Cavernosal

Arteriolar	functional or anatomic
	helicine vessel abnormalities
	blood pressure medication
Fibrosis	Post-priapic; drug injection
Peyronie's Disease	Deformity invading cavernous smooth muscle
	Venous leakage through tunica albuginea
Refractory smooth muscle	Hormonal: prolactinemia, low testosterone level
	Blood pressure medication
	Metabolic: diabetes, uremia

Venous Leakage

| Acquired | Abnormal tunica albuginea; traumatic lesions |
| Congenital | Isolated leakage from corpora into the spongiosum |

Arterial

Aortoiliac atherosclerosis
Steal due to external iliac disease

Occlusive disease of pudendal arteries ⎫
                                        ⎬   atherosclerotic
Occlusive disease of penile arteries   ⎭

                                             idiopathic proliferative

Atheroembolization

---

segment. In our experience, decreased arterial perfusion has been observed in almost half of the men presenting with this complaint. Arterial inflow problems, in turn, condition venous leakage. Our group has observed that up to 23% of men with suspected venous leakage as a sole etiology were found to have unsuspected arterial insufficiency when highly selective angiograms were done. Alcohol and other drug abuses cause impotence, while psychogenic factors can always complicate organic impotence. However, many more cases of impotence are now found to have an organic component than were previously appreciated. Mechanisms of vasculogenic impotence of particular interest to surgeons are listed in Table 1.

Cavernosal Malfunction

Cavernosal causes of impotence have been listed first; these account for many men presenting with the chief complaint of impotence. The specific nature of arteriolar dysfunction has not been elucidated; possibly, it relates to the action of certain drugs, not only upon the arterioles, but on the cavernosal smooth mus-

cle itself. Fibrosis follows episodes of priapism or drug injection; Peyronie's disease, when extensive, invades the corpora cavernosum and affects vascular filling due to the intrinsic fibrosis, as well as causing venous leakage through an inflamed tunica albuginea. Most important, among the cavernosal factors is refractory smooth muscle. The author has noted erectile failure to be common in diabetics with poor control of their disease. Under these circumstances, intracavernous injection of vasoactive agents will fail to elicit an erection. An important mechanism of impotence has been demonstrated in that electrically-elicited, nonadrenergic, noncholinergic relaxation is impaired in diabetic men with impotence, but not in nondiabetic men with impotence.[12] These diabetics also often exhibit abnormalities in neural and vascular function. About 28% of all men screened by us for impotence exhibit one or more abnormalities[13] in pudendal-evoked potentials, or bulbocavernous reflex times.

Venous or Cavernosal Leakage

Venous leakage is probably the most common manifestation of erectile failure; it is to be recalled, however, that full erection requires virtual cessation of venous outflow, so that almost any erectile failure is associated with venous leakage. In early diagnostic workups of impotent men, this phenomenon was confusing, so that the venous leakage syndrome was overdiagnosed. True isolated venous leakage can occur with trauma to the tunica albuginea, e.g., penile fracture, or be due to isolated congenital defects. The pathophysiology of idiopathic acquired cavernosal leakage is poorly understood. Clinical studies[7,8] have demonstrated that the most favorable pattern for surgical interruption occurs when a dorsal vein or superficial venous leakage predominates, as opposed to diffuse crural or spongiosal leakages. In young men who have never had an adequate erection, congenital venous leakage might be found. This history is quite characteristic of a defect, causing depressurization of the corpora into the spongiosum, which can be surgically corrected.

Arteriogenic Impotence

Aortoiliac atherosclerosis is associated with a high incidence of impotence when its repair uses older techniques. In a well-documented series of conventional aortoiliac operations described by Fredberg and Mouritzen,[14] 55% of men with aneurysms were impotent before surgery, whereas 95% (19 of 20) were impotent after surgery. With occlusive disease, 31% (15 of 48) were impotent before surgery, and 60% (29 of 48) were impotent after surgery. In contrast, using techniques which avoid neural autonomic damage and maintain internal iliac flow, the author[6] has observed that about 3% of men might become impotent, particularly with internal iliac artery aneurysms. Age is an important factor in whether or not a man will be impotent either before and after aortoiliac procedures. In the author's experience, approximately 40% of men will be impotent before and after surgery; these men have an average age of 65 years, whereas a little over half of the men with an average age of 57 years become potent postoperatively.

Such clinical information, and other data obtained through our noninvasive screening sequence studies, indicate that decreasing potency with aging does not appear to be related to arterial occlusion per se.[15,16] The average age of men complaining of impotence, with or without decreased arterial perfusion determined noninvasively, is about 55 years. Dramatic age-related decreases in nocturnal penile tumescence, frequency, duration, and degree are correlated with sexual desire, arousal, and coital frequency.[17] The aging factor makes long-term postoperative evaluation of revascularization procedures difficult in that decrements in erectile function do not appear to be linearly related to decrements in arterial inflow.

Hemodynamics of Normal Erection

Considerable data have been gathered concerning the hemodynamics of erection by invasive studies using techniques such as dynamic infusion cavernosometry and cavernosography (DICC),[2] as well as angiography and duplex scanning. Pioneering studies by Michal and Pospichal[18] showed that in the flaccid state, there was a balance between venous outflow and penile inflow. During erection, intracavernous pressure increases from a resting pressure of 10 to 15 mm of mercury to levels ranging from 80 to 90 mm of mercury. During full erection, cavernosal artery flow virtually ceases—a very important factor in interpreting arteriograms, particularly after intracavernous injection of vasoactive agents. Physiologically, it is impossible to generate suprasystolic pressures in any organ by ordinary blood flow phenomena. However, suprasystolic pressures are generated within the penis by perineal muscle contraction, as these obstruct venous outflow and hydraulically compress the closed corporal spaces. Such involuntary muscular contractions are found in preceding erections during sleep when nocturnal penile tumescence is monitored.

Phases in the erectile process are depicted in Figure 1. In the flaccid stage, the smooth muscle of the corpus cavernosum is contracted, as is the deep cavernosal artery. The emissary and pudendal veins are open, and the intracavernous pressure ranges from 10 to 15 mm of mercury. In the next stage of erection, intracavernous pressure increases to 80 to 90 mm of mercury, as arterial inflow increases along with smooth muscle relaxation; the veins become occluded. At a later or rigid stage, the cavernosal artery pressure equilibrates with intracavernous pressure. Finally, suprasystolic pressures and rigidity occur with perineal muscle contraction. The pressure at which cavernosal artery occlusion (CAOP) occurs is detected by a Doppler probe placed at the base of the penis during artificial erection, using roller pump infusion of warm saline with monitoring of intracavernous pressure. As with other measurements, the pressure at which the signal returns as pump flow is gradually reduced is taken as CAOP. Generally, CAOP ranges between 80 to 90 mm of mercury with a gradient not greater than 30 mm of mercury, as compared to simultaneously obtained brachial pressure.[2,16] CAOP measurements obtained during DICC are an indirect measure of the adequacy of arterial inflow. These tests are important when planning microvascular procedures which might involve operations on penile arteries or veins.

Color flow Doppler ultrasound, after injection of an intracavernous vasoactive agent such as prostaglandin E_1 (PGE-1), along with visual sexual stimulation, has quantified control values for normal erectile function in middle-aged men.[19] Mean peak blood flow ve-

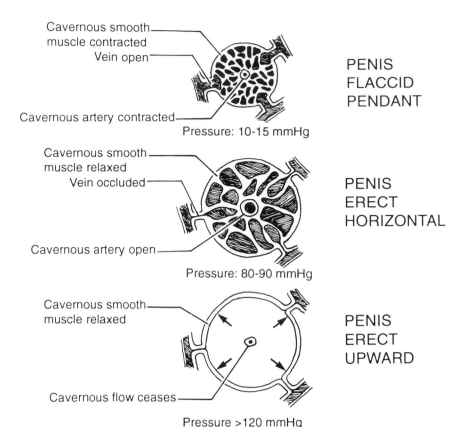

Figure 1. Stages in penile erection emphasizing cavernous smooth muscle relaxation and perineal contraction.

locity in cm per second in the cavernous artery and the ultimate rigidity of erection are directly correlated. The normal changes consist of a 70% increase in deep cavernous artery diameter, systolic peak flow velocity greater than 30 cm per second, and more than 10 mL per minute of blood flow volume. It is interesting that the smooth muscle of the penis, in contrast to that of most organ systems, functions at markedly varying PO_2 levels. In the flaccid state, PO_2 is that of mixed venous blood, increasing to arterial PO_2 values during erection.[20]

Penile Innervation

In 1863, Eckhart[21] made the first observations on penile innervation. He described pelvic nerves in dogs that produced erection upon electrical stimulation. These he called the *nervi erigente*. These nerves, which also serve as efferents for the urinary tract, bladder, colon, rectum, and penis, contain both sympathetic and parasympathetic fibers.[22] When neural elements become diseased or injured, erection is often one of the disturbed functions. Failure of ejaculation, retrograde ejaculation, and anorgasmia also occur. There are no methods of testing these autonomic nerves directly in humans. Autonomic function is indirectly estimated by

measurement of the somatic equivalents in nerves which also carry these autonomic fibers. The bulbocavernosus reflex time and pudendal-evoked potentials are measured by stimulation of the glans penis and detection of contraction of the ischiocavernous muscle, in the case of the former, and the arrival of nerve impulses in the cortex and spinal cord directly, in the case of the latter. These reflect the sacral reflex arc and the integrity of the transmission to the central nervous system respectively.

Lue et al[23] have shown that the spinal nuclei for control of erection in men are located in the anteromediolateral gray matter of the cord at S2 to S4 and at the T10 to L2 cord levels. Thus, two distinct neural pathways relate to erection.[24] The first occurs via the central nervous system to impulses which are integrated in the thoracolumbar cord. The second is a reflexogenic mechanism mediated by the sacrospinal center involving direct stimulation or enteroceptive stimuli of the bladder and rectum. The duality of these systems causes contrasting modes of erection. For example, in certain cases of spinal cord injury, where reflex stimuli are not perceived, erection can be produced by purely psychogenic stimulation. Experiments[25] have been done in cats which reveal that even when the male lumbosacral cord is excised, stimulation by exposure to a female in estrous can cause erection, but direct genital stimuli fail to elicit erection. A second transection in the lower thoracic area will subsequently abolish erection, as will resection of the feline inferior mesenteric ganglion and hypogastric nerves.

In men, the pelvic nerve plexus is a rectangular plate of nerve fibers spreading over the lateral aspect of the rectum, innervating the rectum, bladder, seminal vesicles, and prostate. These nerves subsequently travel with blood vessels into the penis. Distal fibers of the plexus encompass the posterolateral aspect of the prostate and pass into the corpora. These nerves are responsible for erection, as demonstrated by the observation that electrical stimulation of the caudal bundles of the pelvic plexus results in sustained erection.[26] As the nerve fibers are applied closely to the aorta, the iliac, the inferior mesenteric artery, and the prostate, nerve-sparing dissections allow for postoperative potency in both vascular[27] and urologic procedures.[28]

As noted, the control of corporal smooth muscle tone is a key factor affecting erection. The final twigs of the autonomic nerves supply the intracavernosal helicine arteries, as well as the erectile tissue of the corpus cavernosum itself. Neurogenic mechanisms of erection involve three neural effector systems,[2] adrenergic (constrictor system), cholinergic (dilator system), and nonadrenergic, noncholinergic system, which is primarily dilator and possibly related to release of endothelium-derived vasoactive relaxing factor. As mentioned previously, NO is released with stimulation in isolated specimens of corporal tissue.[4] Under normal circumstances, overriding adrenergic tone keeps the smooth muscle constricted and the penis in a flaccid state. This constricted state is reversed by intracavernous injection of alpha-blocking agents such as phentolamine,[29] or a nonspecific muscle relaxant such as papaverine.[30] The discovery of the actions of these agents on the corporal smooth muscle was an important advance in the understanding of erectile physiology. More recently, PGE-1 has been shown to produce a similar effect. Men with spinal cord transection, or any form of neurologic damage, e.g., diabetic neuropathy, are exquisitely sensitive to the injection of small doses of these agents, in contrast to decreased sensitivity when vascular causes predominate.

Arterial Anatomy

The anterior divisions of both internal iliac arteries give rise to the internal pudendal arteries. This arterial anatomy has not been considered in detail by vascular surgeons. The most common arrangement is shown in Figure 2. Each pudendal artery passes out of the pelvis, crosses the ischial spine externally, and reenters the ischiorectal space through the lesser sciatic foramen. It then passes to the base of the penis along the lateral wall to the ischiorectal fossa, emerging from Alcock's canal into the perineum about 4 cm anterior to the lower margin of the ischial tuberosity. Pelvic or perineal injuries can interrupt the penile artery blood supply and cause arteriogenic impotence. The distal branches of the common penile artery consist of the deep cavernosal and dorsal penile, and urethral or spongiosal arteries (Figure 3). The deep cavernosal arteries, in the main, carry blood to the corporate cavernosa. In some instances, the dorsal artery emits branches that pierce the tunica albuginea and enter into intracavernosal spaces as accessory cavernosal arteries. The dorsal arteries supply mainly the glans; however, branches from the spongiose portion of the glans penis also have been shown recently to pierce the cavernosum distally.[31] Considerable descriptive[32,33] literature exists on the angiographic appearances and function of the penile arteries. While emphasizing the dominance of the deep cavernosal artery in erectile function, the role of the dorsal artery has recently been stressed.[31] The many variations in the distal penile arteries still require better characterization. In order to visualize these vessels arteriographically, a small intracorporal injection of vasoactive material is given, not enough to produce full erection, but enough to produce tumescence. The fine anatomy of these arteries can then be viewed in a dilated state.

At this time, it is difficult to relate angiographic absence, for example, of one cavernosal artery or a minor occlusion on one side, as contributing to erectile dysfunction, unless objective data supporting a hemodynamic problem are rigorously documented. As in the extremities, arterial anatomy does not absolutely correlate with arterial perfusion or function. The cavernosal arteries divide into fine branches, some opening directly into cavernosal spaces, which contain smooth muscle and endothelium. Some exhibit a tendril-like appearance forming convoluted and somewhat dilated vessels called helicine arteries. In addition to opening into the cavernosal spaces, small capillary branches nourish the trabecular smooth muscle structure of the corpus cavernosum, which constitutes most of the bulk of the penis. The helicine vessels are most numerous proximally where the deep arterial supply is also most abundant.

Venous Drainage

Figure 4 shows the penile veins. These consist of the superficial, intermediate, and deep vessels with associated emissary circumflex and communicating vessels. The superficial veins, usually seen just beneath the skin, form a superficial dorsal vein which is forked or paired. Distention of this vein does not relate to venous insufficiency; its prominence is rarely relevant.

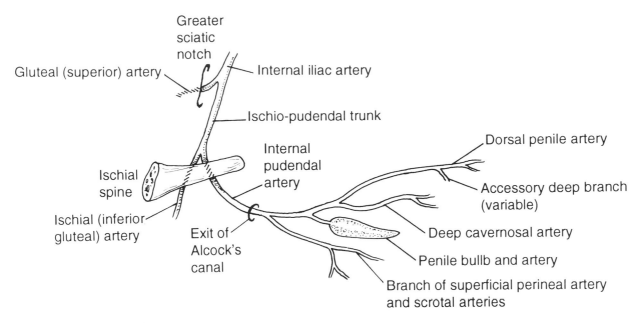

Figure 2. Right oblique schematic of the internal iliac artery and penile branches as seen on angiography with pertinent bony landmarks. Note accessory cavernosal branch from dorsal penile artery (not present in all instances).

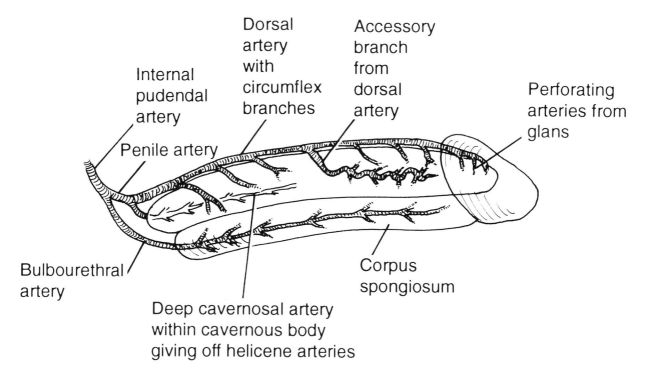

Figure 3. Penile arterial supply. Note accessory cavernosal artery and small perforating branches at the glans arising from dorsal artery.

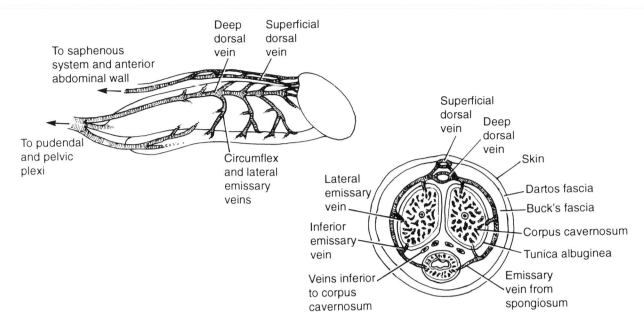

Figure 4. Penile venous drainage in longitudinal and cross-sectional views.

The superficial dorsal vein usually empties into the left saphenous vein, the right saphenous vein and, less commonly and occasionally, into the femoral or epigastric veins. When two prominent trunks exist, each usually empties into the saphenous veins. The intermediate veins lie deep to Buck's fascia and just above the tunica. The most important and prominent is the deep dorsal vein, which is formed by the confluence of 15 or 16 straight veins draining from the glans and forming a retrocoronal plexus. The deep dorsal vein is found in the sulcus between the two corpora cavernosa in close relationship to the paired dorsal nerves and arteries. This vein exhibits a thick muscular coat; proximally, it is also joined by emissary veins draining from the corpus cavernosum and circumflex veins, which pass into the spongiosum.

Multiple veins exiting the penile base merge with several trunks which enter the pudendal vein or plexus. Valves are present at this confluence; usually, three also exist along the course of the dorsal vein. These valves are arranged in a conventional fashion to facilitate blood flow toward the heart while preventing distal reflux, just as arranged in the extremities. The cavernous spaces have no deep veins. One to four large veins exit the proximal end of each crura comprising the proximal venous drainage of the cavernous spaces. These empty ultimately into the pudendal veins or plexus. Although the crura of the corpus cavernosa drain into the deep proximal veins, the corpora distal to the arcuate ligament also empty into the deep dorsal vein circumflex vessels and other veins just posterior to the corporis cavernosum. Conventional valves are also seen at the junction of the lateral vesicle, pudendal, and obturator venous plexus, and at the origin of the internal iliac vein.

Occasionally, thrombophlebitis or occlusion of the internal iliac vein produce priapism which occurs when the patient stands, but disappears during recumbency. Fitzpatrick[34] postulated that the special muscular circumferential venous valves delay venous drainage from the corpora to assist in maintaining erection. However, the main mechanism is dominated by relaxation of the corporal smooth muscle, then arterial pressurization of the corpora with occlusion of venous drainage by the subalbuginal smooth muscle and the albuginea itself. Unique anatomic features in the penile veins also suggest a functional role in maintaining erection, but these do not, in all probability, relate to conventional valves. While certain cases of primary impotence are caused by abnormal congenital connections between corpora cavernosum and spongiosum, these are, in fact, quite rare. As noted in the section on hemodynamics, effective venous occlusion is conditioned by smooth muscle relaxation. When examinations are done to detect venous leak, impotence of any etiology can be related to venous leakage, if the cavernous smooth muscle does not relax or if arterial inflow is inadequate. Every flaccid penis exhibits a venous leak; the anatomic findings of venous leakage must be correlated with physiologic and arteriographic data.

Diagnostic Methods

This section considers diagnostic methods including penile brachial blood pressure indices (PBPI), penile plethysmography, neurologic testing, artificial erection, DICC, CAOP, and arteriography. The last decade has seen important advances in methods of diagnosis, with attempts to standardize and better define physiologic abnormalities. Standards continue to evolve, particularly as related to quantitative data obtained from DICC and CAOP measurements, the various flow changes that occur on high resolution color ultrasonography with time, and, finally, with highly selective arteriography. Each of these modalities will be briefly discussed.

Noninvasive Sequence

The author and his associates[15,16] have used a testing sequence for impotence, beginning with measurement of penile brachial blood pressure indices and penile plethysmographic pulse recording in a flaccid state. It has long been known that a PBPI of less than .6 is generally related to occlusions in the major vessels and is associated with erectile failure. However, PBPI is calculated based on measurements in the flaccid state; it does not convey a pressure ultimately available for erection. Adequate pressure may be obtained in certain men with time after injection of vasoactive agents. A PBPI of .6 to .75 may or may not be associated with impotence. Such values can relate to lesions of the distal vessels, such as the internal pudendal and the proper penile arteries. With PBPIs in this range, penile plethysmography (PVR) is quite useful.[35] This is performed in the author's laboratory using a cuff inflated to diastolic pressure plus one third of systemic pressure. Recordings are made of the penile pulse volume on a polygraph chart with the speed of 25 mm per second and sensitivity setting of 1. As with other plethysmographic recordings, the duration of systolic upstroke, including time to reach peak crests, along with characteristics and amplitude of the pulse waves, are measured.

Normally, penile wave forms are similar to those of the normal lower extremity. A characteristic pattern exhibits a rapid upstroke and wave form resembling a normal pulse, a pressure wave often with a dicrotic notch. The upstroke usually is completed by .2 seconds (5 mm), and the normal wave form amplitude varies from 5 to 30 mm in height. This recording reflects the total volume change in the penis with each pulsation of all arteries as it is compressed by the cuff; such wave forms are affected by ventricular/ejection, blood pressure, vasomotor tone, muscularity or tissue turgor and, finally, cuff position. We believe that it is important to use a pressure transducer within the cuff and applied to the dorsum of the penis. The sensitivity and specificity of this testing has been determined, as compared to arteriography.[16] The combination of PVR and

Table 2
Control Data for Pudendal-Evoked Potentials and Bulbo-Cavernosal Reflex Times

	Mean ± SD	± 3 SD
Lumbar potential	13.2 ± 0.96	16.1
Cortical potential	40.1 ± 1.9	45.9
Central condition time	27.0 ± 1.7	32.1
Bulbocavernous reflex time	30.6 ± 1.9	36.2

The control group, ages 22–54 years (mean 33 years), consisted of 21 subjects reporting normal potency. Data are expressed in milliseconds + standard deviation.

PBPI is 85% sensitive and predicting an abnormal pudendal arteriogram, whereas the specificity or percent of true negatives was 70%.

The author recommends measurement of bulbo cavernos reflex time after dorsal penile nerve stimulation, and also observation of pudendal-evoked responses over the lumbar cord and somatosensory cortex prior to reconstructions for impotence. Such testing will detect spinal or sacral nerve root disorders contributing to impotence. These are particularly important in patients with diabetes or with a history of lumbar disc disease. Normal values determined by Emsellem et al[13] are shown in Table 2. Among 209 impotent men evaluated by us,[13] at least 28% exhibited one or more neural abnormalities, which may or may not coexist with vascular impairment. The detection of neural defects is important as a contraindication to vascular reconstruction and also as an important guide before using intracorporal injections for artificial erection. Nerve damage causes enhanced sensitivity to papaverine, phentolamine, or PGE-1 injections, increasing the likelihood of a priapic episode.

Artificial Erection

With the data from the noninvasive laboratory in hand, and after a directed history and physical examination, intracavernosal injection of pharmacologic agents is used to test erectile function in the clinic setting. Papaverine and alpha-blockers, such as phentolamine, were the first commonly used agents; these have been replaced by PGE-1.[36] Papaverine is a nonspecific muscle relaxant, phentolamine acts by blocking neurotransmitters, while PGE-1, a nonspecific smooth muscle relaxant, probably acts by fixation onto smooth muscle receptors. PGE-1 appears to be safer than the other agents in that it is metabolized more rapidly and causes fewer episodes of priapism. A few patients complain of an aching pain in the corpora after injection, but in this author's experience, the occurrence of priapism requiring reversal is a distinctly rare event after PGE-1 injection.

The intracavernous dosage of PGE-1 now routinely used varies between 10 to 30 mcg. The erectile response is studied over a 1–hour period. Ultrasonography can be used at varying intervals after injection. If this injection is successful, the patient can be treated by self-administration of PGE-1 with appropriate clinical monitoring. A normal erection often occurs with some degree of arterial insufficiency, but its onset may just be slower. A normal erection after injection of appropriate doses of intracavernosal agents suggests that the cavernosal muscle is capable of relaxing, and that ultimately, arterial inflow and venous occlusion are sufficient under these circumstances. An erection with intracorporal pressures of 80 to 90 mm Hg is sufficient for vaginal penetration.

Intracavernous injections of various agents and doses are used for angiography and for DICC. When doing pudendal angiograms, the patient has already failed to respond to increasing injections of vasoactive agents. A small dose, e.g., 15 to 30 mg of papaverine intracavernosally, half an hour before selective pudendal angiography will allow better visualization of the penile arteries. For venous leakage, prior to DICC, larger doses of papaverine, e.g., 60 mg and 2 mg of phentolamine are given a half an hour before testing. The attempt here is to achieve maximum relaxation of the smooth muscle so that a venous leak, if present, can be quantified and visualized. All patients receiving intracavernosal injections must be observed carefully in the clinic and given warnings to return immediately for reversal if erection persists or recurs at home. Occasionally, as a result of such testing, priapism occurs. If the erection does not subside in 2 to 3 hours, or if it becomes painful, reversal is obtained by the use of intracorporal injections of sympathomimetic agents such as dilute phenylephrine or epinephrine. Reversal is an important aspect of artificial erection.

Dynamic Infusion Cavernosometry and Cavernosography

After injecting a standard intracavernous dose of vasoactive agents, these tests measure intracavernous pressure by insertion of fine needles into the cavernous bodies. Erection is stimulated by the roller pump infusion of warmed heparinized saline into the corporis cavernosum. Cavernosal artery flow signals can be detected by a Doppler continuous wave pressure probe placed at the base of the penis and directed respectively toward each crura. CAOP is the intracavernous pressure measured at the moment during erection when the deep cavernosal arterial flow disappears and then reappears as pressure falls slowly. This indicates the pressure available through each of the deep cavernosal arteries for erection. CAOP should not be less than 90 mm of mercury, nor exhibit a gradient of 30 mm mercury or more compared to brachial pressure. False low levels of CAOP may be obtained when the venous leakage is massive, i.e., the intracorporal pressure cannot be raised sufficiently to occlude cavernous flow.

Our techniques for assessment of venous leakage and CAOP were modified from those described by Bookstein et al[37] and Goldstein,[38] using an automated pump specifically designed for this study.[16] Two sets of data are generated: the rate of saline infusion or flow to maintain erection and the rate of fall of cavernosal pressure from suprasystolic erection, which is believed to be less than 1 mm Hg/sec in normal subjects. More importantly, we consider that a flow to maintain erection of greater than 40 mL per minute is abnormal and is diagnostic of venous leakage. Cavernosography with injection of a nonionic contrast medium is then used to visualize the site or sites of leakage after cavernosometry is completed.

Before accepting even these results of DICC as an indication for venous interruption, we now recommend selective arteriography in all cases. We have observed that the predicted value of our screening sequence for vascular disease was 68%, and for venogenic impotence it was 55%. In 44 men screened for venous insufficiency, based on normal PBPI and plethysmography, and findings of venous leakage on DICC, 23% showed an unsuspected proximal arterial stenosis of significant degree.[39] Arterial visualization is, therefore, important before venous interruption not only because of issues of diagnostic accuracy, but also because certain procedures employ the dorsal vein itself as a site of revascularization.

Ultrasonography

High resolution ultrasonography can be used to visualize responses of the dorsal and deep cavernosal arteries at time intervals after intracavernosal injection. The normal values of vessel diameter and flow velocities have been mentioned. We do not use this test routinely. It is useful postoperatively to visualize grafts and to study cavernosal abnormalities such as Peyronie's plaques, or to detect the presence of fibrosis within the corporis cavernosum. Lue et al[40] have used ultrasonography as a screening method, and detected a prevalence of abnormal arterial perfusion in men complaining of impotence of 46%; this value is quite similar to that observed by us using our noninvasive sequence.[15]

Arteriography must be tailored to the patient's needs. In screening over 1000 men complaining of impotence, 9 aortic aneurysms have been detected. Under these circumstances, arteriography should be done in a conventional manner to minimize catheter manipulation. Here, it is important to find large vessel stenoses and to observe the internal iliac arteries. It is not advisable to detail runoff into the penile arteries with severe aortoiliac atheromatous disease. The presence of atheromatous debris makes highly selective internal iliac artery catheterization dangerous. Our technique of highly selective pudendal angiography uses sequential exposures of up to 20 per second after pressure injection. A variety of angiographic techniques have been described, but with the use of nonionic contrast media, it is not necessary to use an anesthetic. Before selective pudendal arteriography, an intracorporal injection of 15 to 30 mg of papaverine is given. It is once again worth reemphasizing that a full erection obliterates cavernosal artery flow.

Nocturnal Penile Tumescence

Penile erections monitored during sleep have traditionally been used to separate psychogenic from organic causes of impotence.[2,41] Changes in penile circumference patterns are detected using strain gauges. However, since circumference is not a precise reflection of penile rigidity, direct observation of the quality of erections must be monitored in some manner. It is interesting to note that response to intracorporal pharmacologic testing does not always separate psychogenic from organic impotence.[42] For this purpose, formal nocturnal tumescence monitoring over a full 3-night period may be required.

Treatment of Vasculogenic Impotence: An Evolving Area

Since the first conference on corpus cavernosal revascularization convened in 1978,[3] there has been spectacular progress in the understanding of the erectile process, and in the development of methods to quantify and test erectile function. The diagnosis and treatment of impotence has evolved into a highly specialized discipline, in which our urologic colleagues have become increasingly active. This is not surprising since cavernosal factors tend to predominate. In this author's experience, 5% to 7% of men presenting with impotence exhibit a situation for direct vascular surgical intervention. This is an important group. Before such intervention, however, initial treatment importantly involves risk factor control such as complete cessation of smoking, control of diabetes mellitus, and switching blood pressure medication to angiotensin-converting enzyme inhibitors when feasible. The author has found oral isoxsuprine 10 mg, taken four times a day, useful; yohimbine HCl is an agent believed to be useful in psychogenic impotence. Many men now successfully self-inject, generally with PGE-1 or other mixtures. The author has observed successful self-injection regimens used for over 5 years. In addition, several types of vacuum constrictor devices are also available.

Surgical techniques which prevent dysfunction or restore sexual function during large vessel reconstruction have been mentioned.[6,10] In a potent man below the age of 60, preservation of the autonomic neural fibers and restoration or maintenance of flow into the internal iliacs will be gratifying in the majority of cases. It is important to avoid dissection of the inferior mesenteric artery and its associated autonomic branches. The orifice of the inferior mesenteric is closed from within the aneurysmal sac. This step also has the advantage of minimizing the complication of left colon ischemia. It is important to discuss, before surgery, the possibility of impotence, as 3% to 4% of patients might become impotent depending on circumstances. This outcome can be a consequence of aging, possibly microembolization, or the need to obliterate an internal iliac artery aneurysm. Transluminal dilation of the common and external iliac arteries is often successful in relieving impotence. The latter improves penile perfusion by relieving steal via the internal iliac and gluteal arteries. Dilation of the internal iliacs or pudendal arteries has not been successful in any case seen by the author.

Small Vessel Reconstruction

We,[10] and others,[11] performed early direct arterialization of the corpora cavernosa, which initially worked spectacularly and shortly failed. These procedures either induced priapism or thrombosed because of fibrosis at the junction of the inferior epigastric artery and the corpus cavernosum. Two types of microvascular bypass are now used. In straightforward cases of trauma or obstruction of the pudendal artery proximally, microvascular bypass into the dorsal artery is performed. The author now prefers to use the inferior epigastric artery with end-to-end anastomoses to the divided dorsal artery with perfusion proximally and distally to take advantage of appropriate runoff. The success of these microvascular operations depends upon the absence of systemic factors, normal neurologic status, and appropriate anatomy as defined by meticulous angiography.

Dorsal vein arterialization has been done when the arteries in the penis are not available for anastomosis. This is a surprisingly common finding in impotence, particularly in men from 30 to 50 years of age. Its cause

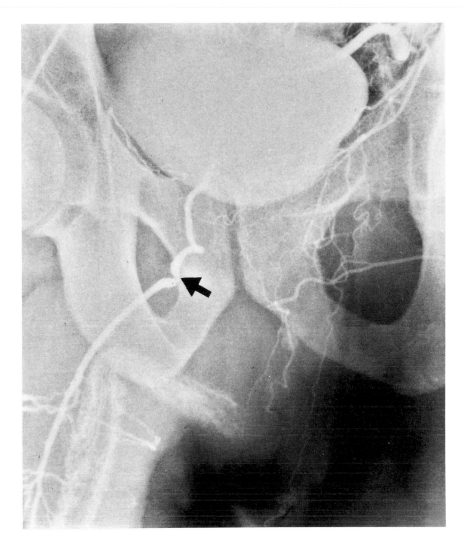

Figure 5. Postoperative angiography of epigastric to deep dorsal vein anastomoses with runoff via the circumflex vessels into the spongiosum. Stenosis at **arrow** was associated with gradual loss of erectile rigidity at 1 year. (Reproduced with permission from Reference 43.)

is unknown, and there appears to be a proliferative or thrombotic process in penile arteries unrelated to atherosclerosis elsewhere. Reported success rates very widely from 20% to 80%; the mechanism of action of deep dorsal vein arterialization is unknown. It was thought, initially, that the arterialized veins fill the corpus cavernosum by retrograde flow through the emissary veins. However, postoperative arteriography[43] and MRI scanning[44] have revealed that the flow is predominantly by circumflex veins into the corpus spongiosum. An arteriogram obtained on a patient a year and a half postoperatively is shown in Figure 5. In spite of this dominant spongiosal flow into the spongiosum, such bypasses do enhance erectile function. Sudden erectile failure has been reported by us and others to relate directly to stenosis or sudden graft occlusion.[44] One serious and specific complication of dorsal vein

arterialization is glans hyperperfusion, which will require distal venous ligation or graft occlusion. This is caused by venous hypertension affecting the glans and distal urethra. If neglected, distal venous hypertension can progress to necrosis of the penile tip with urinary obstruction. The necessity for a cystotomy has been reported. This complication might occur months after dorsal vein arterialization, presumably because of increased collateral development in the retrocoronal plexus; it is usually seen, however, within weeks of the procedure.

Venous Interruption

Success rates for venous interruption vary from 28% to 73%[2]; this wide variation implies the difficulties in patient selection, as well as possible technical inadequacies. In the author's opinion, unfavorable results relate to excision of veins in cases selected solely by DICC. Excision of the dorsal vein and its associated retropubic venous complex is successful[8] while excision of the distal crural veins or spongiolysis have not been successful. We now recommend a routine repeat DICC 3 months after all operations for venous leakage. We have found, in almost all instances, that values for flow to maintain erection have improved.[45] On occasion, additional embolization for new leaks detected at this time can be done by the radiologist using coils. Frequently, men who have not been able to function at all with self-injection can function with self-injection after a venous ligation procedure. Overall, about 70% of these procedures are successful, if one counts those now successful with self-injection.

Prosthetics

Modern penile prosthetics offer an almost immediate prospect for coital sufficiency; however, conventional prostheses destroy normal cavernosal architecture, and vascular reconstructive procedures are foreclosed. New prostheses, such as those recently described by Subrini,[46] also allow erection or vascular tumescence around a very soft prosthesis. Because of medicolegal problems associated with the prosthetic devices, they have been recommended less often in the United States in recent years, but remain an important option when medical treatment, self-injection, or vascular surgery fail.

Summary

The anatomy and physiology of normal erectile function can be better understood by considering the pathogenesis of impotence and the physiologic assumptions underlying neurovascular tests of erectile function. As these become better characterized and more specific, it is highly probable that the treatment of impotence will improve. Further evolution of treatment, based on better and more specific surgical techniques, will apply for these men who fail medical therapy.

References

1. DePalma RG: Mechanisms of vasculogenic impotence. In: White RA, Hollier LH (eds). *Vascular Surgery: Basic Science and Clinical Correlations*. Philadelphia: JB Lippincott Company; 1994.
2. Krane RG, Goldstein I, DeTejada IS: Impotence. *N Engl J Med* 321:1948, 1989.
3. Zorginiotti AW, Rossi G (eds). *Vasculogenic Impotence*. Springfield, IL: Charles C. Thomas Publishers, 1980.
4. Rajfer J, Aronson WJ, Bush PA, et al: Nitric oxide as a mediator of relaxation of the corpus cavernosum in response to nonadrenergic, noncholinergic neurotransmission. *N Engl J Med* 326:90, 1992.
5. Leriche R: Des obliterations arterielle hautes (obliteration de la terminasion de l'aorte) comme cause de insuffiances circulartoires des membres inferieurs. *Bull Mem Soc Chir* 49:1404, 1923.
6. DePalma RG, Edwards CM, Schwab FJ, et al: Sexual dysfunction in aortoiliac disease. In: Bergan JJ, Yas JST (eds). *New Findings in Arterial Surgery*. Orlando, FL: Grune and Stratton; 337, 1987.
7. Lewis RW: Venous surgery for impotence. *Urol Clin North Am* 15:115, 1988.
8. DePalma RG, Schwab F, Druy EM, et al: Experience in the diagnosis and treatment of impotence caused by cavernosal leak syndrome. *J Vasc Surg* 10:117, 1989.
9. Virag R: Syndrome d'erection instabile pour insuffisance veineuse. *J Mal Vasc* 6:121, 1981.
10. DePalma RG, Kedia K, Persky L: Vascular operations for preservation of sexual function. In: Bergan JJ, Yao JST (eds): *The Surgery of the Aorta and Its Body Branches*. New York: Grune and Stratton; 277, 1979.
11. Michal V, Kramar R, Pospichal J: Femoro-pudendal bypass, internal iliac thromboendarterectomy, and direct anastomosis to the cavernous body in the treatment of erectile impotence. *Bull Soc Int Chir* 33:343, 1974.
12. Saenz de Tejada I, Goldstein I, Azudzoi k, et al: Impaired neurogenic and endothelium-mediated relaxation of penile smooth muscle from diabetic men with impotence. *N Engl J Med* 320:1025, 1989.
13. Emsellem HA, Bergsrud DW, DePalma RG, et al: Pudendal-evoked potentials in the evaluation of impotence (abstr). *J Clin Neurophysiol* 5:349, 1988.
14. Fredberg U, Mouritzen C: Sexual dysfunction as a symptom of arteriosclerosis and as a complication to reconstruction in the aortoiliac segment. *J Cardiovasc Surg* 29:149, 1988.
15. DePalma RG, Emsellem HA, Edwards CA, et al: A screening sequence for vasculogenic impotence. *J Vasc Surg* 5:228, 1987.
16. DePalma RG, Schwab FJ, Emsellem HA, et al: Noninvasive assessment of impotence. *Surg Clin North Am* 70:119, 1990.
17. Schiavi RC, Schreiner-Engel P, Mandeli J, et al: Healthy aging and male sexual function. *Ann J Psychiat* 147:766, 1990.
18. Michal V, Pospichal: Phalloarteriography in the diagnosis of erectile impotence. *World J Surg* 2:239, 1978.
19. Lee B, Sikka SC, Randrup ER, et al: Standardization of penile blood flow parameters in normal men using intracavernous prostaglandin E_1 and visual sexual stimulation. *J Urol* 149:49, 1993.
20. Broderick GA, Gordon D, Krasnopolsky L, et al: Anoxia and corporal smooth muscle dysfunction. *Surg Forum* 44:750, 1993.
21. Eckhart C: Intersuchunger uber die erection des penis beim hund. *Beitr Anat Physiol* 3:123, 1863.
22. Pick J: *The Autonomic Nervous System*. Philadelphia: JB Lippincott; 439, 1970.
23. Lue TF, Zeineh SJ, Schmidt RA, et al: Neuroanatomy of penile erection: its relevance to iatrogenic impotence. *J Urol* 131:273, 1984.
24. Weiss HD: The physiology of human penile erection. *Ann Intern Med* 76:793, 1972.

25. Root WS, Bard D: The mediation of feline erection through sympathetic pathways. *Ann J Physiol* 151:80, 1947.

26. Lue TF, Schmidt RA, Tanagho EA: Electrostimulation and penile erection. *Urol Int* 40:60, 1985.

27. DePalma RG, Levine SB, Feldman S: Preservation of erectile function after aortoiliac reconstruction. *Arch Surg* 113:958, 1978.

28. Walsh PC, Donker PJ: Impotence following radical prostatectomy: insight into etiology and prevention. *J Urol* 128:492, 1982.

29. Brindley GS: Cavernosal alpha-blockade: a new technique for investigating and treating erectile impotence. *Brit J Psychiat* 143:332, 1983.

30. Virag R: Intracavernous injection of papaverine for erectile failure. *Lancet* 2:1982, 1982.

31. Garibyan H, Lue TF, Tanagho EA: Anastomotic network between the dorsal and cavernous arteries in the penis. *Int J Impot Res* 4:36A, 1992.

32. Ginestic JF, Romieu: *A Radiologic Exploration of Impotence.* The Hague: Martimus Nijoff; 1978.

33. Juhan CM, Hughet JF, Clerissa JA, et al: Classification of internal pudendal artery lesions in one hundred cases. In: Zorgniotti AW, Rossi G (eds). *Vasculogenic Impotence.* Springfield, IL: Charles C. Thomas Publishers; 169, 1980.

34. Fitzpatrick TJ: The penile intercommunicating venous valvular system. *J Urol* 127:1099, 1982.

35. Stauffer D, DePalma RG: A comparison of penile brachial index (PBI) and penile pulse volume recordings (PVR). *Bruit* 17:29, 1983.

36. Stackl W, Hasun R, Marberger M: Intracavernous injection of prostaglandin E₁ in impotent men. *J Urol* 140:66, 1988.

37. Bookstein JJ, Fellmeth B, Moreland S, et al: Pharmacoangiographic assessment of the corpora cavernosa. *Cardiovasc Intervent Radiol* 11:218, 1988.

38. Goldstein I: Overview of types of results of vascular surgical procedures for impotence. *Cardiovasc Intervent Radiol* 11:240, 1988.

39. DePalma RG, Dalton CM, Gomez CA, et al: Predictive value of a screening sequence for venogenic impotence. *Int J Impot Res* 4:143, 1992.

40. Lue TF, Hricak H, Marich KW, et al: Vasculogenic impotence evaluation by high resolution ultrasonography and pulse Doppler spectrum analysis. *Radiology* 155:777, 1985.

41. Ware JC: Monitoring erections during sleep. In: Kryger MG, Roth T, Dement WC (eds). *Principles and Practice of Sleep Medicine.* Philadelphia: WB Saunders Company; 689, 1989.

42. Allen RP, Brendler: Nocturnal penile tumescence monitoring predicting response to intracorporal pharmacologic erection testing. *J Urol* 140:518, 1988.

43. DePalma RG, Olding MJ: Surgery for vasculogenic impotence. In: Greenhalgh RM (ed). *Vascular Surgical Techniques: An Atlas.* London: WB Saunders Company; 171, 1988.

44. Sohn MH, Sikora RR, Bohndorf KK, et al: Objective follow-up after penile revascularization. *Int J Impot Res* 4:73, 1992.

45. Yu GW, Schwab FJ, Melograna FS, DePalma RG, et al: Preoperative and postoperative dynamic cavernosography and cavernosometry: objective assessment of venous ligation for impotence. *J Urol* 147:618, 1992.

46. Subrini L: Restoration of erectile function using new soft penile implants. *Int J Impot Res* 4:129A, 1992.

CHAPTER 33

Skeletal Muscle Ischemia and Reperfusion:

Mechanisms of Injury and Intervention

Michael M. Farooq, MD; Julie A. Freischlag, MD

Introduction

A primary objective of vascular surgery has been the salvage of limbs threatened by acute or chronic ischemia. However, the decision to reestablish blood flow in a limb with a prolonged acute ischemic interval yields unpredictable and sometimes intractable consequences. Initial local changes subsequent to delayed limb reperfusion include edema, thrombosis, myonecrosis, nerve damage and, at times, limb loss. Varying degrees of systemic changes may ensue, collectively named by Haimovici as the myonephropathic-metabolic syndrome.[1,2] Findings include hyperkalemia, metabolic acidosis, myoglobinuria, and changes in the host inflammatory response. This results in multisystem organ dysfunction manifested by acute renal failure, myocardial and circulatory depression, pulmonary edema, and even death.[3]

Only in recent years have we begun to uncover the underlying pathophysiology of ischemia/reperfusion (I/R) phenomena. In the evolution of vascular surgery and other surgical disciplines, such "basic science" aspects of particular disease processes have become increasingly incorporated into the armamentarium of the surgeon. Ischemia and its counterpart, reperfusion, are established entities now in a spotlight of new scientific illumination, with ultimate hopes for the development of novel or improved interventions to attenuate or perhaps reverse I/R complications.

The current understanding of skeletal muscle I/R mechanisms, and those of their interventional counter-parts, is emphasized in this chapter. Pathophysiologic events in I/R are reviewed at the cellular level. Emphasis is placed on derangements in cell energy metabolism and pathophysiologic mechanisms of inflammatory activation at the microcirculatory level. Neutrophils, endothelium, and participating humoral factors including prostaglandins, cytokines, and complement are discussed as they interplay in the complex pathways of skeletal muscle I/R. Finally, interventional regimens targeting these pathways are described. Gross changes in skeletal muscle morphology, circulation, and function are not stressed, yet may be reviewed through provided references.

Definitions and Overview

The following definitions and overview serve as points of reference to facilitate a basic understanding of I/R pathophysiology.

Complete Versus Partial Ischemia

Complete ischemia is a state of anoxia, resulting from a cessation of oxygen and metabolic substrate delivery due to interrupted arterial blood flow. Subsequently, toxic metabolic by-products accumulate, perhaps adding insult upon the affected tissues. Partial ischemia (or partial perfusion), as seen in shock, is a state of hypoxia involving a diminished delivery of oxygen and substrates due to reduced blood flow. In this

From *The Basic Science of Vascular Disease.* Edited by Sidawy AN, Sumpio BE, and DePalma RG. Armonk, NY: Futura Publishing Company, Inc.; © 1997.

instance, the removal of waste products continues to some degree. This is not to say that complete ischemia of similar duration necessarily produces more tissue dysfunction or injury. To the contrary, limited partial perfusion states are known to exhibit prolonged energetic and membrane potential derangements after reperfusion relative to their completely ischemic counterparts.[4,5] The reasons for these differences are not clear. Despite the nature of the ischemic insult, it is clear that energy depletion initiates functional and structural cellular derangements. These alterations facilitate the activation of secondary tissue injury mechanisms when blood flow is restored.

Reperfusion

In current clinical practice, reperfusion is the reestablishment of unimpeded, normoxic blood flow from a preexisting condition of ischemia. It is during reperfusion that most tissue injury occurs, due largely to the pathophysiologic activation of neutrophils in the reperfusion blood by the ischemic tissue environment. Therapeutic interventions made during reperfusion are being developed in attempts to attenuate this injury. Interventions include physical manipulation of the reperfusion conditions and/or administration of pharmacologic agents. Some physical methods under consideration include graded increases in oxygen content, blood pressure, temperature and/or the absence of blood or specific blood cell elements. These include perfluorocarbon oxygen carriers or leukopenic reperfusion, respectively. Pharmacologic agents often permit the selective targeting of specific inflammatory activation products.

Baseline Conditions

An appreciation of the different degrees of baseline muscle temperature, contractile activity, perfusion, and subsequent reperfusion is necessary when interpreting outcomes between different clinical situations or laboratory models. Temperature variation alters some aspects of tissue energy metabolism, which may make it suitable as an intervention. Muscle tissue subjected to ongoing contraction during ischemia, for instance with tetanic stimulation, exhibits degenerational changes at earlier time points compared to the resting state. This is a situation not usually encountered clinically.[6] For purposes of discussion, ischemia and subsequent reperfusion will occur in tissue at a baseline normothermic, resting state, undergoing complete ischemia and full reperfusion. This more closely parallels conditions seen in clinical cases of acute limb ischemia, and facilitates a basic understanding of I/R pathophysiology.

Overview of Tissue Injury in Skeletal Muscle I/R

Tissue injury in skeletal muscle I/R is a multifactorial process. Injury can occur during ischemia, reperfusion, or both, depending on the duration of ischemia. Critically prolonged or "irreversible" ischemia produces primary cell membrane disruption due to energy reserve exhaustion. This occurs due to adenosine triphosphate (ATP)-dependent ionic pump failure, a consequent failure of ionic and osmotic cell membrane gradients leading to cellular swelling, and a global failure of any cellular processes dependent upon ATP as a driving force. All of these events occur with critically prolonged ischemia alone, prior to reperfusion. Ischemia of relatively short duration demonstrates no significant tissue injury prior to or after reperfusion.

Ischemia of "intermediate" duration may demonstrate relatively preserved tissue at its conclusion. However, it may manifest variable degrees of tissue injury or recovery upon reperfusion, dependent upon the relative duration of preceding ischemia. This may be due in part to failed cell energy regeneration caused by reperfusion washout of energy metabolites formed during ischemia. Ischemia-induced pathophysiologic activation of the inflammatory response seems to cause a majority of the tissue injury witnessed with reperfusion. Ischemia-induced activation of the endothelium is thought by some to be responsible for this "reperfusion injury" through mechanisms of endothelium-derived free radical production and subsequent signal-mediated inflammatory activation.

Endothelial cells exposed to sufficient ischemia manifest changes in critical metabolic enzymes, which then produce oxygen-derived free radicals upon reperfusion. This local production of free radicals may then interact with molecules in the endothelial cell membrane and surrounding milieu sufficient to initiate the production and release of several chemical mediators responsible for neutrophil activation. Specific mediators acting in this capacity include complement, prostaglandins, cytokines, and platelet activating factor, all of which induce neutrophil activation and chemoattraction. Activated neutrophils increase appropriate cell adhesion molecule (CAM) activity to facilitate endothelial cell binding and emigration. This results in injury to the endothelium and subjacent myocytes through neutrophil free radical and lytic enzyme release.

Endothelial injury is reflected by increased vascular permeability, endothelial cell swelling, and increased vascular tone. These changes result from direct endothelial cell injury. Tonic changes occur from diminished basal level release and survival of the endothelium-derived vasodilator substance nitric oxide (NO). Diminished NO release is a reflection of endothelial cell injury, while decreased NO survival is due to its direct reaction with free radicals. At this point, microvascular flow may stop entirely when neutrophils adhere in regions where vessel caliber is already narrowed by endothelial cell swelling and increased vascular tone, a condition known as "no-reflow." This situation permits ongoing ischemic injury to tissues distal to the point of obstruction.

Microvascular and parenchymal tissue injuries are distinct, yet related processes in terms of etiology and time sequence. Ischemic intervals in the intermediate range impact on overall tissue survival based on the degree of microvascular derangement incurred prior to reperfusion. Parenchymal cell injury may occur consequent to dysfunctional endothelial processes, culminating in endothelium-activated reperfusion injury, as well as no-reflow-induced ischemic degeneration.

In summary, prior to reperfusion, the amount of tissue injured is dictated by the degree of ischemia. Brief ischemia does not cause primary tissue injury, or pathophysiologic inflammatory activation. Critically prolonged ischemia, however, results in widespread primary tissue injury due to profound energy depletion, as well as secondary injury from pathologic reperfusion sequelae. Intermediate ischemia demonstrates time-dependent increases in cellular energy deficits and tissue damage. Pathophysiologic alterations occur in this ischemic range which promote chemical mediator release. This incites an injurious inflammatory response with reperfusion.

At present, few laboratory-based therapeutic regimens have become clinically applicable. Useful interventions will arise only with the ability to accurately identify the time course of a given ischemic event and its particular suitability for intervention.

Assessment of Tissue Injury in Skeletal Muscle I/R

Numerous methods have been utilized to define and quantitate tissue injury in I/R.[7,8] Histologic assessment has included light and electron microscopic observation, as well as vital dye uptake and scintigraphy to determine cell viability in concert with microscopic tissue appearance.[9-12] Functional status has been evaluated through the serial assessment of induced tetanic contractile states.[13-15] Circulatory changes such as shunting, reactive hyperemia, and occlusion have been defined through studies of regional blood flow, as well as by imaging techniques.[8,16] Biochemical evidence of cellular injury includes elevated serum levels of potassium, myoglobin, creatine phosphokinase, and cell membrane lipid breakdown products such as the conjugated dienes.[17-19]

Other studies have focused on changes occurring at the microcirculatory and cellular levels. Endothelial injury has been assessed in studies of increased permeability, as reflected through gross tissue weight gain during reperfusion. Endothelial dysfunction has been observed during in vitro assessment of endothelium-dependent vessel relaxation in organ bath chambers. Neutrophil tissue infiltration has been used as an indicator of reperfusion injury duration and severity, as determined through the quantification of neutrophil myeloperoxidase tissue concentrations.

I/R-induced pathophysiologic interactions between neutrophils and endothelial cells have been assessed by a variety of means, including measurement of serum cytokines, complement, and prostaglandins. The expression of CAM is largely defined through binding studies with monoclonal antibodies in cell culture, and through in vivo microscopy. Free radical sources have been identified and quantitated through the administration of enzyme inhibitors, inactivators, and free radical-scavenging compounds.

Cell energy metabolism, or, more precisely, cell energy charge, is the focal point around which ischemia mounts its attack. Laboratory methods have been developed to quantitate cellular metabolic derangements. These can be correlated with the degree of tissue ischemia and any subsequent injury from prolonged ischemia or reperfusion. If reperfusion is successful, signs of gradual recovery can also be assessed in this manner. Studies of cellular energy charge may prove useful as clinical diagnostic tools to better define the extent of ischemia, the indications for aggressive intervention, and the efficacy of that intervention against any resultant injury due to I/R. The freeze-clamp method quantitates the various cellular energy metabolites, defined below, in frozen skeletal muscle biopsies. Direct cell transmembrane electropotential measurement has also been evaluated, and is felt to be more sensitive to the degree of cell dysfunction during early ischemia than metabolite measurements.[5,20] Nuclear magnetic resonance (NMR) spectroscopy has shown promise due to its ability to measure the various metabolite concentrations and pH noninvasively. Some NMR data have shown ATP depletion to progress several hours earlier than has been shown by the freeze-clamp method.[21,22] Surface pH measurements can quantitate the degree of tissue acidosis, which correlates with the degree of tissue ischemia. This method has superceded lactate as a marker of acidosis, due to error caused by washout of the latter during reperfusion.[20,23]

Normal Skeletal Muscle Energy Metabolism

Maintenance of the cellular ATP pool ensures proper cell function. A fundamental aspect of ATP utilization is the stabilization of ionic gradients across membranes of the cell wall and subcellular organelles, such as the calcium-sequestering sarcoplasmic reticulum in skeletal muscle cells. With adequate tissue oxygen delivery, ATP production is accomplished by mitochondrial oxidative phosphorylation, in association with glycolysis, the Krebs cycle, and the electron-transport chain. However, in situations where quick bursts of contraction are required, work can be performed despite the insufficient delivery of oxygen. This is probably why skeletal muscle tolerates ischemia better than some tissues. There are several provisions in skeletal muscle that explain this tolerance. First, myoglobin is present, which is similar to hemoglobin, but with a higher affinity for oxygen. In addition, two types of energy reserves are present: creatine phosphate (CP) and glycogen. The enzyme creatine phosphokinase facilitates the transfer of a terminal high energy phosphate molecule from CP to adenosine diphosphate (ADP), thereby rapidly replenishing ATP after a sudden energy expenditure. Glycolysis is the other means of ATP production, which can function in the absence of oxygen although at much lower efficiency.[24]

Skeletal Muscle Energy Metabolism During Ischemia

In the presence of ischemia, oxygen-dependent oxidative phosphorylation cannot maintain ATP levels. In this situation, these levels are first maintained by utilizing CP reserves. This process continues for about 3 hours, after which CP stores are exhausted. Glycolysis continues as a final means toward ATP restoration, but at the cost of progressive metabolic acidosis due to lactate production. At this point, ATP levels begin to decline due to the much lower efficiency of ATP production by glycolysis. After 6 hours, failing cell charge, compounded by metabolic acidosis, take their toll and result in cell death. When this occurs, solely due to ongoing ischemia, it is deemed "irreversible," implying that intervention at this point cannot reverse the cellular necrosis already incurred. However, some areas may remain marginally viable within larger areas of necrosis.[17,19,25–28]

Skeletal Muscle Energy Metabolism During Reperfusion

Cell energy charge restitution with reperfusion depends on the duration of preceding ischemia and concomitant degree of energy depletion incurred. The ability of reperfusion to restore cell energy charge diminishes after longer ischemic intervals. This may occur in part because the phosphorylated nucleotide breakdown sequence of ATP to ADP proceeds to smaller, lipid-soluble precursors, which are washed away upon reperfusion (Figure 1). All compounds after inosine monophosphate (IMP) are dephosphorylated, rendering them lipid-soluble. Indeed, the preservation of IMP during ischemia seems to play a pivotal role in the successful repletion of ATP with reperfusion.[27] This and other intermediates participate in the regeneration of ATP through denovo or salvage pathways. Each of these pathways functions to a greater or lesser extent dependent on the condition of the cellular milieu and the muscle fiber type.[6,19,26,27]

One hour of reperfusion incompletely restores ATP deficits incurred during ischemic episodes of 5 hours duration.[19] However, CP levels are significantly repleted in this same setting. This may reflect a deficiency in ATP precursors due to their washout, rather than mitochondrial failure which is responsible for CP and ATP maintenance.[26] After 6 hours of ischemia, irreversible cellular and mitochondrial damage has been noted, along with a complete failure to resynthesize ATP or CP upon reperfusion.[27]

Longer periods of reperfusion also yield incomplete ATP regeneration. In the study by Rubin et al,[19] ATP levels after 1 hour of reperfusion did not improve by increasing the reperfusion interval to 48 hours. A variable increase in tissue necrosis was noted during this prolonged reperfusion phase. It was not clear why this variation occurred. However, it was noted that necrosis correlated with the degree of metabolite degradation. Greater numbers of lipid-soluble metabolic products were being formed concomitantly with increasing necrosis. Tissue, restratified according to the degree of necrosis, demonstrated some recovery of ATP levels only in tissue with mild degeneration. It was thought that the washout of soluble precursors prevented restoration of ATP stores, thereby exacerbating tissue injury during reperfusion. However, Rubin et al[29] have also demonstrated that much of the tissue injury in this same model is attenuated by reperfusion with blood depleted of complement and neutrophils. This suggests that a combination of metabolic and inflammatory insults accounts for the injury seen in reperfusion after intermediate periods of ischemia.

In summary, it seems that skeletal muscle ischemia, in the range of 3 to 5 hours, permits formation of lipid-soluble ATP precursors which are subsequently washed out during reperfusion. After 1 hour of reperfusion, tissue salvage is limited by incomplete ATP restoration. Longer reperfusion intervals result in progressive tissue injury, rather than energy repletion and tissue salvage. This "reperfusion injury" may be due, in part, to failed ATP restitution resulting in global cellular degeneration. However, injury due to ischemia-induced pathophysiologic inflammatory activation is largely contributory.

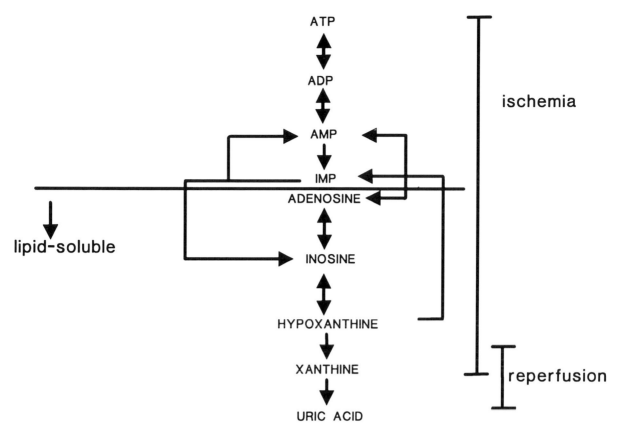

Figure 1. Sequence of phosphorylated nucleotide degradation and resynthesis in skeletal muscle ischemia and reperfusion. A **horizontal line** separates insoluble phosphorylated nucleotides from dephosphorylated lipid-soluble breakdown products. **Brackets** indicate that the conversion of xanthine to uric acid occurs only during reperfusion. Several of the degradation pathways occur irreversibly, which is reflected by alternate routes of adenosine triphosphate (ATP) resynthesis. Adenosine monophosphate (AMP) is irreversibly converted to inosine monophosphate (IMP). IMP is dephosphorylated to inosine during ischemia, or converted to AMP under appropriate reperfusion conditions. AMP is reversibly dephosphorylated to adenosine dependent upon the prevailing perfusion state. Hypoxanthine is a source for the resynthesis of IMP under appropriate reperfusion conditions. ADP = adenosine diphosphate.

Pathophysiologic Inflammatory Activation During Ischemia

There are observations that link the early derangements seen with cell energy metabolism in skeletal muscle ischemia to the inflammatory activation witnessed during reperfusion. There is evidence to support a pathophysiologic enzyme modification which results in the formation of free radicals by endothelial cells exposed to sufficient ischemia. These free radicals may, themselves, produce some local tissue injury. More importantly, they may set off a cascade of intercellular signaling between endothelial cells and neutrophils. This endothelial cell-neutrophil interaction results in further tissue destruction and skeletal muscle death. There are three potential sources of tissue injury which predominate during reperfusion: 1) endogenous free radical production by postischemic endothelial cells; 2) recruitment and activation of neu-

trophils wielding free radicals and lytic enzymes; and 3) continued ischemic injury due to occlusion of microvascular beds (no-reflow phenomenon) secondary to a possible combination of endothelial cell swelling, perivascular tissue edema, failed endothelium-dependent vessel relaxation, adherence of activated neutrophils, and microvascular thrombosis.

Free Radicals

A free radical is a molecule with an unpaired electron in its outer orbit. This renders the molecule unstable and highly reactive (Figure 2). In I/R, superoxide anion is produced by an electron reduction of molecular oxygen by endothelial xanthine oxidase (XO), or neutrophil nicotinamide adenine dinucleotide phosphate (NADPH) oxidase. Superoxide anion converts to hydrogen peroxide (H_2O_2) by spontaneous means,

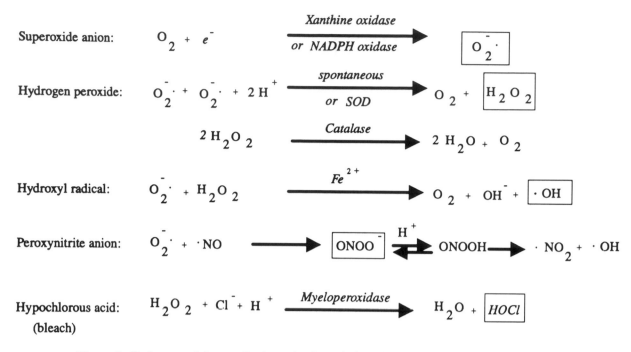

Figure 2. Pathways of free radical synthesis and degradation. Respective products are enclosed in **boxes**. Superoxide anion is produced by xanthine oxidase (XO) in endothelial cells, and by nicotinamide adenine dinucleotide phosphate (NADPH) oxidase in neutrophils. The interaction of two superoxide anion molecules results in the spontaneous production of hydrogen peroxide (H_2O_2). In the presence of iron (Fe_2^+), H_2O_2 combines with superoxide anion yielding hydroxyl radical (OH). Neutrophils convert H_2O_2 to hypochlorous acid (bleach, HOCl) through actions of the enzyme myeloperoxidase. Peroxynitrite anion is formed when superoxide anion combines with nitric oxide (NO). Peroxynitrite anion possesses its own oxidative powers, as well as the ability to form additional free radical species. Superoxide dismutase (SOD) is a naturally occurring enzyme which rapidly catalyzes the conversion of superoxide anion to H_2O_2. Catalase, also endogenously produced, further catalyzes the conversion of H_2O_2 to water. These latter two reactions limit the subsequent production of highly reactive OH and HOCl.

or more rapidly through the action of superoxide dismutase (SOD). Hydroxyl radical (OH) is generated by the iron-catalyzed Fenton reduction of H_2O_2. It is this highly reactive, short-lived free radical that is felt to be responsible for much of I/R tissue injury.[30] In the neutrophil, H_2O_2 reacts with chloride ions, catalyzed by myeloperoxidase, forming hypochlorous acid (HOCl-bleach), which is another potent oxidant. A third injurious free radical route occurs through formation of an intermediate known as peroxynitrite anion, which is postulated to form through the combination of NO and superoxide anion. In addition to direct sulfhydryl oxidation, it can rearrange to yield a hydroxyl radical.[31] Free radicals propagate through interaction with nonradical molecules, or terminate by reacting directly with another free radical. They react with cell membrane phospholipids which produces fatty acid peroxy radicals, a mechanism thought to be responsible for much of actual cell membrane damage.[32]

Several pharmacologic agents have been employed to attenuate free radical-induced reperfusion injury. This may occur by inhibiting or inactivating the

radical-forming enzymes, or through direct reaction with the free radical in question. The relative contributions of pertinent free radicals in I/R have been determined through the selective use of such chemical agents.[33] Free radical scavengers are compounds which chemically react with free radicals, disabling them without perpetuating the free radical chain reaction. Mannitol and dimethylsulfoxide (DMSO) are two such agents. Free radicals can be enzymatically converted into nontoxic molecules, a method employed in many biologic systems (Figure 2). SOD converts superoxide anion into H_2O_2. Although this reaction takes place spontaneously, SOD increases the conversion rate. This is beneficial because superoxide anion can otherwise react with H_2O_2, forming highly reactive hydroxyl radicals through the iron-catalyzed Fenton reduction. Catalase is a second enzyme in this pathway which converts H_2O_2 into water. SOD and catalase are available for exogenous administration.[34] Deferoximine is a clinically approved iron-chelator which inhibits the Fenton-based formation of hydroxyl radicals.[30] Enzymes responsible for free radical production can be chemically inactivated or inhibited. It is known that xanthine oxidase relies on a molybdenum metal core for activity. A molybdenum-poor, tungsten-rich diet effectively inactivates XO, as reflected by attenuated tissue injury in a corresponding I/R model.[35,36] Allopurinol and its metabolite, oxypurinol, are structural analogs of hypoxanthine. They diminish superoxide anion production through the inhibition of XO activity. At higher concentrations, these two compounds can act as free radical scavengers as well, although this mechanism is not encountered at XO inhibitory levels.[37]

Free radicals occur normally in many biologic systems. NO is one such free radical which acts as an important intercellular messenger in virtually all organ systems of the body. In I/R pathophysiology, NO is destroyed by oxygen-derived free radicals, and its endothelial cell production is diminished upon endothelial cell injury. Superoxide anion also provides a beneficial service when produced by neutrophils fighting infection. However, the redeeming features of its production by XO are less clear.

Xanthine Oxidase–Derived Free Radicals

In the cascade of phosphorylated nucleotide degradation, the irreversible breakdown of xanthine to uric acid occurs only in the presence of reperfusion. The preceding series of degradations can occur during ischemia (Figure 1). The significance of this observation relates to the enzyme xanthine dehydrogenase (XD). This enzyme typically converts hypoxanthine to xanthine, and xanthine to uric acid in the presence of the electron-acceptor nicotinamide adenine dinucleotide (NAD). These reactions do not appear to generate uric acid during skeletal muscle ischemia.[27] During ischemic cell injury, an increased flux of calcium into the cytosol is hypothesized to augment protease-mediated modification of XD to XO.[38] In fact, this "D to O conversion" has been shown to occur quite rapidly in response to a number of substances including tumor necrosis factor (TNF), interleukin-1 (IL-1), interleukin-3 (IL-3), complement, mitogens, endotoxin, and oxidants.[39] With reperfusion, XO converts xanthine to uric acid; however, molecular oxygen must serve as the electron-acceptor rather than NAD. This results in the formation of superoxide anion and uric acid supported by abundant levels of hypoxanthine, xanthine, and molecular oxygen (Figure 3).

Bulkley has proposed an evolutionarily conserved mechanism where D to O conversion is of endothelial antibacterial significance. In this model, detection of

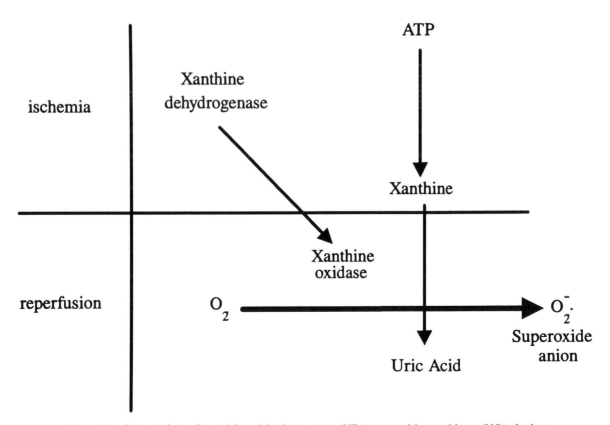

Figure 3. Conversion of xanthine dehydrogenase (XD) to xanthine oxidase (XO) during ischemia and reperfusion (I/R). Molecular oxygen reintroduced upon reperfusion is converted to superoxide anion by XO. Xanthine facilitates this reaction due to its abundance after prolonged ischemia. ATP = adenosine triphosphate.

an invading organism would result in D to O conversion, superoxide anion production, and rapid signal activation of the inflammatory response. Superoxide anion may accomplish this through free radical modification of complement and cell membrane phospholipids which can then act as the mediators.[40–42] The presence of XO in and on the endothelium puts it in an optimal location for bacterial encounters and signal release. In this light, D to O conversion during ischemia would then be considered a pathophysiologic variant of a formerly normal antibacterial mechanism.[43] In addition, participation of such a signaling system could occur with relatively low concentrations of XO, a common theme in signal amplification cascades. The detection of small or trace amounts of XO in skeletal muscle tissue homogenates had led some investgators to question its relevance in skeletal muscle I/R.[44] In a subsequent rat hindlimb model of I/R, significant levels of XD and XO were demonstrated, as well as a marked degree of D to O conversion evidenced during 2 hours of ischemia.[30] These findings, in combination with a cascade effect as described above, may be compatible with activation of the inflammatory system.

Endothelial Free Radical Production in Skeletal Muscle I/R

The participation of endogenous free radicals in skeletal muscle tissue injury may include direct attack and signal-mediated inflammatory (neutrophil) activation. XO has been localized on and in microvascular endothelium utilizing immunohistochemical stain techniques.[45,46] Cultured endothelial cell monolayers subjected to periods of anoxia and reoxygenation demonstrate marked free radical production and cell injury. The addition of XO inhibitor/free radical scavenger allopurinol or oxypurinol, and free radical neutralizing enzymes SOD and catalase, inhibit free radical production and cell injury in this in vitro model.[47,48] In skeletal muscle I/R, the presence of allopurinol, the XO inactivator tungsten, the free radical scavenger DMSO, or SOD and catalase, all decrease contractile and microvascular permeability derangements in reperfusion.[35,36,49] It is arguable that the effects of free radical scavengers, such as allopurinol or DMSO, could result from nonspecific scavenging of neutrophil-derived free radicals. However, the action of allopurinol is more likely one of XO enzyme inhibition, because serum levels in the above studies were felt to be too low for it to act in a scavenging capacity.[37] It has been difficult to determine the primary site of action with the in vivo administration of SOD and catalase. They may effectively inactivate superoxide anion derived from neutrophils, as well as XO. The observation with tungsten most directly supports endothelial superoxide anion

production as a participating mechanism for in vivo skeletal muscle I/R, due to its strict mechanism of XO inactivation.

Neutrophils in Skeletal Muscle I/R

It is well established that neutrophils contribute significantly to skeletal muscle injury during reperfusion. Moreover, their corresponding absence in leukopenic reperfusion demonstrates significant injury attenuation.[29,50–56] Such evidence has prompted many investigators to conclude that neutrophils are the primary means of injury during skeletal muscle reperfusion. Neutrophil sequestration is rapid in canine muscle tissue reperfused after 5 hours of ischemia. In fact, neutrophil infiltration escalates as reperfusion continues. Although tissue damage increases with longer reperfusion intervals, much of the damage caused by neutrophils occurs in the first hour of reperfusion, despite continued infiltration thereafter.[29] In vitro assessment of rabbit neutrophils subjected to in vivo I/R demonstrates significant activation of chemotaxis, phagocytosis, and free radical production after 2 hours of ischemia and 1 hour of reperfusion, a model demonstrating no tissue injury. However, increasing the ischemic interval to 3 hours followed by 1 hour of reperfusion, a model demonstrating tissue injury, reveals diminished free radical production by neutrophils, although chemotaxis and phagocytosis are still activated. This concurs with the findings of tissue injury in the above in vivo necrosis/infiltration data.[29] Neutrophils participating in reperfusion sufficient to cause tissue injury expend much of their free radical-producing capabilities early in reperfusion. Additional, although diminished, tissue injury occurs with continued reperfusion, reflected by ongoing neutrophil infiltration, chemotaxis, and phagocytosis.[57–59]

Mechanisms of Neutrophil Activation

Several lines of investigation support a role for superoxide anion in skeletal muscle I/R neutrophil activation and attraction (Figure 4). The addition of SOD and catalase to human umbilical vein or bovine microvascular endothelial cell cultures reduces neutrophil adhesion.[60,61] In vivo microscopic studies in skeletal muscle show diminished leukocyte rolling and adherence to postcapillary venules. A reduction in microvascular leakage consequent to SOD and allopurinol administration during reperfusion has been demonstrated as well.[62] A number of normally present intercellular signaling mechanisms have been shown to participate in I/R, some consequent to free radical activation.

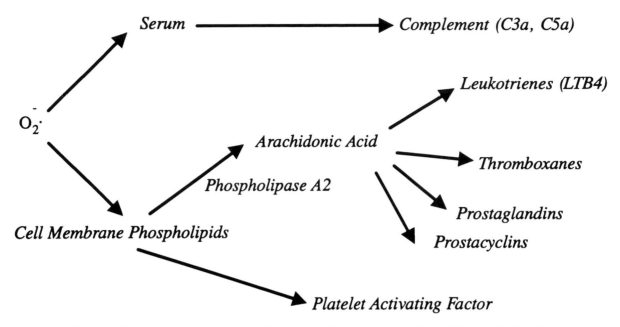

Figure 4. Superoxide anion produced by endothelial xanthine oxidase (XO) may indirectly incite the activation and attraction of neutrophils. This is feasible through the oxidative conversion of chemical mediator substrates present in the cell membrane and extracellular plasma proteins. This may explain the participation of neutrophil-activating compounds such as platelet activating factor, leukotrienes, thromboxanes, and complement.

Complement

Superoxide anion has been causally linked to neutrophil chemoattraction through the activation of complement.[40] Indeed, the complement alternative pathway is shown to be activated during skeletal muscle I/R, possibly facilitating the formation of the complement-derived membrane attack complex. Factors C3a and C5a are also present, directly increasing microvascular permeability and attracting neutrophils.[63,64] Complement depletion reduces permeability changes and neutrophil sequestration in skeletal muscle I/R.[29,55]

Arachidonic Acid Metabolites

Arachidonic acid (AA) metabolites contribute to skeletal muscle I/R. Free radical lipid peroxydation of endothelial cell membranes may induce production of AA metabolites through phospholipase A2 activation.[41] Such metabolites may directly incite permeability changes in endothelial cells, or injure them by attracting neutrophils.[65] Lipoxygenase products facilitate local and distant tissue injury by activating neutrophils within the milieu of the postischemic muscle, as well as in the systemic circulation.[66] Leukotriene B4 (LTB4) is a 5-lipoxygenase product known to incite potent degranulatory, chemoattractive, and endothelial adhesive responses by neutrophils.[67–69]

Thromboxane synthetase products activate neutrophils systemically, but still contribute to some of the local tissue changes.[66,70] Neutrophil free radical production in skeletal muscle I/R is induced by thromboxane B2.[71,72] Leukotrienes and thromboxanes are interdependent and may be synergistic for many of these observed effects. LTB4 is a known inducer of thromboxane production in neutrophils and endothelium, while thromboxane is also required for some of LTB4 actions.[73,74]

Prostacyclins are yet a third major division of AA metabolites, well known for their activity against thromboxanes in mechanisms of vasoreactivity and platelet aggregation. In skeletal muscle I/R, they may play a therapeutic role as defenders against inflammatory activation, again in part antagonized by thromboxanes. Prostacyclin and its stable analog, iloprost, exhibit potent in vitro inhibition of neutrophil activation, enzyme release, and free radical production, as well as skeletal muscle I/R-induced neutrophil adhesiveness to vascular endothelium.[75,76] Iloprost administered prior to ischemia and continued through reperfusion yields diminished tissue necrosis. Studies disagree as to whether iloprost lessens this necrosis through neutrophil inhibitory effects versus other lesser known mechanisms. Iloprost administered during reperfusion alone fails to attenuate muscle injury, suggesting its importance as an onset-inhibitor of inflammatory activation.[77–79]

Platelet Activating Factor

Platelet activating factor (PAF) is a phospholipid-conjugated glycerol derivative which is known to participate in signal activation of the inflammatory response. It is synthesized in phagocytes and endothelial cells, and participates in both immune and ischemia-mediated events.[80] Oxidant-mediated PAF synthesis by cultured endothelial cells augments their adhesion to neutrophils. PAF may be produced through free radical-mediated lipid peroxidation of cell membranes.[42] In vitro studies demonstrate chemically-induced endothelial PAF production occurring prior to or concomitantly with that of prostacyclin, while neutrophil PAF production coincides with that of LTB4. PAF receptor antagonists inhibit production of these products in both cell types, as well as free radical production by neutrophils. These findings support a second messenger role for PAF in intercellular signaling, pertinent to I/R phenomena.[81] Exogenous administration of PAF facilitates leukocyte adherence and permeability changes in intestinal postcapillary venules.[82] Leukocyte adherence and extravasation in bowel I/R are reduced by pretreatment with PAF receptor antagonists.[83] Although these experiments have not yet been performed in skeletal muscle I/R, PAF participation is likely due to the fundamental nature of its production and interactions with neutrophils, endothelium, and other mediators.

Cytokines

Cytokines are soluble polypeptide mediators originally described in pro-inflammatory processes caused by infection and injury, and traditionally known as the acute phase reaction. They are produced by leukocytes and endothelial cells in response to their own feedback stimulation, as well as by other intercellular messengers. In general, cytokines augment inflammatory responses in neutrophils and endothelial cells.[84]

Cytokines IL-1 and TNF in particular have been shown to exhibit changes consistent with I/R phenomena. Vascular permeability is directly increased by IL-1 and TNF.[85] These same two cytokines also upregulate the intercellular adhesiveness of neutrophils and endothelial cells.[86–88] TNF induces neutrophil superoxide anion production.[89] In endothelial cells, it inhibits production of endothelium-derived relaxing factor (NO).[90] In skeletal muscle I/R, significant elevation of postreperfusion venous effluent levels of IL-1, but not TNF, are seen. Such studies are said to be difficult to interpret, due to the fleeting nature of these chemical messengers.[91,92]

Of recent interest is the polypeptide known as transforming growth factor-beta. It has been shown to exhibit endothelial protective effects in cardiac and mesenteric ischemia. Produced by many cell types, its mode of action in ischemia may be through an anti-TNF effect, as reflected in its preservation of endothelium-dependent relaxation and its inhibition of neutrophil free radical production.[90,93] Similar studies in skeletal muscle I/R have yet to be performed.

Cell Adhesion Molecules

Circulating neutrophils become activated through contact with various endothelium-elaborated chemical messengers during I/R. This sets the stage for neutrophil binding, emigration, and subsequent toxic damage. All of these activities are facilitated through the interactions of CAMs. There are three pertinent families of CAMs in I/R: selectins, integrins, and members of the immunoglobulin superfamily (IgCAMs) (Table 1).[94–98]

Selectins are transmembrane glycoproteins found on endothelial cells, neutrophils, and platelets which facilitate intercellular attachment through identification of specific carbohydrate ligands on the receiving cell surface. Neutrophil L-selectin is constitutively expressed, but may undergo activity modulation during cellular activation. Endothelial cells exhibit inducible E-selectin cell-surface expression upon stimulation by IL-1 or TNF in a matter of hours.

Unlike selectins, integrins and IgCAMs bind to one another in the process of intercellular adhesion. Integrins reside on neutrophils, and IgCAMs on endothelium. Integrins are heterodimeric molecules, consisting of a variable heavy alpha-chain noncovalently bound to a conserved light beta-chain. Neutrophils express three types of integrins: CD11a/CD18 (LFA-1), CD11b/CD18 (Mac-1), CD11c/CD18 (p150,95), all designated in the order of the alpha/beta-chain, respectively. The first two are known to be participatory in I/R. Neutrophil adhesive capacity is modulated through qualitative and quantitative changes in the cell surface integrins, mediated by exposure to PAF, LTB4, and IL-8, an endothelium-derived cytokine released in response to endothelial contact with IL-1 or TNF.

IgCAMs are transmembrane glycoproteins comprised of variable numbers of extracellular immunoglobulin domains. Two IgCAMs, intercellular adhesion molecule-1 and -2 (ICAM-1, -2), are expressed on endothelial cells. Each one is interactive with different subsets of the neutrophil integrins mentioned above. ICAM-1 is constitutively expressed by the endothelium in low concentrations. It also exhibits slow, yet prolonged inducible expression to higher levels with IL-1 or TNF exposure. ICAM-2 exhibits constitutive expression only. It is known that a significant amount of neutrophil-related tissue injury occurs in the first

Table 1
Cell Adhesion Molecules

Type	Cell Expression	Expression/Regulation	Target Cell (Counter-receptor)
Selectins			
L-selectin	neutrophils	constitutive expression	activated endothelium (carbohydrate sites)
E-selectin	endothelium	IL-1, TNF inducible (hours)	neutrophils (carbohydrate sites)
Integrins			
CD11a/CD18	neutrophils	constitutive expression	endothelium (IgCAMs)
CD11b/CD18	neutrophils	1) constitutive (low levels) 2) PAF, LTB4, IL-8 inducible expression/adhesiveness	endothelium (IgCAMs)
IgCAMs			
ICAM-1	endothelium	1) constitutive (low levels) 2) IL-1, TNF (slow, but progressive induction)	neutrophils (integrins)
ICAM-2	endothelium	constitutive expression	neutrophils (integrins)

hour of reperfusion, whereas neutrophil infiltration continues for some time thereafter.[29] This implies that the constitutively expressed forms of CAMs are of perhaps primary importance in mediating early I/R adhesion and injury events. Chemically-mediated receptor upregulation may play a role in prolonged reperfusion.

Monoclonal antibodies in concert with in vivo microscopy have helped to define the role of CAMs in I/R. These studies have been performed in skeletal muscle, and extensively in the hamster cheek pouch preparation.[99–102] There are three general phases to neutrophil-endothelial interaction: rolling, attachment, and emigration. Upon reperfusion, circulating inactive neutrophils encounter postischemic venular endothelium, where blood flow in the adjacent physical milieu has slowed adequately to allow prolonged contact between neutrophil and endothelial cells. Constitutively expressed neutrophil L-selectin is thought to be responsible for initial endothelial cell binding, resulting in a microscopy-related observation known as "rolling." At this point, it is thought that the neutrophil first samples the "microenvironment" lining the postischemic endothelium, where a myriad of chemical messengers are then encountered. Neutrophil activation ensues, including free radical and lytic enzyme release, further chemical messenger elaboration, and increased expression/activity of the neutrophil integrins, which are felt to establish stationary intercellular attachments with endothelial IgCAMs. Successful integrin/IgCAM binding is required to facilitate subsequent neutrophil emigration into the extravascular tissues.[103]

In skeletal muscle I/R, monoclonal antibodies directed at several CAMs differentially attenuate neutrophil sequestration and vascular permeability in local tissues, as well as the systemically-exposed lung.[55] Antibodies targeting neutrophil CD18 and CD11b decrease neutrophil sequestration and endothelial damage in muscle and lung. Those antibodies directed against CD11a or ICAM-1 reduce these changes only in the lung. In myocardial I/R, the prereperfusion administration of monoclonal antibodies directed at endothelial ICAM-1 demonstrates a significant reduction in MPO levels, enhanced endothelium-derived relaxing factor (EDRF) activity, and decreased tissue necrosis.[104] Similarly, monoclonal antibodies directed against the neutrophil CD18 subunit demonstrate improved blood flow and decreased neutrophil infiltration.[105] However, overall tissue necrosis failed to differ significantly.

Nitric Oxide

In 1980, Furchgott and Zawadzki first described endothelium-dependent vascular smooth muscle relaxation by acetylcholine.[106] Seven years later, the identity of EDRF and NO was determined: a short-lived, lipid-soluble free radical now known as an intercellular messenger of diverse action and ubiquitous distribution.[107–109]

Vascular tone is modulated in part by a continuous basal release of NO from the endothelium.[110] It is also produced by platelets and neutrophils, acting as an autacoid feedback inhibitor of their cellular activation processes.[111–113] Intercellular actions of NO between endothelium, neutrophils, and platelets have been described subsequent to its initial discovery in the vessel wall.[114–116]

In vitro, EDRF activity is destroyed upon exposure to free radicals, and preserved with the addition of free radical scavengers.[117,118] EDRF activity in the superficial femoral artery of the rabbit has been evaluated in a model of skeletal muscle I/R.[119] Rabbit superficial femoral arterial segments subjected to in vivo I/R demonstrate a persistent deficit regarding in vitro endothelium-dependent vessel relaxation. These same vascular ring segments still relax completely with exposure to nitroprusside, an NO-bearing compound. This suggests that the endothelium alone is sufficiently damaged, such that NO production and release is diminished in a protracted fashion. In myocardial I/R, SOD administration prevents derangements to in vivo coronary endothelium-dependent relaxation.[120] The same investigator noted that basal NO levels are diminished 10 minutes after coronary reperfusion, followed by neutrophil adherence 20 minutes later.[121] The administration of SOD during reperfusion attenuates this neutrophil adherence. These studies suggest that diminished basal NO activity, through its destruction or decreased production, may facilitate neutrophil adherence by loss of its inhibition. Administration of transforming growth factor-beta in this same model also attenuates dysfunctional vasoconstriction, implicating TNF as a contributor to this type of endothelial injury.[90]

A sydnonimine class of compound (SIN-1) has recently been studied which acts as an NO donor. This agent is of interest because compounds such as nitroglycerin exhibit unpredictability, instability, and the potential development of physiologic tolerance. SIN-1 decomposes nonenzymatically to NO. Administration of SIN-1 during the reperfusion phase of feline cardiac I/R demonstrates a significant reduction in EDRF derangements and tissue necrosis.[122] Interestingly, tissue neutrophil accumulation was not attenuated, which suggests that NO-induced neutrophil inhibition was not the primary deterrent of tissue injury. This study reveals a potential means of reversing microvascular derangements secondary to NO deficiencies known to occur during I/R.

In conclusion, there are two probable mechanisms of I/R-induced dysfunction of endothelium-dependent relaxation: direct NO destruction by free radicals, and diminished NO release by injured endothelial cells. The above series of observations make it possible to envision a situation where free radical release during reperfusion could effectively inactivate NO in the microenvironment adjacent to neutrophils and endothelium, thus allowing neutrophil activation and concomitant vessel constriction. The endothelium, injured by direct attack, fails to release the usual basal levels of NO, exacerbating this pathologic vasoconstriction. Neutrophil adherence to this swollen, constricted microvasculature results in "plugging," commonly

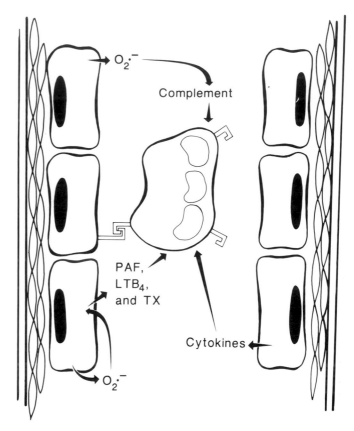

Figure 5A. Longitudinal representation of a microvascular segment in an early phase of reperfusion after a prolonged ischemic episode. Activated endothelium produces xanthine oxidase-derived superoxide anions. These reactive molecules initiate the release of chemical mediators from the cell membrane and serum proteins, which then cause neutrophil activation and attraction. A neutrophil is "rolling" along the vessel wall through the binding activity of constitutively expressed neutrophil L-selectin cell adhesion molecules. PAF = platelet activating factor; LTB4 = leukotriene B4; Tx = thromboxanes.

referred to as the no-reflow phenomenon. Indeed, changes in endothelial permeability and the onset of no-reflow have been observed to precede parenchymal tissue injury in skeletal muscle I/R.[123,124] This implies that microvascular injury may be distinct from and responsible for a substantial amount of gross tissue injury (Figures 5A, 5B, and 5C).

Theoretical Interventional Outline

The clinical presentation of prolonged acute limb ischemia implies that two uncontrolled events have occurred: 1) ATP depletion with the concomitant production of lipid-soluble metabolites; and 2) D to O conversion with the readiness to produce superoxide anion upon the reintroduction of molecular oxygen. Because ATP resynthesis during reperfusion is hampered due to

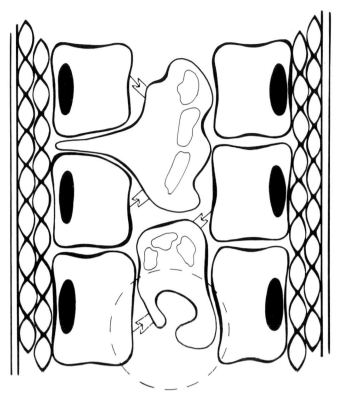

Figure 5B. The same microvascular segment as depicted in Figure 5A, now in a later phase of reperfusion. Endothelial injury results in microvascular leakage, endothelial cell swelling, and a failure of endothelium-dependent basilar relaxation depicted by constricted smooth muscle layers. These processes result in a narrowed vascular lumen, which is now occluded by adherent neutrophils (no-reflow phenomenon). Endothelial cell IgCAMs are firmly bound to neutrophil integrins, which facilitates the emigration of neutrophils into the extravascular space. IgCAMs = immunoglobulin-associated cell adhesion molecules.

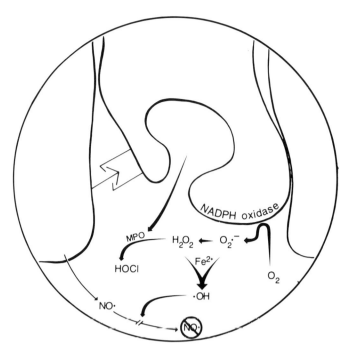

Figure 5C. Expanded view of Figure 5B inset. Neutrophil-derived superoxide anion is converted to hydrogen peroxide (H_2O_2). This acts as a substrate for the production of neutrophil-derived hypochlorous acid (HOCl) or iron-catalyzed hydroxyl radical. Nitric oxide (NO) present in the surrounding milieu is destroyed by these free radicals, which disables NO-dependent processes of vasodilation and neutrophil feedback inhibition. NADPH-icotinamide adenine dinucleotide phosphate; MPO-yeloperoxidase.

the washout of needed precursors, a portion of cellular reperfusion injury occurs secondary to ongoing ionic gradient imbalance, consequent cell swelling, and global cellular dysfunction, due to the interruption of ATP-dependent processes. Since D to O conversion has also occurred, reperfusion results in endothelial cell production of superoxide anion, the consequent elaboration of inflammatory activation mediators, and subsequent tissue destruction by activated neutrophils. Therapeutic interventions are limited to the reperfusion phase in this clinical scenario. Therefore, it seems logical that these two ischemia-induced derangements be focal points toward which therapy is first directed.

Therapeutic intervention might progress as follows: 1) a facilitation of ATP resynthesis; and 2) chemical inhibition of XO superoxide anion release, or superoxide anion elimination with free radical scavengers. In the event that these early interventions yield inadequate tissue salvage, additional targets could be sought further downstream in the activation cascade: 1) inhibi-

tion of chemical mediator release or blockade of their recipient binding sites (i.e., phospholipase A2 inhibition, or PAF antagonist, respectively); 2) administration of chemical mediators which act to oppose the effects of adverse mediators (i.e., iloprost); 3) administration of CAM-blocking antibodies to prevent neutrophil adhesion and emigration; 4) administration of free radical scavengers to diminish neutrophil destructive power; and 5) supplementation of NO to normalize derangements caused by its absence.

Other interventions are of a more mechanical nature including: 1) graded reperfusate oxygenation to delay the rate of free radical formation; 2) graded reperfusion pressure also resulting in gradual reoxygenation; 3) local hypothermia during reperfusion to slow tissue metabolic rate; and 4) leukocyte-depleted reperfusion with blood or a physiologic fluid substitute (i.e., crystalloid, or perfluorocarbon solution).

A combination of the above interventions may lead to an optimal therapeutic outcome in skeletal muscle I/R. The following discussions will focus on interventions targeting some of the salient aspects of I/R pathophysiology. The multitude of antagonists regarding the inflammatory mediator pathways have been described in appropriate sections. Their roles in skeletal muscle I/R therapy may be of potential benefit in combination with the following regimens.

Metabolic Salvage

In crystalloid-perfused heart preparations, ATP resynthesis is facilitated by inhibiting the enzymatic breakdown of ATP to lipid-soluble metabolites, such as adenosine and inosine. This results in improved functional recovery after periods of myocardial I/R through the preservation of intracellular phosphorylated nucleotides needed for ATP regeneration.[125,126] Unfortunately, this metabolic strategy requires the addition of chemical inhibitors prior to the onset of ischemia, which is not an option in clinical cases of acute limb ischemia.

The exogenous administration of adenosine prior to and throughout cardiac I/R demonstrates functional improvements by providing an intracellular precursor source for ATP resynthesis.[127] Again, preischemia administration makes this time course of adenosine application unavailable for limb ischemia. However, because adenosine is a precursor in ATP formation, rather than an inhibitor of ATP degradation, it can be effective as an agent administered strictly during reperfusion. Interestingly, in addition to its role as an ATP precursor, adenosine acts as an intercellular messenger pertinent to several I/R pathways. These include the inhibition of neutrophil-free radical release, neutrophil extravasation, platelet aggregation, and enhanced vasodilation.[128,129] This makes adenosine tenable as a reperfusion phase intervention for both metabolic and inflammatory pathways. In rat intestinal I/R, the topical application of adenosine to the bowel after ischemia demonstrates improvement in ATP restoration, vascular EDRF activity, and tissue salvage.[130] The role of adenosine as an intravascular agent added strictly during the reperfusion phase has yet to be assessed. In addition, the systemic vasodilatory effects of an agent such as adenosine may preclude its use in clinical situations of limb reperfusion.

Pentoxyfylline (PTX) is one of the agents used to inhibit enzymatic degradation of ATP to adenosine and/or inosine.[126] It is a methylxanthine derivative, lending it a structure similar to compounds such as xanthine, adenosine, caffeine, and theophylline. Like adenosine, PTX has effects on the inflammatory response including neutrophil inhibition, decreased production of cytokines, augmentation of prostaglandin synthesis, and initiation of its own EDRF activity.[131–134] Its utility in skeletal muscle I/R is promising, but has yet to be assessed.

Reperfusion with magnesium chloride-adenosine triphosphate (MgCl2-ATP) in a canine gracilis I/R model demonstrates improved skeletal muscle salvage.[135] However, this occurred without a concomitant repletion of ATP levels. Tissue salvage was felt to be derived from the neutrophil inhibitory effects of MgCl2-ATP. A reduction in I/R-induced skeletal muscle vascular permeability is obtained with administration of MgCl2-ATP.[136] In this same study, the in vitro production of neutrophil superoxide anion was diminished with exposure to MgCl2-ATP. This implicates it as a protector of microvascular integrity and function, perhaps affording a diminished no-reflow component. These observations are consistent with the notion that phosphorylated nucleotide compounds are not lipid-soluble and, therefore, are not useful for cell energy repletion when exogenously administered. However, with MgCl2-ATP, beneficial effects are still obtained through its actions of neutrophil inhibition and consequent microvascular protection.

Inhibition of Free Radical Production During Reperfusion

The prevention of free radical release by XO enzymatic inhibition may offer a potential method to diminish the degree of neutrophil activation. In addition, the subsequent production of neutrophil-derived free radicals may be eliminated by the same free radical-targeting agents. The addition of allopurinol, SOD, or deferoximine during reperfusion demonstrates significant amelioration of compartment pressures, and improved muscle perfusion in a rabbit model of hindlimb compartment syndrome produced by acute arterial occlusion.[137] This model was designed to resemble the clinical situation of reversible arterial ischemia, causing a distal extremity compartment syndrome. The neutralization of free radicals by SOD or deferoximine support their application in a clinical reperfusion regimen. Moreover, the concomitant administration of allopurinol in this setting may augment the degree of tissue salvage achieved.

The relative contribution of neutrophils in this type of model has not been concomitantly defined. However, their attraction by chemical mediators invoked through XO-derived superoxide anion is likely to be contributory. In vivo microscopic studies in skeletal muscle show diminished leukocyte rolling and adherence to postcapillary venules, as well as a reduction in microvascular leakage consequent to SOD and allopurinol administration during reperfusion.[62]

Graded Reoxygenation During Reperfusion

A significant reduction in muscle necrosis is observed in a canine gracilis muscle model after 5 hours of ischemia, 1 hour of graded reoxygenation, and 48 hours of systemic reperfusion.[138] This model employed graded reoxygenation which involved a gradual reintroduction of systemic blood and the addition of free radical-targeting agents. Graded reoxygenation consisted of reperfusion with an albumin-based Krebs-Henseleit crystalloid solution which was administered over 1 hour. During this time, oxygen concentration was increased with a membrane oxygenator. Concomitantly, oxygenated systemic blood was gradually added to this crystalloid solution in several aliquots. After 1 hour, systemic circulation was reestablished. Interestingly, the degree of tissue necrosis was further reduced with the addition of SOD, catalase, and mannitol. It is felt that initial reperfusion with an asanguinous crystalloid solution may facilitate the washout of elaborated inflammatory mediators, while simultaneously supplying needed oxygen. The addition of free radical-targeting agents is thought to aid in suppressing XO-derived superoxide anion during this initial phase.

In a rat skeletal muscle I/R model, 4 hours of room-temperature ischemia followed by "controlled" reperfusion resulted in restoration of ATP stores, minimized tissue swelling, and resolved some muscle contractile function.[139] Reperfusion was conducted using an oxygenated Krebs-Henseleit crystalloid solution containing hydroxyethyl starch to balance osmotic pressures, glucose, aspartate and glutamine as energy substrate, 2-mercaptopropionylglycine (MPG) as a free radical scavenger, and diltiazem as a calcium channel blocker. Calcium channel blockade is thought to reduce cellular injury due to massive calcium influx. Reperfusion conditions included normal body temperature and 50 mm of mercury (mm Hg) perfusion pressure for 30 minutes followed by 100 mm Hg for 30 minutes. This study demonstrates the utility of combining several interventional strategies to reduce reperfusion injury. Unfortunately, the control phase of reperfusion was not followed by the reintroduction of systemic blood, which would establish whether elements such as the neutrophil might still inflict damage. It remains to be seen if delaying blood-based reperfusion with the above regimen might minimize overall reperfusion injury. Possible mechanisms in this regard might include normalized metabolic function, quelled XO free radical production, washout of elaborated chemical mediators, and an overall reduction of neutrophil activation.

Leukopenic Reperfusion

A significant reduction in tissue necrosis was achieved by a brief, initial reperfusion interval with leukocyte-poor and complement-poor reperfusate.[29] This was achieved by passing arterial blood through a process of centrifugation, washing, and passage through a leukocyte filter. The effluent was then resus-

pended in hydroxyethyl starch. After 5 hours of ischemia, this modified reperfusion was conducted for 40 minutes, followed by 48 hours of full, systemic reperfusion. This modified reperfusion resulted in a reduction in myeloperoxidase (MPO) activity and overall tissue necrosis. However, the ultimate degree of neutrophil infiltration was not affected. This study suggests that neutrophil activation and injury occur early in reperfusion. The temporary removal of neutrophils and complement during initial reperfusion attenuates much of the injury seen during this period. Neutrophil tissue infiltration continues beyond this period of increased injury, suggesting that mediators of inflammatory activation then become less effective.

Perfluorocarbon emulsion (PFE) is a nonhematogenous, acellular blood substitute capable of significant oxygen-carrying capacity. It consists of a fluosol emulsion responsible for oxygen binding, and a physiologic electrolyte solution needed to balance ionic and osmotic gradients. Simple bubbling of 100% oxygen through this solution achieves full oxygenation. The administration of PFE during reperfusion in a canine gracilis muscle model demonstrated a significant reduction in overall tissue necrosis.[140] Six hours of ischemia were followed by 40 minutes of oxygenated PFE reperfusion. Full systemic blood reperfusion was then carried out for the next 48 hours. MPO activity increased significantly after the prolonged reperfusion phase, although this did not impact on tissue necrosis. This model provides another method of leukocyte-free reperfusion. Oxygen delivery is maintained during the brief period of asanguinous reperfusion. The subsequent reestablishment of normal systemic blood flow is then possible since the window for maximal neutrophil-related tissue damage has passed.

Hypothermia During Reperfusion

In organ preservation, it is well known that hypothermia prolongs tissue viability in organs destined for transplantation. From a metabolic perspective, it is known that enzymatic activity is reduced by half for every 10°C decrement in temperature.[141] In simple terms, the slowing of cellular enzymatic activity by cooling is felt to decrease the rate at which ischemic tissue derangements occurs. In clinical limb ischemia, metabolic processes in the anoxic limb are operating at ambient temperatures. This differentiates it from applications of hypothermia in harvested organs which are cooled prior to the initiation of ischemia. Any tissue injury incurred by prolonged ischemia alone is obviously not reversible by cooling applied during reperfusion. The goal of hypothermia in limb salvage is to minimize reperfusion injury.

The whole limb application of hypothermia is conveniently accomplished by external wrapping with cold gel packs. This method has successfully maintained intramuscular temperatures at 13°C below normal body temperature.[142] Amputated extremities wrapped in plastic and submerged in ice water maintain a temperature of 4°C. This technique might prove more difficult for ischemic limb therapy. In a canine gracilis muscle model, hypothermia was accomplished by pouring cold saline over the isolated muscle pedicle. This resulted in a significant reduction in postreperfusion edema, but not in overall necrosis.[143] Interstitial muscle pH was significantly improved. This effect is thought to be derived from a reduction in enzymatic lactate production. Difficulty was encountered in this model regarding specific temperature and timing variables. It was necessary to initiate cooling to a temperature of 21°C during the final hour of a 6-hour ischemic period. This temperature was then continued through a 1-hour reperfusion phase. Unfortunately, normothermic reperfusion was not initiated at the conclusion of the hypothermic reperfusion event. This may have better demonstrated the model's applicability to clinical therapy by establishing any possible long-term benefits (or morbidity). The combination of this intervention with others may prove beneficial.

Current Clinical Interventions

In clinical practice, the application of laboratory-derived reperfusion regimens has yet to be realized. Techniques have been limited to a combination of arterial repair, thromboembolectomy, mannitol, fibrinolysis, and heparinization. The following discussions review the potential salutary mechanisms of these clinical applications.

In patients with thromboembolic arterial occlusion, fibrinolysis acts as a primary means of therapy, as well as a valuable adjunct to operative intervention. Aside from thrombi responsible for large vessel occlusion, it is argued that thrombi also form in the microcirculation as sequelae to reperfusion.[144] It is felt that investigators who have not observed this phenomenon experimentally may have inadvertently prevented microvascular thrombus formation through the addition of heparin to the preparation prior to the onset of ischemia.

In a rabbit hindlimb model of I/R, 5 hours of ischemia followed by 2 hours of reperfusion demonstrate marked vascular occlusion.[144] This is demonstrated by the absence of distal arterial Doppler flow, microscopic evidence of red cell sludging and thrombi in arterioles, venules, and capillaries, and no recovery of contractile function. The addition of urokinase concomitantly with the reestablishment of systemic blood flow for 2 hours demonstrates the presence of Doppler flow and sporadic evidence of sludging or thrombi. However, this group failed to show any improvement in contractile function. Systemic blood was then infused at a nonhyperemic rate following neutrophil and platelet filtering. This also failed to demonstrate improved flow characteristics. The investigators feel that fibrin deposition is responsible for small vessel occlusion during reperfusion, with the secondary trapping of neutrophils which may then incite additional injury. The long-term implications of this initial urokinase reperfusion intervention are unknown, since a longer phase of reperfusion was not assessed.

Short-term heparinization during and after successful vascular flow restoration is commonplace. This rationale is typically based upon the anticoagulant effects of heparin. Anticoagulation is thought to protect against rethrombosis of a vessel whose intima has recently been damaged by thromboembolic ischemia and subsequent mechanical manipulation. It also prevents the propagation of clots into more distal vasculature.

Preischemic heparinization in a canine gracilis muscle model exposed to 6 hours of ischemia followed by 1 hour of reperfusion demonstrates a marked reduction in vascular permeability and tissue necrosis which is felt to be unrelated to its anticoagulant activity.[145] No significant differences were noted in reperfusion blood flow rates, which suggested that anticoagulant activity was not contributory. Interstitial acidosis was significantly lower at end-ischemia in the heparinized group, although the recovery of normal tissue pH at the end of reperfusion was not significantly different. The dose of heparin was consistent with that used clinically. Though its mechanism of action was not known, it was hypothesized that heparin may act to diminish I/R-induced tissue necrosis through a reduction of cumulative tissue acidosis consequent to the slowing of ischemic metabolic activity.

The addition of heparin during the reperfusion phase of skeletal muscle I/R was assessed regarding its effects on EDRF activity in the rat hindlimb.[146] After 60 minutes of ischemia, addition of heparin concomitantly with the reestablishment of systemic blood flow resulted in normalization of EDRF activity in response to acetylcholine during 30 minutes of reperfusion. Because nitroprusside administration achieved appropriate relaxation responses regardless of intervention, the salutary effect of heparin was determined to be of an endothelium-protective nature. The mechanism of action in this model is not known, but in general it is speculated to be a combination of endothelial membrane stabilization, SOD elaboration, and perhaps TNF expressive modulation. The effects of this intervention on long-term limb function and survival are not known.

Interestingly, both urokinase and heparin are known to inhibit neutrophil phagocytosis and chemotaxis in vitro.[147] Heparin effectively reduced chemotaxis even at low concentrations. Neutrophil superoxide anion production was not affected by either agent. The in vivo effects of urokinase and heparin on skeletal muscle I/R neutrophil activity are unknown. These observations serve as a reminder that even commonly used clinical agents may possess beneficial (or harmful) effects which are not initially appreciated.

Summary

Ischemia is the one variable out of the surgeon's control. When of brief duration, therapy consists of simple blood flow restoration; but if unduly prolonged, limb salvage with reperfusion may be less likely because of the profound, irreversible tissue damage incurred during the ischemic event. In addition, reperfusion at this point would be prohibitive because of life-threatening systemic reperfusion sequelae. Therefore, only cases of an ill-defined, intermediate-duration ischemic insult may benefit from any type of intervention.

Current goals of laboratory investigation need to include the development of a highly reliable means of ischemic assessment. Criteria should then be applied based on this assessment. If a patient falls into a zone of potential salvage, an interventional regimen ideal for that patient's situation would be employed.

The use of cell energy charge as an estimate of tissue extremis may be of utility when measured during the ischemic phase. However, this modality becomes erratic during reperfusion, likely due to extrinsic attack upon the cell by the inflammatory response, as well as the washout of ATP precursors. In addition, the methods of tissue energy assessment need be quick and relatively noninvasive. Freeze-clamp biopsy analysis is a prolonged process, while NMR analysis of a muscle biopsy specimen is completed in 15 minutes.[22]

At present, only the relative duration of an ischemic event is known. Uncertainty exists with regard to the amount of ischemic tissue injury incurred. Precision in this area is necessary. It is not known if the amount of ischemic injury is of sufficient quantity to preclude attempting revascularization and, rather, pursue amputation. To make such a decision would require knowing the profundity of reperfusion sequelae and the likelihood of limb salvage predicted by a given degree of ischemic injury. Laboratory observations that demonstrate a statistically significant improvement of an intervention over the control experiment do not necessarily imply an overwhelming difference suggesting its utility in a clinical regimen. The fantasy of developing a "reperfusion cocktail" which can be administered intra-arterially prior to reperfusion needs to be tempered by the analysis of certain clinical settings in which limbs may have progressed beyond the point of salvage.

References

1. Haimovici H: Arterial embolism with acute massive ischemic myopathy and myoglobinuria. *Surgery* 47(5): 739–747, 1960.
2. Haimovici H: Muscular, renal, and metabolic complications of acute arterial occlusion: myonephropathic-metabolic syndrome. *Surgery* 85:461–468, 1979.
3. Blaisdell, FW: The reperfusion syndrome. *Microcirc Endothelium Lymphatics* 5(3–5):127–141, 1989.
4. Eklof B, Neglen P, Thompson D: Temporary incomplete ischemia of the legs caused by aortic clamping in man: improvement of skeletal muscle metabolism by low-molecular dextran. *Ann Surg* 193:89, 1981.
5. Roberts JP, Perry MO, Harari RJ, et al: Incomplete recovery of muscle cell function following partial but not complete ischemia. *Circ Shock* 17:253–258, 1985.
6. Jennische E, Amundson B, Haljamae H: Metabolic response in feline "red" and "white" skeletal muscle to shock and ischemia. *Acta Physiol Scand* 106:39, 1979.
7. Messina LM, Faulkner JA: The skeletal muscle. In: Zelenock GB (ed). *Clinical Ischemic Syndromes: Mechanisms and Consequences of Tissue Injury*. St. Louis: Mosby-Year Book, Inc.; 457, 1990.
8. Barie PS, Mullins RJ: Experimental methods in the pathogenesis of limb ischemia. *J Surg Res* 44:284–307, 1988.
9. Novikoff AB, Shin WY, Drucker J: Mitochondrial localization of oxidative enzymes: staining results with two tetrazolium salts. *J Biophys Biochem Cytol* 9:47, 1961.
10. Blebea J, Kerr JC, Shumko JZ, et al: Quantitative histochemical evaluation of skeletal muscle ischemia and reperfusion injury. *J Surg Res* 43:311–321, 1987.
11. Blebea J, Kerr JC, Franco CD, et al: Technetium 99m pyrophosphate quantitation of skeletal muscle ischemia and reperfusion injury. *J Vasc Surg* 8:117–124, 1988.
12. Pedowitz RA, Gershuni DH, Friden J, et al: Effects of reperfusion intervals on skeletal muscle injury beneath and distal to a pneumatic tourniquet. *J Hand Surg* 17A(2):245–255, 1992.
13. Fish JS, McKee NH, Pynn BR, et al: Isometric contractile function recovery following tourniquet ischemia. *J Surg Res* 47:365–370, 1989.
14. Chervu A, Moore WS, Homsher E, et al: Differential recovery of skeletal muscle and peripheral nerve function after ischemia and reperfusion. *J Surg Res* 47: 12–19, 1989.
15. Colburn MD, Quinones-Baldrich WJ, Gelabert HA, et al: Standardization of skeletal muscle ischemic injury. *J Surg Res* 52: 309–313, 1992.
16. Granger HJ, Goodman AH, Granger DN: Role of resistance and exchange vessels in local microvascular control of skeletal muscle oxygenation in the dog. *Circ Res* 38(5):379–385, 1976.
17. Harris K, Walker PM, Mickle D, et al: Metabolic response of skeletal muscle to ischemia. *Am J Physiol* 250:H213-H220, 1986.
18. Lindsay T, Walker PM, Mickle DAG, et al: Measurement of hydroxy-conjugated dienes after ischemia-re-

perfusion in canine skeletal muscle. *Am J Physiol* 254: H578-H583, 1988.

19. Rubin B, Liauw S, Tittley J, et al: Prolonged adenine nucleotide resynthesis and reperfusion injury in postischemic skeletal muscle. *Am J Physiol* 262:H1538-H1547, 1992.

20. Jennische E: Relationship between membrane potential and lactate in gastrocnemius and soleus muscle of the cat during tourniquet ischemia and postischemic reflow. *Pflugers Arch* 349:329, 1982.

21. Newman RJ: Metabolic effects of tourniquet ischemia studied by nuclear magnetic resonance spectroscopy. *J Bone Joint Surg Am* 66B:434, 1984.

22. Eckert P, Schnackerz K: Ischemic tolerance of human skeletal muscle. *Ann Plast Surg* 26(1):77–84, 1991.

23. Perry MO, Shire GT, Albert SA: Cellular changes with graded limb ischemia and reperfusion. *J Vasc Surg* 1: 536, 1984.

24. Guyton, AC: Contraction of skeletal muscle. In: Guyton, AC (ed). *Textbook of Medical Physiology.* Philadelphia: WB Saunders Co.; 74, 1991.

25. Walker PM, Lindsay T, Liauw S, et al: The impact of energy depletion on skeletal muscle. *Microcirc Endothelium Lymphatics* 5(3–5):189–206, 1989.

26. Lindsay TF, Liauw S, Romaschin AD, et al: The effect of ischemia/reperfusion on adenine nucleotide metabolism and xanthine oxidase production in skeletal muscle. *J Vasc Surg* 12(1):8–15, 1990.

27. Idstrom JP, Soussi B, Elander A, et al: Purine metabolism after in vivo ischemia and reperfusion in rat skeletal muscle. *Am J Physiol* 258:H1668-H1673, 1990.

28. Walker PM: Ischemia/reperfusion injury in skeletal muscle. *Ann Vasc Surg* 5(4):399–402, 1991.

29. Rubin B, Tittley J, Chang G, et al: A clinically applicable method for long-term salvage of postischemic skeletal muscle. *J Vasc Surg* 13:58–68, 1991.

30. Smith JK, Carden DL, Grisham MB, et al: Role of iron in postischemic microvascular injury. *Am J Physiol* 256: H1472-H1477, 1989.

31. Radi R, Beckman JS, Bush KM, et al: Peroxynitrite-induced membrane lipid peroxidation: the cytotoxic potential of superoxide and nitric oxide. *Arch Biochem Biophys* 288(2):481–487, 1991.

32. Reilly PM, Schiller HJ, Bulkley GB: Pharmacologic approach to tissue injury mediated by free radicals and other reactive oxygen metabolites. *Am J Surg* 161: 488–503, 1991.

33. Schiller HJ, Reilly PM, Bulkley GB: Antioxidant therapy. *Crit Care Med* 21:S92-S102, 1993.

34. Greenwald RA: Superoxide dismutase and catalase as therapeutic agents for human diseases: a critical review. *Free Radic Biol Med* 8:201–209, 1990.

35. McCutchan HJ, Schwappach JR, Enquist EG, et al: Xanthine oxidase-derived H_2O_2 contributes to reperfusion injury of ischemic skeletal muscle. *Am J Physiol* 258:H1415-H1419, 1990.

36. Smith JK, Carden DL, Korthius RJ: Role of xanthine oxidase in postischemic microvascular injury in skeletal muscle. *Am J Physiol* 257:H1782-H1789, 1989.

37. Zimmerman BJ, Parks DA, Grisham MB, et al: Allopurinol does not enhance antioxidant properties of extracellular fluid. *Am J Physiol* 255:H202-H206, 1988.

38. McCord, J: Oxygen-derived free radicals in postischemic tissue injury. *N Engl J Med* 312(3):159–163, 1985.

39. Freidl HP, Till GO, Ryan US, et al: Mediator-induced activation of xanthine oxidase in endothelial cells. *FASEB J* 3:2512–2518, 1989.

40. Carden DL, Grisham MB, Korthius RJ: Neutrophil chemotactic activity generated in canine plasma by superoxide. *FASEB J* 6:A2071, 1992.

41. Otamiri T, Lindahl M, Tagesson C: Phospholipase A2 inhibition prevents mucosal damage associated with small intestinal ischemia. *Gut* 29:489–494, 1988.

42. Lewis MS, Whatley RE, Cain P, et al: Hydrogen peroxide stimulates the synthesis of platelet activating factor by endothelium and induces endothelial cell-dependent neutrophil adhesion. *J Clin Invest* 82:2045–2055, 1988.

43. Bulkley GB: Endothelial xanthine oxidase: a radical transducer of inflammatory signals for reticuloendothelial activation. *Br J Surg* 80:684–686, 1993.

44. Parks DA, Granger DN: Xanthine oxidase: biochemistry, distribution and physiology. *Acta Physiol Scand Suppl* 548:87–99, 1986.

45. Jarasch ED, Grund C, Bruder G, et al: Localization of xanthine oxidase in mammary-gland epithelium and capillary endothelium. *Cell* 25:67, 1981.

46. Vickers S, Hildreth J, Kujada F, et al: Immunohistoaffinity localization of xanthine oxidase in the microvascular endothelial cells of porcine and human organs. *Circ Shock* 31:87, 1990.

47. Ratych RE, Chuknyiska RS, Bulkley GB: The primary localization of free radical generation after anoxia/reoxygenation in isolated endothelial cells. *Surgery* 102: 122–131, 1987.

48. Zweier JL, Kuppusamy P, Lutty GA: Measurement of endothelial cell free radical generation: evidence for a central mechanism of free radical injury in postischemic tissues. *Proc Natl Acad Sci USA* 85:4046–4050, 1988.

49. Korthius RJ, Granger DN, Townsley MI, et al: The role of oxygen-derived free radicals in ischemia-induced increases in canine skeletal muscle vascular permeability. *Circ Res* 57:599–609, 1985.

50. Belkin M, LaMorte WL, Wright JG, et al: The role of leukocytes in the pathophysiology of skeletal muscle ischemic injury. *J Vasc Surg* 10:14–19, 1989.

51. Smith JK, Grisham MB, Granger DN, et al: Free radical defense mechanisms and neutrophil infiltration in postischemic skeletal muscle. *Am J Physiol* 256:H789-H793, 1989.

52. Sirsjo A, Lewis DH, Nylander G: The accumulation of polymorphonuclear leukocytes in postischemic skeletal muscle in the rat, measured by quantitating tissue myeloperoxidase. *Int J Microcirc* 9:163–173, 1990.

53. Walden DL, McCutchan HJ, Enquist EG, et al: Neutrophils accumulate and contribute to skeletal muscle dysfunction after ischemia-reperfusion. *Am J Physiol* 259: H1809-H1812, 1990.

54. Cambria RA, Anderson RJ, Dikdan G, et al: Leukocyte activation in ischemia-reperfusion injury of skeletal muscle. *J Surg Res* 51:13–17, 1991.

55. Seekamp A, Ward PA: Ischemia-reperfusion injury. *Agents Actions Suppl* 41:137–152, 1993.

56. Korthius RJ, Grisham MB, Granger DN: Leukocyte depletion attenuates the vascular injury associated with ischemia/reperfusion. *Am J Physiol* 254:H823-H827, 1988.

57. Freischlag JA, Hanna D: Superoxide anion release (O2-) after ischemia and reperfusion. *J Surg Res* 50: 565–568, 1991.

58. Freischlag JA, Hanna D: Neutrophil (PMN) phagocytosis and chemotaxis after 2 hours of ischemia. *J Surg Res* 50:648–652, 1991.

59. Freischlag JA, Hanna D: Neutrophil (PMN) phagocyto-

sis and chemotaxis after reperfusion injury. *J Surg Res* 52:152–156, 1992.

60. Suzuki M, Inauen W, Kvietys PR, et al: Superoxide mediates reperfusion-induced leukocyte-endothelial cell interactions. *Am J Physiol* 257:H1740-H1745, 1989.

61. Palluy L, Morliere L, Gris JC, et al: Hypoxia/reoxygenation stimulates endothelium to promote neutrophil adhesion. *Free Rad Biol Med* 13:21–30, 1992.

62. Menger MD, Pelikan S, Steiner D, et al: Microvascular ischemia-reperfusion injury in striated muscle: significance of "reflow paradox." *Am J Physiol* 263:H1901-H1906, 1992.

63. Rubin B, Smith A, Romaschin A, et al: Participation of the complement system in ischemia/reperfusion injury. *Microcirc Endothelium Lymphatics* 5:207–221, 1989.

64. Rubin BB, Smith A, Liauw S, et al: Complement activation and white cell sequestration in postischemic skeletal muscle. *Am J Physiol* 259:H525-H531, 1990.

65. Shasbi DM, Shasbi SS, Peach MJ: Polymorphonuclear leukocyte: arachidonate edema. *J Appl Physiol* 59:47–55, 1985.

66. Cambria RA, Anderson RJ, Dikdan G, et al: The influence of arachidonic acid metabolites on leukocyte activation and skeletal muscle injury after ischemia and reperfusion. *J Vasc Surg* 14:549–556, 1991.

67. Goetzl EJ, Picket WC: The human PMN leukocyte chemotactic activity of complex hydroxyeicosatetraenoic acids (HETEs). *J Immunol* 125:1789, 1980.

68. Goldman G, Welbourn R, Paterson IS, et al: Ischemia-induced neutrophil activation and diapedesis is lipoxygenase dependent. *Surgery* 107:428–433, 1990.

69. Lehr HA, Guhlmann A, Nolte D, et al: Leukotrienes as mediators in ischemia-reperfusion injury in a microcirculation model in the hamster. *J Clin Invest* 87:2036–2041, 1991.

70. Lelcuk S, Alexander F, Valeri CR, et al: Thromboxane A2 moderates permeability after limb ischemia. *Ann Surg* 202:642–646, 1985.

71. Paterson IS, Klausner JM, Goldman G, et al: Thromboxane mediates the ischemia-induced neutrophil oxidative burst. *Surgery* 106:224–229, 1989.

72. Cambria RA, Anderson RJ, Dikdan G, et al: Thromboxane synthetase inhibition decreases polymorphonuclear leukocyte activation following hindlimb ischemia. *Am Surgeon* 57(2):76–79, 1991.

73. Dunham B, Shepro D, Hechtman HB: Leukotriene B4 induction of TxB2 in cultured bovine aortic endothelial cells. *Inflammation* 8:313–321, 1984.

74. Welles SL, Shepro D, Hechtman HB: Eicosanoids modulation of stress fibers in cultured bovine endothelial cells. *Inflammation* 9:439–450, 1985.

75. Fantone JC, Marasco WA, Elgas LJ, et al: Stimulus specificity of prostaglandin inhibition of rabbit polymorphonuclear leukocyte lysosomal enzyme release and superoxide anion production. *Am J Pathol* 115:9–16, 1984.

76. Belch JTF, Saniabadi A, Dickson R, et al: Effect of iloprost (ZK 36374) on white cell behavior. In: Grygleswki RJ, Stock G, (eds). *Prostacyclin and Its Stable Analog Iloprost*. Berlin: Springer-Verlag; 97–102, 1987.

77. Belkin M, Wright GJ, Hobson RW: Iloprost infusion decreases skeletal muscle ischemia-reperfusion injury. *J Vasc Surg* 11:77–83, 1990.

78. Blebea J, Cambria RA, DeFouw D, et al: Iloprost attenuates the increased permeability in skeletal muscle after ischemia and reperfusion. *J Vasc Surg* 12:657–666, 1990.

79. Mohan C, Marini C, Gennaro M: The value and limitation of iloprost infusion in decreasing skeletal muscle necrosis. *J Vasc Surg* 16:268–273, 1992.

80. Ward PA, Warren JS, Varani J, et al: PAF, cytokines, toxic oxygen products and cell injury. *Molec Aspects Med* 12:169–174, 1991.

81. Stewart AG, Dubbin PN, Harris T, et al: Platelet-activating factor may act as a second messenger in the release of eicosanoids and superoxide anions from leukocytes and endothelial cells. *Proc Natl Acad Sci USA* 87:3215–3219, 1990.

82. Kubes P, Suzuki M, Granger DN: Platelet-activating factor-induced microvascular dysfunction: role of adherent leukocytes. *Am J Physiol* 258:G158-G163, 1990.

83. Kubes P, Ibbotson G, Russel J, et al: Role of platelet-activating factor in ischemia/reperfusion-induced leukocyte adherence. *Am J Physiol* 259:G300-G305, 1990.

84. Mantovani A, Dejana E: Cytokines as communication signals between leukocytes and endothelial cells. *Immunol Today* 10(11):370–375, 1989.

85. Royall JA, Berkow RL, Beckman JS, et al: Tumor necrosis factor and interleukin 1 alpha increase vascular endothelial permeability. *Am J Physiol* 257:399–410, 1989.

86. Gamble JR, Harlan JM, Kelbanoff SJ, et al: Stimulation of adherence of neutrophils to umbilical vein endothelium by human recombinant tumor necrosis factor. *Med Sci* 82:8667–8671, 1985.

87. Bevilacqua MP, Pober JS, Wheeler ME, et al: Interleukin 1 acts on cultured human vascular endothelium to increase the adhesion of polymorphonuclear leukocytes, monocytes, and related leukocyte lines. *J Clin Invest* 77:2003–2011, 1986.

88. Pober JS, Bevilacqua MP, Mendrick DL, et al: Two distinct monokines, interleukin 1 and tumor necrosis factor, each independently induce biosynthesis and transient expression of the same antigen on the surface of cultured human vascular endothelial cells. *J Immunol* 136:1680–1687, 1986.

89. Shalaby MR, Aggarwal BB, Rinderknecht E, et al: Activation of human polymorphonuclear neutrophil functions by interferon gamma and tumor necrosis factors. *J Immunol* 135:2069–2073, 1985.

90. Lefer AM, Ma X: Cytokines and growth factors in endothelial dysfunction. *Crit Care Med* 21:S9-S14, 1993.

91. Ascer E, Mohan C, Gennaro M, et al: Interleukin-1 and thromboxane release after skeletal muscle ischemia and reperfusion. *Ann Vasc Surg* 6:69–73, 1992.

92. Ascer E, Gennaro M, Cupo S, et al: Do cytokines play a role in skeletal muscle ischemia and reperfusion? *J Cardiovasc Surg* 33:588–592, 1992.

93. Lefer AM, Tsao P, Aoki N, et al: Mediation of cardioprotection by transforming growth factor-B. *Science* 249:61–64, 1990.

94. Bevilacqua MP: Endothelial-leukocyte adhesion molecules. *Annu Rev Immunol* 11:767–804, 1993.

95. Smyth SS, Joneckis CC, Parise LV: Regulation of vascular integrins. *Blood* 81(11):2827–2843, 1993.

96. Kubes P: Polymorphonuclear leukocyte-endothelium interactions: a role for pro-inflammatory and anti-inflammatory molecules. *Can J Physiol Pharmacol* 71:88–97, 1993.

97. Smith CW: Endothelial adhesion molecules and their role in inflammation. *Can J Physiol Pharmacol* 71:76–87, 1993.

98. Welbourn R, Goldman G, Kobzik L, et al: Neutrophil

adherence receptors (CD18) in ischemia. *J Immunol* 145(6):1906–1911, 1990.

99. Messina LM: In vivo assessment of acute microvascular injury after reperfusion of ischemic tibialis anterior muscle of the hamster. *J Surg Res* 48:615, 1990.

100. Richardson M, Berker A, Roberts A, et al: In vivo microscopy of rat skeletal muscle after ischemia using labeled neutrophils (PMN). *J Surg Res* 53:563–567, 1992.

101. von Andrian UH, Arfors KE: Neutrophil-endothelial cell interactions in vivo: a chain of events characterized by distinct molecular mechanisms. *Agents Actions Suppl* 41:153–164, 1993.

102. Winn RK, Vedder NB, Mihelcic D, et al: The role of adhesion molecules in reperfusion injury. *Agents Actions Suppl* 41:113–126, 1993.

103. Furie MB, Tancinco MCA, Smith CW: Monoclonal antibodies to leukocyte integrins CD11a/CD18 and CD11b/CD18 or intercellular adhesion molecule-1 inhibit chemoattractant-stimulated neutrophil transendothelial migration in vitro. *Blood* 78:2089–2097, 1991.

104. Ma XL, Lefer DJ, Lefer AM, et al: Coronary endothelial and cardiac protective effects of a monoclonal antibody to intercellular adhesion molecule 1 in myocardial ischemia and reperfusion. *Circulation* 86:937–946, 1992.

105. Tanaka M, Brooks SE, Richard VJ, et al: Effect of anti-CD18 antibody on myocardial neutrophil accumulation and infarct size after ischemia and reperfusion in dogs. *Circulation* 87:526–535, 1993.

106. Furchgott RF, Zawadzki JV: The obligatory role of endothelial cells in the relaxation of arterial smooth muscle by acetylcholine. *Nature* 288:373–376, 1980.

107. Palmer RMJ, Ferrige AG, Moncada S: Nitric oxide release accounts for the biological activity of endothelium-derived relaxing factor. *Nature* 327:524–526, 1987.

108. Ignarro LJ, Buga GM, Wood KS, et al: Endothelium-derived relaxing factor produced and released from artery and vein is nitric oxide. *Proc Natl Acad Sci USA* 84:9265–9269, 1987.

109. Palmer RMJ, Ashton DS, Moncada S: Vascular endothelial cells synthesize nitric oxide from L-arginine. *Nature* 333:664–666, 1988.

110. Vallance P, Collier J, Moncada S: Effects of endothelium-derived nitric oxide on peripheral arteriolar tone in man. *Lancet* 2:997–1000, 1989.

111. Radomski MW, Palmer RMJ, Moncada S: An L-arginine:nitric oxide pathway present in human platelets regulates aggregation. *Proc Natl Acad Sci USA* 87:5193–5197, 1990.

112. Clancy RM, Lesczczyuska-Piziak J, Abramson SB: Nitric oxide, an endothelial cell relaxation factor, inhibits neutrophil superoxide anion production via a direct action on the NADPH oxidase. *J Clin Invest* 90(3):1116–1121, 1992.

113. Riesco A, Caramelo C, Blum G, et al: Nitric oxide generating system as an autocrine mechanism in human polymorphonuclear leucocytes. *Biochem J* 292(3):791–796, 1993.

114. Azuma H, Ishikawa M, Sekizaki S: Endothelium-dependent inhibition of platelet aggregation. *Br J Pharmacol* 88:411–415, 1986.

115. Salvemini D, De Nucci G, Gryglewski RJ, et al: Human neutrophils and mononuclear cells inhibit platelet aggregation by releasing a nitric oxide-like factor. *Proc Natl Acad Sci USA* 86:6328–6332, 1989.

116. Kubes P, Suzuki M, Granger DN: Nitric oxide: an endogenous modulator of leukocyte adhesion. *Proc Natl Acad Sci USA* 88(11):4651–4655, 1991.

117. Gryglewski RJ, Palmer RMJ, Moncada S: Superoxide anion is involved in the breakdown of endothelium-derived vascular relaxing factor. *Nature* 320(3):454–456, 1986.

118. Rubanyi GM, Vanhoutte PM: Superoxide anions and hyperoxia inactivate endothelium-derived relaxing factor. *Am J Physiol* 250:H822-H827, 1986.

119. Summers ST, Zinner MJ, Freischlag JA: Production of endothelium-derived relaxing factor (EDRF) is compromised after ischemia and reperfusion. *Am J Surg* 166:216–220, 1993.

120. Tsao PS, Lefer AM: Time course and mechanism of endothelial dysfunction in isolated ischemic- and hypoxic-perfused rat hearts. *Am J Physiol* 259:H1660-H1666, 1990.

121. Lefer AM, Ma XL, Weyrich A, et al: Endothelial dysfunction and neutrophil adherence as critical events in the development of reperfusion injury. *Agents Actions Suppl* 41:127–135, 1993.

122. Siegfried MR, Erhardt J, Rider T, et al: Cardioprotection and attenuation of endothelial dysfunction by organic nitric oxide donors in myocardial ischemia-reperfusion. *J Pharmacol Exp Ther* 260(2):668–675, 1992.

123. Duval WD, Duran WN, Boric MP, et al: Microvascular transport and endothelial cell alterations preceding skeletal muscle damage in ischemia and reperfusion injury. *Am J Surg* 154:211–218, 1987.

124. Sternbergh WC III, Adelman B: The temporal relationship between endothelial cell dysfunction and skeletal muscle damage after ischemia and reperfusion. *J Vasc Surg* 16(1):30–39, 1992.

125. Bolling SF, Bies LE, Gallagher KP, et al: Augmenting intracellular adenosine improves myocardial recovery. *Thorac Cardiovasc Surg* 99:579–584, 1990.

126. Bolling SF, Olszanski DA, Bove EL, et al: Enhanced myocardial protection during global ischemia with 5'-nucleotidase inhibitors. *Thorac Cardiovasc Surg* 103(1):73–77, 1992.

127. Ely SW, Mentzer RM, Lasley RD, et al: Functional and metabolic evidence of enhanced myocardial tolerance to ischemia and reperfusion with adenosine. *J Thorac Cardiovasc Surg* 90:549–556, 1985.

128. Grisham MB, Hernandez LA, Granger DN: Adenosine inhibits ischemia-reperfusion-induced leukocyte adherence and extravasation. *Am J Physiol* 257:H1334-H1339, 1989.

129. Ely SW, Berne RM: Protective effects of adenosine in myocardial ischemia. *Circulation* 85(3):893–904, 1992.

130. Kaminski PM, Proctor KG: Extracellular and intracellular actions of adenosine and related compounds in the reperfused rat intestine. *Circ Res* 71:720–731, 1992.

131. Bessler H, Gilgal R, Djaldetti M, et al: Effect of pentoxyfylline on the phagocytic activity, cAMP levels, and superoxide anion production by monocytes and polymorphonuclear cells. *J Leukocyte Biol* 40:747–754, 1986.

132. Strieter RM, Remick DG, Ward RN, et al: Cellular and molecular regulation of tumor necrosis factor-alpha production by pentoxyfylline. *Biochem Biophys Res Com* 155(3):1230–1236, 1988.

133. Nowick WJ Jr, Sullivan G, Mandell G: New pharmacological studies with pentoxyfylline. *Biorheology* 27:449–454, 1990.

134. Berkenboom G, Fang ZY, Unger P, et al: Endothelium-

dependent effects of pentoxyfylline in rat aorta. *Eur J Pharm* 193:81–86, 1991.

135. Hayes PG, Liauw S, Smith A, et al: Exogenous magnesium chloride-adenosine triphosphate administration during reperfusion reduces the extent of necrosis in previously ischemic skeletal muscle. *J Vasc Surg* 11:441–447, 1990.

136. Korthius RJ, Grisham MB, Zimmerman BJ, et al: Vascular injury in dogs during ischemia-reperfusion: improvement with ATP-MgCl2 pretreatment. *Am J Physiol* 254(4pt2):H702-H708, 1988.

137. Perler BA, Tohmeh AG, Bulkley GB: Inhibition of the compartment syndrome by the ablation of free radical-mediated reperfusion injury. *Surgery* 108:40–47, 1990.

138. Walker PM, Lindsay TF, Labbe R, et al: Salvage of skeletal muscle with free radical scavengers. *J Vasc Surg* 5:68–75, 1987.

139. Beyersdorf F, Matheis G, Kruger S, et al: Avoiding reperfusion injury after limb revascularization: experimental observations and recommendations for clinical application. *J Vasc Surg* 9:757–766, 1989.

140. Mohan C, Gennaro M, Marini C, et al: Reduction of the extent of ischemic skeletal muscle necrosis by perfusion with oxygenated perfluorocarbon. *Am J Surg* 164:194–198, 1992.

141. Southard JH: Temperature effects and cooling. In: Zelenock GB (ed). *Clinical Ischemic Syndromes: Mechanisms and Consequences of Tissue Injury.* St. Louis: Mosby-Year Book, Inc.; 303, 1990.

142. Swanson AB, Livengood LC, Sattel AB: Local hypothermia to prolong safe tourniquet time. *Clin Ortho Rel Res* 264:200–208, 1991.

143. Wright JG, Araki CT, Belkin M, et al: Postischemic hypothermia diminishes skeletal muscle reperfusion edema. *J Surg Res* 47:389–396, 1989.

144. Quinones-Baldrich WJ, Chervu A, Hernandez JJ, et al: Skeletal muscle function after ischemia: "no reflow" versus reperfusion injury. *J Surg Res* 51:5–12, 1991.

145. Hobson RW II, Wright JG, Fox D, et al: Heparinization reduces endothelial permeability and hydrogen ion accumulation in a canine skeletal muscle ischemia-reperfusion model. *J Vasc Surg* 7(4):585–590, 1988.

146. Sternbergh WC III, Makhoul RG, Adelman B: Heparin prevents postischemic endothelial cell dysfunction by a mechanism independent of its anticoagulant activity. *J Vasc Surg* 17:318–327, 1993.

147. Freischlag JA, Colburn MD, Quinones-Baldrich, et al: Heparin, urokinase, and ancrod alter neutrophil function. *J Vasc Surg* 16(4):565–574, 1992.

CHAPTER 34

Spinal Cord Ischemia Associated with High Aortic Clamping:

Methods of Protection

David Whitley, MD; Peter Gloviczki, MD

Introduction

Paraplegia caused by ischemic and reperfusion injury to the spinal cord is a severe complication following repair of an aneurysm involving the thoracoabdominal aorta. Patients who survive with this complication have significant permanent disability and major deterioration in health-related quality of life.

At the turn of the century, Alexis Carrel[1] emphasized the importance of protecting the spinal cord during cross-clamping of the thoracic aorta. He recognized that, "the main danger of the aortic operation does not come from the heart or from the aorta itself, but from the central nervous system." For his experiment, he devised an aorto-aortic shunt using a paraffinized tube. An aorto-aortic shunt to protect the cord was used in 1954 by Etheredge[2] during the first successful operation in a patient to treat a thoracoabdominal aortic aneurysm. Since then, several different adjuncts, such as shunts, hypothermia, cerebrospinal fluid (CSF) drainage, and various pharmacologic agents have been employed to prevent the deleterious effects of temporary aortic clamping. None of these adjuncts, however, has provided complete protection for the spinal cord.

In this chapter, we review the pathophysiology of spinal cord ischemia and reperfusion following high aortic cross-clamping, and discuss the effectiveness of current experimental and clinical methods of spinal cord protection.

The Development and Anatomy of the Blood Supply to the Spinal Cord

The blood supply to the spinal cord begins in the embryo in a segmental pattern. There are 31 segmental radicular arteries associated, sending branches in an afferent direction along the developing spinal nerves. Each artery divides into a dorsal and ventral branch forming a superficial capillary network over the surface of the developing spinal cord. Longitudinal anastomotic channels become more differentiated, and they form a single anterior spinal artery and bilateral posterior spinal arteries (Figure 1). As the embryo develops, the vertebral column elongates more rapidly than the cord and the origins of the radicular arteries are displaced. During later intrauterine and early postnatal life, most of the segmental branches atrophy, leaving the adult with only about 6 to 8 radicular arteries that supply the anterior spinal artery and between 10 and 23 that perfuse the posterior spinal arteries.

The anterior spinal artery originates from the intracranial segment of both vertebral arteries and supplies the anterior and lateral columns and the gray mat-

From *The Basic Science of Vascular Disease*. Edited by Sidawy AN, Sumpio BE, and DePalma RG. Armonk, NY: Futura Publishing Company, Inc.; © 1997.

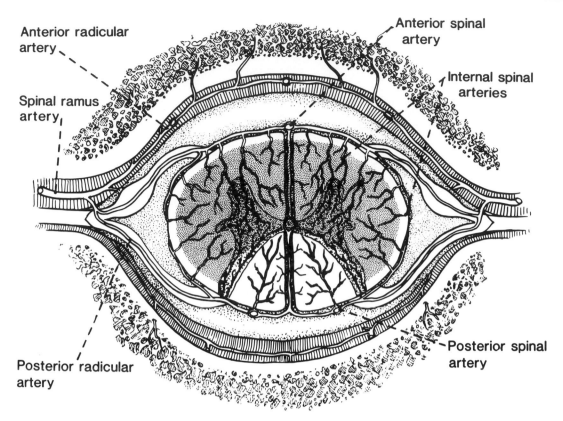

Figure 1. Cross-section of the distal thoracic cord with blood supply. (Reproduced with permission from the Mayo Foundation.)

ter of the spinal cord, except the posterior portion of the posterior horn. The anterior spinal artery in humans and higher primates runs continuously cephalad-to-caudad along the spinal cord.[3] It is the major source of blood supply to the spinal cord and is supplied by the intercostal and lumbar arteries in the thoracolumbar region. The most developed radicular artery arises in the thoracolumbar region and has been called the arteria radicularis magna, or great radicular artery, or the artery of Adamkiewicz (Figure 2). This is the most important artery supplying the distal thoracic and lumbar cord; it arises from the T8 to the T12 level in 75% of patients, from T5 to T8 in 15%, and from L1 to L2 in 10%.[4]

There is variation in the level of origin and the number of arteries supplying the spinal cord. In some cases, a cervical radicular artery may arise from branches of the left subclavian artery. When the artery of Adamkiewicz arises below T12, there is usually an additional radicular artery originating at the level of T7 or T8.[3]

The Pathophysiology of Spinal Cord Ischemia and Reperfusion

Permanent injury to the cord is a consequence of multiple interdependent variables. These include: a)

the severity of neuronal ischemia; b) the rate of neuronal metabolism during ischemic periods; and c) the extent of postischemic reperfusion injury caused by oxygen-derived free radicals and by both direct and complement-mediated leukocytes. Cellular mechanisms, such as calcium influx during reperfusion and cell swelling, also play a role in late neuronal injury.

Hemodynamic Changes

Clamping of the thoracic aorta distal to the left subclavian artery results in a marked reduction in the distal aortic pressure and a decrease in spinal cord blood flow. Subsequent systemic hypotension, due to intraoperative blood loss, may further reduce spinal cord blood flow. CSF pressure increases following aortic clamping, leading to further decreases in spinal cord perfusion pressure. These changes predispose the spinal cord to permanent ischemic injury.

Ischemic Injury

Spinal cord ischemia following high aortic clamping almost always is "incomplete," since blood flow persists in an amount insufficient to maintain normal aerobic metabolism.[5,6] Continued metabolism under

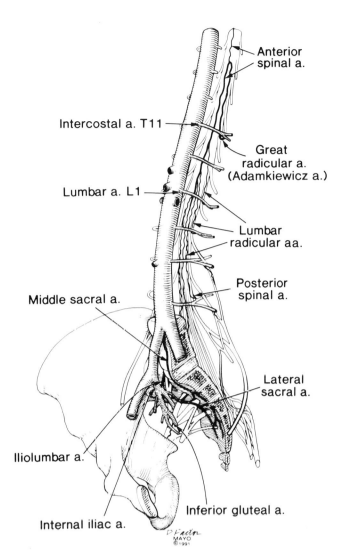

Anterior spinal a.

Intercostal a. T11

Great radicular a. (Adamkiewicz a.)

Lumbar a. L1

Lumbar radicular aa.

Posterior spinal a.

Middle sacral a.

Lateral sacral a.

Iliolumbar a.

Inferior gluteal a.

Internal iliac a.

Figure 2. Blood supply to the spinal cord. (Reproduced with permission from: Gloviczki P, Cross SA, Stanson AW, et al: Ischemic injury to the spinal cord or lumbosacral plexus after aortoiliac reconstruction. *Am J Surg* 162:131–136, 1991.)

hypoxic conditions results in the production of toxic by-products, such as oxygen-derived free radicals. Acidosis may be aggravated by high glucose loads and increased metabolic activity in the hypoxic state.[5,6]

A subtle indicator of ischemic injury to a tissue is enhanced capillary permeability. Increased permeability results in edema formation. Edema is caused by an increase in intracellular sodium due to decreased sodium pumping by the Na $\pm$ K + ATPase; eventual extravasation may occur.

Reperfusion Injury

Oxygen-derived free radicals cause injury to cell membranes during reperfusion through chain reaction peroxidation of lipids within the membrane structure

and by enzyme inactivation (Figure 3). Cellular injury and edema are induced by the xanthine oxidase/hypoxanthine ADP-Fe^{3+} system which produces free radicals at reflow. Hypoxanthine, a by-product of ATP degradation, is the natural substrate for xanthine oxidase. In the absence of oxygen during ischemia, this reaction does not go forward; however, at the moment of reperfusion, with oxygen again present and with correction of acidosis, the reaction goes to completion, with formation of uric acid and the oxygen-free radical, superoxide. Other possible mechanisms for superoxide free radical production at the moment of reperfusion include production by the electron transport chain in part as a result of injury occurring during ischemia, from white cell activation within the ischemic tissue,[7] and oxidation of catecholamines (a burst of catecholamine release is known to occur at the moment of reperfusion) (Figure 3).

Another free radical that can cause tissue injury during reperfusion is the hydroxyl radical (OH^-). Superoxide (O_2-) is converted to the very active hydroxyl radical by iron-requiring reactions, namely the Haber-Weiss and the Fenton reactions (Figure 4). Iron-binding agents, such as deferroxamine, could be useful by reducing free iron for these reactions, as well as blocking local cytokine production which may contribute to secondary cellular injury.[7-9]

Reperfusion injury appears to be a complex mechanism of injury. Membrane injury, cellular enzyme dysfunction, and edema occur during the ischemic period. At reperfusion, further membrane and enzyme injuries occur abruptly, probably due to free radical generation. Enzymes responsible for calcium extraction from the cell become dysfunctional. Sodium entry continues to occur with each depolarization, contributing to further calcium entry. Leukocytes become trapped within endothelial cells resulting in microvascular plugging, leading to focal ischemia and causing further free radical injury.

Delayed Onset Paraplegia

Although spinal cord dysfunction after thoracic aortic occlusion develops in most patients during or immediately after cross-clamping, delayed-onset paraplegia may occur up to 1 to 5 days postoperatively. The cause has been attributed to embolization or thrombosis of the anterior spinal artery, or episodes of postoperative hypotension. Additional mechanisms of spinal cord injury may include edema, leukocyte infiltration and cytotoxic destruction of microglia, and vasoconstriction or delayed free radical injury.[10-14]

Methods of Protection

Theoretically, paraplegia could be prevented if adequate perfusion to the spinal cord could be maintained

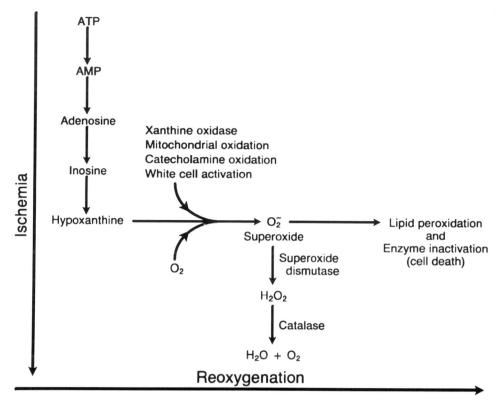

Figure 3. Diagram of sources of oxygen-free radicals during ischemia/reperfusion injury and intrinsic mechanisms of defense against free radical injury within cells. (Adapted with permission from McCord JM: Oxygen-derived free radicals in postischemic tissue injury. *N Engl J Med* 312:159–163, 1985.)

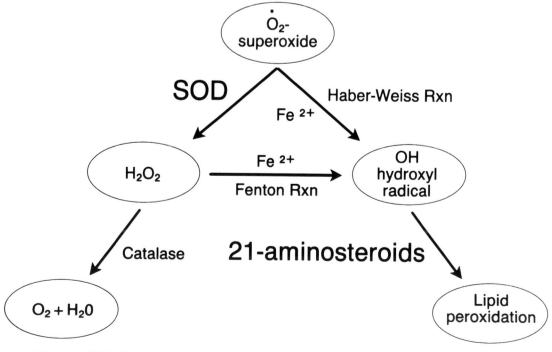

Figure 4. This diagram shows the role of iron reactions in the production of hydroxyl radicals. (Adapted with permission from Reference 7.)

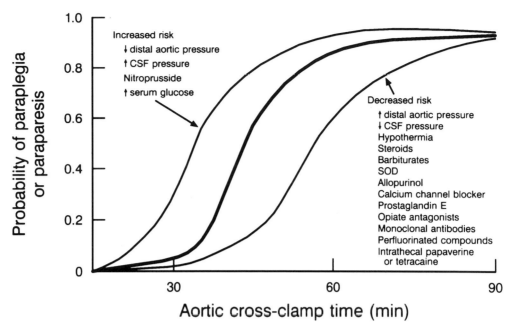

Figure 5. The probability of ischemic spinal cord injury during occlusion of the thoracic aorta. (Adapted with permission from Svensson LG, Loop FD: Prevention of spinal cord ischemia in aortic surgery. In: Bergan JJ, Yao JST (eds). *Arterial Surgery: New Diagnostic and Operative Techniques.* Orlando, FL: Grune & Stratton, Inc.; 273–285, 1988.)

during aortic grafting, and the cord is revascularized following placement of the graft. Since perfusion to the cord is frequently not possible, pharmacologic or hypothermic protection of the cord is required to prevent ischemic injury during prolonged aortic cross-clamping and injury during reperfusion. In addition, circulation to the cord has to be reestablished after aortic repair, either through the great radicular artery, or through intercostal, lumbar, or pelvic collaterals.

Factors Influencing Paraplegia

Extensive research at our institution and other centers has revealed factors that influence ischemia tolerance of the spinal cord. The probability of ischemic spinal cord injury during occlusion of the thoracic aorta increases with prolonged aortic cross-clamp time, decreased distal aortic perfusion,[15] increased CSF pressure,[16–18] failure to revascularize critical intercostal arteries,[19,20] excessive use of sodium nitroprusside,[21] or perioperative hyperglycemia[5,22] (Figure 5).

The risk of spinal cord injury decreases, at least in experiments, by improving the distal aortic pressure,[15] decreasing CSF pressure,[6,16–18,23] using hypothermia,[24–28] or drugs such as steroids,[29,30] barbiturates,[31] superoxide dismutase,[32–34] calcium channel blockers,[35–37] prostaglandins,[33] intrathecal papaverine,[38] MK-801,[39,40] intrathecal tetracaine,[41] monoclonal anti-

bodies,[42] opiate antagonists,[43] or perfluorinated compounds.[44] The canine model used in our laboratory to evaluate the effects of spinal fluid drainage, hypothermia, and drugs on experimental spinal cord ischemia is shown in Figure 6.

Experimental Results of Spinal Cord Protection

Cerebrospinal Fluid Drainage

The spinal cord injury that occurs after thoracic aortic occlusion (Figure 7) is probably caused by several factors such as embolism or thrombotic occlusion of critical intercostal arteries, permanent interruption of a major nutrient vessel, and prolonged spinal cord ischemia during the period of aortic clamping because of inadequate collateral circulation. Experimental studies have documented an increase in CSF pressure during the aortic occlusion period (Figure 8).[16,17,45]

The technique of spinal cord fluid drainage was first described as a method of preventing spinal cord damage following occlusion of the thoracic aorta by Miyamoto et al.[16] This technique was developed following the observation that CSF pressure was elevated after crossclamping the thoracic aorta in dogs. Using the technique of withdrawing CSF to keep the pressure less than 30 cm H_2O, these investigators lowered the paraplegia rate from 75% to 5% after clamping the tho-

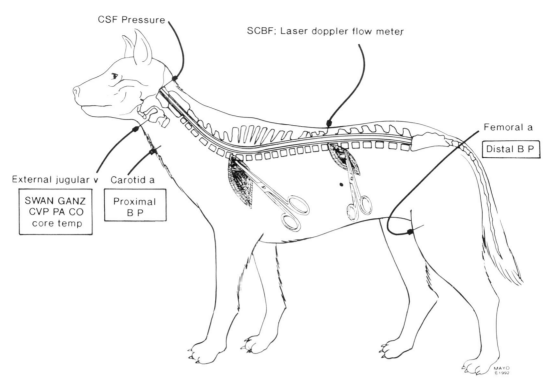

Figure 6. Canine model used to evaluate the effects of drugs, hypothermia, and spinal fluid drainage on experimental spinal cord ischemia. CVP = central venous pressure; PA = pulmonary artery pressure; CO = cardiac output; temp = temperature; BP = blood pressure; SCBF = spinal cord blood flow; a = artery; v = vein.

racic aorta for 1 hour. Blaisdell and Cooley[17] followed with a similar study in which they were able to lower the rate of paraplegia from 50% to 8% in surviving animals by withdrawing CSF and, thus, lowering CSF pressure after occluding the thoracic aorta for 1 hour. One group of animals had their CSF pressure artificially elevated, and CSF pressure equal to or exceeding distal aortic pressure correlated with a 100% paraplegia rate.[17] Other studies have demonstrated the benefit of CSF withdrawal in preventing spinal cord injury during an ischemic insult.[6,18,23,34,46,47]

The mechanism of the protection provided by CSF drainage remains controversial. Many studies have attempted to implicate increased venous pressure as a result of increased CSF pressure as the sole mechanism for the phenomenon of decreased spinal artery perfusion with increasing CSF pressure.[48–50] Griffiths and colleagues performed an eloquent study using hydrogen clearance techniques, demonstrating a local autoregulatory response which increased spinal cord blood flow as CSF pressure increased to a perfusion pressure of 50 mm Hg (perfusion pressure = distal aortic pressure − CSF pressure).[51] Fifty mm Hg perfusion pressure appeared to be the lower limit of autoregulation to maintain normal spinal cord blood flow. They were able to elevate CSF pressure without significantly ele-

vating intracranial pressure and, thus, avoided the Cushing response which has complicated other studies.[51] Their studies implicated a transluminal arterial effect rather than simple venous congestion.[51] Oka and Miyamoto[45] demonstrated that maintaining a relative spinal perfusion pressure of 15 mm Hg by withdrawing spinal fluid completely prevented neurologic injury in their dog model. Mantainence of 0 mm Hg relative spinal perfusion pressure resulted in 100% paralysis after 20 minutes of aortic cross-clamp.

Other studies have not been able to demonstrate the significant benefits of CSF drainage. Wadouh et al[52] did not demonstrate any significant improvement in neurologic outcome in pigs with CSF drainage versus those without drainage. Svensson et al[38] demonstrated no benefit of CSF drainage in a multiple arm study in baboons during aortic cross-clamping. In this study, CSF drainage was effected by performing a laminectomy and allowing the CSF to escape freely. There is some concern that a locally invasive procedure such as a laminectomy alters local autoregulation and may cause vasospasm which would skew results.

Grubbs et al[53] demonstrated that CSF drainage increases spinal cord perfusion pressure from 9.4 to 21.8 mm Hg and significantly decreases neurologic injury in the dog. McCullough et al[46] were able to demon-

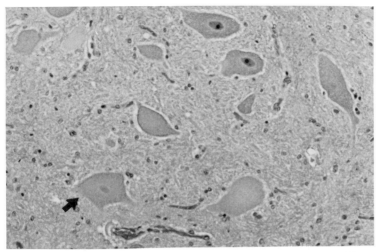

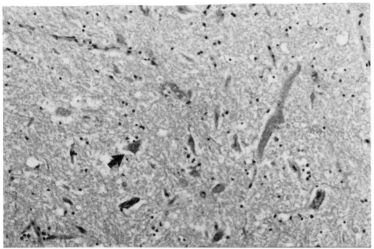

Figure 7. **Top**: light micrograph of a dog's normal lumbar spinal cord gray matter. **Bottom**: light micrograph of lumbar spinal cord gray matter of a paraplegic dog after 60 minutes of thoracic aortic occlusion. Histologically, there is anterior horn cell degeneration with ischemia of surrounding neural tissue. (Hematoxylin-eosin stain; original magnification × 400.) (Reproduced with permission from Reference 15.)

strate that drainage of CSF before thoracic aortic occlusion significantly increased spinal cord perfusion pressure (22 to 30 mm Hg) and decreased paraplegia in the dog. There were no differences in distal aortic pressures between the two groups (30 versus 28 mm Hg). Bower et al[18] showed that CSF drainage not only decreased neurologic injury, but improved blood flow in the spinal cord. Using microspheres, they demonstrated a reduction of flow from 23.1 to 4.0 mL/100 gm/min after aortic cross-clamping. The addition of CSF drainage improved flow to 11.3 mL/100 gm/min in the gray matter of the lower thoracic cord. CSF drainage prevented significant reperfusion hyperemia after removal of the aortic cross-clamp (Figure 9). The magnitude of the hyperemic reflow response may reflect the degree to which the vascular autoregulatory mechanisms have been affected by the ischemic insult. CSF drainage, while improving neurologic outcome after an ischemic insult, has not provided complete protection in all experiments. This probably implicates the involvement of multiple factors in development of an ischemic lesion. For these reasons, studies have com-

bined CSF drainage with other treatment modalities in an attempt to reduce the ischemic insult. Granke et al[34] combined polyethylene glycol-conjugated superoxide dismutase parenterally as a free radical scavenger with CSF drainage in dogs undergoing aortic cross-clamping. There was no paraplegia in the groups with CSF drainage alone, or in the group combining CSF drainage with a free radical scavenger. Francel et al[54] had the lowest paraplegia rate in the group which combined the free radical scavenger 21-aminosteroid with CSF drainage (20%) compared with control (70%) after aortic cross-clamping in the dog.

In experimental animals, it is clear that CSF drainage does not return spinal cord blood flow to normal or provide complete neurologic protection during ischemic periods; however, it may provide significant protection that may allow longer ischemic periods with fewer neurologic insults.

Hypothermia

The mechanism of hypothermic protection of neural tissue appears to be multifactorial. Early research

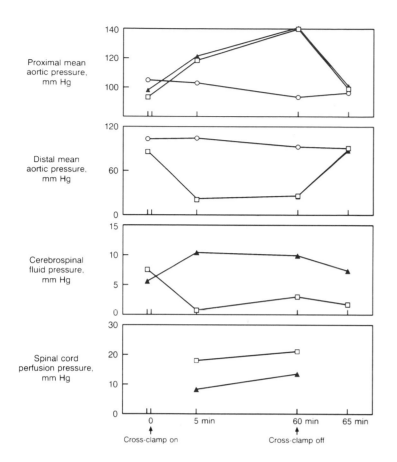

Figure 8. Hemodynamic measurements before, during, and after thoracic aortic occlusion. O————O, group I (control); △————△, group II (cross-clamp); □————□, group III (cross-clamp plus CSF drainage). (Reproduced with permission from Reference 18.)

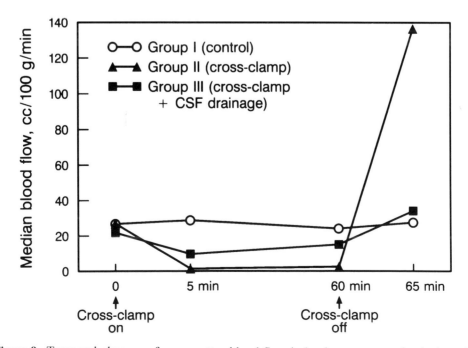

Figure 9. Temporal changes of gray matter blood flow in lumbar segment of spinal cord; marked decrease in local reperfusion hyperemia in dogs submitted to aortic cross-clamp plus CSF drainage. (Reproduced with permission from Reference 18.)

focused on the reduction in metabolic and oxygen requirements which reduce the energy requirements at the tissue level and increase the time that tissue can survive the energy-deficient state.[55–57] Later investigations have further demonstrated that hypothermia decreases the loss of ATP,[58,59] phosphocreatinine with subsequent accumulation of lactate, and nicotinamide adenine dinucleotide phosphate (NADPH).[57] Hypothermia may also reduce the amount of spinal cord edema.[60,61] Much of the theory related to the cellular effects of hypothermia are extrapolated from cerebral ischemia and spinal cord injury studies.

More recent studies have suggested that profound degrees of hypothermia may not be required for protection against ischemia. Decreases in body temperature as little as 3°C may reduce the loss of ATP and phosphocreatinine,[62,63] as well as reduce the release of neurotransmitters such as glutamate which can mediate reperfusion injury.[64] Moderate hypothermia (28°C) appears to significantly elevate spinal cord blood flow as measured in the rat with carbon-14 flow studies.[65] Other studies suggest that mild hypothermia may provide protection in spinal cord models as well.[66]

Systemic Hypothermia

The use of hypothermia as a means of reducing oxygen requirements of target tissues was first investigated in 1950 by Bigelow et al.[67,68] This group eloquently described physiologic effects of graduated systemic cooling in an animal model in order to perform cardiac surgery. They determined that mammals could be cooled to 20°C and survive rewarming; however, if systemic temperature fell to 15°C the animals would not survive rewarming. Following this study, the protective effects of hypothermia were demonstrated by other investigators.[69–73]

The use of profound hypothermia was first introduced in experimental surgery in 1950[67] and first applied clinically in 1952 by Lewis and Tavic.[69] They reported on a 5-year-old child who had an atrial septal defect repaired with 5 minutes of complete inflow occlusion with a core temperature of 26°C. The child survived the operation with no neurologic impairment. The use of hypothermia gained widespread use for the treatment of congenital heart disease and for aneurysms of the aortic arch and some of the thoracoabdominal aorta.[74] The use of hypothermia to protect against spinal cord ischemia during thoracic aortic cross-clamping was first reported by Beattie and Adovasio in 1953.[70] They were able to demonstrate that systemic hypothermia significantly protected against paralysis in animals systemically cooled with blankets to below 30°C. Ventricular fibrillation was a persistent problem in this and many other early experiments.

Pontius et al,[71] using a systemic hypothermia model, were able to demonstrate significant protection against paralysis in canines after aortic cross-clamping and intercostal ligation at multiple levels. Although surgical mortality was significant in both groups, there was no paralysis in the hypothermic group, compared with 65% in the normothermic animals. Cooley and DeBakey[75] used systemic hypothermia with rectal temperatures down to 30°C in 10 patients undergoing descending aortic resection. Four patients died, but none of the six survivors developed paraplegia. Other animal studies to address the problems associated with hypothermia were performed in the rabbit[76] and baboon.[77] Profound hypothermia continued to be associated with arrhythmias and bleeding complications, in particular with platelet dysfunction,[77–79] and with dysfunction of the abdominal viscera and skeletal muscle. In vivo and in vitro studies have demonstrated that production of thromboxane B_2 by platelets is temperature dependent and correlates with a reversible platelet dysfunction. For these reasons, more recent interest focused on the use of mild systemic hypothermia (32° to 34°C). Cooley et al[80] carried out a prospective study comparing deep hypothermia (12° to 16°C) followed by circulatory arrest with moderate systemic hypothermia (24° to 26°C) with only peripheral circulatory arrest. They found significantly improved survival in the latter group.

Hypothermic Perfusion

Hyopothermic regional perfusion for protection of the spinal cord during ischemic periods was first described by Colon et al.[25] They used a proximal and distal aortic clamp with 30 minutes of hypothermic perfusion of the thoracic aorta. This system required a roller pump with heat exchanger to control perfusate temperature. The hypothermic solution perfused the intercostal arteries including, presumably, the one supplying the ARM. None of the 10 treated pigs developed neurologic symptoms. All of the controls sustained neurologic injury. Later studies attempted to apply concepts of organ preservation pioneered in the transplantation field to develop appropriate perfusion solutions. Adenosine was added to the solution because of its properties as a neural depressant,[81] inhibitor of platelet adherence and white cell accumulation in ischemic tissues,[82,83] and because of its ability to enhance regeneration of high-energy phosphates.[84] By adding adenosine to the perfusion solution, Seibel et al[85,86] were able to demonstrate a significant improvement in neurologic outcome, compared with infusion of hypothermic saline alone in an animal model. Other investigators have added various compounds to the perfusion solution including steroids, mannitol, and vitamins, with evidence of improved outcome.[87] The lower the temperature of the infusion solution, the better the neurologic outcome was in the rabbit model.[88] Others have attempted to determine if perfusion of hypothermic solutions alters reperfusion and metabolism. Allen et al[89] have demonstrated that hypothermic perfusion preserves intracellular concentrations of ATP, glucose, glutamate, and aspartate in a rabbit model. Ueno et al[90] compared hypothermic perfusion with percutaneous cooling of the spinal cord and found that the latter was superior in providing sustained lowering of the cord temperature (23° versus 32°C) in the rabbit model. Animal studies have demonstrated that hypothermic perfusion provides excellent neurologic protection. However, this technique is difficult to use in patients because of the variations in blood supply to the cord, and because atherosclerotic occlusion of many of the intercostal arteries makes consistant perfusion of the cord questionable. The use of this technique in patients with acute dissections and rupture is not possible. There is additional concern of embolism of loose atherosclerotic debris into intercostal arteries from the aneurysm. This technique was useful to provide an excellent model for the study of the protective mechanisms provided by hypothermia. It has also led to current investigations of topical regional cooling.

Regional Cooling

Topical regional cooling of the cord by cannulating the epidural and subarachnoid spaces has been performed with good initial results and low morbidity. The theoretical advantage of this technique is that we can benefit from all of the advantages of cord hypothermia without the systemic side effects. The greatest experience with topical regional spinal cord cooling has been in the field of spinal trauma, although its use remains controversial.[91,92] In experiments we placed epidural catheters in dogs for perfusion cooling of the distal spinal cord with iced saline solution, and used CSF drainage to compensate for the elevated CSF pressure. This technique used by Dzsinich in our laboratory comfirmed the benefit of hypothermia, although complete protection was not obtained in all of our animals. Berguer et al[27] developed a model of regional hypothermia by perfusing the subarachnoid space with saline solution at 5°C. They were able to lower cord temperatures to 14° to 19°C while only slightly lowering rectal temperatures. Neurologic outcome in this and other subarachnoid perfusion models was excellent.[93,94] Investigators later were able to institute regional cord hypothermia by infusing solutions into the epidural space in multiple animal models.[95–97]

There is definite evidence that hypothermia can reduce neurologic injury after thoracic aortic occlusion. Further studies into the mechanism and methods must be performed before we can take full advantage of this technique clinically.

Barbiturates

Barbiturates appear to have a protective effect both in cerebral ischemia and spinal cord ischemia.[98–101] In the model of cerebral ischemia, it has been necessary to administer the pharmocologic agent prior to or up to 30 minutes after the ischemic insult.[99–102] This has limited the clinical use of barbiturates to episodes of planned ischemia such as would be seen during temporary surgical occlusion of a feeding artery. Operations on the aorta would lend themselves well to this sort of planned pretreatment.

There are several commonly accepted mechanisms by which barbiturates provide neurologic protection. Barbiturates produce a dose-dependant reduction in cellular metabolism and, thus, oxygen consumption. Cerebral oxygen consumption is reduced by as much as 53% to 55%[103,104] and cerebral blood flow is redirected and reduced.[104,105] These cannot, however, be the only protective effects of barbiturates, as other anesthetic agents that reduce metabolism such as halothane are not protective.[31] Neuronal edema appears to have an important role in the irreversibility of ischemic neuronal injury.[105–107] Pentobarbital reduces the amount of cerebral edema in dogs, while fluoridated hydrocarbon anesthetics do not.[108] In addition, barbiturates function as free radical scavengers, thus minimizing the destructive effects of free radicals and stabilizing the cellular membrane as demonstrated by Demopulos et al.[109] The microcirculation and the endothelium is protected by reduction of peroxidation of free fatty acids.[110,111]

Administration of thiopental before infrarenal aortic occlusion in rabbits resulted in a reduction in paraplegia from 10% to 40% compared with controls.[101] Nylander et al[31] pretreated dogs with thiopental 30 minutes prior to permanently occluding the infrarenal aorta and found a significant reduction in paraplegia in the treated animals (30%) compared with controls (90%). Thiopental penetrates the central nervous system (CNS) easily, and it is the preferred agent because of its lipid solubility which is 15 to 20 times greater than that of pentobarbital.[112]

Kirshner and colleagues[113] studied barbiturates alone and in combination with cold perfusion and superoxide dismutase. These investigators found that only the combination treatment was effective in preventing neurologic deficit after aortic clamping. Aortic cross-clamp time could be extended only if multiple effector pathways were inhibited.

It appears in patients that the greatest effect of short-acting barbiturates will be achieved by using them in combination with other agents.

Superoxide Dismutase (SOD)

Superoxide anions (O_2^{-}), hydrogen peroxide (H_2O_2), and hydroxyl radicals (•OH) are produced in cells by the reduction of oxygen and are highly reactive.[114] Oxygen-free radicals may have a role in the pathology of cerebral, spinal,[115–120] myocardial,[121,122] and kidney ischemia,[123] as well as other tissues. They appear to have an important role in the ischemic lesion in the nervous system affecting both neurons and glia.[124]

Free radicals are capable of peroxidating the lipid portion of cellular membranes and starting a propagating chain reaction that causes injury to adjacent cells and, thus, causes large areas of injury.[125,126] Free radicals are also capable of inducing dramatic changes in vascular permeability both inside and outside of the CNS.[118,127] In regions of extensive damage, the products of peroxidation spill outside of the cell and influence leukocyte chemotaxis.[119] Reductions in local free radicals may diminish local cytokine production, thus limiting secondary cell-mediated injury.[8] Lipid peroxidases inhibit the synthesis of prostacyclin by the vascular endothelium and result in platelet-induced occlusion of the microvasculature because of the unopposed action of thromboxane A_2.[118]

Oxygen radicals are too toxic to remain in living tissue, and mechanisms for removal and control of these products are present within the cellular apparatus. The majority of oxygen-derived free radicals are reduced by cellular enzyme cytochrome oxidase. A variety of SODs catalytically scavenge O_2^{-} as well. SOD, first discovered by McCord and Fridovich,[128] catalyzes the dismutation of O_2^{-} to $H_2O_2 + O_2$ (Figure 4). Although the levels of these scavengers in the cell are low, they appear to provide significant protection against lipid rancidification. The additions of free radical scavengers and antioxidants have provided a degree of protection against the injuries seen with ischemia/reperfusion when added during or immediatly after ischemia.[119,127]

Lim et al[32] used SOD for intra-aortic infusion in a model of thoracic aortic occlusion in dogs and noted significantly less paraplegia in those animals compared with controls. The production of free radicals was not measured. Several investigators[129–131] used a model of infrarenal aortic occlusion in rabbits and found that SOD infused before and during reperfusion reduced the degree of neurologic injury. Again, there was no measurement of free radical formation.

Granke et al[34] used SOD alone and in combination with CSF drainage. Although SOD alone reduced the amount of neurologic injury in dogs after aortic occlusion, the greatest effect was seen in combination with CSF drainage.

In conclusion, SOD may have a preserving effect on the endothelium of spinal vessels during the reperfusion period, which may prevent nervous tissue necrosis.[132] SOD may mediate an inhibition of hyperemia seen after an ischemic period,[133] thus, altering the distribution of blood flow in the ischemic tissue. Further studies correlating the reduction of intraspinal free radicals to treatment with SOD are needed in the future.

Calcium Channel Blockers

Calcium channel blockers have been studied extensively in neural tissue, and have shown promise in promoting dilation of cerebral vessels, and increasing cerebral and spinal cord blood flows in normal and pathologic states.[134–137]

Calcium is the link between electrical stimulation and physiologic response in a number of cells. The cellular plasma membrane is selectively permeable to calcium and achieves an extracellular to intracellular gradient of 10,000 to 1. Calcium entry into the cell can occur through voltage or receptor-operated channels.[138] Voltage-dependent channels are present on neurons and glia.[139] Calcium antagonists inhibit the movement and binding of calcium or facilitate calcium movement.[140]

Profound changes in tissue calcium concentrations have been found in cerebral ischemia.[141] Calcium may play a role in changes that ultimately result in cellular death. The calcium antagonists are able to inhibit neurologic damage secondary to ischemia either by dilatation of supplying vessels, or by preventing calcium influx into the cellular compartment. For this reason, calcium antagonists have been studied extensively in models of cerebral ischemia and have been shown to decrease postischemic hypoperfusion.[142] Nimodipine (dihydropyridine) is a special class of calcium antagonist that has been extensively studied and found to have some specificity toward receptors on cerebral and coronary arteries.[143]

Nimodipine appears to have the ability to attenuate the neurologic deficit resulting from cerebral ischemia in multiple experimental studies. Allen et al[134] treated arterial spasm secondary to subarachnoid hemorrhage with nimodipine and found a significant reduction in the severity of ischemic neurologic deficits from arterial spasm compared with placebo treatment. They noticed no adverse side effects from the agent. Steen et al[137] found that nimodipine improved cerebral blood flow and eventual neurologic recovery after cerebral ischemia in dogs. Mohamed et al[135] found that nimodipine increased cerebral blood flow at lower doses and lowered blood flow at higher doses possibly secondary to systemic hypotension. Meyer and colleagues[142] found that treatment with nimodipine after long periods of cerebral ischemia resulted in improved blood flow, elevation of brain pH, and relief of small vessel spasm in rabbits.

Faden and colleagues in 1984[35] were unable to demonstrate any benefit of nimodipine in attenuating the neurologic injury in a model of spinal ischemia after infrarenal aortic occlusion in a rabbit model. Other investigators[36] using verapamil in a model of spinal ischemia after placement of a thoracic aortic cross-clamp were able to demonstrate spinal cord protection in dogs. A study in rats[144] using the lipophilic calcium channel blocker flunarizine demonstrated an attenuation of the neurologic injury after occlusion of the thoracic aorta with a balloon catheter for up to 1 hour. Guha et al[37] demonstrated increases in spinal blood flow using hydrogen clearance techniques after treatment with low doses of nimodipine. Higher doses did not increase spinal blood flow, but did decrease systemic pressure by 37%. In our own laboratory, Rhee and associates (unpublished data) failed to demonstrate a significant neurologic benefit when nimodipine was administered prior to thoracic aortic clamping in dogs. In this study, nimodipine reduced the postischemic reperfusion hyperemia in the spinal cord as measured with laser-Doppler flowmetry. Reduced hyper-

perfusion significantly correlated with eventual clinical outcome (Figure 10).

Clinical use of calcium channel blockers to attenuate the neurologic sequelae of ischemia is limited. The largest study[145] examined 186 patients with an acute ischemic stroke treated in a double blind fashion with nimodipine. Survival and functional outcome were improved in patients in the nimodipine arm of the study. There appears to be a narrow therapeutic window in which blood flow to neuronal tissue is increased before systemic blood pressure is adversely affected. The evidence that treatment with calcium channel blockers in patients attenuates the neurologic sequelae of spinal ischemia is lacking at this time; however, it may be considered as an adjunct to a multimodality approach to prevention of spinal cord ischemia.

Prostaglandins

Prostaglandins were discovered in the 1930s by Goldblatt[146] and von Euler.[147] The prostaglandins thromboxane A_2 and prostaglandin I_2 (PGI$_2$) have opposing biologic actions on platelets and vessel walls

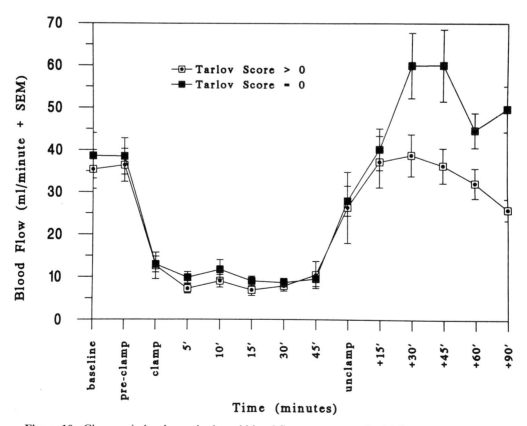

Figure 10. Changes in lumbar spinal cord blood flow as measured with laser-Doppler flowmetry during thoracic aortic cross-clamping: Tarlov 0 vs Tarlov > 0. (Reproduced from Rhee RY, Gloviczki P, Cambria RA, et al: The effects of nimodipine on ischemic injury of the spinal cord during thoracic aortic cross-clamping. Unpublished).

and have been implicated in thrombotic disorders.[148] PGI_2, formed in the endothelium, is a potent vasodilator and inhibitor of platelet aggregation and appears to balance the vasoconstrictive and platelet aggregating effects of thromboxane A_2, which is formed in the platelets.

Prostaglandin E_1 (PGE_1) has been used with some success as an intra-arterial infusion in severely ischemic extremities in patients unable to undergo revascularization procedures.[149–151] In an experimental model of spinal cord ischemia in dogs, treatment with PGE_1 provided significant reductions in neurologic deficit compared with controls.[33] The protection was improved with the addition of SOD.

Papaverine

Papaverine is an inhibitor of phosphodiesterase[152] and stimulates calcium binding to intracellular stores, as well as blocking slow influx calcium channels,[153] thus making it a potent vasodilator. It may have other protective effects including inhibition of superoxide formation[154] and inhibiting aerobic oxidation of substrates in the Krebs cycle.[155] It has been used successfully in dilating mesenteric vessels[156] and saphenous veins.[157]

Intrathecal papaverine significantly elevated spinal cord blood flow during thoracic aortic cross-clamping in baboons.[38] The incidence of postoperative neurologic injury was significantly reduced by the placement of shunts which perfused the ARM and by instillation of intrathecal papaverine. The ASA is continuous in baboons and humans; however, the segment just above the entrance of the ARM is narrow with high resistance, which tends to shunt blood into the lumbar region.[158] Papaverine presumably dilated the ASA above the entrance of the ARM so that blood would flow also into the thoracic region instead of perfusing into the lumbar segment alone.[38] Papaverine is a vasodilatory agent which selectively relieves cerebral vasospasm.[159]

Svensson et al[160] safely used intrathecal papaverine in a few patients[11] undergoing thoracoabdominal surgery. Experiments in our laboratory have shown that papaverine in the usual concentration precipitates in the CSF. In their study, Svensson et al[160] used a 1% (30 mg) preservative-free papaverine hydrochloride in 10% dextrose water solution which was infused over a 5-minute period. Intrathecal papaverine had no significant effect on systemic blood pressure, CSF pressure, and CSF pH. There were no postoperative neurologic deficits in the animal or human groups.[38,160,161] The technique of intrathecal papaverine infusion appears safe in a limited number of studies and may extend the safe cross-clamp period.

MK-801 (N-Methyl-D-Aspartate Antagonist)

Excitatory neurotransmitters, particularly glutamate, have been implicated in cellular injury in ischemic neural tissue.[162–165] Glutamate and aspartate are the primary excitatory neurotransmitters in the brain. Glutamate activity is mediated by several discrete receptor populations, though most studies have focused on the N-methyl-D-aspartate (NMDA) receptor subtype.[40] Excessive levels of glutamate are neurotoxic,[162,164–166] and local and systemic injections will cause focal neuronal degeneration which can be blocked by the receptor antagonist NMDA.[167–169] Prolonged activation of NMDA receptors produces cellular swelling, influx of sodium, chloride, and water, with eventual osmotic lysis and nerve cell death.[170] Activation of the NMDA receptor initiates an influx of calcium which triggers calcium-dependent processes within the cell that are cytotoxic, similar to processes which may be responsible for damage seen with ischemia.[171,172]

MK-801 is a noncompetitive antagonist of the NMDA receptor, which has excellent penetration of the CNS after systemic administration.[173] This antagonist appears to provide significant neuroprotective effects in cerebral ischemia.[40,173–175]

In a model of hypersensitivity-induced spinal cord ischemia in rats, MK-801 pretreatment prevented the occurrence of allodynia.[39] There was significant negative correlation with delay of treatment after onset of the ischemic event. In a model of spinal ischemia secondary to aortic occlusion, MK-801 was effective in reducing the ischemic damage if given 5 minutes after the onset of injury. However, if the treatment was delayed to 10 minutes after the ischemic injury, neuroprotection was not noted in rabbits.[40,173] Similar results were seen in a model of cerebral ischemia.[40] Yum et al[176] treated rabbits with spinal ischemia with MK-801 5 minutes after the ischemic event and found that it significantly decreased neurologic injury compared with controls. The neuroprotective effect of MK-801 does not appear to be related to hypothermia, as body temperature was consistently elevated after treatment with this agent.[40] MK-801 has strong sedative and anticonvulsant properties; however, its role in neuroprotection is unclear.

Monoclonal Antibodies

The appearance of leukocytes in injured tissues has traditionally been thought to be a physiologic response to a pre-existing injury. More recent data, however, suggest that neutrophils are important in the pathogenesis and eventual extension of the injurious process.[177–180] Leukocytes affect ischemic tissues by adhering to the endothelium of capillaries and causing eventual microvascular occlusion.[177] They infiltrate the CNS tissue causing cytotoxic injuries.[178,179,181] The role of leukocytes in ischemia-reperfusion injury is further illustrated by a reduction in the extent of observed injury in neutrophil-depleted animals.[177–182] Once within ischemic tissue, activated neutrophils release oxygen radicals, proteases, and phospholipases, all of which can result in endothelial injury and loss of vascular integrity.[177]

Dramatic insights into the mechanisms of leukocyte-endothelial interactions have been elucidated in the last decade. To gain entrance into ischemic tissue, activated leukocytes must first adhere to and traverse the endothelium bordering capillaries and small vessels. During inflammation or ischemia, a family of adhesion receptors on the leukocyte (CD 18) are upregulated as are their endothelial ligands, the intercellular adhesion molecules (ICAM).[183–185] When both of these binding receptors are activated, the leukocytes become "sticky" and bind to the endothelium, and then migrate into the ischemic/inflamed tissue. If the leukocytes are not able to traverse the endothelium after binding, they may cause plugging of the vessel, leading to the "no-reflow" phenomenon as described by Ames et al.[186] This phenomenon results in inadequate flow to ischemic tissues upon flow restoration.

Recent studies by Clark et al[42,187] have demonstrated that pretreatment with monoclonal antibody directed toward the CD-18 receptor on leukocytes reduced the postoperative neurologic injury in rabbits in a model of aortic occlusion. In a model of cerebral ischemia caused by microsphere injection, pretreatment with anti- CD-18 did not demonstrate any changes in postoperative neurologic outcome.[42,187]

Experiments in our laboratory using a canine model of spinal cord ischemia did not demonstrate any benefit in eventual neurologic outcome after treatment with monoclonal antibodies directed against CD-18. There were no differences in spinal cord blood flow or histology compared with the control group after 1 hour of thoracic and lumbar aortic cross-clamp.

Fluosol-DA

The unique oxygen carrying properties of perfluorochemicals were first recognized and investigated by Clark and colleagues in 1966.[188] Fluosol-DA has been the most effective substance to date. Production of Fluosol-DA involves mixing the oxygen-carrying component perfluorodecalin with perfluorotripropylamine which is then emulsified. It is eventually combined with glycerol, intralipids, and fatty acids. The final particle size is 0.1 m². The surface area available for oxygen exchange is 100 to 170 times that of blood, with

the exchange occurring twice as fast as hemoglobin. Fluosol elimination is primarily through the lungs and urine.[189,190] Small animals have been exchange transfused to a hematocrit of 1% for as long as 24 hours with subsequent normal survival.[190] By decreasing blood viscosity, increasing the availability of O_2 to the tissues, and removing some waste products, it was postulated that these compounds would provide superior characteristics compared with blood during ischemia. For these reasons, Fluosol-DA has been investigated as a blood substitute in ischemic models.

In a model of spinal ischemia in rabbits using an infrarenal aortic cross-clamp, there was no improvement in neurologic outcome compared with controls.[191] In a model of cerebral ischemia in cats, treatment with Fluosol-DA improved neurologic outcome.[190] However, another study using the same model failed to demonstrate any benefit.[192] Fluosol-DA was perfused into the thoracic aorta prior to aortic cross-clamping in a dog model.[44] Distal aortic pressure significantly increased and the rate of postoperative paraplegia decreased when compared with controls.[44] Because of conflicting reports in the literature, however, at present it is not clear that Fluosol-DA provides any benefit compared to blood during periods of ischemia. Further work on the mode of action of Fluosol-DA must be conducted.

Opiate Antagonists

Endogenous opioids are released after ischemic or traumatic CNS injury[193] and are thought to play a role in secondary injury processes.[193–195] The opiate antagonist naloxone was observed to improve neurologic outcome in multiple ischemic and trauma models.[193,196,197]

In a canine model of spinal ischemia, ligation of the infrarenal aorta resulted in persistent elevations of B-endorphins in the CSF of treated dogs compared with controls.[198] Plasma B-endorphins were elevated in the sham operated dogs. Other workers[196,197] have noted elevations of plasma B-endorphins in models of spinal cord injury which may be released secondary to spinal shock.

The mechanism of action by which opiates influence neurologic function during ischemia is not clearly understood. It was noted that increasing doses of morphine decrease cerebral oxygen consumption in dogs.[199] In addition, infusions of intraventricular endorphin resulted in catatonic behavior in rats.[200] Opiates depressed the firing of neurons by eliciting membrane hyperpolarization and depressing acetylcholine turnover.[198,201] Given these points, it is likely that elevation of endorphins further deranges neuron function within the ischemic area. For these reasons, extensive investigations of opiate antagonists have been carried out in CNS ischemic and trauma models.

Naloxone, an opiate antagonist, has been used for spinal cord protection in ischemic and trauma studies. It appears that naloxone increases spinal cord blood flow, inhibits lipid peroxidation, inhibits proteolysis, and improves derangements in calcium flux across cell membranes.[202] In models of spinal injury with subsequent spinal shock, naloxone antagonizes the cardiodepressant effects of endogenous opioids.[203,204] Naloxone appears to increase cardiac contractility by vagal and dopaminergic pathways.[205,206] Naloxone decreases cell death,[207] improves electrophysiologic activity,[208] and eventual neurologic outcome in models of spinal cord ischemia and trauma.[196,208,209] Higher doses of opiate antagonists may also affect naloxone-insensitive receptors, such as the delta or kappa receptors.

Nalmefene is a pure opiate-receptor antagonist with a longer half-life than naloxone (8.6 hours) and enhanced activity at kappa opiate receptors.[43] In a spinal cord injury model, nalmefene given intrathecally significantly improved neurologic recovery and reduced tissue damage. However, when given intravenously there was no improvement over controls.[43] In another model of spinal ischemia in rabbits, nalmefene improved neurologic and histologic outcome compared with control animals.[176] Further studies to clarify the different mechanisms of action in intravenous and intrathecal use, as well as further delineation of drug dosages, are needed.

Aminosteroids

21-Aminosteroid is a novel nonglucocorticoid steroid which has been shown to inhibit iron-dependent lipid peroxidation (Figure 4) and, thus, reduce neurologic injury in brain and spinal cord injury models.[210–212] Fowl et al[29] demonstrated significant reductions in neurologic injury after occluding the aorta in rabbits during treatment with U-74006F. 21-Aminosteroids were developed to recreate the antioxidant effect of glucocorticoids without the glucocorticoid side effects of immunosuppression, hyperglycemia, and muscle wasting. The earliest efforts at synthesizing these compounds resulted in steroid analogs of methylprednisolone which required high doses to inhibit lipid peroxidation.[213] Later efforts produced the 21-aminosteroids (lazaroids) which were synthesized in 1985. Nearly 400 compounds have been tested for activity to date.[116] U74500A and U74006F (trilazad mesylate) are commonly used agents in models of cerebral and spinal cord ischemia. These compounds have been found to inhibit lipid peroxidation by scavenging lipid peroxyl radicals, thus inhibiting the propagation of in-

jury to surrounding tissues in a manner similar to vitamin E.[214] U74006F appears to compete with vitamin E and slow its degradation in injured and ischemic tissue.[210,211] These compounds appear to react with hydroxyl radicals and decrease their concentration in vivo.[116] The only demonstrated neuroprotective mechanism of 21–aminosteroids is their ability to block lipid peroxidation.

Clinical Results of Spinal Cord Protection

The incidence of ischemic spinal cord injury following thoracoabdominal aortic reconstruction varies from 0% to 40%. In the monumental experience of Crawford, a 7% incidence of paraplegia and a 9% incidence of paraparesis was noted in 1509 patients who underwent thoracoabdominal reconstructions.[215] In this series, 276 patients (18%) had dissection and 820 (54%) had extensive type I or type II thoracoabdominal aneurysms. Hollier reported on 150 consecutive patients with thoracoabdominal reconstructions, with 6 (4%) dissections, and 58 (39%) type I and type II aneurysms with the incidence of neurologic injury of 4%.[216]

The incidence of paraparesis and paraplegia in 181 patients (109 males, 72 females, mean age: 68.1 years, range: 33 to 88 years), who were operated on at the Mayo Clinic between January 1, 1980, and April 30, 1992, for thoracoabdominal aneurysms, was 8% (15/181) (Table 1). Fifty-three (29%) of our patients had type I or type II aneurysms, 16 (9%) had dissections, and 29 (16%) underwent emergency repair for symptomatic or ruptured aneurysm. The 30-day mortality rate was 19% (elective repair: 14%, 21/152, emergency repair: 48%, 14/29). Correct assessment of the neurologic status of 26 patients who died within the first 24 hours could not be performed. Therefore, we predict that the risk of neurologic injury was likely higher than the 8% we report here. The highest rate of paraplegia was observed with type II aneurysms (29%), the lowest with type IV (2%) (Table 1).

Aortic Cross-Clamp Time

Numerous clinical and experimental studies have suggested a relationship between the duration of aortic cross-clamp and the production of paraplegia.[217–219] Paraplegia may occur in some patients after even brief cross-clamp intervals,[220] whereas other patients with increased collateral circulation associated with arteriosclerosis may tolerate much longer ischemia without permanent neurologic damage.[217,218]

The maximum safe aortic cross-clamp time not incurring ischemic injury to the spinal cord in patients is not known. Clinical data of Katz et al,[221] who studied

Table 1

Spinal Cord Complications After Repair of
Thoracoabdominal Aortic Aneurysms in 181
Patients Operated at the Mayo Clinic

	Paraplegia/ Paraparesis*	
	No.	%
Type I		
Nondissecting (n = 34)	2	6
Dissecting (n = 2)	0	0
Total (n = 36)	2	6
Type II		
Nondissecting (n = 12)	2	17
Dissecting (n = 5)	3	60
Total (n = 17)	5	29
Type III		
Nondissecting (n = 55)	5	9
Dissecting (n = 9)	2	22
Total (n = 64)	7	11
Type IV		
Nondissecting (n = 64)	1	2
Dissecting (n = 0)	0	0
Total (n = 64)	1	2
Types I–IV		
Nondissecting (n = 165)	10	6
Dissecting (n = 16)	5	31
Total (n = 181)	15	8

* Unable to assess in 26 patients because of death within
<24 hours.

the influence of partial cardiopulmonary bypass or shunt on risk of paraplegia following repair of acute aortic transections, indicated a significant increase in spinal cord injury at approximately 30 minutes after descending thoracic aortic cross-clamping in patients without protection of the distal circulation. Jex et al,[222] from the Mayo Clinic, found a sudden increase in paraplegia if aortic cross-clamping exceeded 45 minutes in patients with dissections of the descending thoracic aorta who did not undergo shunting.

Laschinger et al,[223] in an experimental study, confirmed the relationship between duration of aortic cross-clamping and neurologic injury in dogs. Monitoring evoked spinal cord potentials, they demonstrated that ischemia severe enough to cause spinal cord dysfunction occurs within 3 to 5 minutes after aortic cross-clamping and results in complete loss of spinal cord conduction after 7 to 9 minutes. Prolongation of this

ischemia for periods as short as 10 minutes after complete loss of SEPs resulted in permanent spinal cord injury in a majority (67%) of animals. However, if reperfusion was established in a shorter interval of time (less than 5 minutes) after SEP loss occured, there was no incidence of permanent spinal cord injury. Although not totally analogous to the human model, these experiments suggest that brief periods of spinal cord ischemia may produce significant neurologic injury in the spinal cord of humans, if collateral circulation is not adequate.

Experience and surgical technique continue to be critical to decrease aortic cross-clamp time. Thoracoabdominal reconstructions, therefore, continue to be the most challenging operation for the vascular surgeon.

Reimplantation of Intercostal Arteries

A major cause of neuromuscular deficits after operations for thoracic and thoracoabdominal aortic aneurysms is presumed to be the failure to successfully reanastomose to the new aortic graft those segmental intercostal or lumbar arteries that supply the spinal cord.[224,225] We believe that delayed paraplegia is primarily due to deprivation of the spinal cord of its oxygen supply, usually by hypotensive episodes reducing collateral flow (when critical segmental arteries have been sacrificed) to areas of tenuous blood supply.

Kieffer and other investigators attempted before operation to localize the segmental intercostal and lumbar arteries that supply the spinal cord with highly selective angiography.[226,227] This method, however, failed to identify the great radicular artery in a substantial number of patients, either because of technical problems or because the main intercostal artery was chronically occluded or stenosed. Collateral blood supply to the cord in these patients is unpredictable. Although preoperative identification of the spinal arterial anatomy would be ideal, arteriography is frequently incomplete and time-consuming. In addition, distal embolization, paraparesis, paraplegia, and death have been reported following angiography both in animals and in humans.[227–229] Svensson et al[230,231] reported a technique for intraoperatively localizing the segmental arteries that supply the spinal cord. This method involves the injection of a saline solution saturated with hydrogen into the segmental artery ostia and then observing if a current is generated from a platinum electrode lying intrathecally alongside the spinal cord. The hydrogen-induced current impulse can then be recorded. In human studies, hydrogen-induced current impulse accurately localized intercostals that are critical to spinal cord blood supply, and allowed safe exclusion of the noncritical intercostals. However, this technique is time-consuming and appears cumbersome. Therefore, reimplantation of intercostal arteries is usually blind, presuming that critical blood supply to the cord comes from the T8-L1 levels. While Hollier[216] advocates reimplantation of all patent intercostal arteries, we attempt to reimplant all arteries at T6-L1 level.

In a prospective randomized study, Crawford failed to confirm the benefit of intercostal reimplantation on postoperative paraplegia.[232] However, analysis of a subset of patients in this study showed that the paraplegia rate was significantly higher if intercostal arteries at T11, T12, or at L1 were found patent and were not reimplanted. We continue to use reimplantation of most intercostal arteries, although the analysis of our material also failed to confirm decreased risk of spinal cord injury with intercostal reimplantation.

Perfection of technology and improvement in imaging techniques in the future are prerequisites to provide the fine anatomic details of the critical blood supply to the spinal cord. Patency of the reimplanted critical vessels in most series, however, was not confirmed postoperatively.

Bypass or Shunt

The usefulness of circulatory support during repair of thoracoabdominal aneurysms is still controversial. Bypass and shunts improve distal aortic blood flow and prevent paraplegia in animal studies,[15] but in patients only some of the physiologic benefits could be quantitated. These methods of hemodynamic support increase time and complexity of thoracoabdominal aortic aneurysm repair, although recent studies demonstrated reduction in risk of spinal cord injury during operation for aortic transection and aortic dissection.[221,222] For repair of chronic atherosclerotic thoracic or thoracoabdominal aneurysms, the use of shunts and bypass reduces risk of postoperative paraplegia; also, paraparesis has not been proved, and many surgeons prefer simple aortic cross-clamping with expeditious graft replacement. Proponents of rapid insertion of the aortic graft with reimplantation of major intercostal arteries and visceral vessels without shunting or bypass[233,234] argue that operative time is shorter, paraplegia rates are equal to, if not better than, paraplegia rates following the use of shunts, and that the hemorrhagic complications associated with distal bypass can be avoided. On the other side, proponents of the use of shunts, from the left ventricle, left atrium, or the proximal thoracic aorta to the distal aorta or femoral vessels,[235,236] argue that proximal aortic hypertension and cardiac workload are decreased and distal perfusion is improved, especially to the spinal cord and kidneys. With the use of heparinized shunts, systemic heparinization is avoided, thus reducing the risk of hemorrhagic complications. Without circulatory support, frequent and large amounts of vasodilators (sodium nitroprusside) during aortic clamping are required to control proximal blood pressure. Normalization of proximal aortic blood pressure, however, may have the unwanted effect of decreasing collateral blood flow to the abdominal viscera, and may be potentially deleterious for spinal cord and renal preservation. Verdant et al[237] recently reported no incidences of paraplegia in 366 consecutive reconstructions for descending thoracic aortic aneurysms over a 20-year period. A Gott shunt was placed in all patients as the only form of spinal protection.

Partial cardiopulmonary bypass or total cardiopulmonary bypass with profound hypothermia is advocated for thoracoabdominal reconstructions by several surgeons.[238–240] Partial bypass is suggested if the critical intercostal or high lumbar arteries originate from the aorta distal to the excluded aortic segment, and total cardiopulmonary bypass with systemic hypothermia and circulatory arrest with reimplantation of intercostal arteries, if these originate from the excluded segment.

In the experience of our institution, the only group of patients who benefited from bypass or shunt were those with acute or chronic dissection of the descending thoracic aorta.[222] In patients with atherosclerotic aneurysms of the descending thoracic aorta, the paraplegia rate did not decrease with the use of shunt or bypass.[241] In our patients with thoracoabdominal aneurysms, the results were similar. The rate of paraplegia/paraparesis was 19% with the use of shunt or bypass, in contrast to a rate of 6% in those patients without bypass.

Although current clinical data do not confirm the benefit of the use of bypass or shunts in decreasing the neurologic injury during operations for thoracoabdominal aortic aneurysms, we believe that distal circulatory support is advantageous in patients with poor left ventricular function, to decrease afterload during aortic clamping. Relative indications include extensive type I or II aneurysms when segmental clamping would permit distal perfusion while performing the proximal anastomosis.

Evoked Potentials

Somatosensory evoked potentials (SEP) were first monitored by Cunningham and associates[19,223,242–244] in an attempt to identify the onset of spinal ischemia during operations on the descending thoracic aorta. Theoretically, if spinal ischemia could be identified intraoperatively, specific technical adjuncts designed to avoid ischemia could be instituted to prevent neurologic injury. SEP traces are generated by stimulating the posterior tibial nerves. The signals are conducted through the posterior columns and monitored via scalp electrodes.[223] SEP has limitations in that it evaluates posterior and lateral spinal column function, while paraplegia secondary to ischemia usually results from anterior column ischemia. In addition, peripheral nerve or cortical dysfunction due either to ischemia or to the effects of anesthetic agents may result in false-positive SEP findings; thus, bypass to maintain distal perfusion for this technique is necessary. Changes in latency and amplitude or complete loss of cortical response signify ischemic damage to the cord.

Laschinger et al[223] have demonstrated that loss of the SEP results after 8.5 minutes of aortic cross-clamping in a dog model. There is return of normal SEP and postoperative neurological function if flow is restored within 5 minutes of SEP loss; however, after that, the length of clamp time correlates with postoperative neurologic injury. Using SEP and distal aortic bypass and perfusion techniques, it was recognized that distal perfusion pressures must exceed 70 mm Hg in order to maintain normal SEP waveforms.[244] Vessels critical to spinal cord blood supply could be identified using SEP.[19]

The clinical experience with SEP monitoring in human studies has been disappointing. Cunningham et al[242] reported on 33 patients undergoing thoracic aortic occlusion in whom 15% developed paraplegia. The SEPs were lost in all 5 patients with paraplegia as well as in 11 other patients who did not become paraplegic. Crawford et al[20] subsequently reported on 198 patients, half of whom had distal perfusion and SEP monitoring. No advantage was found in the groups where SEP was used. The incidence of a false negative SEP was 13% and the false positive rate was 67%. Localization of critical spinal arteries for implantation was not possible using SEPs.[20]

Because of SEPs limitation in monitoring the anterior spinal cord, motor evoked potentials (MEP) have been investigated to monitor the motor tracts during aortic surgery.[243,245] This technique produces a signal in the descending spinal cord motor tract by stimulating the cerebral cortex.[243,245] Experimental work by Laschinger et al[243] showed loss of MEPs in dogs undergoing 20 minutes of thoracic aortic cross-clamping.

In an experimental study from our institution,[246] MEPs stimulated in the cortex and recorded from the distal thoracic level of the cord had low overall accuracy (59%) and low sensitivity (45%) in predicting neurologic outcome. The low sensitivity of MEPs in our study was probably related to the method used to stimulate and record these potentials. The MEPs recorded over the low thoracic and proximal lumbar spine are potentials that are transmitted in the axons of the descending corticospinal tracts. The cell bodies of these neurons lie within the cerebral cortex, making their fibers in the spinal white matter more resistant to ischemia than anterior horn cells and interneurons whose cell bodies lie within the ischemic cord. Our data suggest that to improve the sensitivity of MEPs, recordings must be made distal to the anterior horn cells (such as lumbosacral cord, cauda equina, peripheral nerve, or muscle). This conclusion is supported by recent work by Svensson et al[231] who reported that MEPs are highly sensitive in predicting paraplegia when stimulations are elicited with an intrathecal electrode and recordings are made from lower extremity muscles. However, the use of muscle relaxants in patients during the operation may interfere with accurate recording of MEPs.

Further refinements in SEP and MEP monitoring techniques are needed to improve our ability to detect spinal cord ischemia in patients in the perioperative period.

Spinal Fluid Drainage

Drainage of CSF reduces spinal pressure and enhances spinal cord perfusion pressure. Hollier[46] introduced routine CSF pressure monitoring and drainage in patients. Using CSF drainage as part of his protocol, which also included complete intercostal artery reimplantation, maintenance of proximal hypertension, moderate hypothermia, high-dose barbiturates, mannitol, steroids, and calcium channel blockers, spinal cord dysfunction was completely avoided in 42 consecutive patients undergoing thoracoabdominal reconstruction.[219]

A prospective randomized study of CSF drainage in high-risk patients with thoracoabdominal aneurysms (type I and II) was performed by Crawford et al.[232] There was no significant improvement in neurologic outcome in the CSF drainage group. However, a maximum of 50 cc CSF was only withdrawn in this study, resulting in only mild decreases in CSF pressure in some of the patients. Svensson et al[247] used CSF drainage in combination with intrathecal papaverine in 11 patients undergoing aortic cross-clamping with no incidence of neurologic deficit.

Although CSF drainage prevented paraplegia in experiments of Bower et al[18] and Elmore et al[15] from our laboratory, we were unable to demonstrate improved neurologic outcome in patients undergoing repair of thoracic or thoracoabdominal aneurysms. CSF drainage was performed in 68 of our 181 patients. The mean amount of CSF withdrawn was 67.2 mL. Paraplegia was 12% in the drainage group and 6% in the group with no drainage (this difference failed to reach significance). Spinal cord injury occurred even if intercostal artery reimplantation was performed in addition to spinal fluid drainage. In a study by Murray et al,[248] CSF drainage (46.9 ± 6.9 mL) was used in 50 of 99 patients to maintain CSF pressure less than 15 mm Hg during aortic cross-clamping. There was no significant decrease in the incidence of paraplegia in this study.

Experimental data have held promise that CSF drainage would be a useful clinical tool to help reduce the incidence of neurologic deficits after aortic surgery; however, clinical studies up to this time have not confirmed this.

Hypothermia

As outlined earlier, substantial experimental data suggest that hypothermia provides significant protection against neurologic impairment during prolonged ischemia; however, clinical experience with hypothermia has been mixed. Experience with hypothermia has followed a chronologic course similar to the experimental studies as outlined, with systemic hypothermia being the first modality used. Cooley et al[80] compared deep systemic hypothermia (12° to 16°C) to moderate hypothermia (24° to 26°C) in the treatment of trans-

verse arch aneurysms and found a significantly higher morbidity associated with profound hypothermia. There was no significant neurologic impairment seen in the four patients surviving the operation after moderate hypothermia. Mahfood and associates[249] had similar findings using profound hypothermia (15°C) in repair of transverse arch aneurysms with no neurologic sequelae in the surviving patients. Massimo et al[250] observed no neurologic impairment in four patients with aortic dissection who survived resections of the arch and descending thoracic aorta following circulatory arrest and hypothermic perfusion (20° to 24°C). Later, Crawford and colleagues[251] used partial cardiopulmonary bypass and hypothermic circulatory arrest (6° to 18°C) in the treatment of 25 patients with thoracic aortic aneurysms with two of the surviving patients developing paraplegia. This technique allowed salvage of patients where aortic clamp placement was problematic or impossible. Kouchoukos et al[239] also used hypothermic cardiopulmonary bypass (15° to 19°C) and circulatory arrest during operations on the thoracoabdominal aorta in five patients at high risk for the development of spinal cord injury. None of the four survivors had a new spinal injury. Frank et al[252] used moderate hypo-

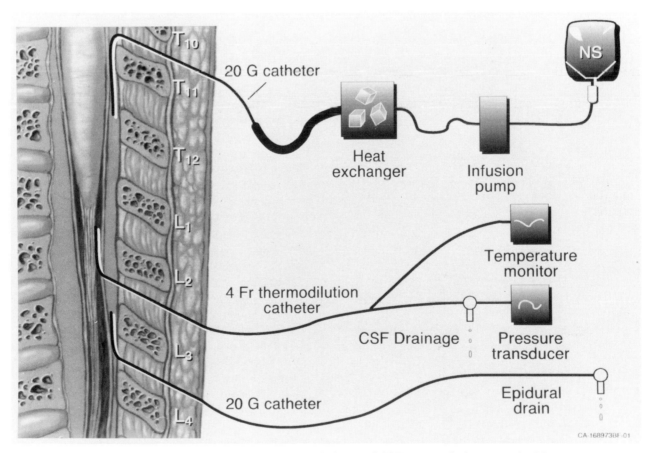

Figure 11. System of epidural cooling and drainage of CSF, currently in use at the Mayo Clinic.

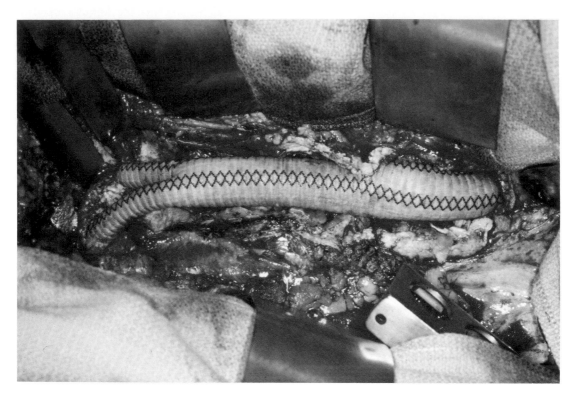

Figure 12. Type III thoracoabdominal aneurysm repaired with a bifurcated gelatin-coated dacron graft. Epidural cooling was used and the patient recovered without ischemic injury to the spinal cord.

thermia (30°C) with partial bypass and segmental repair to minimize the amount of ischemic time for each vascular bed in the repair of thoracoabdominal aneurysms in 18 patients. Sixteen of the 18 patients survived without a neurologic deficit.

Only recently have clinical studies on regional spinal cord hypothermia commenced, with Davison and associates[28] examining regional spinal cord hypothermia during thoracoabdominal aneurysm repair. Eight patients were studied without any postoperative neurologic deficits noted. Initiation of cord hypothermia was carried out by placing inflow catheters into the epidural space through which iced saline (4°C) flowed until CSF temperature was decreased (25° to 28°C) prior to aortic cross-clamping. A catheter was placed in the subarachnoid space to measure temperature and remove CSF to control spinal pressure. They noted only slight decreases in core temperature and increases in spinal pressures. We have been using a similar technique (Figure 11) at the Mayo Clinic for the past 9 months with excellent early results (unpublished data)(Figure 12). As described, systemic deep hypothermia and circulation arrest is not without side effects. It is for these reasons that local hypothermic techniques appear to hold the greatest promise for future clinical utility.

Conclusions

Paraplegia continues to be the most significant complication of thoracoabdominal reconstruction. It is multifactorial and it is unlikely that a single method will ever be successful to prevent paraplegia. At the Mayo Clinic, we continue to use combined methods of protection that include expeditious operation, reimplantation of all or most intercostal arteries, maintenance of proximal hypertension, cerebrospinal fluid pressure monitoring and drainage, mild systemic hypothermia, selective use of atriofemoral bypass, and measurements of evoked potentials. We have recently started to use regional epidural cooling with success. Our pharmacologic support includes judicious use of nitroprusside, the use of steroids, and mannitol. The most important goal of perioperative fluid management is the maintenance of hemodynamic stability, using crystalloids, albumin, packed cells, and blood products.

The goals of further research in the area of spinal cord protection should be the following. We should continue to search for the most effective drugs to prolong ischemia tolerance and decrease reperfusion injury of the cord. We should develop the best technique of regional spinal cord cooling. Finally, a safe method of preoperative or intraoperative identification of critical blood supply to the spinal cord must be developed that would permit identification of critical intercostal and lumbar arteries that need to be spared or reattached.

References

1. Carrel A: The experimental surgery of the thoracic aorta and the heart. *Ann Surg* 52:83–95, 1910.
2. Etheredge SN, Yee J, Smith JV, et al: Successful resection of a large aneurysm of the upper abdominal aorta and replacement with homograft. *Surgery* 38:1071–1081, 1955.
3. Kieffer E: The role of spinal cord arteriography before descending thoracic/thoracoabdominal aneurysmectomy. *Semin Vasc Surg* 5:141–145, 1992.
4. Djindjian R, Favre C: Spinal cord injury during aortography (in French). *J Belge Radiol* 50:207–213, 1967.
5. Lundy EF, Ball TD, Mandell MA, et al: Dextrose administration increases sensory/motor impairment and paraplegia after infrarenal aortic occlusion in the rabbit. *Surgery* 102:737–742, 1987.
6. Hollier LH: Protecting the brain and spinal cord. *J Vasc Surg* 5:524–528, 1987.
7. Weisfeldt ML: Reperfusion and reperfusion injury. *Clin Res* 35:13–20, 1987.
8. Whitley WD, Hancock WW, Kupiec-Weglinski JW, et al: Iron chelation suppresses mononuclear cell activation, modifies lymphocyte migration patterns, and prolongs rat cardiac allograft survival in rats. *Transplantation* 56(5):1182–1188, 1993.
9. Whitley D, Hancock W, Kupiec-Weglinski J, et al: The role of iron in rejection of vascularized organ allografts. *Surg Forum* 41:394, 1990.
10. Chen ST, Hsu CY, Hogan EL, et al: Thromboxane, prostacyclin, and leukotrienes in cerebral ischemia. *Neurology* 36:466–470, 1986.
11. North RJ: Concept of activated macrophage. *J Immun* 121:806–809, 1978.
12. Giulian D: Ameboid microglia as effectors of inflammation in the central nervous system. *J Neurosci Res* 18:155–171, 1987.
13. Norris DA, Weston WL, Sams WM: The effect of immunosuppression and anti-inflammatory drugs upon monocyte function in vitro. *J Lab Clin Med* 90:569–580, 1977.
14. Moore WM Jr, Hollier L: The influence of severity of spinal cord ischemia in the etiology of delayed-onset paraplegia. *Ann Surg* 213:427–431, 1991.
15. Elmore JR, Gloviczki P, Harper CM, Jr et al: Spinal cord injury in experimental thoracic aortic occlusion: investigation of combined methods of protection. *J Vasc Surg* 15:789–799, 1992.
16. Miyamoto K, Ueno A, Wada T, et al: A new and simple method of preventing spinal cord damage following temporary occlusion of the thoracic aorta by draining the cerebrospinal fluid. *J Cardiovasc Surg* 16:188–197, 1960.
17. Blaisdell FW, Cooley DA: The mechanism of paraplegia after temporary thoracic aortic occlusion in its relationship to spinal fluid pressure. *Surgery* 51:351–355, 1962.
18. Bower TC, Murray MJ, Gloviczki P, et al: Effects of thoracic aortic occlusion and cerebrospinal fluid drain-

19. age on regional spinal cord blood flow in dogs: correlation with neurologic outcome. *J Vasc Surg* 9:135–144, 1989.
19. Laschinger JC, Cunningham JN Jr, Baumann FG, et al: Monitoring of SEP during surgical procedures on the thoracoabdominal aorta: III. Intraoperative identification of vessels critical to spinal cord blood supply. *J Thorac Cardiovasc Surg* 94:271, 1987.
20. Crawford ES, Mizrahi GM, Hess KR, et al: The impact of distal aortic perfusion and somatosensory evoked potential monitoring on prevention of paraplegia after aortic aneurysm operation. *J Thorac Cardiovasc Surg* 95:357–367, 1988.
21. Shine T, Nugent M: Sodium nitroprusside decreases spinal cord perfusion pressure during descending thoracic aortic cross-clamping in the dog. *J Cardiothorac Anesth* 4:184–193, 1990.
22. LeMay DR, Neal S: Paraplegia in the rat induced by aortic cross-clamping: model characterization and glucose exacerbation of neurologic deficit. *J Vasc Surg* 6:383–390, 1987.
23. Aadahl P, Saether OD, Stenseth R, et al: Microcirculation of the spinal cord during proximal aortic cross-clamping. *Eur J Vasc Surg* 4:5–10, 1990.
24. Coles JG, Wilson J, Sima A, et al: Intraoperative management of thoracic aortic aneurysm: experimental evaluation of perfusion cooling of the spinal cord. *J Thorac Cardiovasc Surg* 85:292–299, 1983.
25. Colon R, Frazier OH, Cooley DA, et al: Hypothermic regional perfusion for protection of the spinal cord during periods of ischemia. *Ann Thorac Surg* 43:639–643, 1987.
26. Rokkas CK, Sundaresan S, Shuman TA, et al: A primate model of spinal cord ischemia: evaluation of spinal cord blood flow and the protective effect of hypothermia. *Surg Forum* 42:265–267, 1991.
27. Berguer R, Porto J, Fedoronko B, et al: Selective deep hypothermia of the spinal cord prevents paraplegia after aortic cross-clamping in the dog model. *J Vasc Surg* 15:62–72, 1992.
28. Davison JK, Cambria RP, Vierra DJ, et al: Epidural cooling for regional spinal cord hypothermia during thoracoabdominal aneurysm repair. *J Vasc Surg* 20(2):304–310, 1994.
29. Fowl RJ, Patterson RB, Gewirtz RJ, et al: Protection against postischemic spinal cord injury using a new 21-aminosteroid. *J Surg Res* 48:597–600, 1990.
30. Woloszyn TT, Marini CP, Coons MS, et al: A multimodality approach lengthens warm ischemic time during aortic cross-clamping. *J Surg Res* 52:15–21, 1992.
31. Nylander WA, Plunkett RJ, Hammon JW, et al: Thiopental modification of ischemic spinal cord injury in the dog. *Ann Thorac Surg* 33:64–68, 1982.
32. Lim KH, Connoly M, Rose D, et al: Prevention of reperfusion injury of the ischemic spinal cord: use of recombinant superoxide dismutase. *Ann Thorac Surg* 42:282–286, 1986.
33. Grabitz K, Freye E, Prior R, et al: Does prostaglandin E1 and superoxide dismutase prevent ischaemic spinal cord injury after thoracic aortic cross-clamping. *Eur J Vasc Surg* 4:19–24, 1990.
34. Granke K, Hollier LH, Zdrahal P, et al: Longitudinal study of cerebral spinal fluid drainage in polyethylene glycol-conjugated superoxide dismutase in paraplegia associated with thoracic aortic cross-clamping. *J Vasc Surg* 13:615–621, 1991.
35. Faden AI, Jacobs TP, Smith MT: Evaluation of the cal-

cium channel antagonist nimodipine in experimental spinal cord ischemia. *J Neurosurg* 60:796–799, 1984.

36. Gelbfish JS, Phillips T, Rose DM, et al: Acute spinal cord ischemia: prevention of paraplegia with verapamil. *Circulation* 74:5–10, 1986.

37. Guha A, Tator CH, Piper I: Increase in rat spinal cord blood flow with the calcium channel blocker, nimodipine. *J Neurosurg* 63:250–259, 1985.

38. Svensson LG, VonRitter CM, Groeneveld HT, et al: Cross-clamping of the thoracic aorta: influence of aortic shunts, laminectomy, papaverine, calcium channel blocker, allopurinol, and superoxide dismutase on spinal cord blood flow and paraplegia in baboons. *Ann Surg* 204:38–47, 1986.

39. Hao JX, Xu XJ, Aldskogius H, et al: The excitatory amino acid receptor antagonist MK-801 prevents the hypersensitivity induced by spinal cord ischemia in the rat. *Exp Neurol* 113:182–191, 1991.

40. Kochhar A, Zivin JS, Mazzarella V: Pharmacologic studies of the neuroprotective actions of a glutamate antagonist in ischemia. *J Neurotrauma* 8:175–186, 1991.

41. Breckwoldt WL, Genco CM, Connoly RJ, et al: Spinal cord protection during aortic occlusion: efficacy of intrathecal tetracaine. *Ann Thorac Surg* 51:959–963, 1991.

42. Clark WM, Madden KP, Rothlein R, et al: Reduction of central nervous system ischemic injury by monoclonal antibody to intercellular adhesion molecule. *J Neurosurg* 75:623–627, 1991.

43. Faden AI, Sacksen I, Noble LJ: Opiate receptor antagonist nalmefene improves neurologic recovery after traumatic spinal cord injury in rats through a central mechanism. *J Pharmacol Exp Ther* 245:742–748, 1988.

44. Del Rossi AJ, Cernaianu AC, Cilley JH, et al: Preventive effect of Fluosol-DA for paraplegia encountered after surgical treatment of the thoracic aorta. *J Thorac Cardiovasc Surg* 99:665–669, 1990.

45. Oka Y, Miyamoto T: Prevention of spinal cord injury after cross-clamping of the thoracic aorta. *Jpn J Surg* 14:159–162, 1984.

46. McCullough JL, Hollier LH, Nugent M: Paraplegia after thoracic aortic occlusion: influence of cerebrospinal fluid drainage. *J Vasc Surg* 7:153–160, 1988.

47. Woloszyn TT, Marini CP, Coons MS, et al: A multimodality approach lengthens warm ischemic time during aortic cross-clamping. *J Surg Res* 52(1):15–21, 1992.

48. Shulman K, Verdier GR: Cerebral vascular resistance changes in response to cerebrospinal fluid pressure. *Am J Physiol* 213:1084–1088, 1967.

49. Ekstrom-Jodal B: Effect of increased venous pressure on cerebral blood flow in dogs. *Acta Physiol Scand* (suppl)350:51–61, 1970.

50. Emerson TE, Parker JL: Effects of local increases of venous pressure on canine cerebral hemodynamics. In: Langfitt TW, McHenry LCJ, Reivich M, et al (eds). *Cerebral Circulation and Metabolism.* New York: Springer-Verlag New York Inc.; 10–13, 1975.

51. Griffiths IR, Pitts LH, Crawford RA, et al: Spinal cord compression and blood flow. I. The effect of raised cerebrospinal fluid pressure on spinal cord blood flow. *Neurology* 28:1145–1151, 1978.

52. Wadouh F, Lindermann EM, Arndt CF, et al: The arteria radicularis magna anterior as a decisive factor influencing spinal cord damage during aortic occlusion. *J Thorac Cardiovasc Surg* 88:1–10, 1984.

53. Grubbs PE Jr, Marini C, Toporoff B, et al: Somatosensory evoked potentials and spinal cord perfusion pressure are significant predictors of postoperative neurologic dysfunction. *Surgery* 104(2):216–223, 1988.

54. Francel PC, Long BA, Malik JM, et al: Limiting ischemic spinal cord injury using a free radical scavenger 21-aminosteroid and/or cerebrospinal fluid drainage. *J Neurosurg* 79(5):742–751, 1993.

55. Rosomoff HL, Holaday DA: Cerebral blood flow and cerebral oxygen consumption during hypothermia. *Am J Physiol* 179:85–88, 1954.

56. Hagerdal M, Welsh FA, Keykhah MM, et al: Protective effects of combinations of hypothermia and barbiturates in cerebral hypoxia in the rat. *Anesthesiology* 49:165–169, 1978.

57. Hagerdal M, Harp J, Niesson L, et al: The effect of induced hypothermia upon oxygen consumption in the rat aorta. *J Neurochem* 24:311, 1975.

58. Kramer RS, Sanders AP, Lesage AM, et al: The effect of profound hypothermia on preservation of cerebral ATP content during circulatory arrest. *J Thorac Cardiovasc Surg* 56:699–709, 1968.

59. Michenfelder JD, Theye RA: The effects of anesthesia and hypothermia on canine cerebral ATP and lactate during anoxia produced by decapitation. *Anesthesiology* 33:430–439, 1970.

60. Green BA, Khan T, Raimondi AJ: Local hypothermia as a treatment of experimentally induced spinal cord contusion: quantitative analysis of benefit effect. *Surg Forum* 24:436–438, 1973.

61. Martinez-Arizala A, Green B: Hypothermia in spinal cord injury. *J Neurotrauma* (suppl 2)9:S497-S505, 1992.

62. Busto R, Dietrich WD, Globus MY, et al: Small differences in intraischemic brain temperature critically determine the extent of ischemic neuronal injury. *J Cereb Blood Flow Metab* 7:729–738, 1987.

63. Dietrich WD, Halley M, Valdes I, et al: Interrelationships between increased vascular permeability and neuronal damage following temperature-controlled brain ischemia. *Acta Neuropathol* 81:615–625, 1991.

64. Busto R, Globus MY, Dietrich WD, et al: Effect of mild hypothermia on ischemia-induced release of neurotransmitters and free fatty acids in rat brain. *Stroke* 20:904–910, 1989.

65. Sakamoto T, Monafo WW: The effect of hypothermia on regional spinal cord blood flow in rats. *J Neurosurg* 70:780–784, 1989.

66. Robertson CS, Foltz R, Grossman RG, et al: Protection against experimental ischemic spinal cord injury. *J Neurosurg* 64:633–642, 1986.

67. Bigelow WG, Lindsay WK, Greenwood WF: Hypothermia—its possible role in cardiac surgery: an investigation of factors governing survival in dogs at low body temperatures. *Ann Surg* 132:849–866, 1950.

68. Bigelow WG, Callaghan JC, Hoops JA: General hypothermia for experimental intracardiac surgery. *Ann Surg* 132:531–537, 1950.

69. Lewis JF, Tavfic M: Closure of atrial septal defect with the aid of hypothermia: experimental accomplishments and the report of one successful case. *Surgery* 33:52–59, 1953.

70. Beattie EJ, Adovasio A, Keshishian JM, et al: Refrigeration in experimental surgery of the aorta. *Surg Gynecol Obstet* 96:711–713, 1953.

71. Pontius RG, Brockman HL, Hardy EG, et al: The use of hypothermia in the prevention of paraplegia following temporary aortic occlusion: experimental observations. *Surgery* 36:33–38, 1954.

72. Marshall SB, Owens JC, Swan H: Temporary circulatory occlusion to the brain of the hypothermic dog. *AMA Arch Surg* 72:98–106, 1956.

73. Rosomoff HL: Hypothermia and cerebrovascular lesions. I. Experimental interruption of the middle cerebral artery during hypothermia. *J Neurosurg* 13:244–255, 1956.

74. Weiss M, Piwnica A, Lenfant C, et al: Deep hypothermia with total circulatory arrest. *Trans Am Soc Artif Intern Organs* 6:227–235, 1960.

75. Cooley DA, DeBakey ME: Hypothermia in the surgical treatment of aortic aneurysms. *Bulletin de la Societe Internationale de Chirurgie* 3:206–215, 1956.

76. Naslund TC, Hollier LH, Money SR, et al: Protecting the ischemic spinal cord during aortic clamping. *Ann Surg* 215:409–416, 1992.

77. Rokkas CK, Sundaresan S, Shuman TA, et al: Profound systemic hypothermia protects the spinal cord in a primate model of spinal cord ischemia. *J Thorac Cardiovasc Surg* 106(6):1024–1035, 1993.

78. Hessel EA, Scher G, Dillard DH: Platelet kinetics during deep hypothermia. *J Surg Res* 28:23–34, 1980.

79. Valeri ED, Feingold H, Cassidy G, et al: Hypothermia-induced reversible platelet dysfunction. *Ann Surg* 205:175–181, 1987.

80. Cooley DA, Ott DA, Frazier OH, et al: Surgical treatment of aneurysms of the transverse aortic arch: experience with 25 patients using hypothermic techniques. *Ann Thorac Surg* 32:260, 1981.

81. Phillis JW: The selective adenosine A2 receptor agonist, CGS 21680, is a depressant of cerebral cortical neuronal activity. *Brain Res* 509:328–330, 1990.

82. Pham HT, Bendahou M, Sourbier P, et al: Adenosine as a modulator of the inflammatory process. *Int J Immuno* 6:19–23, 1990.

83. Kitakaze M, Hori M, Sato H: Endogenous adenosine inhibits platelet aggregation during myocardial ischemia in dogs. *Circ Res* 69:1402–1407, 1991.

84. Wyatt DA, Ely SW, Lasley RD, et al: Purine-enriched asanguineous cardioplegia retards adenosine triphosphate degradation during ischemia and improves postischemic ventricular function. *J Thorac Cardiovasc Surg* 97:771–778, 1989.

85. Seibel PS, Theodore P, Kron IL, et al: Regional adenosine attenuates postischemic spinal cord injury. *J Vasc Surg* 18(2):153–158, 1993.

86. Herold JA, Kron IL, Langenburg SE, et al: Complete prevention of postischemic spinal cord injury by means of regional infusion with hypothermic saline and adenosine. *J Thorac Cardiovasc Surg* 107(2):536–542, 1994.

87. Ueno T, Furukawa K, Katayama Y, et al: Spinal cord protection: development of a paraplegia-preventive solution. *Ann Thorac Surg* 58(1):116–120, 1994.

88. Ueno T, Itoh T, Hirahara K, et al: Protection against spinal cord ischaemia: one-shot infusion of hypothermic solution. *Cardiovasc Surg* 2(3):374–378, 1994.

89. Allen BT, Davis CG, Osborne D, et al: Spinal cord ischemia and reperfusion metabolism: the effect of hypothermia. *J Vasc Surg* 19(2):332–340, 1994.

90. Ueno T, Furukawa K, Itoh T: Protection against ischemic spinal cord injury: one-shot perfusion and percutaneous topical cooling. *J Vasc Surg* 19(5):882–887, 1994.

91. Wells JD, Hansebout RR: Local hypothermia in experimental spinal cord trauma. *Surg Neurol* 10:200, 1978.

92. Hansebout RR, Tanner JA, Romero-Sierra C: Current status of spinal cord cooling in the treatment of acute spinal cord injury. *Spine* 9:508, 1984.

93. Wisselink W, Becker MO, Nguyen JH, et al: Protecting the ischemic spinal cord during aortic clamping: the influence of selective hypothermia and spinal cord perfusion pressure. *J Vasc Surg* 19(5):788–796, 1994.

94. Salzano RPJ, Ellison LH, Altonji PF, et al: Regional deep hypothermia of the spinal cord protects against ischemic injury during thoracic aortic cross-clamping. *Ann Thorac Surg* 57(1):65–71, 1994.

95. Tabayashi K, Niibori K, Konno H, et al: Protection from postischemic spinal cord injury by perfusion cooling of the epidural space. *Ann Thorac Surg* 56(3):494–498, 1993.

96. Vanicky I, Marsala M, Galik J, et al: Epidural perfusion cooling protection against protracted spinal ischemia in rabbits. *J Neurosurg* 79(5):736–741, 1993.

97. Marsala M, Vanicky I, Galik J, et al: Panmyelic epidural cooling protects against ischemic spinal cord damage. *J Surg Res* 55(1):21–31, 1993.

98. Hoff JT, Smith AL, Hankinson HL, et al: Barbiturate protection from cerebral infarction in primates. *Stroke* 6:28, 1975.

99. Michenfelder JD, Milde JH, Sundt TM: Cerebral protection by barbiturate anesthesia: use after middle cerebral artery occlusion in Java monkeys. *Arch Neurol* 33:345–350, 1976.

100. Smith AL, Hoff JT, Nielsen SL, et al: Barbiturate protection in acute focal cerebral ischemia. *Stroke* 5:1, 1974.

101. Oldfield EH, Plunkett RJ, Nylander WA, et al: Barbiturate protection in acute experimental spinal cord ischemia. *J Neurosurg* 56:511–516, 1982.

102. Bleyaert AL, Nemoto EM, Safar P, et al: Thiopental amelioration of brain damage after global ischemia in monkeys. *Anesthesiology* 49:390–391, 1978.

103. Nordstrom H, Calderini G, Rehncrona S, et al: Effects of phenobarbital anesthesia on postischemic cerebral blood flow and oxygen consumption in the rat. *Acta Neurol Scand* (suppl 64)56:146–147, 1977.

104. Pierce EC Jr, Lambertson CJ, Deutsch S: Cerebral circulation and metabolism during thiopental anesthesia and hyperventilation in man. *J Clin Invest* 41:1664–1671, 1962.

105. Simeone FA, Frazer G, Lawner P: Ischemic brain edema: comparative effects of barbiturates and hypothermia. *Stroke* 10:8–12, 1979.

106. Meyer JS, Taraura T, Marx P, et al: Brain swelling due to experimental cerebral infarction. *Brain* 95:833, 1972.

107. Sundt TM, Grant WC, Garcia JH: Restoration of middle cerebral artery flow in experimental infarction. *J Neurosurg* 31:311, 1969.

108. Smith AL, Marque JJ: Anesthetics and cerebral edema. *Anesthesiology* 45:64, 1974.

109. Demopoulos HB, Flamm E, Seligman ML, et al: Antioxidant effect of barbiturates in model membranes undergoing free radical damage. In: Ingura D, Lassen N (eds). *Cerebral Function, Metabolism and Circulation*. Copenhagen: Munksgaard; 152–153, 1977.

110. Majewska MD, Stroznajder J, Lazarewicz J: Effect of ischemic anoxia and barbiturate anesthesia on free radical oxidation of mitochondrial phospholipids. *Brain Res* 158:423–434, 1978.

111. Flamm ES, Demopoulos HB, Seligman ML, et al: Possible molecular mechanism of barbiturate-mediated protection in regional cerebral ischemia. *Acta Neurol Scand* (suppl 64)56:150–151, 1977.

112. Mark LC, Burns JJ, Brand L, et al: The passage of thiobarbiturates and their oxygen analogs into brain. *J Pharmacol Exp Ther* 123:70–73, 1958.

113. Kirshner DL, Kirshner RL, Heggeness LM, et al: Spinal cord ischemia: an evaluation of pharmacologic agents in minimizing paraplegia after aortic occlusion. *J Vasc Surg* 9:305–308, 1989.

114. Chan PH, Schmidley JW, Fishman RA, et al: Brain injury, edema and vascular permeability changes induced by oxygen-derived free radicals. *Neurology* 34:315–320, 1984.

115. Buckley GB: Pathophysiology of free radical-mediated reperfusion injury. *J Vasc Surg* 5:512–517, 1987.

116. Hall ED, Broughler JM, McCall JM: Antioxidant effects in brain and spinal cord injury. *J Neurotrauma* 9(1):5165, 1992.

117. Wei EP, Koutas HA, Dietrich WD, et al: Inhibition by free radical scavengers and by cyclo-oxygenase inhibitors of pial arteriolar abnormalities from concussive brain injury in cats. *Circ Res* 48:95 1981.

118. Demopoulos HB, Flamm FS, Pietronigro DD, et al: The free radical pathology and the microcirculation in the major nervous system disorder. *Acta Physiol Scand* (suppl)492:91–119, 1980.

119. Del Maestro R: An approach to free radicals in medicine and biology. *Acta Physiol Scand* (suppl)492:153–168, 1980.

120. Milvy P, Kakaii S, Campbell JB, et al: Paramagnetic species and radical products in cat spinal cord. *Ann NY Acad Sci* 222:1102, 1973.

121. Jacobs TP, Kempski O, McKinley D, et al: Blood flow and vascular permeability during motor dysfunction in a rabbit model of spinal cord ischemia. *Stroke* 23:367–373, 1992.

122. Zweier JL, Flaherty JT, Weisfeldt ML: Direct measurement of free radical generation following reperfusion of ischemic myocardium. *Proc Nat Acad Sci USA* 84:1404–1407, 1987.

123. Bayati A, Hellberg O, Odling B, et al: Prevention of ischemic acute renal failure with superoxide dismutase and sucrose. *Acta Physiol Scand* 130:367–372, 1987.

124. Chan PH, Fishman RA: Alterations of membrane integrity and cellular constituents by arachidonic acid in neuroblastoma and glioma cells. *Brain Res* 284:151–157, 1982.

125. Demopoulos HB, Flamm ES, Seligman ML, et al: Molecular pathology of lipids in CNS membranes. In: Jobis FF (ed). *Oxygen and Physiological Function*. Dallas TX: Professional Information Library; 491–508, 1977.

126. Bulkley GB: The role of oxygen free radicals in human disease processes. *Surgery* 94:407–411, 1983.

127. Korthuis RJ, Granger DN, Townsley MI, et al: The role of oxygen-derived free radicals in ischemia-induced increases in canine skeletal muscle vascular permeability. *Circ Res* 57:599–609, 1985.

128. McCord JM, Fridovich I: Superoxide dismutase: an enzymatic function for erythrocuprein (hemocuprein). *J Biol Chem* 244:6049–6055, 1969.

129. Çuevas P, Carceller-Benito F, Reimers D: Administration of bovine superoxide dismutase prevents sequelae of spinal cord ischemia in the rabbit. *Anat Embryol* 179:251–255, 1989.

130. Cuevas P, Reimers D, Carceler F, et al: Ischemic reperfusion injury in rabbit spinal cord: protective effect of superoxide dismutase on neurological recovery and spinal infarction. *Acta Anat* 137:303–310, 1990.

131. Agee JM, Flanagan T, Blackbourne LH, et al: Reducing postischemic paraplegia using conjugated superoxide dismutase. *Ann Thorac Surg* 51(6):911–914, 1991.

132. Plum F: What causes infarction in ischemic brain? *Neurology* 33:222–233, 1983.

133. Cerchiari EL, Hoel TM, Safar P, et al: Protective effects of combined superoxide dismutase and deferoxamine on recovery of cerebral blood flow and function after cardiac arrest in dogs. *Stroke* 18:869–878, 1987.

134. Allen GS, Ahn HS, Preziosi TJ, et al: Cerebral arterial spasm: a controlled trial of nimodipine in patients with subarachnoid hemorrhage. *N Engl J Med* 308:619–624, 1983.

135. Mohamed AA, McCulloch J, Mendelow AD, et al: Effect of the calcium antagonist nimodipine on local cerebral blood flow: relationship to arterial blood pressure. *J Cereb Blood Flow Metab* 4:206–211, 1984.

136. Nowicki JP, MacKenzie CT, Young AR: Brain ischemia, calcium and calcium antagonists. *Pathol Biol* (Paris) 30:282–288, 1982.

137. Steen PA, Newberg LA, Milde JH, et al: Nimodipine improves cerebral blood flow and neurologic recovery after complete cerebral ischemia in the dog. *J Cereb Blood Flow Metab* 3:38–43, 1983.

138. Bolton TB: Mechanisms of action of transmitters and other substances on smooth muscle. *Pharmacol Rev* 59:67–72, 1979.

139. Grotta JC, Creed-Pettigrew L, Lockwood AH, et al: Brain extraction of a calcium channel blocker. *Ann Neurol* 21:171–175, 1987.

140. Vanhoutte PM: The expert committee of the world health organization on classification of calcium antagonists: the viewpoint of the raporteur. *Am J Cardiol* 59:3A-8A, 1987.

141. Harris RJ, Symon L: Extracellular pH, potassium, and calcium activities in progressive ischaemia of rat cortex. *J Cereb Blood Flow Metab* 4:178–186, 1984.

142. Meyer FB, Anderson RE, Yalsh TL, et al: Effect of nimodipine on intracellular brain pH, cortical blood flow and EEG in experimental focal cerebral ischemia. *J Neurosurg* 64:617–626, 1986.

143. Andersson KE: Pharmacodynamic profiles of different calcium channel blockers. *Acta Pharmacol Toxicol* 58(II):31–42, 1986.

144. Morrell RM, Park A, Jacobs AL, et al: Experimental spinal cord ischemia in rats: effects of flunarizine (calcium entry blocker). *Neurology* (suppl I)36:323, 1986.

145. Gelmers HJ, Gorter K, de Weerdt CJ, et al: A controlled trial of nimodipine in acute stroke. *N Engl J Med* 318:203–207, 1988.

146. Goldblatt MW: Properties of human seminal plasma. *J Physiol* (Lond) 84:208–218, 1935.

147. Von Euler US: On the specific vasodilating and plain muscle stimulating substances from accessory genital glands in man and certain animals (prostaglandin and vesiglandin). *J Physiol* (Lond) 88:213–234, 1936.

148. Halushka PV, Dollery CT, MacDermot J: Thromboxane and prostacyclin in disease: a review. *Q J Med* 208:461–470, 1983.

149. Carlson LA, Eriksson I: Femoral-artery infusion of prostaglandin E1 in severe peripheral vascular disease. *Lancet* 1:155–156, 1973.

150. Carlson LA, Olsson AG: Intravenous prostaglandin E1 in severe peripheral vascular disease. *Lancet* 2:810, 1976.

151. Setai GK, Scott SM, Takaro T: Effect of intra-arterial infusion of PGE1 in patients with severe ischemia of lower extremity. *J Cardiovasc Surg* 21:185–192, 1980.

152. Triner L, Vulliemoz Y, Schwartz I, et al: Cyclic phosphodiesterase activity and the action of paperine. *Biochem Biophys Res* 40:64–69, 1970.

153. Imai S, Kitagawau T: A comparison of the differential effects of nitroglycerin, nifedipine and papaverine on contractures induced in vascular and intestinal smooth muscle by potassium and lanthanum. *Jpn J Pharmacol* 31:193–199, 1981.

154. Kukovetz WR, Poch G: Inhibition of cyclic 3',5'-nucleotide phosphodiesterase as a possible mode of action of papaverine and similarly acting drugs. *Arch Pharmacol* 267:189–194, 1970.

155. Plageman PGW, Wohlhueter RM: Inhibition of the transport of adenosine, other nucleosides and hypoxanthine in novikoff rat hepatoma cells by methylxanthines, papaverine, N6–Cyclohexyladenosine and N6–Phenylisopropyladenosine. *Biochem Pharmacol* 31: 1783–1788, 1984.

156. Boley SJ, Sprayregan S, Siegelmann SS, et al: Initial results from an aggressive roentgenological and surgical approach to acute mesenteric ischemia. *Surgery* 82: 848–855, 1977.

157. LoGerfo FW, Haudenschild CC, Quist WC: A clinical technique for prevention of spasm and preservation of endothelium in saphenous vein grafts. *Arch Surg* 119: 1212–1214, 1984.

158. Svensson LG, Klepp P, Hinder RA: Spinal cord anatomy of the baboon: comparison with man and implications for spinal cord blood flow during thoracic aortic cross-clamping. *S Afr J Surg* 24:32–34, 1986.

159. Ogata M, Marshall BM, Lougheed WM: Observations on the effect of intrathecal papaverine in experimental vasospasm. *J Neurosurg* 38:20–25, 1973.

160. Svensson LG, Grum DF, Bednarski M, et al: Appraisal of cerebrospinal fluid alterations during aortic surgery with intrathecal papaverine administration and cerebrospinal fluid drainage. *J Vasc Surg* 11:423–429, 1990.

161. Svensson LG, Stewart RW, Cosgrove DM, et al: Preliminary results and rationale for the use of intrathecal papaverine for the prevention of paraplegia after aortic surgery. *S Afr J Surg* 26:153–159, 1988.

162. Jorgensen MB, Diemer NH: Selective neuron loss after cerebral ischemia in the rat: possible role of transmitter glutamate. *Acta Neurol Scand* 66:536–546, 1982.

163. Meldrum BS: Excitatory amino acids and anoxic/ischemic brain damage. *Trends Neurosci* 8:47–48, 1985.

164. Greenamyre JT: The role of glutamate in neurotransmission and in neurologic disease. *Arch Neurol* 43: 1058–1063, 1986.

165. Rothman SM, Olney JW: Glutamate and pathophysiology of hypoxic-ischemic brain damage. *Ann Neurol* 19: 105–111, 1986.

166. Benveniste H, Drejer J, Schousboe A, et al: Elevation of the extracellular concentrations of glutamate and aspartate in rat hippocampus during transient cerebral ischemia monitored by intracerebral microdialysis. *J Neurochem* 43:1369–1374, 1984.

167. Olney JW, Ho OL, Rhee V: Cytotoxic effects of acidic and sulphur containing amino acids on infant mouse central nervous system. *Exp Brain Res* 14:61–76, 1971.

168. Mangano RM, Schwarcz R: Chronic infusion of endogenous excitatory amino acids into the rat striatum and hippocampus. *Brain Res Bull* 290:372–375, 1983.

169. Olney JW: Brain lesions, obesity, and other disturbances in mice treated with monosodium glutamate. *Science* 164:719–721, 1969.

170. Rothman SM: The neurotoxicity of excitatory amino acids is produced by passive chloride influx. *J Neurosci* 5:1483–1489, 1985.

171. Schanne FAX, Dane A, Young EE, et al: Calcium dependence of toxic death: a final common pathway. *Science* 206:700–702, 1979.

172. Siesjo BK: Calcium and ischemic brain damage. *Eur Neurol* 25:45–56, 1986.

173. Kochhar A, Zivin JA, Lyde PD, et al: Glutamate antagonist therapy reduced neurologic deficits produced by focal central nervous system ischemia. *Arch Neurol* 45: 148–153, 1988.

174. Park CK, Nehls DG, Grahan DI, et al: The glutamate antagonist MK 801 reduces focal ischemic brain damage in the rat. *Ann Neurol* 24:543–551, 1988.

175. Benveniste H, Jorgensen MB, Diemer NH, et al: Calcium accumulation by glutamate receptor activation is involved in hippocampal cell damage after ischemia. *Acta Neurol Scand* 78:529–536, 1988.

176. Faden AI, Yum SW: Comparison of the neuroprotective effects of the N-methyl-D-Aspartate antagonist MK 801 and the opiate-receptor antagonist nalmefene in experimental spinal cord ischemia. *Arch Neurol* 47: 277–281, 1990.

177. Horlon J: Neutrophil-mediated vascular injury. *Acta Med Scand* 715:123–129, 1985.

178. Engler R: Consequence of activation and adenosine-mediated inhibition of granulocytes during myocardial ischemia. *Fed Proc* 46:1407–2412, 1987.

179. Mehta J, Nichols W: Neutrophils as potential participants in acute myocardial ischemia: relevance to reperfusion. *J Am Coll Cardiol* 11:1309–1316, 1988.

180. Ramson JL, Hook BG, Luchesi B: Reduction of the extent of ischemic myocardial injury by neutrophil depletion in the dog. *Circulation* 67:1016–1023, 1983.

181. Engler RL, Dahlgren MD, Morris DD, et al: Role of leukocytes in response to acute myocardial ischemia and reflow in dogs. *Am J Physiol* 251:H314-H322, 1986.

182. Ramson JL, Hook BG, Kunkel SL, et al: Role of leukocytes in response to acute myocardial ischemia and reflow in dogs. *Circulation* 67:1016–1023, 1983.

183. Whitley D, Miyasaka M, Tamatami T, et al: Adhesion molecules in acute and chronic allograft rejection. *Surg Forum* 42:368, 1991.

184. Hancock WH, Whitley WD, Tullius SG, et al: Cytokines, adhesion molecules, and the pathogenesis of chronic rejection of rat renal allografts. *Transplantation* 56(3):643–650, 1993.

185. Hancock WW, Whitley WD, Baldwin WM 3d, et al: Cells, cytokines, adhesion molecules, and humoral responses in a rat model of chronic renal allograft rejection. *Transplant Proc* 24(5):2315–2316, 1992.

186. Ames A, Wright L, Masayoshi K, et al: Cerebral ischemia: the no-reflow phenomenon. *Am J Pathol* 52: 437–443, 1968.

187. Clark WM, Madden KP, Rothlein R, et al: Reduction of central nervous system ischemic injury in rabbits using leukocyte adhesion antibody treatment. *Stroke* 22: 877–883, 1991.

188. Clark LC, Gollan F: Survival of mammals breathing organic liquids equilibrated with oxygen at atmospheric pressure. *Science* 152:1755–1756, 1966.

189. Okamoto H, Iwai M, Tsudo Y, et al: Changes of particle size of perfluorochemical emulsion in circulation. Proceedings of the Postcongress Symposium/Xth International Congress of Nutrition on Perfluorochemical Artificial Blood. Kyoto, Japan: 73–82, 1975.

190. Peerless SJ, Ishikamo R, Peerless MJ: Protective effect

of Fluosol-DA in acute cerebral ischemia. *Stroke* 12: 558–563, 1981.

191. Kolluri S, DeGirolami U, Heros RC, et al: Fluosol and experimental spinal cord ischemia. *Acta Neuropathol* 75:491–494, 1988.

192. Kolluri S, Heros RC, Vonsattel JP, et al: Failure of fluosol to influence the incidence of cerebral infarction or mortality in gerbils subjected to temporary carotid occlusion. *Surg Neurol* 23:553–556, 1986.

193. Faden AI, Hallenbeck JM, Brown CQ, et al: Treatment of experimental stroke: comparison of naloxone and thyrotropin-releasing hormone. *Neurology* 32: 1083–1087, 1982.

194. Hosobuchi Y, Baskin WS, Woo SK, et al: Reversal of induced ischemic neurologic deficit in gerbils by the opiate antagonist naloxone. *Science* 215:63–71, 1982.

195. Faden AI, Jacobs TP, Zivin JA, et al: Comparison of naloxone and a delta-selective antagonist in experimental spinal "stroke." *Life Sci* (suppl 1)33:707–710, 1983.

196. Faden AI, Jacobs TP, Holaday JW: Opiate antagonists improve neurologic recovery after spinal injury. *Science* 211:493–494, 1981.

197. Faden AI, Jacobs TP, Mougey E, et al: Endorphins in experimental spinal injury: therapeutic effect of naloxone. *Ann Neurol* 10:326–332, 1981.

198. DeRiu PL, Petruzzi V, Palmieri G, et al: B-endorphin in experimental canine spinal ischemia. *Stroke* 20: 253–258, 1989.

199. Takeshita H, Michenfelder JD, Theye RA: The effects of morphine and N-allymorphine on canine cerebral metabolism and circulation. *Anesthesiology* 37:605–612, 1972.

200. Bloom JD, Segal D, Ling N, et al: Endorphins: profound behavioral effects in rats suggest new etiological factors in mental illness. *Science* 194:630–632, 1976.

201. Moroni F, Cheney DL, Costa E: B-endorphin inhibits ACh turnover in nuclei of rat brain. *Nature* 267: 267–268, 1977.

202. Long JB, Martinez-Arizala JM, Petras JM, et al: Endogenous opioids in spinal cord injury: a critical evaluation. *Cen Nerv Sys Trauma* 3:295–315, 1986.

203. Faden A, Holaday J: Endorphin in traumatic spinal injury: pathophysiologic studies and clinical implications. In: Emrich H (ed). *The Role of Endorphins in Neuropsychiatry (Modern Problems of Pharmacopsychiatry)*. Basel, Switzerland: Karger Publishing Co.; 158EP-174, 1981.

204. Holaday JW, Faden AI: Naloxone acts at central opiate receptors to reverse hypotension, hypothermia, and hypoventilation in spinal shock. *Brain Res* 189:295–299, 1980.

205. Faden AI, Jacobs TP, Holaday JW: Endorphin-parasympathetic interaction in spinal shock. *J Autonom Nerv Sys* 2:295–304, 1980.

206. Faden AI, Jacobs TP, Feuerstein G, et al: Dopamine partially mediates the cardiovascular effects of naloxone after spinal injury. *Brain Res* 213:415–421, 1981.

207. Faden AI, Jacobs TP, Smith MP, et al: Naloxone in experimental spinal cord ischemia: dose response studies. *Eur J Pharmacol* 103:115–120, 1984.

208. Young W, Flamm ES, Demopoulos HB, et al: Naloxone ameliorates posttraumatic ischemia in experimental spinal contusion. *J Neurosurg* 55:209–219, 1981.

209. Flamm ES, Young W, Demopoulos HB, et al: Experimental spinal cord injury: treatment with naloxone. *Neurosurgery* 10:227–231, 1982.

210. Hall ED, Pozara KE, Broughler JM: Effect of tirilazad mesylate on postischemic lipid peroxidation and recovery of extracellular calcium in gerbils. *Stroke* 22:361, 1991.

211. Hall ED, Yonkers PA, Horan KL, et al: Correlation between attenuation of posttraumatic spinal cord ischemia and preservation of vitamin E by the 21-aminosteroid U-74006F: evidence for an in vivo antioxidant mechanism. *J Neurotrauma* 6:169, 1989.

212. Braughler JM, Pregenzer JF, Chase RL, et al: Novel 21-aminosteroid as potent inhibitors of iron-dependent lipid peroxidation. *J Biol Chem* 262:10438–10440, 1987.

213. Hall ED, McCall JM, Chase RL, et al: A nonglucocorticoid steroid analog of methylprednisolone duplicates its high-dose pharmacology in models of central nervous system trauma and neuronal membrane damage. *J Pharmacol Exp* 242:137–142, 1987.

214. Broughler JM, Pregenzer JF: The 21-aminosteroid inhibitors of lipid peroxidation: reactions with lipid peroxyl and phenoxyl radicals. *Free Radicol Biol Med* 7: 125, 1989.

215. Svensson LG, Crawford ES, Hess KR, et al: Experience with 1509 patients undergoing thoracoabdominal aortic operations. *J Vasc Surg* 17:357–370, 1993.

216. Hollier LH, Money SR, Naslund TC, et al: The risk of spinal cord dysfunction in patients undergoing thoracoabdominal aortic replacement. *Am J Surg* 164(2): 210–214, 1992.

217. Crawford ES, Rubio PA: Reappraisal of adjuncts to avoid ischemia in the treatment of aneurysms of descending thoracic aorta. *J Thorac Cardiovasc Surg* 66: 693–703, 1973.

218. Crawford ES, Waler HSJ III, Saleh SA, et al: Graft replacement of aneurysm in descending thoracic aorta: results without bypass or shunting. *Surgery* 89:73–85, 1981.

219. Najafi H, Javid H, Hunter J, et al: Descending aortic aneurysmectomy without adjuncts to avoid ischemia. *Ann Thorac Surg* 30:326–335, 1980.

220. Adams HD, Van Geertruyden HH: Neurologic complications of aortic surgery. *Ann Surg* 144:574–610, 1956.

221. Katz NM, Blackstone EH, Kirklin JW, et al: Incremental risk factors for spinal cord injury following operation for acute traumatic aortic transection. *J Thorac Cardiovasc Surg* 81:669–674, 1981.

222. Jex RK, Schaff HV, Piehler JM, et al: Early and late results following repair of dissections of the descending thoracic aorta. *J Vasc Surg* 3:226–237, 1986.

223. Laschinger JC, Cunningham JN, Cooper MM, et al: Monitoring of somatosensory evoked potentials during surgical procedures on the thoracoabdominal aorta. I. Relationship of aortic cross-clamp duration, changes in somatosensory evoked potentials, and incidence of neurologic dysfunction. *J Thorac Cardiovasc Surg* 94: 260–265, 1987.

224. Svensson LG, Stewart RW, Cosgrove DM, et al: Intrathecal papaverine for the prevention of paraplegia after operations on the thoracic or thoracoabdominal aorta. *J Thorac Cardiovasc Surg* 93:823–829, 1988.

225. Crawford ES, Palamara AE, Saleh SA, et al: Aortic aneurysms: current status of surgical treatment. *Surg Clin North* Am 59:597–636, 1979.

226. Fereschetian A, Kadir S, Kaufman SL, et al: Digital subtraction spinal cord angiography in patients undergoing thoracic aneurysm surgery. *Cardiovasc Intervent Radiol* 12:7–9, 1989.

227. Kieffer E, Richard T, Chivos J, et al: Preoperative spinal cord arteriography in aneurysmal disease of the

descending thoracic and thoracoabdominal aorta: preliminary results in 45 patients. *Ann Vasc Surg* 3:34–46, 1989.

228. DiChiro G, Fried LC, Doppman JL: Experimental spinal cord angiography. *Br J Radiol* 43:19–30, 1970.

229. Szilagyi DE, Hagemen JH, Smith RF, et al: Spinal cord damage in surgery of the abdominal aorta. *Surgery* 83:38–56, 1978.

230. Svensson LG, Patel V, Coselli JS, et al: Preliminary report of localization of spinal cord blood supply by hydrogen during aortic operations. *Ann Thorac Surg* 49:528–536, 1990.

231. Svensson LG, Patel V, Robinson MF, et al: Influence of preservation of intraoperatively identified spinal cord blood supply on spinal motor evoked potentials and paraplegia after aortic surgery. *J Vasc Surg* 13:355–365, 1991.

232. Crawford ES, Svensson LG, Hess KR, et al: A prospective randomized study of cerebrospinal fluid drainage to prevent paraplegia after high-risk surgery on the thoracoabdominal aorta. *J Vasc Surg* 13:36–46, 1990.

233. Livesay JJ, Cooley DA, Ventemiglia RA, et al: Surgical experience in descending thoracic aneurysmectomy with and without adjuncts to avoid ischemia. *Ann Thorac Surg* 39:37–45, 1985.

234. Hollier LH, Symmonds JB, Pairolero PC, et al: Thoracoabdominal aortic aneurysm repair: analysis of postoperative morbidity. *Arch Surg* 123:871–875, 1988.

235. Donahoo JS, Brawley RK, Gott VL: The heparin-coated vascular shunt for thoracic aortic and great vessel procedures: a 10-year experience. *Ann Thorac Surg* 23:507–513, 1977.

236. Carlson DE, Karp RB, Kouchoukos NT: Surgical treatment of aneurysms of the descending thoracic aorta: an analysis of 85 patients. *Ann Thorac Surg* 35:58–67, 1983.

237. Verdant A, Cossette R, Page A, et al: Aneurysms of the descending thoracic aorta: 366 consecutive cases resected without paraplegia. *J Vasc Surg* 21(3):385–391, 1995.

238. Laschinger JC, Izumoto H, Kouchoukos NT: Evolving concepts in prevention of spinal cord injury during operations on the descending thoracic and thoracoabdominal aorta. *Ann Thorac Surg* 44:667–674, 1987.

239. Kouchoukos NT, Wareing TH, Izumoto H, et al: Elective hypothermic cardiopulmonary bypass and circulatory arrest for spinal cord protection during operations on the thoracoabdominal aorta. *J Thorac Cardiovasc Surg* 99:659–664, 1990.

240. Cunningham JN Jr, Laschinger JC, Spencer FC: Monitoring of SEP during surgical procedures on the thoracoabdominal aorta: IV. Clinical observations and results. *J Thorac Cardiovasc Surg* 94:275, 1987.

241. Cartier R, Orszulak TA, Pairolero PC: Circulatory support during cross-clamping of the descending thoracic aorta: evidence of improved organ perfusion. *J Thorac Cardiovasc Surg* 99:1038–1047, 1990.

242. Cunningham JN Jr, Laschinger JC, Merkin MA, et al: Measurement of spinal cord ischemia during operations upon the thoracic aorta: initial clinical experience. *Ann Surg* 196:285–296, 1982.

243. Laschinger JC, Owen J, Rosenbloom M, et al: Direct noninvasive monitoring of spinal cord motor function during thoracic aortic occlusion: use of motor evoked potentials. *J Vasc Surg* 7:161–171, 1988.

244. Laschinger JC, Cunningham JN Jr, Baumann FG, et al: Monitoring of SEP during surgical procedures on the thoracoabdominal aorta. II. Use of SEP to assess adequacy of distal aortic bypass and perfusion following thoracic aortic cross-clamping. *J Thorac Cardiovasc Surg* 94:266, 1987.

245. Konrad PE, Tacker WA, Levy WJ, et al: Motor evoked potentials in the dog: effects of global ischemia on spinal cord and peripheral nerve signals. *Neurosurgery* 20:117–124, 1987.

246. Elmore JR, Gloviczki P, Harper CM, et al: Failure of motor evoked potentials to predict neurologic outcome in experimental thoracic aortic occlusion. *J Vasc Surg* 14:131–139, 1991.

247. Svensson LG, Grum DF, Bednarski M, et al: Appraisal of cerebrospinal fluid alterations during aortic surgery with intrathecal papaverine administration and cerebrospinal fluid drainage. *J Vasc Surg* 11(3):423–429, 1990.

248. Murray MJ, Bower TC, Oliver WC Jr, et al: Effects of cerebrospinal fluid drainage in patients undergoing thoracic and thoracoabdominal aortic surgery. *J Cardiothorac Vasc Anesth* 7:266–272, 1993.

249. Mahfood S, Qazi A, Garcia J, et al: Management of aortic arch aneurysm using profound hypothermia and circulatory arrest. *Ann Thorac Surg* 39:412–417, 1985.

250. Massimo CG, Poma AG, Viligiard RR, et al: Simultaneous total aortic replacement from arch to bifurcation: experience with six cases. *J Tex Heart Inst* 13:147–151, 1986.

251. Crawford ES, Coselli JS, Safi HJ: Partial cardiopulmonary bypass, hypothermic circulatory arrest, and posterolateral exposure for thoracic aortic aneurysm operation. *J Thorac Cardiovasc Surg* 94:824–827, 1987.

252. Frank SM, Parker SD, Rock P, et al: Moderate hypothermia, with partial bypass and segmental sequential repair for thoracoabdominal aortic aneurysm. *J Vasc Surg* 19(4):687–697, 1994.

CHAPTER 35

Arteriovenous Hemodialysis Access

Bruce A. Jones, MD; Anton N. Sidawy, MD

Introduction

The arteriovenous fistula has provided therapeutic benefit as a form of hemodialysis access for nearly 4 decades. The Scribner and other external shunts provided access for hemodialysis prior to 1966. However, because of their high complication rates, another option was sought. In 1966, Brescia, Cimino, and colleagues developed the technique of a peripheral subcutaneous arteriovenous fistula. It was obvious that the complications of external shunts, including infection and poor patency rates due to thrombosis, could be improved upon by the use of the autogenous Brescia-Cimino subcutaneous arteriovenous fistula. Since 1966, other techniques have been developed and all appear to have their own unique advantages and disadvantages.

Many characteristics of congenital arteriovenous communications also apply to the peripheral arteriovenous fistula created for hemodialysis. Blood flow patterns, pressure gradients, and resistance can all be altered with considerable physiologic variation in the various types of arteriovenous hemodialysis access (AVHA). By varying the material the fistula is created from, the size of the fistula, the proximity to central circulation, as well as many other factors, the fistula can show unique characteristics and be valuable in various clinical circumstances.

History

Long before AVHAs were first utilized for hemodialysis, the congenital and traumatic arteriovenous communications were recognized as clinical entities.

Many of the same principles apply when AVHAs are discussed. The introduction of long-term hemodialysis access by Quinton, Scribner, and colleagues, in 1960, parallels the development of the hemodialysis machine and treatment of end-stage renal failure. The Scribner shunt provided easier and more long-term access for the chronic dialysis patient without the unwelcome need for repetitive venipuncture and cutdown techniques.

The Scribner shunt is an external silastic cannula shunt forming an arteriovenous communication. Because of its external nature, infectious complications are not uncommon and thrombotic complications are seen with regularity.

Recognizing that the Scribner shunt has its limitations, others were spurred to investigate viable alternatives. In 1966, Brescia and Cimino described arteriovenous access by the use of a completely internalized fistula anastomosing the cephalic vein to the radial artery.[1] Immediately, it gained overwhelming approval and popularity, as it was considerably more convenient and the complications of infection and thrombosis seen in the external shunt were markedly decreased. To date, the Brescia-Cimino fistula remains the access of choice in many clinical situations.

Since 1966, other investigators have provided alternatives for AVHA. The Brescia-Cimino fistula does have its associated complications, and the long-term dialysis patient may develop thrombosis of the cephalic vein and/or radial artery. Because of this, alternative techniques for fistula formation were required.

Subsequent techniques employed the use of more proximal vessels in the upper extremities, saphenous vein autografts as straight or looped fistulas in both

From *The Basic Science of Vascular Disease.* Edited by Sidawy AN, Sumpio BE, and DePalma RG. Armonk, NY: Futura Publishing Company, Inc.; © 1997.

the upper and lower extremities, and lastly the use of prosthetic materials. Early prosthetic materials have included bovine heterograft, human umbilical cord vein grafts (HUVG), and Dacron.

In 1976, expanded polytetrafluoroethylene (e-PTFE) was introduced for use as an alternative means of arteriovenous bridge fistula construction. Since then, e-PTFE has gained extraordinary popularity and is the favored material for use in arteriovenous fistula construction when an autogenous fistula cannot be created. It has gained its popularity due to the ease of handling, no preclotting requirement, its resistance to kinking and external pressure, and its ease of revision following infection or thrombosis.

Anatomy

The upper extremity should be evaluated for highly accessible vessels. The artery should have a strong, easily palpable pulse, and the vein should be patent and of adequate size to obtain a good functioning access. In natural fistulas, when the vein itself serves as the conduit, the vein should be superficial in the subcutaneous tissue to be easily accessible for dialysis. When a superficial vein is not available, a prosthetic conduit such as e-PTFE is used to connect the artery with the vein and it is then placed subcutaneously to be easily accessible. In another option, the deeply seated basilic vein can be dissected in its entirety in the arm region, then placed in a subcutaneous tunnel, and anastomosed to the brachial artery.

The natural fistula needs a minimum of 3 to 4 weeks for maturation and thickening of the vessel wall to occur in order to sustain repeated venipuncture. A prosthetic graft should be allowed at least 2 weeks to incorporate in the tissue before it is used for venipuncture. This will decrease complications such as perigraft hematomas, infection, and thrombosis.

Arterial system evaluation should be taken very seriously, as distal ischemia is reported and happens not infrequently when collateral blood supply is not adequate. The radial artery is preferentially chosen because the ulnar artery usually provides adequate collateral supply to the hand and distal tissues. Arteriography has been described in the past for preoperative evaluation.[2] However, this is rarely done when an adequate clinical exam exists.

Brachial, axillary, and femoral vessels have all been described as access vessels and all are viable options in the right circumstances.[3,4] Jendrisak and Anderson have also described arterial access from axillary artery branches.[5]

Graft failure is eventual in most grafts; revision is then indicated. If revision is not successful, the more proximal vessels in the same arm may be utilized. Use of the brachial artery is discouraged by many as a first line procedure because of the less abundant collateral circulation compared to the radial/ulnar artery situation. However, the possibility of limb loss after brachial artery ligation appears to be anecdotal. Lally and colleagues examined a 5-year series of brachial artery ligation in children for insertion of Scribner shunts. Their mean follow-up occurred at 15.8 years and identified no limb loss or growth abnormalities. There was, however, a diminished resting pressure and mildly decreased exercise tolerance.[6] The brachial artery fistula does have a higher blood flow than the more distal fistulas and this may enhance its longevity.[7] However, because of its more proximal nature, the likelihood of the steal phenomenon increases.

A hemodialysis access fistula contains three features common to all types of fistulas constructed. These three elements include the arterial inflow, the venous outflow, and the conduit. The figure shows the possible upper extremity AVHA designs that are clinically used.

Despite problems with the autogenous forearm fis-

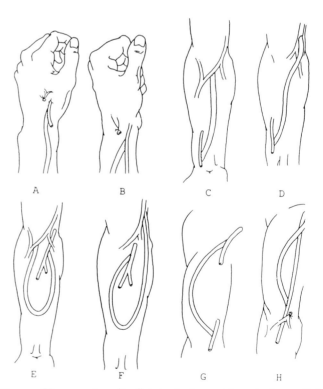

Figure. Upper extremity fistula designs: **A)** posterior radial branch artery to cephalic vein (**snuff-box fistula**); **B)** radial artery to cephalic vein (**Brescia-Cimino fistula**); **C)** radial artery to antecubital vein (**straight graft**); **D)** radial artery to basilic vein-above elbow (**straight graft**); **E)** brachial artery-below elbow to antecubital vein (**loop graft**); **F)** brachial artery-below elbow to basilic vein-above elbow (**loop graft**); **G)** brachial artery-above elbow to axillary vein (**C-shaped graft**); **H)** brachial artery-above elbow to basilic vein-above elbow (**basilic transposition**).

tula, it remains the access with the lowest incidence of thrombosis, infection, or pseudoaneurysm formation. Therefore, it remains the most frequently utilized.

When forearm vessels are not available for autogenous use, another form of access is needed. Construction of more proximal fistulas is a viable option with 2-year patency rates of nearly 75%.[8] The brachiobasilic and brachiocephalic AVHAs are most frequently used as they are easy to access, have few complications, and are technically easy to construct.[8] The other option available is the bridge fistula. Bridge arteriovenous fistulas with prosthetic material are the best alternative to autogenous arteriovenous fistulas. Bridge fistulas may be constructed with various materials, although e-PTFE has become the most commonly used material.

A bridge AVHA may be constructed between virtually any artery/vein combination, provided arterial inflow and venous outflow are adequate. Either a straight graft or loop graft can be utilized. The loop graft may provide a larger access for venipuncture. It also has the advantage of diminished venous hypertension when compared to a straight graft. Lavigne and colleagues point out that the high pressure in the arterial end of the fistula rapidly dissipates across the loop fistula to equal systemic venous pressure on the venous side of the fistula.[9] This lower incidence of venous hypertension is due to the increased length of the loop graft and not the configuration.

Regardless of vessels utilized, the configuration of autogenous fistulas is of four basic types: 1) side of vein to side of artery anastomosis; 2) end of vein to side of artery anastomosis; 3) side of vein to end of artery anastomosis; and 4) end of vein to end of artery anastomosis.

Physiology

Resistance

The new AVHA shows a pattern of decreased peripheral resistance, due to bypassing the peripheral arteriolar and capillary network of the vascular tree. Nearly 90% of vascular resistance to flow is from the artery and capillary network, whereas venous flow accounts for the remaining 10% of vascular resistance. Blood will follow the path of least resistance, and when it reaches the fistula, it preferentially flows into the low resistance venous system, rather than the distal arterial network with its associated higher resistance.[10]

Velocity and Volume

There is also an increase in blood flow velocity across the fistula due to the loss of resistance. The size of the fistula determines the change in resistance, with an inverse ratio noted between fistula size and resistance. Poiseuille's law describes the energy losses that occur across this system; however, the principles of a Newtonian fluid, that being laminar flow in a straight cylindrical tube, must be met in order to strictly apply this law. This is not the case with an arteriovenous fistula. However, in a more simplified approach, the concept of blood flow can be seen as:

$$Pressure = Flow \times Resistance$$

Again, the fistula has bypassed 90% of the vascular bed resistance and, thus, an associated drop in pressure is seen. Because of this, one can appreciate the increase in blood flow that occurs.

It has been shown in the canine model that proximal arterial flow is in direct relation to the fistula size, with increasing proximal flow seen in progressively increasing fistula size up to a point. Beyond this point, further increases in the size of the fistula do not increase the proximal arterial blood flow. This pattern is shown in Table 1.[11]

Dialysis treatment is enhanced with a minimum blood flow volume of 200 mL/min and an optimal minimum of 400 mL/min. Blood flow volume is critically dependent upon location of the access. Forearm accesses generally carry a lower blood flow volume when compared to the upper arm accesses. The inclusion of estimated blood flow volume (EBFV) in the evaluation of AVHAs enhances the diagnosis of fistula complications, as it adds a physiologic value to any anatomic findings already obtained.

By using a peripheral vascular duplex ultrasound system, the authors have determined blood flow volumes for five different access types in a series of 90 patients. These findings are shown in Table 2. Notably, the flow rates are highest for the thigh grafts followed by upper arm grafts and, lastly, forearm grafts provide the lowest flow rates.[12] This does not, however, imply that the larger, more proximal fistulas are preferred. A forearm graft with an adequate flow rate is the preferred choice to alleviate any potential problems of the steal phenomenon that may be associated with the larger, more proximal fistulas.

Flow Patterns

The normal laminar concentric flow of blood is altered in an arteriovenous fistula with resultant turbulent flow predominating. As explained by Zierler, the transition to turbulent flow depends upon the diameter of the tube (in this case, diameter of the fistula), velocity across the tube, the fluid density, and viscosity.[13] The Reynold's number acts as a measure of turbulence and represents these forces acting on a fluid. The prop-

Table 1
Effects of Fistula Diameter on Proximal Femoral Artery Flow

Fistula Diameter (min)	Proximal Femoral Artery Flow* (mL. min.$^{-1}$ Kg.$^{-1}$)		Change in Flow (mL. min.$^{-1}$ Kg.$^{-1}$)
	Fistula Closed	Fistula Open	
2	5.7 ± 0.6	6.8 ± 0.5†	1.1 ± 0.4‡
4	5.2 ± 1.3	28.1 ± 5.7§	22.9 ± 6.1‡
8	4.1 ± 0.4	40.2 ± 5.2§	36.1 ± 5.5‡
16	4.1 ± 0.3	35.3 ± 0.8§	31.2 ± 0.5‖

* Mean ± S.E.
† Not significantly different from control, $P > 0.05$.
‡ Significantly different from all other values in column, $P < 0.01$, except as noted.
§ Significantly different from control, $P < 0.05$.
‖ Not significantly different from vertically preceding value in column. $P > 0.05$.
(Reprinted from Lavigne JE, Messina LM, Golding MR, et al: Fistula size and hemodynamic events within and about canine femoral arteriovenous fistulas. *J Thorac Cardiovasc Surg* 74:551–556, 1977.)

erties of an AVHA are manifested by each of these features, and the degree of turbulence can be estimated by the equation shown below describing the ratio of inertial to viscous forces. Because the characteristics of the vessel walls and of pulsatile flow have not been taken into account, the Reynold's number can only be used as an estimation:

$$Re = \frac{\delta \overline{V} \rho}{\eta}$$

The Reynold's Equation. The point of transition between laminar and turbulent flow depends upon: 1) δ, tube diameter; 2) $\overline{V}$, mean velocity; 3) ρ, specific gravity of the fluid; 4) η, fluid viscosity. The Reynold's number is the ratio of inertial forces to viscous forces acting on the fluid. (Reproduced with permission from Zieler RE, Strandness DE: Hemodynamics for the vascular surgeon. In: More WS (ed). *Vascular Surgery: A Comprehensive Review.* Philadelphia: WB Saunders, Co.; 161–203, 1986.)

Energy Changes

The sum total of energy in any system is defined as the summation of kinetic energy (E_K) + potential energy (E_P). The kinetic energy can be shown in the following equation:

$$E_K = \frac{1}{2}\rho v^2$$

Kinetic energy in a fluid system: ρ = specific gravity of the fluid; v^2 = square of fluid velocity (cm/sec). (Reproduced with permission from Zieler RE, Strandness DE: Hemodynamics for the vascular surgeon. In: More WS (ed). *Vascular Surgery: A Comprehensive Review.* Philadelphia: WB Saunders, Co.; 161–203, 1986.)

The increased velocity change, as well as the change in direction of flow affecting the velocity, will be seen as a kinetic energy loss.

With the density and viscosity of the blood and diameter of the fistula remaining constant, the turbu-

Table 2
Dialysis Fistula Estimated Blood Flow Volume (EBFV)

Access Type	n	Location	EBFV (mL/min)
Natural fistula	30	Forearm	814 ± 66.5
Natural fistula	9	Upperarm	1425 ± 215.5
Prosthetic graft	35	Forearm	798 ± 54.0
Prosthetic graft	10	Upperarm	1221 ± 96.5
Prosthetic graft	6	Thigh	1697 ± 179.7

Table 3
Factors Affecting an Arteriovenous Communication Hemodynamics

Fistula resistance
Collateral development
Anatomic configuration
Blood flow velocity
Blood flow pressure
Blood flow turbulence

lent flow across a fistula is directly proportional to the velocity change. Already having established that the velocity change is given off as kinetic energy, this kinetic energy can, thus, be quantified by estimating the degree of turbulent flow. By using color flow doppler imaging of the perivascular tissues, the degree of turbulence is estimated by the amount of tissue vibration seen and, thus, the kinetic energy loss is quantified.[14]

Pathophysiology

All fistulas must perform in a constantly changing physiologic environment. Blood flow alterations, changes in peripheral resistance, variations in systemic arterial pressure, and anatomic changes, such as collateral development, all contribute to a dynamic range of physiologic factors affecting AVHA. Although not inclusive of all factors, Table 3 lists the important factors contributing to the hemodynamic alterations seen in AVHA.

Local Hemodynamics/Pathophysiology

The typical features of a side-to-side AVHA include a proximal and distal artery, as well as a proximal and distal vein. Their description and nomenclature is based upon their relation to the fistula.

The Proximal Artery

Degeneration of the proximal artery is almost universal. Histologically, an increase in collagenous tissue, a decrease in elastic tissue, and atrophy of the smooth muscle are seen. This is more consistent with thinning or atrophy, rather than the changes seen in atherosclerosis, namely, intimal proliferation and mural thickening.[15] In an experimental arteriovenous fistula in the sheep model, it has been shown that the proximal artery also has glycosaminoglycan content alterations. In particular, the chondroitin sulphate content is elevated.[16]

The etiology of this arterial wall degeneration and reorganization is yet to be determined. In 1970, Ingebrigtsen and colleagues examined the longitudinal stretching of the artery proximal to the fistula in a canine arteriovenous fistula model. A large pressure diminution was noted after fistula construction. With this pressure drop, the stretching force was also naturally reduced. They theorized that the dilatation of this vessel can be attributed to the turbulence of flow that is seen.[17] Both concentric and longitudinal dilatation occur. Although the dilatation of the vessel will cause thinning of the wall, the atrophy of the smooth muscle component is likely caused by the decrease in stretching force that is demonstrated.[18,19]

Regardless of the etiology, the consequences of this degeneration may manifest in several different ways. The structural changes seen may be as simple as arterial dilatation, or as complex as aneurysm development. The degenerative changes seen in the proximal artery are felt to be contributory to early graft failure in dialysis fistulas.[18]

The structural changes that develop in the proximal artery are well known to lead to aneurysm formation.[18,20] The size and nature of these aneurysms may be striking. The histologic changes described earlier, with an increase in collagenous tissue, a decrease in elastic tissue, and atrophy of the smooth muscle, are similar to what is seen in aneurysm formation of most medium-sized muscular arteries not associated with arteriovenous fistulas.[18,21]

Lastly, the development of collateral circulation takes place. The increased blood flow velocity is considered the primary etiology to its development.[22] The one resounding factor behind collateral development is the importance of the distal artery and its contribution to resistance.

The Distal Artery

The pressure in the distal artery is reduced in direct relation to the size of the fistula opening. Flow distally is decreased with each increase in fistula size.[11] This takes place until a fistula diameter of four times that of the distal artery occurs, at which time retrograde flow from the distal artery is seen.[11,23] This was nicely demonstrated by Lavigne and associates in 1977 and can be seen in Table 4.

The local consequence of this flow reversal is the steal phenomenon. This may be represented by early findings of effort fatigue and ischemic pain, to the more advanced findings of tissue loss and potentially limb loss. To counteract this steal phenomenon, the ischemia seen in distal tissue beds produces vasodilation and may lead to the eventual development of collateral circulation. The high flow velocity in the proximal ar-

Table 4
Effects of Fistula Diameter on Distal Femoral Artery Flow

Fistula Diameter (min)	Proximal Femoral Artery Flow (mL. min.⁻¹ Kg.⁻¹)		Change in Flow† (mL. min.⁻¹ Kg.⁻¹)
	Fistula Closed	Fistula Open	
2	5.4 ± 0.4	2.5 ± 0.5‡	−3.1 ± 0.3
4	5.3 ± 1.0	3.0 ± 1.2§	−2.3 ± 0.6
8	4.4 ± 0.2	2.1 ± 1.4§	−2.3 ± 1.6
16	4.0 ± 0.4	−4.6 ± 0.3‖	−8.6 ± 0.5¶

* Mean ± S.E.

† Values in this column do not differ significantly, $P > 0.05$, except as noted.

‡ Significantly different from control, $P < 0.025$.

§ Significantly different from control, $P < 0.05$.

‖ Significantly different from control, $P < 0.001$.

¶ Significantly different from other values in column, $P > 0.05$, except as noted.

(Reprinted with permission from Lavigne JE, Messina LM, Golding MR, et al: Fistula size and hemodynamic events within and about canine femoral arteriovenous fistulas. *J Thorac Cardiovasc Surg* 74:551–556, 1977.)

tery, the low peripheral resistance, and the reversal of flow in the distal artery all contribute to the formation of collateral circulation.[24] A decrease in the size of the distal artery may also occur, likely secondary to a decrease in flow and pressure.[24]

The Proximal Vein

Venous flow changes by varying the size of the fistula. Increases in flow are seen in the vein proximal to the fistula as the fistula size increases. However, only a minimal elevation in pressure can be appreciated.[24] This is due to the venous distension and large venous capacitance of the central circulation.

This distension of the proximal (outflow) vein also leads to histologic changes. Degeneration of the internal elastic lamina, intimal-medial hyperplasia, collagen deposition, and aneurysm development all occur.[25,26] The intimal-medial hyperplasia appears to be most prominent adjacent to the toe of the anastomosis.[27,28] The venous endothelial injury has also been described by Fallon and Stehbens to include an increased turnover of endothelial cells, and the formation of multinucleated endothelial cells characteristic of endothelial regeneration. This finding is predominantly seen directly across from the high flow arterial stream. At this point a "jet lesion" is described consisting of a thin deposit of mural thrombi over a denuded endothelium.[29]

As early as 1967, Fry developed a canine model to study the effect of increased blood velocity on the vascular endothelium.[30] Although this was conducted on an arterial endothelial model, he was able to define the shear stresses seen in the endothelium exposed to higher blood velocities. Marked endothelial deterioration was seen as early as 1 hour after an acute yield stress value of 379 ± 85 dynes/cm² was surpassed. This value corresponds to the level of blood velocity at which a "normal" endothelial cell population density is maintained. From these findings, one can anticipate the same changes in the proximal vein endothelium after increased blood velocity is established from the construction of an AVHA.

More recently, Kohler et al studied the effects of tangential wall stress on venous endothelium when jugular vein grafts were interposed in the carotid arteries of rabbits.[31] By providing external support with a wrapped PTFE graft around the venous graft, it was hypothesized that a decreased wall area would be exposed to increased pressures and wall stress. Due to the decreased wall area, exposed venous distension and, thus, tangential wall stress were diminished. In their tightly wrapped segments, smooth muscle proliferation and matrix deposition were diminished on cross-sectional examination.[31] These findings are important from the aspect of the intimal hyperplasia, seen in the high pressure system of the proximal vein after arteriovenous fistula construction. Ultrastructural examination by electron microscopy confirms that the hyperplasia seen in the proximal vein is almost exclusively that of smooth muscle cells.[27] In contrast to atherosclerotic plaques, a paucity of lipid vacuoles, foam cells, and extracellular matrix is observed. Lymphocytes and macrophages are also absent. From a more clinical standpoint, the venous outflow obstruction will eventually lead to fistula failure. The high pressure ostial blood flow through the fistula affects the vein wall opposite this flow, and may be the site of subsequent bacterial endarteritis.[32]

Venous aneurysm development involving the vein proximal to the fistula is a rare entity. In contrast to Moosa and associates, finding of proximal venous aneurysm development 8 months after surgical placement of a hemodialysis fistula,[26] most aneurysms develop after a prolonged exposure to arterial flow. In fact, Thompson and Lindenauer reviewed their series of 11 aneurysms proximal to a traumatic arteriovenous fistula, and reported that the aneurysms were late developments and had been present for at least 20 years.[33]

The Distal Vein

In a new hemodialysis fistula, the vein distal to the fistula has a markedly elevated pressure with a subsequent decrease in distal venous flow. With a larger fistula size, the distal venous pressure is proportionally increased.[23] A level of venous hypertension is eventually reached that causes distal venous flow to reverse. Lavigne demonstrated this flow reversal with larger fistula sizes.[11] Associated with venous hypertension, edema, varicose veins, and venous ulcers may follow, especially if the outflow vein becomes occluded and the fistula remains patent.

The high volume, high velocity, and high pressure blood flow through the fistula eventually lead to the same histologic destruction seen in the proximal vein, namely, degeneration of the internal elastic lamina, collagen deposition, and, albeit reduced, some degree of intimal-medial hyperplasia.[19] This leads to dilatation and stretching of the vessel wall with subsequent valvular incompetence. With the valvular incompetence, retrograde flow occurs. This retrograde flow and proximal venous obstruction are the major stimuli for the development of venous hypertension if adequate collateral circulation is not formed.

Systemic Hemodynamics/Pathophysiology

With few exceptions, the systemic hemodynamic manifestations seen with AVHAs are generally limited. The surgically created hemodialysis access fistula can manifest all of these findings in certain clinical and pathologic circumstances.

The development of significant cardiac failure is the ultimate manifestation and most dire consequence of an AVHA. The degree to which this develops depends upon multiple factors including: 1) the ostial size of the AVHA; 2) the proximity of the AVHA to the central circulation; and 3) the age of the AVHA.

The central physiologic finding that is common to all the systemic manifestations is the drop in total pe-

ripheral resistance. All subsequent characteristics and pathophysiologic alterations of the AVHA can be attributed to this one concept. Homeostatic regulation requires that this fall in total peripheral resistance be addressed and certain changes take place. With a fall in peripheral resistance, there is a concomitant fall in systemic blood pressure. To maintain essential organ perfusion, an increase in cardiac output can be appreciated almost immediately.[34,35]

With the use of radioactive microspheres, Huang and colleagues have shown an appreciable elevation in cardiac output in the rat model when an aorta to vena cava fistula was created.[36,37] By measuring the flow of microspheres to the lungs, an estimate of shunt flow was determined. They found cardiac index increased 40%, 107%, 129%, and 307% compared to control animals in 1-hour, 1-day, 1-week, and 5-week measurements. Baroreceptor reflexes are activated and a tachycardia response increases the cardiac output. An augmentation in stroke volume through the increased cardiac inotropy also occurs.[38] With time and adaptation, the accelerated cardiac rate eventually nears prefistula values as other mechanisms, such as the increased stroke volume, are recruited to maintain the elevated cardiac output.[38] Interestingly, occlusion of the fistula or the artery proximal to the fistula will result in the reduction of heart rate as described by Nicoladoni in 1875 (known as Branham's sign or Branham-Nicoladoni's sign).

The inotropic effect seen is due to sympathetic nervous discharge and an elevation in circulating endogenous catecholamines. The increase in the sympathathetic and adrenal discharge initially causes a peripheral vasoconstriction in an attempt to maintain an adequate blood pressure and adequate blood flow to essential organs. These mechanisms are only partially successful and other mechanisms are required.[39] An increase in stroke volume augments the cardiac output and is thought to be the primary mechanism responsible. With the development of an AVHA, there is an abrupt rise in central venous return. This elevated venous return causes elevated cardiac pressures, most importantly the end-diastolic pressure. The left ventricle adapts to this acute volume overload by the use of inotropic, chronotropic, and Starling reserves.[40]

Preferential blood flow through a large, more proximal fistula may also indirectly threaten renal blood flow and decrease renal perfusion. This decreased renal perfusion activates the renin-angiotensin-aldosterone system and leads to sodium and water reabsorption.[41–43] An expanded plasma volume is accomplished and with the addition of protein mobilization, the oncotic pressure increases to preserve the expanded intravascular volume. Elevated blood volume may be the underlying cause of any subsequent congestive heart failure. Johnson and Boucher described their experience in a patient with an AVHA. They note that the left ventricular ejection fraction was normal. When the fistula was repaired, the heart failure was relieved. From these findings, they surmised that volume overload rather than impaired systolic function was the etiology for this patient's heart failure.[44]

This highly efficient system of blood volume elevation is even more remarkable when closure of AVHA is accomplished. A rapid diuresis and natruresis occurs, with reports of a 40- to 60-pound weight loss following repair of an aortovena caval fistula.[45] The importance of the elevated blood volume cannot be adequately emphasized. If maintenance of peripheral perfusion cannot be upheld, a significant "steal phenomenon" will ensue with debilitating consequences to other organ systems.[24]

Cardiomegaly can eventually develop over several months.[40–44,46] The degree of cardiac enlargement is variable with relation to AVHA size. Whether this is a true cardiomegaly from cardiac hypertrophy, or from cardiac dilatation, has been a topic of much discussion. Experimental evidence in the canine model shows both hypertrophy and dilatation.[47] More recently, in the rat model, it has been shown that compensatory hypertrophy may be more important. Liu et al have shown that the shape of the myocyte changes, consistent with normal physiologic growth.[48] The ultimate consequence that may occur is cardiac failure. The degree to which this happens, and when this occurs, depend as much upon the patient's cardiac status and cardiac reserve as they do on the characteristics of the AVHA. With increased cardiac output and increased circulatory load, a vicious cycle may develop where expansion of a communication may lead to further expanded intravascular volume to accommodate for further increases in cardiac output. Cardiac decompensation may eventually develop in this scenario.

Interestingly, these complications of cardiac decompensation are seen primarily in acquired arteriovenous connections (AVCs). Quite rarely will cardiac failure be seen in a congenital AVC, unless it is exceedingly large, or manifests early in the neonatal period. Lastly, cardiac failure is rare with the construction of a distal peripheral hemodialysis fistula.[24]

Complications

There are many complications that may eventually lead to graft failure. The primary complications include infection, thrombosis, and pseudoaneurysm formation.[49–54] In addition, the dialysis-associated steal syndrome (DASS) has been noted, as well as the reflex sympathetic dystrophy syndrome (RSDS),[55] skin erosion, serous fluid collections, and distal edema. Ultimately, the elevated cardiac output that may be experienced can eventually lead to cardiac failure.

Thrombosis

The most common cause of late thrombosis is due to venous outflow obstruction. Localized intimal hyperplasia of the vein most frequently causes this venous outflow obstruction. This is usually found just proximal to the vein-graft anastomosis.[52,56] Late thrombosis may also occur due to repeated trauma from accessing the fistula.

The inherent characteristics of an AVHA fistula namely, flow turbulence, mechanical mismatch, and wall shear stress are all thought to contribute to the establishment of intimal hyperplasia. In addition, the endothelial cell is known to produce many mitogenic growth factors including platelet-derived growth factor (PDGF), insulin-like growth factor-1 (IGF-1), and endothelin-1 (ET-1).[57,58] PDGF is mitogenic to both smooth muscle cells and fibroblasts. The ultimate pathologic event is endothelial cell injury leading to subsequent smooth muscle cell proliferation.

Smooth muscle cell proliferation begins in the media followed by migration to the luminal surface. PDGF is known to bind to these smooth muscle cells and is likely responsible for their migration from the media to the intima. Growth factors binding to smooth muscle cells cause their proliferation and, ultimately, connective tissue elements are elaborated.[59]

Palder et al identified venous outflow stenosis as the most common cause of recurrent graft thrombosis in their 4-year review of the experience at Brigham and Women's Hospital.[60] In Rizzuti's 7-year review of 189 expanded polytetrafluoroethylene grafts, 42% of their graft thrombosis events were related to venous outflow stenosis secondary to intimal hyperplasia.[61]

The canine arteriovenous loop graft has been extensively studied. Fillinger et al have shown that flow turbulence is a major contributor in the development of intimal-medial hyperplasia in the loop graft. By banding the proximal artery to reduce flow rates to 50% of original, they noted a decrease in velocity, a decrease in pulsatility, a decrease in pressure, as well as a decrease in turbulence. The decreased turbulence was reflected in a lower Reynold's number. The banded grafts showed a statistically significant decrease in the development of intimal-medial hyperplasia.[62]

Further studies also indicate that the geometry of loop grafts shows correlation to intimal-medial hyperplasia. By using tapered and untapered grafts, Fillinger was able to show that the intimal-medial hyperplasia was significantly reduced following a 4 to 7 mm taper graft, as opposed to a 7 to 4 mm taper graft, or an untapered graft. Color flow Doppler imaging was used to measure the volume of the vibration signal (a measure of turbulence) at the distal anastomosis of the loop graft. The volume of the vibration signal was significantly decreased at the 4 to 7 mm taper graft, and this variable showed significant correlation with venous intimal-medial hyperplasia.[28]

Postoperative hemodynamics can be accessed with color flow duplex monitoring, venous phase angiography, and pulse oximetry.[63] Prior to the widespread use of duplex ultrasonography, pneumatic plethysmography was used for evaluation.[64]

Evaluation of poor fistula function can be very adequately done with noninvasive testing. By using quantitative Doppler spectrum analysis, Tordoir and colleagues obtained diagnostic accuracies of 86% and 81% in graft arteriovenous fistulas and Brescia-Cimino arteriovenous fistulas respectively.[65] The gold standard, however, remains angiography.

The dysfunction in rapid hemodialysis can also be evaluated by recirculation methods.[66,67] By measuring urea recirculation during hemodialysis, Collins et al were able to identify venous stenoses. When the stenoses were corrected, a significant improvement in urea recirculation was seen (36 $\pm$ 3% to 21 $\pm$ 3%).[66]

Infection

Infection, as a complication of arteriovenous hemodialysis fistulas in the chronic renal-failure patient, may be life-threatening. Manifestations may vary from cellulitis to suppuration of the anastomosis site and fulminant sepsis. In a large study of 499 operations in 230 patients for permanent hemodialysis access, Zibari et al reported an overall infectious complication rate of 6%.[54] This included both autogenous and prosthetic fistulas. Other reports indicate higher infection rates near 35%.[53]

Multiple accessing contributes to infectious complications. A recent study of 2131 access procedures revealed a puncture infection rate of 5% per year. A second puncture infection was seen at a rate of 12% per year.[68] The vascular access site is, by far, the primary reason for septic episodes in the dialysis patient.

The dialysis patient manifests a poor host immune response, in addition to poor wound healing, which increase the incidence of infection.[69] Brock et al recently demonstrated higher infectious complication rates in patients who were HIV positive.[70]

It has also been postulated that the mechanism of dialysis itself may lead to wound morbidity because of a decrease in subcutaneous tissue oxygen tension. It has been shown that the subcutaneous oxygen tension can decrease nearly 50% during dialysis.[71]

Femoral access sites are more prone to infection than upper extremity sites. Also, synthetic conduits are more likely to become infected than autogenous tissue. Perioperative antibiotics are beneficial, and the proper use of aseptic technique during accessing cannot be adequately emphasized.

Gram-positive organisms continue to be the most common bacteria involved in hemodialysis fistula infections. Either *Staphylococcus aureus* or *Staphylococcus epidermidis* were present in all culture-positive puncture infections in one recent series.[70] In fact, S. aureus was positive in 71% of their cultures and S. epidermidis was positive in 10%. Gram-negative organisms remain a minor contributor to fistula infection.

Treatment of infected grafts typically requires removal of the entire graft, as well as antibiotic therapy. Cellulitis may be responsive to antibiotic coverage alone. With localized infections, antibiotics and drainage may be appropriate.

Steal Syndrome

Dialysis-associated steal syndrome (DASS) occurs due to the preferential blood flow proceeding through a fistula, with the subsequent hypoperfusion and potential ischemia in the distal tissues. As described earlier, the distal arterial flow is a function of fistula size. Directly proportional to the fistula size is the fistula flow rate. With a large fistula, the preferential blood flow is "stolen" from the distal arterial needs.

Dialysis-associated steal syndrome is manifested by a painful, cold, numb hand.[72–74] The diabetic patient appears to manifest the vascular steal syndrome more frequently than the nondiabetic patient. DASS is also more frequently seen in the more proximal arteriovenous fistula. Anastomotic construction, with the end artery to side of vein technique, rarely produces dialysis associated steal syndrome.

When evaluating vascular steal syndrome, one must be cognizant of other diagnostic possibilities. Included should be neuropathies of uremia or diabetes, symptoms from secondary hyperparathyroidism, and carpal tunnel syndrome.[75]

Preservation of a functioning arteriovenous fistula has become an increasingly important goal. Fistula ligation was originally touted as the procedure of choice to correct for vascular steal. However, over the past 2 decades more refined techniques have become commonplace. External banding of grafts has been the most common technique applied for treatment of dialysis-associated steal syndrome. This, unfortunately, presents another piece of foreign material and it is not always easy to balance fistula flow with distal perfusion.

For the treatment of dialysis-associated steal syndrome and peripheral ischemia, Schanzer and associates describe the technique of ligation of the first artery just distal to the arteriovenous fistula, along with arterial bypass from the artery proximal to the takeoff of the arteriovenous fistula, to the artery distal to the ligation.[56,76] Their 1-year arteriovenous fistula patency and arterial bypass patency rates were both 100%. All but one of their original patients noted subjective relief of symptoms.

Narrowing of the conduit, just distal to the anastomosis, can provide symptomatic relief of steal. By incising the conduit, just distal to the arterial anastomosis, it can then be narrowed uniformly by closure over a small diameter arterial dilator.[77] Banding of the conduit can be done without foreign material by utilizing a crescent shaped plication suture.[78]

Evaluation of steal syndrome can be done with intraoperative blood flow measurements with duplex ultrasonography.[7] The information provided can lead to the appropriate modifications in technique if necessary. Digital photoplethysmography has also been used as a guide to ascertain the appropriate amount of graft narrowing during construction of a fistula.[79]

Pseudoaneurysm Formation

Pseudoaneurysm formation is usually the result of a graft infection and typically occurs at the suture line of the fistula. Traumatic access, with subsequent hematoma formation, may also play a role in the etiology and can occur anywhere along the fistula.[80] Histologically, a hematoma will develop beneath the fibrous scarring seen in the healing process. With continued pressure from the arterial lumen, the hematoma expands and a fibrous capsule forms leading to the pseudoaneurysm. Because of the higher incidence of subsequent infection and thrombosis, surgical excision is recommended.[80]

Venous Hypertension

Distal venous hypertension may result in severe edema of the hand and be extremely disabling.[81,82] Proximal venous obstruction with a patent fistula is the underlying factor most consistent with venous hypertension. This appears to be most common with side-to-side autogenous fistulas and can be alleviated by correcting the cause of venous outflow occlusion.

References

1. Brescia MJ, Cimino JE, Appel K, Hurwich BJ: Chronic hemodialysis using venipuncture and a surgically created arteriovenous fistula. *N Engl J Med* 275:1089–1092, 1966.
2. Gothlin J, Lindstedt E: Angiographic features of Cimino-Brescia fistulas. *AJR* 125(3):582–590, 1975.
3. Polo JR, Sanabia J, Garcia-Sabrido JL, et al: Brachial jugular polytetrafluoroethylene fistulas for hemodialysis. *Am J Kidney Dis* 16(5):465–468, 1990.
4. Freedman BI, Anderson RL, Tuttle AB, et al: The Thomas shunt revisited. *Am J Kidney Dis* 19(1):45–48, 1992.
5. Jendrisak MD, Anderson CB: Vascular access in patients with arterial insufficiency. *Ann Surg* 212(2):187–193, 1990.
6. Lally KP, Foster CE III, Chwals WJ, et al: Long-term follow-up of brachial artery ligation in children. *Ann Surg* 212(2):194–196, 1990.
7. Anderson CB, Etheredge EE, Harter HR, et al: Local blood flow characteristics of arteriovenous fistulas in the forearm for dialysis. *Surg Gynecol Obstet* 144:531–533, 1977.
8. Cantelmo NL, LoGerfo FW, Menzoian JO: Brachiobasilic and brachiocephalic fistulas as secondary angioaccess routes. *Surg Gynecol Obstet* 155:545–548, 1982.
9. Lavigne JE, Brown CS, Fewel J, et al: Hemodynamics within a canine femoral arteriovenous fistula. *Surgery* 77(3):439–443,1975.
10. Lin TV, Boody RJ: Arteriosclerotic abdominal aortic aneurysm: spontaneous rupture into the inferior vena cava. *JAMA* 186:218–220, 1963.
11. Lavigne JE, Messina LM, Golding MR, et al: Fistual size and hemodynamic events within and about canine femoral arteriovenous fistulas. *J Thorac Cardiovasc Surg* 74(4):551–556, 1977.
12. Sidawy AN, et al: Blood flow volumes for angioaccess. Unpublished Data.
13. Zierler RE, Strandness DE Jr: Doppler techniques of lower extremity arterial diagnosis. In: Zwiebel WJ (ed). *Introduction to Vascular Ultrasonography*. 2nd ed. New York: Grune & Stratton, Inc.; 305–331, 1986.
14. Simkins TE, Stehbens WE: Vibrations recorded from the adventitial surface of experimental aneurysms and arteriovenous fistulas. *J Vasc Surg* 8:153–166, 1974.
15. Stehbens, WE: Hemodynamic production of lipid deposition, intimal tears, mural dissection, and thrombosis in the blood vessel wall. *Proc Roy Soc Series B* 185:357, 1974.
16. Rogers KM, Merrilees MJ, Stehbens WE: The effect of haemodynamic stress on the glycosaminoglycan content of blood vessel walls of experimental aneurysms and arteriovenous fistulae. *Artherosclerosis* 58:139–148, 1985.
17. Ingebrigtsen R, Fonstelien E, Solberg LA: Measurement of forces producing longitudinal stretching of the arterial wall examined in the artery proximal to an arteriovenous fistula. *Acta Chir Scand* 136:569–573, 1970.
18. Shumacker HB: Aneurysm development and degenerative changes in dilated artery proximal to arteriovenous fistula. *Surg Gynecol Obstet* 130:636–640, 1970.
19. Stehbens WE: Blood vessel changes in chronic experimental arteriovenous fistulas. *Surg Gynecol Obstet* 127:327–338, 1968.
20. Graham JM, McCollum CH, Crawford ES, et al: Extensive arterial aneurysm formation proximal to ligated arteriovenous fistula. *Ann Surg* 191(2):200–203, 1980.
21. Sako Y, Varco RL: Arteriovenous fistula: results of management of congenital and acquired forms, blood flow measurements, and observations on proximal artery degeneration. *Surgery* 67:40, 1970.
22. John HT, Warren R: The stimulus to collateral circulation. *Surgery* 49:14, 1961.
23. Lough FC, Giordano JM, Hobson RW: Regional hemodynamics of large and small femoral arteriovenous fistulas in dogs. *Surgery* 79(3):346–349, 1976.
24. Sumner DS: Hemodynamics and pathophysiology of arteriovenous Fistulas. In: Rutherford RB (ed). *Vascular Surgery*. Philadelphia: WB Saunders, Co.; 1007–1032.

25. Stehbens WE, Karmody AM: Venous atherosclerosis associated with arteriovenous fistulas for hemodialysis. *Arch Surg* 110:176–180, 1975.

26. Moosa HH, Johnson RR, Julian TB: Venous aneurysm after polytetrafluoroethylene arteriovenous dialysis fistula. *J Vasc Surg* 9(6):825–827, 1989.

27. Swedberg SH, Brown BG, Sigley R, et al: Intimal fibromuscular hyperplasia at the venous anastomosis of PTFE grafts in hemodialysis patients. *Circulation* 80(6): 1726–1736, 1989.

28. Fillinger MF, Reinitz ER, Schwartz RA: Graft geometry and venous intimal-medial hyperplasia in arteriovenous loop grafts. *J Vasc Surg* 11(4):556–566, 1990.

29. Fallon JR, Stehbens WE: Venous endothelium of experimental arteriovenous fistulas in rabbits. *Circ Res* 31: 546–556, 1972.

30. Fry DL: Acute vascular endothelial changes associated with increased blood velocity gradients. *Circ Res* 32: 165–197, 1968.

31. Kohler TR, Kirkman TR, Clowes AW: The effect of rigid external support on vein graft adaptation to the arterial circulation. *J Vasc Surg* 9(2):277–285, 1989.

32. Lindenauer SM: Vascular malformation and arteriovenous fistula. In: Greenfield LJ, Mulholland MW, Oldham KT, Zelenock GB (eds). *Surgery: Scientific Principles and Practice.* Philadelphia: JB Lippincott; 1741–1755, 1993.

33. Thompson NW, Lindenauer SM. Central venous aneurysms and arteriovenous fistulas. *Ann Surg* 170:852–856, 1969.

34. Nakano J, DeSchryver C: Effects of arteriovenous fistula on systemic and pulmonary circulations. *Am J Physiol* 207:1319–1324, 1964.

35. Longo T, Brusoni B, Merlo L, et al: Haemodynamics at rest and under effort in chronic arteriovenous fistulae (AVFs). *J Cardiovasc Surg* 18:509–517, 1977.

36. Huang M, Hester RL, Guyton AC: Hemodynamic changes in rats after opening an arteriovenous fistula. *Am J Physiol* 262(3 Pt 2):H846–851, 1992.

37. Huang M, Hester RL, Guyton AC, et al: Hemodynamic studies in DOCA-salt hypertensive rats after opening of an arteriovenous fistula. *Am J Physiol* 262(6 Pt 2): H1802–1808, 1992.

38. Gupta PD, Singh M: Neural mechanism underlying tachycardia induced by nonhypotensive A-V shunt. *Am J Physiol* 236:H35–41, 1979.

39. Romero, JC. Cardiovascular manifestations of hypertension. In: Brandenburg RO, Fuster V, Giuliani ER, McCoon DC (eds). *Cardiology: Fundamentals and Practice.* Chicago: Year Book Medical Publishers, Inc.; 1738–1747, 1987.

40. Alyono D, Ring WS, Anderson MR, et al: Left ventricular adaptation to volume overload from large aortocaval fistula. *Surgery* 96(2):360–366, 1984.

41. Davis JO, Urquhart J, Higgins JT, et al: Hypersecretion of aldosterone in dogs with a chronic aortic-caval fistula and high output heart failure. *Circ Res* 14(6):471–485, 1964.

42. Spielman WS, Davis JO, Gotshall RW: Hypersecretion of renin in dogs with a chronic aortic-caval fistula and high-output heart failure. *Proc Soc Exp Biol Med* 143: 479–482, 1973.

43. Humphreys MH, Al-Bander H, Eneas JF, et al: Factors determining electrolyte excretion and renin secretion after closure of an arteriovenous fistula in the dog. *J Lab Clin Med* 98(1):89–98, 1981.

44. Johnson RA, Boucher CA: Normal left ventricular ejection fraction in systemic arteriovenous fistuli: implications for the use of noninvasive methods in differential diagnosis of heart failure. *Chest* 79(5):607–609, 1981.

45. Eiseman B, Hughes RH: Repair of an abdominal aortic-vena caval fistula caused by rupture of an atherosclerotic aneurysm. *Surgery* 39:498, 1956.

46. Holman E: Abnormal arteriovenous communications: great variability of effects with particular reference to delayed development of cardiac failure. *Circulation* 32: 1001–1009,1965.

47. Taylor RR, Covell JW, Ross J: Left ventricular function in experimental aorto-caval fistula with circulatory congestion and fluid retention. *J Clin Invest* 47: 1333–1342, 1968.

48. Liu Z, Hilbelink DR, Crockett WB, et al: Regional changes in hemodynamics and cardiac myocyte size in rats with aortocaval fistulas: developing and established hypertrophy. *Circ Res* 69(1):52–58, 1991.

49. Ballard JL, Bunt TJ, Malone JM: Major complications of angioaccess surgery. *Am J Surg* 164:229–232, 1992.

50. Cheek RC, Messina JJ, Acchiardo SR, et al: Arteriovenous fistulas for hemodialysis: experience with 100 cases. *Ann Surg* 42:386–389, 1976.

51. Haimov M, Baez A, Neff M, et al: Complications of arteriovenous fistulas for hemodialysis. *Arch Surg* 110: 708–712, 1975.

52. Kherlakian GM, Roedersheimer LR, Arbaugh JJ, et al: Comparison of autogenous fistula versus expanded polytetrafluoroethylene graft fistula for angioaccess in hemodialysis. *Am J Surg* 152:238–243, 1986.

53. Raju S: PTFE grafts for hemodialysis access. *Ann Surg* 206(5):666–673, 1987.

54. Zibari GB, Rohr MS, Landreneau MD, et al: Complications from permanent hemodialysis vascular access. *Surgery* 104(4):681–686, 1988.

55. Weise WJ, Bernard DB: Reflex sympathetic dystrophy syndrome of the hand after placement of an arteriovenous graft for hemodialysis. *Am J Kidney Dis* 18(3): 406–408, 1991.

56. Schanzer H, Skladany M, Haimov M: Treatment of angioaccess-induced ischemia by revascularization. *J Vasc Surg* 16(6):861–866, 1992.

57. Vane JR, Anggard EE, Botting RM: Regulatory functions of the vascular endothelium. *N Engl J Med* 323(1): 27–36, 1990.

58. Limanni A, Fleming T, Molina R, et al: Expression of genes for platelet-derived growth factor in adult human venous endothelium: a possible nonplatelet dependent cause of intimal hyperplasia in vein grafts and perianastomotic areas of vascular prostheses. *J Vasc Surg* 7:10–20, 1988.

59. Chevru A, Moore WS: An overview of intimal hyperplasia. *Surg Gynecol Obstet* 171:433–447, 1990.

60. Palder SB, Kirkman RL, Whittemore AD: Vascular access for hemodialysis. *Ann Surg* 202(2):325–239, 1985.

61. Rizzuti RP, Hale JC, Burkart TE: Extended patency of expanded polytetrafluoroethylene grafts for vascular access using optimal configuration and revisions. *Surg Gynecol Obstet* 166:23–27, 1988.

62. Fillinger MF, Reinitz ER, Schwartz RA: Beneficial effects of banding on venous intimal-medial hyperplasia in arteriovenous loop grafts. *Am J Surg* 158:87–94, 1989.

63. Halevy A, Halpern Z, Negri M, et al: Pulse oximetry in the evaluation of the painful hand after arteriovenous fistula creation. *J Vasc Surg* 14(4):537–539, 1991.

64. Bussell JA, Abbott JA, Lim RC: A radial steal syndrome

with arteriovenous fistula for hemodialysis. *Ann Int Med* 75(3):387–394, 1971.

65. Tordoir JHM, deBruin HG, Hoeneveld H, et al: Duplex ultrasound scanning in the assessment of arteriovenous fistulas created for hemodialysis access: comparison with digital subtraction angiography. *J Vasc Surg* 10(2): 122–128, 1989.

66. Collins DM, Lambert MB, Middleton JP, et al: Fistula dysfunction: effect on rapid hemodialysis. *Kidney Int* 41: 1292–1296, 1992.

67. Windus DW, Audrain J, Vanderson R, et al: Optimization of high-efficiency hemodialysis by detection and correction of fistula dysfunction. *Kidney Int* 38:337–341, 1990.

68. Taylor B, Sigley RD, May KJ: Fate of infected and eroded hemodialysis grafts and autogenous fistulas. *Am J Surg* 165:632–636, 1993.

69. Hill SL, Donato AT: Complications of dialysis access: a six-year study. *Am J Surg* 162:265–267, 1991.

70. Brock JS, Sussman M, Wamsley M, et al: The influence of human immunodeficiency virus infection and intravenous drug abuse on complications of hemodialysis access surgery. *J Vasc Surg* 16(6):904–910, 1992.

71. Jensen JA, Goodson WH, Omachi RS, et al: Subcutaneous tissue oxygen tension falls during hemodialysis. *Surgery* 101(4):416–421, 1987.

72. Fee HJ, Golding AL: Lower extremity ischemia after femoral arteriovenous bovine shunts. *Ann Surg* 183(1): 42–45, 1976.

73. Lindstedt E, Westling H: Effects of an antebrachial Cimino-Brescia arteriovenous fistula on the local circulation in the hand. *Scand J Urol Nephrol* 9:119–124, 1975.

74. Kinnaert P, Struyven J, Mathieu J, et al: Intermittent claudication of the hand after creation of an arteriovenous fistula in the forearm. *Am J Surg* 139:838–843, 1980.

75. Mattson WJ: Recognition and treatment of vascular steal syndrome to hemodialysis prostheses. *Am J Surg* 154: 198–201, 1987.

76. Schanzer H, Schwartz M, Harrington E, et al: Treatment of ischemia due to ''steal'' by arteriovenous fistula with distal artery ligation and revascularization. *J Vasc Surg* 7(6):770–773, 1988.

77. Khalil IM, Livingston DH: The management of steal syndrome occurring after access for dialysis. *J Vasc Surg* 7(4):572–573, 1988.

78. Rivers SP, Scher LA, Veith FJ: Correction of steal syndrome secondary to hemodialysis access fistulas: a simplified quantitative technique. *Surgery* 112(3):593–597, 1992.

79. Odland MD, Kelly PH, Ney AL, et al: Management of dialysis-associated steal syndrome complicating upper extremity arteriovenous fistulas: use of intraoperative digital photoplethysmography. *Surgery* 110(4):664–670, 1991.

80. Dawkins HG, Vargish T, James PM: Comparative hemodynamics of surgical arteriovenous fistulae in dogs. *J Surg Res* 18:169–175, 1975.

81. Delpin EAS: Swelling of the hand after arteriovenous fistula for hemodialysis. *Am J Surg* 132:373–376, 1976.

82. Mindich B, Dunn I, Frumkin E, et al: Proximal venous thrombosis after side-to-side arteriovenous fistula. *Arch Surg* 108:227–229, 1974.

CHAPTER 36

Arterial and Vascular Graft Infection

Marsel Huribal, MD; John J. Ricotta, MD

Infection of a prosthetic graft is one of the most devastating complications of vascular surgery and carries with it high morbidity and mortality rates. The overall incidence of graft infection varies from 1% to 3% of all vascular operations (Table 1). The cumulative incidence may be as high as 5% to 6%, if both early and late infections are considered.[1]

Aortic graft infection has been reported to carry a mortality rate of 40% to 50%, and in some series mortality rates as high as 75% have been reported (Table 2). Although the mortality rate of infrainguinal graft infection is lower, approximately 20%, the amputation rate in these infrainguinal grafts has been reported to be as high as 80%. Despite the low incidence of graft infection, it is clear that the surgical management of this complication continues to be a challenge for vascular surgeons.

Human graft infection is a complex problem without any diagnostic "gold standard" or uniform principles of management. With the continued use of prosthetic grafts, it is important for vascular surgeons to have a clear concept of the definition of graft infection and an effective management plan in order to deal with this complication. This chapter discusses the definition and pathobiology of graft infection, as well as evaluates the principles that influence the diagnoses and management of this condition.

Definition of Graft Infection

An infected graft is by definition one with established bacterial colonization and growth of an organism within the graft itself. This distinction between wound colonization and invasion of an organism is determined by the quantity and the virulence of the organism, adhesive capacity of the organism to the graft, host defenses, and immune reaction, as well as the graft material used. Initially, it is important to differentiate contamination from invasive graft infection. Graft contamination usually occurs in the immediate postoperative period associated with superficial wound infection. In fact, this situation usually represents a soft tissue wound infection with graft exposure rather than invasive graft infection. Attention to the soft tissue infection with antimicrobial prophylaxis and early wound closure is often sufficient treatment in these cases.

Wound contamination may become the initial step of graft infection. Whether a graft infection follows microbial contamination will depend on the quantity, virulence, and the adhesive capability of the organism. This process may be compared to thermal burn wound infection. Contamination of burn wounds is common and easily dealt with, while invasive sepsis requires aggressive surgical debridement and systemic antibiotics. A parallel exists with graft contamination and graft infection. The quantitative innoculum and the microbiology of the organism are major determinants of outcome. Similar to burn wound sepsis, a graft infection can be defined as a graft with microbial colonization and active invasion of the organism into viable tissue.

The natural history of graft infection is unpredictable. Graft infection may manifest early or remain dormant for several years. The infection may be restricted to the perigraft tissues or actively involve the vessel wall. The patient is at serious risk when the infection begins to invade the natural vessel wall causing anastomotic breakdown, false aneurysm, hemorrhage and

From *The Basic Science of Vascular Disease.* Edited by Sidawy AN, Sumpio BE, and DePalma RG. Armonk, NY: Futura Publishing Company, Inc.; © 1997.

Table 1
Incidence of Vascular Graft Infection in the Literature

Author	Year	Location	Graft Infection Incidence
Humphries[61]	1965	Aorta/Iliac/Fem	2.2
Fry & Lindenauer[62]	1967	Aorta/Iliac	1.3
Szilagyi[4]	1972	Aorta/Fem	1.6
		Fem/Pop	3.0
Goldstone & Moore[31]	1974	Aorta/Fem	1.5
Jamieson[63]	1975	Aorta/Iliac/Fem	2.3
Martin-Paredero[64]	1983	Aorta/Iliac/Fem	2.4
Lorentzen[8]	1985	Aorta/Iliac	0.0
		Aorta/Fem	3.5
		Fem/Pop	3.5
O'Hara[65]	1986	Aorta/Iliac	0.4
		Aorta/Fem	1.3
Szilagyi[66]	1986	Aorta/Iliac/Fem	0.8
Durham[7]	1987	Fem/Pop	2.8
Edwards[67]	1988	Fem/Pop/Tib	2.9

Table 2
Mortality and Morbidity of Aortic Graft Infection

Author	Date	No. Patients	Mortality (%)	Amputation (%)
Fry[62]	1966	12	75	9
Goldstone[31]	1974	27	35	37
Jamieson[63]	1975	15	47	7
Liekweg[68]	1977	84	49	8
Casali[69]	1980	14	64	21
Turnipseed[70]	1983	20	40	15
Martin-Paredero[64]	1983	16	44	31
Fulenwider[71]	1983	21	14	29
Lorentzen[8]	1985	45	29	22
O'Hara[65]	1986	84	28	29
Reilly[18]	1987	101	16	23
Edwards[63]	1988	18	39	0
Yeager[72]	1990	38	26	21
Ricotta[56]	1991	32	25	13

thrombosis, and/or erodes into adjacent organs causing significant hemorrhage, sepsis, and death. Therefore, it is important to identify the different clinical presentations of graft infection, as well as the specific pathogen causing the graft infection itself.

If the graft is colonized by a pathogen of low virulence, such as Staphylococcus epidermis at low levels (10^2, 10^3), the organism may remain dormant for several years prior to the production of a clinically evident graft infection. This explains the occurrence of late graft infection, which can occur up to 7 years after the initial procedure.[2] Even at low concentrations, Staphylococcus epidermis can still stimulate the human immune response and cause activation of macrophages and neutrophils. This local inflammatory response causes production of cytokines and proteases which then damage the perigraft tissues and results in the production of perigraft fluid. This reaction will initially lead to lack of graft incorporation (which may be the only initial findings of graft infection), and eventually

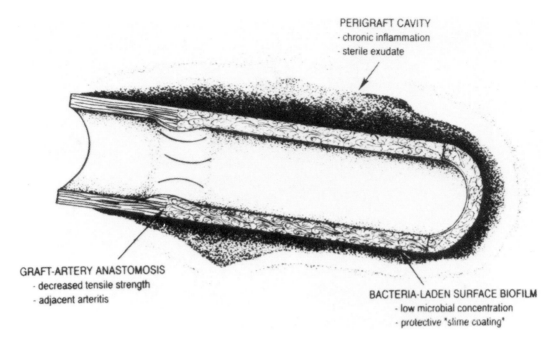

PERIGRAFT CAVITY
- chronic inflammation
- sterile exudate

GRAFT-ARTERY ANASTOMOSIS
- decreased tensile strength
- adjacent arteritis

BACTERIA-LADEN SURFACE BIOFILM
- low microbial concentration
- protective "slime coating"

Figure 1. Schematic of the anatomic and microbiologic characteristics of vascular prosthesis. (Adapted with permission from Reference 23.)

is capable of causing anastomotic destruction and fistulization to the skin or other organs (Figure 1). Infection with more virulent organisms (especially gram negative) will lead to earlier presentation and is more frequently associated signs of systemic sepsis, tissue destruction, and hemorrhage.

Etiologic Factors

Bacterial contamination at the time of graft implantation remains the major cause of infection.[3] This graft contamination may occur because of inadequate sterilization of the graft, contact with the patient's skin, seeding from any disrupted lymphatics draining from an infected source (i.e., ulcer, gangrene), transient bacteremia, or the presence of bacteria within the arterial wall or thrombus. Contamination by organisms from the skin of the patient's perineum is the most common cause of graft infection. Presence of a groin incision is one of the factors most strongly associated with graft infection. Staphylococci are the most common skin organisms and the most frequent isolate from infected grafts.[4] The incidence of S. epidermis positive body surface cultures from patients admitted for arterial revascularization may be as high as 50%.[5] This bacterium may also be cultured at the time of surgery from the thrombus or atheroma in the native vessel in up to 43% of cases.[6] While bacterial colonization within thrombus does not assure graft infection, studies have shown that when preoperative cultures are positive, the risk of de-

veloping graft infection is approximately 10%.[7] Another source of graft infection may be interrupted lymphatics containing bacteria draining from an infected lower extremity lesion. Lorentzen et al[8] demonstrated that 55% of the patients had developed a graft infection, due to an identifiable source of infection preoperatively. While intraoperative cultures from the groin lymphatics are not always positive, groin wounds are the most common sites of graft infection.

A final mechanism of graft infection is seeding from transient bacteremia in the postoperative period. Moore et al[9] have shown this quite elegantly in the dog model. Susceptibility of grafts to infection seems to be related to their degree of tissue incorporation. Although documentation of vascular graft infection by this mechanism remains anecdotal in humans, experience with bacterial endocarditis and endarteritis after bacteremia is a strong argument that this mechanism is operative in some cases.

Microbiology and Immunology

Most common organisms causing graft infection are staphylococci; the most common individual organism is S. aureus, followed closely by S. epidermis. The general use of prophylactic antibiotics has resulted in a relative increase in the incidence of gram negative organisms, which in general are more virulent and invasive and are often not covered by routine antibiotic prophylaxis. There are also several reported cases of

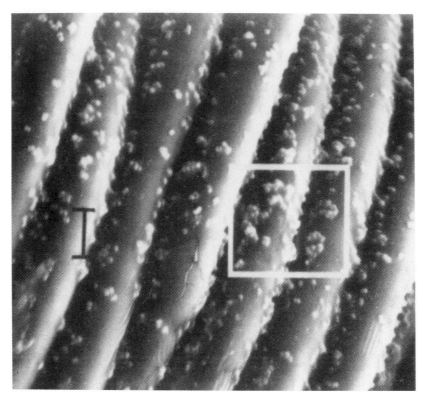

Figure 2. Scanning electron micrograph of knitted Dacron graft colonized in vitro with slime-producing S. epidermidis shows numerous adherent bacterial microcolonies enclosed within a surface biofilm. Area delineated by insert (**A**) is shown at higher magnification in (**B**) (**bar indicates 10 μm**). (Adapted with permission from Reference 16.)

fungi, mycoplasm, and myobacteria.[10–12] As mentioned previously, bacterial adherence is one of the major determinants of graft infection. The type of prosthetic materials influence the degree of bacterial adherence. There are several published data to support the fact that, there is a ten to one-hundredfold decrease in bacterial adherence to polytetrafluoroethylene (PTFE) compared to Dacron.[13] However, long-term follow-up is still needed to determine whether the incidence of late infections can be reduced by the use of PTFE. Currently, there are several animal and human studies looking at the outcome of in situ replacement of infected Dacron grafts, with PTFE in a localized graft infection caused by organisms of low virulence[14,15] In a canine model developed by Bergamini and associates,[16] they studied the efficacy of graft replacement as treatment for vascular prostheses infection from S. epidermis (Figure 2). In this study, while replacement of dacron prostheses infected with S. epidermis with PTFE resulted in early graft healing, bacterial colonization persisted in one third of replacement grafts, which indicates that recurrent clinical infection remains a risk. A second component of bacterial adherence to the graft depends on the inherent abilities of the organism itself. In general, an organism that is invasive will have an enhanced adherence to the graft itself. Therefore, bacteria such as pseudomonas and other gram negative organisms are more likely to adhere to a graft than gram positive bacteria or fungi. Although S. aureus is a gram positive bacteria, it has several unique pathologic factors which make it an invasive pathogen. Three components of this organism's cell wall increase its pathogenicity: peptidoglycan, teichoic acid, and protein A. The peptidoglycan component is capable of inhibiting leukocyte migration, thereby, allowing bacterial proliferation. Teichoic acid activates complement cascade. The cell surface properties of protein A facilitate binding to the Fc component of the IgG molecule, so that it is not available for binding Fc receptor of phagocytes.

Bandyk et al[17] and others[18] have demonstrated that S. epidermis produce an extracellular polysaccharide glycocalyx (mucin, slime) that promotes adherence to the graft as well and protects the bacteria by inhibiting antibiotic penetration.[14] There are also data showing that this mucin may cause T cell suppression,[19] neutrophil suppression,[20] and inhibition of phagocytosis. This organism is characteristically found in smoldering late graft infection. S. epidermis is categorized as a bacteria of low virulence; however, it does

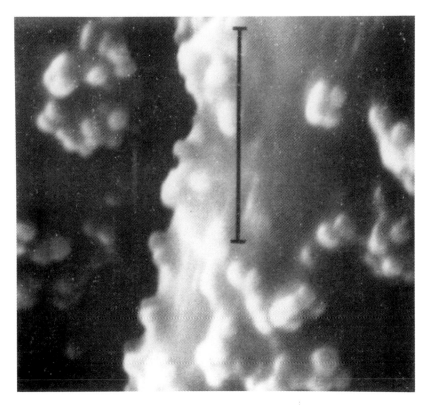

Figure 2B. *(continued)*

activate the human immune system (via macrophage and neutrophils), causing cellular breakdown with inhibition of graft incorporation and formation of perigraft fluid. This fluid may be the only sign in patients presenting with late graft infection caused by S. epidermis. Due to its low virulence, S. epidermis usually does not cause systemic leukocytosis, fever, sepsis, or an increase in erythrocyte sedimentation rate. Routine aspiration, or gram stain swab cultures, may not identify this organism. The best method for identifying S. epidermis may be to culture part of the graft material in glucose supplemented tryptic soy broth solution, then subject the graft's surface to disruption techniques using tissue grinding or oscillation to break down the protective mucin and, thereby, release the organism into the culture medium.[21] In a canine model of aortic graft infection caused by dacron prostheses colonized in vitro with S. epidermis, the recovery rate for the organism 4 weeks after implantation was 30% with agar media, 72% with broth media alone, and 83% with broth media plus biofilm disruption.[21]

The abilities of S. epidermis to adhere, colonize, and produce a bacterial biofilm infection may also be dependent upon the presence of an altered immune status of the patient at the time of graft implantation. Alteration of host defenses are felt to be important determinants of S. epidermis infection in central venous access, arteriovenous shunts, and peritoneal dialysis catheters. Dasgupta et al[22] have shown a higher incidence of peritonitis, due to S. epidermis in patients on peritoneal dialysis with a low peritoneal fluid immunoglobin G concentration. Treating these patients with increasing doses of highly purified immunoglobulin G into the peritoneal dialysis solution has been shown to give a threefold increase in the opsonic capacity of the peritoneal fluid for S. epidermidis and to significantly decrease the peritonitis rate. Patients with high incidence of peritonitis have been also shown to have a decreased production of gamma interferon by peritoneal lymphocytes and decreased secretion of interleukin-1 by the macrophages. The overall outcome of this immunocompromize results is a decrease in the cellular response against S. epidermidis. Similarly, in patients undergoing major vascular reconstruction, emergency procedures and ruptured aneurysm have also been shown to have a depression of both humoral and cellular immune defense system secondary to factors such as surgery, anesthesia, blood transfusion, and stress, which can predispose them to S. epidermis infection at the time of presentation. In a recent study, Bandyk et al[23] demonstrated that almost in one third of patients who presented with delayed S. epidermidis infection had severe systemic infection or ruptured aneurysm at the initial graft implantation.

Bergamini et al[24] have also demonstrated the effect of systemic immunosupression in a rat model on the effectiveness of the animal defending itself against graft infection with S. epidermidis. It has been previously documented that immunosupression of the mouse with the use of steroids, cyclophosphamide, cyclosporine, and malnutrition interferes with the host defense mechanism against bacterial challenge by interfering with the host macrophage, T-cell, and B-cell activity. In this study, Bergamini and associates were able to demonstrate that immunosupression of the host at the time of graft colonization with S. epidermidis does predispose to bacterial growth and the formation of graft infection, as long as the immune supression is severe enough to decrease Ia (immune associated antigen) expression from both lymphocytes and monocytes for at least 24 hours. Ia is a class II major histocompatibility complex antigen in mice that binds and presents foreign antigen to T-helper lymphocytes to initiate the immune response.

Besides systemic immunosupression due to the factors described previously seen in patients undergoing major vascular surgery that predisposes them to S. epidermidis infection, the organism itself can cause local immunosupression. As described previously, the production of the "slime" by the organism can further decrease opsonic capacity, phagocytosis, bacterial killing by neutrophils, and T-cell function.

Unlike S. epidermidis, more virulent strains of bacteria, such as pseudomonas and other gram negative organisms, more readily penetrate the perigraft tissue. They accomplish this by releasing proteases and lysins which cause the breakdown of elastin, and collagen, as well as cell necrosis. This process can weaken the native vessel wall causing pseudoaneurysm or anastomotic breakdown with significant hemorrhage. The combination of aneurysmal dilatation, bacteria, and thrombus deposition may result in development of septic embolization. In contrast to infection with S. epidermidis, patients with infection due to organisms of high virulence more often present with pseudoaneurysm or hemorrhage, and systemic signs of sepsis such as leukocytosis, elevated erythrocyte sedimentation rate and fever, or septic emboli.

Classification

Classification of early graft infection has been described by Szilagyi et al[4] based on the depth of the wound. When only the dermis was affected, the infection was classified as Grade I; when the infection extended into the subcutaneous region but did not invade the graft it was classified as Grade II; and when the infection invaded the graft, it was classified as Grade III. Bunt et al[25] have classified aortic graft infections, differentiating between graft enteric erosion, a graft enteric fistula, or an aortic stump sepsis. These classifica-

tions are both primarily concerned with intra-abdominal procedures. Samson et al[26] have expanded on Szilagyi's classification in evaluating graft infections in the extremities as follows:

I) Cellulitis
II) Subcutaneous infection not involving the graft.
III) Infection involving the body of the graft only.
IV) Infection involving the whole graft including the anastomosis, but no evidence of bleeding.
V) Infection causing an anastomotic bleeding, thrombosis, or systemic sepsis.

Clinical Presentation

The clinical manifestations of a particular graft infection is dependent on the anatomic location of the graft, the type of graft used, and the nature of the infecting organism itself. Thus, it is very important to have a detailed history of the patient, including all previous operative reports, pre- and postoperative complications (such as bacteremia, UTI, pneumonia, sepsis), as well as recent dental, gastrointestinal, and GU procedures. There are several clinical situations which increase the risk of graft infection, including: emergency surgery, diabetes, uremia,[27] unrelated infection at the time of initial surgery,[8] obesity, presentation with hematoma, multiple groin punctures,[28] lymphocele, and perioperative bacteremia or septicemia.[29] Trauma patients presenting with penetrating visceral injuries or patients who present with ischemic bowel following aortic bypass may also be at high risk for developing graft infection.

Infected aortic grafts may present with sepsis, abdominal distention, fever of unknown origin, development of pulsatile mass, a tender fluctuating groin mass, or a draining groin sinus. One of the most dramatic complications of aortic graft infection is severe gastrointestinal hemorrhage secondary to aortoenteric fistula. This process must be suspected in any patient who presents with unexplained gastrointestinal hemorrhage with a history of previous aortic bypass. Gastrointestinal bleeding associated with aortic graft infection may be present without frank aortoenteric fistula formation. Goldstone et al[30] identified two mechanisms of gastrointestinal bleeding in aortic graft infection: direct fistula formation with bleeding, and bleeding from mucosal irritation without a direct fistula. In the latter instance, the bleeding may even be subclinical, while in the former, it is often catastrophic.

Patients may present with false aneurysm at an anastomotic site as the initial symptom of graft infection with or without any signs of sepsis. Some authors[31] believe that the presence of false aneurysm should always suggest the possibility of a graft infection. Draining sinus at the level of the groin may be another indication of late graft infection. As discussed previously, patients who are infected with any of the highly virulent organisms such as pseudomonas, S. auerus, E. coli, and other gram negative bacteria, usually present early with overt signs of sepsis. These may include fever, leukocytosis, increased sedimentation rate, graft thrombosis, pseudoaneurysm, anastomotic breakdown, hemorrhage, and septic embolization downstream of the infected prosthesis.

Patients whose presentation is more remote and associated with anastomotic breakdowns, thrombosis of a graft limb, or chronic draining sinus with minimal signs of sepsis are often infected with organisms of low virulence such as S. epidermis. As described before, diagnoses of this organism requires cultures of the graft wall with disruption of the mucin in order to release the organism into the culture.

Clinical presentation of a femoropopliteal bypass graft infection is usually recognized more readily than an intra-abdominal infection because of its more superficial location. These are characterized by cellulitis, sinus tract, abscess, fluctuant mass, expanding pulsatile mass, thrombosis, bacteremia, and/or sepsis.

Diagnostic Evaluation

Careful evaluation of clinical presentation and laboratory data are important in the diagnosis of graft sepsis, but may often be nonspecific. Proper management requires knowledge of accurate anatomic details of the extent of graft involvement. One or more anatomic imaging such as duplex ultrasonography, computed tomography (CT) scan, magnetic resonance imaging (MRI), or by angiography, as well as radionucleotide scans are usually necessary to identify the location and the extent of the graft infection.

Duplex ultrasonography is the one most commonly used modality to evaluate peripheral sites of graft infection. Ultrasonography can readily determine whether there is perigraft fluid, hematoma, abscess, or pseudoaneurysm at or distal to the groin level. Duplex evaluation produces good flow imaging, as well as delineating the intraluminal disease process. The availability, low cost, and portability of ultrasound imaging has made this modality a mainstay of early diagnosis in accessible sites. However, this technique is not as widely applicable in intra-abdominal or intrathoracic sites.

CT can be helpful in making the diagnosis of graft infection, particularly when all or part of the graft is intra-abdominal. CT is the preferred modality for identifying intra-abdominal graft abnormalities such as lack of graft incorporation, perigraft fluid or air, intestinal thickening, and inflammatory changes. CT scan can

also show the extent of the graft infection (Figure 3 and 4). In the early postoperative period, perigraft air for up to 6 weeks, perigraft air,[32] and perigraft fluid may be present up to 12 weeks.[1] At later time intervals, however, the presence of either perigraft air or fluid is highly suspicious for graft infection and should be correlated with clinical presentation. Ultrasonography and CT scan can both be useful in directing percutaneous needle aspiration of perigraft fluid in selected situations for identifying the infecting organism. This technique can be helpful in selected cases, but may not be definitive since failure to recover an organism does not rule out graft infection. This is particularly true in patients on antibiotics, or those with chronic or subacute infections. As a result of the potential dangers of hemorrhage or contamination, we use perigraft aspiration only in cases where the diagnosis is in doubt.

MRI has a potential advantage as a modality for identifying graft infection, due to its better resolution of the soft tissue and fat involvement. Hansen et al[33] have shown enhanced accuracy in identifying graft infection and the extent of involvement using STIR [axial spin echo (ST) and short (TI) inversion recovery] MRI in 9 patients compared to contrast CT. MRI may also be used to provide angiographic detail (MRA) which would avoid the need to give intravenous contrast to patients that may already have compromised renal function.

Nuclear medicine techniques are often employed to identify graft infection. There have been several studies comparing the gallium scan to CT scan for defining graft infection at different locations.[34,35] These studies rely on the ability of the imaging radionuclide (e.g., Gallium) to localize in areas of inflammation. Johnson et al[36] have shown that gallium scans have a sensitivity of 78% compared to CT scans (100%), although the specificity of this technique is better than that of CT (94% versus 74%). In general, gallium scans have a high positive predictive value. However, the lack of sensitivity of these studies continues to remain a major drawback. Other practical objections to this technique include the length of time to get the results (>24 hours), as well as the difficulty of interpreting results in the early postoperative period. A variety of unrelated inflammatory processes and nonspecific bowel uptake can produce both false positive and false negative results.

The indium 111-labeled white blood cell scan also has value in identifying perigraft inflammation. The sensitivity of this method has been reported higher than that of gallium imaging.[37] However, like the gallium scan it may be difficult to interpret in the immediate postoperative period, due to the inflammatory changes associated with surgery and the increased uptake by the healing cells resulting in false positive results.

There are also several studies describing the use of

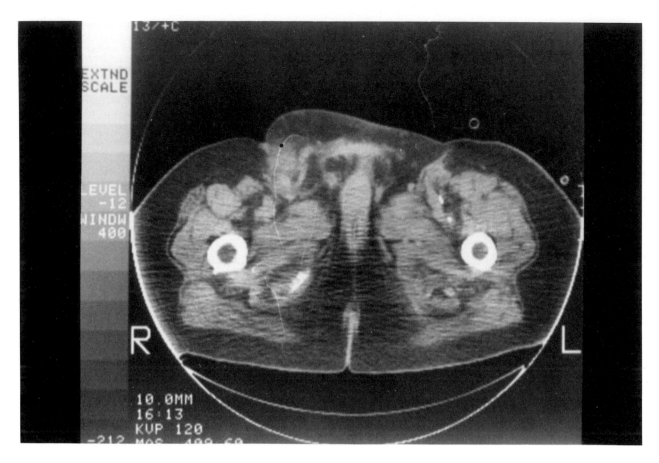

Figure 3 and 4. CT scan shows a right groin abscess extending to the femoral-femoral bypass graft (**1**). The infection appears to involve the proximal portion of the graft, which is still patent (**2**).

[123]I-labeled antigranulocyte antibody scintiography.[38] Again, like other labeling techniques, this test takes >24 hours. Although, it has a sensitivity of 94% and specificity of 75%, it is limited in the early postoperative period due to increased uptake by the granulocytes that accumulate in hematomas.

Arteriography is often used in evaluating a suspected graft infection. Arteriography can demonstrate anastomotic disruption, location of a pseudoaneurysm, and thrombosis of a graft. More importantly, arteriography produces information relevant to the status of the proximal and distal runoff vessels. This information is essential to allow the surgeon to determine the technique of revascularization and to decide whether partial excision of the graft is possible. For the latter reason, we believe every patient should have arteriography whenever feasible.

Endoscopy is utilized when aortoenteric erosion is of concern. When a patient presents with massive gastrointestinal hemorrhage with a previous history of aortic bypass, endoscopy should be done if possible. In cases of significant active hemorrhage, endoscopy may be performed in the operating room. Visualization of the graft or significant bleeding, or ulceration at the fourth portion of the duodenum is diagnostic of an aortoenteric fistula. Endoscopy is helpful in excluding other sources of hemorrhage, such as ulcer and gastritis. Negative endoscopy does not rule out an aortoenteric fistula. Indeed, upper gastrointestinal hemorrhage in the absence of an identifiable endoscopic source in the esophagus, stomach, or proximal duodenum is highly suggestive of aortoenteric fistula.

Prevention

Morbidity and mortality of graft infection has decreased over the last few years due to the use of prophylactic antibiotics, improved perioperative management, and increased sensitivity of diagnostic techniques. However, the most important mechanism to further decrease the incidence of graft infection is prevention. Preventive measures can be effective before, during, and after surgery. All patients, particularly those at high risk for infection, should have their underlying medical problems stabilized prior to sur-

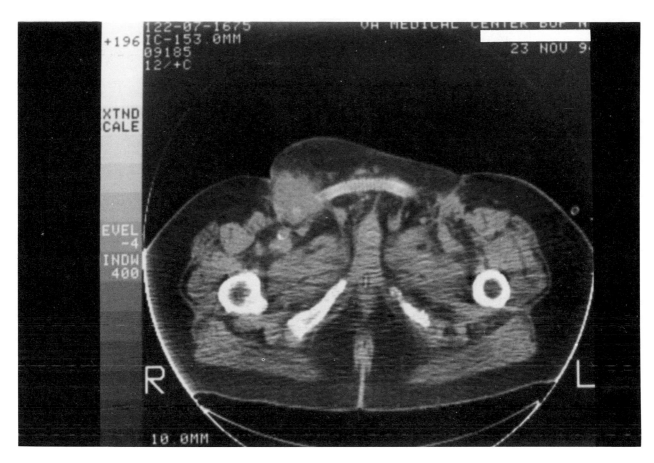

Figure 4. *(continued)*

gery. The most common location for a graft infection is the groin. Therefore, it is best to avoid this area if all possible. Several studies have shown that intra-abdominal aortic procedures have significantly less incidence of graft infection than aortobifemoral by-pass.[39,8] Preoperative bathing with chlorhexidine and intraoperative betadine cleansing have been shown to reduce the rate of infection.[40] Shaving should also be avoided as this increases the chance wound infection;[41] use of clippers is preferred, and should be done as close to the procedure time as possible. With the increase use of invasive radiology for arteriograms, angioplasty, and stenting for short segment stenosis, there is an increased incidence of bacterial contamination and hematoma formation at the groin level. Landreneau et al[28] have demonstrated that there is an increased incidence of groin infection if the surgery is done less than 24 hours after an angioplasty. Therefore, they recommended, that if all possible, surgical procedures should be performed 1 week or more after angioplasty. In the face of large hematoma, elective surgery should be delayed.

The majority of graft contamination occurs at the time of surgery. This is a multifactoral problem that may involve the operating room environment, inadequate graft sterilization, a breakdown in sterile technique, and/or contamination by the patient's skin or intra-abdominal organs. Therefore, adequate patient preparation and draping is necessary. It is also advisable to avoid excessive dissection, disruption of the tissue planes, creation of hematomas, or interruption of the lymphatics. Careful attention to the coverage of vascular grafts after insertion is mandatory. Meticulous closure of the retro-peritoneum and groin wounds is important in preventing late infectious complications.

A cornerstone of preoperative prevention is the use of prophylactic antibiotics. Randomized trials have clearly shown that in every vascular procedure utilizing prophylactic antibiotic treatment, the incidence of graft infection is greatly reduced. Kaiser et al[42] in a prospective randomized study of 462 patients undergoing elective vascular procedure, has demonstrated a wound infection rate of 6.8% in a placebo group compared to 0.9% in patients who received a preoperative cefazolin. Animal studies looking at antibiotic prophylaxis of late bacteremic vascular graft infection have demonstrated that a single dose of ceftriaxone given before a bacteremic challenge (5×10^8 S. aureus) is sufficient to prevent late vascular graft infection.

There is no clear consensus on the choice of antibiotic or its duration of use. However, it is logical to employ antibiotics that will cover the most common causes of graft infection, namely Staphylococcus (aureus and epidermidis) and gram negative organisms. Cephalosporins are the most commonly used antibiotics in elective surgery, even though their sensitivity against S. epidermidis is questionable. If a patient is in a high risk group, vancomycin offers excellent coverage for gram positive organism (including S. epidermidis). If the patient has a hematoma, or is a candidate for reoperative procedure or emergency surgery, gentamicin offers excellent gram negative coverage and should be added to gram positive coverage.

All antibiotics should be given immediately prior to skin incision, and a second dose may be needed if there is excessive blood loss or extended operative time. Pitt et al[43] and others have shown that irrigation with an antibiotic solution of the wound decreases wound infection over saline alone.[44] This is not practiced by all surgeons; however, there seems to be little to lose and much to gain by adopting this practice.

There is no clear consensus on the appropriate length of time that antibiotic therapy should be used postoperatively. However, several studies suggest a range of antibiotic coverage from 24 hours to 3 to 5 days, or even longer.[43,45] Some investigators feel that as long as there are indwelling catheters (foley, central venous pressure, Swan Ganz catheter) present, patients are at risk for experiencing transient bacteremia and should have antibiotic coverage. It is also recommended that patients with remote infections and those with positive arterial wall cultures should be treated with intravenous antibiotics for 10 to 14 days, followed by oral antibiotics for up to 2 months.[46]

Prosthetic vascular grafts should be treated in the same way as cardiac prosthetic valves by patients, dentists, and other medical professionals with regard to prophylactic antibiotic therapy prior to dental extraction, gastrointestinal, or genitourological procedures. While the incidence of graft infection by hematogenous spread is low, it is still present with these procedures.[7]

Bonding antibiotics to vascular grafts has been shown to reduce incidence of infection in animal studies. Ney et al[47] have demonstrated that a suspension of fibrin glue and antibiotic coated on to a PTFE graft resisted infection in a dog model when the animal was exposed to systemic E. coli and S. aureus. When the animals were sacrificed at day 7, there was no evidence of anastomotic breakdown in the treated group. Auramovic et al[48] using a sheep model have demonstrated that rifampicin treatment of protein-sealed Dacron graft combined with intravenous cefoxitin provided more protection from contamination by S. aureus than intravenous cefoxitin alone. Continued improvements in graft protection, patient prophylaxis, and adequate postoperative antibiotic coverage, as well as the use of better antibiotic bonded graft material, may further decrease the incidence of graft infection.

Management

Management of graft infection is a complex problem that must be individualized. There are certain surgical principles that also must be maintained. These include eradication of all infectious processes and maintenance of adequate distal circulation. Whether one should remove, replace, or retain the infected vascular graft depends on the location of the infection, the extent of the graft involvement, and the virulence of the organism. Major management decisions focus on timing of surgery (emergent versus elective), the extent of resection, and the need for revascularization. These decisions will depend on the patient's clinical presentation and location of the graft.

Emergency Procedure

Life-threatening hemorrhage from aortoenteric fistula, rupture of a false aneurysm, and acute limb ischemia from an infected thrombus are the primary complications of aortic vascular graft infection that require emergency intervention. Anastomotic breakdown and rupture of a pseudoaneurysm are urgent complications of both the aorta and peripheral arterial graft infectious process. During surgery, one must initially address the acute problem of controlling the hemorrhage. This can be achieved by direct pressure, balloon, or clamp control of the aorta proximal to the dehisced graft and distally at the level of the iliac and/or femoral vessels. When the hemorrhage is under control, then three therapeutic options should be considered. The initial and the most frequent option is excision of the infected graft with debridement and closure of the area. This is usually followed by immediate extra anatomic bypass. The second option is excision of the infected graft and in situ insertion of an autogenous or a prosthetic material for revascularization. The third option is to remove the portion of the aortic graft that appears to be infected (partial excision) with wide debridement of the retroperitoneum combined with in situ, or an extra-anatomical graft placement for revascularization and lifelong antibiotic coverage.

In managing acute limb ischemia from an infected thrombus, the initial procedure is the thrombectomy of the distal vessel and reconstitution of distal blood flow. The above therapeutic options can then be applied in order to treat the underlying infective cause.

Aortic Graft Infection

Most aortic graft infection can be treated as an urgent rather than emergent problem, thus, allowing adequate time for evaluation and patient preparation. An aortoiliac graft infection is one of the most complex problems to deal with in vascular surgery. Despite adherence to the principles of surgical management dealing with graft infection (eradicate all infective processes and revascularization of limbs), the morbidity and the mortality rates still remain significant. The basic principles include total excision of all infected or thrombosed prosthetic graft with wide debridement of periaortic tissue and the native vessels until a healthy tissue bed is achieved. In early series, revascularization followed graft removal and resulted in a high mortality rate of 50% to 75% with an amputation rate of up to 40%. These rates have decreased significantly over the years (25% mortality and 7% morbidity) by performing a staged procedure beginning with extra-anatomical bypass,[18] followed by total excision of the infected graft, wide debridement of periaortic tissues and the native vessels, oversewing the aortic and the iliac stumps in two layers and, if necessary, protecting these vessels with muscle, omentum, or even a serosal patch.

The early reports of high mortality with total excision and extra anatomic bypass prompted several authors toward more conservative surgery by limiting the extent of graft excision. This has been employed most often when infection is limited to one groin and the graft is patent.[40,50] The successful treatment with the use of intravenous antibiotic and local irrigation with antibiotics solution has been reported in 7 of 10 patients with aortic graft infection by Morris et al[51] These authors have managed to achieve a survival rate of 67% in 3 years with no amputation, in a very selective series limited to early graft infection without any anastomotic breakdown or fistula formation. Nielson et al[52] have used gentamicin beads in the treatment of localized infection with essentially a marginal outcome (3 out of 10 patients). The rationale being that if the treatment fails in this localized segment, one could still do the surgical resection and the appropriate revascularization.

In situ aortic replacement has also been undertaken using both autogenous and prosthetic materials. Ehrenfeld et al[53] have reported a mortality of only 13% in 24 patients using autogenous graft, such as greater saphanous vein or internal iliac artery into the debrided retroperitoneum. Walker et al[54] and Bandyk et al[23] have described successful excision of infected grafts, debridement, and in situ replacement with PTFE grafts in patients with late aortic graft infection. These patients presented without signs of sepsis and usually had bland draining sinuses or perigraft collection with a lack of graft incorporation and negative bacterial cultures or S. epidermis as the only organism isolated. This procedure can only be done in a select group of patients and still carries a mortality rate estimated at around 17% by Walker's group.[54] Treatment of the canine aortic graft infection by graft excision and in situ graft replacement commonly resulted in early graft healing; however, persistent colonization of 22% of the replacement grafts with S. epidermidis signified that recurrent infection remained at risk.[16] Similarly, the follow-up of the study by Bandyk and associates showed that out of 17 initially resected infected graft segments, perigraft fluid adjacent to the replacement graft in two patients and persistent perigraft fluid surrounding the unresected aortofemoral graft limb, proximal to the replacement graft in three patients indicating persistent colonization of S. epidermidis in 29% of the patients in this study,[55] again signified that future infectious complications remained a risk in humans.

In managing aortic graft infection, we recommend that any patient with bleeding needs urgent surgery, with control of the hemorrhage and excision of the infected graft with wide debridement of the surrounding tissue. All wounds are then closed prior to extra-anatomic revascularization. Hemodynamically stable patients who present with sepsis, aortoenteric fistula, infection involving proximal anastomosis, an anastomotic breakdown, or with septic embolization should have initial medical/surgical stabilization that includes appropriate antibiotic coverage. Patients should have an extra-anatomic bypass tunneled through an uninfected tissue plane and then the following:

1. Total excision of the infected graft.
2. Periaortic tissue debridement with an appropriate graft culture using a gram stain.
3. Debridement of the aorta and iliac vessels until a healthy vessel is visualized.
4. Oversewing the vessels with double row closure techniques.
5. Omental pedicle around the aortic stump if necessary to avoid a delayed rupture.
6. Copious irrigation of the wound with warm saline.

We prefer to perform the reconstruction first, and remove the graft at a second operation when possible. This limits lower extremity ischemia and reduces the cardiovascular changes associated with aortic ligation. These surgical procedures can be accomplished in most patients, since aortic graft infections will present urgently, but rarely emergently. With this approach, we have been able to achieve a mortality rate of 17% and amputation rate of 13% in 18 patients.[56]

In selective situations, such as when a patient presents with periaortic fluid accumulation with negative cultures or S. epidermis contamination, they can be treated by removal of the infected graft followed by a local debridement with an in situ placement of an antibiotic bound-PTFE graft. While we have no experience with this approach, several authors have demonstrated results equivalent to total excision and bypass in carefully selected cases.[54,23]

Other alternatives have been considered in patients who present with distal limb local graft contamination or a localized graft infection in a patent well-incorporated graft without any anastomotic breakdown. These patients can be treated by wide local debridement with infusion of an intravenous antibiotic, followed by the coverage of the exposed graft with a muscle flap or a skin graft after adequate granulation is achieved. Proximal graft infection must be excluded before this approach is undertaken.

In local graft infection involving a thrombosed limb, poor incorporation or evidence of anastomotic breakdown, the patient should at least have a resection of that limb, and wide debridement and limb revascularization by an extra-anatomical approach (lateral, obturator, cross femoral). Any time one contemplates resection of an infected graft at the groin involving iliac and/or femoral vessels, attention to the pelvic circulation is required since adequate blood flow to the pelvis is needed in order to avoid further ischemic complications.

Femoropopliteal Graft Infection

Most infrainguinal graft infections present with cellulitis, abscess formation, or drainage of purulent material from a sinus or thrombosis of the graft itself. Due to the location of these bypass grafts, they are more readily found by the patients and more easily diagnosed by the physician. Ultrasonography has been used extensively in order to identify para-anastomotic involvement of the infection, formation of a pseudoaneurysm, or to determine the extent of the graft incorporation. Treatment of infrainguinal graft infection will depend on the extent of soft tissue and graft involvement, as well as on the type of graft conduit implicated.

Superficial wound infection and soft tissue infection require immediate soft tissue debridement, intravenous antibiotics, and aggressive local wound care. Infections extending to the graft, but not invading the graft or the artery-graft anastomosis can be successfully treated with wide debridement of all infected tissue, local wound care, and protecting the graft with a local muscle flap or skin grafting. Calligaro et al[57] have demonstrated in patients who present with patent infected infrainguinal grafts and who also have an intact anastomosis with a complete lack of systemic sepsis, that it is possible to excise all necrotic, infected tissue, and that they were able to achieve complete graft preservation in approximately two thirds of this population.

However, in patients where infections have invaded the vascular graft causing an anastomotic breakdown and thrombosis, complete graft excision and autologous bypass grafting to maintain adequate blood flow to maintain limb viability procedures are required. If the graft is replaced in situ, these patients should have a coverage of their graft with a muscle flap or with skin grafting. An increase of tissue oxygenation, improved phagocytic activity, and simultaneously a decrease of bacterial counts after muscle flap coverage has been reported[58] as well as the excellent delivery of antibiotics into a fibrotic cavity filled with muscle.[59] If a muscle flap or skin grafting is not possible, a porcine xenograft (pigskin) has been reported to be quite useful.[60] While the pigskin undergoes some dissolution, it can be changed every 2 to 3 days until the patient has recovered or is stable enough to undergo more extensive procedures.

Infections involving the autogenous vein may lead to dissolution of the graft. When the autogenous vein graft is exposed to purulent material, the safest procedure is debridement of the wound, placement of the irrigation catheter, and closure of the skin over the graft. Again, pigskin can be used if the defect is too large for primary closure. The patient should be maintained under close observation due to the high risk of a graft rupture.

All patients with infrainguinal graft infection should have a noninvasive evaluation, in order to determine the appropriate management should the patient require a total excision of the graft. An extra-anatomical lateral approach tunneled in the uninfected area is the preferred mode of revascularization. While the mortality rate is only around 20%, the infected infrainguinal bypass carries a high amputation rate. This amputation rate appears to be related to an inability to successfully revascularize the ischemic limb. Therefore, every attempt should be made for early diagnosis with aggressive debridement of the soft tissue and total protection of the graft. The lower extremities must be well studied to insure that the appropriate bypass at the appropriate level will be performed.

References

1. Freischlag JA, Moore WS: Infection on prosthetic vascular grafts. In: Rutherford RB, Johnson G, Kempczinski RF (eds). *Vascular Surgery*, 3rd Ed. Philadelphia: WB Saunders Co.; 510–522, 1989.
2. Bunt TJ: Synthetic vascular graft infections. I. Graft infections. *Surgery* 93:733–746, 1983.
3. Goldstone J, Effeney DJ: Prevention of arterial graft injections. In: Bernhard VM, Towne JB (eds). *Complication in Vascular Surgery*. New York: Grune and Stratton Inc., 487–494, 1980.
4. Szilagyi DE, Smith RF, Elliott JP, Vrandedic NP: Infection in arterial reconstruction with synthetic grafts. *Ann Surg* 176:321–333, 1972.

5. Levy MF, Schmitt DD, Edniston CE, et al: Sequential analysis of staphylococcal colonization of body surface cultures on patients undergoing vascular surgery. *J Clin Microbiol* 28:664–669, 1990.
6. Macbeth GA, Rubin JR, McIntyre KE Jr, Goldstone J, Malone JM: The relevance of arterial wall microbiology to the treatment of prosthetic graft infections: graft vs arterial infections. *J Vasc Surg* 1:750–756, 1984.
7. Durham JR, Malone JM, Bernhard VM: The impact of multiple operation on the importance of arterial wall cultures. *J Vasc Surg* 5:160–169, 1987.
8. Lorentzen JE, Neilsen M, Arendrup et al: Vascular graft infection: an analysis of sixty two graft infection in 2411 consecutive implanted synthetic vascular grafts. *Surgery* 98:81–86, 1985.
9. Moore WS, Malone JM, Keovun K: Prosthetic arterial grafts material: influence on neointimal healing and bacteremic infectability. *Arch Surgery* 115:1379–1383, 1990.
10. Doscher W, Krishnasasty KV, Deckoff S: Fungal infection: case report and a review of the literature. *J Vasc Surg* 6:398–402, 1987.
11. Dale BAS, McCormick JSH: Mycoplasma hominis wound infection following a aortobifemoral bypass. *Eur J Vasc Surg* 5:213–214, 1981.
12. Goldstone J: The infected infra-renal aortic graft. *Acta Chir Scand* 538:72–86, 1987.
13. Schmitt DD, Bandyk DF, Pequet AS, et al: Bacterial adherence to vascular prostheses: a determinant of graft infection. *J Vasc Surg* 6:476–481, 1987.
14. Jacobs M, Reul G, Gregoric I, Cooley D: In-situ replacement and extra-anatomic bypass for the treatment of infected prosthetic grafts. *Eur J Vasc Surg* 5:83–86, 1991.
15. Walker WE, Cooley DA, Duncan JM, Hallman GL, Ott DA, Reul GJ: The management of aorta duodenal fistula by in-situ replacement of the infected abdominal aortic graft. *Ann Surg* 205:727–732, 1987.
16. Bergamini TM, Bandyk DF, Govostis D, Kaebnick HW, Towne JB: Infection of vascular prostheses caused by bacterial biofilms. *J Vasc Surg* 7:21–30, 1988.
17. Bandyk DF, Berni GA, Thiele BL, et al: Aortofemoral graft infection due to staphylococcus epidermis. *Arch Surg* 119:102–108, 1984.
18. Reilly LM, Stoney RJ, Goldstone J, et al: Improved management of aortic graft infections: the influence of operation sequence and staging. *J Vasc Surg* 421–426, 1987.
19. Greg ED, Peters G, Verlsgen M: Effect of extracellular slime substance on the human cellular immune response. *Lancet* 1:365–367, 1984.
20. Johnson GM, Lee GA, Regelman WE: Interference with granulocyte function by staphylococcus epidermis slime. *Infect Immun* 54:13–20, 1986.
21. Bergamini TM, Bandyk DF, Govostis D, Vetsch A, Towne J: Identification of staphylococcus epidermis vascular graft infections: a comparison of culture techniques. *J Vasc* 2:92–98, 1985.
22. Desgupta MK, Costerton JW: Significance of biofilm-adherent bacterial microcolonies on tenckhoff catheters of CAPD patients. *Curr Concepts of CAPD Blood Purif* 7:144–155, 1989.
23. Bandyk DF, Bergamini TM, Kinney et al: In situ replacement of vascular prostheses infected by bacterial biofilm. *J Vasc Surg* 13:575–583, 1991.
24. Bergamini TM, Corpus RA, Hoeg KL, Brittian KR, Peyton JC, Cheadle WG: Immune regulation of bacterial biofilm graft infection. *ASAIO J* 39:219–226, 1994.
25. Bunt TJ: Synthetic vascular graft infections II. *Surgery* 93:733–746, 1983.
26. Samson RH, Veith FJ, Janko GS, Gupta SK, Scher LA: A modified classification and approach to the management of infections involving peripheral arterial prosthetic grafts. *J Vasc Surg* 8:147, 1988.
27. O'Brien T, Collin J: Prosthetic vascular graft infection [review]. *Br J Surg* 79:1262–1267, 1982.
28. Landreneau MD, Ragu S: Infections after elective bypass surgery for lower limb ischemia: the influence of pre-operative transcutaneous arteriography. *Surgery* 90:956–961, 1981.
29. White JV, Freda BA, Kozan R: Does bacteremia pose a direct threat to synthetic vascular grafts? *Surgery* 102:402–408, 1987.
30. Golstone J: Infected prosthetic arterial grafts. In: Haimovici H, Callow AD, DePalma RG, Ernst CB, Hollier LH (eds). Vascular Surgery Principals and Techniques. New York: McGraw-Hill; 564–574, 1984.
31. Goldstone J, Moore WS: Infection in vascular prostheses: clinical manifestation and surgical management. *Am J Surg* 128:225–233, 1974.
32. O'Hara PJ, Barkowski GP, Hertzer NR, et al: Natural history of perigraft air on computerized axial tomographic examination of the abdomen following AAA repair. *J Vasc Surg* 1:429–433, 1984.
33. Hansen ME, Yucel EK, Waltman AC: STIR imaging of synthetic vascular graft infection. *Cardiovasc Intervent Radiol* 16:30–36, 1993.
34. Banzo I, Quince R, Serrano J, et al: GA-67 Citrate scan in vascular graft infection. *Ann Nucl Med* 6:235–239, 1992.
35. LaMuraglia GM: Chronic prosthetic vascular graft infection visualization with gallium-67 (editorial: comment). *J Nucl Med* 32:1427–1428, 1991.
36. Johnson KK, Russ PD, Bair JH, Friefeld GD: Diagnosis of synthetic vascular graft infection: comparison of CT and gallium scan. *Amer J Roentgenology* 154:405, 1990.
37. Chung CJ, Hicklin OA, Pagan JM, Gordon L: Indium III-labeled leukocyte scan in detection of synthetic vascular graft infection: the effect of antibiotic treatment. *J Nucl Med* 32:13–15, 1991.
38. Cordes M, Hepp W, Longer R, Pannhorst J, Hierholzer J, Felix R: Vascular graft infection: detection by 123I-labeled antigranulocyte antibody (Anti-NCA95) scintigraphy. *Nucl Med* 30:173–177, 1991.
39. Szilagyi DE, Elliott JP, Smith RF, Hageman JH, Sood RK: Secondary arterial repair: the management of late failures in reconstructive arterial surgery. *Arch Surg* 110:485–493, 1975.
40. Berry AR, Watt B, Goldacre MJ, Thompson JWW, McNair TJ: A comparison of the use of povidone iodine and chlorohexidine in the prophylaxis of postoperative wound infection. *J Hosp Infection* 3:55–63, 1982.
41. Cruse PJ, Foord R: A ten-year prospective study of 62939 wounds: the epidemiology of wound infection. *Surg Clin North Am* 60:27–40, 1980.
42. Kaiser AB, Clayson KR, Mulherin JL, et al: Antibiotic prophylaxis in vascular surgery. *Ann Surg* 188:283–289, 1978.
43. Pitt H, Postier RG, MacGowan WA, et al: Prophylactic antibiotics in vascular surgery—topical, systemic, or both? *Ann Surg* 192:356–364, 1980.
44. Lord JW, Rossi G, Daliance M: Intraoperative antibiotic wound lavage: an attempt to eliminate postoperative infection in arterial and clean general surgical procedures. *Ann Surg* 185:634–38, 1977.
45. May ARL, Darling RC, Brewster DC, and Darling CS:

A comparison of the use of cephalotin and oxacillin in vascular surgery. *Arch Surg* 115:56, 1980.

46. Bandyk DF, Esses GE: Prosthetic graft infection. *Surg Clin North Am* 74(3):571–590, 1994.

47. Ney Al, Kelley PH, Tsukayama DT, Bubrick MP: Fibrin glue-antibiotic suspension in the prevention of prosthetic graft infection. *J Trauma* 30(8):1000–1006, 1990.

48. Auramovic J, Fletcher JP: Prevention of prosthetic vascular graft infection by rifampicin impregnation of a protein-sealed Dacron graft in combination with parental cephalosporin. *J Cardiovasc Surg* 33:70–74, 1992.

49. Kwaan JHM, Connoly JE: Successful management of prosthetic graft infection with continuous povidone-iodine irrigation. *Arch Surg* 116:716–719, 1981.

50. Popovsky J, Singer S: Infected prosthetic grafts: local therapy with graft preservation. *Arch Surg* 115:203–205, 1980.

51. Morris GE, Friend PJ, Vassalo DJ, et al: Antibiotic irrigation and conservative surgery for major aortic graft infection. *J Vasc Surg* 20:88–95, 1994.

52. Nielson DM, Noer HH, Jorgensen LG, Lorentzen JE: Gentamicin beads in the treatment of localized vascular graft infection: long-term results in 17 cases. *Eur J Vasc Surg* 5:283–557, 1991.

53. Ehrenfeld WK, Wilbur BG, Olcot CNIV, Stoney RJ: Autogenous tissue reconstruction in the management of infected prosthetic grafts. *Surgery* 85:82–92, 1979.

54. Walker WE, Cooley DA, Duncan JM, Hallmer GL, Ott DA, Reul GJ: The management of aorta duodenal fistula in situ replacement of the infected abdominal aortic graft. *Ann Surg* 205:727–732, 1987.

55. Bergamini TM, Corpus RA, Brittian KR, Peyton JC, Cheadle WG: The natural history of bacterial biofilm graft infection. *J Surg Resc* 56:393–396, 1994.

56. Ricotta JJ, Faggioli GL, Stella A, Curl GR, et al: Total excision and extra-anatomic bypass for aortic graft infection. *Am J Surg* 162:145–149, 1991.

57. Calligaro KD, Veith FJ, Schwartz ML, et al: When is it safe to leave an infected prosthetic arterial graft in place? *Current Critical Problems in Vascular Surgery.* In: Frank J. Veith FJ (ed). Quality Medical Publishing; St Louis: 56:365–370, 1992.

58. Chang N, Mathes SJ: Comparison of the effect of bacterial inoculation in musculocutaneous and random patterns flaps. *Plast Reconstr Surg* 70:1–8, 1982.

59. Gosain A, Chang N, Mathes S, et al: A study of relationship between blood flow and bacterial inoculation in musculocutaneous and fasciocutaneous flaps. *Plast Reconstr Surg* 86:1152–1159, 1990.

60. Ledgerwood AM, Lucas CE: Biological dressing for exposed vascular grafts: a reasonable alternative. *J Trauma* 15:567, 1975.

61. Humphries AW, Young JR, DeWolfe VG, LeFevre FA: Complications of abdominal aortic surgery. I. Aortoenteric fistulas. *Arch Surg* 86:43–50, 1963.

62. Fry WJ, Lindenauer SM: Infection complicating the use of plastic arterial implants. *Arch Surg* 94:699–709, 1967.

63. Jamieson GG, DeWeese JA, Rob CG: Infected arterial grafts. *Ann Surg* 181:850–852, 1975.

64. Martin-Paredero V, Busuttil RW, Dixon SM, et al: Fate of aortic graft removal. *Am J Surg* 146:194–197, 1983.

65. O'Hara PJ, Hertzer NR, Beven EG, Krajewski LP: Surgical management of infected abdominal aortic grafts: review of 25 years experience. *J Vasc Surg* 3:725–731, 1986.

66. Szilagyi DE, Elliot JP, Smith RE, et al: A thirty year survey of the reconstructive surgical treatment of aortoiliac occlusive disease. *J Vasc Surg* 3:421–436, 1986.

67. Edwards MJ, Richardson JD, Klamer TW: Management of aortic prosthetic infections. *Am J Surg* 155:327–330, 1988.

68. Liekweg WG, Greenfield LJ: Vascular Prosthetic infections: collected experience and results of treatment. *Surgery* 81:335–342, 1977.

69. Casali RE, Tucker WE, Thompson BW, Read RC: Infected prosthetic grafts. *Arch Surg* 115:577–580, 1980.

70. Turnipseed WD, Berkoff HA, Detmer DE, et al: Arterial graft infections: delayed vs. immediate vascular reconstruction. *Arch Surg* 118:410–414, 1983.

71. Fulenwider JT, Smith RB, Johnson RW, et al: Reoperative abdominal arterial surgery: a ten year experience. *Surgery* 93:20–27, 1983.

72. Yeager RA, Moneta GL, Taylor LM, et al: Improving survival and limb salvage in patients with aortic graft infections. *Am J Surg* 159:466–469, 1990.

CHAPTER 37

Neuropathic and Biomechanical Etiology of Foot Ulceration in Diabetics

Rhonda Lee Travaglino-Parda, MD
Christopher E. Attinger, MD
Anton N. Sidawy, MD

It is estimated that 11 million people in the United States have diabetes mellitus, 90% of whom have the non-insulin-dependent type.[1] The most common disabling chronic complication of diabetes mellitus is neuropathy. Although death seldom occurs from neuropathy alone, a great deal of morbidity and reduced quality of life can be attributed to the consequences of diabetic neuropathy.

Diabetes mellitus is the most common cause of peripheral neuropathy in industrialized countries.[2] The prevalence of neuropathy increases with the duration of diabetes, from 8% at the time diabetes is diagnosed, increasing to 50% by 25 years of duration of diabetes.[3] Neuropathy, peripheral vascular disease, and infection with poor wound healing are the three major pathophysiologic factors responsible for pedal ulceration; thus, this complication has important socioeconomic implications in the growing diabetic population. While not as dramatic in presentation as vascular insufficiency, the insidious development of neuropathy in diabetics is associated with considerable morbidity and disability. Neuropathy causes more diabetic foot problems, and more days of hospitalization, than any other complication of the disease.[4] Fifteen percent of all diabetics will have some form of foot complication in their lifetimes. Furthermore, it is estimated that more than half of all nontrauma-related amputations done in the United States are performed on diabetics. Diabetic patients face a fifteenfold increased risk of major lower extremity amputation. Studies have shown that once one limb has been amputated, the prognosis for the other limb is poor.[5] Prevention of this sequence poses a major challenge to physicians.

Although it was long believed that small vessel disease was responsible for lower limb problems in diabetic patients, it is now well-recognized that the majority of wounds to the plantar aspect of the diabetic foot are not due to angiopathy. Rather, they are a consequence of trauma which is not recognized by patients due to neuropathy.[6] Loss of protective sensation results in a number of biomechanical conditions conspiring to cause injury. While neuropathy is a major permissive factor, plantar ulcers develop at areas of high plantar pressure. It is generally believed that diabetes mellitus alters both musculoskeletal and soft tissue mechanics in a manner that increases plantar pressure in certain areas of the foot, making tissue damage more likely. Plantar ulceration has been linked in several retrospective studies and in one prospective study to high plantar pressures.[7-11] Diabetes, especially when accompanied by neuropathy, is associated with higher than normal plantar pressures.[9,12]

From *The Basic Science of Vascular Disease*. Edited by Sidawy AN, Sumpio BE, and DePalma RG. Armonk, NY: Futura Publishing Company, Inc.; © 1997.

Understanding the pathogenesis of peripheral neuropathy, and recognizing its clinical features and biomechanical sequelae, can help in the identification and treatment of high-risk patients and, therefore, reduce the morbidity of diabetic foot disease. This chapter discusses neuropathy and its sequelae, biomechanical changes in the foot, and the interaction between neuropathy and these changes in the formation of foot ulcers in diabetic patients.

Diabetic Neuropathy

Classification

The diabetic neuropathies have been classified by their degree of symmetry, type of nerve fiber affected, anatomic distribution, clinical symptoms, and known associated etiologic mechanisms.[13] While a classification system suggests discrete clinical categories, a system should not imply full understanding of these entities. Classification is hindered by the clinical variability and overlap of syndromes which may occur in any one individual.[14] Presently, it is unclear whether this variability reflects different etiologic mechanisms, or merely different manifestations of one process whose variable expression depends on host risk factors. An ideal classification would be based on clinical and pathologic features, but until our understanding of the pathogenesis is complete, a simple clinical classification system can be used.[15] A clinical classification, as described by Boulton, is presented; this system subdivides diabetic neuropathies into mononeuropathies and polyneuropathies (Table).[16]

Mononeuropathies

Isolated and Multiple

Mononeuropathies comprise the neural deficits corresponding to the distribution of single or multiple

Table
Classification of Diabetic Neuropathy

I. Mononeuropathies
  1. Isolated and multiple
  2. Cranial
II. Polyneuropathies
  1. Diabetic sensory polyneuropathy
    A. Acute sensory neuropathy
    B. Chronic sensorimotor neuropathy
  2. Proximal motor polyneuropathy
  3. Autonomic neuropathy

(Adapted with permission from Reference 16.)

peripheral nerves. The mononeuropathies are represented by focal and multifocal peripheral nerve abnormalities. Boulton terms these as isolated mononeuropathies and mononeuritis multiplex, which is the involvement of more than one nerve in the same patient. They tend to be sudden in onset and in most cases are self-limited. Although relatively uncommon, recognition of the mononeuropathies is important because they comprise the nerve dysfunction which may be treatable or reversible. The nerves most commonly affected are the peroneal and median nerves.[15,17] Involvement of the peroneal nerve presents with foot drop. The foot drop may require splinting until its spontaneous resolution. Involvement of the median and ulnar nerves usually present as entrapment neuropathies which can be treated surgically with decompression or transposition. Just as in nondiabetic patients, repetitive use and chronic trauma are factors in the development of carpal tunnel syndrome, but diabetics have been found to have greater than average risk of developing the syndrome.[18] This increased risk probably represents an increased susceptibility of diabetic nerves to mechanical or ischemic injury.

Cranial

Mononeuropathies involving most of the cranial nerves have been described, but the most common are the extraocular mononeuropathies with the oculomotor (3rd cranial nerve) being the most common, followed in frequency by cranial nerves 6 and 4. These tend to occur in the older type II diabetic patients and may be associated with pain in the orbit. Pupillary function is usually spared in oculomotor mononeuropathies, but exclusion of other causes, for example, aneurysms or other cerebral vascular event, is essential before diagnosing this condition. As with other mononeuropathies, the treatment is supportive with the prognosis for recovery good.[15]

Polyneuropathies

The most common form of diabetic neuropathy is a symmetrical distal sensory polyneuropathy.[15] While diabetes does not selectively affect sensory nerves, sensory neuropathies are the most common and, hence, more widely recognized by clinicians.[15,19,20] Boulton divides these into two forms, acute and chronic, differing in presentation, associated findings, and prognosis.[16]

Diabetic Sensory Polyneuropathies

Acute Sensory Neuropathy. This clinical entity is less common and is associated with pain as a principal component. The onset is sudden and is often precipitated by sudden change in metabolic state, such as ketoacidosis or the institution of insulin treatment, in newly diagnosed diabetics. In contrast to the severe symptoms, there are few clinical signs. Electrophysiologic studies show only minor abnormalities. The prognosis for this acute neuropathy is good, normally resolving within 1 year of onset.[16]

Chronic Sensorimotor. Over 20% of neuropathic patients have this form of neuropathy. The onset of symptoms is gradual with no obvious precipitating events. The usual presenting complaints are pain, paresthesias, or numbness. Examination reveals abnormalities of both sensory and motor function. The sensory deficits usually have a stocking-glove distribution; in addition, there are signs of small muscle wasting and loss of deep tendon reflexes. Electrophysiologic assessment confirms mixed sensory or motor nerve abnormalities. The prognosis of this type of neuropathy must be guarded, with the majority of patients affected being at great risk for neuropathic ulceration. Patients with this type of neuropathy are more likely to have evidence of other microvascular complications, such as retinopathy and nephropathy, than those with mononeuropathies.[15]

Proximal Motor Polyneuropathy

Pain, proximal muscle wasting, and weakness are the primary features of this condition which is more common in males and generally affects older type II diabetic patients. The onset may be either abrupt or more subacute (day to weeks) with deep aching constant pain in one or both thighs with associated wasting and weakness of affected muscles.[19] Another associated finding is weight loss; therefore, it is important to exclude malignancy as the underlying pathology. The distribution may be symmetrical or asymmetrical. The sum of evidence of this neuropathy indicates an ischemic etiology. The wasting is a prominent feature and follows weakness by an interval of 2 to 3 weeks. Most commonly affected are the quadriceps group, the iliopsoas muscles, and the great adductors of the thigh. The prognosis for recovery is generally good with most patients regaining some, but not all, muscle strength.[16]

Autonomic Neuropathies

Autonomic neuropathies can impair any function modulated by the autonomic nervous system in diabetic patients. Neuropathy produces diffuse clinical autonomic nervous system dysfunction, usually confined to one or two organ systems.[14] Up to 40% of diabetics have autonomic derangements,[21] as determined by cardiovascular reflex tests. Autonomic

symptoms begin insidiously and may progress over a period of years.

Etiology

Despite the advances in our understanding of the pathophysiology of neuropathic symptoms and signs, our knowledge of the pathogenesis of peripheral neuropathies remains incomplete. Metabolic and structural factors are both implicated in the sequence of pathologic events in nerve tissue, which result in diabetic nerve dysfunction. Symptomatic neuropathy usually occurs after many years of diabetes mellitus, and the incidence of neuropathy increases with the duration of this disease.[2] Because prolonged hyperglycemia precedes the development of neuropathy in diabetics, it is believed that hyperglycemia plays a prominent role in causing metabolic derangements in neural tissue. This relationship is supported by the finding that diabetic neuropathy is more severe and more frequent in patients who have poor metabolic control, and that improved diabetic control improves nerve function.[14] Also, type I diabetics with decreased nerve conduction velocities may improve with insulin during the initial months of treatment.[19] Diabetes of short duration with neuropathy exhibits slowed nerve conduction velocities in the absence of anatomic abnormalities. Whether the metabolic changes affect the nerve directly, or by altering perineural microvasculature, remains to be elucidated, and is central to the debate between those who believe that metabolic abnormalities, including those of the polyol pathway, are the principal cause and those who favor microvascular disease as the cause.[17] Both mechanisms are likely to be at work in a single individual and indeed the two may be related.[22]

Evidence for a metabolic defect in diabetic nerve tissue has been found in human diabetic polyneuropathy and experimental nerve studies.[23,24] Greene and Sima hypothesized that persistent hyperglycemia increases the glucose concentration in peripheral nerve endoneurium. A flux of glucose through the polyol pathway occurs, activated by the enzyme aldose reductase, that leads to sorbitol production (Figure 1). Unlike glucose, which does not require insulin to enter

$$D - Glucose + NADPH + H \cdot \xrightarrow{\text{Aldose Reductase}} Sorbitol + NADP$$

$$Sorbitol + NAD \xrightarrow{\text{Sorbitol Dehydrogenase}} D - Fructose + NADH + H$$

Figure 1. The polyol pathway. Aldose reductase inhibitors prevent the conversion of glucose to sorbitol. (Reproduced with permission from Reference 15.)

nerve cells, sorbitol cannot pass freely through cell membranes. In addition, sorbitol dehydrogenase is absent in nerve cells; therefore, sorbitol accumulates within the cell.[25–27] In experimental studies, activation of the polyol pathway with increased sorbitol tissue accumulation led to decreased nerve conduction velocity.[25,28] Tissue levels of sorbitol were found to be elevated and were associated with the severity of neuropathy.[29] These findings set the stage for the study of sorbinil and other aldose reductase inhibitors, such as tolrestat and statil, to determine if the therapeutic use of an aldose reductase inhibitor could arrest, prevent, or even reverse diabetic polyneuropathy.[30] Studies have shown that taking sorbinil daily for 1 year reduced the elevated nerve content of sorbitol toward normal. Sima et al also found that the decrease in sorbitol was associated with a burst of regenerative activity in the follow-up sural nerve biopsies of patients treated with sorbinil.[31,32]

Sorbitol accumulation is also thought to cause osmotic swelling of tissues, which can lead to ischemia and cell damage. Using magnetic resonance spectroscopy, Griffey et al showed that the water content of sural nerve fibers from diabetics with neuropathy was increased, compared to diabetics with neuropathy who had been treated with aldose reductase inhibitors.[33] These findings may provide a link between metabolic and ischemic theories for the etiology of diabetic neuropathy.[34]

Sorbitol accumulation is also thought to cause increased glycosylation of proteins that may be involved in the thickening of basement membranes.[29,35,36] The thickness of basement membranes in endoneurial microvessels is greater in diabetics with neuropathy than in controls, and is statistically associated with severity of neuropathy of myelinated fibers.[37]

Another key feature of the activated polyol pathway theory is that there is inhibition of myoinositol uptake by the nerve and, therefore, neural levels of myoinositol are decreased. Myoinositol is an important precursor of phosphoinositides, which are the parts of the cell membrane necessary for nerve conduction (Figures 2 and 3). A decrease in myoinositol levels in nerve tissue is hypothesized to cause a sequence of

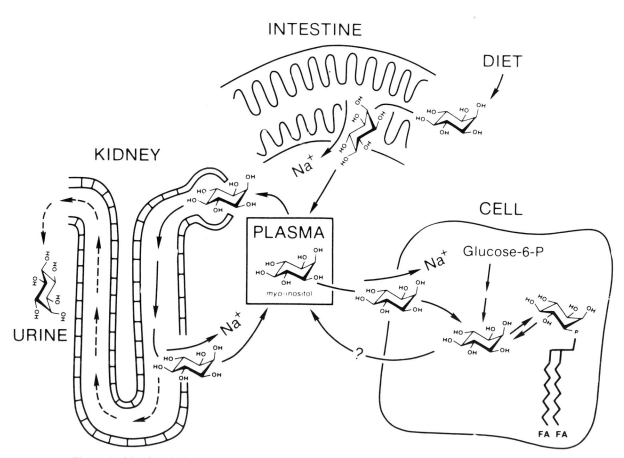

Figure 2. Myoinositol metabolism. Myoinositol is reversibly incorporated into inositol containing phospholipids, the phosphoinositides. Glucose competitively inhibits sodium-dependent myoinositol transport in the intestine, kidney, and nerve. (Reproduced with permission from Reference 13.)

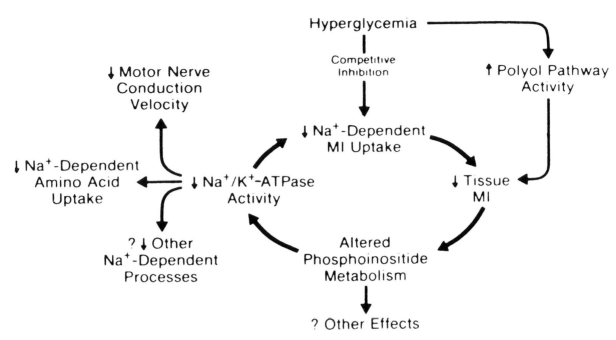

Figure 3. Decreased myoinositol levels are hypothesized to cause a protein kinase C mediated reduction in axolemmal sodium-potassium-ATPase activity and altered axolemmal sodium permeability, thereby altering nerve conduction. (Reproduced with permission from Reference 40.)

events leading to a protein kinase C (PKC)-mediated reduction in axolemmal sodium-potassium-ATPase activity, altered axolemmal sodium permeability, and structural changes at the nodes of Ranvier, beginning with axo-glial dysjunction.[23,24,38–41] Contradicting this thesis, Dyck et al found mean nerve levels of myoinositol not to be decreased in diabetic patients with or without neuropathy, and were not associated with any of the end points of neuropathology in diabetics. If confirmed, this observation would cast considerable doubt on the primary role of myoinositol depletion in the pathogenesis of diabetic polyneuropathy.[29,42]

The pathogenesis of diabetic polyneuropathy is obviously multifactorial, with hyperglycemia playing a prominent role.[2] Many believe that interposed in the sequence between metabolic disturbances and pathologic alterations of nerve fibers are tissue alterations, namely microvascular changes. In addition to hyperglycemia and associated metabolic abnormalities, new evidence implicates changes in perineural vasculature and resultant ischemia in the development of diabetic polyneuropathy. Dyck et al formulated criteria for ischemic nerve damage based on pathologic studies of experimental ischemic neuropathy.[43] They contend that if these criteria are met in a disease of unknown cause, it is reasonable to infer ischemia as the etiology for the pathologic process.[43] Based on extensive postmortem and sural nerve biopsy studies, they believe there is strong evidence for an ischemic basis for dia-

betic neuropathy. Biopsies of sural nerves taken from neuropathic diabetic patients show features of microangiopathy, including basement membrane thickening and endothelial hyperplasia.[22]

Two recent carefully performed autopsy studies of nerve trunks from diabetics concluded that ischemia of the nerve is crucial in the pathogenesis of diabetic polyneuropathy.[44,45] Altered nerve metabolism may lead to "dying-back" axonopathy, also known as centripetal gradient. This axonopathy pattern shows fiber loss to be more progressive distally than proximally (Figure 4). There is loss of both myelinated and unmyelinated fibers. Multifocal ischemic lesions may also be contributory.[2] Multifocal fiber loss is consistent with ischemic polyneuropathy.[19]

In assessing endoneurial microvessels and sural nerves from diabetics, endothelial hyperplasia and excessive capillary closure correlated with the severity of neuropathy. The fiber loss was multifocal, which is also consistent with ischemic polyneuropathy. These changes are thought to be primary and not secondary to neural fiber degeneration, because they are characteristic of pathologic changes in other vessels in diabetic patients. The severity of the vessels and fiber pathology are statistically associated. Such vessel alterations have not been described as secondary to fiber degeneration.[37] These changes could cause nerve fiber damage. Mechanisms to consider are ischemia, decreased oxygen transport and exchange, and altered

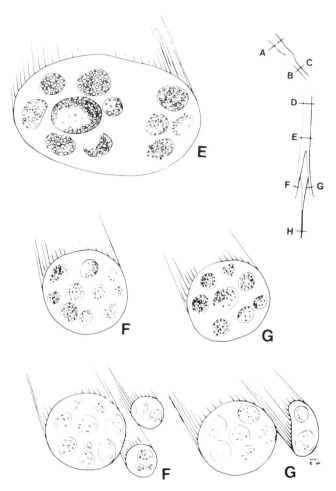

Figure 4. Spatial distribution of fiber loss in diabetic polyneuropathy. Proximally in the sciatic nerve, fiber loss is multifocal and becomes greater distally. In addition, in the more distal nerve segments, new multifocal regions of damage are seen. These changes are consistent with multifocal ischemic injury along the length of the nerve. (Reproduced with permission from Reference 43.)

capillary permeability. Multifocal ischemia might be caused by capillary closure, which has been observed in diabetics. Altered capillary permeability is suggested by the finding of increased endoneurial albumin content in diabetic nerves compared to controls.[37]

Other views of the pathogenesis are emerging. There is evidence for hyperglycemia-related nonenzymatic glycosylation of tissue affecting primarily the vasoneurosom and the endoneural matrix; chronic changes in these could lead to ischemic changes in the nerves of diabetic patients.[29,42]

Others argue that the focus is to find a factor associated with diabetes mellitus which damages nerves. They assert that diabetic neuropathy is actually associated with a diabetes-related factor that slows nerve regeneration.[46] This hypothesis is supported by several studies that have found an association between dia-

betic neuropathy and alterations in the endogenous content of trophic factors in animal models of diabetes mellitus.[47] Insulin, whose total or relative deficiency is the cause of diabetes, is a peptide that shares several chemical and functional properties with nerve growth factor. Nerve growth factor is essential for the survival and maintenance of sympathetic and peripheral sensory neurons. In diabetic neuropathy, sympathetic and sensory neurons are affected while the rest of the cellular elements of the central nervous system are usually spared.[47] Faradji and Sotelo demonstrated that the levels of nerve growth factor in the serum of patients with long-standing diabetes with peripheral neuropathy were low. Electrophysiologic studies further showed that the decrease in the levels of nerve growth factor was closely related to the severity of the neuropathy.[48]

Foot Changes as They Relate to Neuropathy

The deleterious changes that occur in the skin, bones, and joints of diabetics are primarily attributable to neuropathy.[49] These changes predispose the foot to potentially limb- and life-threatening complications such as ulceration, osteoarthropathy, and gangrene, especially when ischemia and sepsis are superimposed.[50]

While most clinicians are fully aware of the sensory deficits and their sequelae, the consequences of motor and autonomic dysfunction are not well recognized. Diabetes does not selectively affect sensory nerves. The most common form of diabetic neuropathy is a distal symmetrical polyneuropathy, with varying degrees of sensory, motor, and autonomic fiber involvement.[19,37,51] The manifestations of diabetic neuropathy range from subclinical alterations of nerve conduction, affecting about 75% of all patients who have diabetes for more than a few years, to extremely severe neuropathy with life-threatening autonomic dysfunction.[2,52] The clinical manifestations of neuropathy vary depending on the classes of nerve fiber involved. Small fiber neuropathy often precedes large and mixed fiber neuropathy. Small fiber disease results in deficits of pain and temperature differentiation, while large fiber involvement results in loss of light touch, proprioception, and vibratory sense. Large fiber involvement also impairs deep tendon reflexes and can be confused with spinal pathology. Vibratory detection thresholds are the most sensitive and, therefore, diminished vibratory sensation is the earliest manifestation of distal symmetrical polyneuropathy to be clinically apparent. The result is a reduction in afferent sensory perception. While the majority of patients will experience foot numbness only, symptoms of discomfort are not uncommon and can occur at any stage of disease.[53] Paradoxically, while patients complain of burning, lancinating, or shooting pain in the foot, physical examination reveals decreased sensation. These symptoms may coincide with episodes of infection, emotional stress, ketoacidosis, or shortly after induction of insulin therapy, giving rise to the term "insulin neuritis."[49,54] Theories for the cause of the discomfort include simultaneous degeneration and regeneration of nerve fibers, and also discrepancies in the ratio of large fiber versus small fiber involvement.

Small fiber disease also leads to aberrations in the autonomic nervous system. Because of the autonomic nerve dysfunction, the diabetic foot undergoes what has been termed an autosympathectomy. Studies have estimated that sympathetic activities were absent in 60% of diabetics with peripheral neuropathy.[55] Three consequences of autonomic neuropathy in the diabetic lower extremity are increased blood flow, artery wall rigidity secondary to medial wall calcification, and decreased skin hydration secondary to decreased sweat gland and sebaceous gland dysfunction. Since autonomic dysfunction is not limited to the lower extremity, systemic symptoms of autonomic dysfunction follow with nocturnal diarrhea, constipation, impotence, early satiety, vomiting, anhydrosis, and syncope. It is very important to elicit this symptomatology because autonomic neuropathy carries the highest morbidity and mortality rates of all the various presentations of diabetic neuropathies.[49] Autonomic dysfunction leads to abnormalities in distribution of blood flow by atrioventricular (AV) shunting. A direct relationship between AV shunts and autonomic neuropathy has been demonstrated.[56–58] Increased AV shunting is supported by findings of increased PO_2 in foot venous blood. Although blood flow is increased, the consequence of this increased blood flow, through AV shunts, is a bypass of capillary nutrient circulation. In experimental animals, AV shunting led directly to ulcer formation.[59,60]

In some patients, even in the absence of peripheral vascular disease, a failure of sympathetic fibers caused by autonomic neuropathy leads to a reduction in toe blood pressure, a parameter often used as an ischemic index.[61] Blood pressure depends not only on blood flow, but on the resistance to flow in the capillary bed, namely, the degree of arteriolar constriction. Irwin et al[62] believe that the drop in pressure from ankle to toe in diabetic patients may simply be caused by a loss of peripheral vascular resistance, and that toe lesions ascribed to peripheral vascular disease in these patients may be a manifestation of severe diabetic autonomic neuropathy. Since the autonomic nervous system supplies sympathetic adrenergic fibers to the smooth muscle in the wall of the arterioles, a failure of sympathetic fibers leads to arteriolar vasodilatation and a resultant decrease in peripheral vascular resistance. Thus, this could explain the reduction of toe

blood pressure in diabetics with autonomic neuropathy.

It is not known why medial wall calcification occurs, but this has also been found in vessels following lumbar sympathectomy.[63] The medial wall calcification is a complication of diabetes for which neuropathy is the only important etiologic factor. The lumen size is not changed, but the vessel loses its flexibility and therefore peripheral blood flow increases.[64] Increased blood flow in the diabetic foot, therefore, results from the opening of AV shunts and rigid arterial wall secondary to medial wall calcification. The involved foot may, therefore, appear warm with an increased temperature compared to the uninvolved foot. This increased blood flow may also cause what has been termed neuropathic edema of the diabetic foot.

Since the autonomic nervous system also supplies the sweat glands and the sebaceous glands of the skin, the loss of sweat gland and sebaceous gland function in the foot results in abnormalities in skin hydration. The foot becomes predisposed to dryness, fissuring, and cracking which can serve as a portal of entry for infection.

Biomechanical Sequelae of Diabetic Neuropathy

In patients with primarily motor neuropathy, foot drop can be the initial presentation. The presence of foot drop may represent a progressive mononeuropathy, or it may be attributable to entrapment of the peroneal nerve at the head of the fibula. More commonly, the motor fibers of the intrinsic foot muscles, the interossei, lumbricals, and extensor digitorum brevis, are affected and give rise to the characteristic foot deformity of diabetic neuropathy. Slow nerve conduction velocity, as well as decreased action potential in these muscles, results in their weakness and eventual wasting. The most common finding of distal motor neuropathy resembles an intrinsic muscle palsy with intrinsic muscle wasting and the characteristic claw toe deformity, with cocked-up toes and plantarly prominent metatarsal heads (Figure 5).[7,65] This appearance is due to weakening of the intrinsic muscles of the foot, which normally act to flex the metatarsal phalangeal joint and extend the proximal interphalangeal joint, a deformity analogous to the claw hand as a result of ulnar nerve pathology. When the intrinsic muscles of the foot are weakened, they can no longer oppose the action of the long extensor muscles of the leg and this leads to metatarsal phalangeal joint hyperextension and proximal interphalangeal joint flexion. These structural changes shift weight bearing from the toes to the metatarsal heads. In addition, the plantar fat pad shifts distally so that

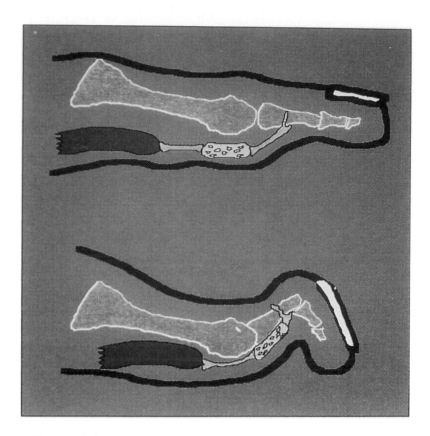

Figure 5. Characteristic claw toe deformity with anterior displacement of plantar fat pad (**yellow**). (Reproduced with permission from Reference 7.)

the metatarsal heads are covered only by skin and subcutaneous tissue, which is less able to withstand direct or shear pressure. This shift in the soft tissue "pad" under this weight-bearing point ultimately leads to subtarsal callus formation and eventual ulceration if unrecognized or untreated. Callus forms in response to excessive tissue pressure and if left untreated contributes to increasing plantar pressure itself, thereby increasing the risk for plantar ulceration. In addition, digital contractures, either claw toe or hammer toe deformities, have an increased potential for skin breakdown on the dorsum secondary to shoe irritation. These digital contractures also predispose to ulceration on the plantar aspect of the metatarsal heads because the deformity increases retrograde plantar flexion forces on the metatarsal heads.[49]

The cavus foot type is most commonly evident in the diabetic, owing to motor involvement in distal symmetrical polyneuropathy. The motor neuropathy affects the balance between the intrinsic and extrinsic muscles. Since the intrinsic muscles are primarily affected, the weakened intrinsics cannot oppose the forces of the long extrinsic muscles, resulting in claw toe and hammer toe deformities and the characteristic high-arched (cavus) foot. The end result is a transfer

of weight-bearing points from the toes to the head of the metatarsals. Impairment of the peroneal muscles is compensated by the extensor muscles functioning to dorsiflex the foot, particularly the extensor hallucis longus, which leads to hyperextension of the hallux.[49] These pathomechanical processes result in deformities that predispose the foot to ulceration.

Weakness of various muscle groups creates dynamic imbalances that either initiate or compound deformities within the foot. Those muscles primarily affected are the anterior thigh (quadriceps), anterior leg (tibialis anterior, extensor hallucis longus, and extensor digitorum longus), and the foot intrinsics.

Muscular imbalance is compounded by inflexibility of the soft tissues secondary to the nonenzymatic glycosylation of proteins, namely collagen. Glucose binds to the collagen and it increases the cross-linkages between molecules resulting in decreased elasticity. The collagen of skin and tendinous structures are both affected and contribute to limited joint mobility, as well as "stiff skin" which is less resilient to shear forces. Biopsies of patients with limited joint mobility confirm increased cross-linking and glycosylation of collagen.[35,66] Nonenzymatic glycosylation of many proteins in the body has been demonstrated in diabetics.[35,67]

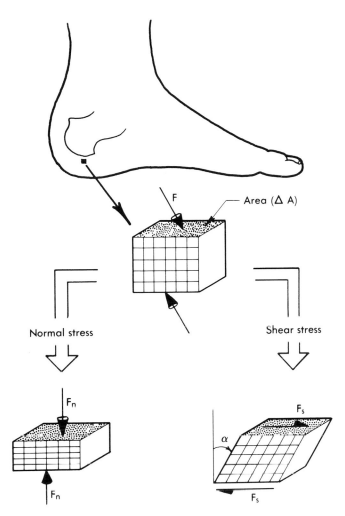

Figure 6. Illustration of normal versus shear stress on heel of foot. (Reproduced with permission from Reference 69.)

Studies in the foot skin have shown that keratin in the stratum corneum is glycosylated compared with nondiabetic skin.[68] This process has been shown to affect the mechanical properties of tissue, usually reducing elasticity. It is postulated that these changes make the skin stiffer and, thus, less able to distribute pressure through deformation. Soft tissue must be able to distribute load, so that excessive stresses do not act on a very small contact area.[69] Stress is defined as the ratio of force to the area on which it acts. The same force applied to the entire surface of the foot will cause only small deformations and no major damage (Figure 6).[69] Figure 7 depicts the different effects of normal pressure on soft tissues with different degrees of elasticity or compliance.[69]

It has been suggested that neuropathy predisposes patients to the production of excessive plantar keratoses.[70] Whether or not this is true, recent evidence has shown that the removal of callus from bony prominences in the forefoot reduces plantar pressure by an average of 29%.[71] In addition, previous ulceration is widely regarded as a leading risk factor for future ulceration.[7] This is reasonable because the initial ulceration represents proof that patients have the combination of other risk factors that produce ulceration. In addition, the wound repair process changes the tissue properties in the area of the healed ulcer, making this tissue clinically stiffer and hence less resilient to deformation forces. Such scar tissue may act in much the same way that callus appears to act by transferring large concentrated loads to the immediately underlying softer tissue.[7]

Foot Biomechanics

Normal Gait

To fully appreciate the abnormalities of the biomechanics of the diabetic foot, one must understand what is required in normal gait. The walking cycle is made up of two phases: the stance phase, also known as the flexor stabilization phase, and the swing phase, also known as the extensor substitution phase (Figure 8).

The Stance Phase of Gait

During normal gait, initial floor contact is at heel strike.[72] Heel strike marks the beginning of the stance phase which is the contact period of gait. Heel strike follows with a short period of double limb support, then an intervening interval of single limb support, until double limb support resumes at the end of the stance phase. Double limb support continues until the toe-off "lift-off" of the swing phase occurs. The stance phase is the contact period of gait (Figure 9). When the foot strikes the ground in gait, Newton's law applies in that there will be equal forces experienced by both the foot and the floor.[7] These forces are known as ground reactive forces.[73] During this phase of the walking cycle, the anterior muscle group serves a critical function in counteracting the ground reactive forces encountered at heel strike. These reactive forces are countered by deceleration of ankle plantar flexion and smoothing the transition of forces from the lateral aspect of the foot to the medial side.[73] Deceleration of ankle plantar flexion is needed to decrease the force in which the forefoot encounters the ground after heel strike. Smoothing the transition of forces from the lateral aspect of the foot to the medial side of the foot requires full mobility at the subtalar joint. Without this transition, the ground reactive forces are transmitted unbuffered to the foot, knee, and lower back, leading to pathology. Buffering

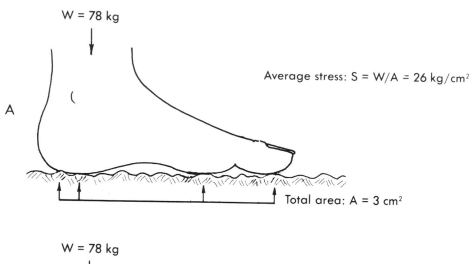

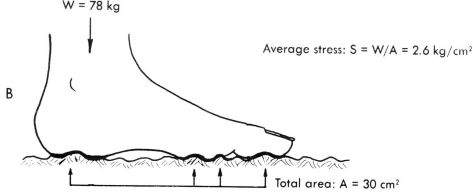

Figure 7. Comparison of stresses (pressure) on different tissue types. **A.** Foot with inelastic "stiff" soft tissue. Stress is concentrated on very few contact areas. **B.** Foot with compliant soft tissue. Stress is distributed over a greater area rather than areas of peak plantar pressure. (Reproduced with permission from Reference 69.)

is achieved through contact phase pronation at the subtalar joint along with smooth ankle plantar flexion.

The Swing Phase of Gait

Near the end of the stance phase, propulsion of forces leads to "toe-off," marking the onset of the swing phase. During the swing phase, ankle dorsiflexion is required. The tibialis anterior begins to contract and dorsiflexes the first metatarsal. This results in the hallux being slightly flexed in relation to the first metatarsal head. This position is stable and helps the toe-off function. Bony and muscular stability are critical in this phase to maintain the foot in a position with the optimum mechanical advantage. Figure 10 summarizes the gait cycle, including position and movement required by different muscles and joints of the lower extremity.[72]

Abnormal Foot Biomechanics

Patients with diabetes mellitus who have anterior muscle group weakness lose the ability to decelerate ankle plantar flexion and cannot counter the ground reactive forces of heel strike; therefore, abrupt "slap" of the forefoot against the ground occurs along with an increase in load under the metatarsal heads.[73] In addition, contact is produced earlier in the gait cycle and for a longer period of time than what is normally expected.[73] Smoothing the transition of forces from the lateral aspect of the foot to the medial side of the foot requires full mobility at the subtalar joint. In diabetics, the subtalar joint is often immobile. Thus, forces are transferred from lateral to medial foot much faster than should be and, as the forces progress medially, they pick up more momentum than normal. Not only does the pressure to the plantar surface of the foot change, but the subtalar joint also meets the point of contact on the calcaneus abruptly which leads to joint remodeling with progressive decrease in the range of motion at this joint. The more immobility at the subtalar joint, the less effective is pronation in absorbing ground forces. When heel rise begins, the weight is shifted onto the metatarsal heads. Because of the anterior compartment muscle weakness in the diabetic leg, the posterior compartment, namely the gastrocnemius and soleus,

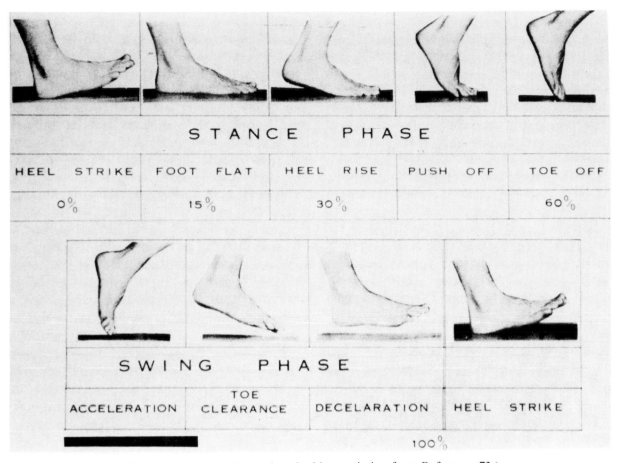

Figure 8. The walking cycle. (Reproduced with permission from Reference 73.)

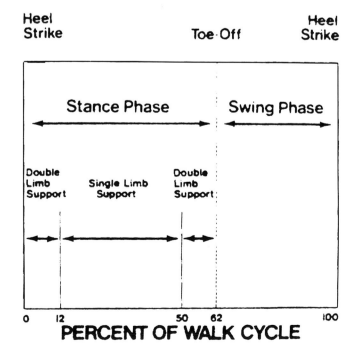

Figure 9. Percent of the walking cycle. (Reproduced with permission from Mann RA: Overview of foot and ankle biomechanics. In: Jahss MH (ed). *Disorders of the Foot and Ankle*. Philadelphia: WB Saunders, Co.; 1991.)

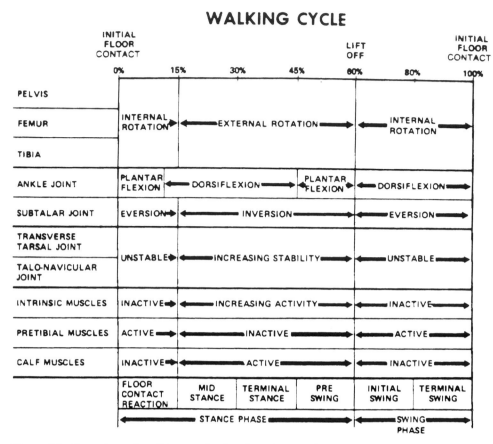

Figure 10. Overview of walking cycle showing phases of cycle with associated actions of musculoskeletal tissues. (Reproduced with permission from Reference 72.)

dominates. These muscles exert an increased plantar flexion pull on the calcaneus, which ultimately results in the equinus deformity. With an equinus deformity, the midtarsal joint is unlocked creating hypermobility within the forefoot. Hence, with propulsion on a forefoot which is unstable, there is an increase in shear forces occurring under the metatarsal heads. This combination of increase in shear forces along with the decreased resiliency of the skin secondary to nonenzymatic glycosylation of collagen in the skin as well as thinning of the plantar fat pads secondary to their migration results in ulceration beneath one of the metatarsal heads.

Diabetics with anterior compartment atrophy pose a problem during the swing phase as well, often exhibiting dragging of the foot. During the swing phase, when dorsiflexion of the ankle and hallux are required, the diabetic foot shows limited mobility of the hallux, in addition to suboptimal dorsiflexion. Therefore, the hallux remains in contact with the ground longer and is subject to ulceration.

Loss of intrinsic muscle function in the foot will permit the development of either stance phase or swing phase deformity of the digit. Digital contracture

may follow loss of sensation of proprioceptive function, where the digits contract to grasp the ground to compensate for a loss of balance. Studies support the findings of increased sway during standing in diabetic patients due to the loss of proprioceptive function. While it would seem that increased uncertainty in gait would also occur, studies have not supported this theory.[74]

Both barefoot and in-shoe plantar measurements can now be made to assess the risk of injury secondary to the abnormal biomechanics of the diabetic foot in relation to the gait cycle (Figures 11, 12, and 13; see color insert).[7] This assessment can then be used to determine preventive measures tailored to the individual. Figure 14 (see color insert) shows the different plantar pressures in one individual with four different types of footwear. This assessment helped to determine the best footwear for ulcer healing.[7]

Charcot Deformity

Any change in the bones and joints of neuropathic feet that causes deformity alters normal foot mechanics.

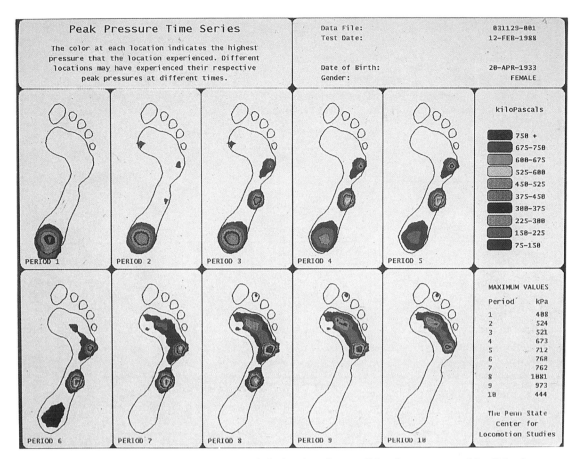

Figure 11. Plantar pressures measured during barefoot walking in a neuropathic diabetic patient. **"Cool" colors** represent low pressures; **"hot" colors** represent high pressures. Note the high pressure zones in the midfoot and under the fifth metatarsal which remain loaded for over 60% of the ground contact time. (Reproduced with permission from Reference 7.)

Multiple factors contribute to the bone and joint destruction seen in diabetic patients. The diabetic Charcot foot represents a progressive process that affects multiple tissues in the lower extremity and is characterized by pathologic fractures with exuberant repair mechanisms.[64] The result is destruction of bones and joints in the foot that ultimately leads to severe deformity.

The theories of the etiology of Charcot foot deformity have varied throughout history, as different diseases have become less or more prominent. The common feature of all these diseases is the presence of neuropathy, with tabes dorsalis and Hansen's disease being the most common examples. Today, Charcot deformity is seen most commonly in patients with diabetes mellitus.[64] Several theories have been espoused as the accepted etiology for Charcot deformity. The neurotraumatic theory stated that the deformity was due to trauma to an insensitive foot; therefore, the bones and joints would be subjected to pressures beyond their capability leading to instability followed by fracture and then repair.[64] Since not all patients showed hyper-

trophic changes and mainly demonstrated extensive bony erosion, it was theorized that these patients had a hypervascular state that led to bone resorption. Peripheral neuropathy with loss of protective sensation, autonomic neuropathy with increased blood flow to bone, and trauma have emerged as the most important factors.[75] The mechanism of destruction may be single injury or repetitive moderate stress applied to the bones and joints of an insensate foot and ankle. Peripheral blood flow is thought to be increased secondary to autonomic neuropathy with AV shunting. The increased blood flow is thought to result in active bone resorption. The result is fractures, effusions, ligamentous laxity followed by erosion of articular cartilage, fragmentation, disintegration, and ultimately collapse of the foot.[75]

Charcot collapse of the midfoot may lead to a "rocker-bottom" foot deformity resulting in hammertoes that increase the risk for dorsal digital ulceration. In addition, the collapsed midfoot becomes vulnerable to plantar ulceration.

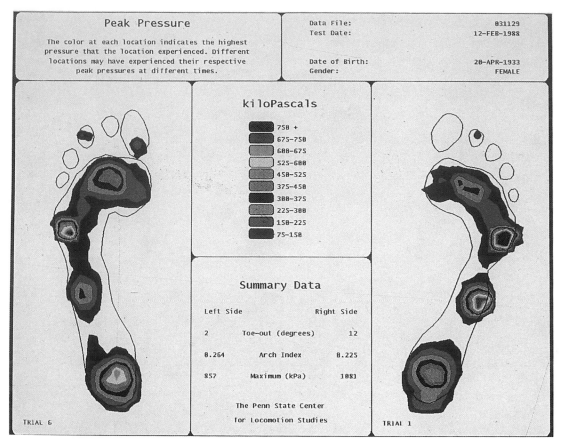

Figure 12. Peak pressure plot summarizing the data in Figure 11. The most pressure at each area on the plantar foot surface is shown on the plot. (Reproduced with permission from Reference 7.)

Biomechanical Changes Caused by Surgery of the Foot

Segmental amputations of the foot can also have a great effect on the biomechanics of foot function. Gait is altered in addition to the obvious structural changes. The more proximal the foot amputation, the shorter the swing phase will be on the amputated side. The remaining portions of the foot take on a greater load for a longer duration, thereby setting the stage for injury and potential ulceration.[73]

The hallux plays a major role in the propulsion toe-off phase of the walking cycle and is responsible for distributing body weight from one limb to the other. Hallux amputation leads to transfer of function to the second toe which is not capable of these functions. The compensatory forces act on the second toe, resulting in hammer toe deformity. In addition, because of the shift in weight bearing to the lateral side of the foot, there is increased potential for ulceration of the lateral foot.

The other toes function mainly in a proprioceptive capacity and so their amputation causes little functional loss. However, toe space-fillers are important postoperatively to prevent hallux valgus with increased risk of ulceration over the medial first metatarsal head.

Transmetatarsal ray amputations lead to transfer ulcerations of the remaining or contralateral segments because of the loss of muscular forces stabilizing flexion/extension and eversion/inversion. Complete transmetatarsal amputations fare better, except for loss of dorsiflexion. For this reason, Achilles lengthening procedures are sometimes needed to improve gait after transmetatarsal amputation.[76] After Lisfranc amputations through the metatarsal-tarsal joint, the foot tends to go into equinovarus because the remaining attachment of the tibialis anterior muscle cannot oppose the intact posterior compartment muscles. The more proximal Chopart amputation at the talonavicular level leaves no extensor muscle to oppose the posterior compartment. In these more proximal amputations, inversion occurs secondary to division of the peroneus longus and brevis muscles. Achilles lengthening in addition to tendon transfers can improve these deformities which usually develop after Lisfranc and Chopart amputations, making these options more useful alternatives in foot salvage.

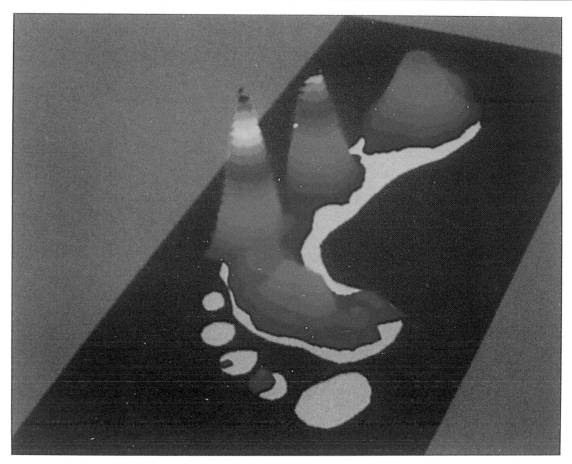

Figure 13. Three-dimensional interpretation of the same peak pressure data shown in Figure 12. (Reproduced with permission from Reference 7.)

Pathophysiology of Diabetic Foot Ulceration

Although it was long believed that the etiology of diabetic foot ulcers was small vessel disease due to occlusion in the microcirculation, studies have shown that diabetics have less occlusive disease in the foot than nondiabetics.[52] The pattern of atherosclerosis in the majority of diabetics shows minimal disease in the aortoiliac vessels, with a tendency toward occlusion in the distal superficial femoral artery and in the tibial-peroneal vessels. Most patients with even severe plantar ulcerations have strong pedal pulses.

Whereas patients who present with ulceration of the forefoot secondary to ischemia complain of rest pain and are found to have a cold foot with absent pulses, patients with ulceration of the foot secondary to neuropathy usually have no symptoms and the ulcer tends to be painless; the foot is warm with or without edema, with a tendency toward dry skin and palpable pulses. The characteristic bone and joint changes which occur with neuropathy have been discussed in other sections of this chapter. Once skin ulceration occurs in the diabetic foot, the risk for amputation is sig-

nificant.[77] While neuropathy plays a major permissive role, ulceration of the diabetic foot does not occur solely because of the presence of neuropathy, but results from some type of trauma to the skin surface. Although acute trauma can harm the skin surface in anyone, most diabetic foot ulcers result from relatively minor trauma. Injury occurs most commonly from poorly fitting footwear and during foot contact in normal daily walking.

There is no clear agreement on the pressure threshold for ulceration; however, it has generally been accepted that forces greater than 10 kg cm^2 acting on the foot during gait will contribute to ulcer formation on the plantar surface of the foot.[73] The development of ulceration depends on several factors including care taken by patients, activity level of patients, as well as a number of tissue characteristics.[7] The specific location of the ulcer is determined by the mechanical problems that preexist within the intrinsic foot type and will vary from patient to patient (Figure 15). Although foot deformity contributes to high plantar pressures, it is important to note that it is the combination of neuropathy and foot deformity which carries the greatest risk for plantar ulceration.[78,79] Masson et al compared pa-

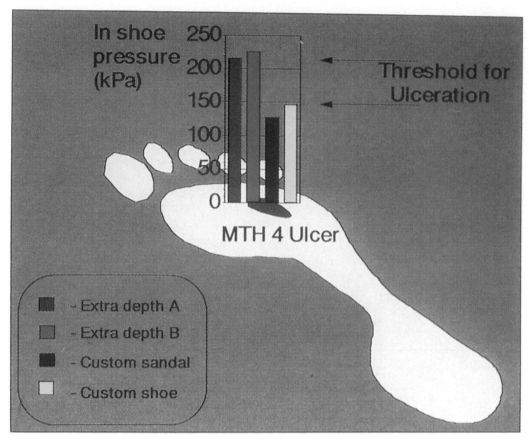

Figure 14. Peak pressure at fourth metatarsal head in one individual with four different types of custom footwear. Ulceration recurred while wearing shoes **A** and **B**. The ulcer remained healed after wearing a reconfigured custom sandal. This sandal was used to pattern a definitive shoe. At 4 months, the ulcer had not recurred. (Reproduced with permission from Reference 7.)

tients with diabetes and rheumatoid arthritis having similar foot deformities and elevated plantar pressures. The incidence of plantar ulceration was 32% in the diabetic group versus none in the rheumatoid group.[79]

While loss of sensation results in failure to perceive damage caused by mechanical trauma, friction, or penetrating heat, the majority of neuropathic ulcers are not caused by accidental trauma or by ischemia from continuing pressure, but from moderate repetitive stress on the same part of the foot.[80] Patients with insensitive feet accept unvarying patterns of repetitive stress on a continuing basis long after a normal foot would have started to feel soreness.[80] The pain in a normal foot, experienced after a few miles of walking, induces an adjustment in gait so that a different part of the soft tissue or a different bone bears the stress, even though the total stress on the whole foot is unchanged. The difference between normal feet and denervated feet is not that normal feet are stronger, but rather that they feel the pain at the stage where inflammation begins to develop, forcing the person to rest or to change the gait to alter the pattern of stress.[80] Stud-

ies done by Brand support this theory (Figure 16; see color insert). The feet of large numbers of rats were tested with a subset of rats having had their feet denervated. Repetitive pressure was applied to a small area of the footpad thousands of times each day. Both the amount of pressure and the pattern of repetition were held constant in any given phase of the experiment. At a pressure of 20 psi, a pressure within the range experienced by rats or humans in normal running, 10,000 repetitions per day were tolerated with only the development of hyperemia, edema, and increase in footpad temperature. After resting, the footpad returned to normal. When the same stresses were repeated to the same area of the footpad the following day, the edema occurred earlier and did not readily resolve. Histologically, the footpad showed inflammatory changes and hyperplasia of the skin. After repeating the experiment daily for 1 week, the inflammatory reaction progressed to focal areas of necrosis by the second and third days, and by the seventh day, the skin had ulcerated and the entire footpad was necrotic. Although this process occurred somewhat earlier in the

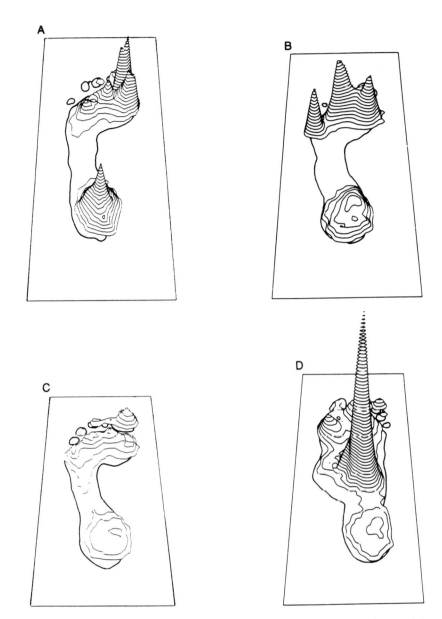

Figure 15. Peak plantar pressure diagrams from four different diabetic patients with varying duration of disease, body mass, and foot deformity. **A.** Three focal areas of increased pressure in medial forefoot. **B.** Focal areas of increased pressure under first, third, and fifth metatarsal heads. **C.** No focal areas of increased pressure. **D.** Extremely high pressure area underneath midfoot deformity in patient with Charcot collapse of midfoot. (Reproduced with permission from Reference 78.)

rats whose feet had been denervated, the actual findings were qualitatively similar. In other phases of this study, the same pressures were given, but the number of repetitions per day were fewer and the rats were rested over the weekend. Ulceration did not occur and the footpad skin became hypertrophied with a thick layer of keratin.

Thus, in causing both loss of protective sensation and structural deformity of the foot, neuropathy is a major permissive factor for diabetic plantar ulceration.

It is paramount for the physician taking care of patients with neuropathy of the foot to understand the role played by these factors not only to treat but, most importantly, to prevent the development of such ulceration. Restoring adequate blood flow to the foot to heal already established tissue loss is not the end of the responsibility of the operating surgeon; it should be the beginning of continuous foot management directed at preventing repetitive injury to the soft tissue of the foot.

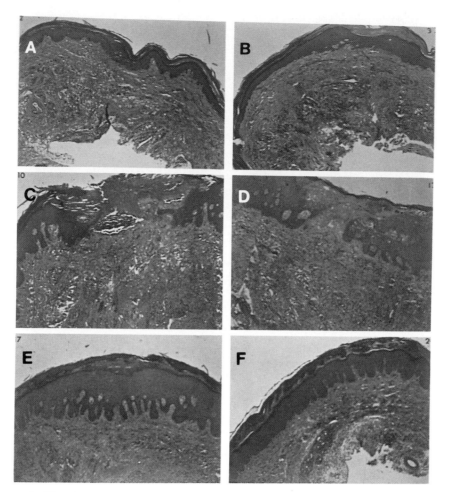

Figure 16. Histologic appearance of rat footpads studied by Brand. **A-C** show results of equal pressure (20 psi) applied 10,000 times each day to same location on footpads. **D-F** show results when repetitions were decreased to 8000 times per day, 5 days per week, for 6 weeks. (See text.)

Experiment 1: **A**. Day 2: Footpad shows edema and a few inflammatory cells. **B**. Day 3: Epithelium shows hyperplasia. Deeper tissue shows marked inflammation and necrosis. **C**. Day 10: Tissue is ulcerated. Deeper tissue is necrotic. **Experiment 2**: **D**. Day 13: Epithelium breaks and on each side of the break hyperplasia occurs. **E**. Day 17: Epithelium with hyperplasia and resorbing blister. **F**. Day 28: No damage seen, but thick epithelial hyperplasia exists. (Reproduced with permission from Reference 80.)

References

1. Perez MI, Kohn SR: Cutaneous manifestations of diabetes mellitus. *J Am Acad Dermatol* 4:519, 1994.
2. Said G, Goulon-Goeau C, Slama G, et al: Severe early onset polyneuropathy in insulin-dependent diabetes mellitus. *N Engl J Med* 326:1257, 1992.
3. Bessman AN, Birke JA, Boulton AJM, Calhoun JH, Campbell DR, Cohen E, et al: In: Frykberg RG (ed). *The High Risk Foot in Diabetes Mellitus*. New York: Churchill Livingstone, Inc.; 1991.
4. Keyser E: Foot wounds in diabetic patients. *Postgr Med* 91:98, 1992.
5. Anonymous Position Statement: Foot care in patients with diabetes mellitus. *Diabetes Care* 16:19, 1993.
6. Edmonds ME: Experience in a multidisciplinary diabetic foot clinic. In: Connor H, Boulton AJM, Ward JD (eds). *The Foot in Diabetes*. New York: John Wiley & Sons; 1987.
7. Cavanagh PR, Ulbrecht JS: Biomechanics of the foot in diabetes mellitus. In: Levin ME, O'Neal LW, Bowker J (eds). *The Diabetic Foot*. St. Louis: Mosby-Year Book, Inc.; 199, 1993.
8. Boulton AJM, Betts RP, Franks CI, et al: The natural history of foot pressure abnormalities in neuropathic diabetic subjects. *Diabetes Res* 5:73, 1987.
9. Boulton AJM, Hardisty CA, Betts RP, et al: Dynamic foot pressure and other studies as diagnostic and management aids in diabetic neuropathy. *Diabetes Care* 6:26, 1983.
10. Ctercteko GC, Dhanendran M, Hutton WC, et al: Vertical forces acting on the feet of diabetic patients with neuropathic ulceration. *Br J Surg* 68:608, 1981.
11. Stokes IAF, Faris IB, Hutton WC: The neuropathic ulcer

and loads on the foot in diabetic patients. *Acta Orthop Scand* 46:839, 1975.

12. Boulton AJM, Betts RP, Franks CI, et al: Abnormalities of foot pressure in early diabetic neuropathy. *Diabetic Med* 4:1987.

13. Dyck PJ, Karnes J, O'Brien PC: Diagnosis, staging, and classification of diabetic neuropathy and associations with other complications. In: Dyck PJ, Thomas PK, Asbury AK, Winegrad AI, Porte D (eds). *Diabetic Neuropathy*. Philadelphia: WB Saunders, Co.; 36, 1987.

14. Greene DA: Neuropathy in the diabetic foot: new concepts in etiology and treatment. In: Levin ME, O'Neal LW (eds). *The Diabetic Foot*. St. Louis: Mosby-Year Book, Inc.; 76, 1988.

15. Boulton, AJM: Diabetic neuropathy. In: Frykberg RG (ed). *The High Risk Foot in Diabetes Mellitus*. New York: Churchill Livingstone, Inc.; 49, 1991.

16. Boulton AJM: Clinical presentation and management of diabetic neuropathy and foot ulceration. *Diabetic Med* 8Spec:s48, 1991.

17. Dyck PJ: New understanding and treatment of diabetic neuropathy. *N Engl J Med* 326:1287, 1992.

18. Asbury AK: Focal and multifocal neuropathies of diabetes. In Dyck PJ, Thomas PK, Asbury AK, Winegrad AI, Porte D (eds). *Diabetic Neuropathy*. Philadelphia: WB Saunders, Co; 45, 1987.

19. Ward KA, Dellacorte MP, Grisafi PJ: Pathophysiology of diabetic neuropathy. *J Am Podiatr Med Assoc* 83:149, 1993.

20. Thomas PK, Brown MJ: Diabetic polyneuropathy. In: Dyck PJ, Thomas PK, Asbury AK, Winegrad AI, Porte D (eds). *Diabetic Neuropathy*. Philadelphia: WB Saunders, Co; 56, 1987.

21. Ewing DJ, Clarke BF: Diabetic autonomic neuropathy: a clinical viewpoint. In: Dyck PJ, Thomas PK, Asbury AK, Winegrad AI, Porte D (eds). *Diabetic Neuropathy*. Philadelphia: WB Saunders, Co.; 66, 1987.

22. Young MJ, Veves A, Walker MG, et al: Correlations between nerve function and tissue oxygenation in diabetic patients: further clues to the etiology of diabetic neuropathy? *Diabetologia* 35:1146, 1992.

23. Vogelstein B, Fearon ER, Hamilton SR, et al: Genetic alterations during colorectal tumor development. *New Engl J Med* 319:525, 1988.

24. Slamon DJ: Proto-oncogenes and human cancers. *New Engl J Med* 317:955, 1988.

25. Frank RN: The aldose reductase controversy. *Diabetes* 43:169, 1994.

26. Gabbay KH, Snider JJ: Nerve conduction defect in galactose-fed rats. *Diabetes* 21:295, 1972.

27. Gabbay KH: Role of sorbitol pathway in neuropathy. In: Camerini-Davalos RA, Cole HS (eds). *Vascular and Neurological Changes in Early Diabetes*. New York: Academic Press, Inc; 417–424, 1972.

28. Gregersen G: Variations in motor conduction velocity produced by acute changes of the metabolic state in diabetic patients. *Diabetologia* 4:273, 1968.

29. Dyck PJ, Zimmerman BR, Vilen TH, et al: Nerve glucose, fructose, sorbitol, myoinositol, and fiber degeneration and regeneration in diabetic neuropathy. *New Engl J Med* 319:542, 1988.

30. Carrier DR, Heglund NC, Earls KD: Variable gearing during locomotion in the human musculoskeletal system. *Science* 265:651, 1994.

31. Friend SH, Dryja TP, Weinberg RA: Oncogenes and tumor-suppressing genes. *New Engl J Med* 318:618, 1988.

32. Gauwerky CE, Hoxie J, Nowell PC, et al: Pre-B-cell leukemia with a t(8;14) and a t(14;18) translocation is preceded by follicular lymphoma. *Oncogene* 2:431, 1988.

33. Griffey RH, Eaton RP, Sibbitt RR, et al: Diabetic neuropathy: structural analysis of nerve hydration by magnetic resonance spectroscopy. *JAMA* 260:2872, 1988.

34. Harati, Y: Diabetic peripheral neuropathy. In: Kominsky SJ (ed). *Medical and Surgical Management of the Diabetic Foot*. St. Louis: Mosby-Year Book, Inc.; 71, 1994.

35. Brownlee M, Cerami A, Vlassara H: Advanced glycosylation end products in tissue and the biochemical basis of diabetic complications. *N Engl J Med* 318:1315, 1988.

36. Gupta R: A short history of neuropathic arthropathy. *Clin Orthop* 296:43, 1993.

37. Yasuda H, Dyck PJ: Abnormalities of endoneurial microvessels and sural nerve pathology in diabetic neuropathy. *Neurology* 37:20, 1987.

38. Greene DA, Lattimer SA: Sodium and energy dependent uptake of myoinositol by rabbit peripheral nerve. *J Clin Invest* 70:1009, 1982.

39. Greene DA, Yagihashi S, Lattimer SA, et al: NA$^+$-K$^+$-ATPase, conduction, and myoinositol in the insulin-deficient BB rat. *Am J Physiol* 247:E534, 1984.

40. Greene DA, Lattimer S, Ulbrecht J, et al: Glucose-induced alterations in nerve metabolism: current perspective on the pathogenesis of diabetic neuropathy and future directions for research and therapy. *Diabetes Care* 8:290, 1985.

41. Sima AAF, Lattimer SA, Yagihashi S, et al: Axo-glial dysjunction: a novel structural lesion that accounts for poorly reversible slowing of nerve conduction in the spontaneously diabetic bio-breeding rat. *J Clin Invest* 77:474, 1986.

42. Asbury A: Understanding diabetic neuropathy. *N Engl J Med* 319:577, 1988.

43. Dyck PJ: Pathology. In: Dyck, PJ, Thomas PK, Asbury AK, Winegrad AI, Porte D (eds). *Diabetic Neuropathy*. Philadelphia: WB Saunders, Co.; 223, 1987.

44. Muschel R, Liotta LA: Role of oncogenes in metastases. *Carcinogenesis* 9:705, 1988.

45. Danes BS, Gardner EJ, Lipkin M: Studies on the identification of genetic risk for heritable colon cancer. *Cancer Detect Prev* 8:349, 1985.

46. Bathgate RH: A model of nerve regeneration in diabetic neuropathy. *Med Hypothesis* 41:63, 1993.

47. Ordonez G, Fernandez A, Perez R, et al: Low contents of nerve growth factor in serum and submaxillary gland of diabetic mice. *J Neurol Sci* 121:163, 1994.

48. Faradji V, Sotelo J: Low serum levels of nerve growth factor in diabetic neuropathy. *Acta Neurol Scand* 81:402, 1990.

49. Weber GA, Cardile M: Diabetic neuropathies. In: *Clinics in Podiatric Medicine and Surgery*. Philadelphia: WB Saunders, Co.; 1–36, 1990.

50. Brooks AP: The neuropathic foot in diabetes part II: Charcot's neuroarthropathy. *Diabetic Med* 3:116, 1986.

51. Brown MJ, Asbury AK: Diabetic neuropathy. *Ann Neurology* 15:2, 1984.

52. LoGerfo FW, Coffman JD: Vascular and microvascular disease of the foot in diabetics. *New Engl J Med* 311:1615, 1984.

53. Veves A, Manis C, Murray HJ, et al: Painful neuropathy and foot ulceration in diabetic patients. *Diabetes Care* 16:1187, 1993.

54. Sharma AK, et al: The effect of insulin treatment on myelinated nerve fiber maturation and integrity and on

body growth in streptozotocin-diabetic rats. *J Neurol Sci* 67:285, 1985.

55. Fagius J, Wallin BG: Sympathetic reflex latencies and conduction velocities in patients with polyneuropathy. *J Neurol Sci* 47:449, 1980.

56. Kida Y, Kashiwagi A, Nishio Y, et al: Is difference of arterial and venous oxygen content a possible marker for diabetic foot? *Diabetes Care* 6:515, 1988.

57. Boulton AJM, Scarpello JMB, Ward JD: Venous oxygenation in the diabetic neuropathic foot: evidence of arteriovenous shunting. *Diabetologia* 22:6, 1981.

58. Uccioli L, Mancini L, Giordano A, et al: Lower limb arteriovenous shunts, autonomic neuropathy, and diabetic foot. *Diab Res Clin Pract* 16:123, 1992.

59. Sima AA, Nathaniel V, Bril V, et al: Histopathological heterogeneity of neuropathy in insulin-dependent and non-insulin-dependent diabetes, and demonstration of axo-glial dysjunction in human diabetic neuropathy. *J Clin Invest* 81:349, 1988.

60. Edmonds ME, Roberts VC, Watkins PJ: Blood flow in the diabetic neuropathic foot. *Diabetologia* 22:9, 1982.

61. Uccioli L, Monticone G, Durola L, et al: Autonomic neuropathy influences great toe blood pressure. *Diabetes Care* 17:284, 1994.

62. Irwin ST, Gilmore J, McGrann S, et al: Blood flow in diabetics with foot lesions due to small vessel disease. *Br J Surg* 75:1201, 1988.

63. Edmunds ME, Watkins PJ: Management of the diabetic foot. In: Dyck PJ, Thomas PK, Asbury AK, Winegrad AI, Porte D (eds). *Diabetic Neuropathy*. Philadelphia: WB Saunders, Co.; 208, 1987.

64. Banks AS, McGlamry ED: Charcot foot. *J Am Podiatr Med Assoc* 79:213, 1989.

65. Elkeles RS, Wolfe JHN: The diabetic foot. *Br Med J* 303:1053, 1991.

66. Brink SJ: Limited joint mobility as a risk factor for diabetic complications. *Clinical Diabetes* 5:122, 1987.

67. Brownlee M, Vlassara H, Cerami A: Nonenzymatic glycosylation and the pathogenesis of diabetic complications. *Ann Intern Med* 101:527, 1984.

68. Delbridge L, Ellis CS, Robertson K: Nonenzymatic glycosylation of keratin from the stratum corneum of the diabetic foot. *Br J Dermatol* 112:547, 1991.

69. Thompson DE: The effects of mechanical stress on soft tissue. In: Levin ME, O'Neal LW (eds). *The Diabetic Foot*. St. Louis: Mosby-Year Book, Inc.; 91, 1988.

70. Sage RA: Diabetic ulcers: evaluation and management. In: Harkless LB, Dennis KH (eds). *Clinics in Podiatric Medicine and Surgery: The Diabetic Foot*. Philadelphia: WB Saunders, Co.; 1987.

71. Cavanagh PR, Derr JA, Ulbrecht JS, et al: Problems with gait and posture in neuropathic patients with insulin-dependent diabetes mellitus. *Diabetic Med* 9:482, 1992.

72. Mann RA: Overview of foot and ankle biomechanics. In: Jahss MH (ed). *Disorders of the Foot and Ankle*. Philadelphia: WB Saunders, Co.; 385, 1991.

73. Schoenhaus HD, Wernick E, Cohen RS: Biomechanics of the diabetic foot. In: Frykberg RG (ed). *The High Risk Foot in Diabetes Mellitus*. New York: Churchill Livingstone, Inc.; 125, 1991.

74. Cavanagh PR, Simoneau GG, Ulbrecht JS: Ulceration, unsteadiness, and uncertainty: the biomechanical consequences of diabetes mellitus. *J Biomechanics* 26:23, 1993.

75. Sanders LJ, Frykberg RG: Diabetic neuropathic osteoarthropathy: the Charcot foot. In: Frykberg RG (ed). *The High Risk Foot in Diabetes Mellitus*. New York: Churchill Livingstone, Inc.; 297, 1991.

76. Frykberg RG, Giurini J, Habershaw G, et al: Prophylactic surgery in the diabetic foot. In: Kominsky SJ (ed). *Medical and Surgical Management of the Diabetic Foot*. St. Louis: Mosby-Year Book, Inc.; 399, 1994.

77. Pecoraro RE, Reiber GE, Burgess EM, et al: Pathways to diabetic limb amputation. *Diabetes Care* 13:513, 1990.

78. Cavanagh PR, Sims DS Jr, Sanders LJ: Body mass is a poor predictor of peak plantar pressure in diabetic men. *Diabetes Care* 14:750, 1991.

79. Masson EA, Hay EM, Stockley I, et al: Abnormal foot pressures alone may not cause ulceration. *Diabetic Med* 6:426, 1989.

80. Brand PW: Repetitive stress in the development of diabetic foot ulcers. In: Levin ME, O'Neal LW (eds). *The Diabetic Foot*. St. Louis: Mosby-Year Book, Inc.; 83, 1988.

Index

C